**Seventh Edition**

# Basic Skills in
# INTERPRETING
# LABORATORY DATA

Christopher J. Edwards and Brian L. Erstad

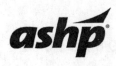

Any correspondence regarding this publication should be sent to the publisher, American Society of Health-System Pharmacists, 4500 East-West Highway, Suite 900, Bethesda, MD 20814, attention: Special Publishing.

The information presented herein reflects the opinions of the contributors and advisors. It should not be interpreted as an official policy of ASHP or as an endorsement of any product.

Because of ongoing research and improvements in technology, the information and its applications contained in this text are constantly evolving and are subject to the professional judgment and interpretation of the practitioner due to the uniqueness of a clinical situation. The editors and ASHP have made reasonable efforts to ensure the accuracy and appropriateness of the information presented in this document. However, any user of this information is advised that the editors and ASHP are not responsible for the continued currency of the information, for any errors or omissions, and/or for any consequences arising from the use of the information in the document in any and all practice settings. Any reader of this document is cautioned that ASHP makes no representation, guarantee, or warranty, express or implied, as to the accuracy and appropriateness of the information contained in this document and specifically disclaims any liability to any party for the accuracy and/or completeness of the material or for any damages arising out of the use or non-use of any of the information contained in this document.

*Vice President, Publishing Office*: Daniel J. Cobaugh, PharmD, DABAT, FAACT
*Editorial Director, Special Publishing*: Lori N. Justice, PharmD
*Editorial Coordinator, Special Publishing*: Elaine Jimenez
*Director, Production and Platform Services, Publishing Operations*: Johnna M. Hershey, BA
*Cover Design*: DeVall Advertising
*Cover Art*: berCheck - stock.adobe.com
*Page Design*: David Wade

Library of Congress Cataloging-in-Publication Data

Names: Edwards, Christopher J. PharmD, editor. | Erstad, Brian, editor. | American Society of Health-System Pharmacists, issuing body.
Title: Basic skills in interpreting laboratory data / [edited by] Christopher J. Edwards, Brian L. Erstad.
Description: Seventh edition. | Bethesda, MD : American Society of Health-System Pharmacists, 2022. | Includes bibliographical references and index. | Summary: "Basic Skills in Interpreting Laboratory Data continues to be the most popular teaching text on laboratory data for pharmacy students as well as the go-to reference for pharmacists in therapeutic practice. Now in its seventh edition, Basic Skills has been expanded and updated to cover new drugs, research, and therapeutic approaches. Edited by new co-editors Christopher J. Edwards, PharmD, BCPS, and Brian L. Erstad, PharmD, FASHP, FCCP, MCCM, BCPS, the seventh edition is a comprehensive, in-depth guide to all aspects of lab work that apply to clinical practice. Written by a team of over 30 established clinicians and pharmacy faculty members and reviewed by additional experts, it is designed to make all information clear and quickly accessible. The seventh edition boasts new minicases that provide clinical scenarios for using tests and managing patients, and quickview charts throughout offer clear interpretations of lab results"—Provided by publisher.
Identifiers: LCCN 2021049621 (print) | LCCN 2021049622 (ebook) | ISBN 9781585286416 (paperback) | ISBN 9781585286423 (adobe pdf) | ISBN 9781585286430 (epub)
Subjects: MESH: Clinical Laboratory Techniques | Reference Values | Clinical Laboratory Services
Classification: LCC RB37 (print) | LCC RB37 (ebook) | NLM QY 80 | DDC 616.07/5—dc23/eng/20211015
LC record available at https://lccn.loc.gov/2021049621
LC ebook record available at https://lccn.loc.gov/2021049622

ISBN: 978-1-58528-641-6 (paperback)
ISBN: 978-1-58528-642-3 (Adobe pdf)
ISBN: 978-1-58528-643-0 (ePub)

10 9 8 7 6 5 4 3 2 1

DOI: 10.37573/9781585286423

# DEDICATION

This book is dedicated to all of the
pharmacy educators helping to shape
the future of our profession.

*Chris Edwards and Brian Erstad*

# CONTENTS

DOI 10.37573/9781585286423.FM

# PREFACE

The publication of this edition of *Basic Skills in Interpreting Laboratory Data* has been made possible by the dedicated chapter authors, reviewers, and the publishing staff at the American Society of Health-System Pharmacists. It has been an honor to serve as the editors and to work with this team.

The seventh edition of this work brings about several major changes. After serving as the sole editor for 5 editions of this work, Mary Lee, PharmD, has relinquished this role to pursue other projects, although she continues to be a chapter author. As the new editors, we are indebted to her for the countless hours she spent developing the foundations upon which this edition was built.

Similarly, with this edition, five new lead authors were invited to update existing chapters due to unavailability of the original chapter authors. Drs. Jason Karnes and Laura Ramsey joined as authors for the chapter on Pharmacogenetics and Molecular Testing. Drs. Jessica DeAngelo and Jacqueline Finger revamped the chapter on Cardiac Function and Related Tests to focus on laboratory values relevant to this aspect of practice. Drs. Michael Katz and Timothy Jacisin also joined to serve as authors for the chapter Hematology: Red and White Blood Cell Tests. Dr. Kimmy Nguyen took the role of lead author for the chapter on Renal Function and Related Tests, and Dr. Raine Ghamrawi stepped into the role of lead author for the chapter on Interpretation of Serum Drug Concentrations. All of the lead authors are established clinicians and/or experienced faculty at colleges of pharmacy or medicine, which enhance the quality of the chapter content.

A new group of reviewers has joined this project, and many reviewers are board-certified or otherwise recognized as established experts. Their specialty knowledge and scrutiny of the chapter content have helped to ensure that each chapter is up-to-date and content is relevant to clinical practice. As you use this book, you will find that the seventh edition includes updated chapter content with references, and almost all of the chapters have at least one new minicase and learning point. In addition, the abbreviations in the front of the book have been expanded for reader convenience.

Significant and notable new chapter content:

1. Pharmacogenomics: Significant expansion to add new information that has become available since the publication of the previous edition.

2. Cardiology: Expanded information about available laboratory testing relevant to cardiology practice.

3. Nutrition Support: A new chapter has been added to discuss laboratory testing pertinent to the assessment and monitoring of patients receiving parenteral nutrition.

4. Infectious Diseases has been divided into two sections given the amount of material relevant to this topic with each section being expanded to include new laboratory tests in each area.

Suggestions for using this book efficiently:

- For a general overview of the laboratory tests for various organ systems or types of diseases, use the table of contents to identify the most appropriate section or chapter(s). The chapters are grouped into three major sections: Basic Concepts and Test Interpretations, System Disorders and Diagnostic Tests, and Tests for Special Populations. By reading the section or a chapter from start to finish, you get a detailed summary of the laboratory tests used to evaluate that organ system or disease, why the test is used, what a normal value range is for the test, and how to interpret an abnormal laboratory test result.

- Minicases guide the reader through common clinical scenarios about ordering appropriate laboratory tests, interpreting results, managing patients, and addressing spurious laboratory tests. Learning points conclude each chapter and highlight key concepts about the laboratory tests. Using the book in this way will be helpful, especially when used as a companion to a disease state management course, a pharmacotherapeutics course, or a course that prepares students for full-time clinical rotations.

- For information on a specific laboratory test, use the alphabetical index to locate the test, and then go to the page(s) to access the following information: the purpose of the test; how the test result relates to the pathophysiology of a disease or the physiologic function of a cell or organ; the normal range for the test; causes for an abnormal test result; and causes of false-positive or false-negative results. This approach will be most useful in the clinical management of a patient.

- Quickview charts are provided for some of the most common laboratory tests. These charts are standardized template presentations of information that allow readers to quickly learn about a specific laboratory test (eg, what the test is used for, what a normal

DOI 10.37573/9781585286423.FM

result is, and causes of an abnormal result). This approach also will be most useful in the clinical management of a patient, but the Quickview content should be supplemented with the in-depth information in the chapters about a particular laboratory test.

The authors, reviewers, and we as editors hope that *Basic Skills in Interpreting Laboratory Data* is useful to your practice.

*Chris Edwards and Brian Erstad*
December 2021

## EDITORS

**Christopher J. Edwards, PharmD, BCPS**
Assistant Professor
Department of Pharmacy Practice & Science
R. Ken Coit College of Pharmacy
University of Arizona
Tucson, Arizona

**Brian L. Erstad, PharmD, FASHP, FCCP, MCCM, BCPS**
Professor and Head
Department of Pharmacy Practice & Science
R. Ken Coit College of Pharmacy
University of Arizona
Tucson, Arizona

## CONTRIBUTORS

**Jason Altman, MD**
Western Mass GI Associates
Springfield, Massachusetts

**Candi C. Bachour, PharmD**
Department of Clinical Pharmacy
University of Tennessee Health Science Center
Memphis, Tennessee

**Jeffrey F. Barletta, PharmD, FCCM**
Professor and Vice-Chair
Department of Pharmacy Practice
Midwestern University College of Pharmacy, Glendale Campus
Glendale, Arizona

**Lindsay Benedik, PharmD, BCPS, BCGP**
Director, Pharmacology Education, Foundations
Assistant Professor, Medical Education & Geriatrics
Write State University, Boonshoft School of Medicine
Dayton, Ohio

**Jill S. Borchert, PharmD, BCACP, BCPS, FCCP**
Professor and Vice-Chair, Pharmacy Practice
Midwestern University College of Pharmacy
Downers Grove, Illinois

**Susan P. Bruce, PharmD, BCPS**
Dean and Professor
Wingate University
School of Pharmacy
Wingate, North Carolina

DOI 10.37573/9781585286423.FM

**Rodrigo M. Burgos, PharmD, MPH**
Clinical Assistant Professor
College of Pharmacy
University of Illinois Chicago
Chicago, Illinois

**Lingtak-Neander Chan, PharmD, BCNSP, FACN**
Professor and Vice Chair
Department of Pharmacy
Interdisciplinary Faculty in Nutritional Sciences
School of Pharmacy & Graduate Program in Nutritional Sciences
University of Washington
Seattle, Washington

**Peter A. Chyka, PharmD, DABAT, FAACT**
Professor Emeritus
College of Pharmacy, Knoxville Campus
The University of Tennessee Health Science Center
Knoxville, Tennessee

**Lisa M. Cillessen, PharmD, BCACP**
Clinical Associate Professor
UMKC School of Pharmacy at MSU
Springfield, Missouri

**Jessica DeAngelo, PharmD, MBA, BCPS**
Clinical Assistant Professor
R. Ken Coit College of Pharmacy
University of Arizona
Cardiology Clinical Pharmacist
Banner – University Medical Center Tucson
Tucson, Arizona

**Lea E. Dela Peña, PharmD, BCPS**
Associate Professor, Pharmacy Practice
Midwestern University Chicago College of Pharmacy
Downers Grove, Illinois

**Sharon M. Erdman, PharmD, FIDP**
Clinical Professor of Pharmacy Practice
Purdue University College of Pharmacy
Infectious Diseases Clinical Pharmacist
Eskenazi Health
Indianapolis, Indiana

**Paul Farkas, MD, AGAF, FACP**
Chief of Gastroenterology
Mercy Hospital
Assistant Clinical Professor of Medicine
Tufts University School of Medicine
Springfield, Massachusetts

**Jacqueline Finger, PharmD, BCCP**
Cardiovascular Critical Care Clinical Pharmacist
Banner – University Medical Center Tucson
Tucson, Arizona

**Riane Ghamrawi, PharmD, BCPS, BCIDP**
Clinical Pharmacy Specialist
Antimicrobial Stewardship/Infectious Diseases
UC Health West Chester Hospital
West Chester Township, Ohio
UC Health Daniel Drake Center for Post-Acute Care
Cincinnati, Ohio

**Paul O. Gubbins, PharmD, FCCP, FIDP**
Associate Dean
Vice Chair and Professor
Division of Pharmacy Practice and Administration
UMKC School of Pharmacy at MSU
Springfield, Missouri

**Timothy C. Jacisin, PharmD**
Clinical Pharmacy Specialist
Newark Beth Israel Medical Center
Newark, New Jersey

**Jessica L. Jacobson, PharmD, BCPS, BCPPS**
Clinical Pharmacy Specialist, Pediatric Intensive Care
Director, PGY2 Pediatric Pharmacy Residency
Rush University Medical Center
Chicago, Illinois

**Min J. Joo, MD, MPH, FCCP**
Professor of Medicine
Department of Medicine
University of Illinois at Chicago
Chicago, Illinois

**Jason H. Karnes, PharmD, PhD, BCPS, FAHA, FCCP**
Associate Professor
Department of Pharmacy Practice and Science
R. Ken Coit College of Pharmacy
University of Arizona
Tucson, Arizona

**Michael D. Katz, PharmD**
Professor
Department of Pharmacy Practice and Science
R. Ken Coit College of Pharmacy
University of Arizona
Tucson, Arizona

**Kathy E. Komperda, PharmD, BCPS**
Professor, Pharmacy Practice
Midwestern University College of Pharmacy
Downers Grove, Illinois

**Donna M. Kraus, PharmD, FAPhA, FCCP, FPPAG**
Associate Professor Emerita of Pharmacy Practice
College of Pharmacy
University of Illinois at Chicago
Chicago, Illinois

**Mary Lee, PharmD, BCPS, FCCP**
Vice President and Special Assistant to the President
Pharmacy and Optometry Education
Midwestern University
Professor, Pharmacy Practice
Midwestern University Chicago College of Pharmacy
Downers Grove, Illinois

**Heather Lyons-Burney, PharmD**
Clinical Associate Professor
UMKC School of Pharmacy at MSU
Springfield, Missouri

**Jasmine S. Mangrum, PharmD, MPH**
Assistant Teaching Professor, Clinical Practice
School of Pharmacy
University of Washington
Seattle, Washington

**Nicholas M. Moore, PhD, D(ABMM), MLS (ASCP)$^{CM}$**
Assistant Director
Division of Clinical Microbiology
Associate Professor
Department of Medical Laboratory Science
Rush University Medical Center
Chicago, Illinois

**Kimmy T. Nguyen, PharmD**
Assistant Professor
Wilkes University
Kingston, Pennsylvania

**Laura B. Ramsey, PhD**
Associate Professor, Department of Pediatrics
University of Cincinnati College of Medicine
Cincinnati Children's Hospital Medical Center
Cincinnati, Ohio

**Keith A. Rodvold, PharmD, FCCP, FIDSA**
Distinguished Professor
Colleges of Pharmacy and Medicine
University of Illinois Chicago
Chicago, Illinois

**Joanna Sampson, MD**
Western Mass GI Associates
Springfield, Massachusetts

**Sarah A. Schmidt, PharmD, BCPS, BCOP**
Clinical Assistant Professor—Hematology/Oncology
University of Oklahoma College of Pharmacy
Oklahoma City, Oklahoma

**Roohollah Sharifi, MD, FACS**
Section Chief of Urology
Jesse Brown Veterans Administration Hospital
Professor of Urology and Surgery
University of Illinois College of Medicine
Chicago, Illinois

**Beth S. Shields, PharmD, BCPPS**
Associate Director, Pharmacy Operations
Clinical Pharmacy Specialist, Pediatrics
Rush University Medical Center
Chicago, Illinois

**Matthew Slitzky, MD**
Western Mass GI Associates
Springfield, Massachusetts

**Karen J. Tietze, PharmD**
Professor of Clinical Pharmacy
Department of Pharmacy Practice and Pharmacy
    Administration
University of the Sciences
Philadelphia College of Pharmacy
Philadelphia, Pennsylvania

**Eva Vivian, PharmD, MS, PhD, FADCES**
Professor, Pharmacy Practice
University of Wisconsin—Madison School of Pharmacy
Madison, Wisconsin

**Lori A. Wilken, PharmD, BCACP**
Clinical Assistant Professor, Pharmacy Practice
University of Illinois at Chicago College of Pharmacy
Chicago, Illinois

**Sharon Wu, PharmD, BCACP**
Assistant Clinical Professor
University of Washington School of Pharmacy
Seattle, Washington

# REVIEWERS

**Nabila Ahmed-Sarwar, PharmD, BCPS, BCACP, CDCES, BC-ADM**
Associate Professor of Pharmacy Practice
Wegmans School of Pharmacy, St. John Fisher College
Rochester, New York

**Rebekah Hanson Anguiano, PharmD, BCPS, BCACP**
Clinical Pharmacist/Assistant Professor
University of Illinois at Chicago, College of Pharmacy
Chicago, Illinois

**Madelyn Batey, PharmD, BCPS**
Clinical Pharmacist in Internal Medicine
Adjunct Clinical Professor in Pharmacy
University of Michigan Medicine
Ann Arbor, Michigan

**Suzanne G. Bollmeier, PharmD, FCCP, BCPS, AE-C**
Professor, Pharmacy Practice
St. Louis College of Pharmacy
St. Louis, Missouri

**Stacy Brown, PhD**
Assistant Professor
Gatton College of Pharmacy
East Tennessee State University
Johnson City, Tennessee

**Dr. Luigi Brunetti, PharmD, MPH**
Associate Professor
Rutgers Ernest Mario School of Pharmacy
Department of Pharmacy Practice and Administration
Piscataway, New Jersey

**Todd W. Canada, PharmD, BCNSP, BCCCP, FASHP, FTSHP**
Regional Director, Galveston/Houston
Clinical Assistant Professor
MD Anderson Cancer Center
Division of Pharmacy
Houston, Texas

**Katie E. Cardone, PharmD, BCACP, FNKF, FASN, FCCP**
PharmD Program Director, Associate Professor
Albany College of Pharmacy and Health Sciences/Albany
    Medical Center
Albany, New York

**Amber B. Cipriani, PharmD, BCOP, CPP**
Precision Medicine Pharmacy Coordinator
University of North Carolina Medical Center
Clinical Assistant Professor
UNC Eshelman School of Pharmacy
Chapel Hill, North Carolina

**Amy C. Donihi, PharmD, BCPS, BC-ADM, FCCP**
Professor, Pharmacy and Therapeutics
Clinical Pharmacist, Inpatient Diabetes Care and Education
University of Pittsburgh School of Pharmacy
Pittsburgh, Pennsylvania

**Christine Eisenhower, PharmD, BCPS**
Clinical Associate Professor
The University of Rhode Island
College of Pharmacy
Kingston, Rhode Island

**Brian L. Erstad, PharmD, FASHP, FCCP, MCCM, BCPS**
Professor and Head
Department of Pharmacy Practice & Science
R. Ken Coit College of Pharmacy
University of Arizona
Tucson, Arizona

**Aaron P. Hartmann, PharmD, BCPS**
Clinical Specialist, Internal Medicine
Department of Pharmacy
Barnes-Jewish Hospital
St. Louis, Missouri

**Michael P. Kane, PharmD, FCCP, BCPS, BCACP**
Professor, Department of Pharmacy Practice
Albany College of Pharmacy and Health Sciences
Clinical Pharmacy Specialist
Albany Medical Center Division of Community
    Endocrinology/The Endocrine Group
Albany, New York

**William M. Kolling, RPh, PhD**
Associate Professor
Schools of Pharmacy and Medicine
Southern Illinois University Edwardsville
Edwardsville, Illinois

DOI 10.37573/9781585286423.FM

**Lauren D. Leader, PharmD, BCPS**
Clinical Pharmacy Specialist
Obstetrics and Gynecology
Michigan Medicine
Ann Arbor, Michigan

**Joel Marrs, PharmD, MPH**
Ambulatory Pharmacy Clinical Coordinator
Billings Clinic
Billings, Montana

**Emily K. McCoy, PharmD, BCACP**
Associate Clinical Professor, Department of
    Pharmacy Practice
Auburn University Harrison School of Pharmacy
Adjunct Assistant Professor, Department of Internal Medicine
University of South Alabama College of Medicine
Mobile, Alabama

**Rick Miller, PharmD, BCPS, BCOP, FASHP**
Clinical Pharmacy Specialist
Ruby Memorial Hospital
Morgantown, West Virginia

**Amanda Munson, PhD**
Associate Professor
Program Director, MS in Pharmacogenomics &
    Personalized Medicine
Department of Pharmacogenomics
Bernard J. Dunn School of Pharmacy
Shenandoah University, ICPH Fairfax
Inova Center for Personalized Health
Fairfax, Virginia

**Frank P. Paloucek, PharmD, FASHP, FAACT, DPLA, DABAT**
Clinical Professor and Director PGY1 Residency Program
University of Illinois at Chicago
Chicago, Illinois

**Brent N. Reed, PharmD, BCPS, BCCP, FCCP**
Associate Professor, Pharmacy Practice and Science
University of Maryland School of Pharmacy
Baltimore, Maryland

**Carrie A. Sincak, PharmD, BCPS, FASHP**
Associate Dean for Clinical Affairs
Professor of Pharmacy Practice
Midwestern University Chicago College of Pharmacy
Downers Grove, Illinois

**Jim Thigpen, PharmD, BCPS**
Associate Professor, Pharmacy Practice
Bill Gatton College of Pharmacy
East Tennessee State University
Johnson City, Tennessee

**Noreen H. Chan Tompkins, PharmD, BCPS-AQ ID**
Clinical Pharmacy Specialist, Pediatric Infectious Disease
Professor, Department of Pharmacy Practice
Loma Linda University Children's Hospital and
    School of Pharmacy
Loma Linda, California

**Tamara L. Trienski, PharmD, BCIDP**
Clinical Pharmacy Specialist, Infectious Diseases
Allegheny General Hospital/Allegheny Health Network
Pittsburgh, Pennsylvania

# CLINICAL PROOFREADERS

**Jared Cavanaugh, PharmD**
Assistant Professor, Clinical and Administrative Sciences
California Northstate University College of Pharmacy
Elk Grove, California

**S. Dee Melnyk Evans, PharmD, MHS**
Consultant
Burlington, North Carolina

**Mort Goldman, PharmD, FCCP, BCPS**
Senior Consultant
Pharmacy Consulting International
Cleveland, Ohio

**Lauren M. Hynicka, PharmD**
Associate Professor
University of Maryland
School of Pharmacy
Baltimore, Maryland

**Allison King, PharmD**
Investigational Drug Pharmacist, Residency Coordinator
Children's Mercy Hospital
Kansas City, Missouri

**Colleen Lauster, PharmD, BCPS, CDE**
Clinical Pharmacy Specialist, Ambulatory Care
Beaumont Hospital – Royal Oak
Royal Oak, Michigan

**Cindy Powers Magrini, PharmD, AAHIVP**
Clinical Pharmacy Specialist, Positive Health Clinic
Allegheny General Hospital
Pittsburgh, Pennsylvania

**Rickey C. Miller, PharmD, BCOP, BCPS, FASHP**
Oncology Clinical Pharmacy Specialist
WVU Medicine – WVU Cancer Institute
Morgantown, West Virginia

**Kimberly J. Novak, PharmD, BCPS, BCPPS, FPPA**
Advanced Patient Care Pharmacist–Pediatric and
   Adult Cystic Fibrosis
Director, PGY2 Pharmacy Residency–Pediatrics
Nationwide Children's Hospital
Department of Pharmacy
Columbus, Ohio

**Song Oh, PharmD, BCCCP**
Assistant Professor
Department of Clinical & Administrative Sciences
California Northstate University College of Pharmacy
Elk Grove, California

**\*R. Laney Owings, PharmD, BCPS, BCPP**
Medication Safety Evaluator
U.S. Food and Drug Administration
Chapel Hill, North Carolina

**Seon Jo Park, PharmD, BCOP**
Hematology Oncology Pharmacy Specialist
Allegheny General Hospital
Pittsburgh, Pennsylvania

**Steven Plogsted, BS, PharmD, BCNSP, CNSC, FASPEN**
Clinical Pharmacy Specialist (ret.)
Nationwide Children's Hospital
Columbus, Ohio

**Tamara Trienski, PharmD, BCIDP**
Clinical Pharmacy Specialist, Infectious Diseases
Allegheny General Hospital/Allegheny Health Network
Pittsburgh, Pennsylvania

**Raynold Yin, PharmD, APh, BCACP, CDE**
Ambulatory Care Pharmacist
Sharp Grossmont Hospital
San Diego, California

**Spencer K. Yingling, PharmD, BCOP**
Oncology Pharmacy Specialist
WVU Medicine
Morgantown, West Virginia

*Dr. Owings' editorial contributions were done in her personal capacity and do not represent the opinions of the Food and Drug Administration, the Department of Health and Human Services, nor the Federal Government.

DOI 10.37573/9781585286423.FM

| | |
|---|---|
| μm | micrometer |
| 1,25-DHCC | 1,25-dihydroxycholecalciferol |
| 17-OHP | 17α-hydroxyprogesterone |
| $^{201}$TI | thallium-201 |
| 2,3 DPG | 2,3-diphosphoglycerate |
| 25-HCC | 25-hydroxycholecalciferol |
| 3SR | self-sustained sequence replication |
| 5HT | serotonin |
| 6-AM | 6-acetylmorphine |
| 6MWT | 6-minute walk test |
| $^{99m}$Tc | technetium-99m |
| $^{201}$Tl | thallium-201 (radio isotope) |
| α$_1$AC | α1-antichymotrypsin |
| A-G6PD | glucose-6 phosphate dehydrogenase variant |
| A1c | glycosylated hemoglobin |
| A2M, α2M | α2-macroglobulin |
| AA | atomic absorption |
| AACE | American Association of Clinical Endocrinologists |
| AAG | α1-acid glycoprotein |
| ABG | arterial blood gas |
| ABW | average body weight |
| ACA | anticentromere antibody |
| ACC | American College of Cardiology |
| ACCF | American College of Cardiology Foundation |
| ACCP | American College of Clinical Pharmacy |
| ACCP | anticyclic citrullinated peptide |
| ACE | angiotensin-converting enzyme |
| ACE-I | angiotensin-converting enzyme inhibitor |
| ACPA | anticitrullinated protein antibody |
| ACR | albumin-to-creatinine ratio; American College of Rheumatology |
| ACS | acute coronary syndrome |
| ACT | activated clotting time; α1-coded testing |
| ACTH | adrenocorticotropic hormone (corticotropin) |
| ADA | American Diabetes Association |
| ADAM | androgen deficiency in aging males |
| ADCC | antibody-dependent cellular cytotoxicity |
| ADH | antidiuretic hormone |
| ADME | absorption, distribution, metabolism, excretion |
| ADP | adenosine diphosphate |
| AEDs | antiepileptic drugs |
| AFB | acid-fast bacilli |
| AFP | α-fetoprotein |
| AG | anion gap |
| AGPA | allergic granulomatosis with polyangiitis |
| AHA | American Heart Association |
| AIDS | acquired immunodeficiency syndrome |
| ALK | anaplastic lymphoma kinase |
| ALL | acute lymphoblastic leukemia |
| ALP | alkaline phosphatase |
| ALT | alanine aminotransferase |
| AMA | antimitochondrial antibody |
| AMI | acute myocardial infarction |
| AML | acute myelogenous leukemia |
| ANA | antinuclear antibody |
| ANCA | antineutrophil cytoplasmic antibody |
| ANF | atrial natriuretic factor |
| ANP | atrial natriuretic peptide |
| anti-HAV IgG IgG | antibody against hepatitis A virus |
| anti-HAV IgM IgM | antibody against hepatitis A virus |
| anti-HBc | antibody to hepatitis B core antigen |
| anti-HbeAg | antibody to hepatitis B extracellular antigen |
| anti-HBs | antibody to hepatitis B surface antigen |
| anti-HCV | antibody against HCV antigen |
| anti-HD | antibody against hepatitis D |
| APC | activated protein C |
| APC | antigen-presenting cell |
| apoB | apolipoprotein B |
| APS | antiphospholipid antibody syndrome |
| aPTT | activated partial thromboplastin time |
| ARB | angiotensin receptor blocker |
| ARNI | angiotensin receptor neprilysin inhibitor |
| ASA | aspirin |
| ASCO | American Society of Clinical Oncology |
| ASCVD | atherosclerotic cardiovascular disease |
| AST | aspartate aminotransferase |
| AT | antithrombin |
| ATP | adenosine triphosphate |
| ATP-K | adenosine triphosphate potassium |
| ATP | Adult Treatment Panel |
| ATP III | Adult Treatment Panel III |
| ATS | American Thoracic Society |
| AUA | American Urological Association |
| AUA-SI | American Urological Association Symptom Index |
| AUC | area under the (serum concentration time) curve |
| AV | atrioventricular |
| AVP | arginine vasopressin |
| B&B | Brown and Brenn |
| B2M | β2-microglobulin |
| BAL | bronchial alveolar lavage; bronchoalveolar lavage |

DOI 10.37573/9781585286423.FM

| | | | |
|---|---|---|---|
| BAMT | blood assay for *Mycobacterium tuberculosis* | CF | complement fixation |
| BBT | basal body temperature | CFTR | cystic fibrosis transmembrane conductance regulator |
| BCG | Bacillus Calmette-Guérin | CFU, cfu | colony-forming units |
| bDNA | branched-chain DNA | CFW | calcofluor white |
| BGMK-hDAF | buffalo green monkey kidney cell line decay accelerating factor | CGE | capillary gel electrophoresis |
| | | CGM | continuous glucose monitoring |
| BHI | brain heart infusion | $CH_{50}$ | complement hemolytic 50% |
| BHR | bronchial hyper-responsiveness | CHD | coronary heart disease |
| BID | twice daily | CHF | congestive heart failure |
| BMI | body mass index | CI | chemical ionization |
| BMP | basic metabolic panel | CIS | combined intracavernous injection and stimulation |
| BNP | brain or B-type natriuretic peptide | | |
| BP | blood pressure | CK | creatine kinase |
| BPH | benign prostatic hyperplasia | CK-BB | creatine kinase isoenzyme BB |
| BPSA | benign form of prostate-specific antigen | CK-MB | creatine kinase isoenzyme MB |
| BPT | bronchial provocation testing | CK-MM | creatine kinase isoenzyme MM |
| BRAF | v-Raf murine sarcoma viral oncogene homolog B1 | CK1 | creatine kinase isoenzyme 1 |
| | | CK2 | creatine kinase isoenzyme 2 |
| BSA | body surface area | CK3 | creatine kinase isoenzyme 3 |
| BSL | biosafety level | CKD | chronic kidney disease |
| BT | bleeding time | CKD-EPI | Chronic Kidney Disease Epidemiology Collaboration |
| BTP | β-trace protein | | |
| BUN | blood urea nitrogen | CLIA-88 | Clinical Laboratory Improvement Amendments of 1988 |
| *C. difficile* | *Clostridium difficile* | | |
| C3 | complement protein 3 | CLIA | Clinical Laboratory Improvement Amendments |
| C4 | complement protein 4 | | |
| CA | cancer antigen | CLL | chronic lymphocytic leukemia |
| CA | carbonic anhydrase | CLSI | Clinical and Laboratory Standards Institute |
| CABG | coronary artery bypass graft | | |
| CAC | coronary artery calcium | cm | centimeter |
| $CA_{corr}$ | corrected serum calcium level | CMA | cornmeal agar |
| CAD | coronary artery disease | $C_{min}$ | minimum concentration (of a drug) |
| CAH | congenital adrenal hyperplasia | CML | chronic myelogenous leukemia |
| CAN2 | chromID Candida agar | CMP | comprehensive metabolic panel |
| cANCA | cytoplasmic antineutrophil cytoplasmic antibody | CMR | cardiac magnetic resonance |
| | | CMV | cytomegalovirus |
| CAP | College of Pathologists | CNA | colistin-nalidixic acid |
| CAP | community-acquired pneumonia | $C_{normalized}$ | normalized total concentration |
| CAT | computerized axial tomography | CNP | c-type natriuretic peptide |
| $CA_{uncorr}$ | uncorrected serum calcium level (or actual measured total serum calcium) | CNS | central nervous system |
| | | CO | carbon monoxide; cardiac output; cyclooxygenase |
| CBC | complete blood count | | |
| CCFA | cycloserine cefoxitin fructose agar | $CO_2$ | carbon dioxide |
| CCNA | cell cytotoxicity neutralization assay | CO-Hgb | carboxyhemoglobin |
| CCP | cyclic citrullinated peptide | COP | colloid osmotic pressure |
| CCR5 | chemokine coreceptor 5 | COPD | chronic obstructive pulmonary disease |
| cCRP | cardiac C-reactive protein | CPE | cytopathic effect |
| CCT | cardiac computed tomography | CPIC | Clinical Pharmacogenetics Implementation Consortium |
| cd | candela | | |
| CD | clusters of differentiation | CPK | creatine phosphokinase |
| CDC | Centers for Disease Control and Prevention | CPPD | calcium pyrophosphate dihydrate |
| | | cPSA | complexed PSA |
| CDR | complementarity-determining regions | CrCl | creatinine clearance |
| CE | capillary electrophoresis | CREST | syndrome characterized by **c**alcinosis, **R**aynaud disease, **e**sophageal motility disorder, **s**clerodactyly, and **t**elangiectasias |
| CEA | carcinoembryonic antigen | | |
| CEDIA | cloned enzyme donor immunoassay | | |
| CETP | cholesteryl ester transfer protein | | |

| | |
|---|---|
| CRH | corticotrophin-releasing hormone |
| CRP | C-reactive protein |
| CSF | cerebrospinal fluid |
| $C_{ss,\,avg}$ | average steady-state concentration (of a drug) |
| CT | computed tomography |
| cTnC | cardiac-specific troponin C |
| cTnI | cardiac-specific troponin I |
| cTnT | cardiac-specific troponin T |
| CVD | cardiovascular disease |
| CX | circumflex |
| CXCR4 | CXC chemokine coreceptor |
| CYP | cytochrome P450 drug metabolizing enzymes |
| CYP2C19 | cytochrome P450 2C19 enzyme |
| CYP2D6 | cytochrome P450 2D6 enzyme |
| CYP3A4 | cytochrome P450 3A4 enzyme |
| CYP450 | cytochrome P450 enzyme |
| CYP4F2 | cytochrome P450 4F2 enzyme |
| CZE | capillary zone electrophoresis |
| D&C | dilation and curettage |
| D5W | 5% dextrose in water |
| DASH | dietary approaches to stop hypertension |
| DAT | direct agglutination test |
| DAT | direct antibody test |
| DCCT | Diabetes Control and Complications Trial |
| DCP | des-gamma-carboxyprothrombin |
| DDAVP | desmopressin |
| dTT | dilute thrombin time |
| DDT | dichlorodiphenyltrichloroethane |
| DEA | desthylamiodarone |
| DFA | direct fluorescent antibody |
| DHA | docosahexaenoic acid |
| DHEA | dehydroepiandrostenedione or dehydroepiandrosterone |
| DHEAS | dehydroepiandrosterone sulfate |
| DI | diabetes insipidus |
| DIC | disseminated intravascular coagulation |
| DIM | dermatophyte identification medium |
| DKA | diabetic ketoacidosis |
| dL | deciliter |
| DLCO | diffusing capacity of the lung for carbon monoxide |
| DM | diabetes mellitus |
| DNA | deoxyribonucleic acid |
| DNP | dendroaspis natriuretic peptide |
| $DO_2$ | oxygen delivery |
| DOAC | direct oral anticoagulant |
| DPD | dihydropyrimidine dehydrogenase |
| DPP-4 | dipeptidyl peptidase-4 |
| dsDNA | double-stranded DNA |
| DST | dexamethasone suppression test |
| DTI | direct thrombin inhibitor |
| DTM | dermatophyte test medium |
| E2 | estradiol |
| EBM | esculin base medium |
| EBV | Epstein-Barr virus |
| ECD | energy coupled dye |
| ECG | electrocardiogram |
| ECMO | extracorporeal membrane oxygenation |
| ECT | ecarin clotting time |
| ECW | extracellular water |
| ED | emergency department |
| EDTA | ethylenediaminetetraacetic acid |
| EGFR | epidermal growth factor receptor |
| eGFR | estimated glomerular filtration rate |
| EF | ejection fraction |
| EI | electron ionization |
| EIA | enzyme immunoassay |
| EIB | exercise- or exertion-induced bronchospasm |
| EKG | electrocardiogram |
| ELISA | enzyme-linked immunosorbent assay |
| ELVIS | enzyme-linked virus-inducible system |
| EM | electron microscopy |
| EMB | eosin methylene blue |
| eMERGE | Electronic Medical Records and Genomics |
| EMIT | enzyme-multiplied immunoassay technique |
| EMR | electronic medical record |
| EOF | electroosmotic flow |
| EPA | eicosapentaenoic acid |
| EPS | expressed prostatic secretions |
| ER | estrogen receptor |
| ERS | European Respiratory Society |
| ERV | expiratory reserve volume |
| ESA | erythrocyte-stimulating agent |
| ESBL | extended-spectrum β-lactamase |
| ESC | European Society of Cardiology |
| ESI | electrospray ionization |
| ESR | erythrocyte sedimentation rate |
| ESRD | end-stage renal disease |
| Etest | epsilometer test |
| ETIB | enzyme-linked immunoelectrotransfer blot |
| EU | ELISA units |
| EUCAST | European Committee on Antimicrobial Susceptibility Testing |
| EULAR | European League Against Rheumatism |
| FA | fluorescent antibody |
| Fab | fraction antigen-binding |
| FAB | fast atom bombardment |
| FAB | French-American-British |
| FACS | fluorescence-activated cell sorting |
| FALS | forward-angle light scattering |
| FANA | fluorescent antinuclear antibody |
| FBG | fasting blood sugar |
| FDA | Food and Drug Administration |
| FDP | fibrin degradation product |
| $FEF_{25-75}$ | forced expiratory flow at 25% to 75% of vital capacity |
| FEF | forced expiratory flow |
| $FE_{Na}$ | fractional excretion of sodium |
| FENO | fractional exhaled nitric oxide |

| | | | | |
|---|---|---|---|---|
| FEV$_1$ | forced expiratory volume in 1 second | | HAAg | hepatitis A antigen |
| FiO$_2$ | fraction of inspired oxygen | | HAP | hospital-acquired pneumonia |
| FISH | fluorescent in situ hybridization | | HAV | hepatitis A virus |
| FITC | fluorescein isothiocyanate | | Hb; hgb | hemoglobin |
| fL | femtoliter | | HbA1c | glycated hemoglobin |
| FM | Fontana-Masson | | HBcAg | hepatitis B core antigen |
| FN | false negative | | HBeAg | hepatitis B extracellular antigen |
| FOB | fecal occult blood | | HBsAg | hepatitis B surface antigen |
| FP | false positive | | HBV | hepatitis B virus |
| FPG | fasting plasma glucose | | hCG | human chorionic gonadotropin |
| FPIA | fluorescence polarization immunoassay | | HCO$_3^-$ | bicarbonate |
| fPSA | free prostate specific antigen | | HCT, Hct | hematocrit |
| FRC | functional residual capacity | | HCV | hepatitis C virus |
| FSC | forward-scattered light | | HDAg | hepatitis D antigen |
| FSH | follicle-stimulating hormone | | HDL | high-density lipoprotein |
| FTA-ABS | fluorescent treponemal antibody absorption | | HDL-C | high-density lipoprotein cholesterol |
| | | | HDV | hepatitis D virus |
| FVC | forced vital capacity | | HER-1 | human epidermal growth factor receptor 1 |
| FWR | framework regions | | | |
| g | gram | | HER-2 | human epidermal growth factor receptor 2 |
| G-CSF | granulocyte colony–stimulating factor | | | |
| G6PD | glucose-6 phosphate dehydrogenase | | HEV | hepatitis E virus |
| GA | gestational age | | HFpEF | heart failure with preserved ejection fraction |
| GAD | glutamic acid decarboxylase | | | |
| GADA | glutamic acid decarboxylase autoantibodies | | HFrEF | heart failure with reduced ejection fraction |
| GAP | group A streptococcus | | HGA | human granulocytic anaplasmosis |
| GAS | group A streptococci | | Hgb | hemoglobin |
| GC | gas chromatography | | HHS | hyperosmolar hyperglycemic state |
| GC-MS | gas chromatography and mass spectrometry | | HIPA | heparin-induced platelet activation |
| | | | HIT | heparin-induced thrombocytopenia |
| GDM | gestational diabetes mellitus | | HIV | human immunodeficiency virus |
| GERD | gastroesophageal reflux disease | | HIV-1 | human immunodeficiency virus type 1 |
| GF | Gridley fungus | | HLA | human leukocyte antigen |
| GFR | glomerular filtration rate | | HLA-B27 | human leukocyte antigen B27 |
| GGT, GGTP | gamma-glutamyl transferase; gamma-glutamyl transpeptidase | | HLA-DQ | human leukocyte antigen coded DQ genes |
| GHB | gamma-hydroxybutyrate | | HLAR | high-level aminoglycoside resistance |
| GI | gastrointestinal | | HME | human monocytic ehrlichiosis |
| GIP | glucose-dependent insulinotropic peptide | | HMG-CoA | 3-hydroxy-3-methyl-glutaryl-coenzyme A |
| GLC | gas liquid chromatography | | HMWK | high-molecular weight kininogen |
| GLIM | Global Leadership Initiative on Malnutrition | | HPA | hypothalamic pituitary axis |
| | | | HPF | high-power field |
| GLP-1 | incretin hormones glucagon-like peptide-1 | | HPLC | high-performance (or pressure) liquid chromatography |
| GLUT | glucose transporter | | HPV | human papillomavirus |
| GM-CSF | granulocyte/macrophage colony-stimulating factor | | HR | heart rate |
| | | | hr | hour |
| GMS | Gomori methenamine silver | | hs-CRP | high-sensitivity C-reactive protein |
| GnRH | gonadotropin-releasing hormone | | HSG | hysterosalpingogram, hysterosalpingography |
| GOLD | Global Initiative for Chronic Obstructive Lung Disease | | | |
| | | | hsTnI | high-sensitivity troponin I |
| gp | glycoprotein | | hsTnT | high-sensitivity troponin T |
| GPA | granulomatosis with polyangiitis | | HSV | herpes simplex virus |
| GTF | glucose tolerance factor | | Ht | height |
| H&E | hematoxylin and eosin | | HTN | hypertension |
| *H. Pylori* | *Helicobacter pylori* | | I | intermediate |

| | | | |
|---|---|---|---|
| IA | immunoassay | $K_{corr}$ | corrected serum potassium level |
| IA-2A | insulinoma-associated-2 autoantibodies | KDIGO | Kidney Disease Improving Global Outcomes |
| IAA | insulin autoantibodies | | |
| IAT | indirect antiglobulin test | kg | kilogram |
| IBW | ideal body weight | KIMS | kinetic interaction of microparticles in solution |
| IC | inspiratory capacity | | |
| $IC_{50}$ | inhibitory concentration 50% | Km | Michaelis constant |
| $IC_{90}$ | inhibitory concentration 90% | KOH | potassium hydroxide |
| ICA | immunochromatographic assay | KRas | V-Ki-ras2 Kirsten rat sarcoma viral oncogene homolog |
| ICA | islet cell cytoplasmic autoantibodies | | |
| ICD | International Classification of Diseases | $K_{uncorr}$ | uncorrected serum potassium level (or actual measured serum potassium) |
| ICTV | International Committee on Taxonomy of Viruses | | |
| | | L | liter |
| ICU | intensive care unit | LA | latex agglutination |
| ICW | intracellular water | La/SSB | La/Sjögren syndrome B |
| ID | immunodiffusion | LAD | left anterior descending |
| IDC | International Diabetes Center | LADA | latent autoimmune disorder |
| IDL | intermediate-density lipoproteins | LBBB | left bundle branch block |
| IDMS | isotope dilution mass spectrometry | LBW | lean body weight |
| IDSA | Infectious Diseases Society of America | LC | liquid chromatography |
| IEF | isoelectric focusing | LCAT | lecithin cholesterol acyltransferase |
| IFA | immunofluorescence assay; indirect fluorescent antibody | LCR | ligase chain reaction |
| | | LDH | lactate dehydrogenase |
| IFE | immunofixation electrophoresis | LDH1 | lactate dehydrogenase isoenzyme 1 |
| IFG | impaired fasting glucose | LDH2 | lactate dehydrogenase isoenzyme 2 |
| IFN-γ | interferon gamma | LDH3 | lactate dehydrogenase isoenzyme 3 |
| IFR | immunofixation electrophoresis | LDH4 | lactate dehydrogenase isoenzyme 4 |
| IgA | immunoglobulin A | LDH5 | lactate dehydrogenase isoenzyme 5 |
| IgD | immunoglobulin D | LDL | low-density lipoprotein |
| IgE | immunoglobulin E | LDL-C | low-density lipoprotein cholesterol |
| IgG | immunoglobulin G | LE | lupus erythematosus |
| IgM | immunoglobulin M | LFT | liver function test |
| IGNITE | Implementing GeNomics In PracTicE | LH | luteinizing hormone |
| IGT | impaired glucose tolerance | LHRH | luteinizing hormone–releasing hormone |
| IHC | immunohistochemistry | | |
| IHD | ischemic heart disease | LIS | laboratory information system |
| IIEF | International Index of Erectile Function | LMP | last menstrual period |
| IIM | idiopathic inflammatory myopathy | LMWH | low molecular weight heparin |
| IMA | inhibitory mold agar | Lp(a) | lipoprotein(a) |
| IM-ADR | immune-mediated adverse drug reaction | $Lp-PLA_2$ | lipoprotein-associated phospholipase $A_2$ |
| | | LPL | lipoprotein lipase |
| INR | international normalized ratio | LSD | lysergic acid diethylamide |
| IP | interphalangeal | LTA | light transmittance aggregometry |
| iPSA | inactive PSA | LUTS | lower urinary tract symptoms |
| IPSS | International Prostate Symptom Score | LVEF | left ventricular ejection fraction |
| IQ | inhibitory quotient | m | meter |
| IRMA | immunoradiometric assay | $m^2$ | meters squared |
| IRV | inspiratory reserve volume | MAbs | monoclonal antibodies |
| ISE | ion-selective electrode | Mac | MacConkey |
| ISI | International Sensitivity Index | MAC | membrane attack complex |
| ITP | idiopathic thrombocytopenic purpura | MAC | *Mycobacterium avium* complex |
| IV | intravenous | MALDI | matrix-assisted laser desorption/ionization |
| J | joule | | |
| JIA | juvenile idiopathic arthritis | MALDI-TOF | matrix-assisted laser desorption ionization time-of-flight |
| JRA | juvenile rheumatoid arthritis | | |
| JVP | jugular venous pressure | MAP | mitogen-activated protein |
| k | constant of proportionality | MAT | microagglutination test |
| K | kelvin | MBC | minimum bactericidal concentration |

| | | | |
|---|---|---|---|
| MBP | mannose-binding protein | NACB | National Academy of Clinical Biochemistry |
| mcg | microgram | NAEPP | National Asthma Education Prevention Program |
| MCH | mean corpuscular hemoglobin | | |
| MCHC | mean corpuscular hemoglobin concentration | NAFLD | nonalcoholic fatty liver disease |
| MCP | metacarpophalangeal | NASBA | nucleic acid sequence-based amplification |
| MCT | medium chain triglycerides | | |
| MCTD | mixed connective tissue disease | NASH | nonalcoholic steatohepatitis |
| MCV | mean corpuscular volume | NCBI | National Center for Biotechnology Information |
| MDMA | 3,4-methylenedioxy-$N$-methamphetamine (Ecstasy) | NCCB | nondihydropyridine calcium channel blocker |
| MDR | multidrug resistant | | |
| MDRD | Modification of Diet in Renal Disease | NCEP | National Cholesterol Education Program |
| MDx | molecular diagnostics | | |
| mEq | milliequivalent | ng | nanogram |
| mg | milligram | NGS | next-generation sequencing |
| MHA | Mueller-Hinton agar | NGSP | National Glycohemoglobin Standardization Program |
| MHA-TP | microhemagglutination *Treponema pallidum* | | |
| | | NHANES | National Health and Nutrition Examination Survey |
| MHC | major histocompatibility complex | | |
| MI | myocardial infarction | NHL | Non-Hodgkin lymphoma |
| MIC | minimum inhibitory concentration | NIH | National Institutes of Health |
| $MIC_{50}$ | MIC value representing 50% of a bacterial population | NK | cells natural killer (T) lymphocytes |
| | | NKDEP | National Kidney Disease Education Program |
| $MIC_{90}$ | MIC value representing 90% of a bacterial population | | |
| | | NKF KDOQI | National Kidney Foundation Kidney Disease Outcomes Quality Initiative |
| MIF | microimmunofluorescence | | |
| min | minute | NLA | National Lipid Association |
| mL | milliliter | nm | nanometer |
| mm | millimeter | NMIBC | non-muscle-invasive bladder cancer |
| $mm^3$ | cubic millimeter | NNRTI | non-nucleoside reverse transcriptase inhibitor |
| mmol | millimole | | |
| mTOR | mammalian target of rapamycin | NNS | number needed to screen |
| moAb | monoclonal antibody | NPV | negative predictive value |
| mo | month | NQO1 | NADPH quinone dehydrogenase 1 |
| mol | mole | NQMI | non Q-wave myocardial infarction |
| mOsm | milliosmole serum osmolality | NRS/CHOL | National Reference System for Cholesterol |
| MOTT | mycobacteria other than tuberculosis | | |
| MPO | myeloperoxidase | NRTI | nucleoside reverse transcriptase inhibitor |
| MPV | mean platelet volume | NSAID | nonsteroidal anti-inflammatory drug |
| MRI | magnetic resonance imaging | NSCLC | non-small-cell lung cancer |
| mRNA | messenger ribonucleic acid | NSTEMI | non-ST-segment elevation myocardial infarction |
| MRO | medical review officer | | |
| MRP1 | multidrug resistant protein 1 | NT-proBNP | N-terminal-proBNP |
| MRP2 | multidrug resistant protein 2 | NTM | nontuberculous mycobacteria |
| MRP3 | multidrug resistant protein 3 | NUDT15 | nudix hydrolase 15 |
| MRSA | methicillin-resistant *Staphylococcus aureus* | NYHA | New York Heart Association |
| | | OA | osteoarthritis |
| MS | mass spectrometry | OAT | organic anion transport |
| MSSA | methicillin-susceptible *Staphylococcus aureus* | OATP1 | organic anion-transporting polypeptide 1 |
| mTOR | mammalian (or mechanistic) target of rapamycin | OATP2 | organic anion-transporting polypeptide 2 |
| MTP | metatarsophalangeal | OCT | organic cation transport |
| N | newton | OGTT | oral glucose tolerance test |
| NA | nucleic acid | OIR | Office of In Vitro Diagnostics and Radiological Health |
| NAAT | nucleic acid amplification test | | |

| | |
|---|---|
| OSHA | Occupational Safety and Health Administration |
| $P_1G_1O_1$ | one live birth, one pregnancy, no spontaneous or elective abortions |
| P-gp | P-glycoprotein |
| Pa | Pascal |
| pAB | polyclonal antibody |
| $PaCO_2$ | partial pressure of carbon dioxide, arterial |
| PAD | peripheral arterial disease |
| PAE | postantibiotic effect |
| PAI1 | plasminogen activator inhibitor 1 |
| pANCA | perinuclear antineutrophil cytoplasmic antibody |
| $PaO_2$ | partial pressure of oxygen, arterial |
| PAS | periodic acid-Schiff |
| PBC | primary biliary cirrhosis |
| PBMC | peripheral blood mononuclear cell |
| PBP | penicillin-binding protein |
| $PC_{20}FEV_1$ | provocation concentration of the bronchoconstrictor agent that produces a 20% reduction in $FEV_1$ |
| PCA | postconceptional age |
| PCI | percutaneous coronary intervention |
| $pCO_2$ | partial pressure of carbon dioxide |
| PCOS | polycystic ovary syndrome |
| PCP | phencyclidine |
| PCR | polymerase chain reaction |
| PCSK9 | proprotein convertase subtilisin/kexin type 9 |
| PD | pharmacodynamic |
| PDA | potato dextrose agar |
| PE | phycoerythrin |
| $Peak_{steady\ state}$ | peak concentration of a drug in serum or plasma at steady state |
| PEA | phenylethyl alcohol |
| PEFR | peak expiratory flow rate |
| PET | positron emission tomography |
| PF3 | platelet factor 3 |
| PF4 | platelet factor 4 |
| PFA | potato flake agar |
| PFGE | pulsed-field gel electrophoresis |
| PFT | pulmonary function test |
| pg | picogram |
| PG | prostaglandin |
| PG2 | prostacyclin |
| PGx | pharmacogenetic |
| pH | power of hydrogen or hydrogen ion concentration |
| PHY | phenytoin |
| Ph | Philadelphia |
| PI | protease inhibitor |
| PICU | pediatric intensive care unit |
| PID | pelvic inflammatory disease |
| PIP | proximal interphalangeal |
| PK | pharmacokinetic |
| PKU | phenylketonuria |

| | |
|---|---|
| PL | phospholipid |
| PMA | postmenstrual age |
| PMN | polymorphonuclear leukocyte |
| PNA | postnatal age |
| PNA-FISH | peptide nucleic acid fluorescent in situ hybridization |
| PO | per os (by mouth) |
| $pO_2$ | partial pressure of oxygen |
| POC | point-of-care |
| POCT | point-of-care testing |
| PPAR | peroxisome proliferator-activated receptor |
| PPD | purified protein derivative |
| PPG | postprandial glucose |
| PPI | proton pump inhibitor |
| PPV | positive predictive value |
| PR | progesterone receptor |
| PR3 | proteinase 3 |
| PRN | as needed |
| PRU | P2Y12 reaction units |
| PSA | prostate specific antigen |
| PSAD | prostate specific antigen density |
| PSADT | prostate specific antigen doubling time |
| PSB | protected specimen brush |
| PSM | patient self-management |
| PST | patient self-testing |
| PT | prothrombin time |
| PTCA | percutaneous transluminal coronary angioplasty |
| PTH | parathyroid hormone |
| q | every |
| Q | perfusion |
| QC | quality control |
| QID | four times daily |
| qPCR | real-time polymerase chain reaction |
| QRS | electrocardiograph wave; represents ventricular depolarization |
| QwMI | Q-wave myocardial infarction |
| R | resistant |
| R-CVA | right cerebral vascular accident |
| RA | rheumatoid arthritis |
| RAAS | renin-angiotensin-aldosterone system |
| RADT | rapid antigen detection test |
| RAEB | refractory anemia with excess blasts |
| RAIU | radioactive iodine uptake test |
| RALS | right-angle light scattering |
| RBC | red blood cell |
| RBF | renal blood flow |
| RCA | right coronary artery |
| RDW | red cell distribution width |
| RF | rheumatoid factor |
| RhMK | rhesus monkey kidney |
| RI | reticulocyte index |
| RIA | radioimmunoassay |
| RIBA | recombinant immunoblot assay |
| RIDTs | rapid influenza diagnostic tests |
| RNA | ribonucleic acid |

| | | | |
|---|---|---|---|
| RNP | ribonucleoprotein | STEMI | ST-segment elevation myocardial infarction |
| Ro/SSA | Ro/Sjögren syndrome A antibody | SV | stroke volume |
| RPF | renal plasma flow | SVC | slow vital capacity |
| RPR | rapid plasma reagin | $SvO_2$ | venous oxygen saturation |
| RR | respiratory rate | $T_3$ | triiodothyronine |
| RSA | rapid sporulation agar | $T_3RU$ | triiodothyronine resin uptake |
| RSAT | rapid streptococcal antigen test | $T_4$ | thyroxine |
| RSV | respiratory syncytial virus | TAT | turnaround time |
| RT | reverse transcriptase; reverse transcription | TB | tuberculosis |
| RT-PCR | reverse-transcriptase polymerase chain reaction | TBG | thyroxine-binding globulin |
| | | TBI | total body irradiation |
| RV | residual volume | TBPA | thyroid-binding prealbumin |
| S | susceptible | TBW | total body water |
| S | Cys C serum cystatin C | TBW | total body weight |
| S:P ratio | saliva:plasma concentration ratio | TC | total cholesterol |
| SA | sinoatrial | TCA | tricyclic antidepressant |
| $SaO_2$ | arterial oxygen saturation | TDM | therapeutic drug monitoring |
| SAMHSA | Substance Abuse and Mental Health Services Administration | TEE | transesophageal echocardiography |
| | | TF | tissue factor |
| SAT | serum agglutination test | TFPI | tissue factor pathway inhibitor |
| SBA | sheep blood agar | TG | triglyceride |
| SBT | serum bactericidal test | THC | total hemolytic complement |
| $Scl_{70}$ | scleroderma-70 or DNA topoisomerase I antibody | TIA | transient ischemic attack |
| | | TIBC | total iron-binding capacity |
| SCr | serum creatinine | TID | three times daily |
| $ScvO_2$ | central venous oxygen saturation | TJC | The Joint Commission |
| SD | standard deviation | TK | tyrosine kinase |
| SDA | Sabouraud dextrose agar | TKI | tyrosine kinase inhibitor |
| SDA | strand displacement amplification | TLA | total laboratory automation |
| sec | second | TLC | therapeutic lifestyle changes |
| SEGA | subependymal giant cell astrocytoma | TLC | thin layer chromatography |
| SGE | spiral gradient endpoint | TLC | total lung capacity |
| SGLT | sodium glucose cotransporters | TMA | transcription mediated amplification |
| SHBG | sex hormone-binding globulin | TN | true negative |
| SI | International System of Units | TnC | troponin C |
| SIADH | syndrome of inappropriate antidiuretic hormone | TNF | tumor necrosis factor |
| | | TnI | troponin I |
| SID | strong ion difference | TnT | troponin T |
| SIG | strong ion gap | TP | true positive; tube precipitin |
| SIHD | stable ischemic heart disease | tPA | tissue plasminogen activator |
| SLE | systemic lupus erythematosus | TPMT | thiopurine methyltransferase |
| Sm | Smith antibody | TPN | total parenteral nutrition |
| SMBG | self-monitoring blood glucose | TR | therapeutic range |
| SNP | single nucleotide polymorphism | TRH | thyrotropin-releasing hormone |
| SNRI | serotonin–norepinephrine reuptake inhibitor | TRUS | transrectal ultrasound of the prostate |
| | | TSB | trypticase soy broth |
| SnRNP | small nuclear ribonucleoprotein particle | TSH | thyroid-stimulating hormone |
| SPECT | single-photon emission computed tomography | TST | tuberculin skin test |
| | | TT | thrombin time |
| SPEP | serum protein electrophoresis | TTE | transthoracic echocardiography |
| SRA | C-serotonin release assay | TTKG | transtubular potassium gradient |
| SSC | side-scattered light | TTP | thrombotic thrombocytopenic purpura; total testing process |
| ssDNA | single-stranded DNA | | |
| SSRI | selective serotonin reuptake inhibitor | TTR | time in therapeutic range |
| STD | sexually transmitted disease | TV | tidal volume |

| | | | |
|---|---|---|---|
| $T_xA_2$ | thromboxane $A_2$ | Vd | volume of distribution |
| type 1 DM | type 1 diabetes mellitus | VDRL | Venereal Disease Research Laboratory |
| type 2 DM | type 2 diabetes mellitus | VISA | vancomycin-intermediate |
| U | urinary creatinine concentration | | *Staphylococcus aureus* |
| $U_1RNP$ | uridine-rich ribonuclear protein | VKOR | vitamin K epoxide reductase |
| UA | unstable angina | VKORC1 | vitamin K epoxide reductase complex |
| UCr | urine creatinine | | subunit 1 |
| UFC | urine-free cortisol | VLDL | very low-density lipoprotein |
| UFH | unfractionated heparin | $V_{max}$ | maximum rate of metabolism |
| UGT1A1 | uridine diphosphate glucuronyl | VPA | valproic acid |
| | transferase | $VO_2$ | oxygen consumption |
| UKPDS | United Kingdom Prospective Diabetes | VRE | vancomycin-resistant enterococci |
| | Study | VTE | venous thromboembolism |
| ULN | upper limit of normal | vWF | von Willebrand factor |
| uNGAL | urine neutrophil gelatinase associated | VZV | varicella zoster virus |
| | lipocalcin | W | watt |
| uPA | urokinase plasminogen activator | WB | western blot |
| U-PGx | Ubiquitous Pharmacogenetics | WBC | white blood cell |
| | Consortium | WHO | World Health Organization |
| UTI | urinary tract infection | wk | week |
| UUN | urinary urea nitrogen | WNL | within normal limits |
| UV | ultraviolet | Wt | weight |
| V | total urine volume collected; | WT | wild type |
| | ventilation; volt | xPOCT | multiplexed point-of-care testing |
| VAP | ventilator-associated pneumonia | yr | year |
| VC | vital capacity | | |

# PART I

## BASIC CONCEPTS AND TEST INTERPRETATIONS

# 1

# Definitions and Concepts

*Karen J. Tietze*

## OBJECTIVES

*After completing this chapter, the reader should be able to*

- Differentiate between accuracy and precision

- Distinguish between quantitative and qualitative laboratory tests

- Define reference range and identify factors that affect a reference range

- Differentiate between sensitivity and specificity, and calculate and assess these parameters

- Identify potential sources of laboratory errors and state the impact of these errors in the interpretation of laboratory tests

- Identify patient-specific factors that must be considered when assessing laboratory data

- Discuss the pros and cons of point-of-care and at-home laboratory testing

- Describe a rational approach to interpreting laboratory results

Laboratory testing is used to detect disease, guide treatment, monitor response to treatment, and monitor disease progression. However, it is an imperfect science. Laboratory testing may fail to identify abnormalities that are present (false negatives [FNs]) or identify abnormalities that are not present (false positives [FPs]). This chapter defines terms used to describe and differentiate laboratory tests and describes factors to consider when assessing and applying laboratory test results.

## DEFINITIONS

Many terms are used to describe and differentiate laboratory test characteristics and results. The clinician should recognize and understand these terms before assessing and applying test results to individual patients.

### Accuracy and Precision

*Accuracy* and *precision* are important laboratory quality-control measures. Laboratories are expected to test analytes (the substance measured by the assay) with accuracy and precision and to document the quality-control procedures. Accuracy of a quantitative assay is usually measured in terms of analytical performance, which includes accuracy and precision. Accuracy is defined as the extent to which the mean measurement is close to the true value. A sample spiked with a known quantity of an analyte is measured repeatedly; the mean measurement is calculated. A highly accurate assay means that the repeated analyses produce a mean value that is the same as or very close to the known spiked quantity. Accuracy of a qualitative assay is calculated as the sum of the true positives (TPs) and true negatives (TNs) divided by the number of samples tested (accuracy = [(TP + TN) ÷ number of samples tested] × 100%). Precision refers to assay reproducibility (ie, the agreement of results when the specimen is assayed many times). An assay with high precision means that the methodology is consistently able to produce results in close agreement.

### Analyte

The *analyte* is the substance measured by the assay. Some substances, such as phenytoin and calcium, are bound extensively to proteins such as albumin. Although the unbound fraction elicits the physiologic or pharmacological effect (bound substances are inactive), most routine assays measure the total substance (bound plus unbound). The free fraction may be assayable, but the assays are not routine. Therefore, the reference range for total and free substances may be quite different. For example, the reference range is 10–20 mcg/mL for total phenytoin, 1–2 mcg/mL for free phenytoin, 9.2–11 mg/dL for total serum calcium, and 4–4.8 mg/dL for free (also called *ionized*) calcium.

Some analytes exist in several forms and each has a different reference range. Results for the total and each form are reported. For example, bilirubin circulates in conjugated and unconjugated subforms as well as bound irreversibly to albumin

*Note: This chapter is based, in part, on the second edition chapter titled "Definitions and Concepts," which was written by Scott L. Traub.*

DOI 10.37573/9781585286423.001

(δ bilirubin). *Direct bilirubin* refers to the sum of the conjugated plus the δ forms (water soluble forms); *indirect bilirubin* refers to the unconjugated form (water insoluble form). Lactate dehydrogenase (LDH) is separated electrophoretically into five different isoenzymes: LDH1, LDH2, LDH3, LDH4, and LDH5. Creatine kinase (CK) exists in three isoforms: CK1 (CK-BB), CK2 (CK-MB), and CK3 (CK-MM).

## Biomarker

A *biomarker* (biological marker) is a marker (not necessarily a quantifiable laboratory parameter) defined by the Food and Drug Administration (FDA) as "A defined characteristic that is measured as an indicator of normal biological processes, pathogenic processes, or responses to an exposure or intervention, including therapeutics interventions."[3] Biomarkers are used to diagnose and stage disease (ie, determine the extent of disease), assess disease progression, and predict or assess response to therapeutic interventions. For example, tumor markers are biomarkers used to identify the presence of some cancers, to stage disease, or to assess patient response to drug and nondrug cancer treatments. Many biomarkers are common laboratory parameters. For example, glycosylated hemoglobin A1c (HbA1c) is used to assess average blood sugar levels over the past three months in patients with diabetes.

## Noninvasive Versus Invasive Tests

A *noninvasive test* is a procedure that examines fluids or other substances (eg, urine and exhaled air) obtained without using a needle, tube, device, or scope to penetrate the skin or enter the body. An *invasive test* is a procedure that examines fluids or tissues (eg, venous blood and skin biopsy) obtained by using a needle, tube, device, or scope to penetrate the skin or enter the body. Invasive tests pose variable risk depending on the method of specimen collection (eg, pain and bruising associated with venipuncture) and are less convenient than noninvasive tests.

## Predictive Value

The *predictive value*, derived from a test's sensitivity, specificity, and prevalence of the disease in the population being tested, is used to assess a test's reliability (**Table 1-1**). As applied to a positive test result, the predictive value indicates the percent of positives that are true positives. For a test with equal sensitivity and specificity, the predictive value of a positive result increases as the prevalence of the disease in the population increases. For example, the glucose tolerance test has a higher predictive value for diabetes in women who are pregnant than in the general population as a result of the higher prevalence of diabetes in pregnancy compared with the general population due to gestational diabetes. A borderline abnormal serum creatinine concentration has a higher predictive value for kidney disease in patients in a nephrology unit than in patients in a general medical unit. The lower the prevalence of disease in the population tested, the greater the chance that a positive test result is

**TABLE 1-1.** Relationship of Sensitivity, Specificity, Disease Prevalence, and Predictive Value of a Positive Test (the predictive value of a positive test increases as the disease prevalence and sensitivity and specificity of the test increase)

| SENSITIVITY AND SPECIFICITY (%) | PREVALENCE (%) | PREDICTIVE VALUE OF POSITIVE TEST (%) |
|---|---|---|
| 95 | 0.1 | 1.9 |
|    | 1   | 16.1 |
|    | 2   | 27.9 |
|    | 5   | 50 |
|    | 50  | 95 |
| 99 | 0.1 | 9 |
|    | 1   | 50 |
|    | 2   | 66.9 |
|    | 5   | 83.9 |
|    | 50  | 99 |

Predictive value of positive test = [TP ÷ (TP + FP)] × 100%.
Predictive value of negative test = [TN ÷ (TN + FN)] × 100%.
Disease prevalence = (TP + FN) ÷ number of patients tested.
TP = diseased persons detected by test (true positives).
FP = nondiseased persons positive to test (false positives).
FN = diseased persons not detected by test (false negatives).
TN = nondiseased persons negative to test (true negatives).

in error. The predictive value may also be applied to negative results. As applied to a negative test result, the predictive value indicates the percent of negatives that are true negatives (refer to **Minicase 1**).

## Qualitative Tests

A *qualitative test* is a test whose results are reported as either positive or negative without further characterization of the degree of positivity or negativity. Exact quantities may be measured in the laboratory but are still reported qualitatively using predetermined ranges. For example, a serum or urine pregnancy test is reported as either positive or negative; a bacterial wound culture is reported as either positive for one or more specific microorganisms or reported as no growth; a urine toxicology drug screen is reported as either positive or negative for specific drugs; a hepatitis C virus (HCV) ribonucleic acid (RNA) test is reported as positive or negative for hepatitis C viral RNA; and an acid-fast stain for *Mycobacterium* is reported as either positive or negative.

# MINICASE 1

## Bladder Urothelial Carcinoma Recurrence Surveillance

Frequent active surveillance is recommended for patients following treatment for nonmuscle-invasive bladder cancer (NMIBC). The gold standard active surveillance monitoring strategies for NMIBC include cystoscopy and urine cytology. For patients with a low risk of recurrence, the American Urological Association/Society of Urologic Oncology recommends patients undergo the first surveillance cystoscopy within three to four months after initial treatment, then six to nine months later, and then annually for five years; more frequent active surveillance is recommended for patients at a greater risk of recurrence.[1] Cystoscopy is an invasive test with well-described risks; a noninvasive active surveillance laboratory test would reduce healthcare costs and patient risk.

The sensitivity and specificity of a new noninvasive Bladder EpiCheck test in 353 subjects with incident or recurrent bladder urothelial carcinoma undergoing active surveillance with cystoscopy and cytology were assessed.[2]

QUESTION: After reviewing the following results, what conclusions can be made about the clinical performance of the Bladder EpiCheck test?

Bladder EpiCheck Results ($n = 353$)

True positives (TP): 30    True negatives (TN): 272

False positives (FP): 37    False negatives (FN): 14

DISCUSSION: Calculate sensitivity, specificity, predictive value of a positive test, and predictive value of a negative test.

Sensitivity = (TP ÷ [TP + FN]) × 100% = (30 ÷ [30 + 14]) × 100% = 68.2%

Specificity = (TN ÷ [TN + FP]) × 100% = (272 ÷ [272 + 37]) × 100% = 88%

Predictive value of positive test = (TP ÷ [TP + FP]) × 100% = (30 ÷ [30 + 37]) × 100% = 44.8%

Predictive value of negative test = (TN ÷ [TN + FN]) × 100% = (272 ÷ [272 + 14]) × 100% = 95.1%

In this study, the noninvasive Bladder EpiCheck urine test had a high overall negative predictive value (NPV), high specificity, and clinically acceptable sensitivity. The clinical application of this test is to surveil for cancer recurrence to determine if a more invasive, but more sensitive, monitoring strategy is necessary. If patients test negative and are truly negative, additional testing is not necessary. A high overall negative predictive value of 95.1% makes this test useful for this application despite a lower predictive value of positive test.

## Quantitative Tests

A *quantitative test* is a test whose results are reported as an exact numeric measurement (usually a specific mass per unit measurement) and assessed in the context of a reference range of values. For example, serum potassium is commonly reported in milliequivalents per liter, creatinine clearance is commonly reported in milliliters per minute, fractional exhaled nitric oxide (FeNO) is commonly reported in parts per billion, and LDH is commonly reported in units per liter. Some test results are reported as titers (dilutions). For example, a serum antinuclear antibody titer of 1:160 is usually associated with active systemic lupus erythematosus (SLE) or other autoimmune diseases, though some patients may have "low titer" disease with titers of 1:40 or 1:80.

## Reference Range

The *reference range* (also known as *the reference interval* or the *reference value*) is a statistically-derived numerical range obtained by testing a sample of individuals assumed to be healthy. The upper and lower limits of the range are not absolute (ie, normal versus abnormal), but rather points beyond which the probability of clinical significance begins to increase. The term *reference range* is preferred over the term *normal range*.[4] The reference population is assumed to have a Gaussian distribution with 68% of the values within one standard deviation (SD) above and below the mean (±1 SD), 95% within ±2 SD, and 99.7% within ±3 SD (**Figure 1-1**).

The reference range for a given analyte is usually established in the clinical laboratory as the mean or average value plus or minus two SDs. Acceptance of the mean ±2 SD indicates that one in 20 normal individuals will have test results outside the reference range (2.5% have values below the lower limit of the reference range and 2.5% have values above the upper limit of the reference range). Accepting a wider range (eg, ±3 SD) includes a larger percentage (99.7%) of normal individuals but increases the chance of including individuals with values only slightly outside of a narrower range, thus decreasing the sensitivity of the test.

Qualitative laboratory tests are either negative or positive and lack a reference range; any positivity is considered abnormal. For example, any amount of serum acetone, porphobilinogen, or alcohol in serum or plasma is considered abnormal. The presence of glucose, ketones, blood, bile, or nitrate in urine is abnormal. The results of the Venereal Disease Research Laboratory (VDRL) test, tests for red blood cell (RBC) sickling, and the malaria smear are either positive or negative.

### Factors That Influence the Reference Range

Many factors influence the reference range. Reference ranges may differ between laboratories depending on analytical technique, reagent, and equipment. The initial assumption that the sample population is normal may be false. For example, the reference range is inaccurate if too many individuals with covert

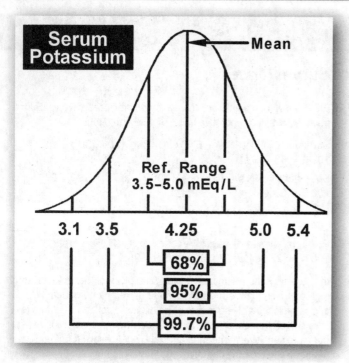

**FIGURE 1-1.** Gaussian (random) value distribution with a visual display of the area included within increments of standard deviation (SD) above and below the mean: ±1 SD = 68% of total values; ±2 SD = 95% of total values; and ±3 SD = 99.7% of total values. (*Source*: Reprinted with permission from Basic Skills in Interpreting Laboratory Data, 6th edition.)

disease (ie, no signs or symptoms of disease) are included in the sample population. Failure to control for physiologic variables (eg, age, gender, ethnicity, body mass, diet, posture, and time of day) introduces factors that may result in an inaccurate reference range. Reference ranges calculated from nonrandomly distributed (non-Gaussian) test results or from a small number of samples may not be accurate.

Reference ranges may change as new information relating to disease and treatments becomes available. For example, the generally accepted upper limit of normal for thyroid-stimulating hormone (TSH) (4.12 milli-international units per liter) is based on data from the National Health and Nutrition Examination Survey (NHANES III).[5] But the availability of more sensitive assays and the recognition that the original reference population data were skewed has led some clinicians to conclude that the upper limit of normal for TSH should be lowered.[6] In contrast, recent data supports extending the upper limit of normal for TSH for patients 80 years and older.[7]

### Critical Value

The term *critical value* refers to a result that is far enough outside the reference range that it indicates impending morbidity (eg, potassium < 2.8 mEq/L). Because laboratory personnel are not in a position to consider mitigating circumstances, a designated member of the healthcare team is notified immediately

on discovery of a critical value test result. Critical values may not always be clinically relevant, however, because the reference range varies for the reasons discussed previously.

## Semiquantitative Tests

A *semiquantitative test* is a test whose results are reported as either negative or with varying degrees of positivity but without exact quantification. For example, urine glucose and urine ketones may be reported as negative or trace, 1+, 2+, 3+, or 4+; the higher numbers represent a greater amount of the measured substance in the urine, but not a specific concentration.

## Sensitivity

The *sensitivity* of a test refers to the ability of the test to identify positive results in patients who actually have the disease (the true positive rate).[8,9] Sensitivity assesses the proportion of true positives disclosed by the test (**Table 1-2**). A test is completely sensitive (100% sensitivity) if it is positive in every patient who actually has the disease. The higher the test sensitivity, the lower the chance of a false negative result; the lower the test sensitivity, the higher the chance of a false negative result. However, a highly sensitive test is not necessarily a highly specific test (see below).

Highly sensitive tests are preferred when the consequences of not identifying the disease are serious; less sensitive tests may be acceptable if the consequence of a false negative is less significant or if low sensitivity tests are combined with other tests. For example, inherited phenylalanine hydroxylase deficiency (phenylketonuria or PKU) results in increased phenylalanine concentrations. High phenylalanine concentrations damage the central nervous system and are associated with intellectual developmental disorder. Intellectual disability is preventable if PKU is diagnosed and dietary interventions are initiated before 30 days of age. The phenylalanine blood screening test, used to screen newborns for PKU, is a highly sensitive test when testing infants at least 24 hours of age.[10] In contrast, the prostate specific antigen (PSA) test, a test commonly used to screen men for prostate cancer, is highly specific but has low sensitivity, especially at low PSA cut-off values of 4–10 ng/mL.[11] Thus, PSA cannot be relied on as the sole prostate cancer screening method.

Sensitivity also refers to the range over which a quantitative assay can accurately measure the analyte. In this context, a sensitive test is one that can measure low levels of the substance; an insensitive test cannot measure low levels of the substance accurately. For example, a digoxin assay with low sensitivity might measure digoxin concentrations as low as 0.7 ng/mL. Concentrations below 0.7 ng/mL would not be measurable and would be reported as "less than 0.7 ng/mL" whether the digoxin concentration was 0.6 ng/mL or 0.1 ng/mL. Thus, this relatively insensitive digoxin assay would not differentiate between medication nonadherence with an expected digoxin concentration of zero and low concentrations associated with inadequate dosage regimens.

**TABLE 1-2.** Calculation of Sensitivity and Specificity[a,b]

| SCREENING TEST RESULT | DISEASED | NONDISEASED | TOTAL |
|---|---|---|---|
| Positive | TP | FP | TP + FP |
| Negative | FN | TN | FN + TN |
| Total | TP + FN | FP + TN | TP + FP + FN + TN |

FN = diseased persons not detected by test (false negatives); FP = nondiseased persons positive to test (false positives); TN = nondiseased persons negative to test (true negatives); TP = diseased persons detected by test (true positives).
[a]Sensitivity = [TP ÷ (TP + FN)] × 100%.
[b]Specificity = [TN ÷ (FP + TN)] × 100%.

## Specificity

*Specificity* refers to the percent of correctly identified negative results in people without the disease (the true negative rate).[8,9] Specificity assesses the proportion of true negatives disclosed by the test (Table 1-2); the lower the specificity, the higher the chance of a false positive result. A test with a specificity of 95% for the disease in question indicates that the disease will be detected in 5% of people without the disease. Tests with high specificity are best for confirming a diagnosis because the tests are rarely positive in the absence of the disease. Several newborn screening tests (eg, PKU, galactosemia, biotinidase deficiency, congenital hypothyroidism, and congenital adrenal hyperplasia) have specificity levels above 99%.[12] In contrast, the erythrocyte sedimentation rate (ESR) is a nonspecific test; infection, inflammation, and plasma cell dyscrasias increase the ESR.

Specificity as applied to quantitative laboratory tests refers to the degree of cross-reactivity of the analyte with other substances in the sample. Quinine may cross-react with or be measured as quinidine in some assays, falsely elevating reported quinidine concentrations. Phenazopyridine interferes with urine ketone tests using sodium nitroprusside (eg, Ketostix).

## Specimen

A *specimen* is a sample (eg, whole blood, plasma, serum, urine, stool, sputum, sweat, gastric secretions, exhaled air, cerebrospinal fluid, or tissues) used for laboratory analysis. Whole blood contains all blood constituents (red blood cells, white blood cells, platelets, and plasma). Plasma is the watery acellular portion of blood. Plasma contains dissolved proteins (eg, albumin, globulins, fibrinogen, enzymes, and hormones), electrolytes (eg, sodium, potassium, chloride, calcium, and magnesium), lipids, carbohydrates, amino acids, and other organic substances (eg, urea, uric acid, creatinine, bilirubin, ammonium ions). Serum is the liquid that remains after the fibrin clot is removed from plasma. While some laboratory tests are performed only on plasma (eg, prothrombin time, activated partial thromboplastin time, D-dimer, and fibrinogen concentrations) or serum (eg, albumin, creatinine, bilirubin, and acetaminophen concentrations), other laboratory tests can be performed on either plasma or serum (eg, glucose, cortisol, electrolytes, and phenytoin concentrations). Some tests are performed on whole blood (eg, blood gases, hemoglobin, hematocrit, complete blood count, and erythrocyte sedimentation rate).

# LABORATORY TEST RESULTS

## Units Used in Reporting Laboratory Results

Laboratory test results are reported with a variety of units. For example, four different units are used to report serum magnesium concentration (1.0 mEq/L = 1.22 mg/dL = 0.5 mmol/L = 12.2 mg/L). Additionally, the same units may be reported in different ways. For example, mg/dL, mg/100 mL, and mg% are equivalent units. Enzyme activity is usually reported in terms of units, but the magnitude varies widely and depends on the methodology. Rates are usually reported in volume per unit of time (eg, creatinine clearance is measured in mL/min or L/hr), but the ESR is reported in mm/hr and coagulation test results are reported in seconds or minutes. This lack of standardization is confusing and may lead to misinterpretation of the test results.

The International System of Units (Système Internationale d'Unités, or SI) was created over 60 years ago to standardize quantitative units worldwide.[13] Seven base units and symbols are designated: length (meter, m), mass (kilogram, kg), time (second, s), electric current (ampere, A), thermodynamic temperature (kelvin, K), luminous intensity (candela, cd) and amount of substance (mole, mol). Twenty-two derived units are designated. However, it is difficult for clinicians to relate to molar concentrations (eg, serum cholesterol 4.14 mmol/L versus 160 mg/dL or HbA1c 10 mmol/L versus 8%). In the United States, most laboratory results are reported in conventional units.

## Rationale for Ordering Laboratory Tests

Laboratory tests are performed with the expectation that the results will:

- Discover occult disease
- Confirm a suspected diagnosis
- Differentiate among possible diagnoses
- Determine the stage, activity, or severity of disease
- Detect disease recurrence
- Assess the effectiveness of therapy
- Guide the course of therapy

**TABLE 1-3.** Comparative Features of Screening and Diagnostic Laboratory Tests[14]

| FEATURE | SCREENING TEST | DIAGNOSTIC TEST |
|---|---|---|
| Simplicity of test | Fairly simple | More complex |
| Target population | Individuals without signs or symptoms of the disease | Individuals with signs or symptoms of the disease |
| Characteristic | High sensitivity | High specificity |
| Disease prevalence | Relatively common | Common or rare |
| Risks | Acceptable to population | Acceptable to individual |

Laboratory tests are categorized as *screening* or *diagnostic* tests. Screening tests, performed in individuals without signs or symptoms of disease, detect disease early when interventions (eg, lifestyle modifications, drug therapy, and surgery) are likely to be effective. Screening tests are performed on healthy individuals and are generally inexpensive, quick and easy to perform, and reliable, but they do not provide a definitive answer. Screening tests require confirmation with other clinical tests. Diagnostic tests, performed on at-risk individuals, are typically more expensive, and are associated with some degree of risk, but they provide a definitive answer.

Comparative features of screening tests are listed in **Table 1-3**. Examples of screening tests include the Papanicolaou smear, human papillomavirus (HPV) deoxyribonucleic acid (DNA) test, lipid profile, PSA, fecal occult blood (FOB), tuberculin skin test, human immunodeficiency virus (HIV) antibody/HIV antigen test, sickle cell tests, fasting blood glucose (FBG), blood coagulation tests, and serum chemistries. Screening tests may be performed on healthy outpatients (eg, ordered by the patient's primary care provider or performed during public health fairs) or on admission to an acute care facility (eg, prior to scheduled surgery). Abnormalities identified during screening are followed by more specific tests to confirm the results.

Screening tests must be cost-effective and population appropriate. The number needed to screen (NNS) is defined as "the number of people that need to be screened for a given duration to prevent one death or one adverse event."[15] For example, 2,726 women between the ages of 20 and 64 years need to be screened for cervical cancer to identify one woman with cancer.[16]

Diagnostic tests are performed in individuals with signs or symptoms of disease, a history suggestive of a specific disease or disorder, or an abnormal screening test. Diagnostic tests are used to confirm a suspected diagnosis, differentiate among possible diagnoses, determine the stage of activity of disease, detect disease recurrence, and assess and guide the therapeutic course. Diagnostic test features are listed in Table 1-3. Examples of diagnostic tests include serum human chorionic gonadotropin (HCG), B-type natriuretic peptide (BNP), FeNO, blood cultures, serum cardiac-specific troponin I and T, kidney biopsy, and the cosyntropin test.

Many laboratories group a series of related tests (screening and/or diagnostic) into a set called a *profile*. For example, the basic metabolic panel (BMP) includes common serum electrolytes (sodium, potassium, and chloride), carbon dioxide content, blood urea nitrogen (BUN), calcium, creatinine, and glucose. The comprehensive metabolic panel (CMP) includes the BMP plus albumin, alanine aminotransferase (ALT), aspartate aminotransferase (AST), alkaline phosphatase (ALP), total bilirubin, and total protein. Grouped together for convenience, some profiles may be less costly to perform than the sum of the cost of each individual test. However, profiles may generate unnecessary patient data. Attention to cost is especially important in the current cost-conscious era. A test should not be done if it is unnecessary, redundant, or provides suboptimal clinical data (eg, non-steady-state serum drug concentrations). Before ordering a test, the clinician should consider the following questions:

- Was the test recently performed and in all probability the results have not changed at this time?

- Were other tests performed that provide the same information?

- Can the needed information be estimated with adequate reliability from existing data? For example, creatinine clearance can be estimated using age, height, weight, and serum creatinine rather than measured from a 24-hour urine collection. Serum osmolality can be calculated from electrolytes and glucose rather than measured directly.

- What will I do if results are positive or negative? For example, if the test result will not aid in clinical decisions or change the diagnosis, prognosis, or treatment course, the benefits from the test are not worth the cost of the test.

## Factors That Influence Laboratory Test Results

Laboratory results may be inconsistent with patient signs, symptoms, or clinical status. Before accepting reported laboratory values, clinicians should consider the numerous laboratory- and patient-specific factors that may influence the results (**Table 1-4**). For most of the major tests discussed in this book, a Quickview chart summarizes information helpful in interpreting results. **Figure 1-2** depicts the format and content of a typical Quickview chart.

## Laboratory-Specific Factors

Laboratory errors are uncommon but may occur. Defined as a test result that is not the true result, laboratory error most appropriately refers to inaccurate results that occur because of an error made by laboratory personnel or equipment. However, laboratory error is sometimes used to refer to otherwise accurate results rendered inaccurate by specimen-related issues. Laboratory errors should be suspected for one or more of the following situations:

- The result is inconsistent with trends in serial test results.
- The magnitude of error is great.
- The result is not in agreement with a confirmatory test result.
- The result is inconsistent with clinical signs or symptoms or other patient-specific information.

True laboratory errors (inaccurate results) are caused by one or more laboratory processing or equipment errors, such as deteriorated reagents, calibration errors, calculation errors, misreading the results, computer entry or other documentation errors, or improper sample preparation. For example, incorrect entry of thromboplastin activity (International Sensitivity Index [ISI]) when calculating the International Normalized Ratio (INR) results in accurately assayed but incorrectly reported INR results.

Accurate results may be rendered inaccurate by one or more specimen-related problems. Improper specimen handling prior to or during transport to the laboratory may alter analyte concentrations between the time the sample was obtained from the patient and the time the sample was analyzed in the laboratory.[17] For example, arterial blood withdrawn for blood gas analysis must be transported on ice to prevent continued in vitro changes in pH, carbon dioxide, and oxygen. Failure to remove the plasma or serum from the clot within 4 hours of obtaining blood for serum potassium analysis may elevate the reported serum potassium concentration. Red blood cell hemolysis elevates the serum potassium and phosphate concentrations. Failure to refrigerate samples may cause falsely low concentrations of serum enzymes (eg, CK). Prolonged tourniquet time may hemoconcentrate analytes, especially those that are highly protein bound (eg, calcium).

## Patient-Specific Factors

Laboratory test values cannot be interpreted in isolation of the patient. Numerous age-related (eg, decreased renal function) and other patient-specific factors (eg, time of day, posture) as well as disease-specific factors (eg, time course) affect lab results. The astute clinician assesses laboratory data in context of all that is known about the patient.

*Time course.* Incorrectly timed laboratory tests produce misleading laboratory results. Disease states, normal physiologic patterns, pharmacodynamics, and pharmacokinetics time courses must be considered when interpreting laboratory values. For example, digoxin has a prolonged distribution phase. Digoxin serum concentrations obtained before tissue distribution is complete do not accurately reflect true tissue drug concentrations. Postmyocardial infarction enzyme patterns are complex and evolve over a prolonged period of time. For example, CK increases about 6 hours following myocardial

**TABLE 1-4.** Factors That Influence Assessment of Laboratory Results

**Assay used and form of analyte**
- Free form
- Bound form

**Clinical situation**
- Acuity of disease
- Severity of disease

**Demographics**
- Age
- Gender
- Ethnicity
- Height
- Weight
- Body surface area

**Drugs**
- Drug–drug interactions
- Drug–assay interactions

**Food**
- Time of last meal
- Type of food ingested

**Nutritional status**
- Well nourished
- Poorly nourished

**Posture**
- Upright
- Supine

**Pregnancy**

**Specimen analyzed**
- Serum
- Plasma
- Whole blood (venous or arterial)
- Cerebrospinal fluid
- Urine
- Stool
- Sputum
- Other (eg, tissue, sweat, gastric contents, effusions, breath)

**Temporal relationships**
- Time of day
- Time of last dose

## QUICKVIEW | Contents of a typical Quickview chart

| PARAMETER | DESCRIPTION | COMMENTS |
|---|---|---|
| **Common reference ranges** | | |
| Adults | Reference range in adults | Variability and factors affecting range |
| Pediatrics | Reference range in children | Variability, factors affecting range, age grouping |
| **Critical value** | Value beyond which immediate action usually needs to be taken | Disease-dependent factors; relative to reference range; value is a multiple of upper normal limit |
| **Inherent activity** | Does substance have any physiologic activity? | Description of activity and factors affecting activity |
| **Location** | | |
| Production | Is substance produced? If so, where? | Factors affecting production |
| Storage | Is substance stored? If so, where? | Factors affecting storage |
| Secretion/excretion | Is substance secreted/excreted? If so, where/how? | Factors affecting secretion or excretion |
| **Causes of abnormal values** | | |
| High | Major causes | Modification of circumstances, other related causes or drugs that are commonly monitored with this test |
| Low | Major causes | |
| **Signs and symptoms** | | |
| High level | Major signs and symptoms with a high or positive result | Modification of circumstances/other related signs and symptoms |
| Low level | Major signs and symptoms with a low result | Modification of circumstances/other related causes |
| **After event, time to...** | | |
| Initial elevation | Minutes, hours, days, weeks | Assumes acute insult |
| Peak values | Minutes, hours, days, weeks | Assumes insult not yet removed |
| Normalization | Minutes, hours, days, weeks | Assumes insult removed and nonpermanent damage |
| **Causes of spurious results** | List of common causes | Modification of circumstances/assay specific |
| **Additional information** | Any other pertinent information regarding the laboratory value of assay | |

**FIGURE 1-2.** Contents of a typical Quickview chart. (*Source*: Reprinted with permission from Basic Skills in Interpreting Laboratory Data, 6th edition.)

infarction (MI) and returns to baseline about 48–72 hours after the MI. Lactate dehydrogenase increases about 12–24 hours following MI and returns to baseline about 10 days after the MI. Troponin increases a few hours following MI and returns to baseline in about 5–7 days. Serial samples are used to assess myocardial damage.

Lab samples obtained too early or too late may miss critical changes and lead to incorrect assessments. For example, cosyntropin (synthetic adrenocorticotropic hormone [ACTH]) tests adrenal gland responsiveness. The baseline 8 a.m. plasma cortisol is compared with the stimulated plasma cortisol obtained 30 and 60 minutes following injection of the drug. Incorrect timing leads to incorrect results. The sputum acid-fast bacilli (AFB) smear may become AFB-negative with just a few doses of antituberculosis drugs, but the sputum culture may remain positive for several weeks. Expectations of a negative sputum culture too early in the time course may lead to the inappropriate addition of unnecessary antituberculosis drugs.

Non-steady-state drug concentrations are difficult to interpret; inappropriate dosage adjustments (usually inappropriate dosage increases) may occur if the clinician fails to recognize that a drug has not reached steady-state concentrations. Although non-steady-state drug concentrations may be useful when assessing possible drug toxicity (eg, overdose situations and new onset adverse drug events), all results need to be interpreted in the context of the drug's pharmacokinetics. Absorption, distribution, metabolism, and elimination may change with changing physiology. For example, increased/decreased hepatic or renal perfusion may affect the clearance of a drug. Some drugs (eg, phenytoin) have very long half-lives; constantly changing hemodynamics during an acute care hospitalization may prevent the drug from achieving steady-state while the patient is acutely ill.

*Age.* Age influences many physiologic systems. Age-related changes are well-described for neonates and young children, but less data is available for the elderly and the very elderly (usually described as ≥ 90 years of age). Age influences some but not all laboratory values; not all changes are clinically significant.

Pediatric reference ranges often reflect physiologic immaturity, with laboratory values approaching those of healthy adults with increasing age. For example, the complete blood count (CBC) (hemoglobin, hematocrit, RBC count, and RBC indices) ranges are greatly dependent on age with different values reported for premature neonates, term neonates, and young children. The fasting blood glucose reference range in premature neonates is approximately 20–65 mg/dL compared with 60–105 mg/dL for children 2 years of age and older and 70–110 mg/dL for adults. The serum creatinine reference range for children 1–5 years of age differs from the reference range for children 5–10 years of age (0.3–0.5 mg/dL versus 0.5–0.8 mg/dL). Reference ranges for children are well-described because it is relatively easy to identify age-differentiated populations of healthy children. Most laboratory reference texts provide age-specific reference values.

Geriatric reference ranges are more difficult to establish because of physiologic variability with increasing age and the presence of symptomatic and asymptomatic disease states that influence reference values. Dental problems and digestive issues may lead to inadequate nutrition influencing some laboratory tests. Some physiologic functions (eg, cardiac, pulmonary, renal, and metabolic functions) progressively decline with age, but each organ declines at a different rate.[18] Other physiologic changes associated with aging include decreased body weight, decreased height, decreased total body water, increased extracellular water, increased fat percentage, and decreased lean tissue percentage; and loss of cell membranes integrity.[18] Published studies sometimes lead to contradictory conclusions due to differences in study methodology (eg, single point versus longitudinal evaluations) and populations assessed (eg, nursing home residents versus general population). Little data is available for the very elderly (≥ 90 years of age).[19,20] Most laboratory reference texts provide age-specific reference values.

Despite the paucity of data and difficulties imposed by different study designs and study populations, there is general consensus that some laboratory reference ranges are unchanged, some are different but of uncertain clinical significance, and some are significantly different in the elderly (**Table 1-5**). For example, decreased lean muscle mass with increased age results in decreased creatinine production. Decreased renal function is associated with decreased creatinine elimination. Taken together, the serum creatinine reference range in the elderly is not different from younger populations though creatinine clearance declines with age. Significant age-related changes are reported for the 2-hour postprandial glucose test, serum lipids, and arterial oxygen pressure (Table 1-5). The 2-hour postprandial glucose increases by about 5–10 mg/dL per decade. Progressive ventilation-perfusion mismatching from loss of elastic recoil with increasing age causes progressively decreased arterial oxygen pressure with increasing age. Total cholesterol and LDL-cholesterol (LDL-C) increase with age then decline in the very old.

***Genetics, ethnicity, and gender.*** Inherited ethnic and/or gender differences are identified for some laboratory tests. For example, the hereditary anemias (eg, thalassemias and sickling disorders such as sickle cell anemia) are more common in individuals with sub-Saharan African, Asian, and Mediterranean ancestry.[28] Glucose-6-phosphate dehydrogenase (G6PD) deficiency is an example of an inherited sex-linked (X-chromosome) enzyme deficiency found primarily in men of African, Asian, Middle Eastern, and Mediterranean ancestry.[29] The A-G6PD variant occurs mostly in Africans and affects about 13% of African-American males and 3% of African-American females in the United States. The Mediterranean G6PD variant, associated with a less common but more severe enzyme deficiency state, occurs mostly in individuals of Greek, Sardinian, Kurdish, Asian, and Sephardic Jewish ancestry.

Other enzyme polymorphisms influence drug metabolism. The genetically linked absence of an enzyme may lead to drug

**TABLE 1-5.** Laboratory Testing: Tests Affected by Aging[18;20-27]

### No Change

Amylase

Lipase

Hemoglobin

Hematocrit

Red blood cell count

Red blood cell indices

Platelet count

White blood cell count and differential

Serum electrolytes (sodium, potassium, chloride, bicarbonate, magnesium)

Coagulation

Total iron binding capacity

Thyroid function tests (thyroxine, $T_3$RU)

Liver function tests (AST, ALT, LDH)

### Some change (unclear clinical significance)

Alkaline phosphatase

Erythrocyte sedimentation rate

Serum albumin

Serum calcium

Serum uric acid

Thyroid function tests (TSH, $T_3$)

### Clinically significant change

Arterial oxygen pressure

2-hr postprandial glucose

Serum lipids (total cholesterol, low-density lipoprotein, triglycerides)

Serum testosterone (in men)

Serum estradiol (in women)

### No change but clinically significant decrease in renal function

Serum creatinine

ALT = alanine aminotransferase; AST = aspartate aminotransferase; LDH = lactate dehydrogenase; TSH = thyroid-stimulating hormone; $T_3$RU = triiodothyronine resin uptake; $T_3$ = triiodothyronine.

toxicity secondary to drug accumulation or lack of drug effect if the parent compound is an inactive prodrug (eg, codeine). The cytochrome P450 (CYP450) superfamily consists of greater than 100 isoenzymes with selective but overlapping substrate specificity. Some individuals are poor metabolizers while some are ultra-rapid metabolizers. Several of the cytochrome P450 phenotypes vary by race. For example, the CYP2D6 poor metabolism phenotype occurs in 5%–10% of Caucasians and the CYP2C19 poor metabolism phenotype occurs in 10%–30% of Asians.[30,31]

Additional enzyme polymorphisms include pseudocholinesterase deficiency, phenytoin hydroxylation deficiency, inefficient *N*-acetyltransferase activity, inefficient or rapid debrisoquine hydroxylase activity, diminished thiopurine methyltransferase activity, partial dihydropyrimidine dehydrogenase inactivity, and defective uridine diphosphate glucuronosyl transferase activity.[32] Other examples of genetic polymorphisms include variations in the β-2 adrenoceptor gene that influence response to sympathomimetic amines and variations in drug transporters such as P-glycoprotein (P-gp), multidrug resistance gene associated proteins (MRP1, MRP2, MRP3), and organic anion transporting peptide (OATP).[32]

***Biologic rhythms.*** Biologic rhythms are oscillatory (cyclical) temporal patterns of varying lengths. The master clock, located in the suprachiasmatic nucleus of the hypothalamus, coordinates timing signals and multiple peripheral clocks.[33] A circadian rhythm is an approximately 24-hour endogenously generated cycle.[34] Ultradian rhythms are shorter than 24-hour; infradian rhythms are longer than 24-hour.[35,36]

Well-described, human circadian rhythms include body temperature, cortisol production, melatonin production, and hormonal production. Platelet function, cardiac function, and cognition also follow a circadian rhythm.[37] Other biologic rhythms include the 8-hour rhythm for circulating endothelin, the approximately weekly (circaseptan) rhythm for urinary 17-ketosteroid excretion, and the seasonal rhythms for cholesterol and 25-hydroxycholecalciferol.[38,39]

Statistically significant circadian rhythms have been reported for CK, ALT, γ glutamyl transferase (GGT), LDH, and some serum lipids.[40,41] Glomerular filtration has a circadian rhythm.[42] Circadian variations in aminoglycoside pharmacokinetics, including netilmicin, amikacin, and gentamicin, have been reported.[43] Though the clinical significance of diurnally variable laboratory results is not well understood, diurnal variability should be considered when assessing laboratory values. Obtaining laboratory results at the same time of day (eg, routine 7 a.m. blood draws) minimizes variability due to circadian rhythms. Different results obtained at different times of the day may be due to circadian variability rather than acute physiologic changes.

***Drugs.*** The four generally accepted categories of drug–laboratory interactions include methodological interference; drug-induced end-organ damage; direct pharmacologic effect; and a miscellaneous category. Many drugs interfere with analytical methodology. Drugs that discolor the urine interfere with fluorometric, colorimetric, and photometric tests and mask abnormal urine colors. For example, amitriptyline and propofol turn the urine a blue–green color, phenazopyridine and rifampin turn the urine an orange–red color, and doxorubicin turns the urine red. Other drugs directly interfere with the laboratory assay. For example, high doses of ascorbic acid (greater than 500 mg/day) cause false negative stool occult blood tests. Some drugs interfere with urinary fluorescence tests for urine catecholamines by producing urinary fluorescence themselves (eg, ampicillin, chloral hydrate, and erythromycin). Monoclonal antibodies interfere with a variety of laboratory tests.[44] For example, daratumumab (Darzalex) FDA-approved in 2015 for treatment of multiple myeloma, interferes with indirect antiglobulin tests (indirect Coombs test), serum protein electrophoresis (SPE), and immunofixation electrophoresis (IFE) assays.[45] Omalizumab (Xolair) complexes with immunoglobulin E (IgE) elevating serum total IgE for up to a year following administration.[46]

Direct drug-induced, end-organ damage (eg, kidney, liver, and bone marrow) change the expected laboratory results. For example, amphotericin B causes renal damage evidenced by increased serum creatinine. Bone marrow suppressants, such as doxorubicin and bleomycin, cause thrombocytopenia. Some drugs alter laboratory results as a consequence of a direct pharmacologic effect. For example, thiazide and loop diuretics increase serum uric acid by decreasing uric acid renal clearance or tubular secretion. Narcotics, such as codeine and morphine sulfate, increase serum lipase by inducing spasms of the sphincter of Oddi. Urinary specific gravity is increased in the presence of dextran. Other examples of drug–laboratory interactions include drugs that cause a positive direct Coombs test (eg, isoniazid, sulfonamides, and quinidine), drugs that cause a positive antinuclear antibody test (eg, penicillins, sulfonamides, and tetracyclines), drugs that interfere with the C-urea breath test (eg, proton pump inhibitors), and drugs that inhibit bacterial growth in blood or urine cultures (eg, antibiotics).

Thyroid function tests are a good example of the complexity of potential drug-induced laboratory test changes. Thyroxine ($T_4$) and triiodothyronine ($T_3$) are displaced from binding proteins by salicylates, heparin, and high-doses of furosemide. Free $T_4$ levels initially increase, but chronic drug administration results in decreased $T_4$ levels with normal TSH levels. Phenytoin, phenobarbital, rifampin, and carbamazepine stimulate hepatic metabolism of thyroid hormone, resulting in decreased serum hormone concentration. Amiodarone, high-dose β-adrenergic blocking drugs, glucocorticosteroids, and some iodine contrast dyes interfere with the conversion of $T_4$ to $T_3$. Ferrous sulfate, aluminum hydroxide, sucralfate, colestipol, and cholestyramine decrease $T_4$ absorption. Somatostatin, octreotide, and glucocorticosteroids suppress TSH production.

**Pregnancy.** Pregnancy is a normal physiologic condition that alters the reference range for many laboratory tests. Normal pregnancy increases serum hormone concentrations (eg, estrogen, testosterone, progesterone, human chorionic gonadotropin, prolactin, corticotropin-releasing hormone (CRH), ACTH, cortisol, and atrial natriuretic hormone). The plasma volume increases by 30%–50%, resulting in a relative hyponatremia (eg, serum sodium decreased by about 5 mEq/L) and modest decreases in hematocrit. The metabolic adaptations to pregnancy include increased RBC mass and altered carbohydrate (eg, 10%–20% decrease in fasting blood glucose) and lipid (eg, 300% increase in triglycerides (TG) and a 50% increase in total cholesterol) metabolism. Pregnancy changes the production and elimination of thyroid hormones, resulting in different reference values over the course of pregnancy.[47] For example, thyroxine-binding globulin increases during the first trimester, but pregnancy-associated accelerated thyroid hormone metabolism occurs later in the pregnancy. Other physiologic changes during pregnancy include an increased cardiac output (increases by 30%–50%), decreased systemic vascular resistance, increased glomerular filtration rate (increases by 40%–50%), shortened prothrombin and partial thromboplastin times, and hyperventilation resulting in compensated respiratory alkalosis and increased arterial oxygenation.[48]

## Other Factors

Organ function, diet, fluid status, patient posture, and altitude affect some laboratory tests.

### Organ Function

Renal dysfunction may lead to hyperkalemia, decreased creatinine clearance, and hyperphosphatemia. Hepatic dysfunction may lead to reduced clotting factor production with prolonged partial thromboplastin times and prothrombin times. Bone marrow dysfunction may lead to pancytopenia.

### Diet

Serum glucose and lipid profiles are best assessed in the fasting state. Unprocessed grapefruit juice down-regulates intestinal CYP3A4 and increases the bioavailability of some orally administered drugs.

### Fluid Status

Hypovolemia is associated with a decreased amount of fluid in the bloodstream; all blood constituents (eg, sodium, potassium, creatinine, glucose, and BUN) become more concentrated. This effect is called *hemoconcentration*. Although the absolute amount of the substance in the body has not changed, the loss of fluid results in an abnormally high concentration of the measured analyte. The converse is true with hemodilution. Relativity must be applied or false impressions may arise (refer to **Minicase 2**).

### Posture

Plasma renin release is stimulated by upright posture, diuretics, and low-sodium diets; plasma renin testing usually occurs after 2–4 weeks of normal sodium diets under fasting supine conditions.

### Altitude

At high altitude, hemoglobin initially increases secondary to dehydration. However, hypoxia stimulates erythropoietin production, which in turn stimulates hemoglobin production,

## MINICASE 2

### Interpretation of Laboratory Parameters in Dehydration

Christopher, a 67-year-old male with a long history of asthma, presented to the emergency department (ED) with a one-day history of sudden onset fever, chills, dry cough, nasal congestion, muscle aches, fatigue, nausea, and diarrhea. On admission to the ED, his temperature was 100.4°F (oral) and he was hypotensive and tachycardic with decreased skin turgor and dry mucus membranes. A BMP and CBC were ordered. The BMP was notable for elevated serum electrolytes, BUN, and serum creatinine. The BUN to creatinine ratio was greater than 20 to 1. The CBC was notable for an elevated white blood cell (WBC) count with an increased percentage of lymphocytes and elevated platelets, hematocrit, and hemoglobin. A rapid influenza diagnostic test was positive. Fluid resuscitation and peramivir (Rapivab) were ordered.

QUESTION: Peramivir (Rapivab) is dosed according to renal function. Dose reduction is required if the estimated creatinine clearance is less than 50 mL/min. The manufacturer provides dosing recommendations based on estimated creatinine clearance using the Cockcroft Gault equation. Is it appropriate to use Christopher's admission creatinine to estimate his creatinine clearance?

DISCUSSION: No. Christopher is severely dehydrated; all laboratory parameters are hemoconcentrated. His admission serum creatinine is high and underestimates his renal function. The regimen for patients with estimated creatinine clearance at least 50 mL/min is a one-time 600 mg dose. Given that Christopher has two risk factors for influenza complications (age ≥ 65 y and chronic pulmonary disease), the peramivir (Rapivab) dose needs to be optimal. The best approach is to recheck the serum creatinine after the couple of hours of rehydration, and then estimate the creatinine clearance.

resulting in increased hemoglobin concentration and increased blood viscosity. Physiologic changes depend on altitude and duration of exposure. Serum hemoglobin reference ranges are adjusted progressively upward for individuals living 1000 m or more above sea level.[49]

## NONCENTRALIZED LABORATORY TESTS

### Point-of-Care Testing

*Point-of-care (POC) testing (POCT)*, also known as *near patient testing*, *bedside testing*, or *extra-laboratory testing*, is clinician-directed diagnostic testing performed at or near the site of patient care rather than in a centralized laboratory.[50] Typically, nonlaboratory healthcare personnel (eg, pharmacists, physicians, physician assistants, nurses, nursing assistants, respiratory therapists, and paramedics) perform POC testing. POC test equipment ranges from small, hand-held devices to table-top analyzers. In vitro, in vivo, and ex vivo POC testing refer to tests performed near the patient (eg, fingerstick blood glucose), in the patient (eg, specialized intra-arterial catheter that measures lactate), and just outside the patient (eg, intra-arterial catheter attached to an external analyzer), respectively. Although POC testing is not a new concept, recent technological advances (eg, microcomputerization, miniaturization, biosensor development, and electrochemical advances) and apps enabled by smart phones, smart watches (wearable testing), and tablets have rapidly expanded the variety of available POC tests beyond the traditional urinalysis dipsticks or fingerstick blood glucose monitors.[51] The availability of multiplexed point-of-care testing (xPOCT), defined as the simultaneous detection of more than one analyte from a single specimen, will expand as technology advances.[52]

The major advantages of POC testing include reduced turnaround time (TAT) and test portability.[53] Reduced TAT is especially advantageous in settings where rapidly available laboratory test results may improve patient care (eg, emergency departments, operating rooms, critical care units, accident scenes, and patient transport). Reduced TAT also enhances patient care in more traditional ambulatory settings by reducing patient and provider time and minimizing delays in initiating therapeutic interventions. Patient care sites without local access to centralized laboratories (eg, nursing homes, rural physician practices, and military field operations) also benefit from POC testing. Other POC advantages include blood conservation (POC tests usually require drops of blood as opposed to the several milliliters required for traditional testing); less chance of preanalytical error from inappropriate transport, storage, or labeling of samples; and overall cost savings. Although the per test cost is usually higher with POC testing, cost analyses must consider the per unit cost of the test as well as other costs such as personnel time, length of stay, and quality of life.

The major disadvantages of POC testing include misuse or misinterpretation of results, loss of centrally-generated epidemiologic data, documentation errors, inappropriate test material disposal, and quality assurance issues.[53] All laboratory testing must meet the minimum standards established by the Clinical Laboratory Improvement Amendments of 1988 (CLIA-88).[54] Under CLIA-88, tests are categorized into one of three groups based on potential public health risk: waived tests, tests of moderate complexity, and tests of high complexity. Waived tests (eg, fecal occult blood test) pose no risk of harm to the patient if used incorrectly or use such simple and accurate methodologies that inaccurate results are unlikely. Many POC tests meet the criteria for waived status but increasingly sophisticated POC tests may be subject to more stringent control. State-specific regulations may be more stringent than federal regulations.

## Home Testing

*Home testing* refers to patient-directed diagnostic and monitoring testing usually performed by the patient or family member at home. Numerous FDA-approved, home-use, nonprescription laboratory test kits are marketed; home glucose and pregnancy testing are among the most popular. The FDA's Office of In Vitro Diagnostics and Radiological Health (OIR) maintains a searchable list of approved home-testing kits. Many non-FDA-approved home testing kits are marketed via the Internet.

Nonprescription home testing kits are available for the screening, detection, and monitoring of a wide range of medical conditions. Home testing laboratory test kits are marketed for pregnancy (HCG), menopause (follicle stimulating hormone [FSH]), ovulation (luteinizing hormone [LH]), drugs of abuse, FOB, breath alcohol, blood glucose, HbA1c, ketones, prothrombin time (PT), carcinoembryonic antigen (CEA), PSA, allergies, thyroid hormones, estrogen, testosterone, urinary tract infections, sexually transmitted infections, group A Streptococcus infection, HIV, hepatitis C, Lyme disease, and paternity and genetic testing. Specimens tested include urine, blood, hair, breath, feces, semen, saliva, and oropharyngeal secretions.

Advantages of home testing include convenience, cost-savings (as compared with physician office visit), quickly available results, and privacy. Home monitoring of chronic drug therapy, such as blood glucose control with insulin therapy, may give the patient a better sense of control over the disease and improve patient outcomes. Disadvantages of home testing include misinterpretation of test results, delays in seeking medical advice, and lack of pre- and posttest counseling and psychological support. In addition, home test kits typically do not provide the consumer with information regarding sensitivity, specificity, precision, or accuracy. Home-use test kits are marketed either as complete test kits (the individual obtains his or her own sample, tests the sample and reads the results) or as collection kits (the individual obtains the sample, mails the sample to the laboratory, and receives the results by mail, Internet, or telephone). Consumers should read and follow the test instructions to minimize testing error.

## GUIDELINES FOR INTERPRETING LABORATORY RESULTS

Laboratory results must be interpreted in context of the patient and the limitations of the laboratory test. However, a laboratory result is only one piece of information; diagnostic and therapeutic decisions cannot be made on the basis of one piece of information. Clinicians typically give more weight to the presence or absence of signs and symptoms associated with the medical problem rather than to an isolated laboratory report. For example, an asymptomatic patient with a serum potassium concentration of 3.1 mEq/L (reference range: 3.5–5.0 mEq/L) does not cause as much concern as a patient who has a potassium concentration of 3.3 mEq/L and is symptomatic. Tests for occult disease, such as colon cancer, cervical cancer, and hyperlipidemia, are exceptions to this logic because, by definition, the patients being tested are asymptomatic. Baseline results, rate of change, and patterns should be considered when interpreting laboratory results.

## Baseline Results

Baseline studies establish relativity and are especially useful when reference ranges are wide or when reference values vary significantly among patients. For example, lovastatin and other hydroxymethyl glutaryl coenzyme A (HMG CoA) reductase inhibitors cause myopathy and liver dysfunction in a small percentage of patients. The myopathy is symptomatic (muscle pain or weakness) and elevates CK concentrations. The drug-induced liver dysfunction is asymptomatic and causes elevated AST and ALT. FDA labeling for statins recommends obtaining liver function tests before starting therapy then as clinically indicated.[55] Baseline laboratory values are also used to establish relative therapeutic goals. For example, the activated partial thromboplastin time (aPTT) is used to assess patient response to heparin anticoagulation. Therapeutic targets are expressed in terms of how much higher the patient's aPTT is compared with the baseline control.

## Laboratory Value Compared with Reference Range

Not all laboratory values above the upper limit of normal (ULN) require intervention. Some elevations may be transient and resolve with continued drug administration. Risk-to-benefit considerations may require that some evidence of drug-induced organ damage is acceptable given the ultimate benefit of the drug. For example, a 6-month course of combination drug therapy, including isoniazid, a known hepatotoxin, is recommended for treatment of latent tuberculosis.[56] The potential benefit of at least 6 months of therapy (ie, lifetime protection from tuberculosis in the absence of reinfection) means that clinicians are willing to accept some evidence of liver toxicity with continued drug therapy (eg, isoniazid is continued until AST is greater than five times the ULN in asymptomatic individuals or greater than three times the ULN in symptomatic patients).[57]

## Rate of Change

The *rate of change* of a laboratory value provides the clinician with a sense of risks associated with the particular signs and symptoms. For example, a patient whose RBC count falls from 5 million/mm³ to 3.5 million/mm³ over several hours is more likely to need immediate therapeutic intervention than if the decline took place over several months.

## Isolated Results Versus Trends

An isolated abnormal test result is difficult to interpret. However, one of several values in a series of results or similar results from the same test performed at two different times suggests a pattern or trend. For example, a random serum glucose concentration of 300 mg/dL (reference range ≤ 200 mg/dL in adults) might cause concern unless it was known that the patient was admitted to the hospital the previous night for treatment of diabetic ketoacidosis with an admission random serum glucose of 960 mg/dL. A series of laboratory values adds perspective to an interpretation but may increase overall costs.

## Spurious Results

A *spurious laboratory value* is a false laboratory value. The only way to differentiate between an actual and a spurious laboratory value is to interpret the value in context of what else is known about the patient. For example, a serum potassium concentration of 5.5 mEq/L (reference range: 3.5–5.0 mEq/L) in the absence of significant electrocardiographic changes (ie, wide, flat P waves, wide QRS complexes, and peaked T waves) and risk factors for hyperkalemia (ie, renal insufficiency) is most likely a spurious value. Possible causes of falsely elevated potassium, such as hemolysis, acidosis, and laboratory error, have to be ruled out before accepting that the elevated potassium accurately reflects the patient's actual serum potassium. Repeat testing of suspected spurious laboratory values increases the cost of patient care but may be necessary to rule out an actual abnormality.

## FUTURE TRENDS

Point-of-care testing will progress and become more widely available as technological advances produce smaller and more portable analytical devices. Real-time, in vivo mobile and wearable POC testing may become standard in many patient care areas. Laboratory test specificity and sensitivity will improve with more sophisticated testing. Genetic testing (laboratory analysis of human DNA, RNA, chromosomes, and proteins) will undergo rapid growth and development in the next few decades; genetic testing will be increasingly used to predict an individual's risk for disease, identify carriers of disease, establish diagnoses, and provide prognostic data. Genetic links for a diverse group of diseases including cystic fibrosis, Down syndrome, Huntington disease, breast cancer, Alzheimer disease, schizophrenia, PKU, and familial hypercholesterolemia are established; genetic links for many additional diseases will be established. Variations in DNA sequences will be well-described and linked to individualized disease management strategies.[58] Nanobiosensor-based POC technology is being developed for the detection, diagnosis, and monitoring of medical conditions such as cancer, diabetes, and HIV.[59] Advances in array-based technologies (ie, simultaneous evaluation of multiple analytes from one sample) will reduce sample volume and cost.

## PATIENT ASSESSMENT

The evaluation of patient laboratory data is an important component of designing, implementing, monitoring, evaluating, and modifying patient-specific medication therapy management plans. Depending on the setting, state laws, and collaborative practice agreements, some pharmacists have the authority to order and assess specific laboratory tests (eg, drug serum concentrations, serum creatinine, liver function tests, serum electrolytes) or to perform POCT (eg, lipid screening profiles, prothrombin time, HbA1c, rapid strep test). Pharmacists in ambulatory clinics and acute care inpatient settings have routine access to the same patient laboratory data as all other members of the healthcare team, but many community-based pharmacists do not have access to patient laboratory data. Though lack of access to laboratory data is currently a barrier, the increasing use of electronic health records will improve pharmacist access to patient laboratory data.

## SUMMARY

Clinical laboratory tests are convenient methods to investigate disease- and drug-related patient issues, especially since knowledge of pathophysiology and therapeutics alone is insufficient to provide high-quality clinical considerations. This chapter should help clinicians appreciate general causes and mechanisms of abnormal test results. However, results within the reference range are not always associated with a lack of signs and symptoms. Many factors influence the reference range. Knowing the sensitivity, specificity, and predictive value is important in selecting an assay and interpreting its results. Additionally, an understanding of the definitions, concepts, and strategies discussed should also facilitate mastering information in the following chapters.

## LEARNING POINTS

1.  *What factors should be considered when assessing a laboratory parameter that is outside the reference range?*

    **ANSWER:** The upper and lower limits of the reference range are not absolute; by definition, some normal results fall outside the reference range. Other factors to consider include the sensitivity and specificity of the test, the critical value for the test, the acuity of the change, drug-drug and drug-test interactions, patient signs and symptoms, laboratory error, specimen handling, patient age, and the timing of the test.

2.  *What factors should be considered when assessing laboratory parameters in a pregnant patient?*

    **ANSWER:** Physiologic changes during pregnancy, including increased plasma volume, increased RBC mass, altered carbohydrate and lipid metabolism, serum hormone changes, increased cardiac output, increased glomerular filtration rates, and acid-base alterations, result in different laboratory reference ranges. Be aware of and check for pregnancy-specific reference values when assessing laboratory parameters in a pregnant patient.

3.  *What factors should be considered when recommending at-home laboratory testing kits?*

    **ANSWER:** Advantages of patient-directed diagnostic and monitoring testing include convenience, cost-savings as compared with a physician office-visit, quickly available results, and privacy. Disadvantages include lack of information regarding sensitivity, specificity, precision, or accuracy; misinterpretation of the test results; the absence of pre- and post-test counseling; and delays in seeking medical advice. Patients who wish to purchase FDA-approved home-testing kits should be cautioned to seek advice before making treatment decisions based solely on home-testing laboratory results.

# REFERENCES

1. Chang SS, Boorjian SA, Chou R, et al. Diagnosis and treatment of non-muscle invasive bladder cancer: AUA/SUO Guideline. *J Urol.* 2016;196(4):1021-1029.PubMed

2. Witjes JA, Morote J, Cornel EB, et al. Performance of the bladder EpiCheck™ methylation test for patients under surveillance for non-muscle-invasive bladder cancer: results of a multicenter, prospective, blinded clinical trial. *Eur Urol Oncol.* 2018;1(4):307-313.PubMed

3. U.S. Department of Health & Human Services/U.S. Food and Drug Administration. The BEST Resource: Harmonizing biomarker terminology. June 2016. https://www.fda.gov/media/99221/download. Accessed May 1, 2020.

4. Whyte MB, Kelly P. The normal range: it is not normal and it is not a range. *Postgrad Med J.* 2018;94(1117):613-616.PubMed

5. Hollowell JG, Staehling NW, Flanders WD, et al. Serum TSH, T$_4$, and thyroid antibodies in the United States population (1988 to 1994): National Health and Nutrition Examination Survey (NHANES III). *J Clin Endocrinol Metab.* 2002;87(2):489-499.PubMed

6. Wartofsky L, Dickey RA. The evidence for a narrower thyrotropin reference range is compelling. *J Clin Endocrinol Metab.* 2005;90(9): 5483-5488.PubMed

7. Cappola AR. The thyrotropin reference range should be changed in older patients. *JAMA.* 2019;322(20):1961-1962.PubMed

8. Lalkhen AG, McCluskey A. Clinical tests: sensitivity and specificity. *Contin Educ Anaesth Crit Care Pain.* 2008;8(6):221-223.

9. Weinstein S, Obuchowski NA, Lieber ML. Clinical evaluation of diagnostic tests. *Am J Roentgenol.* 2005;184(1):14-19.PubMed

10. van Wegberg AMJ, MacDonald A, Ahring K, et al. The complete European guidelines on phenylketonuria: diagnosis and treatment. *Orphanet J Rare Dis.* 2017;12(1):162.PubMed

11. Holmström B, Johansson M, Bergh A, et al. Prostate specific antigen for early detection of prostate cancer: longitudinal study. *BMJ.* 2009;339:b3537. PubMed

12. Kwon C, Farrell PM. The magnitude and challenge of false-positive newborn screening test results. *Arch Pediatr Adolesc Med.* 2000;154(7):714-718.PubMed

13. Bureau International des Poids et Mesures. The International System of Units (SI). 9th edition. 2019. https://www.bipm.org/utils/common /pdf/si-brochure/SI-Brochure-9-EN.pdf. Accessed May 1, 2020.

14. Boardman LA, Peipert JF. Screening and diagnostic testing. *Clin Obstet Gynecol.* 1998;41(2):267-274.PubMed

15. Rembold CM. Number needed to screen: development of a statistic for disease screening. *BMJ.* 1998;317(7154):307-312.PubMed

16. Landy R, Castanon A, Hamilton W, et al. Evaluating cytology for the detection of invasive cervical cancer. *Cytopathology.* 2016;27(3):201-209. PubMed

17. Plebani M. Quality indicators to detect pre-analytical errors in laboratory testing. *Clin Biochem Rev.* 2012;33(3):85-88.PubMed

18. Rughwani N. Normal anatomic and physiologic changes with aging and related disease outcomes: a refresher. *Mt Sinai J Med.* 2011;78(4): 509-514.PubMed

19. Vásárhelyi B, Debreczeni LA. Lab test findings in the elderly. *EJIFCC.* 2017;28(4):328-332.PubMed

20. Tietz NW, Shuey DF, Wekstein DR. Laboratory values in fit aging individuals–sexagenarians through centenarians. *Clin Chem.* 1992;38(6): 1167-1185.PubMed

21. Favaloro EJ, Franchini M, Lippi G. Aging hemostasis: changes to laboratory markers of hemostasis as we age - a narrative review. *Semin Thromb Hemost.* 2014;40(6):621-633.PubMed

22. Edwards N, Baird C. Interpreting laboratory values in older adults. *Medsurg Nurs.* 2005;14(4):220-229, quiz 230.PubMed

23. Fraser CG. Age-related changes in laboratory test results. Clinical implications. *Drugs Aging.* 1993;3(3):246-257.PubMed

24. Duthie EH Jr, Abbasi AA. Laboratory testing: current recommendations for older adults. *Geriatrics.* 1991;46(10):41-50.PubMed

25. Kelso T. Laboratory values in the elderly. Are they different? *Emerg Med Clin North Am.* 1990;8(2):241-254.PubMed

26. Tietz NW, Wekstein DR, Shuey DF, Brauer GA. A two-year longitudinal reference range study for selected serum enzymes in a population more than 60 years of age. *J Am Geriatr Soc.* 1984;32(8):563-570.PubMed

27. Siest G. Study of reference values and biological variation: a necessity and a model for Preventive Medicine Centers. *Clin Chem Lab Med.* 2004;42(7):810-816.PubMed

28. Iolascon A, De Franceschi L, Muckenthaler M, et al. EHA research roadmap on hemoglobinopathies and thalassemia: an update. *Hemasphere.* 2019;3(3):e208.

29. Howes RE, Piel FB, Patil AP, et al. G6PD deficiency prevalence and estimates of affected populations in malaria endemic countries: a geostatistical model-based map. *PLoS Med.* 2012;9(11):e1001339. PubMed

30. Caraco Y. Genes and the response to drugs. *N Engl J Med.* 2004;351(27): 2867-2869.PubMed

31. Nguyen A, Desta Z, Flockhart DA. Enhancing race-based prescribing precision with pharmacogenomics. *Clin Pharmacol Ther.* 2007;81(3): 323-325.PubMed

32. Prandota J. Advances of molecular clinical pharmacology in gastroenterology and hepatology. *Am J Ther.* 2010;17(5):e137-e162.PubMed

33. Sollars PJ, Pickard GE. The neurobiology of circadian rhythms. *Psychiatr Clin North Am.* 2015;38(4):645-665.PubMed

34. Edery I. Circadian rhythms in a nutshell. *Physiol Genomics.* 2000;3(2): 59-74.PubMed

35. Laje R, Agostino PV, Golombek DA. The times of our lives: Interaction among different biological periodicities. *Front Integr Neurosci.* 2018;12:10. PubMed

36. Kooman JP, Usvyat L, van der Sande FM, et al. 'Time and time again': oscillatory and longitudinal time patterns in dialysis patients. *Kidney Blood Press Res.* 2012;35(6):534-548.PubMed

37. Rivkees SA. Mechanisms and clinical significance of circadian rhythms in children. *Curr Opin Pediatr.* 2001;13(4):352-357.PubMed

38. Otsuka K, Cornélissen G, Halberg F. Circadian rhythms and clinical chronobiology. *Biomed Pharmacother.* 2001;55(suppl 1):7s-18s.PubMed

39. Singh R, Sharma PK, Malviya R. Review on chronotherapeutics: a new remedy in the treatment of various diseases. *Eur J Bio Sci.* 2010;2(3): 67-76.

40. Rivera-Coll A, Fuentes-Arderiu X, Díez-Noguera A. Circadian rhythms of serum concentrations of 12 enzymes of clinical interest. *Chronobiol Int.* 1993;10(3):190-200.PubMed

41. Rivera-Coll A, Fuentes-Arderiu X, Díez-Noguera A. Circadian rhythmic variations in serum concentrations of clinically important lipids. *Clin Chem.* 1994;40(8):1549-1553.PubMed

42. Wuerzner G, Firsov D, Bonny O. Circadian glomerular function: from physiology to molecular and therapeutical aspects. *Nephrol Dial Transplant.* 2014;29(8):1475-1480.PubMed

43. Beauchamp D, Labrecque G. Chronobiology and chronotoxicology of antibiotics and aminoglycosides. *Adv Drug Deliv Rev.* 2007;59(9-10): 896-903.PubMed

44. Zhang Z, Hu W, Li L, et al. Therapeutic monoclonal antibodies and clinical laboratory tests: when, why, and what is expected? *J Clin Lab Anal.* 2018;32(30):e22307.

45. Darzalex [package insert]. Horsham, PA: Janssen Pharmaceutical Companies; 2015. Revised September 2019.

46. Xolair [package insert]. South San Francisco, CA: Genentech, Inc.; 2003. Revised May 2019.

47. McNeil AR, Stanford PE. Reporting thyroid function tests in pregnancy. *Clin Biochem Rev*. 2015;36(4):109-126.PubMed

48. Costantine MM. Physiologic and pharmacokinetic changes in pregnancy. *Front Pharmacol*. 2014;5:65 10.3389/fphar.2014.00065.PubMed

49. World Health Organization. Haemoglobin concentrations for the diagnosis of anaemia and assessment of severity. Vitamin and Mineral Nutrition Information System. Geneva, World Health Organization, 2011 (WHO/NMH/NHD/MNM/11.1). https://www.who.int/vmnis/indicators /haemoglobin.pdf. Accessed May 1, 2020.

50. Gutierres SL, Welty TE. Point-of-care testing: an introduction. *Ann Pharmacother*. 2004;38(1):119-125.PubMed

51. Wang P, Kricka LJ. Current and emerging trends in point-of-care technology and strategies for clinical validation and implementation. *Clin Chem*. 2018;64(10):1439-1452.

52. Dincer C, Bruch R, Kling A, et al. Multiplexed point-of-care testing: xPOCT. *Trends Biotechnol*. 2017;35(8):728-742.PubMed

53. Shaw JLV. Practical challenges related to point of care testing. *Pract Lab Med*. 2015;4:22-29.PubMed

54. Centers for Disease Control and Prevention. CLIA Law and Regulations. https://www.cdc.gov/clia/law-regulations.html. Accessed May 1, 2020.

55. Food and Drug Administration. FDA drug safety communication: important safety label changes to cholesterol-lowering statin drugs. https://www.fda.gov/drugs/drug-safety-and-availability/fda-drug-safety -communication-important-safety-label-changes-cholesterol-lowering -statin-drugs Accessed May 1, 2020.

56. Nahid P, Dorman SE, Alipanah N, et al. Executive summary: official American Thoracic Society/Centers for Disease Control and Prevention/Infectious Diseases Society of America clinical practice guidelines: treatment of drug-susceptible tuberculosis. *Clin Infect Dis*. 2016;63(7):853-867.PubMed

57. Saukkonen JJ, Cohn DL, Jasmer RM, et al. An official ATS statement: hepatotoxicity of antituberculosis therapy. *Am J Respir Crit Care Med*. 2006;174(8):935-952.PubMed

58. Pene F, Courtine E, Cariou A, Mira JP. Toward theragnostics. *Crit Care Med*. 2009;37(1)(suppl):S50-S58.PubMed

59. Noah NM, Ndangili PM. Current trends of nanobiosensors for point-of-care diagnostics. *J Anal Methods Chem*. 2019. Oct. 23;2019:2199718.

## BIBLIOGRAPHY

Bakerman S, Bakerman P, Strausbauch P. *Bakerman's ABC's of Interpretive Laboratory Data*. 5th ed. Scottsdale, AZ: Interpretive Laboratory Data Inc; 2014.

Fischbach FT, Dunning MB III. *A Manual of Laboratory and Diagnostic Tests*. 10th ed. Philadelphia, PA: Lippincott Williams & Wilkins; 2017.

Jacobs DS, Oxley DK, DeMott WR. *Laboratory Test Handbook Concise with Disease Index*. 3rd ed. Hudson, OH: Lexi-Comp Inc; 2004.

Jacobs DS, DeMott WR, Oxley DK. *Laboratory Test Handbook with Key Word Index*. 5th ed. Hudson, OH: Lexi-Comp Inc; 2001.

Kraemer HC. *Evaluating Medical Tests*. Newbury Park, CA: Sage Publications; 1992.

Laposata M. *Laboratory Medicine: The Diagnosis of Disease in the Clinical Laboratory*. 3rd ed. New York, NY: McGraw-Hill Companies Inc; 2018.

Sacher RA, McPherson RA. *Widmann's Clinical Interpretation of Laboratory Tests*. 11th ed. Philadelphia, PA: FA Davis Company; 2000.

Speicher CE. *The Right Test: A Physician's Guide to Laboratory Medicine*. 3rd ed. Philadelphia, PA: WB Saunders; 1998.

Williamson MA, Snyder LM. *Wallach's Interpretation of Diagnostic Tests*. 10th ed. Philadelphia, PA: Lippincott Williams & Wilkins; 2015.

# 2 Introduction to Common Laboratory Assays and Technology

*Nicholas M. Moore*

## OBJECTIVES

*After completing this chapter, the reader should be able to*

- Discuss the current and developing roles of laboratory testing in accurately diagnosing diseases

- Describe the basic elements of photometry and the major components of a spectrophotometer

- Explain the principles of turbidimetry and nephelometry as applied to laboratory testing

- Review the analytic techniques of electrochemistry based on potentiometry, coulometry, voltammetry, and conductometry

- Describe the major electrophoresis techniques and their applications

- Describe the major analytic techniques of chromatography and compare gas- and high-performance liquid chromatography with respect to equipment and methodology

- Explain the basic principles of immunoassays and compare the underlying principles, methods, and tests performed involving radioimmunoassay, enzyme-linked immunosorbent assay, enzyme-multiplied immunoassay, fluorescent polarization immunoassay, and agglutination enzyme-linked immunoassay tests

- Identify the basic components of a mass spectrometry system

- Explain the basic principles of the commonly used cytometry systems

*(continued on page 20)*

## THE CHANGING ROLE OF THE LABORATORY IN THE DIAGNOSIS OF DISEASE

Traditionally, the physician bases a clinical diagnosis and patient management protocol on the patient's family and medical history, clinical signs and symptoms, and data derived from laboratory and imaging diagnostic procedures. An accurate history and physical examination of the patient are still considered among the most informative procedures in establishing accurate diagnoses of disease, with clinical laboratory test results playing important roles in confirming and ruling out certain diseases.

Pharmaceutical companies have developed drugs based on these collective observations and known disease mechanisms. Some common examples include medications for high cholesterol, which modify the absorption, metabolism, and generation of cholesterol. Agents have been developed that are aimed at improving insulin release from the pancreas and sensitivity of the muscle and fat tissues to insulin action. Antibiotics are based on the observation that microbes produce substances, which inhibit other species. Hypotensive medications that lower blood pressure have typically been designed to act on physiologic pathways involved in hypertension (such as renal salt and water absorption, vascular contractility, and cardiac output). This has often been a reactive approach, with appropriate treatments and therapy starting after the signs and symptoms appear.

The past 30 years have seen remarkable progress in the role of the laboratory in personalizing medicine, a consequence of the advances in human and medical genetics. These advances have enabled a more detailed understanding of the impact of genetics in disease and have led to new disciplines: genomics, epigenetics, proteomics, and metabolomics. It is anticipated that further discoveries in these newly emerging domains will have profound impact on the practice of medicine into a more personalized medicine approach impacted through the use of precision diagnostics.

Many of the traditional laboratory procedures and tests that are described in the following parts of this chapter will create the framework upon which these potential advances will be based: researchers are simplifying them and improving throughput and analytic performance in real time. Because these tests have become more automated, they will take their place alongside current testing procedures. In the United States alone, approximately 12 billion laboratory assays are performed in clinical laboratories annually. Although most laboratory testing is not performed by clinicians themselves, it is essential that they have an understanding of the more common, as well as newer, emerging methods and techniques used to generate this clinical data. This understanding is essential for the proper utilization of the correct diagnostic assay and, most importantly, the correct interpretation of test results. This chapter provides an introduction to these methods and techniques.

Clinical laboratory testing represents a vast array of diverse procedures, ranging from the microscopic examination of tissue specimens (histopathology) to the measurement of cellular components to the amplification and detection of nucleic acids, such as the detection of a gene mutation or fusion for malignancies or the identification of antimicrobial resistance genes in bacteria. A consideration of all diverse methodologies used in these procedures is beyond the scope of this chapter, but all share some of the common characteristics of automation and mechanization. The two

DOI 10.37573/9781585286423.002

## OBJECTIVES

- Describe the impact of genomics, epigenetics, and proteomics on the personalization of medical practice and the newer roles that laboratory tests will play in the future
- Review the basic principles of molecular diagnostics
- Diagram the basic techniques of the polymerase chain reaction

often intertwine; automation commonly involves the mechanization of basic manual laboratory techniques or procedures, such as those described throughout this chapter. The common goals of total laboratory automation (TLA) result in increased efficiency and throughput, which leads to decreased turnaround times, reduced errors, and the ability to integrate various quality assurance and improvement processes in the laboratory.

## AUTOMATION IN THE HOSPITAL AND CLINICAL LABORATORY

This trend toward automation in the hospital and clinical laboratory is, in part, motivated by the drive toward higher productivity and cost efficiency.[1] Another key driver clinical laboratories face is the federal government. According to a report issued from the U.S. Department of Health and Human Services, the Office of the Inspector General (OIG) stated that Medicare could have saved $910 billion (38%) on laboratory test reimbursement if they lowered the reimbursement rate for the top 20 laboratory tests.[2] A final conclusion from this report was the OIG should consider reintroducing competitive bidding and adjusting the reimbursement rate for these laboratory tests. Clinical laboratories, like many other departments in hospitals and other healthcare facilities, are facing the pressure of providing more services while maintaining high-quality standards with a reduced revenue stream. In its most comprehensive sense, TLA encompasses all procedures from receipt of the specimen to the reporting of results. System designs and functionality can vary depending on the specific application and manufacturer. They can involve consolidated analyzers, individual or integrated, and automated devices that address specific tasks, coupled to specimen processing and transportation systems, as well as process control software (ie, middleware) that automates each stage of the system. One plausible vision of the future is that the centralized hospital and clinical laboratory will consist mainly of automated laboratory systems capable of performing high-volume and esoteric testing operated by skilled medical laboratory scientists.[3,4]

Laboratory automation involves a variety of steps and generally begins with processes that are manual in nature: obtaining the specimen, identifying a patient, transporting, and conducting any preanalytic specimen processing. Once in the laboratory, a quality control (QC) process begins with a check of the pre-ordered specimen to ensure that specimens have correct identification labels and bar codes, the correct tube was used for the blood test ordered, and the appropriate quality and adequate quantity of material is provided for the testing requested. The TLA systems are currently capable of performing only some of the previously listed preanalytic checks. Determining whether, for example, a specimen is grossly hemolyzed, icteric, or lipemic usually requires examination by a laboratory scientist.

In many divisions of the centralized laboratory, three major areas (eg, chemistry analyzers, hematology analyzers, and automated microbial identification systems) generate information in almost completely automated ways. Using the example of a chemistry analyzer, introduction of a specimen begins with aspiration of the sample into a continuous-flow system. Each specimen passes through the same continuous stream and is subjected to the same various analytical reactions. In some systems, the use of repeated flushing and washing steps of probes within the systems prevents carryover between specimens, while other systems use discrete specimen sampling through the use of disposable pipet tips. Many results generated by automated chemistry analyzers rely on reactions based on principles of photometry, which will be discussed later in this chapter. In addition to the more commonly requested serum or plasma chemistry analytes, enzymes, therapeutic drugs, hormones, and other substances can also be measured using these techniques.

All modern automated analyzers rely on computers and sophisticated software to perform these sample processing functions. Calculations (statistics on patient or control values), monitoring (linearity and QC), and display (acquisition and collation of patient results and warning messages and $\delta$ checks) functions are routinely performed by these instruments once the specimen has been processed. Automation does not end at this stage. Many centralized laboratories have electronic interfaces that link separate analyzers to the laboratory information system (LIS). In turn, the LIS is interfaced with the hospital electronic medical record system. This interface allows for vital two-way connectivity between the two systems. Laboratory orders are automatically sent to the LIS from the electronic medical record. This type of automation can prevent errors when a manual requisition system is utilized. Also, laboratory diagnostic information can be immediately uploaded into the patient chart for review by the clinician once results are verified manually by a medical laboratory scientist or through the use of automated rule systems developed by the laboratory. Then, based on the results generated, some laboratories have created electronic rules that can automatically order repeat and reflex testing, track samples and results through the system, and manage storage and, when necessary, retrieval of specimens for repeat or additional testing.

Standardization within the laboratory automation arena is an essential means of assuring QC and quality assurance for the diagnostic data. The Clinical and Laboratory Standards Institute is an organization that uses a consensus-based approach in developing a series of comprehensive standards and guidelines that serves as the "gold standard" for laboratory operation and automation.[5]

The discipline of informatics is a parallel component of laboratory automation. As generators and collectors of a large volume of information, laboratories provide relevant clinical information to a wide network of physicians and other healthcare professionals in an efficient manner. Informatics in the laboratory involves the use of collected data for the purposes of healthcare decision making. Modern LISs have the capability of analyzing data in a variety of ways that enhance patient care. The ability to transmit and share such information over the Internet is becoming as indispensable a function of the laboratory as performing the tests themselves. Some laboratories and healthcare systems have implemented patient access portals where patients can have limited access to their healthcare information, including laboratory test results after physicians have reviewed these results. The portals will become centers of information management for hospital-based medicine practice as well as for the community. In parallel with the development of the highly automated core laboratory, technological advances in the miniaturization of analyzers continue to enhance point-of-care (POC) testing platforms. Further progress in this area will allow greater opportunities for community engagement and outreach by laboratories and integrated health systems that are attempting to increase access to essential healthcare services and diagnostics in communities where health inequities exist.

# PHOTOMETRY

*Photometry* is the measurement of light. Light is how we define the visible radiant energy from the ultraviolet (UV) and visible portions of the electromagnetic spectrum. The wavelength of light is often expressed in nanometers (nm). Humans can only naturally perceive a limited range of about 380 to 750 nm (**Table 2-1**). Modern clinical laboratory instruments, however, can accurately measure the absorbance or emittance between 150 (the low UV) and 2,500 nm (the near infrared region).[7] These instruments are classified by the source of light as well as whether the light is absorbed or emitted. Four types of photometric instruments are currently in use in laboratories: molecular absorption, molecular emission (fluorometers), atomic emission (flame photometers), and atomic absorption (AA) spectrophotometers.

## Molecular Absorption Spectrophotometers

*Molecular absorption spectrophotometers*, usually referred to as *spectrophotometers*, are commonly employed in conjunction with other methodologies, such as nephelometry, which is discussed below, and enzyme immunoassay (EIA). In spectrophotometry, analyzers measure the intensity of light at selected wavelengths. Spectrophotometers are easy to use, have relatively high specificity, produce highly accurate results, and can generate both qualitative and quantitative data. The high specificity and accuracy are obtained by isolated analytes reacting with various substances that produce colorimetric reactions.

The basic components of two types of spectrophotometers (single and double beam) are depicted in **Figure 2-1**. Single-beam instruments have a light source (I) (eg, a tungsten bulb or laser), which passes through an entrance slit that minimizes stray light. Specific wavelengths of light are selected using a monochromator (II). Light of a specific wavelength then passes through the exit slit and illuminates the contents of the analytical cell or cuvette (III). After passing through the test solution, the light strikes a detector, usually a photomultiplier tube (IV). This tube amplifies the electronic signal, which is then sent to a recording device (V). The result is then compared with a standard curve to yield a specific concentration of analyte.

The double-beam instrument, similar in design to single-beam instruments, is designed to compensate for changes in absorbance of the reagent blank and light source intensity. It utilizes a mirror (VI) to split the light from a single source into two beams, one passing through the test solution and one through the reagent blank. By doing so, it automatically corrects optical errors that may be introduced in the blank as the wavelength changes.

Most measurements are made in the visible range of the spectrum, although sometimes measurements in the UV and

**TABLE 2-1.** Wavelength Characteristics of Ultraviolet, Visible, and Infrared Light

| WAVELENGTH (NM) | COLOR OBSERVED | REGION |
|---|---|---|
| <380 | Invisible | Ultraviolet |
| 390–440 | Violet | Visible |
| 440–500 | Blue | Visible |
| 500–580 | Green | Visible |
| 580–600 | Yellow | Visible |
| 600–620 | Orange | Visible |
| 620–750 | Red | Visible |
| >800 | Not visible | Infrared |

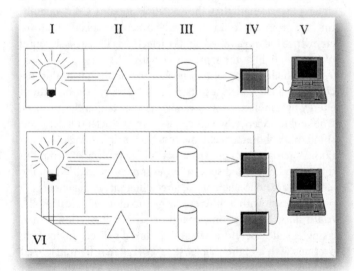

**FIGURE 2-1.** Schematic of single-beam (upper portion) and double-beam (lower portion) spectrophotometers. I = radiant light source; II = monochromator; III = analytical cuvette; IV = photomultiplier; V = recording device; VI = mirror.

infrared ranges are employed. The greatest sensitivity is achieved by selecting the wavelength of light in the range of maximum absorption. If substances are known to interfere at this wavelength, measurements may be made at a different wavelength in the absorption spectrum. This modified procedure allows detection or measurement of the analyte with minimal interference from other substances.

## Molecular Emission Spectrophotometers

*Molecular emission spectrophotometry* is usually referred to as *fluorometry*. The technology found in these instruments is based on the principle of luminescence: an energy exchange process that occurs when electrons absorb electromagnetic radiation and then emit this excited energy at a lower level (eg, longer wavelength). An atom or molecule that fluoresces is termed a *fluorophore*. Three types of photoluminescence techniques—fluorescence, phosphorescence, and chemiluminescence—form the principle on which these sensitive clinical laboratory instruments operate.

*Fluorescence* results from a three-stage process that occurs in fluorophores. The first stage involves the absorption of radiant energy by an electron in the ground state creating an excited singlet state. During the very short lifetime of this state (order of nanoseconds), energy from the electronic-vibrational excited state is partially dissipated through a radiationless transfer of energy that results from interactions with the molecular environment and leads to the formation of a relaxed excited singlet state. This is followed by relaxation to the electronic ground state by the emission of radiation (fluorescence). Because energy is dissipated, the energy of the emitted photon is lower and the wavelength is longer than the absorption photon. The difference between these two energies is known as *Stokes shift*. This principle is the basis for the sensitivity of the different fluorescence techniques because the emission photons can be detected at a different wavelength than the excitation photons. Consequently, the background is lower than with absorption spectrophotometry where the transmitted light is detected against a background of incident light at the same wavelength.[7]

The phenomenon of *phosphorescence* is similar to fluorescence because it also results from the absorption of radiant energy by a molecule; however, it is also a competitive process. Unlike fluorescence, which results from a singlet-singlet transition, phosphorescence is the result of a triplet-singlet transition. When a pair of electrons occupies a molecular orbital in the ground or excited state, a *singlet state* is created. When the electrons are no longer paired, three different arrangements are possible, each with a different magnetic moment, creating the *triplet state*. The electronic energy of a triplet state is lower than a singlet state; therefore, when the relaxed excited singlet state overlaps with a higher triplet state, energy may be transferred through a process called *intersystem crossing*. As in the case of an excited singlet state, energy may be dissipated through several radiationless mechanisms to the electronic ground state; however, when a triplet-singlet transition occurs, the result is phosphorescence. The probability of this type of transition is much lower than a singlet-singlet transition (fluorescence), and the emission wavelength and decay times are also longer than for

fluorescence emission. Because the various forms of radiationless energy transfer compete so effectively, phosphorescence is generally limited to certain molecules, such as many aromatic and organometallic compounds, at very low temperatures or in highly viscous solutions.[8,9]

The phenomenon of *chemiluminescence* is also similar to that of fluorescence in that it results from light emitted from an excited singlet state. However, unlike both fluorescence and phosphorescence, the excitation energy is caused by a chemical or electrochemical reaction. The energy is typically derived from the oxidation of an organic compound, such as luminol, luciferin, or an acridinium ester. Light is derived from the excited products that are formed in the reaction.

Different instruments have been developed that use these basic principles of luminescence. These devices use similar basic components along the following pathway: a light source (laser or mercury arc lamp), an excitation monochromator, a sample cuvette, an emission monochromator, and a photodetector.[7] Although the principles of these instruments are relatively straightforward, various modifications have been developed for specific applications.

An important example is fluorescent polarization in fluorometers. Fluorescent molecules (fluorophores) become excited by polarized light when the plane of polarization is parallel to their absorption transition vector, provided the molecule remains relatively stationary throughout the excited state. If the molecules rotate rapidly, light will be emitted in a different plane than the excitation plane. The intensity of light emitted by the molecules in the excitation polarization plane and at 90° permits the fluorescence polarization to be measured. The degree to which the emission intensity varies between the two planes of polarization is a function of the mobility of the fluorophore. Large molecules move slowly during the excited state and will remain highly polarized. Small molecules that rotate faster will emit light that is depolarized relative to the excitation plane.[11]

One of the most common applications of fluorescence polarization is competitive immunoassays, used to measure a wide range of analytes, including therapeutic and illicit drugs, hormones, antigens, and antibodies. This important methodology involves the addition of a known quantity of fluorescent-labeled analyte molecules to a serum antibody (specific to the analyte) mixture. The labeled analyte will emit depolarized light because its motion is not constrained. However, when it binds to an antibody, its motion will decrease, and the emitted light will be more polarized. When an unknown quantity of an unlabeled analyte is added to the mixture, competitive binding for the antibody will occur and reduce the polarization of the labeled analyte. By using standard curves of known drug concentrations versus polarization, the concentration of the unlabeled analyte can be determined.[9]

## Atomic Emission and Atomic Absorption Spectrophotometers

*Atomic absorption (AA) spectrophotometry* has limited use in most modern clinical laboratories, and AA spectrophotometry procedures are currently associated mainly with toxicology laboratories where poisonous substances, such as lead and arsenic, need to be identified. In this technique, the element is dissociated from its chemical bonds (atomized) and placed into an unexcited ground state (neutral atom). In this state, the element is in its lowest energy state and capable of absorbing energy in a narrow range that corresponds to its line spectrum.[10] Generally speaking, AA spectrophotometry methods have greater sensitivity compared with flame emission methods. Furthermore, due to the specificity of the wavelength from the cathode lamp, AA methods are much more specific for the element being measured.[31]

## TURBIDIMETRY AND NEPHELOMETRY

When light passes through a solution, it can be either absorbed or scattered. The basis for measuring light scatter has been applied to various immunoassays for specific proteins or haptens. *Turbidimetry* is the technique for measuring the percent of light absorbed. In this method, the turbidity of a solution decreases the intensity of the incident light beam as it passes through particles in a solution. A major advantage of turbidimetry is that measurements can be made with laboratory instruments (eg, a spectrophotometer) used for other procedures in laboratory testing. Errors associated with this method usually involve sample and reagent preparation. For example, because the amount of light blocked depends on both the concentration and size of each particle, differences in particle size between the sample and the standard is one cause of error. The length of time between sample preparation and measurement, another cause of error, should be consistent because particles settle to varying degrees, allowing more or less light to pass. Large concentrations are necessary because this test measures small differences in large numbers.

*Nephelometry*, which is similar to turbidimetry, is a technique that is used for measuring the scatter of light by particles. The main differences are that (1) the light source is usually a laser and (2) the detector, used to measure scattered light, is at a right angle to the incident light. Beam light scattered by particles is a function of the size and number of the particles. Nephelometric measurements are more precise than turbidimetric ones as the smaller signal generated for low analyte concentrations is more easily detected against a very low background.[11] Because antigen–antibody complexes are easily detected by this method, it is commonly employed in combination with EIAs. Nephelometers are routinely used in clinical microbiology laboratories to prepare a standardized inoculum of a bacterium used in the performance of antimicrobial susceptibility testing.

## REFRACTOMETRY

*Refractometry* measurements are based on the principle that light bends as it passes through different media. The ability of a liquid to bend light depends on several factors: wavelength of the incident light, temperature, physical characteristics of the medium, and solute concentration in the medium. By keeping the first three parameters constant, refractometers can measure the total solute concentration of a liquid. This procedure is particularly useful, especially as a rapid screening test because no chemical reagents and reactions are involved.[7]

Refractometers are commonly used to measure total dissolved plasma solids (mostly proteins) and urine specific gravity. In the refractometer, light is passed through the sample and then through a series of prisms. The refracted light is projected on an eyepiece scale. The scale is calibrated in grams per deciliter for serum protein, and in the case of urine, for specific gravity. In the eyepiece, a sharp line of demarcation is apparent and represents the boundary between the sample and distilled water. In the case of plasma samples, the refraction angle is proportional to the total dissolved solids. Although proteins are the predominant chemical species, other substances such as electrolytes, glucose, lipids, and urea contribute to the refraction angle. Therefore, measurements made on plasma do not correlate exactly to the true protein concentrations, but as the nonprotein solutes contribute to the total solutes in a predictable manner, accurate corrections are possible.[12]

## OSMOMETRY

In the clinical laboratory, *osmometer* readings are interpreted as a measure of total concentration of solute particles and are used to measure the osmolality of biological fluids such as serum, plasma, or urine. When osmotically active particles are dissolved in a solvent (water, in the case of biological fluids), four physical properties of the water are affected: the osmotic pressure and the boiling point are increased, and the vapor pressure and the freezing point are decreased. Because each property is related, they can be expressed mathematically in terms of the others (colligative properties) and to osmolality. Osmolarity is the number of solute particles per liter of solvent. Osmolality is also the number of solute particles per kilogram of solvent. Consequently, several methods can be used to measure osmolality, with freezing-point depression and vapor pressure osmometry being used most routinely.[13]

The most commonly used devices to measure osmolality or other colligative properties of a solution are freezing-point depression osmometers. In these analyzers, the sample is rapidly cooled several degrees below its freezing point in the cooling chamber. The sample is stirred to initiate freezing of the supercooled solution. When the freezing point of the solution is reached (the point where the rate of the heat of fusion released by ice formation comes into equilibrium with the rate of heat removal by the cooling chamber), the osmolality can be calculated.[7]

In certain situations, it is important to measure the colloid osmotic pressure (COP), a direct measure of the contribution of plasma proteins to the osmolality. Because of the large molecular weight of plasma proteins, their contribution to the total osmolality is very small as measured by freezing-point depression and vapor pressure osmometers. Because a low COP favors a shift of fluid from the intravascular compartment to the interstitial compartment, measuring the COP is particularly important in monitoring intravascular volume and useful in guiding fluid therapy in different circumstances to prevent peripheral and pulmonary edema.

The *COP osmometer*, also known as a *membrane osmometer*, consists of two fluid-filled chambers separated by a semipermeable membrane. One chamber is filled with a colloid-free physiologic saline solution that is in contact with a pressure transducer. When the plasma or serum is placed in the sample chamber, fluid moves by osmosis from the saline chamber to the sample chamber, thus causing a negative pressure to develop in the saline chamber. The resultant pressure is the COP.[13]

# ELECTROCHEMISTRY

In the clinical laboratory, analytic electrochemical techniques involve the measurement of the current or voltage produced by the activity of different types of ions. These analytic techniques are based on the fundamental electrochemical phenomena of potentiometry, coulometry, voltammetry, and conductometry.

## Potentiometry

*Potentiometry* involves the measurement of electrical potential differences between two electrodes in an electrochemical cell at zero current flow. This method is widely used in both laboratory-based analyzers and POC analyzers to measure pH, $pCO_2$, and electrolytes in whole blood samples. This electrochemical method is based on the Nernst equation, which relates the potential to the concentration of an ion in solution, to measure analyte concentrations.[14] Each electrode or half-cell in an electrochemical cell consists of a metal conductor that is in contact with an electrolyte solution. One of the electrodes is a reference electrode with a constant electric potential; the other is the measuring or indicator electrode. The boundaries between the ion conductive phases in the cell determine the type of potential gradients that exist between the electrodes and are defined as redox (oxidation reduction), membrane, and diffusion potentials.

A redox potential occurs when the two electrolyte solutions in the electrochemical cell are brought into contact with each other by a salt bridge so that the two solutions can achieve equilibrium. A potentiometer may be used to measure the potential difference between the two electrodes. This is known as the *redox potential difference* because the reaction involves the transfer of electrons between substances that accept electrons (oxidant) and substances that donate electrons (reductant). Junctional potentials rather than redox potentials occur when either a solid state or liquid interface exists between the ion conductive phases. These produce membrane or diffusion potentials, respectively. In each case the concentration of an ion in solution can be measured using the Nernst equation, which relates the electrode potential to the activity of the measured ions in the test solution[7]:

$$E = E^0 - (0.059/z)\log (C_{red}/C_{ox})$$

where $E$ = the total potential (in mV), $E^0$ = is the standard reduction potential, $z$ = the number of electrons involved in the reduction reaction, $C_{red}$ = the molar concentration of the ion in the reduced form, and $C_{ox}$ = the molar concentration of the ion in the oxidized form.

Ion-selective electrodes (ISEs) consisting of a membrane that separates the reference and test electrolyte solutions are very selective and sensitive for the ions that they measure. For this reason, further discussion on potentiometry will focus on these types of electrodes. The ISE method, having comparable or better sensitivity than flame photometry, has become the principal test for determining urine and serum electrolytes in the clinical laboratory. Typically, ion concentrations such as sodium, potassium, chloride, calcium, and lithium are measured using this method (**Table 2-2**).

The principle of ISE involves the generation of a small electrical current when a particular ion makes contact with an electrode. The electrode selectively binds the ion to be measured. To measure the concentration, the circuit must be completed with a reference electrode. The three types of electrodes are ion-selective glass membranes, solid-state electrodes, and liquid ion-exchange membranes. As shown in **Figure 2-2**, ion-selective glass membranes preferentially allow hydrogen ($H^+$), sodium ($Na^+$), and ammonium ($NH_4^+$) ions to cross a hydrated outer layer of glass. The $H^+$ glass electrode or pH electrode is the most common electrode for measuring $H^+$. Electrodes for $Na^+$, potassium ($K^+$), lithium ($Li^+$), and $NH_4^+$ are also available. An electrical potential is created when these ions diffuse across the membrane.

Solid-state electrodes consist of halide-containing crystals for measuring specific ions. An example is the silver–silver chloride electrode for measuring chloride.[7] Liquid ion-exchange membranes contain a water-insoluble, inert solvent that can dissolve an ion-selective carrier. Ions outside the membrane produce a concentration-related potential with the ions bound to the carrier inside the membrane.[7] The electrodes are separated from the sample by a liquid junction or salt bridge. Because the liquid junction generates its own voltage at the sample interface, it is a source of error. This error is overcome by adjusting the composition of the liquid junction.[15] Overall, this method is simple to use and more accurate than flame photometry for samples having low plasma water due to conditions such as hyperlipoproteinemia.[16]

Compared with other techniques, such as flame photometry, ISEs are relatively inexpensive and simple to use and have an extremely wide range of applications and wide concentration range. They are also very useful in biomedical applications because they measure the activity of the ion directly in addition to the concentration.

## Coulometry

*Coulometry* is an analytical method for measuring an unknown concentration of an analyte in solution by completely converting the analyte from one oxidation state to another. This is accomplished through a form of titration where a standardized concentration of the titrant is reacted with the unknown analyte, requiring no chemical standards or calibration. The point at which all of the analyte has been converted to the new oxidation state is called the *endpoint* and is determined by some type of indicator that is also present in the solution.

This technique is based on the Faraday law, which relates the quantity of electric charge generated by an amount of substance produced or consumed in the redox process and is expressed as $znF = It = Q$, where $z$ is the number of electrons involved in the reaction, $n$ is the quantity of the analyte, $F$ is the Faraday constant (96,487 C/mol), $I$ is the current, $t$ is time, and $Q$ is the amount of charge that passes through the cell.

**TABLE 2-2.** Common Laboratory Tests Performed with Various Assays

| ASSAY | ANALYSIS TIME (MIN) | COMMON TESTS | USE |
|---|---|---|---|
| ISE | 6–18 | Electrolytes, (sodium potassium, chloride, calcium, lithium, total carbon dioxide) | Primary testing method |
| GC | 30 | Toxicologic screens, organic acids, drugs (eg, benzodiazepines and TCAs) | Primary testing method |
| HPLC | 30 | Toxicologic screens, vanilmandelic acid, hydroxy-vanilmandelic acid, amino acids, drugs (eg, indomethacin, anabolic steroids, cyclosporin) | Primary and secondary or confirmatory testing methods |
| ELISA | 0.1–0.3 | Serologic tests (eg, ANA, rheumatoid factor, hepatitis B, cytomegalovirus, and human immunodeficiency virus antigens/antibodies) | Primary testing method |
| EMIT | 0.1–0.3 | Therapeutic drug monitoring, (eg, aminoglycosides, vancomycin, digoxin, antiepileptics, antiarrhythmics, theophylline), toxicology/drugs of abuse testing (acetaminophen, salicylate, barbiturates, TCAs, amphetamines, cocaine, opiates) | Primary testing method |
| FPIA | 0.5–2 | Therapeutic drug monitoring (eg, aminoglycosides, vancomycin, antiepileptics, antiarrhythmics, theophylline, methotrexate, digoxin, cyclosporine), thyroxine, triiodothyronine, cortisol, amylase, cholesterol, homocysteine | Primary testing method |
| PCR | 20–60 | Microbiologic and virologic markers of organisms and genetic markers | Primary testing method |

ANA = antinuclear antibody; ELISA = enzyme-linked immunosorbent assay; EMIT = enzyme-multiplied immunoassay technique; FPIA = fluorescent polarization immunoassay; GC = gas chromatography; HPLC = high-performance liquid chromatography; ISE = ion-selective electrode; PCR = polymerase chain reaction; TCAs = tricyclic antidepressants.

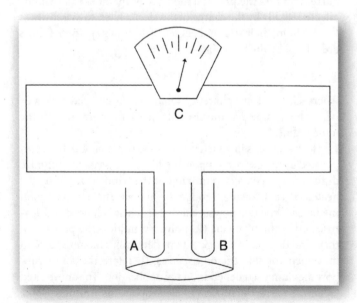

**FIGURE 2-2.** The pH meter is an example of a test that uses ISE to measure the concentration of hydrogen ions. An electric current is generated when hydrogen ions come in contact with the ISE (A). The circuit is completed using a reference electrode (B) submerged in the same liquid as the ISE (also known as the *liquid junction*). The concentration can then be read on a potentiometer (C).

Coulometry is often used in clinical applications to determine the concentration of chloride in clinical samples. The chloridometer is used to measure the chloride ion ($Cl^-$) concentration in sweat, urine, and cerebrospinal fluid samples.[7] The device uses a constant current across two silver electrodes. The silver ions ($Ag^+$) that are generated at a constant rate react with the $Cl^-$ ions in the sample. The reaction that produces insoluble AgCl ceases once excess $Ag^+$ ions are detected by an indicator and reference electrodes. Because the quantity of $Ag^+$ ions generated is known, the quantity of $Cl^-$ ions may be calculated using the Faraday law.

## Voltammetry

*Voltammetry* encompasses a group of electrochemical techniques in which a potential is applied to an electrochemical cell with the simultaneous measurement of the resulting current. By varying the potential of an electrode, it is possible to oxidize and reduce analytes in a solution. At more positive potentials, the electrons within the electrode become lower in energy and the oxidation of species in a solution becomes more likely. At lower potentials, the opposite occurs. By monitoring the current of an electrochemical cell at varying electrode potentials, it is possible to determine several parameters, such as concentration, reaction kinetics, and thermodynamics of the analytes.[13]

This technique differs from potentiometry in several important ways. Voltammetric techniques use an externally applied force (potential) to generate a signal (current) in a way that would not normally occur, whereas in potentiometric techniques, the analytical signal is produced internally through a redox reaction. The electrode arrangement is also quite different between the two techniques. To analyze both the potential and the resulting current, three electrodes are employed in voltammetric devices. The three electrodes include the working, auxiliary, and reference electrodes, which (when connected through a voltmeter) permit the application of specific potential functions. The measurement of the resulting current can yield results about ionic concentrations, conductivity, and diffusion. The ability to apply different types of potential functions or waveforms has led to the development of different voltammetric techniques: linear potential sweep polarography, pulse polarography, cyclic voltammetry, and anode stripping voltammetry.[7] These analytical methods, though not commonly used in clinical laboratories, are very sensitive (detection limits as low as the parts per billion range) and can identify trace elements in patient tissues such as hair and skin.

## Conductometry

*Conductometry* is the measurement of current flow (proportional to conductivity) between two nonpolarized electrodes of which a known potential has been established. Clinical applications include urea estimation through the measurement of the rate-of-change of conductance that occurs with the urease-catalyzed formation of $NH_4^+$ and bicarbonate ($HCO_3^-$). The technique is limited at low concentrations because of the high conductance of biological fluids. Perhaps the most important application of impedance (inversely proportional to conductance) measurements in the clinical laboratory involves the Coulter principle for the electronic counting of blood cells. This method is discussed in detail in the cytometry section.

# ELECTROPHORESIS

*Electrophoresis* is a common laboratory technique, with applications in various clinical laboratory disciplines. Routine diagnostic applications of electrophoresis technology exist for infectious diseases, malignancies, genetic diseases, paternity testing, forensic analysis, and tissue typing for transplantation. Electrophoresis involves the separation (ie, migration) of charged solutes or particles based on its size. Briefly, samples are applied to an electric field in a solution or in a support medium (ie, agarose gel) and exposed to a current electric field for a set duration of time. The migration of molecules within the support medium when exposed to the electrical field is dependent on the overall molecular charge, shape, and size of the molecule being studied.[17] Because most molecules of biologic importance are both water-soluble and charged, this analytical tool is one of the most important techniques for molecular separation in the clinical laboratory. The main types of electrophoresis techniques used in both clinical and research laboratories include cellulose acetate, agarose gel, polyacrylamide gel, isoelectric focusing (IEF), two-dimensional, and capillary electrophoresis (CE). Because of many clinical applications, electrophoresis apparatus, cellulose acetate and agarose gels, and reagents are available from commercial suppliers for each of these specific applications.

The primary application of electrophoresis is the analysis and purification of very large molecules such as proteins and nucleic acids. Electrophoresis also can be applied to the separation of smaller molecules, including charged sugars, amino acids, peptides, nucleotides, and simple ions. Through the proper selection of the medium for electrophoretic separations, extremely high resolution and sensitivity of separation can be achieved. Electrophoretic systems are usually combined with highly sensitive detection methods to monitor and analyze the separations that suit the specific application.[18]

The basic electrophoresis apparatus consists of a high voltage direct power supply that provides the electrical current, electrodes, a buffer, and a support for the buffer or a capillary tube. The support medium used provides a matrix that facilitates separation of the particles. Common support matrices include filter paper, cellulose acetate membranes, agarose, and polyacrylamide gels. When an electrostatic force is applied across the electrophoresis apparatus, the charged molecules will migrate to the anode or the cathode of the system depending on their charge. The force that acts on these molecules is proportional to the net charge on the molecular species and the applied voltage (electromotive force). This relationship is expressed as $F = qE/d$, where $F$ is the force exerted on the charged molecule, $q$ is its net charge, $E$ is the electromotive force, and $d$ is the distance across the electrophoretic medium.[13]

Although the basic principles are simple, procedures employed in the electrophoresis process are considerably more complex. For molecules to be separated, they must be dissolved in a buffer that contains electrolytes, which carry the applied current and fix the pH. The mobility of the molecules will be affected locally by the charge of the electrolytes, the viscosity of the medium, their size, and degree of asymmetry. These factors are related by the following equation:

$$\mu = q/6\eta r$$

where $\mu$ is the electrophoretic mobility of the charged molecule, $q$ is its net charge, $\eta$ is the viscosity of the medium, and $r$ is the ionic radius.[19]

The conditions in which this process occur are further complicated by the use of a support medium, necessary to minimize diffusion and convective mixing of the bands (caused by the heated current flowing through the buffer). The most common media used include polysaccharides such as cellulose and agarose and synthetic media (ie, polyacrylamide). The porosity of these media will, to a large extent, determine the resistance to movement for different ionic species. Therefore, the type of support medium used depends on the application. The above cited factors affecting the process of electrophoresis are controllable and provide optimal resolution for each specific application.

## Gel Electrophoresis
### Cellulose Acetate and Agarose Gel Electrophoresis

*Cellulose acetate* and *agarose gel electrophoresis* are methods commonly used in many clinical laboratories for both serum protein and hemoglobin separations. Serum protein electrophoresis is often used as a screening procedure for the detection of disease states, such as inflammation, protein loss, monoclonal gammopathies, and other dysproteinemias. When the molecules have been separated into bands, specific stains can then be used to visualize them. Densitometry is typically used to quantify each band. When a monoclonal immunoglobulin (Ig) pattern is identified, another technique, immunofixation electrophoresis, is used to quantify IgG, IgA, IgM, IgD, and IgE that are present in the specimen. Once these proteins are separated on an agarose gel, specific antibodies are directed at the immunoglobulins. The sample is then fixed and stained to visualize and quantify the bands.[20] Separation of proteins may also be accomplished with IEF where the proteins migrate through a stable pH gradient with the pH varying in the direction of migration. Each protein moves to its isoelectric point (ie, the point where the protein's charge becomes zero and migration ceases). This technique is often used for separating isoenzymes and hemoglobin variants.

Hemoglobin electrophoresis is the most common method for the screening for the presence of abnormal hemoglobin protein variants (hemoglobinopathies), of which more than 1,000 have been described. These variant forms of hemoglobin are often the result of missense mutations in the various globin genes (α, β, γ, or δ) due to a single nucleotide substitution. Many of these abnormal hemoglobin variants are benign without any clinical signs or symptoms and are identified only accidentally. However, certain mutations can have different manifestations, including altering the structure, stability, synthesis, or function of the globin protein. Hemoglobin S disease (sickle cell disease) is the most common hemoglobinopathy that is caused by a single nucleotide substitution of valine for glutamic acid at the sixth position of the β globin chain. Hemoglobin S disease results in changes that affect the shape and deformability of red blood cells, which ultimately leads to veno-occlusive disease and hemolysis.

Normal adult hemoglobin is composed of two α-subunits and two β-subunits (α2β2) and comprises approximately 97% of the total hemoglobin. Hemoglobin proteins are separated on a cellulose acetate membrane at an alkaline pH (8.6) initially and then on an agarose gel at an acid pH (6.2). Electrophoresis at both pH conditions is performed for optimal resolution of comigrating hemoglobin bands that occur at either of the pH conditions. For example, hemoglobin S, which causes patients to have sickle cell disease or sickle cell trait, comigrates with hemoglobins D and G at pH 8.6, but it can be separated at pH 6.2. The choice of support media is determined by the resolution of the hemoglobin bands that are achieved. Following electrophoresis, the bands are stained for visualization and the relative proportions of the hemoglobins are obtained by densitometry.[21]

Electrophoresis is also an important technique used in the laboratory to separate deoxyribonucleic acid (DNA), ribonucleic acid (RNA), and protein fragments. Three common techniques used are Southern, northern, and western blots. These techniques differ in the target molecules that are separated. Southern blots separate DNA that is cut with restriction endonucleases and then identified with a labeled (usually radioactive) DNA probe. Northern blots separate fragments of RNA that are probed with labeled DNA or RNA. Western blots separate proteins that are probed with radioactive or enzymatically tagged antibodies. The initial confirmation of human immunodeficiency virus (HIV) infection in patients that were repeatedly sero-reactive for HIV antibodies were performed using western blots (**Figure 2-3**). Western blots are largely no longer performed in clinical laboratories, but confirmatory assays employ the same targets in an immunochromatographic assay.

Each method involves a series of steps that leads to the detection of the various targets. Following electrophoresis, typically performed with an agarose or polyacrylamide gel, the molecules are transferred to a solid stationary support during the probe hybridization, washing, and detection stages of the assay. The DNA, RNA, or protein in the gel may be transferred onto nitrocellulose paper through electrophoresis or capillary blotting. In the former method, the molecules, by virtue of their negative charge, are transferred by electrophoresis. The latter method involves layering the gel on wet filter paper with the nitrocellulose paper on top. Dry filter paper is placed on the nitrocellulose paper and the molecules are transferred with the flow of buffer from the wet to dry filter paper via capillary action. Following the transfer, the nitrocellulose paper is soaked in a blocking solution containing high concentrations of DNA, RNA, or protein. This prevents the probe from randomly sticking to the paper during hybridization. During the hybridization stage, the labeled DNA, RNA, or antibody is incubated with the blot where binding with the molecular target occurs. The probe-target hybrids are detected following a wash step to remove any unbound probe.

## Two-Dimensional Electrophoresis

*Two-dimensional electrophoresis* is a powerful and widely used method in proteomics for the analysis of complex protein mixtures extracted from cells, tissues, or other biological samples. Proteins are sorted according to two independent properties: IEF, which separates proteins according to their isoelectric points, and sodium dodecylsulfate–polyacrylamide gel electrophoresis, which separates proteins according to their molecular weights. Each spot on the resulting two-dimensional array corresponds to a single protein species in the sample.[22] Using this technique, thousands of different proteins can be separated through the use of Coomassie dyes, silver staining, radiography, or fluorographic analysis; quantified; and characterized. Additionally, this technology can be used to explore protein families and search for differences, either genetic or disease based.

## Capillary Electrophoresis

*Capillary electrophoresis* (CE) includes diversified analytical techniques, such as capillary zone electrophoresis (CZE), capillary gel electrophoresis (CGE), capillary chromatography, capillary IEF, micelle electrokinetic capillary chromatography, and capillary isotachophoresis. Currently, only the first two in the previous list have practical applications in the clinical laboratory. Although historically a research tool, CE is being adapted for various applications in the clinical laboratory because of its rapid and high-efficiency separation power, diverse applications, and potential for automation. The possibility of CE becoming an important technology in the clinical laboratory is illustrated by its use in the separation and quantification of a wide spectrum of biological components ranging from macromolecules (proteins,

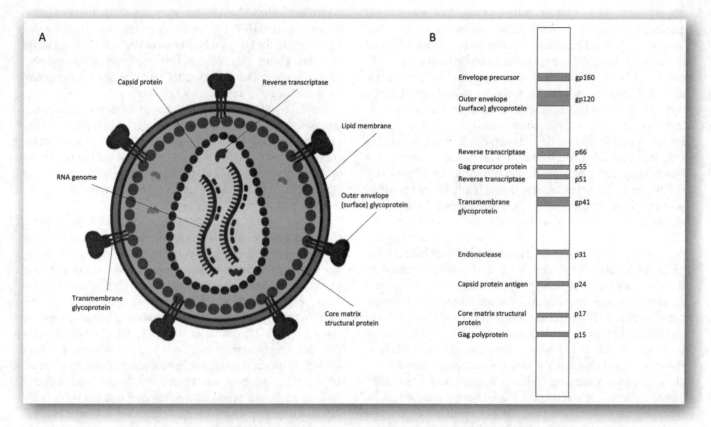

**FIGURE 2-3.** HIV-1 viral structure. (A) The complete structure of a single HIV virion is shown labeling key portions of the virus. (B) A diagram of the HIV western blot confirmatory ELISA assay. HIV-1 separated proteins are transferred from the gel to a nitrocellulose membrane. If antibodies specific to viral antigens are present, they will bind to the membrane and will remain visible following a series of wash steps and application of a conjugate and a horseradish peroxidase, which results in the appearance of bands seen visually on the nitrocellulose strip. Created with BioRender.com.

lipoproteins, and nucleic acids) to small analytes (amino acids, organic acids, or drugs).

The CE apparatus consists of a small-bore, silica-fused capillary (25 to 75 μm), approximately 50 to 100 cm in length, connected to a detector at one end, and via buffer reservoirs to a high-voltage power supply (25 to 35 kV) at the other end.[23] Because the small capillaries efficiently dissipate the heat, high voltages can be used to generate intense electric fields across the capillary to produce efficient separations with short separation times. In a CE separation, a very small amount of the sample (0.1 to 10 nL) is required. When the sample solution is injected into the apparatus, the molecules in the solution migrate through the capillary due to its charge in an electric field (electrophoretic mobility) or due to electroosmotic flow (EOF). The negatively charged surface of the silica capillary attracts positive-charged ions in the buffer solution, which in turn migrate toward the cathode and carry solvent molecules in the same direction. The overall movement of the solvent is called *EOF*. The separated proteins are eluted from the cathode end of the capillary. Quantitative detectors such as fluorescence, absorbance, electrochemical detectors, and mass spectrometry (MS) can be used to identify and quantify the proteins in the solution in amounts as little as 10 to 20 mol of substance in the injected

volume.[23] Two major advantages of using CE platforms include the ability to apply higher voltages than traditional electrophoresis platforms and its ease of automation.

## Capillary Zone Electrophoresis

*Capillary zone electrophoresis* (CZE) is the most widely used type of CE and is used for the separation of both anionic and cationic solutes, usually in a single analysis. In CZE, the anions and cations migrate in different directions, but they both rapidly move toward the cathode due to EOF, which is usually significantly higher than the solute velocity. Therefore, all molecules, regardless of their charge, will migrate to the cathode. In this way the negative, neutral, and positive species can be detected and separated. Common clinical applications include high-throughput separation of serum and urine protein and hemoglobin variants. In the future, other applications will become more commonplace. However, these systems are expensive, and currently, conventional methods are used.

## Capillary Gel Electrophoresis

*Capillary gel electrophoresis* (CGE) is the CE analog of traditional gel electrophoresis and is used for the size-based separation of biological macromolecules such as oligonucleotides, DNA restriction fragments, and proteins. The separation is performed by filling the capillary with a sieve-like matrix such as polyacrylamide or agarose to reduce the EOF. Therefore, larger molecules such as DNA will move more slowly resulting in better separation. Although CGE electrophoresis is primarily used in research, clinical applications are being developed.

## Pulsed-Field Gel Electrophoresis

In *pulsed-field gel electrophoresis* (PFGE), the current is alternately applied to different pairs of electrodes so that the electric field is cycled through different directions. As the field adjusts direction, molecules reorient themselves to the new field before migration continues through the agarose gel. This technique has been widely used to permit the separation of very large molecules, such as DNA fragments larger than 50 kb. Also, PFGE has been used for typing various strains of bacterial DNA after the genetic material has been cut with a particular restriction enzyme (the cut DNA provides a unique bacterial fingerprint). In the past, PFGE was commonly used to assess bacterial strain relatedness in the setting of outbreak investigations when investigators are attempting to determine if multiple bacterial isolates arise from a common source.[24] More recently, whole genome sequencing (discussed later) has largely replaced PFGE for outbreak investigations.

## DENSITOMETRY

*Densitometry* is a specialized form of spectrophotometry used to evaluate electrophoretic patterns. Densitometers can perform measurements in an absorbance optical mode and a fluorescence mode, depending on the type of staining of the electrophoretic pattern. An absorbance optical system consists of a light source, filter system, a movable carriage to scan the electrophoretic medium, an optical system, and a photodetector (silicon photocell) to detect light in the absorbance mode. When a densitometer is operated in the absorbance mode, an electrophoretic pattern located on the carriage system is moved across a focused beam of incident light. After the light passes through the pattern, it is converted to an electronic signal by the photocell to indicate the amount of light absorbed by the pattern. The absorbance is proportional to the sample concentration. The filter system provides a narrow band of visible light to provide better sensitivity and resolution of the different densities. This mode of operation is commonly used to evaluate hemoglobin and protein electrophoresis patterns and applications of molecular diagnostics (MDx), including one- and two-dimensional, DNA, RNA, and polymerase chain reaction (PCR) gel electrophoresis bands; dot blots; slot blots; image analysis; and chromosome analysis.

The fluorescence method is used in the case of electrophoretic patterns that fluoresce when radiated by UV light (340 nm). Densitometers used in this mode include a UV light source and a photomultiplier tube instead of the silicon photocell. When the pattern located on the carriage moves across a focused beam of UV light, the pattern absorbs the light and emits visible light. The light is focused by a collection of lenses onto a UV-blocking filter and then to a photomultiplier tube, where the visible light is converted into an electronic signal that is proportional to the intensity of the light. In each case, the electrophoretic patterns are evaluated by comparison of peak heights or peak areas of the sample and the standards. Current densitometry systems employ sophisticated software to provide analysis of the signal intensities with high resolution and sensitivity.[7]

## CHROMATOGRAPHY

*Chromatography* is another method used primarily for separating and identifying various compounds. In this procedure, components (solutes) from a mixture are separated by the differential distribution between mobile and stationary phases. In routine clinical practice, paper chromatography has been replaced by three other types of chromatography: thin layer chromatography (TLC), gas chromatography (GC), and high-performance (or pressure) liquid chromatography (HPLC). Chromatographic assays require more time for specimen preparation and performance; they are usually performed only when another assay type is not available or when interferences are suspected with an immunoassay. Chromatographic assays do not require premanufactured antibodies and, therefore, afford better flexibility than an immunoassay.

### Thin Layer Chromatography

*Thin layer chromatography* (TLC) is commonly used for drug screening and analysis of clinically important substances such as oligosaccharides and glycosaminoglycans (eg, dermatan sulfate, heparin sulfate, and chondroitin sulfate). In this method, a thin layer of gel (sorbent) is applied to glass or plastic, forming the stationary phase. The sorbent may be composed of silica, alumina, polyacrylamide, or starch. The choice of sorbent depends on the specific application because compounds have different relative affinities for the solvent (mobile phase) and the stationary phase. These factors affect the separation of a mixture into the different components. Silica gel is the most commonly used sorbent because it may be used to separate a broad range of compounds, including amino acids, alkaloids, sugars, fatty acids, lipids, and steroids.

Used for identification and separation of multiple components of a sample in a single step, TLC is also used in initial component separation prior to analysis by another technique. Quantification of various substances is possible with TLC; each spot can be scraped off and analyzed individually.[7] Although TLC is a useful screening technique, it has lower sensitivity and resolution than either gas or high-performance chromatography. Another disadvantage, as with gas and high-performance chromatography, is that someone with skill and expertise must interpret the results.

### Gas Chromatography

*Gas chromatography* (GC) is a subtype of column chromatography. This technique is used to identify and quantify volatile substances, such as alcohols, steroids, and drugs in the picogram range (Table 2-1). This technique is also based on the principles of paper and TLC, but it has better sensitivity. Instead of a solvent, GC uses an inert gas (eg, nitrogen or helium) as a carrier in the mobile phase for the volatile substance being analyzed.

A column packed with inert material, coated with a thin layer of a liquid phase, is substituted for paper or gel. The sample is injected into the column (contained in a heated compartment) where it is immediately volatilized and picked up by the carrier gas. Heating at precise temperature gradients is essential for good separation of the analytes. The gas carries the sample through the column where it contacts the liquid phase, which has a high boiling point. Analytes with lower boiling points migrate faster than those with higher boiling points, thus fractionating the sample components. When the sample leaves the column, it is exposed to a detector. The most common detector consists of a hydrogen flame with a platinum loop mounted above it. When the sample is exposed to the flame, ions collect on the platinum loop and generate a small current. This current is amplified by an electrometer, and the signal is sent on to an integrator or recorder. The recorder produces a chromatogram with various peaks being recorded at different times. Because each sample component is retained for a different length of time, the peak produced at a particular retention time is characteristic for a specific component (**Figure 2-4**). The amount of each component present is determined by the area of the characteristic peak or by the ratio of the peak heights calibrated against a standard curve.

This technique has many advantages, including high sensitivity and specificity. However, it requires sophisticated and expensive equipment. In addition, one or more compounds may produce peaks with the same retention time as the analyte of interest. In cases of such interference, the temperature and composition of the liquid phase can be adjusted for better peak resolution.

## High-Performance Liquid Chromatography

*High-performance liquid chromatography* (HPLC) is widely used, especially in forensic laboratories for toxicologic screening and to measure various drugs (Table 2-2). This is the most widely utilized form of liquid chromatography in clinical laboratories. Its basic principles are similar to those of GC, but it is useful for nonvolatile or heat-sensitive substances.

Instead of gas, HPLC utilizes a liquid solvent (mobile phase) and a column packed with a stationary phase, usually with a porous silica base. The mobile phase is pumped through the column under high pressure to decrease the assay time. The sample is injected onto the column at one end and migrates to the other end in the mobile phase. Various components move at different rates, depending on their solubility characteristics and the amount of time spent in the solid versus liquid phases. As the mobile phase leaves the column, it passes through a detector that produces a peak proportional to the concentration of each sample component. The detector is usually a spectrophotometer with variable wavelength capability in the UV and visible ranges. A signal from the detector is sent to a recorder or integrator, which plots peaks for each component as it elutes from the column (**Figure 2-5**). Each component has its own characteristic retention time, so each peak represents a specific component. As with GC, interferences may occur with compounds of similar structure or solubility characteristics; the peaks may fall on top of each other. Better resolution can be obtained by using a column packing with different characteristics or by changing the composition and pH of the mobile phase. Compounds are identified by their retention times and quantified either by computing the area of the peak or by comparing the peak height or area to an internal standard to obtain a peak height or peak area ratio. This ratio is then used to calculate a concentration by comparison with a predetermined standard curve.

Although HPLC offers both high sensitivity and specificity, it requires specialized equipment and personnel. Furthermore, because the substance being determined is usually in a body fluid (eg, urine or serum), one or more extraction steps are needed to isolate it. Another concern is that because many assays require a mobile phase composed of volatile and possibly toxic solvents, Occupational Safety and Health Administration guidelines must be followed. In addition, assays developed for commercial use may be costly as modifications to published methods are almost always required.

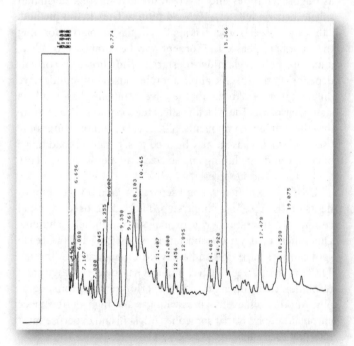

**FIGURE 2-4.** Gas chromatogram. The area under the curve or peak height of an analyte (eg, drug or toxin) is compared with the area under the curve or peak height of an internal standard, and then the ratio is calculated. This ratio is compared with a standard curve of peak area ratios to give the concentration of the analyte.

## IMMUNOASSAYS

*Immunoassays* are based on a reaction between an antigenic determinant (ie, hapten) and a labeled antibody.[25] The label may consist of a radioisotope, an enzyme, enzyme substrate, a fluorophore, or a chromophore. The reaction may be measured by several detection methods, including liquid scintillation,

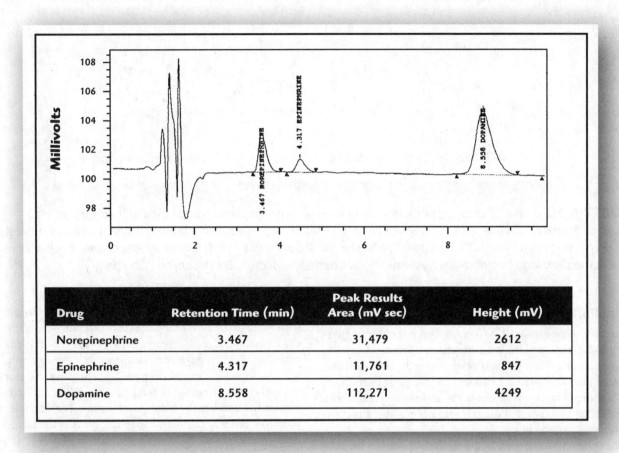

| Drug | Retention Time (min) | Peak Results Area (mV sec) | Height (mV) |
|---|---|---|---|
| Norepinephrine | 3.467 | 31,479 | 2612 |
| Epinephrine | 4.317 | 11,761 | 847 |
| Dopamine | 8.558 | 112,271 | 4249 |

**FIGURE 2-5.** High-performance liquid chromatography chromatogram. The appearance of this chromatogram is similar to the gas chromatogram, and the area or peak height ratio is used to quantify the analyte in a sample.

UV absorbance, fluorescence, fluorescent polarization, and turbidimetry or nephelometry. The immunoassay method is commonly used for determination of drug concentrations in serum.

Immunoassays can be divided into two general categories: *heterogeneous* and *homogeneous*. In heterogeneous assays, the free and bound portions of the determinant must be separated before either or both portions can be assayed. This separation can be accomplished by various methods, including protein precipitation, double antibody technique, adsorption of free drug, and removal by immobilized antibody on a solid phase support. Homogeneous assays do not require a separation step and, therefore, can be easily automated. The binding of the labeled hapten to the antibody alters its signal in a way (color change or reduction in enzymatic activity) that can then be used to measure the analyte concentration.

Early immunoassays used polyclonal antibodies (pAbs), generated as a result of an animal's natural immune response. Typically, an antigen is injected into an animal. The animal's immune system then recognizes the material as foreign and produces antibodies against it. These antibodies are then isolated from the blood. Many different antibodies may be generated in response to a single antigen. The numbers as well as the specificities of the antibodies depend on the size and number of antigenic sites on the antigen. In general, the larger and more complex the antigen

(eg, cell or protein), the more antigenic sites (epitopes) it has and the greater the variety of antibodies formed.

Although pAbs have been used successfully, both specificity and response may vary greatly because of their heterogeneous nature. The result is a high degree of cross-reactivity with similar substances. This cross-reactivity difficulty was eliminated with the development of monoclonal antibodies (moAbs). Prior to 1975, the only moAbs available were from patients suffering from multiple myeloma, a cancer of the blood and bone marrow in which uncontrolled numbers of malignant plasma cells are produced. Usually, these tumor cells produce a single (monoclonal) type of antibody. In 1975, a technique was developed to make moAbs in the laboratory.[26] The technique is based on the fusion of (1) genetic material from plasma cells that produce an antibody but cannot reproduce, and (2) myeloma cells that do not produce an antibody but can reproduce limitlessly. The plasma cells and myeloma cells are cultured together, resulting in a mixture of both parent cells and hybrid cells. This hybrid cell produces the specific antibody and reproduces indefinitely. The mixture is incubated in a special medium, which kills the parent cells and leaves only the hybrid antibody-producing cells alive. The hybrid cells can then be grown using conventional cell culture techniques, resulting in large amounts of the moAb. The development of moAbs has allowed for high sensitivity and specificity in immunoassay technology.

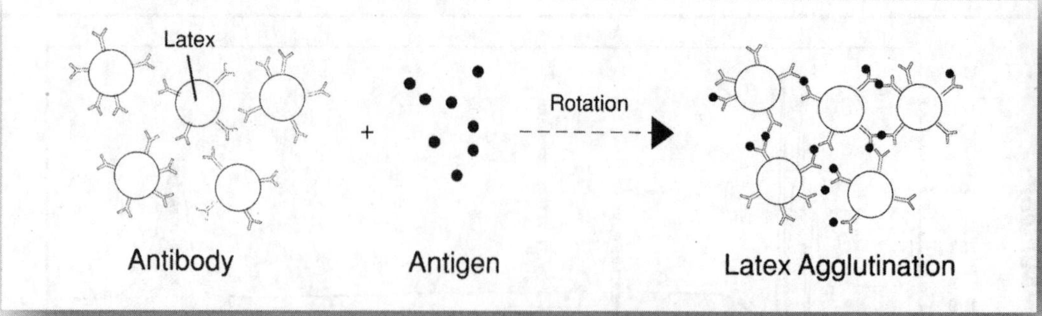

**FIGURE 2-6.** Schematic of latex agglutination immunoassay. The specimen (cerebrospinal fluid, serum, etc.) contains the analyte (in this case, antigens to bacteria) that causes an easily readable reaction. (*Source:* Adapted with permission from Power DA, McCuen PJ, eds. *Manual of BBI Products and Laboratory Procedures.* Cockeysville, MD: Becton Dickinson Microbiology Systems; 1998. Courtesy ©Becton, Dickinson, and Company.)

## Radioimmunoassay

Today *radioimmunoassay* (RIA) is rarely used in the clinical laboratory and is discussed from a historical perspective. A heterogeneous immunoassay, RIA was developed in the late 1950s and has been primarily used for endocrinology testing purposes.[27] This technique takes advantage of the fact that certain atoms can be either incorporated directly into the analyte's structure or attached to antibodies.

The primary atoms used in the clinical laboratory fall into two classes: γ-*emitters* and β-*emitters.* The γ-emitters ($^{125}$I and $^{57}$Co) are generally incorporated into compounds such as thyroid hormone and cyanocobalamin (vitamin $B_{12}$).[11] These types of isotopes can be counted directly with standard γ-counters that utilize a sodium iodide–thallium crystal. When the γ-ray hits the crystal, it gives off a flash of light. This light, in turn, stimulates a photomultiplier tube to amplify the signal. The β-emitters ($^{14}$C and $^{3}$H) are primarily used to measure steroid concentrations.[6] Because endogenous substances tend to absorb the radiation, β-rays cannot be counted directly. Therefore, this technique requires a scintillation cocktail with an organic compound capable of absorbing the β-radiation and reemitting it as a flash of light. This light is then amplified by a photomultiplier tube and counted.

Extremely sensitive, RIA has been made more specific with the introduction of moAbs. Unfortunately, this technique also has several significant disadvantages[11]: a short shelf-life for labeled reagents, lead shielding, waste disposal, monitoring of personnel for radiation exposure, strict record keeping, and special licensing. Because enzyme-linked immunoassays have none of these problems and can perform essentially the same tests as RIA, the clinical use of RIA has decreased in recent years.

## Agglutination

The simplest immunoassay is *agglutination.* Typical tests that can be performed using this assay include tests for human chorionic gonadotropin, rheumatoid factor, antigens from infectious agents, such as bacteria and fungi, and antinuclear antibodies. The agglutination reaction, used to detect either antigens or antibodies, results when multivalent antibodies bind to antigens with more than one binding site. This reaction occurs through the formation of cross linkages between antigen and antibody particles. When enough complexes form, clumping results and a visible mass is formed (**Figure 2-6**). Because the reaction depends on the number of binding sites on the antibody, the greater the number the better the reaction. For example, IgM produces better agglutination than IgG because the former has more binding sites.

The agglutination reaction is also affected by other factors[25]: avidity and affinity of the antibody; number of binding sites on the antigen as well as the antibody; relative concentrations of the antigen and antibody; Z-potential (electrostatic interaction that causes particles in solution to repel each other); and viscosity of medium. The two types of agglutination reactions are direct and indirect. *Direct agglutination* occurs when the antigen and antibody are mixed together, resulting in visible clumping. An example of this reaction is the test for *Salmonella typhi* antibody. *Indirect agglutination* (also known as *passive* or *particle agglutination*) uses a carrier for either the antibody or antigen. Originally, erythrocytes were selected as the carrier (as described for hemolytic anemia tests). However, latex-coated particles are now commonly used, and the latex agglutination method is simpler and less expensive than the erythrocyte immunoassay. In addition, latex particles allow titration of the amount of antibody bound to the latex particle, thus reducing variability. Other advantages include a rapid performance time with no separation step, allowing full automation. Disadvantages include expensive equipment and lower sensitivity than either RIA or EIA. The use of an automated particle counter increases the sensitivity of the test 10 to 1,000 times.[28]

## Enzyme Immunoassays

*Enzyme immunoassays* (EIAs) employ enzymes as labels for specific analytes. When antibodies bind to the antigen-enzyme complex, a defined reaction occurs (eg, color change, fluorescence, radioactivity, or altered activity). This altered enzyme activity is used to quantitate the analyte. The advantages of

EIAs include commercial availability at a relatively low cost, long shelf life, good sensitivity, automation, and none of the specific requirements mentioned for RIA.

## Enzyme-Linked Immunosorbent Assay

*Enzyme-linked immunosorbent assay* (ELISA) is a heterogeneous EIA. This assay employs the same basic principles as RIA except that enzyme activity rather than radioactivity is measured. The ELISA is commonly used to determine antibodies directed against a wide range of antigens, such as rheumatoid factor, hepatitis B antigen, and bacterial and viral antigens in the serum (Table 2-2).

In a competitive ELISA assay, the specific antibody is adsorbed to a solid phase. Enzyme-labeled antigen is incubated together with the sample containing unlabeled antigen and the antibodies attached to the solid phase. After a specified time, equilibrium is reached between the binding of the enzyme-labeled and unlabeled antigens to the solid phase antibody, and the solid phase is washed with buffer. The remaining product is measured with a spectrophotometer or fluorometer. The amount of the reaction product will be inversely proportional to the amount of unlabeled antigen in the sample because an increasing amount of unlabeled antigen will displace enzyme-labeled antigen from antibody binding.

## Enzyme-Multiplied Immunoassay

*Enzyme-multiplied immunoassay technique* (EMIT) is a homogeneous EIA; the enzyme is used as a label for a specific analyte (eg, a drug). Many drugs commonly assayed using EMIT are also measured by fluorescence polarization immunoassay (FPIA) (eg, digoxin, quinidine, procainamide, *N*-acetylprocainamide, and aminoglycoside antibiotics) (Table 2-2). With the EMIT assay, the enzyme retains its activity after attaching to the analyte. For example, to determine a drug concentration, an enzyme is conjugated to the drug and incubated with antidrug antibody.

As shown in **Figure 2-7**, the test drug is covalently bound to an enzyme that retains its activity and acts as a label. When this complex is combined with antidrug antibody, the enzyme is inactivated. If the antibody and enzyme-bound drug are combined with serum that contains unbound drug, competition occurs. Because the amount of antidrug antibody is limited, the free drug in the sample and the enzyme-linked drug compete for binding to the antibody. When the antibody binds to the enzyme-linked drug, enzyme activity is inhibited. The result is that the serum drug concentration is proportional to the amount of active enzyme remaining. Because no separation step is required, this assay has been automated.

## Fluorescent Polarization Immunoassay

*Fluorescent polarization immunoassay* (FPIA), the most common form of immunoassay, is used to measure concentrations of many serum analytes, such as blood urea nitrogen and creatinine. It is also commonly employed for determining serum drug concentrations of aminoglycoside antibiotics, vancomycin, and theophylline (Table 2-2).

Molecules having a ring structure and a large number of double bonds, such as aromatic compounds, can fluoresce when

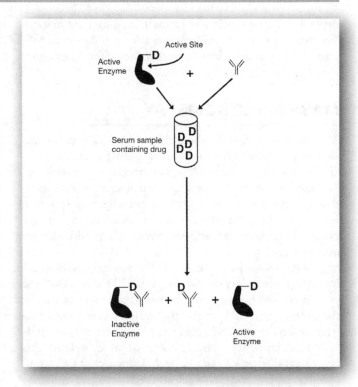

**FIGURE 2-7.** Enzyme-multiplied immunoassay technique. This assay is used in quantifying the drug concentration in a serum sample, as described in the text.

excited by a specific wavelength of light. These molecules must have a particular orientation with respect to the light source for electrons to be raised to an excited state. When the electrons return to their original lower energy state, some light is reemitted as a flash with a longer wavelength than the exciting light. Fluorescent immunoassays take advantage of this property by conjugating an antibody or analyte to a fluorescent molecule. The concentration can be determined by measuring either the degree of fluorescence or, more commonly, the decrease in the amount of fluorescence present.[11,28] In FPIA, a polarizing filter is placed between the light source and the sample and between the sample and the detector. The first filter assures that the light exciting the molecules is in a particular orientation; the second filter assures that only fluorescent light of the appropriate orientation reaches the detector.

The fluorescent polarization of a small molecule is low because it rotates rapidly and is not in the proper orientation long enough to give off an easily detected signal. To decrease this molecular motion, the molecule is complexed with an antibody. Because this larger complex rotates at a slower rate, it stays in the proper orientation to be excited by the incident light. When unlabeled analyte is mixed with a fixed amount of antibody and fluorescent-labeled analyte, a competitive binding reaction occurs between the labeled and unlabeled analytes. The result is a decrease in fluorescence. Thus, the concentration of unlabeled analyte is inversely proportional to the amount of fluorescence.[28]

Because of their simplicity, automation, and low cost, assays have been developed with relatively high sensitivity for many drugs (eg, antiepileptics, antiarrhythmics, and antibiotics). The primary difficulty is interference from endogenous substances (lipids and bilirubin) or metabolites of the drugs within the patient specimen.

# MASS SPECTROMETRY

*Mass spectrometry* (MS) involves the fragmentation and ionization of molecules in the gas phase according to their mass to charge ratio (m/z). The resulting mass fragments are displayed on a mass spectrum, or a bar graph, that plots the relative abundance of an ion versus its m/z ratio. Because the mass spectrum is characteristic of the parent molecule, an unknown molecule can be identified by comparing its mass spectrum with a library of known spectra.

A wide array of MS systems has been developed to meet the increasing demands of the biomedical field. However, the basic principles and components of mass spectrometers are essentially the same. These include an inlet unit, an ion source, a mass analyzer, an ion detector, and a data/recording system. Compounds introduced into a mass spectrometer must first be isolated. This is accomplished with separation techniques such as GC, liquid chromatography, and CE, which are used in tandem with mass spectrometers. In a GC/MS system, an interface between the GC and MS components that restricts the gas flow from the GC column into the mass spectrometer is required to prevent a mismatch in the operating pressures between the two instruments. The unit must also be heated to maintain the volatile compounds in the vapor state and remove most of the carrier gas from the GC effluent entering the ion source unit.[29]

## Ionization Methods

The ionization of the molecules introduced into MS is accomplished by several methods. In each case, the ion sources are maintained at high temperatures and high vacuum conditions necessary for ionizing vaporized molecules. The *electron ionization* (EI) method, a form of gas-phase ionization, consists of a beam of high-energy electrons that bombard the incoming gas molecules. The energy used is sufficiently high to not only ionize the gas molecules, but also cause them to fragment through the breaking of their chemical bonds. This process yields ion fragments in addition to intact molecular ions that appear in the mass spectra. The EI method is most useful for low molecular weight compounds (<400 Da) because of problems with excessive fragmentation and thermal decomposition of large molecules during vaporization.[30,31] Therefore, EI is typically used in GC/MS systems that are suitable for applications, including the analysis of synthetic organic chemicals, hydrocarbons, pharmaceutical compounds, organic acids, and drugs of abuse.

*Chemical ionization* (CI) is another form of gas-phase ionization. Because the sample molecule is ionized by a reagent such as methane or ammonia that is first ionized by an electron beam, CI is a less energetic technique than EI. Less fragmentation is produced by this method, making it useful for determining the molecular weights of many organic compounds and for enhancing the abundance of intact molecular ions.

*Electrospray ionization* (ESI), a form of atmospheric pressure ionization, generates ions directly from solution, permitting it to be used in combination with HPLC and CE systems. This method involves the creation of a fine spray in the presence of a strong electric field. As the droplets become declustered, the force of the surface tension of the droplet is overcome by the mutual repulsion of like charges, allowing the ions to leave the droplet and enter the mass analyzer. This technique will yield multiple ionic species, especially for high molecular weight ions that have a large distribution of charge states, thus making it a very sensitive technique for small, large, and labile molecules.[32] This ionization method is well-suited for the analysis of peptides, proteins, carbohydrates, DNA fragments, and lipids. Other common ionization techniques include *fast atom bombardment*, which uses high velocity atoms such as argon to ionize molecules in a liquid or solid, and *matrix-assisted laser desorption/ionization* (MALDI), which uses high energy photons to ionize molecules embedded on a solid organic matrix.[32]

## Mass Analyzers

Following ionization, the gas phase ions enter the *mass analyzer*. This component of the mass spectrometer separates the ions by their m/z ratios. Commonly used mass analyzers include the double-focusing magnetic sector analyzer, quadrupole mass spectrometers, quadrupole ion trap mass spectrometers, and tandem mass spectrometers.

The *double-focusing magnetic sector* analyzer uses a magnetic field perpendicular to the direction of the ion motion to deflect the ions into a circular path with a radius dependent on the m/z ratio and the velocity of the ion. The detector will then separate the ions by their m/z ratios. However, because the kinetic energy (or velocity) of the molecules leaving the ion source is not necessarily constant, the path radii will become dependent on the velocity and the m/z ratio. To enhance the resolution, an electrostatic analyzer or electric sector is used to allow molecules with only a specific kinetic energy to pass through its field. That is, for a particular kinetic energy, the radius of curvature is directly related to the m/z ratio. This type of analyzer is commonly used in combination with EI and fast atom bombardment ionization systems.

*Quadrupole mass spectrometers* act as a filter for molecules or fragments with a specific m/z ratio. This is accomplished by using four equally spaced parallel rods with direct current (DC) and radio frequency (RF) potentials on opposing rods of the quadrupole. The field produced is along the x- and y-axis. The RF oscillation causes the ions to be attracted or repelled by the rods. Only ions with a specific m/z ratio will have a trajectory along the z-axis, allowing them to pass to the detector, while others will be trapped by the rods of the quadrupole. By varying the RF field, other m/z ranges are selected, thus resulting in the mass spectrum.[31] The quadrupole mass spectrometer, commonly combined with the EI ionization system, is perhaps the most commonly used type of mass spectrometer because of its relatively low cost, ability to analyze m/z ratios up to 3,000, and compatibility with ESI ionization systems.

The *ion trap analyzer* is another form of a quadrupole mass spectrometer, consisting of a ring electrode to which an RF voltage is applied to two end caps at ground potential. This arrangement generates a quadrupole field trapping ions that are injected into the chamber or are generated within it. As the RF field is scanned, ions with specific and successive m/z ratios are ejected from the trap to the ion detector through holes in the caps.[31] The quadrupole ion trap mass spectrometer is notable for its high sensitivity and compact size.

*Tandem mass spectrometers* use multiple stages of mass analysis on subsequent generations of ion fragments. This is accomplished by preselecting an ion from the first analysis and colliding it with an inert gas, such as argon or helium, to induce further fragmentation of the ion. The next stage involves analyzing the fragments generated by an earlier stage. The abbreviation $MS^n$ is applied to the stages, which analyze fragments beyond the initial ions (MS) to the first generation of ion fragments ($MS^2$) and subsequent generations ($MS^3$, $MS^4$, etc.). These techniques can be tandem in space (two or more instruments) or tandem in time. In the former case, many combinations have been used for this type of analysis. In the later cases, quadrupole ion trap devices are often used and can achieve multiple $MS^n$ measurements.[33] Tandem mass analysis is primarily used to obtain structural information such as peptides sequences, small DNA/RNA oligomers, fatty acids, and oligosaccharides. Other mass analyzers, such as time-of-flight and Fourier transform mass spectrometers, are not commonly used for clinical applications.

## Ion Detector

The *ion detector* is the final element of the mass spectrometer. Once an ion passes through the mass analyzer, a signal is produced in the detector. The detector consists of an electron multiplier that converts the energy of the ion into a cascade of secondary electrons (similar to a photomultiplier tube), resulting in about a million-fold amplification of the signal. Due to the rapid rate at which data are generated, computerized data systems are indispensable components of all modern mass spectrometers. The introduction of rapid processors, large storage capacities, and spectra databases has led to automated high throughput. Miniaturization of components has also led to the development of bench-top systems practical for routine clinical laboratory analysis. Clinical applications include newborn screening for metabolic disorders, hemoglobin analysis, drug testing, and microbial identification. Pharmaceutical applications include drug discovery, pharmacokinetics, and drug metabolism. Clinical microbiology has seen a radical shift in the last decade in the approach used to identify microorganisms. Traditional identification had been based on biochemical testing and relies on well-isolated colonies from microbiologic media for testing. These methods are time-consuming, and much progress has been made to reduce the turnaround time to provide clinicians with more rapid identification to provide more targeted antimicrobial chemotherapy. Some laboratories have adopted the use of MALDI-TOF (time of flight) to provide more rapid bacterial or yeast identification of clinical pathogens. There are two current FDA-cleared MALDI-TOF systems available for use in clinical laboratories. Both systems have robust databases capable of identifying a variety of aerobic and anaerobic bacteria and yeasts. Identification of more complex organisms, including mycobacterial species and molds are possible, and

both companies continue to add new improve their systems by adding more spectra to their databases to improve identification.

In this application, a colony from an agar plate or an aliquot directly from a positive blood culture bottle is applied to a card and is overlaid with a matrix and allowed to dry on the plate. The plate is loaded onto the analyzer where a laser ionizes the sample. The mass of the ions generated from the ionization process is analyzed using a flight tube, which detects the lighter ions that travel faster than the heavier, slower traveling ions. The result of the detection of the ionized targets (typically bacterial ribosomal proteins) is the generation of a unique mass spectrum. In this spectrum, the mass-to-charge ratio is plotted against the signal intensity. Therefore, the system only detects highly abundant proteins that are of low mass and readily ionized by the laser. In effect, the mass profile generated is a bacterial fingerprint. The spectrum is compared with a comprehensive database of spectra for well-characterized bacterial or fungal pathogens. Depending on the similarity of the peaks, laboratories can accurately identify a colony to the genus or species level.[34]

# CYTOMETRY

*Cytometry* is defined as a process of measuring physical, chemical, or other characteristics of (usually) cells or other biological particles. Although this definition encompasses the fields of flow cytometry and cellular image analysis, many additional methods are now used to study the vast spectrum of cellular properties. Consequently, the term *cytomics* has been introduced. Cytomics is defined as the science of cell-based analysis that integrates genomics and proteomics with dynamic functions of cells and tissues. The technology used includes techniques discussed in this chapter, such as flow cytometry and MS, and others that are beyond the scope of this chapter.

## Flow Cytometry

*Flow cytometry* is the technology used to measure properties of cells as they move or flow in liquid suspension.[35] It is a technique used to measure multiple characteristics of individual cells within heterogeneous populations. Instruments generally referred to as *flow cytometers* are based on the principles of laser-induced fluorometry and light scatter. The terminology can become confusing as various conventions have taken root over the years. However, regardless of the principles of detection or measurement, the term *flow cytometry* may in general be applied to technologies that rely on cells moving in a fluid stream for analysis.

The hematology analyzer, an instrument employing flow cytometry, also incorporates the principles of impedance, absorbance, and laser light scatter to measure cell properties and generate a complete blood count laboratory report. The basis of cell counting and sizing in hematology analyzers is the Coulter principle, which relates counting and sizing of particles to changes in electrical impedance across an aperture in a conductive medium (created when a particle or cell moves through it). The basic system consists of a smaller chamber within a larger chamber, both filled with a conductive medium and each with one electrode across in which a constant DC is applied. The fluids within each chamber communicate through a small aperture (100 μm) or sensing zone. When a nonconductive particle or cell passes through the aperture, it displaces an equivalent volume of conductive fluid. This increases the conductance and creates a voltage pulse for each cell counted, the intensity of which is proportional to the cell volume.[14]

In hematology analyzers, blood is separated into two samples for measurement. One volume is mixed with a diluent and delivered to a chamber where platelet and erythrocyte counts are performed. Particles with volumes between 2 and 20 femtoliter (fL) are counted as platelets, and particles with volumes >36 fL are counted as erythrocytes. The other volume is mixed with a diluent, and an erythrocyte lysing reagent is used to permit leukocyte (>36 fL) counts to be performed. The number of cells in this size range may be subtracted from the erythrocyte count performed in the other chamber.

Modern hematology analyzers employ additional technologies to enhance the resolution of blood cell analysis. The RF energy is used to assess important information about the internal structure of cells such as nuclear volume. Laser light scatter is used to obtain information about cell shape and granularity. The combination of these and other technologies—such as light absorbance for hemoglobin measurements—provide accurate blood cell differentials, counts, and other important blood cell indices. These basic principles are common to many hematology analyzers used in clinical laboratories. However, each uses different proprietary detection, measurement and software systems, and ways of displaying the data.

Flow cytometers incorporate the principles of fluorometry and light scatter to the analysis of particles or cells that pass within a fluid stream. This technology provides multiparametric measurements of intrinsic and extrinsic properties of cells. Intrinsic properties, including cell size and cytoplasmic complexity, are properties that can be assessed directly by light scatter and do not require the use of any type of probe. Extrinsic cellular properties, such as cell surface or cytoplasmic antigens, enzymes or other proteins, and DNA/RNA, require the use of a fluorescent dye or probe to label the components of interest and a laser to induce the fluorescence (older systems used mercury arc lamps as a light source) to be detected.

The basic flow cytometer consists of four types of components: fluidics, optics, electronics, and data analysis. Fluidics refers to the apparatus that directs the cells in suspension to the flow cell where they will be interrogated by the laser light. Fluidics systems use a combination of air pressure and vacuum to create the conditions that allow the cells to pass through the flow chamber in single file. The optical components include the laser (or other light source), flow chamber, monochromatic filters, dichroic mirrors, and lenses. These are used to direct the scattered or fluorescent light to detectors, which measure the signals that are subsequently analyzed.[35]

The light scattered by the cell when it reaches the flow chamber is used to measure its intrinsic properties. *Forward-scattered light* (FSC) is detected by a diode and reflects the size of the passing cell. *Side-scattered light* (SSC) is detected by a photomultiplier tube at an angle approximately 90 degrees to the laser beam. The SSC is a function of the cytoplasmic complexity of the cell, including the granularity of the cell. The correlated measurements and analysis of FSC and SSC can allow for differentiation among cell types (ie, leukocytes) and can be depicted on a scattergram.

The analysis of extrinsic properties is more complicated. The measurement of DNA or RNA, for example, requires the use of intercalating nucleic acid dyes such as propidium iodide. The detection of antigenic determinants on cells can be performed with fluorescent-labeled moAbs directed at these antigens. In each case, the principle of detection involves the use of laser light to excite the fluorescent dye and detect its emitted signal. Fluorescent dyes are characterized by their excitation (absorption) and emission wavelength spectra and by the difference between the maxima of these spectra or Stokes shift (discussed in the spectrophotometry section). These properties permit the use of multiple fluorescent probes on a single cell.

To illustrate the operation of a flow cytometer, consider a four-color, six-parameter (FSC and SSC) configuration (**Figure 2-8**).[36] An argon gas laser with a wavelength of 488 nm is commonly used because it simultaneously excites several different dyes that possess different emission wavelengths. Fluorochromes conjugated with moAbs that may be used include fluorescein isothiocyanate, phycoerythrin (PE), energy-coupled dye, and Cy5PE (tandem dye composed of the carbocyanine derivative Cy5 and PE) with peak emission wavelengths of approximately 520, 578, 613, and 670 nm, respectively. The emitted light at each of these wavelengths is detected at an angle of 90 degrees. The array of optical filters selects light in each wavelength region and directs it to a different photomultiplier tube where it is detected, amplified, and converted into an electronic signal. This measurement can be made on thousands of cells in a matter of seconds. The result is a histogram that identifies distinct cell populations based on light scatter and extrinsic properties. In the case of blood, a histogram will distinguish lymphocytes, monocytes, and granulocytes by light scatter. The B cell, T cell, T-cell subsets, and natural killer cell populations can all be distinguished.

This important method of cell analysis has found many applications in medicine, making it a relatively common clinical laboratory instrument. Flow cytometry analysis is routinely used to assist in classifying the type of leukemia and lymphoma, derive prognostic information in these and other malignancies, monitor immunodeficiency disease states such as HIV/AIDS, enumerate stem cells by cluster differentiation (CD34), and assess various functional properties of cells.

## Image Cytometry

*Image cytometry*, more commonly known as *histology*, is a laboratory method that uses instruments and techniques to analyze tissue specimens. Examining individual cells, rather than the collection of cells that make up a tissue, is referred to as *cytology*. The basic components of an image cytometry system may include a microscope, camera, computer, and monitor. Variations and complexity of these systems exist, which are beyond the scope of this chapter. However, the essence of these instruments is the ability to acquire images in two or three (confocal microscopy) dimensions to study the distribution of various components within cells or tissues. The high optical resolution

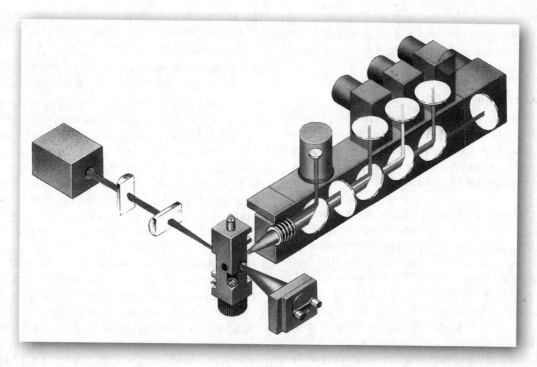

**FIGURE 2-8.** Schematic of a four-color flow cytometry system. The laser beam is focused onto the flow cell through which the cell suspension is directed. Scattered light is detected by the forward and side scatter detectors. Emitted light from specific moAb labeled with fluorochromes are detected. Appropriate dichroic long pass filters direct the specific wavelength of light through a narrow band pass filter and then to the appropriate PMT. (Courtesy of Beckman Coulter.)

of these systems is an important determinant in obtaining morphometric information and precise data about cell and tissue constituents through the use of fluorescence/absorbance-based probes, as in flow cytometry.[37] Specific applications of image cytometry generally involve unique methods of cell or tissue preparation and other modifications. This lends to the versatility of this technology, which yields such applications as the measurement of DNA content in nuclei to assess prognosis in cancer and the detection of specific nucleic acid sequences to diagnose genetic disorders.

## In Situ Hybridization

Among the methods of image cytometry, *in situ hybridization* is perhaps the most commonly used in the clinical laboratory, particularly in molecular cytogenetics laboratories. In situ hybridization is used to localize nucleic acid sequences (entire chromosomes or parts, including genes) in cells or tissues through the use of probes, which consist of a nucleic acid sequence that is complementary to the target sequence and labeled in some way that makes the hybridized sequence detectable. These principles are common to all methods of in situ hybridization, but they differ in the type of probe that is used. Fluorescent probes, which provide excellent spatial resolution, have become a preferred method of in situ hybridization for many applications. (Radioactive probes are also used for this application. However, because their spatial resolution is limited, detection and artifacts are often produced.)

*Fluorescent in situ hybridization* (FISH) is a powerful molecular cytogenetics technique used for detecting genes and genetic anomalies and monitoring different diseases at the genetic level. These assays are more sensitive and can detect chromosomal abnormalities that cannot be appreciated by routine chromosome analysis (ie, karyotyping). Typically, metaphase chromosomes or interphase nuclei are denatured on a slide along with a fluorescent labeled DNA probe. The probe and chromosomes are hybridized, and the slide is washed, counterstained, and analyzed by fluorescent microscopy. There are various types of FISH probes that can be utilized, such as DNA probes to detect nick translations or RNA probes that can detect in vitro transcription. An appropriate arrangement of filters is used to direct the relevant wavelength of light from the light source to excite the fluorescent molecule on the probe. All but the emission wavelength of light is blocked with a special filter permitting the signal from the probe to be visualized.[38] In molecular cytogenetics, these assays are commonly used to identify gene fusions or translocations.

## MOLECULAR DIAGNOSTICS

*Molecular diagnostics* (MDx) were initially introduced into the clinical laboratories as manual, labor-intensive techniques. This discipline has experienced an overwhelming period of maturation in the past several years. Testing has moved quickly from highly complex, labor-intensive procedures to more user-friendly, semiautomated protocols, and the application potential of MDx continues to evolve. Nucleic acid amplification technologies are among the procedures that have most revolutionized MDx testing.

## Nucleic Acid Amplification

*Polymerase chain reaction* (PCR) is the most frequently used of these technologies. Other amplification techniques that are used in clinical laboratory procedures include ligase chain reaction, transcription mediated amplification, branched DNA amplification, isothermal amplification, and nucleic acid sequence-based amplification.

The PCR technology is used principally for detecting microbiologic organisms and genetic diseases (Table 2-2). Examples of microorganisms identified by this process include chlamydia, cytomegalovirus, Epstein-Barr virus, HIV, mycobacteria, and herpes simplex virus. As PCR amplifies nucleic acid sequences, if one knows the sequence of interest, then an assay can be developed and optimized for use in patient testing. While the list of cleared and approved targets is limited to the most commonly encountered microorganisms, new assays are being developed by many diagnostic companies. PCR can often identify organisms with greater speed and sensitivity than conventional methods. For clinical microbiology laboratories, PCR methods are attractive because they are rapid, sensitive, and specific. Many laboratories have moved from culture-based methods to molecular amplification methods for the rapid identification of patients that may be colonized with multidrug-resistant organisms, such as *Clostridioides difficile,* methicillin-resistant *Staphylococcus aureus*, or vancomycin-resistant enterococci. Rapid identification of these patients is crucial in healthcare settings that often place these patients on contact precautions to try and reduce the spread of these organisms. The PCR applications in microbiology can also be used to identify organisms carrying antibiotic resistance genes, such as the *Klebsiella pneumoniae* carbapenemase *bla*$_{KPC}$ gene that confers resistance to all β-lactam antibiotics among members of the *Enterobacterales* and other gram-negative bacilli.

Genetic diseases diagnosed using PCR include α-1 antitrypsin deficiency, cystic fibrosis, sickle cell anemia, fragile X syndrome, Tay-Sachs disease, drug-induced hemolytic anemia, and Von Willebrand disease. In addition, cancer research has benefited from PCR through the diagnosis of various cancers (eg, chronic myeloid leukemia and pancreatic and colon cancers) as well as through the detection of residual disease after treatment.[39] This technique is used to amplify specific DNA and RNA sequences enzymatically.

In addition, PCR takes advantage of the normal DNA replication process. In vivo, DNA replicates when the double helix unwinds and the two strands separate. A new strand forms on each separate strand through the coupling of specific base pairs (eg, adenosine with thymidine and cytosine with guanosine). The PCR cycle is similar and consists of three separate steps (**Figure 2-9**)[28]:

1. Denaturation: The reaction tube is heated causing the double stranded DNA to separate.

2. Primer annealing: Sequence-specific primers are allowed to bind to opposite strands flanking the region of interest by decreasing the temperature.

3. Primer extension: DNA polymerase then extends the hybridized primers, generating a copy of the original DNA template.

The efficiency of the extension step can be increased by raising the temperature. Typical temperatures for the three steps are 201.2°F (94°C) for denaturation, 122°F to 149°F (50°C to 65°C) for annealing, and 161.6°F (72°C) for extension. Note that cycle temperatures are influenced by the specific enzyme used, the primer sequence, and the genomic sample. Because one cycle is typically completed in less than three minutes, many cycles can occur within a short time, resulting in the exponential production of millions of copies of the target sequence.[40] The genetic material is then identified by agarose gel electrophoresis.

One potential disadvantage of this method is contamination of the amplification reaction with products of a previous PCR (carryover), exogenous DNA, or other cellular material. Contamination can be reduced by prealiquoting reagents, using dedicated positive-displacement pipettes, and physically separating the reaction preparation from the area where the product is analyzed. In addition, multiple negative controls are necessary to monitor for contamination. Also common in clinical laboratories are instrument platforms that can perform real-time (q) PCR as well as multiplex PCR, which allows amplification of two or more products in parallel in a single reaction tube.[40] In real-time detection methods, a labeled oligonucleotide probe containing a fluorophore on the 5′ end and a quencher on the 3′ end bind to the DNA template. With the probe bound, the quencher prevents the fluor from emitting light. During DNA synthesis, the extending forward primer causes strand displacement. As the activity of the DNA polymerase enzyme continues reading along the template, the exonuclease activity of the polymerase enzyme cleaves the probe, resulting in the generation of light that is detected by the instrument. As each cycle of PCR continues, more fluorescent molecules are released, resulting in increasing fluorescence proportional to the amount of amplicon present. Several in vitro diagnostic companies such as BD Diagnostics, BioFire, Cepheid, and Nanosphere have U.S. Food and Drug Administration (FDA)-approved platforms that can allow for simultaneous detection of multiple microorganism targets. Use of these multiplex assays is attractive because they require minimal sample volumes to generate multiple results. These tests are typically referred to as syndromic panels—named as such for the most common samples tested, which include upper and lower respiratory tract specimens, stool, blood, and cerebrospinal fluid to detect CNS infections. Other companies are developing similar panels that can aid in the detection of prosthetic joint infections, which are routinely diagnosed using culture methods, but those suffer from decreased analytic sensitivity.

## GENOMICS, EPIGENETICS, PROTEOMICS, AND METABOLOMICS

Newly developed techniques capable of examining the DNA, messenger RNA (mRNA), and proteins of cells have provided a

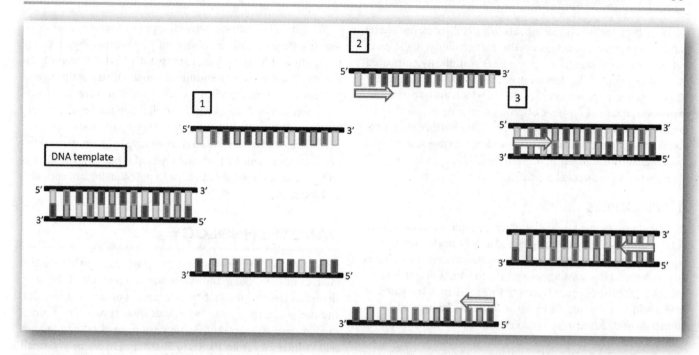

**FIGURE 2-9.** Stages of a single PCR reaction cycle. Beginning with your DNA template, the sample is added into a microtube with DNA polymerase, forward and reverse sequence specific primers that will bind to and amplify the region of interest within the template, and excess amounts of deoxynucleotide triphosphates (dNTP). During Step 1 (denaturation), the sample is heated between 93°C and 96°C to separate the double-stranded DNA into two single stranded templates. During Step 2 (annealing), the forward and reverse sequence specific primers will bind to complementary sequences within the template to facilitate replication. Annealing occurs between 50°C and 70°C. During Step 3, extension of the template occurs at 68°C and 75°C. During extension, DNA polymerase will catalyze the addition of complementary dNTP to the primer using the sample DNA as the template. This completes one cycle of the PCR reaction yielding two copies of the amplified region of interest.

framework for detailed molecular classifications and treatments of diseases. Genetic analysis of cystic fibrosis, for example, has shown the disease to be the result of more than 1,500 different mutations in the gene cystic fibrosis transmembrane conductance regulator.[41] The most common mutation accounts for two-thirds of cystic fibrosis cases. Several related developments, especially in the areas of tumor classifications, are based on the fields of genomics, epigenetics, and proteomics. The most important laboratory procedures are array-based comparative genomic hybridization and the data derived from these studies—bioinformatics.

## Genomics

The study of all the genes of a cell, its DNA sequences, and the fine-scale mapping of genes is the science of *genomics*. A genome is the sum total of all genes of an individual organism. Knowledge of full genomes has created multiple possibilities, mainly concerned with patterns of gene expression associated with various diseases.[42,43]

## Epigenetics

*Epigenetics* refers to modifications of the genome that are functionally relevant but do not involve a change in the nucleotide sequence. Histone deacetylation and DNA methylation are examples of such changes, both of which serve to suppress gene expression without altering the sequence of the silenced genes. Such changes may continue to exist for many cell divisions and even the remainder of the cell's life, as well as for future generations of cells. However, because there is no change in the underlying DNA sequence of the organism, nongenetic factors cause the organism's genes to express themselves differently.[44]

## Proteomics

The study of the full complement of proteins in a cell or tissue is called *proteomics* and includes the comprehensive analysis and characterization of all proteins, including their structure and function that are encoded by the human genome. Protein-based assays were among the first assays to be approved by the FDA, mostly using immunohistochemistry techniques. Most important biological functions are controlled by signal transduction, which are processes governed by the enzyme activities of proteins. Diseases such as cancer, while fundamentally the result of genomic mutations, manifest as dysfunctional protein signal transduction. Many pharmaceuticals are now being developed to aim at modulating the aberrant protein activity, not the genetic defect.[45-47]

Proteomics will eventually have a great impact in the practice of medicine. Although the genome is the source of basic cellular information, the functional aspects of the cell are controlled by and through proteins, not genes. The main challenge to the study of proteomics is due to the proteome's complexity compared with the genome. The human genome encodes approximately 23,000 genes, approximately 21,000 of which encode proteins. However, the total number of proteins in human cells is estimated to be between 250,000 and 1 million. Furthermore, proteins are dynamic and constantly undergo changes, synthesis, and breakdown. Currently, most of the FDA-approved targeted therapeutics are directed at proteins and not genes.

## Metabolomics

Similar to proteomics, metabolomics is a rapidly emerging field that combines multiple strategies and techniques to identify and quantify metabolites. Metabolites are small molecule substrates (ie, intermediates substances and the products of our metabolism). Like the Human Genome Project, which launched in 1990 and was completed in April 2003, the Human Metabolome Project, funded by Genome Canada, was launched in 2005 to describe and understand the complete collection of small molecules in a sample, including endogenous and exogenous compounds. The project led to the development of the Human Metabolome Database (https://hmdb.ca/) a freely available web-accessible database that contains detailed information about small molecule metabolites found in the human body. To date, the database contains more than 114,000 metabolite entries with links to more than 5,700 protein sequences associated with the metabolites. Metabolomics is useful for future identification biomarkers that could be used as diagnostic or prognostic of any number of diseases.

## ARRAY-BASED COMPARATIVE HYBRIDIZATION

Molecular profiles of cells can now be determined using *array-based comparative hybridization*.[48] This technique is especially useful in profiling tumor cells. Until recently, changes occurring in cancer cells were studied one at a time or in small groups in small sets of tumors. New array comparative hybridization or microarray technology ("gene chips") has enabled investigators to simultaneously detect and quantify the expression of large numbers of genes (potentially all genes) in different tumors using mRNA levels. In this technique, samples are obtained from tissues embedded in paraffin blocks, and serve as the sources to prepare new blocks that may contain up to thousands of tissue fragments. These multiple samples are then used to test the expression of potential tumor markers by mRNA expression profiling. The mRNA levels, however, do not always correspond to changes in tumor cell proteins. The quantity of protein within a cell depends not only on the amount and rate of transcription and translation, but also on protein breakdown and the rate of transport out of the cell. Although tissue used for mRNA profiling may include both tumor and stromal cells, by adding immunohistochemistry methods, specific proteins in tissue sections originating from both normal as well as tumor cells can be identified.

As a specific example, several types of breast cancer cells, which were previously identified only by morphology, are now being studied by array-based comparative hybridization techniques. Combined with immunohistochemistry staining and protein expression levels, new subtypes that were not previously well defined have been identified (eg, the basal-like carcinomas).[49] As a consequence, new treatment modalities have been developed. Array-based comparative hybridization methods have also identified new subtypes of other tumors, such as lymphomas and prostate cancer with potential for susceptibility and prognosis.[50]

## NANOTECHNOLOGY

*Nanotechnology* refers to the emerging science that studies interactions of cellular and molecular components at the most elemental level of biology, typically clusters of atoms, molecules, and molecular fragments. Nanoscale objects have dimensions smaller than 100 nm. At this dimension, smaller than human cells (which vary from 10,000 to 20,000 nm in diameter), small clusters of molecules and their interactions can be detected. Nanoscale devices smaller than 50 nm can easily enter most cells, while those smaller than 20 nm can move out of blood vessels, offering the possibility that these devices will be able to enter biological chambers, such as the blood–brain barrier or the gastrointestinal epithelium, and identify tumors, abnormalities, and deficiencies in enzymes and cellular receptor sites. Within these biological chambers, they will be able to interact with an individual cell in real time and in that cell's native environment.

Despite their small size, nanoscale devices can also hold tens of thousands of small molecules, such as a magnetic resonance imaging contrast agent or a multicomponent diagnostic system capable of assaying a cell's metabolic state. A good example of this approach will capitalize on existing "lab-on-a-chip" and microarray technologies developed at the micron scale. Widely used in biomedical research and to a lesser extent for clinical diagnostic applications today, these technologies will find new uses when shrunk to nanoscale. (In some instances, nanotechnology has already taken advantage of previous clinically relevant technological developments on larger scales.)

Currently, innovative testing is available for many different viruses, mutation analysis, and hematologic and solid tumors. With continuing advances and developments in nanotechnology, it is impossible to speculate as to what this new area of testing holds for the future of the clinical laboratory.

## SUMMARY

This chapter presents a brief overview of the more common and some emerging laboratory methodologies, including their potential advantages and pitfalls. Some historical methods have been discussed to provide a basis and description of the simple principles on which the more complex methods are based. A summary of some of the most common assay methods performed for routine laboratory tests is provided in Table 2-2.

Because of its simplicity and improved sensitivity, ISE has replaced flame photometry as the principal method for measuring serum and urine electrolytes in clinical specimens. Some methods, including turbidimetry, nephelometry, and spectrophotometry, are used in conjunction with other tests such as immunoassays. With these methods, concentrations of substances such as immune complexes are able to be determined.

Mass spectrometry is the gold standard for the identification of unknown substances, including drugs of abuse. Many of the newest designer drugs and bath salts are only identifiable based on this technique, as no other methodologies exist to detect them in clinical specimens. The two principal forms of chromatography are liquid and gas. Both types are similar in that they depend on differences in either solubilities or boiling points, respectively, to separate different analytes in a sample. Another group of important tests are the immunoassays: EIA, EMIT, ELISA, and FPIA. These methods depend on an immunologically mediated reaction that increases sensitivity and specificity over RIA. These assays are commonly used to determine routine clinical chemistries and drug concentrations. PCR and other nucleic acid amplification techniques are used to amplify specific DNA and RNA sequences, primarily in the areas of microbiology and detection of genetic diseases. Finally, with the potential advances envisioned in the area of nanotechnology, the laboratory will be able to provide clinicians with information and access to the patient's cellular and molecular environments, thus providing the ability to target therapies at the exact site of the pathologic process.

The rapid technological advancement of laboratory instrumentation has led to the implementation of new and enhanced clinical laboratory methodologies, including MS, cytometry, laboratory automation, and POC testing. Although laboratory medicine endeavors to keep pace with the burgeoning developments in biomedical sciences, especially with an increase in the sophistication of the tests, it is essential that today's clinicians have a basic understanding of the more common and esoteric tests to select the most appropriate one in each case. All of these developments will translate directly into improved patient care.

## REFERENCES

1. Smith T. Quality automated. In: *Advance for Administrators of the Laboratory.* King of Prussia, PA: Merion Publications Inc; 2007:44-48.

2. US Department of Health and Human Services, Office of the Inspector General. Comparing lab test payment rates: Medicare could achieve substantial savings. http://oig.hhs.gov/oei/reports/oei-07-11-00010.pdf (accessed 2015 October 1).

3. Felder RA. Automation: survival tools for the hospital laboratory. Paper presented at The Second International Bayer Diagnostics Laboratory Testing Symposium. New York; 1998 Jul 17.

4. Felder RA, Graves S, Mifflin T. Reading the future: increasing the relevance of laboratory medicine in the next century. *MLO Med Labs Obs.* 1999; 31:20-21, 24-26.

5. Clinical and Laboratory Standards Institute. Standards documents for automation and informatics. http://shop.clsi.org/automation-documents/ (accessed 2015 Oct 20).

6. Imants RL. Microfabricated biosensors and microanalytical systems for blood analysis. *Acc Chem Res.* 1998;31:317-324.

7. Nguyen A. Principles of instrumentation. McPherson RA, and Pinkus MR, eds. *Henry's Clinical Diagnosis and Management by Laboratory Method.* 21st ed. Philadelphia: WB Saunders; 2006:60-79.

8. Wehry EA. Molecular fluorescence and phosphorescence spectrometry. Settle FA, ed. *Handbook of Instrumental Techniques for Analytical Chemistry.* Upper Saddle River, NJ: Prentice-Hall; 1997:507-539.

9. Tiffany TO. Fluorometry, nephelometry, and turbidimetry. Burtis CA, and Ashwood ER, eds. *Tietz Fundamentals of Clinical Chemistry.* 5th ed. Philadelphia: WB Saunders; 2001:74-90.

10. Evenson MA. Photometry. Burtis CA, and Ashwood ER, eds. *Tietz Fundamentals of Clinical Chemistry.* 5th ed. Philadelphia: WB Saunders; 2001:56-73.

11. Moore RE. Immunochemical methods. McClatchey KD, ed. *Clinical Laboratory Medicine.* Baltimore: Williams & Wilkins; 1994:213-238.

12. George JW, O'Neill SL. Comparison of refractometer and biuret methods for total protein measurement in body cavity fluids. *Vet Clin Pathol.* 2001;30(1):16-18.PubMed

13. Freier ES. Osmometry. Burtis CA, and Ashwood ER, eds. *Clinical Chemistry.* 2nd ed. Philadelphia: WB Saunders; 1994:184-190.

14. Durst RA. Siggaard-Andersen. Electrochemistry. Burtis CA, and Ashwood ER, eds. *Tietz Fundamentals of Clinical Chemistry.* 5th ed. Philadelphia: WB Saunders; 2001:104-120.

15. Burnett W, Lee-Lewandrowski E, Lewandrowski K. Electrolytes and acid-base balance. McClatchey KD, ed. *Clinical laboratory medicine.* Baltimore: Williams & Wilkins; 1994:331-354.

16. Ladenson JH, Apple FS, Koch DD. Misleading hyponatremia due to hyperlipemia: a method-dependent error. *Ann Intern Med.* 1981;95(6):707-708.PubMed

17. Southern EM. Detection of specific sequences among DNA fragments separated by gel electrophoresis. *J Mol Biol.* 1975;98(3):503-517.PubMed

18. Hoefer Scientific Instruments. *Protein Electrophoresis Applications Guide—Hoefer.* San Francisco: Hoefer Scientific Instruments; 1994.

19. Christenson RH, Azzazy HME. Amino acids and proteins. Burtis CA, and Ashwood ER, eds. *Tietz Fundamentals of Clinical Chemistry.* 5th ed. Philadelphia: WB Saunders; 2001:300-351.

20. Chang R. *Physical Chemistry With Applications to Biological Systems.* New York: MacMillan; 1977.

21. Fairbanks VF, Klee GG. Biochemical aspects of hematology. Burtis CA, and Ashwood ER, eds. *Clinical Chemistry.* 2nd ed. Philadelphia: WB Saunders; 1994:1974-2072.

22. Görg A, Postel W, Günther S. The current state of two-dimensional electrophoresis with immobilized pH gradients. *Electrophoresis.* 1988;9(9):531-546.PubMed

23. Karcher RE, Nuttall KL. Electrophoresis. Burtis CA, and Ashwood ER, eds. *Tietz Fundamentals of Clinical Chemistry.* 5th ed. Philadelphia, PA: WB Saunders; 2001:121-132.

24. Tenover FC, Arbeit RD, Goering RV, et al. Interpreting chromosomal DNA restriction patterns produced by pulsed-field gel electrophoresis: criteria for bacterial strain typing. *J Clin Microbiol.* 1995;33(9):2233-2239. PubMed

25. Slagle KM. Immunoassays: tools for sensitive, specific, and accurate test results. *Lab Med.* 1996;27:177.

26. Köhler G, Milstein C. Continuous cultures of fused cells secreting antibody of predefined specificity. *Nature.* 1975;256(5517):495-497. PubMed

27. Berson SA, Yalow RS, Bauman A, et al. Insulin-I131 metabolism in human subjects: demonstration of insulin binding globulin in the circulation of insulin treated subjects. *J Clin Invest.* 1956;35(2):170-190. PubMed

28. Ashihara Y, Kasahara Y, Nakamura RM. Immunoassays and Immunochemistry. In: McPherson RA, Pinkus MR, eds. *Henry's Clinical Diagnosis and Management by Laboratory Methods.* 21st ed. Philadelphia, PA: WB Saunders; 2001.

29. Kitson FG, Larsen BS, McEwen CN. *Gas Chromatography and Mass Spectrometry: A Practical Guide*. San Diego: Academic Press; 1996.

30. Siuzdak G. *Mass Spectrometry for Biotechnology*. San Diego: Academic Press; 1996.

31. Bowers LD, Ullman MD, Burtis CA. Chromatography. Burtis CA, and Ashwood ER, eds. *Tietz Fundamentals of Clinical Chemistry*. 5th ed. Philadelphia: WB Saunders; 2001:133-156.

32. Van Bramer SE. An introduction to mass spectrometry (1997). http://science.widener.edu/svb/massspec/massspec.pdf (accessed 2015 Oct 18).

33. Busch KL, Glish GL, McLuckey SA. *Mass Spectrometry/Mass Spectrometry: Techniques and Applications of Tandem Mass Spectrometry*. New York: VCH Publishers Inc; 1988.

34. van Veen SQ, Claas EC, Kuijper EJ. High-throughput identification of bacteria and yeast by matrix-assisted laser desorption ionization-time of flight mass spectrometry in conventional medical microbiology laboratories. *J Clin Microbiol*. 2010;48(3):900-907.PubMed

35. Melnick SJ. Acute lymphoblastic leukemia. *Clin Lab Med*. 1999;19(1):169-186.PubMed

36. Alamo AL, Melnick SJ. Clinical application of four and five-color flow cytometry lymphocyte subset immunophenotyping. *Cytometry*. 2000;42(6):363-370.PubMed

37. Raap AK. Overview of fluorescent in situ hybridization techniques for molecular cytogenetics. *Current Protocols in Cytometry*. 1997; 8.1.1-8.1.6.

38. Wilkinson DG. The theory and practice of in situ hybridization. Wilkinson DG, ed. *In Situ Hybridization—A Practical Approach*. Oxford: Oxford University Press; 1992:1-13.

39. Erlich HA, Gelfand D, Sninsky JJ. Recent advances in the polymerase chain reaction. *Science*. 1991;252(5013):1643-1651.PubMed

40. Remick DG. Clinical applications of molecular biology. McClatchey KD, ed. *Clinical Laboratory Medicine*. Baltimore: Williams & Wilkins; 1994:165-174.

41. Ratjen F, Döring G. Cystic fibrosis. *Lancet*. 2003;361(9358):681-689. PubMed

42. Bloom MV, Freyer GA, Micklos DA. *Laboratory DNA Science: An Introduction to Recombinant DNA Techniques and Methods of Genome Analysis*. Menlo Park, CA: Addison-Wesley; 1996.

43. Russo VEA, Martienssen RA, Riggs AD. *1996 Epigenetic Mechanisms Of Gene Regulation*. Plainview, NY: Cold Spring Harbor Laboratory Press; 1996.

44. Anderson NL, Anderson NG. Proteome and proteomics: new technologies, new concepts, and new words. *Electrophoresis*. 1998;19(11):1853-1861.PubMed

45. Blackstock WP, Weir MP. Proteomics: quantitative and physical mapping of cellular proteins. *Trends Biotechnol*. 1999;17(3):121-127.PubMed

46. Wilkins MR, Pasquali C, Appel RD, et al. From proteins to proteomes: large scale protein identification by two-dimensional electrophoresis and amino acid analysis. *Biotechnology (N Y)*. 1996;14(1):61-65.PubMed

47. Shinawi M, Cheung SW. The array CGH and its clinical applications. *Drug Discov Today*. 2008;13(17-18):760-770.PubMed

48. Peppercorn J, Perou CM, Carey LA. Molecular subtypes in breast cancer evaluation and management: divide and conquer. *Cancer Invest*. 2008;26(1):1-10.PubMed

49. Rosenwald A, Wright G, Chan WC, et al. The use of molecular profiling to predict survival after chemotherapy for diffuse large-B-cell lymphoma. *N Engl J Med*. 2002;346(25):1937-1947.PubMed

50. Eeles RA, Kote-Jarai Z, Giles GG, et al. Multiple newly identified loci associated with prostate cancer susceptibility. *Nat Genet*. 2008;40(3):316-321.PubMed

# 3

# Primer on Drug Interferences with Test Results

*Mary Lee*

Through a variety of mechanisms, drugs can interfere with laboratory test results. If the clinician who has ordered the laboratory test is not aware that the drug has altered the results of the test, inappropriate management of the patient may follow, including unnecessary hospitalization, extra office visits, or additional laboratory or clinical testing—all of which may increase the cost of healthcare. This chapter addresses this situation and provides resources that health professionals can use to better interpret laboratory tests when a drug is suspected to interfere with test results.

## IN VIVO AND IN VITRO DRUG INTERFERENCES WITH LABORATORY TESTS

When a drug interferes with a laboratory test result, it alters the laboratory value. Mechanisms for drug interference of clinical laboratory tests can be classified as either in vivo or in vitro.[1] *In vivo drug interferences* can also be called physiologic and can be subclassified as pharmacological or toxicological. In vivo drug interferences account for most effects of drugs on laboratory tests.[2] In contrast, the term *in vitro drug interferences* is used synonymously with analytical or methodological interferences.

### In Vivo Interference

An in vivo interference is an actual change in the analyte concentration or activity prior to specimen collection and analysis. The assay measurement is actual and accurate and reflects a change in the measured substance that has occurred in the patient. Therefore, an in vivo interference will always change a laboratory test result, independent of the assay methodology. A drug can produce an in vivo interference in several ways. By a direct extension of its pharmacological effects, a drug can produce changes in some laboratory test results. For example, thiazide and loop diuretics will commonly cause increased renal elimination of potassium. Therefore, decreased serum potassium levels can occur in treated patients. In these patients, hypokalemia is actual and accurate. Similarly, β adrenergic antagonists decrease renin and aldosterone secretion, which can lead to increased serum potassium levels.[2]

Other drugs produce changes in laboratory test results by producing in vivo toxicological effects. As the drug damages a particular organ system, abnormal laboratory tests may be one of the first signs of the problem. For example, as isoniazid and rifampin produce hepatotoxicity, elevated hepatic transaminases will signal the onset of liver inflammation. Similarly, as a prolonged course of high-dose aminoglycoside antibiotic causes acute proximal tubular necrosis, serum creatinine and serum trough aminoglycoside levels will increase steadily if the antibiotic is not stopped or if the antibiotic dose is not reduced. In the face of cyclophosphamide-induced bone marrow suppression, neutropenia will become evident 10 to 14 days after a dose has been administered.

### In Vitro Interference

Drugs in a patient's body fluid or tissue can directly interfere with a clinical laboratory test during the in vitro analytical process. This type of drug–laboratory test interaction is highly dependent on the laboratory test methodology, as the reaction may occur with one specific assay method but not another. In vitro drug-laboratory test interactions are

DOI 10.37573/9781585286423.003

common with radioimmunoassays for which cross reactions can occur because of drug metabolites or drugs that are chemically similar to the parent drug, or because of heterophilic antibodies that are similar to endogenous antibodies. False high or false low laboratory test results occur.[2-5] For example, serum digoxin levels are commonly determined using a radioimmunoassay, a fluorescent polarization immunoassay, or a TDx assay. However, these assays are based on the three-dimensional structure of the digoxin molecule, and many other drugs with a similar chemical structure to digoxin (eg, spironolactone, estrogen replacement products, cortisol, digoxin metabolites) can cross-react with the assay.[6] A falsely increased or decreased serum digoxin level can result. To determine the true serum digoxin level in this situation, another assay technique (eg, high-pressure liquid chromatography [HPLC]) may be used. In addition, substances that are prepackaged in or added to the in vitro system before or after sample collection can cause laboratory test interference in vitro. As an example, test tubes sometimes contain lithium heparin or sodium fluoride. Heparin can interfere with aminoglycoside assays, and fluoride can cause false increases in blood urea nitrogen (BUN) when measured by the Ekatchem assay.

Alternatively, a drug may cause discoloration of the body fluid specimen, which may interfere with colorimetric, photometric, or fluorometric laboratory-based assay methods. For example, phenazopyridine causes an orange-red discoloration of urine that may be mistaken for blood. Nitrofurantoin may cause a brown discoloration of the urine that may alarm the patient. These types of drug interference with laboratory testing can be detected visually and appropriate attribution of the abnormality should be made by knowledgeable clinicians and clinical laboratory staff.

Other common mechanisms by which drugs cause in vitro interferences with laboratory tests include the following:

- A drug alters the specimen pH (usually urine) so that reagent reactions are inhibited or enhanced. For example, acetazolamide produces an alkaline urinary pH that causes false-positive proteinuria with reagent dip strips.

- A drug chelates with an enzyme activator or reagent used in the in vitro laboratory analysis. For example, large doses of biotin, as are included in some over-the-counter nutritional supplements, can compete for the biotin-streptavidin complex which is a component of many radioimmunoassays.[3,7-9] Also, daptomycin interacts with rabbit or human thromboplastin, which is associated with a dose-dependent prolongation of prothrombin time and international normalized ratio.[10,11]

- A drug absorbs at the same wavelength as the analyte. For example, methotrexate interferes with analytic methods using high performance liquid chromatography and an absorbance range of 340 to 410 nm.

- A drug reacts with reagent to form a chromophore (eg, cefoxitin or cephalothin) with the Jaffe-based creatinine assay.

In addition to the parent drug, other drug-related components may cause significant interferences with laboratory tests. Metabolites can cross-react with the parent drug in an assay, such as in the case with cyclosporine. Its metabolites cross-react with the parent drug in HPLC assays and can produce a falsely high measurement of the concentration of cyclosporine.[12] Contaminants in herbal products, which are subject to less regulation than medications in the United States, may interfere with some laboratory tests.[7] Inactive ingredients of some drug products, which includes excipients such as lactose or starch, preservatives, colorants, or flavoring agents, may influence assay results. Although most manufacturers do report the inactive ingredients in their products, little systematic research has been performed to assess the impact of these substances on laboratory tests. Compounding these factors, many laboratory test interferences are concentration related, and many drug metabolites and their usual plasma concentrations have yet to be identified. Therefore, systematic study of all of these potential causes of interactions is difficult to conduct and is not available in many cases.[13]

## Simultaneous In Vivo and In Vitro Effects

Some drugs can affect an analyte both in vivo and in vitro. In these situations, interpretation is extremely difficult because the degree of impact in each setting cannot be determined easily. For example, when a drug produces hemolysis in a patient with glucose-6-phosphate dehydrogenase deficiency who is exposed inadvertently to ciprofloxacin, hemolytic anemia may result. Hemolyzed red blood cells produce a red discoloration of the plasma or serum. The hemoglobin released from the damaged red blood cells can interfere with analysis of alkaline phosphatase or γ-glutamyl transferase, both of which can be assayed using a spectrophotometric analysis that depends on color changes after a chemical reaction.[13,14] Simultaneous in vivo and in vitro drug interferences with laboratory tests can also occur commonly when drugs increase bilirubin or when a drug causes lipemia.[15]

# IDENTIFYING DRUG INTERFERENCES

## Incidence of Drug Interferences

The true incidence of drug interferences with laboratory tests is unknown. This is because many situations probably go undetected. However, as the number of laboratory tests and drugs on the U.S. commercial market increase, it is likely that the number of cases of in vivo interferences will also increase. As a reflection of this, consider the number of drug–laboratory test interferences reported by D. S. Young, author of one of the classic literature references on this topic. In the first edition of *Effects of Drugs on Clinical Laboratory Tests,* published in the journal *Clinical Chemistry* in 1972, 9,000 such interactions were included.[16] In the second edition of the same publication, which was published in 1975, 16,000 such interactions were reported.[17] In 1997, this resource, which had been converted to an online searchable database, included more than 135,000 interactions.[18] In 2014, this resource included 171,000 interactions.[19]

As for in vitro interferences, the number of drug–laboratory test interferences may be moderated over time because of newer, more specific laboratory test methodologies that minimize cross-reactions with drug metabolites or drug effects on reagents or laboratory reactions.[14,18] In addition, manufacturers of commonly used laboratory equipment systematically study the effects of drugs on assay methods.[17] Therefore, this information is often available to clinicians who confront problematic laboratory test results in patients. This increased awareness reduces the number of patients who are believed to have experienced newly reported drug–laboratory test interferences.

## Suspecting a Drug Interference

A clinician should suspect a drug–laboratory test interference when an inconsistency appears among related test results or between test results and the clinical picture. Specifically, clinicians should become suspicious when the following occurs:

- Test results do not correlate with the patient's signs, symptoms, or medical history.
- Results of different tests—assessing the same organ anatomy or organ function, or the drug's pharmacologic effects—conflict with each other.
- Results from a series of the same test vary greatly over a short period of time and for no apparent reason.
- Serial test results are inconsistent.

### No Correlation with Patient's Signs, Symptoms, or Medical History

As emphasized elsewhere in this book, when an isolated test result does not correlate with signs, symptoms, or medical history of the patient, the signs and symptoms should be considered more strongly than the test result. This rule is particularly true when the test result is used to confirm suspicions raised by the signs and symptoms in the first place or when the test result is used as a surrogate marker or indirect indicator of underlying pathology.

For example, serum creatinine is used in various formulae to approximate the glomerular filtration rate, which is used to assess the kidney's ability to make urine. However, actual urine output and measurement of urinary creatinine excretion is a more accurate method of assessing overall renal function. If a patient's serum creatinine has increased from a baseline of 1 mg/dL to 5 mg/dL over a three-day period, but the patient has had no change in urine output, urinary creatinine excretion, or serum electrolyte levels, then the serum creatinine level may be elevated because of a drug interference with the laboratory test. Similarly, if a patient has a total serum bilirubin of 6 mg/dL, but the patient is not jaundiced or does not have scleral icterus, then a drug interference with the laboratory test should be considered.

### Conflicting Test Results

Occasionally, pharmacological or toxicological effects of a drug produce conflicting results of two tests that assess the same organ function. For example, a presurgical test screen shows a serum creatinine of 4.2 mg/dL in an otherwise healthy 20-year-old patient with a BUN of 8 mg/dL. Usually, if a patient had true renal impairment, BUN and serum creatinine would be elevated in tandem. Thus, in this patient, a drug interference with the laboratory test is suspected. Further investigation revealed that the patient received cefoxitin shortly before blood was drawn for the laboratory test. Cefoxitin can falsely elevate serum creatinine concentrations. Thus, the elevated serum creatinine is likely due to drug interference with the laboratory test and not to renal failure. To confirm that this is the case, cefoxitin should be discontinued and the serum creatinine repeated after that. If it is due to the drug, the elevated serum creatinine should return to the normal range.[20]

### Varying Serial Test Results Over a Short Time Period

Typically, the results of a specific laboratory test should follow a trend in a patient. However, in the absence of a new onset of medical illness or worsening of existing disease, a sudden change in the laboratory test result trend should cause examination of a possible drug interference with a laboratory test. For example, prostate specific antigen (PSA) is a tumor marker for prostate cancer. It is produced by glandular epithelial cells of the prostate. The normal serum level is <4 ng/mL in a patient without prostate cancer, and the level is typically elevated in patients with prostate cancer. However, it is not specific for prostate cancer. Elevated PSA serum levels are also observed in patients with benign prostatic hyperplasia, prostatitis, or following instrumentation of the prostate. A 70-year-old male patient with metastatic prostate cancer has a PSA of 30 ng/mL and has decided not to undergo treatment. Four serial PSA tests over the course of one year and done at three-month intervals show no change. Despite the absence of any changes on pelvic computerized axial tomography, bone scan, or chest radiograph, his PSA is 10 ng/mL at his most recent office visit. After a careful interview of the patient, the urologist discovers that the patient has been treated for androgenetic alopecia for the past six months with finasteride. The patient received the prescription from another physician for lower urinary tract voiding symptoms, and finasteride lowered the PSA level.[21]

### Serial Test Results That Are Inconsistent with Expected Results

Generally, repeated laboratory test results should show little change over time assuming that the status of the medical condition or treatment for the medical condition in an individual patient stays the same. However, when serial test results are inconsistent with expected results, a drug–laboratory test interference should be suspected. For example, leuprolide, a luteinizing hormone-releasing hormone (LHRH) agonist, is useful in the management of prostate cancer, which is an androgen dependent tumor. Persistent use of leuprolide causes down-regulation of pituitary LHRH receptors, decreased secretion of luteinizing hormone, and decreased production of testicular androgens. A patient with prostate cancer treated with leuprolide should experience a sustained reduction in serum testosterone levels from normal (280 to 1,100 ng/dL) to castration levels (<50 ng/dL) after 2 to 3 weeks. The serum testosterone level should remain below 50 ng/dL as long as the patient continues treatment with leuprolide, and as long as he makes returns to the clinic for repeated doses on schedule. However, one of the adverse effects of leuprolide is decreased libido and erectile dysfunction, which

## MINICASE 1

### How can a vitamin cause any problems?

Annie J., a 30-year-old female patient, developed multiple sclerosis and began taking a biotin nutritional supplement in a dose of 300 mg by mouth daily. The patient has heard that biotin can slow disease progression. Two months later, during an annual physical examination, a full set of clinical laboratory tests was obtained that showed significantly elevated serum free thyroxine ($FT_4$), elevated free triiodothyronine ($FT_3$), and low thyroid stimulating hormone (TSH). Upon reviewing these laboratory test results, the physician scheduled the patient for a follow-up clinic visit. A physical examination showed a normal size thyroid gland with no nodules on palpation, a normal heart rate, no tachycardia, and normal blood pressure. The patient did not have exophthalmos. In review of systems, the patient had no reports of weight loss, palpitations, hyperactivity, nervousness, or mood swings. A medication history showed that the only new medication started prior to the blood drawing was biotin. Because the efficacy of biotin for multiple sclerosis has not been proven, the physician asked the patient to discontinue biotin and to have thyroid function tests repeated in 1 week.

QUESTION: Assume that biotin caused a drug-laboratory test interference. Was the interference an in vitro or an in vivo interference? What is the mechanism by which biotin most likely caused the interference?

DISCUSSION: Biotin causes an in vitro drug-laboratory test interaction with thyroid function tests. $FT_4$, $FT_3$, and TSH testing are commonly performed by radioimmunoassay, which employs a streptavidin-biotin complex. Exogenous biotin in the patient's blood sample, which resulted from oral administration of biotin, interfered with the streptavidin-biotin complex's binding with thyroid hormones and led to false assay measurements.[3,7-9]

Although the patient's $FT_4$ and $FT_3$ suggest that patient has hyperthyroidism, the patient has no symptoms consistent with the disease. Moreover, the onset of the abnormal laboratory tests appears to be temporally related to the start of biotin, and normalization of thyroid function tests should occur after biotin is discontinued. These all suggest that the patient has a biotin-induced laboratory test interference.

---

is a direct extension of the drug's testosterone-lowering effect. Such a patient may seek medical treatment of sexual dysfunction, and he may be inappropriately prescribed depot testosterone injections. Thus, in this case, depot testosterone injections will cause a change in serum testosterone levels in the wrong direction. If serum testosterone levels increase, this should be a signal that the patient has serial test results, which are inconsistent with expected results of leuprolide, and an investigation should be done as to the cause (**Minicase 1**).[22]

## MANAGING DRUG INTERFERENCES

When a drug is suspected to interfere with a laboratory test, the clinician should collect appropriate evidence to confirm the interaction by taking the following steps:

1. Establishing a temporal relationship between the change in the laboratory test and drug use and ensuring that the change in the laboratory test occurred after the drug was started or after the drug dose was changed

2. Ruling out other drugs as causes of the laboratory test change

3. Ruling out concurrent diseases as causes of the laboratory test change

4. If possible, discontinuing the causative agent and repeating the test to see if dechallenge results in a correction of the abnormal laboratory test

5. Choosing another laboratory test that will provide assessment of the same organ's function, but is unlikely to be affected by the drug (the clinician can compare the new results against the original laboratory test result, and check for dissimilarity or similarity of results)

6. Finding evidence in the medical literature that documents the suspected drug–laboratory test interference

7. Contacting the head of diagnostic labs who maintains or has access to computerized lists of drugs that interfere with laboratory tests (the person would also provide assistance in interpreting aberrant laboratory test results)[13]

For any particular patient case, it is often not possible to obtain information on all seven of the previously listed items. The first four items are crucial in any suspected drug–laboratory test interference. With the availability of highly accessible, electronic databases—which can scour the literature quickly for drug–laboratory test interactions—and more electronic cross-talk between databases for clinical laboratory tests and those for medications, clinicians can easily find published information about drug interferences with laboratory tests; consult with a clinical laboratory specialist, if necessary, and then take the appropriate steps in managing the patient (**Minicase 2**).[23,24]

## LITERATURE RESOURCES

A systematic search of the medical literature is essential for providing the appropriate evidence to confirm the drug–laboratory test interaction. This search will ensure that a complete and comprehensive review—necessary in making an accurate assessment—has been done. When searching the literature, it is recommended to use the method originally described by Watanabe et al and, subsequently, modified by C. F. Kirkwood.[25,26] Using this technique, the clinician would search tertiary, secondary, and then primary literature. Although there

## MINICASE 2

### Trimethoprim–Sulfamethoxazole-Induced Hypoprothrombinemia

Sally S., a 65-year-old female patient, is started on trimethoprim-sulfamethoxazole 800/160 mg by mouth twice daily for an upper urinary tract infection due to *Escherichia coli*. Antibiotic treatment will continue for 14 days. She has atrial fibrillation and is also taking digoxin 0.125 mg by mouth daily and warfarin 2.5 mg by mouth daily. She has been on warfarin for years and says that she is fully aware of all the DOs and DON'Ts of taking warfarin. Her International Normalized Ratio (INR) regularly and consistently is 2.5, which is therapeutic. She has no history of liver disease and appears healthy and well nourished. Prior to the start of the trimethoprim-sulfamethoxazole, her serum sodium was 137 mEq/L, potassium 4 mEq/L, BUN 10 mg/dL, creatinine 1 mg/dL, and INR 2.5. After 3 days of trimethoprim-sulfamethoxazole, a repeat INR is 5.2, and she reports persistent nose bleeding, which stops for a few hours but then restarts again.

QUESTION: What do you think is causing the laboratory abnormality? How should this patient's condition be managed?

DISCUSSION: Trimethoprim–sulfamethoxazole inhibits cytochrome 2C9, the principal hepatic enzyme that catabolizes warfarin, decreases vitamin K–producing bacteria in the gastrointestinal tract, and displaces warfarin from its plasma protein-binding sites. A search of the medical literature documents multiple cases of enhanced warfarin effect when trimethoprim–sulfamethoxazole is taken concurrently.[29,30]

In this patient, the drug interaction occurred after trimethoprim-sulfamethoxazole was started. She is not taking any other medications that could cause the drug–laboratory test interaction and has no history of vitamin K deficiency or liver disease, which could be causing hypoprothrombinemia. To confirm that trimethoprim–sulfamethoxazole is causing the drug interaction, the physician could discontinue the drug and then see if her INR returns to the range of 2 to 3. However, because the trimethoprim-sulfamethoxazole–warfarin interaction is well known, a better approach might be to continue antibiotic treatment, hold warfarin until the INR has decreased to 2.5, and then resume warfarin at a reduced daily dose while the patient is taking antibiotic.

---

are slight variations in the types of publications included in each category, a brief description of each literature category follows.

*Tertiary literature* includes reference texts, monograph databases, and review articles which provide appropriate foundational content and background material essential for understanding basic concepts and historical data relevant to the topic. *Secondary literature* is a gateway to primary literature, and it includes indexing and abstracting services (eg, PubMed). *Primary literature* includes case reports, experimental studies, and other non-review types of articles in journals about the topic. These represent the most current literature on the topic. By systematically scanning the literature in this order, the clinician can be sure to have identified and analyzed all relevant literature, which is crucial in developing appropriate conclusions for these types of situations.

### Tertiary Literature

Tertiary literature, which contains useful information about drug–laboratory test interferences, includes the *Physicians' Desk Reference*. Each complete package insert included in this book contains a precautions section that includes information on drug–laboratory test interferences. However, it is important to note that the *Physicians' Desk Reference* does not include package inserts on all commercially available drugs, nor does it include complete package inserts for all of the products included in the text. Also, manufacturers often do not update package insets with findings from current literature.[27] Thus, additional resources will need to be checked (eg, DailyMed by the National Institutes of Health [http://dailymed.nlm.nih.gov/dailymed/]). DailyMed includes more than 95,000 package inserts. Also, the drug monographs in the *AHFS Drug Information*, published by the American Society of Health-System Pharmacists, include a section on laboratory test interferences. Although the information provided is brief, it can be used as an initial screen. This resource is available electronically by subscription from the American Society of Health-System Pharmacists (www.ahfsdruginformation .com) or from other online databases including First Databank (www.fdbhealth.com) or Lexicomp (www.wolterskluwer.com /en/solutions/lexicomp).

A variety of other books about clinical laboratory tests are provided (**List 1**). Some are comprehensive references while others are handbooks. All of them provide information about drug–laboratory test interferences. However, the reference texts are more complete than the handbooks. In addition, several comprehensive review articles include current information about drug–laboratory test interferences.

Micromedex Solutions, DynaMed Plus, Drugs.com, Facts and Comparisons, and Lexicomp, are all online searchable databases (**List 2**). For every drug included in the system, information is available in a drug monograph format, and any information about drug–laboratory test interferences is included in the monograph. Although not always listed separately as a laboratory test interference, the information may be included in the adverse reaction, warning, or monitoring section of the monograph. In addition, for some drugs, drug information questions and answers are included. To access relevant information, the clinician can search information using the name of the drug or the laboratory test. Often, the drug–laboratory test interference is assigned a severity rating (eg, major or minor interference) as an indication of its clinical significance, and references to primary literature are available so that the reader can learn more. These online databases vary in content completeness and ease of use.[28]

## LIST 1. Tertiary Resources

### Books and Handbooks

Rifai N, Horvath AR, Wittwer CT. *Tietz Fundamentals of Clinical Chemistry and Molecular Diagnostics.* 8th ed. St. Louis, MO: Elsevier; 2019.

DasGupta A, Hammett-Stabler CA, eds. *Herbal Supplements: Efficacy, Toxicity, Interactions with Western Drugs and Effects on Lab Tests.* Hoboken, NJ: Wiley; 2011.

Laposata M, ed. *Laboratory Medicine: The Diagnosis of Disease in the Clinical Laboratory.* New York, NY: McGraw Hill Medical; 2018.

McPherson RA, Pincus MR, eds. *Henry's Clinical Diagnosis and Management by Laboratory Methods.* 23rd ed. Philadelphia, PA: Elsevier WB Saunders; 2017.

Rao LV, Snyder LM. *Wallach's Interpretation of Diagnostic Tests: Pathways to Arriving at a Clinical Diagnosis.* 11th ed. Philadelphia, PA: Wolters Kluwer; 2021.

Young DS. *Effects of Preanalytic Variables on Clinical Laboratory Tests.* 3rd ed. Washington, DC: American Association for Clinical Chemistry; 2007.

Young DS. *Effects of Drugs on Clinical Laboratory Tests.* 5th ed. Washington, DC: American Association for Clinical Chemistry; 2000.

### Review Articles

- DasGupta A, Bernard DW. Herbal remedies: effects on clinical laboratory tests. *Arch Pathol Lab Med.* 2006; 130(4):521-528.

  This review summarizes literature from 1980 to 2005 on herbal drug interactions with laboratory tests. Mechanisms include (1) herbal agent-induced in vivo toxic effects, (2) direct assay interference by the herbal agent, or (3) contaminant in the herbal agent produces in vivo or in vitro effects that produce changes in laboratory test results. The effect of Chan su on digoxin blood levels and St. John's wort on blood levels of cyclosporine, digoxin, theophylline, and protease inhibitors are just some of the herbal agent–laboratory test interactions discussed. This is a follow-up to the author's first article on the topic, which was published in the *American Journal of Clinical Pathology* in 2003. As of 2021, this review has not been updated.

- Kroll MH, Elin RJ. Interference with clinical laboratory analyses. *Clin Chem* 1994; 40(11 Pt 1):1996-2005.

  This is an excellent overview of drug–laboratory test interactions. The article describes how drugs, metabolites, and additives (eg, heparin and ethylenediamine tetra-acetic acid) can produce significant interactions and discrepancies during in vitro analytic procedures. It also provides a summary of useful references (although outdated) on the topic. In addition, a suggested approach to drug–laboratory test interactions is described.

- Lopez A, Fraissinet F, Lefebvre H, et al. Pharmacological and analytical interference in hormone assays for diagnosis of adrenal incidentaloma. *Ann Endocrinol* 2019; 80(4):250-258.

  This is an excellent overview of patient-related factors, medications, and analytical factors that can interfere with laboratory tests for metanephrines, aldosterone, renin, cortisol, or corticosteroid binding globulin.

- Montanelli L, Benvenga S, Hegedus L, et al. Drugs and other substances interfering with thyroid function. In: Vitti P, Hegedus L, eds. *Thyroid Diseases.* Chaim, Switzerland: Springer International Publishing; 2018:733-761. 10.1007/978-3-319-45013-1_27.

  This review discusses drugs that interfere with regulation of the hypothalamic-pituitary-thyroid axis and drugs that interfere with thyroid function. For each medication class included, the mechanism of the drug-laboratory test interaction is provided and, when available, the frequency of the interaction in treated patients, whether the interaction appears to be dose related, and the timeline for the interaction.

- Sher PP. Drug interferences with clinical laboratory tests. *Drugs* 1982; 24(1):24-63.

  This useful reference provides many tables of drugs known to interfere with various laboratory tests. The data are arranged by laboratory test. For many common laboratory tests, summary tables of drugs known to interfere with the particular laboratory tests are provided. Also, mechanisms for the in vivo and in vitro interactions are described. Although this reference is dated and is not useful for newer drugs, it is an excellent resource for older drugs.

- Sonntag O, Scholer A. Drug interference in clinical chemistry: recommendation of drugs and their concentrations to be used in drug interference studies. *Ann Clin Biochem.* 2001;38(Pt 4):376-385.

  In 1995, 18 clinical laboratory test experts identified 24 commonly used drugs known to interfere with laboratory tests. Usual therapeutic and toxic drug concentrations were identified. Both concentrations of each drug were added in vitro to blood and urine specimens and then various laboratory tests were run on the specimens. Laboratory testing was duplicated in three different laboratories. This review article summarizes drug–laboratory test interactions for more than 70 different laboratory tests.

- Yao H, Rayburn ER, Shi Q, et al. FDA-approved drugs that interfere with laboratory tests: a systematic search of U.S. drug labels. *Crit Rev Clin Lab Sci* 2017;54(1):1-17.

  This includes two extensive listings of medications that affect urine and blood-based assays along with the authors' review of the package labeling of more than 65,000 single ingredient medications. It is a useful reference.

## LIST 2. Databases and Websites to Access Databases*

| | |
|---|---|
| American Hospital Formulary Service Drug Information | www.ahfsdruginformation.com |
| DailyMed | https://dailymed/nlm.nih.gov/ |
| DynaMed Plus | www.dynamed.com |
| Facts and Comparisons | www.factsandcomparisons.com |
| Lexicomp | www.wolterskluwer.com/en/solutions/lexicomp |
| Micromedex Solutions | http://www.micromedex.com |
| Prescribers' Digital Reference | http://www.pdr.net |

*A subscription may be required to access the resource.

List 1 includes websites of commonly used databases for drug laboratory test interactions. In addition, some local clinical laboratory websites (eg, http://www.mayocliniclabs.com /test-info) may be convenient to access and use.[25]

### Secondary and Primary Literature

For secondary literature, the main indexing or abstracting service that should be used is PubMed. This allows the clinician to check the literature from thousands of biomedical journals from 1946 to the present. Due to improvements in search capabilities, clinicians can search using text words (ie, words as they might appear in the title or abstract of a journal article). The database will automatically convert that text word to official medical subject headings or accepted indexing terms. As a result, search output is optimized despite the lack of proficiency or experience of the searcher. In addition, the database provides links enabling clinicians to locate related articles or order articles online, which enhance search capabilities and convenience in obtaining relevant primary literature articles.

This chapter does not allow a complete tutorial on developing search strategies, conducting PubMed searches, and evaluating primary literature. However, the reader is encouraged to develop expertise in this area so that he or she can identify current, relevant literature efficiently. A wide variety of tutorials and webcasts are available free of charge (https://www.ncbi.nlm.nih .gov/pubmed/).

## SUMMARY

Although the number of drug–laboratory test interferences increases as the number of commercially available drugs increases, improved literature resources that compile information on this topic and improved assay methodologies have helped clinicians in dealing with suspected cases of this problem. Most drug–laboratory test interferences are due to in vivo effects of drugs; that is, the drug's pharmacological or toxic effects produce specific alterations in laboratory values. A drug–laboratory test interference should be suspected whenever a laboratory test result does not match the signs and symptoms in a patient, when the results of different tests that assess the same organ function or drug effect conflict with each other, or when serial laboratory test values vary greatly over a short period of time or are inconsistent with expected results.

To determine if a drug is interfering with a drug–laboratory test, the clinician should, at a minimum, establish a temporal relationship between the change in the laboratory test and drug use; rule out other drugs and diseases as the cause; and discontinue the drug and repeat the laboratory test to see if dechallenge corrects the abnormal laboratory test. The literature should be checked to see if documentation of the drug–laboratory test interference can be found. The literature search should be systematic to ensure retrieval of the most comprehensive and current information. Therefore, the clinician should proceed from the tertiary to the secondary and then to the primary literature and use a variety of resources to arrive at a conclusion.

## LEARNING POINTS

1. *What are the differences between an in vivo and an in vitro drug interference with a laboratory test?*

   ANSWER: An in vivo interaction is characterized by an actual change in measured analyte concentration or activity prior to specimen collection and analysis. That is, the change in the measured analyte occurred in the patient and the laboratory test abnormality is true. An in vitro interaction is characterized by a drug's physical presence in a body fluid or tissue specimen, which interferes with clinical laboratory testing during the analytical process. The interference occurs outside the patient's body and after the specimen is collected from the patient.

2. *What type of laboratory test is prone to in vitro drug interferences? If a drug laboratory test interaction is suspected, what options are available?*

   ANSWER: Radioimmunoassays are prone to in vitro drug interferences when cross reactions occur between the measured analyte and other substances in the specimen, which could include a drug's metabolites, other chemically similar drugs, or heterophilic antibodies. If a drug-laboratory test interference is suspected, the clinician can explore the option of performing the laboratory test using a different assay method (eg, high performance liquid chromatography).

3. **What key information should a clinician collect to confirm that a drug is causing a laboratory test interaction?**

**ANSWER:** The four key criteria in confirming the presence of a drug–laboratory test interaction include the following:

Ensuring that the change in the laboratory test occurred after the drug was started

Ruling out other drugs as causes of the laboratory test change

Ruling out concurrent medical illness(es) as causes of the laboratory test change

Stopping the drug and seeing if the laboratory test result returns to the predrug value

4. **What type of literature resource should a clinician access first to review foundational information on a drug's adverse reaction profile and the likelihood that it could be causing an in vivo laboratory test abnormality?**

**ANSWER:** Tertiary literature, which includes reference texts, review articles, and searchable databases, will provide good background information on medications. This information is helpful in understanding the primary literature on the topic.

## REFERENCES

1. Sher PP. Drug interferences with clinical laboratory tests. *Drugs.* 1982;24(1):24-63.PubMed

2. Funder JW, Carey RM, Mantero F, et al. The management of primary aldosteronism: case detection, diagnosis, and treatment: An Endocrine Society clinical practice guidelines. *J Clin Endocrinol Metab.* 2016;101(5):1889-1916.PubMed

3. Odhaib SA, Mansour AA, Haddad NS. How biotin induces misleading results in thyroid bioassays: case series. *Cureus.* 2019;11(5):e4727. PubMed

4. Tsoi V, Bhayana V, Bombassaro AM, et al. Falsely elevated vancomycin concentrations in a patient not receiving vancomycin. *Pharmacotherapy.* 2019;39(7):778-782.PubMed

5. Yao H, Rayburn ER, Shi Q, et al. FDA-approved drugs that interfere with laboratory tests: a systematic search of US drug labels. *Crit Rev Clin Lab Sci.* 2017;54(1):1-17.PubMed

6. Steimer W, Müller C, Eber B. Digoxin assays: frequent, substantial, and potentially dangerous interference by spironolactone, canrenone, and other steroids. *Clin Chem.* 2002;48(3):507-516.PubMed

7. Gifford JL, de Koning L, Sadrzadeh SMH. Strategies for mitigating risk posed by biotin interference on clinical immunoassays. *Clin Biochem.* 2019;65:61-63.PubMed

8. Avery G. Biotin interference in immunoassay: a review for the laboratory scientist. *Ann Clin Biochem.* 2019;56(4):424-430.PubMed

9. Bowen R, Benavides R, Colón-Franco JM, et al. Best practices in mitigating the risk of biotin interference with laboratory testing. *Clin Biochem.* 2019;74:1-11.PubMed

10. Smith SE, Rumbaugh KA. False prolongation of International Normalized Ratio associated with daptomycin. *Am J Health Syst Pharm.* 2018;75(5):269-274.PubMed

11. Saito M, Hatakeyama S, Hashimoto H, et al. Dose-dependent artificial prolongation of prothrombin time by interaction between daptomycin and test reagents in patients receiving warfarin: a prospective in vivo clinical study. *Ann Clin Microbiol Antimicrob.* 2017;16(1):27.PubMed

12. Steimer W. Performance and specificity of monoclonal immunoassays for cyclosporine monitoring: how specific is specific? *Clin Chem.* 1999;45(3):371-381.PubMed

13. Dimeski G. Interference testing. *Clin Biochem Rev.* 2008;29(suppl 1): S43-S48.PubMed

14. Lippi G, Salvagno GL, Montagnana M, et al. Influence of hemolysis on routine clinical chemistry testing. *Clin Chem Lab Med.* 2006;44(3): 311-316.PubMed

15. Punja M, Neill SG, Wong S. Caution with interpreting laboratory results after lipid rescue therapy. *Am J Emerg Med.* 2013;31(10):1536.e1-1536.e2. PubMed

16. Young DS, Thomas DW, Friedman RB, Pestaner LC. Effects of drugs on clinical laboratory tests. *Clin Chem.* 1972;18(10):1041-1303.PubMed

17. Young DS, Pestaner LC, Gibberman V. Effects of drugs on clinical laboratory tests. *Clin Chem.* 1975;21(5):1D-432D.PubMed

18. Young DS. Effects of drugs on clinical laboratory tests. *Ann Clin Biochem.* 1997;34(Pt 6):579-581.PubMed

19. Young DS. AACC effects on clinical laboratory tests: drugs, disease, herbs and natural products. http://clinfx.wiley.com/aaccweb/aacc/. Accessed August 12, 2020.

20. Grötsch H, Hajdu P. Interference by the new antibiotic cefpirome and other cephalosporins in clinical laboratory tests, with special regard to the "Jaffé" reaction. *J Clin Chem Clin Biochem.* 1987;25(1):49-52.PubMed

21. D'Amico AV, Roehrborn CG. Effect of 1 mg/day finasteride on concentrations of serum prostate-specific antigen in men with androgenic alopecia: a randomised controlled trial. *Lancet Oncol.* 2007;8(1):21-25. PubMed

22. de Jong IJ, Eaton A, Bladou F. LHRH agonists in prostate cancer: frequency of treatment, serum testosterone measurement and castrate level: consensus opinion from a roundtable discussion. *Curr Med Res Opin.* 2007;23(5):1077-1080.PubMed

23. ten Berg MJ, Huisman A, van den Bemt PM, et al. Linking laboratory and medication data: new opportunities for pharmacoepidemiological research. *Clin Chem Lab Med.* 2007;45(1):13-19.PubMed

24. Hickner J, Thompson PJ, Wilkinson T, et al. Primary care physicians' challenges in ordering clinical laboratory tests and interpreting results. *J Am Board Fam Med.* 2014;27(2):268-274.PubMed

25. Watanabe AS, McCart G, Shimomura S, Kayser S. Systematic approach to drug information requests. *Am J Hosp Pharm.* 1975;32(12):1282-1285. PubMed

26. Sheehan AH, Jordan JK. Formulating an effective response; a structured approach. In: Malone PM, Malone MJ, Park SK, eds. *Drug Information: A Guide for Pharmacists.* 6th ed. New York, NY: McGraw-Hill Education; 2018:33-58.

27. Geerts AF, De Koning FHP, Egberts TC, et al. Information comparison of the effects of drugs on laboratory tests in drug labels and Young's book. *Clin Chem Lab Med.* 2012;50(10):1765-1768.PubMed

28. Shields KM, Park SK. Drug information resources. In: Malone PM, Malone MJ, Park SK, eds. *Drug Information: A Guide for Pharmacists.* 6th ed. New York, NY: McGraw-Hill Education; 2018:59-112.

29. Lane MA, Zeringue A, McDonald JR. Serious bleeding events due to warfarin and antibiotic co-prescription in a cohort of veterans. *Am J Med.* 2014;127(7):657-663.e2.PubMed

30. Baillargeon J, Holmes HM, Lin YL, et al. Concurrent use of warfarin and antibiotics and the risk of bleeding in older adults. *Am J Med.* 2012;125(2):183-189.PubMed

# 4

# Point-of-Care Testing

*Lisa M. Cillessen, Heather Lyons-Burney,*
*and Paul O. Gubbins*

## OBJECTIVES

*After completing this chapter, the reader should be able to*

- Identify resources for Clinical Laboratory Improvement Amendments–waived point-of-care testing options

- Interpret the performance characteristics of common point-of-care tests

- Describe clinical opportunities for point-of-care testing in an outpatient pharmacy setting for both population- and patient-specific applications

- Identify potential resources for maintaining good laboratory practices

- Discuss the limitations for Clinical Laboratory Improvement Amendments–waived point-of-care testing

The pharmacist's role in the healthcare system is continually evolving. Over time, the pharmacist's role has shifted from being product focused to delivering patient-oriented pharmaceutical care. Today, pharmacists are on the frontline of providing patient-centered care and wellness, and their role in delivering care as a member of the healthcare team is essential. Pharmacists are highly trained, accessible healthcare professionals who are second only to registered nurses in terms of the number of practicing professionals. They are also underutilized in the U.S. healthcare delivery system.[1] However, when working in collaboration with physicians and other healthcare professionals, pharmacists' roles and their ability can be expanded to deliver quality patient-centered care and improve public health.[1]

Working in collaboration with other providers and public health officials, pharmacists can leverage their knowledge and accessibility to offer point-of-care testing (POCT) services that are waived under the Clinical Laboratory Improvement Amendments of 1988 (CLIA-88) (CLIA-waived POCT).[2] Such services are offered to manage chronic diseases, improve access to healthcare services, rapidly initiate appropriate therapy, and screen for diseases of public health significance.[2] Chapter 1 defines POCT, differentiates it from home testing, and provides an overview of the advantages and disadvantages of these testing paradigms. The objective of this chapter is to describe and illustrate opportunities to perform CLIA-waived POCT in outpatient pharmacy settings. This chapter focuses on POC tests and POCT by expanding on the overview of common CLIA-waived POC tests provided in Chapter 1; in addition, this chapter discusses available tests, reviews their performance measures and practical limitations, discusses their use in current practice, and identifies potential future applications for their use in practice.

## FEDERAL AGENCIES INVOLVED WITH CLINICAL LABORATORY IMPROVEMENT AMENDMENTS– WAIVED POINT-OF-CARE TESTS AND TESTING

The U.S. Food and Drug Administration (FDA) and the Centers for Medicare and Medicaid Services (CMS) are the federal agencies charged with oversight of CLIA. The Centers for Disease Control and Prevention (CDC) supports the CLIA program by serving as a resource for analytical, research, and technical information on CLIA and POCT.

The FDA regulates test manufacturers and classifies their tests by a premarket authorization process. During this authorization process, the FDA uses criteria in the CLIA regulations to classify tests according to their level of complexity (high, moderate, or waived) and potential for risk to public health. Waived tests are low-complexity methods that are simple to use, and their risk of producing erroneous results is negligible or poses no reasonable risk of harm to the patient if performed incorrectly.[3] In public health emergencies, like the COVID-19 pandemic, the FDA commissioner can authorize the use of medical products, including diagnostic tests, before they undergo the normal review and classification process using an Emergency Use Authorization (EUA).[4] Since an EUA allows use of a diagnostic test before it has been classified according to its complexity, the authorization must specify the

DOI 10.37573/9781585286423.004

test can be performed in a patient care setting (ie, at the POC), or else it must be performed in a laboratory capable of carrying out moderate to high complexity tests.[4]

CMS regulates facilities that conduct laboratory testing, including all POC tests, on human specimens for health assessment, diagnosis, prevention, or treatment of disease. Waived laboratories, such as community pharmacies or ambulatory care clinics, can only perform waived tests and are not subject to regular inspections, personnel requirements, or proficiency testing. To perform such tests, these sites must obtain a CLIA Certificate of Waiver from CMS, pay applicable fees biannually, and follow the manufacturers' testing instructions. In most states, the process is similar; however, CMS has exempted New York and Washington from CLIA so some of the processes and regulations to perform CLIA-waived tests are different. More information on how to apply for a CLIA Certificate of Waiver can be found at the CMS website (https://www.cms.gov/Regulations -and-Guidance/Legislation/CLIA/How_to_Apply_for_a _CLIA_Certificate_International_Laboratories.html).

## Resources

The market for CLIA-waived POC tests continually and rapidly grows and changes. Therefore, a pharmacist who has a CLIA waiver must be aware of the most current information on the available tests. The FDA, CMS, and CDC websites provide useful and current information on CLIA-waived tests (**Table 4-1**).[5,6]

**TABLE 4-1.** Resources for CLIA-Waived POCT

| AGENCY | RESOURCE | SITE | COMMENTS |
|--------|----------|------|----------|
| FDA | Searchable list of analytes used in waived laboratory test systems | http://www.accessdata.fda.gov /scripts/cdrh/cfdocs/cfClia /analyteswaived.cfm | • Select an analyte to display a list of waived test systems for it, with hyperlinks to regulatory information and documentation<br>• Updated frequently<br>• Contains more regulatory information than clinicians need |
| | Website with information on EUAs issued for emergencies (eg, COVID-19, H1N1) | https://www.fda.gov/medical-devices /emergency-situations-medical -devices/emergency-use-authorizations | • Information on EUAs for diagnostic, nondiagnostic, and therapeutic medical devices<br>• Information on diagnostics tests for a given disease includes date EUA was issued, manufacturer, hyperlink to authorizing letter, technology, authorized setting, hyperlinks to authorizing documents |
| CMS | A listing of tests that have been granted a waived status under CLIA | https://www.cms.gov/Regulations-and -Guidance/Legislation/CLIA/Downloads /waivetbl.pdf | • List is organized by CPT code<br>• Contains less information than the U.S. FDA website<br>• Provides basic information (eg, CPT code, test name, and manufacturer) in an easy-to-read tabular format, which clinicians may find useful |
| CDC | CLIA website | https://www.cdc.gov/clia/default.aspx | • Good resource with professional information and educational resources regarding the analytical and technical aspects of a test for a given analyte |
| | Website for CLIA-waived POC tests | https://www.cdc.gov/labquality /waived-tests.html | • Contains hyperlinks to documents that outline good laboratory practices for sites performing waived tests and a booklet detailing the practical considerations for performing CLIA-waived POCT or developing CLIA-waived POCT services[5,6] |

CPT = current procedural terminology; FDA = Food and Drug Administration.

# PERFORMANCE CHARACTERISTICS OF CLINICAL LABORATORY IMPROVEMENT AMENDMENTS–WAIVED POINT-OF-CARE TESTS AND THEIR APPLICATION

Like any test, CLIA-waived POC tests have random and systemic error associated with their use. Thus, pharmacists should be aware of the variability of POC tests when interpreting their results. A given test's performance characteristics will be included in the manufacturer's test literature. In addition, such information may be gleaned from the literature or the manufacturers' websites.

Most CLIA-waived POC tests for chronic disease management that are applicable to outpatient pharmacy settings are either qualitative or quantitative. All CLIA-waived POC tests for infectious diseases that are applicable to outpatient pharmacy settings are qualitative. CLIA-waived POC tests can be described in terms of several performance characteristics introduced in Chapter 1, including accuracy/bias, precision, specificity, sensitivity, negative predictive value (NPV), and positive predictive value (PPV).

## Accuracy and Bias

The terms *accuracy* and *bias* are often used synonymously. Accuracy, the percentage of true results, is a performance measure of qualitative CLIA-waived POC tests. In contrast, bias, how close the mean test measurement is to the true value, is a performance measure for quantitative CLIA-waived POC tests. The accuracy of a qualitative CLIA-waived POC test can be affected by many variables, including errors in sample collection, environmental conditions (eg, temperature, humidity), operator error (ie, not following test manufacturer instructions), improper instrument operation, and maintenance. Likewise, depending on the analyte, negative or positive bias associated with a quantitative CLIA-waived POC test may necessitate confirmatory lab-based testing for values that exceed a certain acceptable threshold.

## Precision

For a CLIA-waived POC test, *precision* characterizes test reproducibility (ie, the degree to which the test performed under constant conditions produces the same measurement each time). For qualitative CLIA-waived POC tests, precision is characterized by PPV, which is the proportion of true positive results relative to all (ie, true and false) positive results. A CLIA-waived POC qualitative test with high precision regularly returns truly positive results. For quantitative CLIA-waived POC tests, precision is characterized by values such as standard deviation, relative standard deviation (coefficient of variance), or standard error of the mean. A CLIA-waived POC quantitative test with high precision regularly produces results that are in close agreement.

## Application of Accuracy/Bias and Precision

Accuracy/bias and precision characterize the quality of a CLIA-waived POC test. These quality measures help the clinician choose the test, by comparing the expected performance of a test across different manufacturers. In addition, using these measures clinicians can evaluate the validity of a test's result, and assess whether it is performing within its expected error limits. These quality measures are determined in studies for regulatory approval, the results of which are included in the manufacturer's provided package insert for the test.

## Specificity and Sensitivity

CLIA-waived POC tests for chronic disease management in an outpatient pharmacy setting evaluate the need for therapy and medication adjustments at a certain treatment threshold. In the case of infectious diseases, they confirm the presence of an infectious disease and aid in its diagnosis. A perfect CLIA-waived POC test for a chronic disease would return the exact value above or below the threshold, whereas one for an infectious disease would produce a positive result in all patients with the infection and a negative result in all patients without it. Unfortunately, like laboratory-based tests, no CLIA-waived POC test is perfect.[7] Thus, when choosing a CLIA-waived POC test, clinicians must consider a test's *specificity* and *sensitivity*, when there is a referenced laboratory standard for comparison, or the analogous respective terms *negative percent agreement* and *positive percent agreement*, in the absence of one.[8]

The *specificity*, or *negative percent agreement*, of a qualitative CLIA-waived POC test represents its ability to not detect the analyte when it is indeed absent (ie, a true negative). The specificity of a quantitative test is dependent on a cutoff value, which is also known as the *limit of detection*.

A qualitative CLIA-waived POC test with 90% specificity will incorrectly detect the presence of the analyte in 10% of those tested when they do not have the analyte of interest (ie, false positives). Thus, when screening for the presence of an infectious disease, using a CLIA-waived POC test with high specificity is desired because it means the test is rarely positive in the absence of the infection. The *sensitivity*, or *positive percent agreement*, of a qualitative CLIA-waived POC test represents its ability to detect the analyte when it is indeed present (ie, a true positive). The sensitivity of a quantitative test is dependent on a predefined cutoff or threshold value so that a diagnosis or therapeutic management decision can be made. A qualitative CLIA-waived POC test with 80% sensitivity will positively detect 80% of those tested who have the analyte of interest, but it will not detect the other 20% who also have it (ie, false negatives). Thus, when screening for an infectious disease that carries a poor prognosis or is highly contagious, using a CLIA-waived POC test with high sensitivity is desired because a false negative result cannot be tolerated.

## Application of Specificity and Sensitivity

*Specificity* and *sensitivity* are performance characteristics that are independent of the population of interest being tested and are considered fixed characteristics of the test.[7] Therefore, without further improvements in the methodology or analytical techniques, their values do not significantly change. Choosing the CLIA-waived POC test with the highest specificity minimizes the chance that someone without the condition or disease will be misidentified as having it. Thus, when using a CLIA-waived POC test to screen for a condition or disease that many of those tested will not have, choose the method with the highest sensitivity to optimize the testing efforts. A highly sensitive test does not often produce a false negative result. By doing so, the chance that someone with the condition or disease goes undetected will be minimized. To assess the value of specificity and sensitivity and relate them to patients in one's clinical setting, the test's NPV and PPV must be considered.[7] By calculating either of these values, clinicians can apply a test's performance to their own clinical setting.

## Negative Predictive and Positive Predictive Value

For a qualitative CLIA-waived POC test, the NPV addresses the likelihood that a given patient *does not* have the condition or disease of interest when the test result is negative. Similarly, for a qualitative CLIA-waived POC, the PPV addresses the likelihood that a given patient *has* the condition or disease of interest when the test result is positive.

## Application of Negative Predictive Values and Positive Predictive Values

The application of these values provides useful insight into how to interpret test results. Unlike specificity and sensitivity, NPVs and PPVs are not fixed characteristics of the test, but they are dependent on the population being tested and are influenced by the prevalence of the disease. Understanding how these values are influenced by disease prevalence can help clinicians use strategies to optimize test performance and mitigate overtesting and thereby improve the usefulness of a CLIA-waived POC test.

The NPV allows the clinician to determine how reassuring to be when answering the question from the patient who tested negative ("How likely is it that I do not have this condition?"), whereas the PPV allows the clinician to answer the question from the concerned patient who tested positive ("How likely is it that I have this condition?").[7]

## Interferences

*Interferences* are a performance characteristic that is not statistically based. Rather, interferences are medical conditions, medications, or other substances that might influence test results positively or negatively. For qualitative tests, interference can cause false negative or false positive results, whereas for quantitative tests, it can obscure the limit of detection. Interferences with CLIA-waived POC tests can occur and often involve cross-reactivity, microbial, or other interfering substances, such as chemicals or certain foods. Information on interferences is included in the manufacturer information included with the tests, which personnel performing the test must read to ensure they have the most up-to-date information.

## SPECIMENS USED IN CLINICAL LABORATORY IMPROVEMENT AMENDMENTS–WAIVED POINT OF CARE

Waived tests are approved for use only with unprocessed specimens that require no manipulation (eg, centrifugation, precipitation, dilution, and extraction). Serum or plasma specimens

require manipulation during sample preparation or training in their handling; thus they are not suitable for use in CLIA-waived POC tests.[9] Clinicians should be aware that some test systems provide instructions for processed and unprocessed specimen types, but waived use is intended only for the testing of unprocessed specimens.

## Specimens Used in Common Clinical Laboratory Improvement Amendments–Waived Point-of-Care Tests for Chronic Disease State Management

In addition, depending on the type of specimen the test analyzes, not all CLIA-waived POC tests used for disease state management are suitable or feasible for use in an outpatient pharmacy setting. The most commonly obtainable specimen types for POCT in disease state management are urine and whole blood.

### Urine

The urine dipstick and tablet reagent urinalysis are common CLIA-waived POC tests found in many outpatient settings. Urine testing may involve a tabletop POC testing device or may be a manually read test kit. The determination of what type of POC testing device to use may factor in cost, time to test, and efficiency to document results.[10] It is important to consider the specificity and sensitivity, and the NPV and PPV, for the POC urine test used at the practice site due to variability between devices.[11] Subsequent therapy or treatment recommendations based on data collected from a POC urine test should be based on the specific device and analyte sampled. Typically, a sample is obtained in a clean container and analyzed promptly. If the time between collection and analysis is delayed more than 4 hours, the sample may be able to be refrigerated.[12] Depending upon the test, an average of 1 to 2 oz may be needed for an accurate analysis. In addition, patients may be asked to obtain a sample in the morning in order for more concentrated urine to be collected.[13] Often, a clean catch urine is necessary, requiring the patient to clean the genital area before collecting the sample to avoid contamination. Patients may be asked to alter sampling technique to obtain a first-void urine or a midstream urine sample.[11] Menstrual period or vaginal secretion effect on certain test results may impact the timing of a test or ability to obtain a clean sample.

### Whole Blood

Pharmacists obtain whole blood samples through a finger stick method for a variety of CLIA-waived POC tests. Blood conservation is one advantage of POC tests; as such, tests analyze whole blood analytes using volumes typically measured in drops of blood rather than milliliters. Each testing device may require varying amounts of a blood sample for a given analyte, making it critical for pharmacists to follow the manufacturer's guidelines for blood sample collection as required by CLIA-waived testing regulations. The minimal amount of blood required by POC tests may also reduce the chance of errors that can occur when using larger volumes. As described in Chapter 1, a quick turnaround time (TAT) is also a major advantage to POCT. The TAT is the time interval from sample collection to test performance, and it is a critical step in ensuring test accuracy for some CLIA-waived POC tests. Outpatient pharmacy settings are often very busy; thus, pharmacists performing CLIA-waived POCT services in these settings must be cognizant of proper sample collection technique and timing information. This information is also found in the manufacturer's guidelines.

## Specimens and Types of Tests Used for Common Clinical Laboratory Improvement Amendments–Waived Point-of-Care Tests for Infectious Diseases Screening and Management

Currently, there are CLIA-waived tests for 17 infectious diseases analytes, but not all these tests have POC applications or are suitable for testing in the outpatient pharmacy setting. The most common obtainable specimen types for POCT for screening or management of infectious diseases are swabbed secretions from nose, nasopharynx, oropharynx, oral mucosal transudate, and whole blood.

### Secretions From the Nose, Nasopharynx, and Oropharynx

Several infectious disease analytes, such as group A streptococci (GAS), severe acute respiratory syndrome coronavirus 2 (SARS-CoV-2), and influenza A and B, cause acute respiratory illnesses. The upper respiratory tract—the nasopharynx, oropharynx, and laryngopharynx—is easily accessible to airborne microorganisms and is colonized throughout life by commensal organisms and potential bacterial pathogens, including GAS, but not by viruses. Collecting lower respiratory tract specimens, such as sputum for diagnostic purposes, often requires invasive procedures, and for this reason, CLIA-waived POC tests for GAS, SARS-CoV-2, and influenza A and B rely on obtaining secretions from the more readily accessible upper respiratory tract. With minimal training, pharmacists can perform nasopharyngeal, nasal, or oropharyngeal swabs to collect specimens that would be suitable for the available CLIA-waived POC tests. Such samples can also be collected by nasopharyngeal aspiration or nasal wash, but these collection methods are technically difficult and not practical for a pharmacist to perform in an outpatient setting.[14,15]

### Oral Mucosal Transudate

To date, human immunodeficiency virus (HIV) -1 and -2 are the only infectious disease analytes measured from oral mucosal transudate specimens for CLIA-waived tests. In 2004, the FDA approved a rapid HIV antibody–based, CLIA-waived POC test—which it had initially approved for finger stick, whole blood, and plasma specimens—for use with specimens of oral mucosal transudate. In 2012, the FDA approved an identical version of the test for sale directly to consumers for in-home use, which cannot be used in clinical outpatient settings. Oral mucosal transudate is more acceptable to patients because of its noninvasive, pain-free specimen collection and its rapid TAT. Moreover, the test enabled the expansion of testing efforts from laboratory-based facilities to outpatient settings, community health and nonclinical outreach testing sites, thereby increasing the availability of HIV testing and allowing more people to get tested and learn their results in a timely manner. The test also enables individuals to get tested at least once as part of routine healthcare.[16] With minimal training, pharmacists can swab a person's oral cavity to obtain oral mucosal transudate and perform the professional version of the CLIA-waived test. In general, POC tests for HIV-1 or HIV-2 using oral mucosal transudate specimens are less technically demanding than methods using blood and minimize the concern for biohazard disposal. Methods using oral mucosal transudate have low sensitivity and may miss more acute HIV infections than CLIA-waived tests that use whole blood specimens.

### Whole Blood

HIV-1, HIV-2, and hepatitis C virus (HCV) are among the common infectious disease analytes measured from whole blood for CLIA-waived POC tests. Like POC tests for chronic disease state management, many pharmacists are comfortable with obtaining whole blood samples through a finger stick method for these CLIA-waived POC tests.[17,18] Unlike the CLIA-waived oral tests for HIV-1 and HIV-2, the CLIA-waived whole blood tests for HIV-1 and HIV-2 require more equipment (eg, lancets) and biohazard waste precautions (eg, sharps containers and gloves). Although a blood sample for HIV-1, HIV-2, and HCV CLIA-waived tests that use whole blood can be obtained by venipuncture, it is easier to obtain the sample via finger stick for POCT purposes in outpatient pharmacy settings. However, HIV-1 and HIV-2 antibodies and p24 antigen concentrations are generally lower in whole blood finger stick samples than from plasma.

### Types of Point-of-Care Tests for Infectious Diseases

The types of tests that exist to detect pathogens are antigen, molecular, and antibody-based methods. These methods differ in what is measured and their role in testing for a given pathogen. Antigen tests detect protein fragments of the pathogen that elicit an immune response; therefore, they may serve as a marker for infection. However, the tests do not distinguish between antigen from a viable pathogen and antigen from a nonviable pathogen, so a positive antigen test does not necessarily mean the patient has an active infection. Antigen tests target protein fragments that are large enough to detect without the use of amplification reactions, often through lateral flow chromatographic enzyme immunoassays or latex agglutination techniques. Such techniques can be performed with little or no training and typically produce a visual readout. However, despite its convenience, visual readouts may be unreliable; thus, for some pathogens, many contemporary antigen tests use an automated reader.[19] Antigen tests typically have lower sensitivity than molecular tests and provide a qualitative result.[19] These tests can be used to detect exposure that may necessitate therapy, and screen for potential outbreaks in institutions or environments with close quarters to develop further preventative strategies.

Molecular methods for detecting pathogens amplify nucleic acids in the viral genome using real-time reverse transcription polymerase chain reaction (rtRT-PCR) or reverse transcription isothermal amplification. The amplification reaction in rtRT-PCR methods requires a series of alternating temperature cycles, which makes their application to a POC platform challenging.

However, technological advances such as the advent of reverse transcription isothermal amplification (ie, RT-loop-mediated isothermal amplification [RT-LAMP]), in which amplification reaction occurs at a constant temperature, have enabled molecular diagnostic tests to be applied to a POC testing platform.[19] Molecular tests are typically highly sensitive, provide a qualitative result or a semiquantitative measure of pathogen burden, and are useful for detecting active infections.

Serological methods detect the presence of immunoglobulin M (IgM) or immunoglobulin G (IgG) antibodies directed against the virus in a whole blood, plasma, or serum sample. These methods typically use enzyme-linked immunosorbent assays (ELISA) techniques. Performing serological tests involve applying a small sample of blood from a finger stick (ie, drops) to a cartridge containing the immunoassay, followed by a couple of drops of a buffer solution. The qualitative results should then be readily displayed within minutes. The initial antibody response to an infection varies for each pathogen and among individuals. The response is comprised of IgM antibodies followed, in time, by IgG antibodies. Thus, a test that detects IgM antibodies would indicate a recently acquired infection, whereas one detecting IgG antibodies would signify that some time had elapsed since acquisition of infection. Serologic methods do not detect active acute infection, and are typically used for diagnosis of chronic infections or public health disease surveillance and epidemiology efforts (ie, HIV, HCV, and COVID-19).

# USES AND APPLICATION OF COMMON CLINICAL LABORATORY IMPROVEMENT AMENDMENTS–WAIVED POINT-OF-CARE TESTS

The use of CLIA-waived POC tests provides another tool for pharmacists practicing in patient-centered, team-based environments to contribute to the appropriate management of chronic diseases. CLIA-waived POCT services are also used in outpatient pharmacy settings to monitor the safety and efficacy of medications as well as provide measurable clinical outcome data consistent with evidence-based guidelines. CLIA-waived POC tests are used in the screening of at-risk patients for certain disease states (eg, diabetes, dyslipidemia) and in their long-term management. Direct pharmacist involvement using CLIA-waived POCT in conjunction with medication therapy services, collaborative practice agreements (CPAs), or collaborative drug therapy management (CDTM) agreements can assist patients in reaching their chronic disease management goals as well as build strong patient and pharmacist relationships demonstrating positive clinical outcomes and return on investment.[1,20] Pharmacists also perform CLIA-waived POC tests to screen for infections of public health interest (eg, HCV, SARS-CoV-2, and influenza), or to aid in the diagnosis and management of an acute infection in an individual patient (eg, influenza, GAS). This section explores common CLIA-waived POCT services provided by pharmacists in the outpatient setting; however, it is not an all-inclusive representation of the pharmacist's role in POCT.

# HgbA1c
## Use in Pharmacy

An estimated 34.2 million Americans have been diagnosed with diabetes mellitus, with an additional 7.3 million remaining undiagnosed.[21] In 2015, it was estimated that 88 million Americans age 18 or older had prediabetes.[21] Measurement of the percent concentration of glycated hemoglobin (HgbA1c) in blood is a useful CLIA-waived POC test for identifying patients with prediabetes and monitoring patients with diabetes during routine follow-up visits. Pharmacists can perform screening for diabetes as part of large community or corporate health and wellness efforts. Individuals identified as being at risk can then be offered counseling on nonpharmacologic lifestyle changes (eg, exercise, dietary adjustments, and smoking cessation) or referred to their provider for additional follow-up. It is important that pharmacists reference national diabetes guidelines when discussing results and determining the appropriate time to refer patients to their primary care provider.

## Determining Appropriate Testing Candidates

Patients at risk for diabetes that do not have current diagnostic testing for diabetes should obtain an initial laboratory-based HgbA1c to determine glycemic status; however, if a validated and regularly monitored CLIA-waived POC test is used for the HgbA1c, it may be acceptable to use that test for diagnosis when associated signs and symptoms are present.[22] For patients with a current diagnosis, CLIA-waived POCT of HgbA1c for monitoring allows for more timely disease management.[23] Immediate feedback from CLIA-waived POCT has demonstrated increased likelihood of medical or pharmaceutical intervention, as well as greater HgbA1c lowering as compared with commercial laboratory testing.[24]

## Application of HgbA1c Point-of-Care Testing in Practice

As part of enhanced pharmacy services, pharmacists in an outpatient setting can build CLIA-waived POCT services into their workflow. Depending on the state board of pharmacy's statutes, the pharmacist engaged in a CPA/CDTM agreement can then follow the protocol to adjust medication dosages, recommend nonpharmacological therapies, or schedule additional testing or physician follow-up (**Minicase 1**).

## Performance Characteristics

Prior to the early 1990s, measurement of HgbA1c was not standardized, so it was used only as a surrogate marker of glycemic control. In the early 1990s, the landmark Diabetes Control and Complications Trial (DCCT) established the correlation between HgbA1c measurement and the risk of developing complications from diabetes; subsequently, target values were created to lower patients' risk of poor outcomes.[25-27] Rigorous standardization was needed because in the DCCT a very small difference, such as 2%, in mean HgbA1c values between treatment groups translated into a significant decrease in the risk for a variety of complications from diabetes.[25] The National Glycohemoglobin Standardization Program (NGSP) was initiated to standardize HgbA1c test results so laboratory results

## MINICASE 1

# Type 2 Diabetes Mellitus and HgbA1C

Stuart M., a 60-year-old man with a 5-year history of type 2 diabetes mellitus, presents to his primary care clinic for a follow-up visit. Although he was diagnosed 5 years earlier, he exhibited symptoms of diabetes for at least 2 years before diagnosis, including nocturia. He reports increased physical activity but has gained 10 lb over the past year with little success in weight loss (weight 190 lb; height 5'10"; BMI 27.3 kg/m²). He reports eating a high-carbohydrate diet with pasta or bread at every dinner. Stuart M.'s medications for diabetes include metformin 500-mg tablets, one tablet twice a day for the past 4 years, and various nutritional supplements that he has tried with no noticeable improvement. His personal blood glucose logs over the past 3 months indicate values ranging throughout the day from 108 to 264 mg/dL. His previous A1C level, tested with the POCT device 3 months ago at the clinic, was 7.8%. The pharmacist performs POC A1C testing based on a CPA. Stuart M.'s vital signs include blood pressure (BP), 128/78 mm Hg;

heart rate (HR), 84 beats/min; respiration rate (RR), 20 breaths/min; and HgbA1C, 8.3%.

QUESTION: What does this A1C level indicate?

DISCUSSION: The rise in A1C level of 0.5% over 3 months indicates that the patient's average blood glucose level is increased, and he is at increased risk for diabetes complications. In addition to the A1C level, the patient's weight gain and report of a high-carbohydrate diet would contribute to the pharmacist's decision to modify therapy. According to the CPA and following therapeutic guidelines, the pharmacist may decide to maximize the metformin therapy and educate the patient on dietary strategies to reduce the amount of carbohydrates consumed and increase physical activity with the goal of weight loss. The pharmacist would also recommend a follow-up visit with a repeat A1C level in 3 months.

were comparable to those in the DCCT.[27] As part of the NGSP, a network of laboratories works with test manufacturers to standardize their methods.[27] Over the years, the rigorous standardization efforts have facilitated the monitoring of HgbA1c with rapid reporting of results, which has demonstrated improved glycemic control in type 1 and insulin-treated type 2 patients with diabetes.[28,29]

The American Diabetes Association recommends that the HgbA1c methods used be NGSP certified.[30] NGSP requires annual manufacturer certification of POC instruments against a secondary reference laboratory with a HgbA1c range of 4% to 10%. The HgbA1c reporting range for certain devices may exceed the NGSP certification of accuracy up to 10%, thus requiring the end user to assess a manufacturer's documentation of calibration at the upper limit of their reportable range.[24] Although the same quality standards apply for laboratory and POC HgbA1c systems, a concern regarding the lack of required proficiency testing for end users performing CLIA-waived POC HgbA1c tests exists.[25,26] Few data characterize how these methods truly perform when conducted in the setting of a CLIA-waived laboratory; thus, their real analytical performance is not known.[25,26] Nonetheless, data indicate that CLIA-waived POC methods for HgbA1c perform no worse than many laboratory-based HgbA1c methods.[25] Moreover, in a series of studies, investigators have demonstrated that the analytical performance of POC instruments for HgbA1c have improved considerably in the last decade.[31,32] Measurement of HgbA1c via CLIA-waived POC tests are based on structural differences among the various types of hemoglobin (Hgb) molecules, using either affinity separation or more specific immunoassays.[26] Affinity separation methods use a boronate matrix to measure "total" glycation and distinguish glycated Hgb from nonglycated Hgb.[26] Based on affinity separation, the analyzers of the CLIA-waived POC tests measure the percentage of HgbA1c.

An advantage to affinity separation methods is a lack of interference by nearly all Hgb variants or derivatives.[26] Immunoassay methods use specific antibodies directed toward the first several amino acids and the glucose molecule of the N-terminal of the β-chain of the Hgb molecule.[26] These methods measure total Hgb through methods including turbidimetric measurement and latex agglutination inhibition.[26] Although most immunoassays do not interfere with common Hgb variants (eg, HbAS, HbAC, HbAD, and HbAE), they are subject to interference with rare Hgb variants resulting from amino acid substitutions.[25] Overestimation of HgbA1c due to variants could result in overly aggressive treatment; thus, it is important for the user to factor in this potential influence.[24]

In evaluating the performance characteristics of CLIA-waived POC, HgbA1c tests bias and measures of imprecision are important.[25] Acceptable levels of accuracy and precision for HgbA1c POCT devices have been suggested by some authors at within 0.2 points of true value and a coefficient of variation <3%.[32] As the measurement of HgbA1c can result in therapy adjustments, consistency between POCT devices, TAT, and methods are important components of a laboratory's policies and procedures. Therefore, using devices meeting NGSP quality measures that are subject to regular monitoring for accuracy will help ensure accurate and standardized results.

## Hemoglobin

### Use in Pharmacy

Anemia is caused by the impaired production or increased destruction of red blood cells, blood loss, or fluid overload. Several CLIA-waived POC tests for Hgb and hematocrit (Hct) using capillary blood samples have been used in critical care settings as well as in outpatient settings to assist with the diagnosis of anemia or its associated morbidities.

### Determining Appropriate Testing Candidates

Patients at risk for anemia include those who have deficiencies in their diet, intestinal disorders, chronic conditions, or genetic disorders as well as those who are menstruating or pregnant. Pharmacists using POC tests for Hgb in outpatient settings can screen for anemia as well as monitor therapies.

### Application of Hemoglobin Point-of-Care Testing in Practice

Hemoglobin POCT devices use relatively small amounts of finger stick blood, allowing for ease of use for trained pharmacists, and quick results. Pharmacists may use results to manage or monitor anemia, providing recommendations to the patient and communicating results or recommendations to the provider. Sickle cell disease is a common genetic disorder worldwide that has used POCT devices for the screening and early diagnosis of the disease. However, a detailed discussion of application to sickle cell disease is outside the scope of this chapter.

### Performance Characteristics

The CLIA-waived POC tests to determine an Hgb level are typically based on either the conductometric method or the spectrophotometric method.[33] The commonly used spectrophotometric method measures the azide-methemoglobin formed by the test reagent mixed with a drop-size sample of capillary, venous, or arterial blood. The conductometric POCT device uses optical absorption photometry to obtain Hgb and Hct from a single drop of blood in less than 1 minute.

In addition to the POCT devices described previously, a noninvasive, multi-wavelength sensor exists that uses a spectrophotometric method to determine Hgb concentration.[34] Another device also uses a sensor that emits wavelengths of light to measure Hgb concentration data based on light absorption through the finger. In a similar manner as conventional pulse oximetry, it uses signal processing algorithms and adaptive filters to translate the absorption data. The proposed advantages of a noninvasive testing device would be no risk of exposure to bloodborne pathogens for the pharmacist and a painless process for the patient.

Physiologic factors can affect Hgb measurement, emphasizing the need for consistency in laboratory procedures and documentation. Identified causes of variation include capillary blood versus venous blood, tourniquet use for longer than 30 seconds, patient position (standing, sitting, or supine), time of day, whether the right or left hand is used, and even which finger is used for a capillary sample.[35]

## Cholesterol

### Use in Pharmacy

Heart disease has a profound effect on the United States population as the leading cause of death among men and women and affects all races and ethnic groups.[36] In 2018, it was estimated that atherosclerotic cardiovascular disease (ASCVD) caused nearly one of every three deaths in the United States.[36] Elevated cholesterol is one of the leading causes of ASCVD. Hyperlipidemia, defined as a total serum cholesterol >200 mg/dL, affects an estimated 95 million adults, although only an estimated 43 million are taking medication(s) to reduce their risk.[37]

Pharmacists perform screening for ASCVD risk as part of large community or corporate health and wellness efforts. Individuals identified as at risk are offered counseling on nonpharmacologic lifestyle changes (eg, exercise, dietary adjustments, blood pressure management, and smoking cessation) or referred to their provider for additional follow-up. Additionally, under a CPA/CDTM agreement, pharmacists can initiate or modify medications to minimize a patient's ASCVD risk.

### Determining Appropriate Testing Candidates

While many workplace health and wellness plans offer annual cholesterol screenings, current clinical guidelines recommend screening adult patients every 4 to 6 years to assess a patient's ASCVD risk.[38] Patients on therapy are often monitored on a routine basis.[38]

### Application of Cholesterol Point-of-Care Testing in Practice

Trained pharmacists applying and properly using CLIA-waived POC tests for the management of chronic diseases provides significant benefits to community health. Chronic disease management for cardiovascular disease and hyperlipidemia, specifically, are areas in which pharmacists have demonstrated a positive impact on outcomes.[1] Managing ASCVD and lowering ASCVD risk often require prescription medication therapies in addition to nonpharmacological lifestyle changes. In addition, clinical management guidelines for ASCVD and the medications used in its treatment recommend regular monitoring of laboratory values to determine appropriate drug dosing. It is important for pharmacists to reference national disease state guidelines when discussing results and determining the appropriate time to refer patients to their primary care provider.

As part of enhanced pharmacy services, pharmacists in an outpatient setting can build CLIA-waived POCT services into their workflow. As described previously, common CLIA-waived POC tests for chronic disease state management require the collection of a small blood sample for the monitoring of cholesterol. Depending on the state board of pharmacy's statutes, the pharmacist engaged in a CPA/CDTM agreement could then follow the protocol to adjust medication dosages, recommend nonpharmacological therapies, or schedule additional testing or physician follow-up. The accessibility of pharmacists enables them to reach large numbers of adults at risk for ASCVD with appropriate cholesterol testing, which may benefit prevention and treatment efforts in a community.

### Performance Characteristics

Historically, the National Cholesterol Education Program's goal to reduce morbidity and mortality caused by ASCVD relied on accurate and precise measurement of the lipid profile. In response to the need to improve cholesterol measurement, the CDC created the Cholesterol Reference Method Laboratory Network to ensure that manufacturers of diagnostic products in meeting the criteria of the National Reference System for Cholesterol (NRS/CHOL).[39] The NRS/CHOL determines the methods and materials for cholesterol testing that are used by research laboratories, which may determine the American College of Cardiology and American Heart Association prevention guidelines for healthcare professionals on the treatment and management of blood cholesterol to reduce ASCVD risk.

Several of the CLIA-waived tests have demonstrated acceptable ranges of specificity and sensitivity when compared with test methods from the Clinical and Laboratory Standards Institute (CLSI).[40] Many waived tests and devices are available for the testing of cholesterol that report results ranging from only total cholesterol to an entire standard lipid panel (eg, total cholesterol, high-density lipoprotein, low-density lipoprotein-calculated, and triglycerides). These tests and devices typically use finger stick capillary or venous blood samples and produce results within a few minutes. There are two common CLIA-waived POC test methodologies, one using combined enzymatic methodology and solid-phase technology and the other using reflectance photometry to produce results in minutes. The procedure manuals for each test provide guidance on proper specimen collection, handling, and quality control (QC) measures. Variants, including day-to-day or seasonal variations, can contribute to the accuracy of a cholesterol level.[41,42] Common variants to consider in interrupting the POC test results include age, gender, diet and alcohol, exercise, medications, fasting, and pregnancy.[41,42]

## Blood Chemistries

### Use in Pharmacy

A wide variety of CLIA-waived POCT devices measure blood chemistry in an outpatient setting. A blood chemistry analyzer uses a whole blood sample and can measure analytes, including ionized calcium, carbon dioxide, chloride, creatinine, glucose, potassium, sodium, and urea nitrogen. In addition, some CLIA-waived blood chemistry analyzers measure other analytes, including alanine amino transferase, aspartate amino transferase, albumin, total bilirubin, alkaline phosphatase, and total protein. Blood chemistry analyzers with these analytical capabilities can be used by a pharmacist practicing under a CPA or CDTM provisions in state regulations or statutes to determine liver and renal function values and assist with any appropriate medication dosing adjustments for chronic conditions, such as diabetes or cardiovascular disease.

Many medications are used in the management of chronic diseases that can lead to electrolyte imbalances. Additionally, most medications' pharmacokinetics are impacted by renal and/or liver function. Blood chemistry panels, such as a complete metabolic panel, can assist pharmacists in understanding a patient's renal and liver function to adjust or monitor the safety of these medications. CLIA-waived POC platforms for blood chemistries have multiple panels, not all of which are CLIA-waived. Measuring blood chemistries in real time can enable the pharmacist to adjust the medications accordingly. It is important that pharmacists understand the performance characteristics of these tests, reference guidelines, and ranges when discussing results and determining the appropriate time to refer patients to their primary care provider.

### Determining Appropriate Testing Candidates

Patients under the supervision of a pharmacist for chronic disease management (eg, hypertension, diabetes) require routine blood chemistry monitoring to ensure the safety and efficacy of their medications. Pharmacists should consult relevant national guidelines and perform necessary basic assessments to determine when to use these tests in the appropriate patient.

### Application of Blood Chemistries Point-of-Care Testing in Practice

Many medications on the market require renal or hepatic dosing adjustments as a patient's renal or liver function declines. Assessing a patient's renal and hepatic function at the POC allows a pharmacist with a CPA/CDTM agreement to adjust the medication dose or modify a patient's treatment to provide safe pharmacological treatment.[43] Several chronic disease medications (eg, diuretics, angiotensin converting enzyme inhibitors) can impact a patient's electrolytes. To safely start and modify these medications, it is essential to assess the patient's electrolytes before and after. Using POCT to monitor the electrolytes allows the pharmacist to make real-time decisions and adjust medications accordingly.

### Performance Characteristics

CLIA-waived POC tests for blood chemistries analyze whole blood samples collected through venipuncture or finger stick, depending on the analyzer and analytes being tested. Analyzers can provide results within minutes from a few drops of blood. To produce readable results, the analyzer conducts chemical reactions between the whole blood and the chemical reagents provided to produce chromophores, which are then measured through photometry. Using absorbed wavelengths, the analyzer can determine the concentration of the desired analyte. In general CLIA-waived POC tests for blood chemistries meet established thresholds for total allowable error for most analytes.[44] However, in different settings, analytes such as sodium, glucose, calcium, and others may demonstrate significant bias, compared with reference methods.[44] Reasons for the bias include differences in analytical methods used by the CLIA-waived POC test and the comparator or improper sample collection technique (eg, failure to properly clean the fingertip prior to obtaining capillary blood).[44,45]

## Urinalysis

### Use in Pharmacy

The urine dipstick and tablet reagent urinalysis are common CLIA-waived POC tests found in many outpatient settings. Urinalysis screens for a variety of different diagnostics (eg, urinary tract infection, pregnancy) and assists in the management of chronic diseases (eg, glucose, ketones, albumin to creatinine ratio). With a CPA/CDTM agreement, pharmacists provide nonpharmacological treatment and antibiotic treatment for a urinary tract infection identified through a CLIA-waived POC urinalysis. Additionally, pharmacists use urinalysis to assess patients with diabetes through monitoring glucose, albumin, and ketones in the urine, providing guidance on adherences and efficacy of medication(s).

### Determining Appropriate Testing Candidates

When considering incorporating urinalysis into the pharmacy workflow, the location for obtaining a urine sample will determine the site's ability to use these POC tests. The site needs to ensure a private area to obtain a urine specimen while ensuring the accuracy of the sample.

### Application of Urinalysis Point-of-Care Testing in Practice

A variety of urinalysis POC tests allow pharmacists to screen for and manage a variety of conditions and disease states. The urinalysis test provides pharmacists with values for bilirubin, glucose, Hgb, ketone, leukocytes, nitrite, pH, protein, and specific gravity. This test can be used to detect an acute urinary tract infection. Additional POC testing for urine albumin concentration or albumin to creatinine ratio for identification of microalbuminuria can assist the pharmacist in the management of diabetes or hypertension.[24] Pharmacists involved with prescribing or administering birth control may benefit from urine human chorionic gonadotropin (hCG) testing to determine a patient's pregnancy status. Outpatient monitoring for proteinuria for pregnant patients during routine prenatal care may aid in identifying patients at risk for preeclampsia.[24,46] The pharmacist involved in a smoking cessation program might use a nicotine detection test. This test detects nicotine and its metabolites in urine and could indicate the smoking status of an individual as a low or high nicotine consumer. Additionally, urine POC tests can also be used for a variety of other screening and diagnostic purposes; however, these uses are beyond the scope of this chapter. It is important that pharmacists reference national disease state guidelines when discussing results and determining the appropriate time to refer patients to their primary care provider.

### Performance Characteristics

Urine POCT studies are limited and, of those available, there is considerable variation in how the urine screening tests are performed: such testing is often in conjunction with other physical assessments, the review of symptoms, and laboratory testing. The interpretation of results depends on proper collection procedures and testing methods. Additionally, it is important to consider specificity and sensitivity and the NPV and PPV for the POC urine test used at the practice site because of variability between devices.[11]

## Hepatitis C Virus

### Use in Pharmacy

An estimated 2.4 million people in the United States are infected with HCV, and nearly half of infected individuals are unaware of their infection because they are asymptomatic.[47-49] The CDC estimates suggest there were nearly 44,700 new infections in 2017.[50] Studies demonstrate that testing adults for HCV is cost effective in a variety of outpatient pharmacy settings and can facilitate linkage to care.[51]

Clinic models that are led by pharmacists or models in which they assist in care provide accessible and effective alternatives for providing outpatient HCV care.[52] Given the accessibility of pharmacists, training pharmacists on the application and proper use of screening for HCV with CLIA-waived POC tests can have a significant impact on public health efforts, increasing the number of people getting tested, especially those at high risk (eg, younger patients using illicit intravenous drugs) who are not receiving care.[17,53] Pharmacist-directed CLIA-waived POCT efforts can increase the linkage to care (eg, follow-up assessment with providers, medicine distribution, and access to medication assistance programs) and expand access to appropriate counseling services and community resources.[17,53] Such efforts can also enhance collection of prevalence and surveillance data to help resources reach targeted at-risk populations.

### Determining Appropriate Testing Candidates

Guidelines for HCV testing have evolved as HCV shifted from a chronic infection to a curable disease. Current guidelines recommend routine, one-time testing for all adults and risk-based testing for patients younger than 18 years. Periodic repeat testing can be performed in all individuals who are at increased risk of or have been exposed to HCV. Pharmacists can identify individuals for testing based upon risk behaviors or exposures and other conditions or circumstances outlined in the national guidelines.[54]

### Application of Hepatitis C Virus Point-of-Care Testing in Practice

In 2013, the CDC recommended that the testing sequence for current active hepatitis C infection begin with testing for the HCV antibody, including use of the rapid POC assay prior to further HCV RNA testing and linkage to care. A positive HCV antibody test does not distinguish whether the patient currently has acute or chronic active HCV infection or a past infection that has resolved. Therefore, to confirm active infection, individuals testing positive must have a follow-up HCV RNA PCR test to detect HCV viremia, which informs management and treatment decisions.[54] Persons with a negative screening are considered not infected and do not need further evaluation unless they have a known risk factor.[54] Thus, CLIA-waived POCT for HCV offers potential savings in healthcare expense as well as the opportunity to educate patients on risk factors.

### Performance Characteristics

Currently, there is one FDA-approved CLIA-waived POC rapid immunoassay test that detects antibodies to HCV from whole blood samples obtained either by venipuncture or finger stick.[55] The results from it can be read between 20 to 40 minutes after the analysis is started, which enables a patient to receive pretest and posttest counseling within a single visit. This test is a noninstrumented, indirect lateral flow immunoassay, and its performance characteristics are summarized in **Table 4-2**. It has excellent sensitivity and specificity using whole blood from a finger stick.[56] In a multicenter study of individuals at risk for HCV infection, the test demonstrated a clinical performance equivalent to laboratory-based tests across all specimen types.[57] In addition, several studies have observed that the specificity of the HCV rapid test with all specimen types is similar to

**TABLE 4-2.** Summary of CLIA-Waived POC Tests for HIV and HCV[a]

| TEST | MANUFACTURER | CLIA WAIVER GRANTED | METHOD | ANALYTE(S) (TYPE OF ABS) | SPECIMEN TYPE | TIME TO RESULTS (MIN) | OVERALL CLINICAL SENSITIVITY (%)[b] | OVERALL CLINICAL SPECIFICITY (%)[b] |
|---|---|---|---|---|---|---|---|---|
| **HIV** | | | | | | | | |
| OraQuick Advance Rapid HIV-1/2 antibody test | OraSure Technologies | June 2004 | Lateral flow | HIV-1/2 Abs (IgG) | OMT, FSWB, VPWB | 20 | HIV-1 Abs 99.3 (OMT) 99.6 (FSWB) | 99.8 (OMT) 100 (VPWB) |
| Uni-Gold Recombigen HIV test | Trinity Biotech | November 2004 | Sandwich | HIV-1/2 Abs (IgG + IgM) | FSWB, VPWB | 10 | 100 | 99.7 |
| Clearview HIV-1/2 Stat-Pak[43] | Chembio | May 2006 | Lateral flow | HIV-1/2 Abs (IgG) | FSWB, VPWB | 15 | HIV-1 Abs = 99.7 HIV-2 Abs = 100 | HIV-1 Abs = 99.9 |
| Sure Check HIV-1/2 | Chembio | March 2011 | Lateral flow | HIV-1/2 Abs (IgG) | FSWB, VPWB | 15 | HIV-1 Abs = 99.7 HIV-2 Abs = 100 | 99.9 |
| DPP HIV-1/2 | Chembio | December 2012 | Dual path flow | HIV-1/2 Abs (IgG) | OMT FSWB VPWB | 25–40 (OMT) 10–25 (FSWB) 10–25 (VPWB) | 98.9 (OMT) 99.8 (FSWB) 99.9 (VPWB) | 99.9 (OMT) 100 (FSWB) 99.9 (VPWB) |
| Determine HIV-1/2 Ag/Ab combo test[43] | Abbott Laboratories | December 2014 | Lateral flow | HIV-1 p24 Ag HIV-1/2 Abs (IgG + IgM) | FSWB | 20 | HIV-1 Abs = 99.9 HIV-2 Abs = 100 | Low risk 100 High risk 98.9 Overall 99.6 |
| INSTI HIV-1/2 antibody test[44] | bioLytical Laboratories | July 2012 | Flow through | HIV-1/2 Abs (IgG + IgM) | FSWB | <2 | 99.8[c] | 99.5 |
| **HCV** | | | | | | | | |
| OraQuick rapid antibody HCV test | OraSure Technologies | February 2011 | Lateral flow | HCV Abs | FSWB VPWB | 20–40 | 100 | 100 |

Abs = antibodies; Ag = antigen; FSWB = whole blood via finger stick; OMT = Oral mucosa transudate; VPWB = whole blood via venipuncture.
[a]Values obtained from product package inserts and/or from manufacturers websites, except where noted.[43,44]
[b]Data for whole blood via finger stick unless otherwise noted, data for whole blood via venipuncture not provided.
[c]Only HIV-1 Abs data provided.

that reported for anti-HCV enzyme immunoassay (EIA).[58] The CLIA-waived POC test to detect antibodies to HCV also has a high degree of interoperator agreement in result interpretation.[59] For these reasons, the initial testing for HCV antibody screening with POC rapid immunoassay is an effective alternative to the third-generation EIA methods.[56]

## Human Immunodeficiency Virus

### Use in Pharmacy

Estimates suggest that nearly 1.2 million individuals in the United States are living with an HIV infection, of whom 161,800, or one in eight (13%), are unaware of their infection.[60] Testing is important because individuals who are unaware of their HIV infection status cannot take advantage of treatments to reduce viral loads and maintain their health; thus, they pose a risk of transmitting the infection to others.[16]

Given the accessibility of pharmacists and a less stigmatizing setting, pharmacies can be effective for the delivery of HIV testing, even though they are underutilized. Data demonstrate that by training pharmacists to perform CLIA-waived POC tests for the screening of HIV, pharmacies can be an effective setting for those who have not previously been tested and increase access to testing, particularly in underserved areas.[61] HIV screening in pharmacies can have significant impact on public health efforts to increase the number of people getting tested, especially those who engage in high-risk behaviors. Pharmacist-directed CLIA-waived POCT efforts could increase the linkage to medical treatment (eg, facilitate medicine distribution and access to medication assistance programs); expand access to appropriate counseling services, community resources, and care; and aid in risk-mitigation efforts (eg, needle exchange programs). Such efforts can also enhance the collection of prevalence and surveillance data to help resources reach targeted at-risk populations quicker. Recognizing these public health benefits, the CDC offers a training program on HIV testing in community pharmacies (https://www.cdc.gov/hiv/effective-interventions/diagnose/hiv-testing-in-retail-pharmacies?Sort=Title%3A%3Aasc&Intervention%20Name=HIV%20Testing%20in%20Retail%20Pharmacies).

### Determining Appropriate Testing Candidates

The CDC recommends that individuals aged 13 to 64 years be tested for HIV at least once as part of routine care and that individuals with risk factors be tested annually.[16] When performing CLIA-waived POCT for HIV, refer to national guidelines to determine who should be tested.[16]

### Application of Human Immunodeficiency Virus Point-of-Care Testing in Practice

Studies show that the accessibility of community pharmacies can be leveraged to successfully offer CLIA-waived POCT services for HIV infection.[18,61-66] Moreover, establishing CLIA-waived POCT services for HIV in a pharmacy practice setting requires a modest amount of staff training, and the costs are similar to other services offered in these settings.[18,63,64,66] Collectively, studies indicate pharmacies can serve as an alternate, highly accessible, and less stigmatizing healthcare facility to perform HIV testing services.[18,62-66] Approximately 1 week is needed for viral infection and replication to produce detectable p24 antigen, which is the first viral protein that can be measured after HIV infection. This antigen is then detectable for approximately 1 to 8 weeks (average within 2 weeks), until there is sufficient antibody production to bind and neutralize it. On average, the onset of symptoms occurs within 1 to 3 weeks of infection and corresponds to seroconversion (ie, the development of antibodies). Seroconversion occurs in most individuals within 4 weeks of potential exposure (ie, infection). Individuals who have not seroconverted by 4 weeks should do so by 12 weeks postexposure. At that point, if seroconversion has not occurred (ie, the test result is negative), the individual is considered HIV negative.

### Performance Characteristics

There are several CLIA-waived POC tests to detect antibodies to HIV-1 and HIV-2 and one test that detects those antibodies plus HIV-1 p24 antigens. Following specimen collection, the time to test results for HIV POC tests ranges from 1 minute to 20 minutes, which enables a patient to receive pretest and posttest counseling within a single visit. These test devices are typically based on a capillary lateral flow design and use whole blood from a finger stick or oral mucosal transudate. The performance characteristics of these tests are summarized in Table 4-2.

The performance characteristics of the CLIA-waived POC tests for HIV are sufficient to detect HIV infection or its absence. In general, the CLIA-waived POC tests for HIV have specificity and sensitivity equivalent to nonwaived HIV screening test kits (eg, ELISA) approved for laboratory use.[67] The performance characteristics of CLIA-waived POC tests for HIV vary depending on the type of test (eg, antigen or antibody-based), whether it detects only one type of immunoglobulin (ie, IgG) or more (ie, IgM and IgG) antibodies, the stage of infection, whether the analyte has achieved measurable concentrations to give a positive result (ie, the window period), and the type of specimen (eg, whole blood or oral mucosal transudate) being analyzed. Acute HIV infection (ie, the period from infection to seroconversion) is difficult to detect with CLIA-waived POC tests because HIV antibody titers are typically low in this stage of HIV infection. Thus, these tests have lower sensitivity than the nonwaived laboratory-based ELISAs and automated systems for detecting seroconversion.[67] This means the window period may be longer for CLIA-waived POC tests for HIV compared with a nonwaived test performed in a laboratory. According to the CDC, laboratory-based antigen/antibody tests can detect HIV infection from venous blood within 18 to 45 days postexposure; the CLIA-waived POC counterpart does so within 18 to 90 days.[68] Tests using oral mucosal transudate are highly accurate but have even lower sensitivity for detecting seroconversion than those using serum, plasma from venous blood, or whole blood from a finger stick because the antibody concentration found in oral mucosal transudate is lower.[69,70] Thus, CLIA-waived POC tests that measure HIV antibody in oral mucosal transudate often fail to detect acute HIV.[67,70] By measuring p24 antigen in addition to antibodies for HIV-1 and HIV-2, the marketed combination CLIA-waived POC test should allow for the detection of acute infection.[71] However, to date, the test does not detect p24 antigen with a high sensitivity; thus its accuracy for detecting acute infection is poor as well.[72,73] In addition to stage of infection, HIV prevalence in the population being tested can impact the oral tests.[69] In high-prevalence settings, the PPVs for either whole blood or oral mucosal transudate are similar; however, in low-prevalence settings, PPVs are much higher for whole blood than oral mucosal transudate specimens.[70] CLIA-waived POC HIV testing will involve an initial HIV test and, if it is reactive, a follow-up HIV test in a moderate to high complexity laboratory. A negative test result in someone after a potential HIV exposure should be repeated after the window period, approximately 12 weeks after the potential exposure.[68]

## Influenza A and B

### Use in Pharmacy

The annual burden of influenza in the United States fluctuates markedly depending on a variety of variables. According to CDC estimates, each year since 2010, influenza infects between 9 and 45 million individuals and results in 140,000 to 810,000 hospitalizations and up to 61,000 deaths.[74] Influenza occurs seasonally and produces symptoms that are often indistinguishable from bacterial respiratory infections. Moreover, the prompt initiation of appropriate cost-effective antiviral therapy is key to hastening the resolution of the infection and limiting its severity.

Using CLIA-waived POC tests to screen for influenza represents a collaborative opportunity for pharmacy and local health departments to improve data sharing that informs disease surveillance efforts.[75] In some cases, such efforts can be combined with technological solutions to improve vaccine and antiviral distribution and perhaps even curtail inappropriate antibacterial use. In addition, POCT for influenza can assist with efforts to distinguish between influenza and COVID-19.

### Determining Appropriate Testing Candidates

The CDC has published useful algorithms to guide interpretation of CLIA-waived POC tests for influenza and clinical decision-making when influenza activity in the community is high (https://www.cdc.gov/flu/professionals/diagnosis /algorithm-results-circulating.htm) or low (https://www .cdc.gov/flu/professionals/diagnosis/algorithm-results-not -circulating.htm).[76] To determine if a patient is an appropriate candidate for testing, pharmacists should perform an appropriate physical assessment to determine if the patient has symptoms consistent with an acute respiratory disease that began within several days of patient presentation. Accordingly, CLIA-waived POCT for influenza should be performed using a highly sensitive and specific test during the influenza season when the disease prevalence is high.[76] Pharmacy researchers developed a physician–pharmacist collaborative management model for influenza based largely on the CDC principles.[77] In that model, pharmacists in a community practice setting provided CLIA-waived POCT services for influenza by screening adult patients for symptoms of an influenza-like illness and using proper nasal swab specimen collection technique to obtain a sample.[77]

The PPV of the tests was maximized by performing these activities only when local influenza activity had been documented by state or federal surveillance and by performing a physical assessment and assessing vital signs (eg, heart rate, blood pressure, respiratory rate, temperature, and oxygen saturation).[77] Only 11% of patients with an influenza-like illness had a positive result. Moreover, because the CPA prevented pharmacists from dispensing oseltamivir or antibacterial therapy to patients who tested negative, the study demonstrated that this practice model can lead to rational use of antivirals and avoid the overuse of unnecessary antimicrobial therapy.[77]

To determine whether influenza is present in a specific patient population and assist providers in diagnosing and treating acute respiratory illnesses, the CDC also recommends that CLIA-waived POCT be done during an acute outbreak of a respiratory disease and in patients with clinical signs and symptoms of influenza during the influenza season.[76]

### Application of Influenza A and B Point-of-Care Testing in Practice

Studies demonstrate that protocol driven CLIA-waived POCT for influenza using antigen or molecular tests can be successfully implemented in the outpatient setting, particularly in community pharmacies.[77-80] These services increase access to care outside of normal clinic hours for patients regardless of their insurance status or whether they have a primary care provider.[77-80] In addition, such services provide patients appropriate therapy without promoting the overuse of antibiotics.[78] By offering CLIA-waived POCT services for influenza in the outpatient setting, pharmacists can also collaborate with public health agencies to improve seasonal surveillance efforts and reduce inappropriate antibacterial use in respiratory illnesses during the influenza season.[2,75,81]

### Performance Characteristics

The results of antigen or molecular CLIA-waived POC tests for influenza depend on viral load, which is influenced by several variables, including patient age and the timing of sample collection relative to symptom onset. Pharmacists should recognize that viral loads are higher in samples obtained from infected children than those obtained from infected adults. Thus, when evaluating literature to select a test with appropriate performance data for their patients, pharmacists should be aware that performance data are typically better when the tests are performed using samples from infected children than samples from infected adults.[19] In addition, viral shedding peaks 24 to 72 hours after symptoms begin. This time interval represents the ideal window to achieve optimal test performance. Therefore, when assessing whether a patient is an appropriate test candidate, pharmacists should establish when symptom onset began. Other variables that pharmacists cannot mitigate that influence viral load (and therefore may affect test performance) include the viral strain, materials used to collect the sample, type of specimen, and, in the case of antigen tests, the volume of viral transport media used in test.[19] In addition, regardless of method, the performance characteristics of these tests can be affected by annual genomic drifts or a shift when it occurs.[82,83]

Historically, CLIA-waived POC tests for influenza virus nucleoprotein antigen have been chromatographic lateral flow immunoassays. Such tests often lacked sensitivity for a variety of reasons, including being based upon immunochromatographic methodology that did not amplify the target antigen and relying on visual detection.[19] However, since 2015, several technological and regulatory developments have led to improvements in the sensitivity of CLIA-waived POC tests for influenza in general. First, with the advent of isothermal nucleic acid amplification methods that enable rapid detection of DNA/RNA, the first molecular test for influenza was authorized by the FDA in 2015.[84] Then, in 2017, the FDA reclassified these tests from class I to class II devices.[85] This reclassification enabled the FDA to impose more rigorous performance thresholds for the antigen tests in 2018. According to the new thresholds, existing and new antigen tests must achieve sensitivity of at least 80% compared with a molecular test and 80% to 90% when compared with viral culture.[85] Tests that could not meet the performance standards are no longer available in the United States.

The performance characteristics of marketed antigen and molecular CLIA-waived POC influenza tests are summarized in **Table 4-3**. The antigen CLIA-waived POC influenza tests are simple to use and provide results within 15 minutes. The tests differ in terms of simple sample processing prior to test, incubation and run times, and throughput capacity.[86] Most tests now use automated, rather than visual, detection to improve sensitivity and performance to meet the FDA thresholds. As stated previously, antigen tests have lower sensitivities to detect influenza viruses in respiratory specimens than molecular tests.[82,83] Thus, negative results of antigen CLIA-waived POC influenza tests should not be used to exclude a diagnosis of influenza.[82,83] For this reason, the Infectious Diseases Society of America (IDSA) recommends the use of molecular CLIA-waived POC influenza tests rather than antigen CLIA-waived POC influenza tests for the detection of influenza viruses in respiratory specimens of outpatients.

Molecular CLIA-waived POC influenza tests use different amplification methods, including isothermic nucleic acid amplification, RT-PCR, and one that uses RT-PCR followed by hybridization to allow for qualitative to be read visually.[19] Unlike antigen CLIA-waived POC influenza tests, molecular tests use samples that require no manipulation (ie, addition of buffers). Molecular tests produce results within 15 to 30 minutes depending on the amplification method. In general, sensitivities of available molecular CLIA-waived POC tests range from 66% to 100%.[82]

# Group A Streptococci
## Use in Pharmacy

Pharmacists can use POC tests for GAS to assist in the acute management of infected patients.[78-80,87-89] GAS causes 5% to 10% of adult acute pharyngitis and 15% to 30% of acute pharyngitis among children.[90] Epidemiologically, GAS pharyngitis occurs primarily in the winter and early spring and afflicts individuals in a narrow age range. Clinically, GAS pharyngitis has a well-recognized presentation and rarely requires confirmation by culture, but its symptoms are often indistinguishable from viral respiratory tract infections. Data from the United States, Canada, and the United Kingdom demonstrate that CLIA-waived POC tests for GAS improve access to care and help ensure that appropriate antibiotic therapy is initiated if warranted, which could hasten infection resolution by 1 to 2 days.[78-80,87-89]

## Determining Appropriate Testing Candidates

GAS is the most common bacterial cause of acute sore throat, but it is difficult to accurately diagnose it as a cause of pharyngitis.[91] On the basis of clinical manifestations alone, GAS pharyngitis is often indistinguishable from viral respiratory tract infections.[91,92] In contrast, to adults, GAS pharyngitis is more common than viral etiologies among children and adolescents (**Minicase 2**). Therefore, to aid in the identification of patients with pharyngitis who have a high likelihood of GAS infection, additional strategies are needed. Performing an appropriate physical exam and applying its results using a validated, age-based clinical prediction rule, such as the Modified Centor Criteria Score, can further assist in identifying patients with pharyngitis who would benefit most from CLIA-waived POCT for GAS.[93] Originally developed in 1981, the Modified Centor Criteria Score was based on the presence of tonsillar exudates, swollen tender anterior cervical nodes, fever, and the lack of cough and was used to estimate the probability of acute GAS pharyngitis in adults with a sore throat.[93] The score was later modified by adding age to the criteria and validated in a large study of adults and children.[94] The Modified Centor Criteria Score ranges from −1 to 5, with testing for GAS recommended in patients with a score of 2 or higher.[92] However, even when using this clinical prediction rule, there is limited success in accurately diagnosing GAS pharyngitis because at the highest Modified Centor Criteria Scores (eg, ≥4), it only helps identify 53% of patients with GAS pharyngitis.[91-95] The Modified Centor Criteria and their interpretation are summarized in **Table 4-4**. In a pilot study, pharmacy researchers developed a physician–pharmacist collaborative management model for GAS based largely on these principles.[87] In that model, pharmacists in a community practice setting used the Modified Centor Criteria to screen 316 patients, of whom 273 were eligible for testing. Only 48 patients (17.5%) had a positive test result and received amoxicillin or azithromycin per their CPA. This pilot project demonstrated that such a practice model can dramatically reduce inappropriate antimicrobial use in the community practice setting.[87] Like influenza, these results were validated by several studies, including one that used a molecular test, in a variety of community pharmacy settings, in multiple states, and several countries.[78-80,87-89]

## Application of Group A Streptococci Point-of-Care in Practice

Performance characteristics of current CLIA-waived POC tests for GAS are sufficiently robust: the current guidelines do not recommend any additional confirmatory tests for adults when results are negative. Although confirmatory testing is currently recommended when CLIA-waived POC test results are negative in children and adolescents, data suggest that such follow-up testing may not be necessary.[91,96]

**TABLE 4-3.** Summary of Performance Characteristics for CLIA-Waived POC Tests for Influenza A and/or B[a,b]

| TEST (MANUFACTURER) | SPECIMEN TYPE | TIME TO RESULTS (MIN) | OVERALL CLINICAL SENSITIVITY (%) A/B | OVERALL CLINICAL SPECIFICITY (%) A/B | PPV (%) A/B | NPV (%) A/B | OVERALL ACCURACY (%) A/B |
|---|---|---|---|---|---|---|---|
| **Antigen-Based Tests** | | | | | | | |
| BD Veritor System for Rapid Detection of Flu A+B (Becton Dickinson)[c] | NPS | 10 | 81.3/77.8[f] | 95.6/100[g] | 89.7/100[h] | 91.7/99.0[h] | 91/99[h] |
| BinaxNOW Influenza A&B Card with Digival 2 (Abbott Laboratories) | NS, NPS | 15 | 84.3/89.5[i] | 94.7/99.4[i] | 83/94.4 | 95.1/98.9[i] | 92.2/98.2[i] |
| QuickVue Influenza A+B Test (Quidel Corporation)[d] | NS, NPS | ≤10 | 81.5/80.9[f,i] | 97.8/99.1[g,i] | 90/89.9[h,i] | 95.6/98.0[h,i] | 94.5/97.3[h,i] |
| Sofia Influenza A+B (Quidel Corporation)[c,e] | NS, NPS | 3–15 | NS 90/89 / NPS 97/90 | NS 95/96 / NPS 95/97 | NS[h] 82/81 / NPS[h] 75/84 | NS[h] 97/98 / NPS[h] 99/98 | NS[h] 94/95 / NPS[h] 95/96 |
| Acucy Influenza A&B Test (Sekisui Diagnostics, LLC) | NPS, NS | 15 | 96.4/82.3[i] | 96.0/98.1[i] | 87.4/89.0[i] | 77.7/84.2[h,i] | 96.1/95.6[h,i] |
| **Molecular Tests[j]** | | | | | | | |
| ID NOW Influenza A & B 2 (Abbott) | NPS, NS | <15 | 92.8/100[i] | 98.5/97.7 | 95.3/81.5[h,i] | 97.6/100[h,j] | 97.0//97.9[h,i] |
| Xpert Xpress Flu (Cephid) | NPS, NS | 20–30 | NS 98.9/98.4 / NPS 97.6/97.3 | NS 97.6/99.3 / NPS 98.2/99.6 | Data not provided | | |
| AcculaTM Flu (Mesa Biotech) | NS | <30 | 97/94 | 94/99 | 83/90 | 76.3/89.3 | 95/98 |
| Cobas RInfluenza A/B Assay (Roche) | NPS | <30 | 100/100 | 96.8/94.1 | Data not provided | | |
| Silaris Influenza A/B (Sekisui Diagnostics, LLC) | NS | <30 | 97/94 | 94/99 | 82/90 | 99/99 | 94.5/98.2 |

A = influenza virus A; B = influenza virus B; NPS = nasopharyngeal swab; NS = nasal swab.
[a]Values obtained from product package inserts and/or from manufacturers websites.
[b]Data for nasal aspirate/nasal wash not included.
[c]Requires separate analyzer or reader device.
[d]Does not distinguish between influenza A and B virus infections when used alone.
[e]Immunofluorescence assay.
[f]Values represent positive percent agreement.
[g]Values represent negative percent agreement.
[h]Values taken from 2 × 2 table of results in package insert.
[i]Clinical study included both specimen types.
[j]Includes only tests that detect influenza A and/or B, not other respiratory pathogens.

## MINICASE 2

## Group A Streptococcal Pharyngitis and Point-of-Care Testing

Maya B., a 10-year-old girl, presents to the community pharmacy in November with her mother. The mother states that Maya B. reported a sore throat, mild cough, and headache after attending a slumber party 2 days earlier. In addition, one of the other girls attending the slumber party tested positive for GAS yesterday. Maya B.'s physical findings include a red throat and tender cervical lymph nodes.

QUESTION: What additional information should the pharmacist obtain to determine if CLIA-waived POCT for GAS would be appropriate in this patient?

DISCUSSION: The pharmacist should obtain vital signs and calculate a Modified Centor Criteria Score as part of the CPA to determine the likelihood of GAS pharyngitis.

Maya's vital signs are as follows: BP 120/70 mm Hg, HR 80 beats/min, RR 20 breaths/min, temperature 101°F, and weight 90 lb.

| Modified Centor Criteria Score[92-95] | Patient's Calculated Score |
|---|---|
| • Absence of cough (+1) | • (0) |
| • Swollen and tender anterior cervical lymph nodes (+1) | • (+1) |
| • Temperature >100.4°F (+1) | • (+1) |
| • Tonsillar exudate or swelling (+1) | • (0) |
| • Age (years):<br>  3 to 14 (+1)<br>  15 to 44 (0)<br>  >45 (–1) | • (+1)<br>• Score = 3; probability of GAS ~28% to 35% |

QUESTION: Based on the pharmacist's findings, how should the pharmacist proceed under CPA?

DISCUSSION: The pharmacist should perform a throat swab and CLIA-waived POCT to verify the presence of GAS. The recommended management of GAS according to the patient's Modified Centor Criteria score would be antibiotics based on the result of the CLIA-waived POC test. In addition, the pharmacist should recommend an analgesic/antipyretic for symptom management.

### Performance Characteristics

CLIA-waived POC tests that detect GAS antigens have been marketed for years and have evolved and improved through several generations. The tests use a variety of antigen detection methods (eg, latex agglutination, ELISAs, lateral flow immunochromatographic assays, and optical immunoassays). In addition, several molecular methods to detect GAS exist that use either rt-PCR or isothermal nucleic acid amplification are now CLIA-waived. The use of antigen POC tests is addressed in the IDSA guideline for the diagnosis and management of GAS pharyngitis.[96] However, the guideline was published before the advent of the CLIA-waived molecular tests, so their use is not addressed. The antigen CLIA-waived POC tests for GAS infection have limited sensitivity; therefore, the IDSA guideline recommends confirming negative results in populations at high risk of developing pharyngitis because of GAS or viral etiologies with a throat culture to reduce the chance of missing a positive case.[96] The specificity associated with CLIA-waived antigen POC tests for GAS infection is high; therefore, positive results do not require a backup culture in a patient, regardless of age.[96] A comprehensive meta-analysis of 48 studies found that sensitivity and specificity across all studies analyzed were 86% and 96%, respectively.[91] Investigators also found that although there was marked variability in sensitivity, specificity varied little across studies.[91] In contrast to the IDSA guideline, overall, the study demonstrated that the sensitivity of POC tests for GAS is sufficiently high and a backup culture is not needed, particularly given the low risk of complications such as acute rheumatic fever

in the United States.[91] Moreover, investigators concluded that the high overall specificity of POC tests for GAS could minimize the overdiagnosis of GAS pharyngitis and prevent unnecessary antibiotic use in such cases.[91] Molecular CLIA-waived POC tests for GAS have much higher sensitivity than the antigen-based tests, which lowers the chance of missing a positive case.[96]

## COVID-19

### Use in Pharmacy

Discovered in late 2019, the novel SARS-CoV-2 is associated with a constellation of mild to life-threatening symptoms, known as COVID-19, and has rapidly spread as a worldwide pandemic. Early in the course of the pandemic, using the EUA provisions, the FDA commissioner accelerated the marketing of POC tests to detect SARS-CoV-2 (COVID-19 POC tests). Shortly thereafter, the Department of Health and Human Services issued a policy permitting licensed pharmacists to order and administer FDA-authorized COVID-19 POC tests.[97] This policy illustrates the important role pharmacists performing POCT can have in providing services that contribute to the health and well-being of their community. The policy extended the legal protections under the Public Readiness and Emergency Preparedness Act to pharmacists performing COVID-19 POC tests so they could collect nasopharyngeal, throat, or nasal swabs from patients with suspected infection and perform assays that have EUA.[97] By leveraging the accessibility of pharmacists, the policy sought to expand the nation's testing capacity, so that if necessary, public

**TABLE 4-4.** Modified Centor Score Criteria and Interpretation[88-91]

| | | TOTAL SCORE | RISK OF GAS INFECTION (%) |
|---|---|---|---|
| • Absence of cough (+1) | | ≥4 | 51–53 |
| • Swollen and tender anterior cervical lymph nodes (+1) | | 3 | 28–35 |
| • Temperature >100.4°F (+1) | | 2 | 11–17 |
| • Tonsillar exudate or swelling (+1) | | 1 | 5–10 |
| • Age (yr): 3–14 (+1) 15–44 (0) ≥45 (–1) | | ≤0 | 1–2.5 |

health mitigation strategies, including contact tracing and isolation, could be employed. Under the policy, pharmacists can also perform FDA-authorized serological COVID-19 tests. However, for a pharmacist to perform a serological COVID-19 test marketed under an EUA, it would need to be CLIA-waived. Such tests that are not CLIA-waived or lack a CLIA classification are considered moderate- or high-complexity tests and are not allowed to be performed outside an appropriately CLIA-certified laboratory.[98] Thus, pharmacists' POCT efforts for COVID-19 entail testing patients for active infection using molecular or antigen-based tests so that they may be linked to care or public health professionals.

### Determining Appropriate Testing Candidates

Decisions regarding who qualifies for testing rest with state and local health departments or healthcare providers. Individuals are encouraged to visit their state or local health department's website for the latest local information on testing in their locale.

### Application of COVID-19 Point-of-Care Testing in Practice

Many antigen or molecular COVID-19 POC tests have been marketed under an EUA, but not all of them are considered waived. Antigen or molecular tests have a variety of uses. They are recommended for diagnosis of acute infection in persons with signs or symptoms of infection.[99] To control transmission, testing is performed with antigen or molecular tests in asymptomatic individuals with recent known or suspected exposure to SARS-CoV-2.[99] In addition, such tests are used for asymptomatic individuals without known or suspected exposure to SARS-CoV-2 to assist in early detection in institutional settings.[99] Antigen and molecular tests are also used to detect the resolution of infection to determine when individuals can end isolation.[99] Lastly, antigen or molecular tests can be used in public health surveillance efforts for SARS-CoV-2.[99]

Serological COVID-19 tests have also been marketed under an EUA, but to date, all but one of them are considered moderate- or high-complexity tests and are not allowed to be performed outside an appropriately CLIA-certified laboratory. These tests are not authorized for diagnosis of COVID-19; rather they are recommended for situations in which it is necessary to determine whether the individual being tested was previously infected.

### Performance Characteristics

Having EUA status means tests can be used in the declared emergency, but the FDA has not thoroughly evaluated them to grant approval. Gaining FDA EUA status requires minimal performance data, and at the time of authorization, typically tests only have data regarding limits of detection from contrived samples. As experience is gained with tests during the evolving pandemic, emerging clinical data, often from small samples, provide estimates of their negative percent agreement and positive percent agreement (ie, specificity and sensitivity, respectively) as well as their NPV and PPV. Initial data contained in the package inserts of the individual tests suggest the specificity COVID-19 that could be performed outside an appropriately CLIA-certified laboratory are similar (98.8% to 98.9%), regardless of the type (eg, antigen, molecular, or serological) test.[100-110] In addition, the overall sensitivity of such tests is high (93.9% to 100%).[100-110] However, though high, the sensitivity of antigen tests varies by test (84% to 98%) and appears to be slightly less sensitive (mean 93.9%) than molecular (99.5%) or serological (100%) tests.[100-110] These initial findings are consistent with other POC tests for respiratory viruses in that molecular tests are typically highly specific and more sensitive than antigen tests. Like other respiratory viruses, the performance characteristics such as NPV and PPV of these tests will likely be influenced by viral load, when and how viral shedding occurs, patient characteristics, and sample type. The effects of annual genomic drifts or a shift should it occur on these tests is unknown.

## GOOD LABORATORY PRACTICES

To provide consistency in the patient care process, it is vital to develop appropriate policies and procedures specific to each CLIA-waived POC test to optimize the ability of the test to produce results that aid in chronic disease state management or detect the analyte of interest without overtesting. For CLIA-waived POC tests in chronic disease state management, pharmacists should specify the frequency of testing as part of the patient-specific care plan in accordance with relevant national clinical guidelines. In addition, frequency of monitoring should be driven by the patient's disease progression and achievement of treatment goals. Although CLIA-waived tests are determined to be simple for the user, it is necessary for a pharmacist to be properly trained on each CLIA-waived device and for the laboratory to follow "good laboratory practices" for waived testing sites per CDC guidelines.[5] These practices include steps that should be taken before initiating or expanding CLIA-waived POCT services and include actions taken during and after the actual performance of test (**Figure 4-1**).[5]

## Before Initiating Services (Preparation Phase)

Recommended practices prior to initiating POCT services involve regulatory, logistic, procedural, and personnel considerations. An initial step toward initiating CLIA-waived POCT services is to identify a qualified individual who will be responsible and accountable for testing operations.[5,9] As described previously, some states have additional requirements that must be met to fulfill this role. Individuals leading and working in a waived laboratory must be familiar with local, state, and federal regulatory requirements. In addition to the CLIA requirements and state pharmacy practice acts, practitioners need to be familiar with state and local regulations governing laboratory operations, federal laws governing privacy (eg, Health Insurance Portability and Accountability Act), Occupational Safety and Health Administration (OSHA) work place safety standards (eg, OSHA standards related to workplace hazards and bloodborne pathogens standards), and information from the CDC and CLSI regarding biosafety and precautions for preventing the transmission of bloodborne pathogens in the workplace.[5,9] Having familiarity with these regulations and resources will help ensure that any CLIA-waived POCT services protect patient confidentiality and are safe for both the patient and testing personnel.[5]

Many factors must be considered prior to initiating services to create a testing space that meets the needs of the practice setting, employees, patients, and the environmental requirements specified in the test manufacturers' package insert. Additional considerations that are addressed include a fiscal assessment of the proposed POCT services and an analysis of offered tests so that all factors required to properly conduct the test(s) of interest can be determined (eg, advantages and disadvantages of the available devices, any additional equipment, and access to ancillary care services).[5]

Developing written policies and procedures that clearly outline the responsibilities and testing instructions for testing personnel and facility directors is a critical process that must occur before testing begins. Procedures should be based on the manufacturer's instructions and be used to train testing personnel.[5] In addition to test performance, the policies and procedures should outline and standardize specimen collection techniques, QC procedures, proper handling and storage of tests and reagents, and documenting and reporting results.[5]

Testing personnel are a critical component to any CLIA-waived POCT service. Because personnel at waived testing sites are not subject to proficiency testing, it is essential that they be trained by a qualified person and be competent in any test they will perform before performing the test.[5] Training should include an observed performance of the trainee performing the test. Many training resources are available through test manufacturers and distributors, professional organizations, and governmental agencies. Training should be documented and reviewed on a regular basis to ensure that all updates or changes are noted. Although proficiency testing is not mandated, including such assessments is recommended as part of any quality assurance program.[5]

## Test Ordering and Sample Collection (Preanalytical Phase)

Considering all aspects in the planning phase helps ensure personnel have the resources, understanding, and skills needed to perform a CLIA-waived POC test properly during the preanalytical phase. Good laboratory practices in this phase include confirming the test has been properly ordered, identifying the patient, labeling the sample collection device to avoid any confusion with other patients, providing the patient with pretest education or information, reviewing the complete test procedure, and preparing the test area and materials.[5]

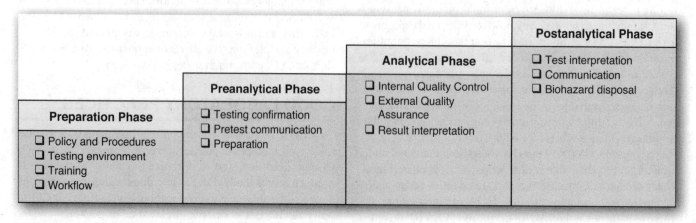

**FIGURE 4-1.** Steps of Good Laboratory Practices

## During Testing (Analytical Phase)

Good laboratory practices in the analytical phase involve QC, test performance, and result interpretation and documentation.[5] The QC measures are important to ensure proper training of the user's technique, the integrity of the testing device, and the overall performance of the POCT analytical device. It is a process that consists of two components: internal QC and external QA. Internal QC requires the analysis of manufacturer-provided QC materials. These materials are imbedded in the test in known concentrations and produce a result that indicates whether the analytical method and the reading device are functioning properly. The purpose of internal QC is to monitor the precision and function of the analytical method over time. In contrast, external QA monitors the testing process from specimen application to result interpretation. External QA requires analyzing patient-like samples comprised of liquid or other materials similar to patient specimens provided by the manufacturer or purchased separately. These patient-like samples can be run before or concurrent with patient samples, and their results are compared across testing personnel to monitor the accuracy of reporting. QC test results should be documented, and any action taken in response to QC tests should be recorded. The CLIA-waived laboratory director should incorporate a QC plan in the site's policy and procedures.[5] The POC test and device manufacturer provides QC materials, which often include internal and external controls. A test site should determine QC testing frequency that fits its operations for each test system, but at a minimum, QC testing should be performed as often as the product insert recommends.[5]

Each CLIA-waived POC test and device can require different techniques for acquiring or testing a sample. Therefore, CLIA requirements stipulate that when personnel perform the tests, they must strictly adhere to the manufacturer's guidelines and follow specific storage conditions for the test and test materials (eg, testing strips, cartridges, cassettes, and reagent). Temperature and humidity may also be critical factors in providing a successful test result. The CLIA-waived POC test results should be interpreted within the manufacturer's specified time period, and the test should be repeated if the results conflict with the available clinical information or are invalid.[5] Once valid test results are obtained, they should be documented according to established policy and procedures in a timely fashion.

## After Testing (Postanalytical Phase)

Good laboratory practices in the postanalytical phase involve issuing test reports, performing supplemental or confirmatory testing, testing area cleanup, disposing biohazard waste, and documenting testing activities. The pharmacist's appropriate interpretation of the test results is a critical part of the postanalytical phase, along with communicating the results to the patient and provider. The pharmacist's discussion of a laboratory result with the patient should be well planned and considerate of the patient's response. When a pharmacist encounters a test result that requires follow-up with a physician for further evaluation, it is important to communicate with the patient's physician and have referral resources ready and available as needed. In some cases, good laboratory practices and state or local statutes mandate that test results for certain infectious diseases also be reported to local or state public health agencies.[5] For all postanalytical phase activities, the testing site should have specific policies and procedures clearly defined and in place.

# LIMITATIONS OF POINT-OF-CARE TESTING

## Legal and Regulatory Barriers to Pharmacists Performing Clinical Laboratory Improvement Amendments–Waived Point-of-Care Tests

Under CLIA requirements, there are no minimum educational or training requirements needed for the director or testing personnel.[3,5] Therefore, in nearly all states, pharmacists can serve in either of these roles and perform a CLIA-waived POC test. However, the ability of pharmacists to use the result of a CLIA-waived POC test to make a therapeutic decision for the management of chronic diseases or acute infections falls under the scope of practice, which is regulated by state agencies and boards of pharmacy.[2] However, studies have identified that legislative and regulatory variability across states may produce confusion among practitioners and represent a barrier to pharmacists' efforts to perform POCT.[2,111] Although performing CLIA-waived POCT may not be explicitly addressed in many pharmacy practice acts, such activities may be permissible under CPA/CDTM agreement provisions in state regulations or statutes.[2] A few states, however, still do not have these provisions in their pharmacy practice acts. There is variability across states with CPA/CDTM agreement provisions in terms of specificity, scope, and structure.[2] For example, some states restrict CPAs/CDTM agreements to written agreements for individual patients, whereby pharmacists can treat a patient for the condition specified in the protocol only if they have advanced authorization from the patient's primary care provider. Such an approach poses a challenge for patients who do not have a primary care provider.[81]

## Lack of Training/Education

According to their classification, CLIA-waived POC tests are simple to perform with low risk for erroneous results or harm to patients if they are performed incorrectly.[3] However, they are not error proof; CLIA regulations explicitly stipulate that individuals who perform the tests must strictly adhere to the manufacturer's instructions.[3] Although CDC and CMS studies indicate that waived laboratories (including pharmacies) generally perform testing correctly, the results of the agencies' surveys also highlight the need for additional education and training for site directors and testing personnel.[5] Because CLIA requirements do not specify any level of education for directors or testing personnel in waived laboratories, lack of education regarding CLIA-waived testing is a gap that exists across all healthcare professional education.[5] Two national surveys of academic pharmacy suggest that education on CLIA-waived POC tests for infectious diseases is generally lacking from professional pharmacy degree programs.[112,113] This is an opportunity for the expansion of core curricula that would enhance pharmacists' participation in POCT services. Training for pharmacists is available through an accredited national certificate training program offered by a national pharmacy professional organization that is designed for community pharmacists to implement testing programs for influenza, GAS, HIV, and HCV.[114] Data suggest that the program can help improve training and expand POCT services.[115]

## Overtesting

Overtesting is a concern with CLIA-waived POC tests for infectious diseases because they are qualitative and detect seasonal pathogens that produce infections with nonspecific symptoms (eg, GAS and influenza) or produce infections that are most prevalent in specific high-risk populations (eg, HIV and HCV); therefore, overtesting is a concern. To optimize the ability of the test to detect the analyte of interest and avoid overtesting, pharmacists should develop practices that enable them to distinguish patients who could benefit from testing. Because low disease prevalence can negatively impact the PPV of qualitative tests, pharmacists can optimize test performance and minimize overtesting by performing relevant physical assessments and gathering additional information to identify those in need of testing. Taking such steps will also enable them to make referrals to physicians for follow-up or make immediate referrals to emergency medical care.

## FUTURE APPLICATIONS FOR CLINICAL LABORATORY IMPROVEMENT AMENDMENTS–WAIVED POINT-OF-CARE TESTS IN OUTPATIENT PHARMACY PRACTICE SETTINGS

With continued transformations in the delivery of healthcare in the United States and advances in technology, there will likely be many more innovative applications of CLIA-waived POC tests for chronic disease state and infectious diseases in outpatient pharmacy practice settings. The growing shortage of primary care providers will lead to an increasing role of pharmacists performing CLIA-waived POC test to screen for and manage chronic diseases. Scientific advances in genetic testing and molecular diagnostics will increase the POC tests on the market. The potential to perform POC pharmacogenomic testing will enable pharmacists to help guide and select therapies based on a patient's genetic make-up, limiting side effects and increasing efficacy. The development of new molecular-based CLIA-waived POC tests or improved current antibody/antigen-based tests may make it more practical to test infectious disease analytes of public health interest (eg, tuberculosis and pathogens responsible for sexually transmitted infections). In addition, in cases such as sexually transmitted infections, molecular-based CLIA-waived POC tests could allow a pharmacist working under a CPA/CDTM agreement to institute prompt therapy under protocol. Adapting to these changes will be vital for pharmacists

to develop workflow processes and financial models to sustain CLIA-waived POCT.

Ongoing reforms to the U.S. healthcare delivery system will continue to raise awareness of pharmacists as ready access points to the healthcare system. To fully realize this potential for POCT services in outpatient pharmacy practice settings, local, state, and federal regulations governing pharmacy practice must continue to evolve so pharmacists can practice to their fullest professional potential. Technological advances in health informatics will ultimately enable the pharmacist to have access to electronic medical records (EMRs) regardless of practice setting. Similarly, pharmacists will transmit CLIA-waived POCT results to a patient's EMRs, their primary provider, and other relevant public health agencies.

## LEARNING POINTS

1. **How have the CLIA-88 created opportunities for pharmacists in outpatient settings?**

   **ANSWER:** Technology has allowed many laboratory tests useful in the detection and management of chronic diseases and infections to be simplified and classified as CLIA-waived. CLIA-waived POCT represents an opportunity for pharmacists in outpatient settings to expand their patient care services.

2. **What must pharmacists know to properly perform CLIA-waived tests in their practice settings?**

   **ANSWER:** To properly perform a CLIA-waived test in outpatient settings, pharmacists must understand the basis of the test, how to handle specimens, and how to perform the test. They must also understand all relevant state and federal regulations related to performing such tests and reporting the results.

3. **What must pharmacists know to provide useful POCT services in their practice settings?**

   **ANSWER:** To provide useful POCT services, pharmacists must understand how to identify patients who would benefit from testing. In addition, they must understand how to evaluate the various performance characteristics and the limitations of the test.

## REFERENCES

1. Giberson S, Yoder S, Lee MP. *Improving Patient and Health System Outcomes Through Advanced Pharmacy Practice. A Report to the US Surgeon General.* Washington, DC: US Public Health Service Office of the Chief Pharmacist; 2011.

2. Gubbins PO, Klepser ME, Dering-Anderson AM, et al. Point-of-care testing for infectious diseases: opportunities, barriers, and considerations in community pharmacy. *J Am Pharm Assoc (2003).* 2014;54(2):163-171. PubMed

3. Clinical Laboratory Improvement Amendments of 1988. 42 U.S.C. 263a PL100-578.

4. U.S. Food and Drug Administation. Emergency use authorization. https://www.fda.gov/emergency-preparedness-and-response/mcm-legal-regulatory-and-policy-framework/emergency-use-authorization. Accessed June 26, 2020.

5. Howerton D, Anderson N, Bosse D, et al. Good laboratory practices for waived testing sites: survey findings from testing sites holding a certificate of waiver under the clinical laboratory improvement amendments of 1988 and recommendations for promoting quality testing. *MMWR Recomm Rep.* 2005;54(RR-13):1-25, quiz CE1-CE4.PubMed

6. Centers for Disease Control and Prevention. To test or not to test: considerations for waived testing. https://www.cdc.gov/clia/Resources /WaivedTests/pdf/15_255581-B_WaivedTestingBooklet_508Final.pdf. Accessed June 1, 2020.

7. Lalkhen AG, McCluskey A. Clinical tests: sensitivity and specificity. *Contin Educ Anaesth Crit Care Pain.* 2008;8:221-223.

8. US Department of Health and Human Services, US Food and Drug Administration. Statistical guidance on reporting results from studies evaluating diagnostic tests. Published March 2007. https://www.fda.gov /regulatory-information/search-fda-guidance-documents/statistical -guidance-reporting-results-studies-evaluating-diagnostic-tests -guidance-industry-and-fda. Accessed September 11, 2020.

9. American College of Physicians. Center for Practice Improvement & Innovation and Medical Laboratory Evaluation Program. Waived testing: doing it right. www.acponline.org/system/files/documents/running _practice/mle/waived-testing-doing-it-right.pdf. Accessed June 23, 2020.

10. Young PE, Diaz GJ, Kalariya RN, et al. Comparison of the time required for manual (visually read) and semi-automated POCT urinalysis and pregnancy testing with associated electronic medical record (EMR) transcription errors. *Clin Chim Acta.* 2020;504:60-63.PubMed

11. McTaggart MP, Price CP, Pinnock RG, et al. The diagnostic accuracy of a urine albumin-creatinine ratio point-of-care test for detection of albuminuria in primary care. *Am J Kidney Dis.* 2012;60(5):787-794. PubMed

12. Pernille H, Lars B, Marjukka M, et al. Sampling of urine for diagnosing urinary tract infection in general practice: first-void or mid-stream urine? *Scand J Prim Health Care.* 2019;37(1):113-119.PubMed

13. Wu HY, Peng YS, Chiang CK, et al. Diagnostic performance of random urine samples using albumin concentration vs ratio of albumin to creatinine for microalbuminuria screening in patients with diabetes mellitus: a systematic review and meta-analysis. *JAMA Intern Med.* 2014;174(7):1108-1115.PubMed

14. Kim C, Ahmed JA, Eidex RB, et al. Comparison of nasopharyngeal and oropharyngeal swabs for the diagnosis of eight respiratory viruses by real-time reverse transcription-PCR assays. *PLoS One.* 2011;6(6):e21610. PubMed

15. Dawood FS, Jara J, Estripeaut D, et al. What is the added benefit of oropharyngeal swabs compared with nasal swabs alone for respiratory virus detection in hospitalized children aged <10 years? *J Infect Dis.* 2015;212(10):1600-1603.PubMed

16. Branson BM, Handsfield HH, Lampe MA, et al. Revised recommenda-tions for HIV testing of adults, adolescents, and pregnant women in health-care settings. *MMWR Recomm Rep.* 2006;55(RR-14):1-17, quiz CE1-CE4.PubMed

17. Dong BJ, Lopez M, Cocohoba J. Pharmacists performing hepatitis C antibody point-of-care screening in a community pharmacy: a pilot project. *J Am Pharm Assoc* 2017;57(4):510-515.e2.

18. Darin KM, Klepser ME, Klepser DE, et al. Pharmacist-provided rapid HIV testing in two community pharmacies. *J Am Pharm Assoc.* 2015;55(1):81-88.PubMed

19. Azar MM, Landry ML. Detection of Influenza A and B viruses and respiratory syncytial virus by use of Clinical Laboratory Improvement Amendments of 1988 (CLIA)-waived point-of-care assays: a paradigm shift to molecular tests. *J Clin Microbiol.* 2018;56(7):e00367-18.

20. Newman TV, San-Juan-Rodriguez A, Parekh N, et al. Impact of community pharmacist-led interventions in chronic disease management on clinical, utilization, and economic outcomes: an umbrella review. *Res Social Adm Pharm.* 2020;16(9):1155-1165.PubMed

21. Centers for Disease Control and Prevention. *National Diabetes Statistics Report. Estimates of Diabetes and Its Burden in the United States, 2020.* Atlanta, GA: US Department of Health and Human Services; 2020.

22. O'Brien MJ, Sacks DB. Point-of-Care hemoglobin A1c. [published online ahead of print, September 12, 2019]. *JAMA.* 2019;322(14):1404-1405. PubMed

23. American Diabetes Association. Classification and diagnosis of diabetes: standards of medical care in diabetes. *Diabetes Care.* 2019;42(suppl 1): S13-S28.PubMed

24. Whitley HP, Yong EV, Rasinen C. Selecting an A1C point-of-care instrument. *Diabetes Spectr.* 2015;28(3):201-208.PubMed

25. Little RR, Rohlfing CL. The long and winding road to optimal HbA1c measurement. *Clin Chim Acta.* 2013;418:63-71.PubMed

26. Lenters-Westra E, Schindhelm RK, Bilo HJ, Slingerland RJ. Haemoglobin A1c: historical overview and current concepts. *Diabetes Res Clin Pract.* 2013;99(2):75-84.PubMed

27. Bode BW, Irvin BR, Pierce JA, et al. Advances in hemoglobin A1c point of care technology. *J Diabetes Sci Technol.* 2007;1(3):405-411.PubMed

28. Cagliero E, Levina EV, Nathan DM. Immediate feedback of HbA1c levels improves glycemic control in type 1 and insulin-treated type 2 diabetic patients. *Diabetes Care.* 1999;22(11):1785-1789.PubMed

29. Ferenczi A, Reddy K, Lorber DL. Effect of immediate hemoglobin A1c results on treatment decisions in office practice. *Endocr Pract.* 2001;7(2): 85-88.PubMed

30. Miller CD, Barnes CS, Phillips LS, et al. Rapid A1c availability improves clinical decision-making in an urban primary care clinic. *Diabetes Care.* 2003;26(4):1158-1163.PubMed

31. Lenters-Westra E, Slingerland RJ. Six of eight hemoglobin A1c point-of-care instruments do not meet the general accepted analytical performance criteria. *Clin Chem.* 2010;56(1):44-52.PubMed

32. Lenters-Westra E, Slingerland RJ. Three of 7 hemoglobin A1c point-of-care instruments do not meet generally accepted analytical performance criteria. *Clin Chem.* 2014;60(8):1062-1072.PubMed

33. Siegrist KK, Rice MJ. Point-of-care blood testing: the technology behind the numbers. *Anesth Analg.* 2019;129(1):92-98.PubMed

34. Shah N, Osea EA, Martinez GJ. Accuracy of noninvasive hemoglobin and invasive point-of-care hemoglobin testing compared with a laboratory analyzer. *Int J Lab Hematol.* 2014;36(1):56-61.PubMed

35. Berkow L. Factors affecting hemoglobin measurement. *J Clin Monit Comput.* 2013;27(5):499-508.PubMed

36. Centers for Disease Control and Prevention, National Center for Health Statistics. Underlying cause of death 1999-2018 on CDC Wonder online database. http://wonder.cdc.gov/ucd-icd10.html. Accessed May 29, 202).

37. Benjamin EJ, Blaha MJ, Chiuve SE, et al. Heart disease and stroke statistics—2017 update: a report from the American Heart Association. Circulation. 2017;135(10):e1-458.

38. Grundy SM, Stone NJ, Bailey AL, et al. 2018 AHA/ACC/AACVPR/ AAPA/ABC/ACPM/ADA/AGS/APhA/ASPC/NLA/PCNA Guideline on the Management of Blood Cholesterol: A Report of the American College of Cardiology/American Heart Association Task Force on Clinical Practice Guidelines. *J Am Coll Cardiol.* 2019;73(24):e285-e350.PubMed

39. Myers GL, Kimberly MM, Waymack PP, et al. A reference method laboratory network for cholesterol: a model for standardization and improvement of clinical laboratory measurements. *Clin Chem.* 2000;46(11):1762-1772.PubMed

40. Rapi S, Bazzini C, Tozzetti C, et al. Point-of-care testing of cholesterol and triglycerides for epidemiologic studies: evaluation of the multicare-in system. *Transl Res.* 2009;153(2):71-76.PubMed

41. Ockene IS, Chiriboga DE, Stanek EJ 3rd, et al. Seasonal variation in serum cholesterol levels: treatment implications and possible mechanisms. *Arch Intern Med.* 2004;164(8):863-870.PubMed

42. Shivappa N, Steck SE, Hurley TG, et al. A population-based dietary inflammatory index predicts levels of C-reactive protein in the Seasonal Variation of Blood Cholesterol Study (SEASONS). *Public Health Nutr.* 2013;10:1-9.PubMed

43. Heringa M, Floor-Schreudering A, De Smet PAGM, Bouvy ML. Clinical decision support and optional point of care testing of renal function for safe use of antibiotics in elderly patients: a retrospective study in community pharmacy practice. *Drugs Aging.* 2017;34(11):851-858. PubMed

44. Murata K, Glaser L, Nardiello M, et al. Analytical performance of the Abaxis Piccolo Xpress point of care analyzer in whole blood, serum, and plasma. *Clin Biochem.* 2015;48(18):1344-1346.PubMed

45. Zaninotto M, Miolo G, Guiotto A, et al. Quality performance of laboratory testing in pharmacies: a collaborative evaluation. *Clin Chem Lab Med.* 2016;54(11):1745-1751.PubMed

46. Henderson JT, Thompson JH, Burda BU, Cantor A. Preeclampsia screening: evidence report and systematic review for the US Preventive Services Task Force. *JAMA.* 2017;317(16):1668-1683.PubMed

47. Hofmeister MG, Rosenthal EM, Barker LK, et al. Estimating prevalence of hepatitis C virus infection in the United States, 2013-2016. *Hepatology.* 2019;69(3):1020-1031.PubMed

48. Holmberg SD, Spradling PR, Moorman AC, Denniston MM. Hepatitis C in the United States. *N Engl J Med.* 2013;368(20):1859-1861. PubMed

49. Denniston MM, Klevens RM, McQuillan GM, Jiles RB. Awareness of infection, knowledge of hepatitis C, and medical follow-up among individuals testing positive for hepatitis C: National Health and Nutrition Examination Survey 2001-2008. *Hepatology.* 2012;55(6):1652-1661. PubMed

50. Centers for Disease Control and Prevention. Viral hepatitis surveillance: United States, 2017. https//:www.cdc.gov/hepatitis/statistics/2017 surveillance/index.htm. Accessed June 14, 2020.

51. AASLD-IDSA. HCV testing and linkage to care. Recommendations for testing, managing, and treating hepatitis C. http://www.hcvguidelines.org /full-report/hcv-testing-and-linkage-care. Accessed June 15, 2020.

52. Naidjate SS, Zullo AR, Dapaah-Afriyie R, et al. Comparative effectiveness of pharmacist care delivery models for hepatitis C clinics. *Am J Health Syst Pharm.* 2019;76(10):646-653.PubMed

53. Isho NY, Kachlic MD, Marcelo JC, Martin MT. Pharmacist-initiated hepatitis C virus screening in a community pharmacy to increase awareness and link to care at the medical center. *J Am Pharm Assoc.* 2017;57(3S):S259-S264.PubMed

54. Centers for Disease Control and Prevention. Testing recommendations for chronic hepatitis C virus infection. http://www.cdc.gov/hepatitis/hcv /guidelinesc.htm. Accessed September 13, 2020.

55. Cha YJ, Park Q, Kang ES, et al. Performance evaluation of the OraQuick hepatitis C virus rapid antibody test. *Ann Lab Med.* 2013;33(3):184-189. PubMed

56. Lee SR, Yearwood GD, Guillon GB, et al. Evaluation of a rapid, point-of-care test device for the diagnosis of hepatitis C infection. *J Clin Virol.* 2010;48(1):15-17.PubMed

57. Lee SR, Kardos KW, Schiff E, et al. Evaluation of a new, rapid test for detecting HCV infection, suitable for use with blood or oral fluid. *J Virol Methods.* 2011;172(1-2):27-31.PubMed

58. Zachary P, Ullmann M, Djeddi S, et al. Evaluation of three commercially available hepatitis C virus antibody detection assays under the conditions of a clinical virology laboratory. *J Clin Virol.* 2005;34(3):207-210, discussion 216-218.PubMed

59. Smith BD, Drobeniuc J, Jewett A, et al. Evaluation of three rapid screening assays for detection of antibodies to hepatitis C virus. *J Infect Dis.* 2011;204(6):825-831.PubMed

60. Centers for Disease Control and Prevention. Estimated HIV incidence and prevalence in the United States, 2014-2018. HIV Surveillance Supplemental Report 25(No.1). Published May 2020. http://www.cdc.gov /hiv/library/reports/hiv-surveillance.html. Accessed June 25, 2020.

61. Collins B, Bronson H, Elamin F, et al. The "No wrong door" approach to HIV testing: results from a statewide retail pharmacy-based HIV testing program in Virginia, 2014-2016. *Public Health Rep.* 2018;133(2 suppl): 34S-42S.PubMed

62. Amesty S, Blaney S, Crawford ND, et al. Pharmacy staff characteristics associated with support for pharmacy-based HIV testing. *J Am Pharm Assoc.* 2012;52(4):472-479.PubMed

63. Calderon Y, Cowan E, Rhee JY, et al. Counselor-based rapid HIV testing in community pharmacies. *AIDS Patient Care STDS.* 2013;27(8):467-473. PubMed

64. Weidle PJ, Lecher S, Botts LW, et al. HIV testing in community pharmacies and retail clinics: a model to expand access to screening for HIV infection. *J Am Pharm Assoc (2003).* 2014;54(5):486-492.PubMed

65. Darin KM, Scarsi KK, Klepser DG, et al. Consumer interest in community pharmacy HIV screening services. *J Am Pharm Assoc (2003).* 2015;55(1):67-72.PubMed

66. Lecher SL, Shrestha RK, Botts LW, et al. Cost analysis of a novel HIV testing strategy in community pharmacies and retail clinics. *J Am Pharm Assoc.* 2015;55(5):488-492.PubMed

67. Arora DR, Maheshwari M, Arora B. Rapid point-of-care testing for detection of HIV and clinical monitoring. *ISRN AIDS.* 2013;2013:287269. PubMed

68. Centers for Disease Control and Prevention. Types of HIV tests. https://www.cdc.gov/hiv/basics/hiv-testing/test-types.html. Accessed September 11, 2020.

69. Wesolowski LG, Mackellar DA, Ethridge SF, et al. Repeat confirmatory testing for persons with discordant whole blood and oral fluid rapid HIV test results: findings from post marketing surveillance. *PLoS One.* 2008;3(2):e1524.PubMed

70. Pai NP, Vadnais C, Denkinger C, et al. Point-of-care testing for infectious diseases: diversity, complexity, and barriers in low- and middle-income countries. *PLoS Med.* 2012;9(9):e1001306.PubMed

71. Masciotra S, Luo W, Youngpairoj AS, et al. Performance of the Alere Determine HIV-1/2 Ag/Ab combo rapid test with specimens from HIV-1 seroconverters from the US and HIV-2 infected individuals from Ivory Coast. *J Clin Virol.* 2013;58(suppl 1):e54-e58.PubMed

72. Duong YT, Mavengere Y, Patel H, et al. Poor performance of the determine HIV-1/2 Ag/Ab combo fourth-generation rapid test for detection of acute infections in a national household survey in Swaziland. *J Clin Microbiol.* 2014;52(10):3743-3748.PubMed

73. Smallwood M, Pant Pai N. Improving the quality of diagnostic studies evaluating point of care tests for acute HIV infections: problems and recommendations [commentary]. *Diagnostics (Basel).* 2017;7(1):13. PubMed

74. Centers for Disease Control and Prevention. Disease burden of influenza. https://www.cdc.gov.flu/about/burden/index.html. Accessed June 18, 2020.

75. Gubbins PO, Klepser ME, Adams A, et al. Potential for pharmacy-public health collaborations using pharmacy-based point of care testing services. *J Public Health Manag Pract.* 2017;23(6):593-600.PubMed

76. Center for Disease Control and Prevention. Guidance for clinicians on the use of rapid influenza diagnostic tests. https://www.cdc.gov/flu /professionals/diagnosis/overview-testing-methods.htm#diagnostic. Accessed June 22, 2020.

77. Klepser ME, Klepser DG, Dering-Anderson AM, et al. Effectiveness of a pharmacist-physician collaborative program to manage influenza-like illness. *J Am Pharm Assoc.* 2016;56(1):14-21.PubMed

78. Klepser DG, Klepser ME, Murry JS, et al. Evaluation of a community pharmacy-based influenza and group A streptococcal pharyngitis disease management program using polymerase chain reaction point-of-care testing. *J Am Pharm Assoc (2003).* 2019;59(6):872-879.PubMed

79. Klepser DG, Klepser ME, Smith JK, et al. Utilization of influenza and streptococcal pharyngitis point-of-care testing in the community pharmacy practice setting. *Res Social Adm Pharm.* 2018;14(4):356-359. PubMed

80. Kirby J, Mousa N. Evaluating the impact of influenza and streptococcus point-of-care testing and collaborative practice prescribing in a community pharmacy setting. *J Am Pharm Assoc.* 2020;60(3S):S70-S75. PubMed

81. Klepser ME, Adams AJ, Klepser DG. Antimicrobial stewardship in outpatient settings: leveraging innovative physician-pharmacist collaborations to reduce antibiotic resistance. *Health Secur.* 2015;13(3):166-173.PubMed

82. Centers for Disease Control and Prevention. Information on rapid molecular assays, RT-PCR, and other molecular assays for diagnosis of influenza virus infection. Published October 21, 2019. https://www.cdc.gov/flu/professionals/diagnosis/molecular-assays.htm. Accessed June 21, 2020.

83. Uyeki TM, Bernstein HH, Bradley JS, et al. Clinical practice guidelines by the Infectious Diseases Society of America: 2018 update on diagnosis, treatment, chemoprophylaxis, and institutional outbreak management of seasonal influenza. *Clin Infect Dis.* 2019;68(6):e1-e47.PubMed

84. Zanoli LM, Spoto G. Isothermal amplification methods for the detection of nucleic acids in microfluidic devices. *Biosensors (Basel).* 2012;3(1):18-43.PubMed

85. US Food and Drug Administration. Microbiology devices: reclassification of influenza virus antigen detection test systems intended for use directly with clinical specimens. *Fed Regist.* 2017;8:3609-3619.

86. Koski RR, Klepser ME. A systematic review of rapid diagnostic tests for influenza: considerations for the community pharmacist. *J Am Pharm Assoc.* 2017;57(1):13-19.PubMed

87. Klepser DG, Klepser ME, Dering-Anderson AM, et al. Community pharmacist-physician collaborative streptococcal pharyngitis management program. *J Am Pharm Assoc.* 2016;56(3):323-329.e1. PubMed

88. Thornley T, Marshall G, Howard P, Wilson APR. A feasibility service evaluation of screening and treatment of group A streptococcal pharyngitis in community pharmacies. *J Antimicrob Chemother.* 2016;71(11):3293-3299.PubMed

89. Papastergiou J, Trieu CR, Saltmarche D, Diamantouros A. Community pharmacist-directed point-of-care group A streptococcus testing: evaluation of a Canadian program. *J Am Pharm Assoc.* 2018;58(4):450-456.PubMed

90. Schroeder BM. Diagnosis and management of group A streptococcal pharyngitis. *Am Fam Physician.* 2003;67(4):880-884.PubMed

91. Lean WL, Arnup S, Danchin M, Steer AC. Rapid diagnostic tests for group A streptococcal pharyngitis: a meta-analysis. *Pediatrics.* 2014;134(4):771-781.PubMed

92. Cohen DM, Russo ME, Jaggi P, et al. Multicenter clinical evaluation of the Novel Alere strep A isothermal nucleic acid amplification test. *J Clin Microbiol.* 2015;53(7):2258-2261.PubMed

93. Pelucchi C, Grigoryan L, Galeone C, et al. Guideline for the management of acute sore throat. *Clin Microbiol Infect.* 2012;18(suppl 1):1-28.PubMed

94. McIsaac WJ, White D, Tannenbaum D, Low DE. A clinical score to reduce unnecessary antibiotic use in patients with sore throat. *CMAJ.* 1998;158(1):75-83.PubMed

95. McIsaac WJ, Kellner JD, Aufricht P, et al. Empirical validation of guidelines for the management of pharyngitis in children and adults. *JAMA.* 2004;291(13):1587-1595.PubMed

96. Shulman ST, Bisno AL, Clegg HW, et al. Clinical practice guideline for the diagnosis and management of group A streptococcal pharyngitis: 2012 update by the Infectious Diseases Society of America. *Clin Infect Dis.* 2012;55(10):1279-1282.PubMed

97. U.S. Department of Health & Human Services. Guidance for licensed pharmacists, COVID-19 testing, and immunity under the PREP Act. Published April 8, 2020. https://www.hhs.gov/sites/default/files/authorizing-licensed-pharmacists-to-order-and-administer-covid-19-tests.pdf. Accessed April 19, 2020.

98. Gibbs JN, Cato ME, Schlanger SJ. New FDA policy significantly limits serological testing. https://bit.ly/2y7KiOf. Accessed April 19, 2020.

99. Centers for Disease Control and Prevention. Overview of testing for SARS-CoV-2. Published June 13, 2020. https://www.cdc.gov/coronavirus/2019-ncov/hcp/testing-overview.html. Accessed June 29, 2020.

100. Xpert Xpress-CoV-2 EUA [package insert]. Sunnyvale, CA: Cepheid. August 2020. https://www.cepheid.com/Package%20Insert%20Files/Xpress-SARS-CoV-2-PI/302-3750%20rev%20C%20PACKAGE%20INSERT%20EUA%20XPRESS%20SARS-COV2.pdf. Accessed September 16, 2020.

101. Cobas SARS-COV-2 & Influenza A/B Nucleic Acid Test [package insert]. Branchburg, NJ: Roche Molecular Systems, Inc. https://www.fda.gov/media/142193/download. Accessed September 16, 2020.

102. ID NOW COVID-19 [package insert]. Scarborough, ME: Abbott Diagnostics Scarborough, Inc. https://www.alere.com/en/home/product-details/id-now-covid-19.html. Accessed September 16, 2020.

103. Accula SARS-CoV-2 [package insert]. San Diego, CA: Mesa Biotech, Inc. https://static1.squarespace.com/static/5ca44a0a7eb88c46af449a53/t/5e8d218517114d6ea7f60dc2/1586307464282/60061+Rev+1+Accula+SARS-CoV-2+IFU.pdf. Accessed September 16, 2020.

104. Cue COVID-19 Test Instructions For Use Document C101. California: Cue Health Inc. https://www.fda.gov/media/138826/download. Accessed September 16, 2020.

105. Xpress X. SARS-CoV-2/Flu/RSV EUA [package insert]. Sunnyvale, CA: Cepheid. https://www.fda.gov/media/142438/download. Accessed September 28, 2020.

106. Binax NOWTM. COVID-19 Ag CARD [package insert]. Scarborough, ME: Abbott Diagnostics Scarborough, Inc. https://www.globalpointofcare.abbott/en/product-details/navica-binaxnow-covid-19-us.html. Accessed September 16, 2020.

107. LumiraDx SARS-CoV-2 Ag Test [package insert]. Waltham, MA: LumiraDx UK Ltd. https://www.lumiradx.com/us-en/. Accessed September 16, 2020.

108. BD Veritor System for Rapid Detection of SARS-CoV-2 [package insert]. Franklin Lakes, NJ: Becton, Dickinson and Company. https://www.fda.gov/media/139755/download. Accessed September 16, 2020.

109. SOFIA 2 SARS Antigen FIA [package insert]. San Diego, CA: Quidel Corporation. https://www.quidel.com/sites/default/files/product/documents/EF1438900EN00_0.pdf. Accessed May 9, 2020.

110. Assure COVID-19 IgG/IgM Rapid Test Device [package insert]. Hangzhou, China: Assure Tech. Co. https://www.fda.gov/media/139792/download. Accessed September 24, 2020.

111. Daunais DM, Klepser ME, Ogrin BJ. Assessment of pharmacy students' and licensed pharmacists' perceived knowledge, application, and interpretation regarding rapid diagnostic tests (RDTs) for infectious diseases. *Curr Pharm Teach Learn.* 2015;7:100-105.

112. Freed SL, Valente CA, Hagerman JK, et al. Assessment of the curricular content devoted to the application and interpretation of rapid diagnostic tests in colleges of pharmacy in the United States. *Pharm Educ.* 2011;11:205-208.

113. Huang V, Klepser ME, Gubbins PO, et al. Quantification of curricular content devoted to point-of-care testing for infectious diseases in schools and colleges of pharmacy in the United States. *Pharm Educ.* 2015;15:1-6.

114. National Association of Chain Drugstores. Community pharmacy-based Point-of-Care Testing Certificate Program. http://nacds.learnercommunity.com/Point-of-Care-Testing-Certificate. Accessed June 30, 2020.

115. Smith MG, Rains L. Evaluation of an accredited training program on implementation of point-of-care testing in community pharmacies. *J Am Pharm Assoc.* 2020. https://www.japha.org/article/S1544-3191(20)30203-X/fulltext. Accessed June 29, 2020.

# 5

# Interpretation of Serum Drug Concentrations

*Riane Ghamrawi and Lindsay Benedik*

The pharmacist is a key member in the therapeutic drug monitoring process. This chapter is designed to review the indications for drug concentration monitoring and discuss how drug concentrations obtained from the clinical laboratory, specialized reference laboratory, or physician's office should be interpreted. General considerations for interpretation are described as well as unique considerations for drugs that commonly undergo therapeutic drug monitoring. Future directions of therapeutic drug monitoring are also discussed.

This chapter is not intended to provide an in-depth review of pharmacokinetic dosing methods; nevertheless, knowledge of certain basic pharmacokinetic terms and concepts is expected. The general phrase *drug concentration* will be used throughout the chapter unless specific references to serum, plasma, whole blood, and saliva are more appropriate. The bibliography lists numerous texts about therapeutic drug monitoring and clinical pharmacokinetic principles with applications to clinical practice.

## THERAPEUTIC DRUG MONITORING

*Therapeutic drug monitoring* is broadly defined as the use of drug concentrations to optimize drug therapy for individual patients.[1] Prior to using drug concentrations to guide therapy, physicians adjusted drug doses based on their interpretation of clinical response. In many cases, drug doses were increased until obvious signs of toxicity were observed (eg, nystagmus for phenytoin or tinnitus for salicylates). The idea that intensity and duration of pharmacologic response depended on serum drug concentration was first reported by Marshall and then tested for the screening of antimalarials during World War II.[2,3] Koch-Weser, in a hallmark paper, described how steady-state serum concentrations of commonly used drugs can vary 10-fold among patients receiving the same dosage regimen.[4] He further described how serum concentrations predict the intensity of therapeutic or toxic effects more accurately than dosage.

Starting in the 1960s, there was rapid improvement in analytical methods used for drug concentration measurements; extensive research correlating serum or plasma drug concentrations with clinical efficacy and toxicity quickly followed. Today, with the emergence of immunoassays that require no specialized equipment, drug concentration measurements can be easily performed in outpatient clinic offices.

The increased availability and convenience of drug assay methods has led to a number of concerns. Is therapeutic drug monitoring being done simply because it is available, rather than because it is clinically necessary? There are numerous reports of suboptimal therapeutic drug monitoring practices that contribute to inappropriate decision-making as well as wasted resources.[5-7] Questions have been raised about whether therapeutic drug monitoring actually improves patient outcomes.[8,9] Alternatively, many clinicians claim that therapeutic drug monitoring is greatly underused and could, if appropriately used, further improve patient care and reduce healthcare costs.[10-12] Clearly, there is a need for more education of all healthcare professionals involved in the therapeutic drug monitoring process to make its use more appropriate and cost-effective. Such education efforts have been shown to effectively reduce the number of inappropriate drug concentration requests.[13]

DOI 10.37573/9781585286423.005

## Goal and Indications for Drug Concentration Monitoring

The primary goal of therapeutic drug monitoring is to maximize the benefit of a drug to a patient in the shortest possible time while minimizing the risk of drug toxicity. The number of hospitalizations or office visits used to adjust therapies or manage and diagnose adverse drug reactions may therefore be reduced, resulting in overall cost savings.

Drug concentration measurements should not be performed unless the result will affect some future action or decision. Monitoring should not be done simply because the opportunity presents itself; it should be used discriminatingly to answer clinically relevant questions and resolve or anticipate problems in drug therapy management.[14] The clinician should always ask, "Will this drug concentration value provide more information to me than sound clinical judgment alone?"[9] The following examples provide clinical situations and clinical questions that drug concentration measurements might be able to impact:

- **Therapeutic confirmation:** A patient is on a regimen that appears to offer the maximum benefit with acceptable side effects. *Question: What drug concentration is associated with a therapeutic effect in this patient for future reference?*

- **Dosage optimization:** A patient has a condition in which the clinical response is not easily measured and has been initiated on a standard regimen of a drug. There is modest improvement, and no symptoms of toxicity are evident. *Question: Can I increase the dose to further enhance the effect? If so, by how much?*

- **Confirmation of suspected toxicity:** A patient is experiencing certain signs and symptoms that could be related to the drug. *Question: Are these signs and symptoms most likely related to a dose that is too high? Can I reduce the daily dose to maintain efficacy and if so, by how much?*

- **Avoidance of inefficacy or toxicity:** A patient is initiated on a standard regimen of an antibiotic that is known to be poorly absorbed in a small percentage of patients. Sustained subtherapeutic concentrations of this drug can lead to drug resistance. *Question: Will a higher daily dose be needed in this patient?* A patient has been satisfactorily treated on a regimen of Drug A. The patient experiences a change in health or physiologic status or a second drug, suspected to interact with Drug A, is added. *Question: Will a regimen adjustment be needed to avoid inefficacy or toxicity?*

- **Distinguishing nonadherence from treatment failure:** A patient has not responded to usual doses and nonadherence is a possibility. *Question: Is this a treatment failure, or does the patient need counseling on adherence?*

## Characteristics of Ideal Drugs for Therapeutic Drug Monitoring

Not all drugs are good candidates for therapeutic monitoring. Those for which drug concentration monitoring will be most useful have the following characteristics[15]:

- **Readily available assays:** Methods for drug concentration measurement must be thoroughly evaluated for sensitivity, specificity, accuracy, and precision and be available to the clinician at a cost to justify the information to be gained. Chromatographic methods are most likely used in laboratory settings and are considered in many cases to be the reference methods. Increased interest in methods for use in ambulatory settings, however, has led to the development of immunoassay systems purported to be fast, reliable, and cost-effective.[16-20]

- **Lack of easily observable, safe, or desirable clinical endpoint:** Clinically, there is no immediate, easily monitored, and predictable clinical parameter to guide dose titration. For example, waiting for arrhythmias or seizures to occur or resume may be an unsafe and undesirable approach to dosing antiarrhythmics and antiepileptics.

- **Dangerous toxicity or lack of effectiveness:** Toxicity or lack of effectiveness of the drug presents a danger to the patient. For example, serum concentrations of the antifungal drug, flucytosine, are not routinely monitored. However, specialized monitoring may be done to ensure that concentrations are less than 100 mg/L to avoid gastrointestinal (GI) side effects, blood dyscrasias, and hepatotoxicity. As another example, specialized monitoring of the protease inhibitors (PIs) may be done to ensure adequate concentrations because rapid emergence of antiviral resistance is observed with sustained exposure to subtherapeutic concentrations.

- **Unpredictable dose–response relationship:** The presence of an unpredictable dose–response relationship, such that a dose rate that produces therapeutic benefit in one patient may cause toxicity in another patient. This would be true for drugs that have significant interpatient variation in pharmacokinetic parameters, drugs with nonlinear elimination behavior, and drugs with pharmacokinetic parameters that are affected by concomitant administration of other drugs. For example, patients given the same daily dose of phenytoin can demonstrate a wide range of serum concentrations and responses.

- **Narrow therapeutic range:** The drug concentrations associated with therapeutic effect overlap considerably with the concentrations associated with toxic effects, such that the zone for therapeutic benefit without toxicity is narrow. For example, the therapeutic range of total serum concentrations of phenytoin is widely accepted to be 10 to 20 mg/L for most patients; the upper limit of the range is only twice the lower limit.

- **Good correlation between drug concentration and efficacy or toxicity:** This criterion must apply if we are using drug concentrations to adjust the dosage regimen of a drug. For example, a patient showing unsatisfactory seizure control with a serum phenytoin concentration of 8 mg/L is likely to show improved control with a serum concentration of 15 mg/L.

Other than availability of an assay, it may not be necessary for a drug to fulfill the previously listed characteristics for drug concentration monitoring to help guide clinical decision-making. Newer drugs that do not yet have clearly defined therapeutic ranges may be monitored only under special circumstances (eg, to ensure adherence). Other drugs may not have a clearly defined upper or lower limit to the therapeutic range but are monitored under special circumstances to ensure efficacy or avoid toxicity. The fact remains, the drug concentration is important for answering a specific clinical question: Will the information provided by this measurement help to improve the patient's drug therapy?

## Information Needed for Planning and Evaluating Drug Concentrations

Drug concentrations should be interpreted in light of full information about the patient, including clinical status. Information surrounding the timing of the sample relative to the last dose is especially critical and is one of the biggest factors making drug concentrations unusable or cost-ineffective.[5,21-23] **Table 5-1** provides a list of the essential information needed for a drug concentration request. Laboratory request forms or computer entry forms must be designed to encourage entry of the most important information. All relevant information should be included on both the request form and the report form to facilitate an accurate interpretation. It is particularly important to verify the time of the sample draw because phlebotomists or computer-generated labels commonly identify samples with the time of the intended draw instead of the actual draw time. Some hospital laboratories have minimized the number of inappropriate samples by refusing to run any samples that are not accompanied by critical information, such as the timing of the sample relative to the last dose; however, this practice can be cumbersome and is not widely used.[5] The laboratory report form should also include the assay used; active metabolite concentration (if measured); and parameters reflecting the sensitivity, specificity, and precision of the method.

Accuracy and completeness of the information provided on a laboratory request form are particularly important in light of the many problems that can occur during the therapeutic drug monitoring process. A drug concentration that seems to be illogical, given the information provided on the form, may be explained by a variety of factors, as shown in **Table 5-2** (**Minicase 1**).

## Considerations for Appropriate Interpretation of Drug Concentrations

To appropriately interpret a drug concentration, it is important to have as many answers as possible to the following questions:

- **Therapeutic range.** What do the studies show to be the usual therapeutic range? How frequently will patients show response at a concentration below the lower limit of the usual range? How frequently will patients show toxicity at a concentration above or even below the upper limit of the usual range? What are the usual signs and symptoms indicating toxicity?

- **Sample timing.** Was the sample drawn at a steady state? Was the sample drawn at a time during the dosing interval (if intermittent therapy) that reflects the intended indication for monitoring (a peak, a trough, a "random" concentration, or an average concentration)? During the dosing interval, when is a peak concentration most likely to occur for the

formulation administered? Does the formulation exhibit a lag time for release, absorption, or distribution such that the lowest concentration will occur into the next dosing interval?

- **Use of concentrations for dose adjustment.** Does the drug display first-order (linear) pharmacokinetic elimination behavior such that an increase in daily dose will produce a proportional increase in the average drug concentration? Will more complex adjustment methods be needed for drugs that display nonlinear elimination behavior? Is the dosage adjustment method focused on attaining specific peaks, troughs, or specific average concentrations?

- **Protein binding, active metabolites, and other considerations.** How are total drug concentrations in serum interpreted in cases of altered serum protein binding? How are concentrations or contributions of active metabolites considered along with parent drug? Is the drug administered as a racemic mixture and if so, do the enantiomers differ in activity and pharmacokinetic behavior? Do certain physiologic or pathologic conditions affect a patient's response to the drug at a given concentration?

Each of these categories is described in general in the section that follows and, more specifically, for each drug or drug class in the Applications section.

## THE THERAPEUTIC RANGE

The *therapeutic range* is also known as the "therapeutic window," "therapeutic reference range," "optimal plasma concentration," and "target range." The therapeutic range is best defined as "ranges of drug concentrations in blood that specify a lower limit below which a drug induced therapeutic response is relatively unlikely to occur and an upper limit above which tolerability decreases or above which it is relatively unlikely that therapeutic improvement may be still enhanced."[1,24-26] Therapeutic reference ranges are population-based averages for which most patients are expected to respond with acceptable side effects. Thus, there will always be some patients who exhibit therapeutic effect at drug concentrations below the lower limit, while others will experience unacceptable toxicity at concentrations below the upper limit. Therefore, a patient's therapy is always best guided by a patient's individual therapeutic concentration and correlated clinical response. It may be most beneficial to measure drug concentrations when a patient has attained the desired clinical response and establish the obtained drug concentration as the optimal concentration for an individual patient.[25,26]

**Figure 5-1** illustrates how the probability of response and toxicity increases with drug concentration for a hypothetical drug and how a therapeutic range might be determined based on these relative probabilities. **Figure 5-2** shows how patterns for response and toxicity can change in two different patients receiving the same drug. If the hypothetical drug in question has an active metabolite that accumulates more than the parent drug in renal impairment and if that metabolite contributes more to toxicity than to efficacy, then the individual therapeutic range in the patient with renal impairment will be narrower. Concentration monitoring of the active metabolite would be especially important in that situation.

**TABLE 5-1.** Information Needed to Order and/or Interpret a Laboratory Value

| TYPE OF DATA | SPECIFIC DATA | WHY NECESSARY |
|---|---|---|
| Patient identification | • Name, address, identification number, and physician name | All blood samples look alike and could easily be switched among patients without appropriate identification |
| Patient demographics and characteristics | • Age, gender, ethnicity, height, weight, and pregnancy | The therapeutic range for a given drug may depend on the specific indication being treated (eg, digoxin for atrial arrhythmias versus heart failure); if there is no history of prior drug concentration measurements, information about concurrent disease states, physiologic status, and social habits may help with initial determination of population pharmacokinetic parameters, in order to determine if the resulting concentration is expected or not; information about renal function and albumin is important if a total drug concentration is being measured for a drug normally highly bound to serum proteins; it is also important to know if any endogenous substances due to diseases will interfere with the assay; electrolyte abnormalities may affect the interpretation of a given concentration (eg, digoxin) |
| History and physical examination | • Condition being treated<br>• Organ involvement (renal, hepatic, cardiac, GI, and endocrine)<br>• Fluid balance and nutritional status<br>• Labs (albumin, total protein, liver function enzymes, INR, bilirubin, serum creatinine or creatinine clearance, thyroid status, and electrolyte abnormalities)<br>• Smoking and alcohol history | |
| Specimen information | • Time of collection<br>• Source of specimen: blood, urine, or other body fluid site of collection<br>• Order of sample, if part of a series<br>• Type of collection tube<br>• Time of receipt by laboratory | Laboratories often retain samples for several days and detailed information will help to find a sample if important pre, post, or random samples are needed; the time of collection relative to the dose is extremely important for proper interpretation (Close to a trough? Closer to a peak?); knowing the type of collection tube is important because of the many interferences that may occur; it is important to know the collection site relative to the administration site, if an IV route is used; if a series of samples is to be drawn, the labeled timing of the collection tubes can get mixed up |
| Drug information | • Name of drug to be assayed<br>• Current dosage regimen, including route<br>• Type of formulation (sustained-release, delayed-release, or prompt-release)<br>• Length of time on current regimen<br>• Time of last dose<br>• Concurrent drug therapy<br>• Duration of IV infusion | It is important to know if the concentration was drawn at a steady state and when the concentration was drawn relative to the last dose; it is also important to know if there are any potential drug interferences with the assay to be used |
| Drug concentration history | • Dates and times of prior concentration measurements<br>• Response and drug regimen schedules associated with prior concentrations | It is important to know what drug concentrations have been documented as effective or associated with toxicity; it is also important to know how drug concentrations have changed as a consequence of dosage regimen |
| Purpose of assay and urgency of request | • Therapeutic confirmation<br>• Suspected toxicity<br>• Anticipated inefficacy or toxicity due to change in physiologic/health status or drug–drug interaction<br>• Identification of drug failure<br>• Suspected overdose | This forces the clinician to have a specific clinical question in mind before ordering a sample; it also aids in the interpretation of results |

GI = gastrointestinal;
INR = International Normalized Ratio.
*Source:* Adapted with permission from references 16 and 17.

**TABLE 5-2.** Common Reasons Why Drug Concentration Results Do Not Make Sense

| CATEGORY OF FACTOR | SPECIFIC EXAMPLES |
|---|---|
| Related to drug administration or blood sampling logistics | • Wrong dose or infusion rate administered<br>• Dose skipped or infusion held for a period of time<br>• Dose given at time other than recorded; blood drawn as ordered<br>• Dose given at right time; blood drawn at time other than recorded<br>• Sample taken through an administration line, which was improperly flushed prior to sample withdrawal<br>• Sample taken from the wrong patient<br>• Improper or prolonged storage prior to delivery to laboratory<br>• Wrong collection tube/device used<br>• Patient was dialyzed between doses |
| Related to pharmacokinetics | • Sample is drawn prior to steady-state attainment<br>• Orders for digoxin samples are not clearly specified to be drawn at least 6 hours postdistribution<br>• Samples are ordered at the wrong times relative to last dose to reflect specific needs (eg, peaks and troughs)<br>• Concentrations of active metabolites are not ordered when appropriate<br>• Concentrations for total drug are ordered for a drug with unusual serum protein binding without recognition that the usual therapeutic range of total drug will not apply<br>• Samples after IV administration are drawn prior to completion of distribution phase (eg, vancomycin, aminoglycosides) |
| Related to the laboratory | • The wrong drug is assayed<br>• Critical active metabolites are not assayed<br>• Interferences or artifacts caused by endogenous substances (bilirubin, lipids, and hemolysis) or concurrent drugs<br>• Improper or prolonged storage prior to assay<br>• Technical errors with the assay |
| Related to the patient | • Patient does not adhere to therapy<br>• Taking interacting medications that may increase or decrease a drug's concentration<br>• Patient-specific laboratory parameters important for a drug's pharmacokinetic profile are altered (eg, albumin) |

*Source:* Adapted with permission from references 17 and 25.

Drug concentration monitoring is often criticized by claims that therapeutic ranges are not sufficiently well defined.[10,11] The lack of clearly defined therapeutic ranges for older drugs is partially attributable to how these ranges were originally determined. Eadie describes the process that was typically used for determination of the therapeutic ranges of the antiepileptic drugs: "These ranges do not appear to have been determined by rigorous statistical procedures applied to large patient populations. Rather, workers seem to have set the lower limits for each drug at the concentration at which they perceived a reasonable (although usually unspecified) proportion of patients achieved seizure control, and the upper limit at the concentration above which overdosage-type adverse effects appear to trouble appreciable numbers of patients, the values then being rounded off to provide a pair of numbers, which are reasonably easy to remember."[14] In an ideal world, studies to define therapeutic ranges for drugs should use reliable methods for measurement of response and should be restricted to patients with the same diseases, age range, and concurrent medications.[1] In recent years, the U.S. Food and Drug Administration (FDA) has recognized the importance of determining concentration versus response relationships early during clinical trials.[27]

Anything that affects the pharmacodynamics of a drug, meaning the response at a given drug concentration, affects the therapeutic range, including the following factors:

• **Indication.** Drugs that are used for more than one indication are likely to be interacting with different receptors. Thus, a different concentration versus response profile might be expected depending on the disease being treated. For example, higher serum concentrations of digoxin are needed for treatment of atrial fibrillation as compared with heart failure. Higher antibiotic drug concentrations may be needed for resistant organisms or to penetrate specific infected tissue sites.

## MINICASE 1

### Importance of Documenting Drug Administration Times

Michael T., an 86-year-old man (95 kg, 178 cm, baseline SCr 0.78), is receiving vancomycin monotherapy for treatment of a gram-positive bacteremia (unknown source). According to the medical chart, he receives four doses of vancomycin 2,000 mg q 12 h infused over 2 hours on a schedule of 7 a.m./7 p.m. The estimated/predicted half-life of vancomycin in Michael T. based on estimated creatinine clearance is 6 hours. A concentration drawn at 6 a.m. the following morning is reported as 16 mg/L. Based on the current information, the regimen of vancomycin 2,000 mg q 12 h is continued. A repeat concentration 3 days later at 6:30 a.m. reveals a vancomycin trough concentration of 27 mg/L. Renal function, as indicated by creatinine clearance, has not changed in this patient. The pharmacist receives a call to assess and interpret this concentration. If accurate, a dosage adjustment will be necessary to avoid toxicities.

QUESTION: What are the possible explanations for apparent changes in serum vancomycin results? Which vancomycin concentration accurately reflects the current dosage regimen?

DISCUSSION: For any drug requiring therapeutic drug monitoring, one must first consider whether the concentrations accurately represent a steady state. With an estimated vancomycin half-life of 6 hours, a steady state should have been reached after four doses or 48 hours. Because vancomycin depends greatly on the kidney for elimination, a second consideration would be renal function. Of note, this patient's creatinine clearance is unchanged. Laboratory errors or assay interference/artifacts could lead to difficulty in interpretation of serum drug concentrations. In the case of aminoglycosides, for example, coadministration of piperacillin–tazobactam may lead to in vitro inactivation, which may lead to falsely subtherapeutic concentrations. However, no such interferences were noted for vancomycin in this case. Finally, it is important to confirm the accuracy of blood sampling or drug administration times. After investigating this patient's medication administration record further, it is discovered that his third vancomycin dose was held, and no adjustment to timing of orders was performed. For this reason, the measured concentration of 16 mg/L was in fact 24 hours after the last dose and therefore did not reflect a true 12-hour trough on the 2,000 mg q 12 h regimen. After analysis of subsequent administration times and doses of vancomycin, the dose is adjusted to 2,000 mg q 24 h. If the first measured concentration had been initially noted to be drawn 24 hours after the previous dose, the clinician could have predicted an elevated vancomycin concentration on the every-12-hour regimen, and a dose adjustment would have been made at that time.

• **Active metabolites.** As shown in Figure 5-2, variable presence of an active metabolite can shift the therapeutic range for that individual patient up or down. These metabolites may behave in a manner similar to the parent drug or may interact with different receptors altogether. In either case, the relationship between parent drug concentration and response will be altered.

• **Concurrent drug treatment.** In a manner similar to active metabolites, the presence of other drugs that have similar pharmacodynamic activities will contribute to efficacy or toxicity but not to measurement of the drug concentration. The therapeutic range will be shifted.

• **Patient's age.** While there is limited information concerning developmental changes in pharmacodynamics in the

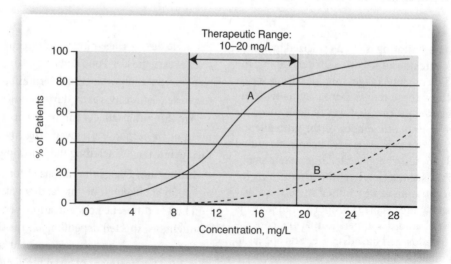

**FIGURE 5-1.** The therapeutic range for a hypothetical drug. Line A is the percentage of patients displaying a therapeutic effect; line B is the percentage of patients displaying toxicity.

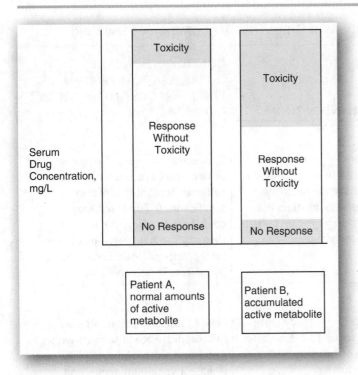

**FIGURE 5-2.** Representation showing how the individual therapeutic range of a hypothetical drug can differ in a patient with renal impairment because of accumulated active metabolite.

pediatric population, it is understood that the numbers and affinities of pharmacologic receptors change with progression of age, particularly into advanced age.[28] Age-related changes in pharmacodynamics and pharmacokinetics would be expected to result in a shift of the therapeutic range.

• **Electrolyte status.** Electrolytes play a critical role in cardiac function and therefore may affect the pharmacodynamics of a given drug. As an example, hypokalemia, hypomagnesemia, and hypercalcemia are all known to increase the cardiac effects of digitalis glycosides and enhance the potential for digoxin toxicity at a given serum concentration.[29]

• **Concurrent disease.** Some disease states may alter the pharmacodynamics and, in some cases, the pharmacokinetics of a given drug and subsequently alter the therapeutic range. As an example, patients with underlying heart disease (cor pulmonale, coronary artery disease) have increased sensitivity to digoxin.[29]

• **Variable ratios of enantiomers.** Some drugs are administered as racemic mixtures of enantiomers, which may have different response/toxicity profiles as well as pharmacokinetic behaviors. Thus, a given concentration of the summed enantiomers (using an achiral assay method) is associated with different concentrations of response or toxicity in patients with different proportions of the enantiomers. This has been extensively studied for disopyramide.[30]

• **Variable genotype.** There is growing evidence that response to certain drugs is genetically determined. For selected drugs, patients may be genotyped before starting drug treatment

to identify them as nonresponders, responders, or toxic responders (see Chapter 6).[31-33] One such drug is bupropion, for which wide patient variability in response is associated with genetic polymorphisms of CYP2B6.[34]

• **Variable serum protein binding.** Theoretically, only the unbound concentration of drug in blood is capable of establishing equilibrium with pharmacologic receptors, thus making it a better predictor of response than total drug concentration. Most drug concentrations in serum, plasma, or blood, however, are measured as the summed concentration of bound and unbound drug. It is likely that some of the patients who show toxicity within the conventional therapeutic range have abnormally low protein (eg, albumin) binding and high concentrations of an unbound drug in blood.[35] Low protein binding of a drug in blood can be the result of either reduced protein concentrations or the presence of other substances in blood that displace the drug from protein binding sites. Phenytoin would be an example of a drug requiring consideration of plasma proteins in evaluation of serum concentrations.

In summary, the therapeutic range reported by the laboratory is only an initial guide and not a guarantee of desired clinical response in any individual patient. Every effort must be made to consider other signs of clinical response and toxicity in addition to the drug concentration measurement. Therapeutic ranges for the most commonly monitored drugs discussed in the Applications section of this chapter are reported in **Table 5-3**.

## SAMPLE TIMING

Incorrect timing of sample collection is the most frequent source of error when therapeutic drug monitoring results do not agree with the clinical picture.[23,36] Warner reviewed five studies in which 70% to 86% of the samples obtained for therapeutic drug monitoring purposes were not usable. In most cases, this was the result of inappropriate sample timing, including lack of attention to the time required to reach a steady state.[23] There are two primary considerations for sample timing: (1) how long to wait after initiation or adjustment of a dosage regimen and (2) when to obtain the sample during a dosing interval.

### At Steady State

When a drug regimen (a fixed dose given at a regularly repeated interval) is initiated, concentrations are initially low and gradually increase until a steady state is reached. Pharmacokinetically, *steady state* is defined as the condition in which the rate of drug entering the body is equal to the rate of its elimination. For therapeutic drug monitoring, a steady state means that drug concentrations have leveled off at their highest and, when given as the same dose at a fixed interval, the concentration versus time profiles are constant from interval to interval. This is illustrated in **Figure 5-3** for a continuous infusion and a chronic intermittent dosage regimen.

Drug concentration measurements should not be made until the drug is sufficiently close to a steady state so that the maximum benefit of the drug is ensured. The time required to reach

**TABLE 5-3.** Data to Aid Interpretation of Concentrations of Drugs That Are Commonly Monitored

| | RECOMMENDED CONCENTRATIONS | RECOMMENDED TIMING | CONSIDERATIONS FOR INTERPRETATION: PROTEIN BINDING, ACTIVE METABOLITES, OTHER FACTORS |
|---|---|---|---|
| **Bronchodilators** | | | |
| Theophylline | Adult: 5–15 mg/L<br>Child: 5–10 mg/L<br>Neonate: 5–10 mg/L | Trough or $C_{ss,avg}$ steady state occurs in 24 hr for an average adult nonsmoker receiving a maintenance infusion, but may take longer for sustained-release products | Concentrations up to 20 mg/L may be necessary in some patients; the caffeine metabolite is of minor significance in adults but may contribute to effect in neonates; theophylline has been replaced by safer bronchodilators in children, and by caffeine in neonates |
| **Antiepileptics** | | | |
| Carbamazepine | 4–12 mg/L | Trough or $C_{ss,avg}$ steady state may require up to 2–3 wk after initiation of full dose rate due to autoinduction | Lower total concentrations may be more appropriate in patients with decreased protein binding (liver disease, hypoalbuminemia, and hyperbilirubinemia), or in patients taking other anticonvulsants |
| Phenobarbital | 10–40 mg/L | Anytime during interval; steady state may require up to 3 wk | Many drug interactions; consider impact on concentration when starting/stopping interacting medications |
| Phenytoin | Based on total phenytoin concentrations:<br>Adult: 10–20 mg/L<br>Infant: 6–11 mg/L<br>Neonate: 8–15 mg/L | Trough or $C_{ss,avg}$ steady state may require up to 3 wk | Measurement of unbound phenytoin concentrations (therapeutic range of 1–2 mg/L) may be preferred in most patients; lower total phenytoin concentrations may be more appropriate in patients with decreased protein binding due to hypoalbuminemia (eg, liver disease, nephrotic syndrome, pregnancy, cystic fibrosis, burns, trauma, malnutrition, AIDS, and advanced age), ESRD, concurrent use of salicylic acid or VPA |
| Valproic Acid (VPA) | Epilepsy: 50–100 mg/L (total)<br>Mania: 50–125 mg/L (total) | Trough or $C_{ss,avg}$<br>Steady state may require up to 5 days | Lower total VPA concentrations may be more appropriate in patients with hypoalbuminemia (liver disease, cystic fibrosis, burns, trauma, malnutrition, and advanced age), hyperbilirubinemia, ESRD, and concurrent use of salicylic acid; VPA shows interpatient variability in unbound fraction because of nonlinear protein binding; total concentrations increase less than proportionately with increases in daily dose, while unbound concentrations increase proportionately |

**TABLE 5-3.** Data to Aid Interpretation of Concentrations of Drugs That Are Commonly Monitored, cont'd

| | RECOMMENDED CONCENTRATIONS | RECOMMENDED TIMING | CONSIDERATIONS FOR INTERPRETATION: PROTEIN BINDING, ACTIVE METABOLITES, OTHER FACTORS |
|---|---|---|---|
| **Antimicrobial Drugs** | | | |
| Amikacin | Traditional dosing: Peaks: 20–30 mg/L Troughs: < 8 mg/L | Traditional dosing: steady state should be based on estimated half-life, particularly in patients with renal impairment<br><br>Extended-interval dosing: per institution specific protocol (consider two-point and patient-specific kinetics)<br><br>Desired peak will depend on infection site (ie, high inoculum infections necessitating higher peaks) | |
| Gentamicin, tobramycin | Traditional dosing: Peaks: 6–10 mg/L Troughs: < 1–2 mg/L | Traditional dosing: steady state should be based on estimated half-life, particularly in patients with renal impairment<br><br>Extended-interval dosing: per institution specific protocol (consider two-point and patient-specific kinetics)<br><br>Desired peak depends on infection site (ie, high inoculum infections necessitating higher peaks) | |
| Vancomycin | AUC-guided monitoring for serious MRSA infections: >400–600 mg × hr/L Troughs/traditional based monitoring: 10–20 mg/L | AUC-guided monitoring: one concentration obtained at 1–2 hr postinfusion ($C_{max}$) and a second concentration obtained at the end of dosing interval (trough, $C_{min}$) once steady state is reached; if using Bayesian software, may obtain trough concentration (at end of dosing interval) only; can be drawn prior to reaching steady state<br><br>Trough-based monitoring: Concentration within 30 min to 1 hr of next dose; steady state may require up to 2–3 days in patients with normal renal function | AUC-guided monitoring is reserved for invasive MRSA infections; there is not enough data to assess which monitoring approach (AUC-guided vs. trough-only monitoring) should be followed in noninvasive MRSA or other infections |

*(continued)*

**TABLE 5-3.** Data to Aid Interpretation of Concentrations of Drugs That Are Commonly Monitored, cont'd

| | RECOMMENDED CONCENTRATIONS | RECOMMENDED TIMING | CONSIDERATIONS FOR INTERPRETATION: PROTEIN BINDING, ACTIVE METABOLITES, OTHER FACTORS |
|---|---|---|---|
| **Antifungal Agents** | | | |
| Itraconazole | Trough concentration >0.5–1 mg/L | Concentration can be drawn at any time during a dosing interval once steady state is reached | Variability in absorption and concentrations noted between different formulations (eg, oral capsules versus oral solution) |
| Posaconazole | Trough >1 mg/L | Concentration can be drawn at any time during dosing interval once steady state is reached at end of first week of therapy | Variability in absorption and concentrations noted between different formulations (eg, oral tablets versus oral suspension) |
| Voriconazole | Lower limit: >1 mg/L Upper limit: <4–6 mg/L | Trough concentration (eg, prior to next dose) within first week of therapy initiation or dosage adjustments<br><br>Steady state may be reached in 1–2 days; however, it is recommended to wait at least 5 days to measure trough concentration | |
| **Cardiac Drugs** | | | |
| Digoxin | 0.5–1.2 mcg/L | NEVER sooner than 6 hr after an oral dose; steady state may require up to 7 days with normal renal function | Toxicity more likely within therapeutic range in patients with hypokalemia, hypomagnesemia, hypercalcemia, underlying heart disease, and hypothyroidism; patients with hyperthyroidism may be resistant at a given digoxin concentration, drug interactions |
| **Cytotoxic Drugs** | | | |
| Methotrexate | Therapeutic levels: variable High-dose regimen: 0.1–1 $\mu$M/L Low-dose regimen: <0.2 $\mu$M/L | Per protocol for determination of leucovorin rescue regimen | Decreased protein binding is observed in some situations, but implications for interpretation of total concentrations are unclear |
| **Immunosuppressant Drugs** | | | |
| Cyclosporine | 100–500 mcg/L (whole blood, using specific assay) | Trough or 2-hr after dose; steady state may require up to 5 days | Highly variable unbound fraction in blood; higher total concentrations may be acceptable in patients with hypercholesterolemia or prior to acute rejection episodes (increased serum binding); lower total concentrations might be acceptable in patients with decreased binding in serum (low cholesterol) |

**TABLE 5-3.** Data to Aid Interpretation of Concentrations of Drugs That Are Commonly Monitored, cont'd

| | RECOMMENDED CONCENTRATIONS | RECOMMENDED TIMING | CONSIDERATIONS FOR INTERPRETATION: PROTEIN BINDING, ACTIVE METABOLITES, OTHER FACTORS |
|---|---|---|---|
| Tacrolimus | Initiation: 20 mcg/L Maintenance: 5–10 mcg/L Goal concentrations may be patient and institution specific | Trough concentrations three times a week initially until concentrations are stabilized; monitoring intervals can be extended with maintenance therapy | Therapeutic range may shift slightly with concomitant immunosuppressant medications and by indication; many drug interactions; consider impact on concentration when starting/stopping interacting medications |
| **Psychotropics** | | | |
| Lithium | Acute management: 0.5–1.2 mEq/L Maintenance: 0.6–0.8 mEq/L | 12 hr after the evening dose on BID or TID schedule; steady state may require up to 1 wk | Monovalent cation, which is not bound to plasma proteins; does not undergo metabolism |

a steady state can be predicted if the drug's half-life is known, as shown here:

| NUMBER OF HALF-LIVES | PERCENTAGE OF STEADY STATE ATTAINED |
|---|---|
| 2 | 75% |
| 3 | 88% |
| 4 | 94% |
| 5 | 97% |

This means the clinician should wait three half-lives at a minimum before obtaining a sample for monitoring purposes.

The clinician also should anticipate that the "usual" half-life in a given patient may actually be longer due to impaired elimination processes, and it may be prudent to wait longer if possible. The half-lives of drugs that are typically monitored are reported in the Applications section, and typical times to steady state are reported in **Table 5-3**.

Sometimes drugs are not given as a fixed dose at a fixed interval, or they may undergo diurnal variations in pharmacokinetic handling.[37,38] Although the concentration-versus-time profiles may differ from each other within a given day, the patterns from day to day will be the same if steady state has been attained. In cases of irregular dosing or diurnal variations, it is important that drug concentration measurements on different visits be obtained at similar times of the day for comparative purposes.

An unusual situation is caused by autoinduction, as exemplified by carbamazepine. The half-life of carbamazepine is longer

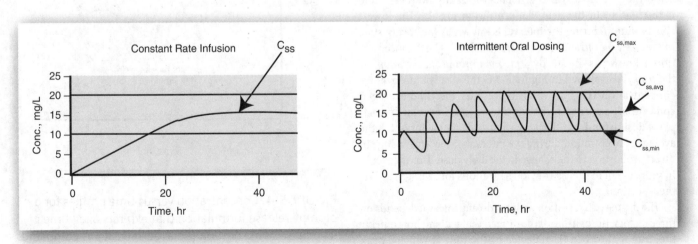

**FIGURE 5-3.** Concentration versus time plots for a constant infusion and intermittent therapy after initiation of therapy, without a loading dose. The half-life for this hypothetical drug is 8 hours. Thus, 88% of the eventual average steady-state concentration ($C_{ss,avg}$) is attained in 24 hours.

after the first dose but progressively shortens as the enzymes that metabolize carbamazepine are induced by exposure to itself.[39] The half-life of carbamazepine during chronic therapy cannot be used to predict the time required to reach a steady state. The actual time to reach a steady state is somewhere between the time based on the first-dose half-life and that based on the chronic-dosing half-life. For this reason, patients are typically started on 25% to 33% of the target total daily dose.[40] Autoinduction has been found to be reversible when carbamazepine is held for 6 or more days.[41]

It is a common misconception that a steady state is reached faster when a loading dose is given. Although a carefully chosen loading dose will provide desired target concentrations after the first dose, the resulting concentration is only an approximation of the true steady-state concentration, and it will still require at least three half-lives to attain a true steady state. Whenever possible, it is best to allow more time for a steady state to be attained than less. This is also important because the average half-life for the population may not apply to a specific patient.

There are some exceptions to the rule of waiting until a steady state is reached before sampling. If there is suspected toxicity early during therapy, a drug concentration measurement is warranted and may necessitate immediate reduction or suspension of a dose. Dosing methods designed to predict maintenance dosage regimens using pre–steady-state drug concentrations are useful when rapid individualization of the dosage regimen is needed.[42-47] For example, a pre–steady-state concentration may be warranted for patients with poor renal function receiving vancomycin in whom supratherapeutic drug concentrations are more likely to occur and cause adverse drug effects.

## Within the Dosing Interval

Figure 5-3 shows typical concentration versus time profiles for a drug given by continuous infusion and a drug given by oral intermittent dosing. Once a steady state is attained, drug concentrations during a continuous infusion remain constant, and samples for drug concentration measurements can be obtained at any time. When a drug is given intermittently, however, there is fluctuation in the drug concentration profile. The lowest concentration during the interval is known as the steady-state *minimum concentration*, or the *trough*. The highest concentration is known as the steady-state *maximum concentration*, or the *peak*. Also shown in Figure 5-3 is the steady-state average concentration ($C_{ss,avg}$), which represents the time-averaged concentration during the dosing interval. An important principle of dosing for drugs that show first-order behavior is that the average concentration during the interval or day will change in direct proportion to the change in the daily dose. This is covered in more detail in the Use of Concentrations for Dosage Adjustment section.

The degree of fluctuation within a dosing interval depends on three factors: the half-life of the drug in that patient; how quickly the drug is absorbed (as reflected by the time at which a peak concentration occurs for that particular formulation); and the dosing interval. The least fluctuation (lowest peak:trough ratio) occurs for drugs with relatively long half-lives that are slowly absorbed or given as sustained-release formulations (prolonged

peak time) in divided doses (short dosing interval). However, drugs with relatively short half-lives that are quickly absorbed (or given as immediate-release products) and given only once daily show the greatest amount of fluctuation within the interval.

The choice of timing for samples within the dosing interval should be based on the clinical question to be addressed. Troughs are usually recommended for therapeutic confirmation, especially if the therapeutic range was formulated based on trough concentrations as is the case for most of the antiepileptic drugs (AEDs).[14] Trough concentrations are also recommended if the indication for concentration monitoring is avoidance of inefficacy (or in case of certain antimicrobials, development of antimicrobial resistance) or distinguishing nonadherence from therapeutic failure. Trough concentrations should also be monitored if the patient tends to experience symptoms of inefficacy before the next dose (in which case a shortening of the dosing interval might be all that is needed). Although it is logical to assume that the lowest concentration during the interval will occur immediately before the next dose, this is not always the case. Some products are formulated as delayed-release products (eg, enteric-coated valproic acid [VPA]) that are designed to be released from the intestine rather than the stomach. As such, they may not begin to be absorbed for several hours after administration, and the concentration of drug from the previous dose continues to decline for several hours into the next interval. It is important to recognize that the predose concentration for those formulations is not the lowest concentration during the interval (**Figure 5-4**).

Peak concentrations are monitored less often for drugs given orally because the time at which peak concentrations occur is

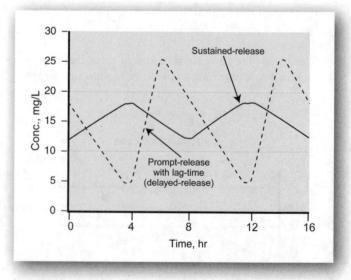

**FIGURE 5-4.** Concentration versus time profiles for a prompt-release formulation that exhibits a lag time in its release or absorption (delayed-release) as compared with a sustained-release formulation without lag time. Note that the lowest concentration during the dosing interval for the delayed-release product occurs at a time that is typically expected for the peak to occur.

difficult to predict. If a peak concentration is indicated, the package insert should be consulted for time to peak concentration of individual products. Peak concentration monitoring would be appropriate if the patient complains of symptoms of toxicity at a time believed to correspond with a peak concentration or in some cases correspond to clinical efficacy. Peaks may also be used for intravenous (IV) drugs (eg, aminoglycosides) because the time of the peak is known to correspond to the end of the infusion. For aminoglycosides, the peak concentration is believed to be a predictor of efficacy.[48]

Sometimes the clinician wishes to get an idea of the average concentration of drug during the day or dosing interval. This is particularly useful when the concentration is to be used for a dose adjustment. Pharmacokinetically, the average concentration equals the area under the curve (AUC) during the dosing interval (requiring multiple samples) divided by the interval. (Note: the AUC during an interval or portion of an interval is used as the monitoring parameter in place of single drug concentration measurements for certain drugs, such as some immunosuppressant and cytotoxic drugs, because it provides a better indication of overall drug exposure.) However, determination of the AUC, or $C_{ss,avg}$, by multiple sampling is not cost-effective for the most commonly monitored drugs. The following alternatives aid in estimating the $C_{ss,avg}$ without multiple samples:

- Look up the expected time to reach a peak concentration for the particular formulation and obtain a sample midway between that time and the end of the dosing interval.[24]

Measure the trough concentration (as close to the time of administration of the next dose as possible) and use that along with the population value for the drug's volume of distribution ($V_d$) to estimate the peak concentration (in the following equation). Then take the average of the trough and the peak to get an estimate of the average steady-state concentration.

$$Peak_{steady-state} = (Dose/V_d) + measured\ trough$$

- If you have reason to believe that there is little fluctuation during the dosing interval, then a sample drawn any time during the interval provides a reasonable reflection of the average concentration.

There are special and extremely important timing considerations for some drugs, such as digoxin. It must reach specific receptors, presumably in the myocardium, to exhibit its therapeutic effect, but this takes several hours after the dose is administered. Early after a digoxin dose, concentrations in serum are relatively high, but the response is not yet evident because digoxin has not yet equilibrated at its site of action. Thus, only digoxin concentrations that are in the postdistribution phase should be monitored and compared with the reported therapeutic range (**Minicase 2**).

The timing of samples for other drugs may be based on the requirements for certain dosing methods. This is true for aminoglycosides and certain lithium dosing methods. Sample timing for drugs such as methotrexate is specified in protocols because

## MINICASE 2

## Importance of Sample Timing for Digoxin

Ruth D., a 93-year-old female patient with heart failure, coronary artery disease, and diabetes mellitus type 2, was recently discharged from the hospital after a heart failure exacerbation that resulted from new-onset atrial fibrillation with rapid ventricular response. During the hospital stay, the patient received IV doses of metoprolol; however, the patient's heart rate remained elevated in the 130s and the decision was made to initiate digoxin upon admission. The patient received a loading dose of digoxin 250 mcg IV every 6 hours for three doses followed by 0.25 mg orally once daily at 9:00 a.m. The patient has arrived for her follow-up cardiology appointment. She reports nausea, vomiting, and a loss of appetite for the past several days. On presentation, she is also noted to have some bradycardia. Because of concern for possible digoxin toxicity, the cardiology nurse practitioner ordered a digoxin concentration and basic metabolic panel at 11:30 a.m., which resulted the following results:

Digoxin: 3.4 mcg/L
Serum creatinine: 0.8 mg/dL
Potassium: 3.8 mmol/L
Magnesium: 1.9 mg/dL
Calcium: 9.1 mg/dL

The cardiology nurse practitioner calls the clinical pharmacy specialist for assistance with digoxin dose adjustment. Ruth D.'s

renal function is stable and there have been no medication changes since her discharge last week.

QUESTION: Are there other possible causes for the patient's GI symptoms? What considerations should be taken into account in the interpretation of this patient's digoxin concentration? What recommendation should be made at this time?

DISCUSSION: Several non–drug-related reasons for the patient's GI symptoms are possible, including infection, constipation, acid reflux, and stress, among others that should be considered in addition to digoxin toxicity. There are no new medications; therefore, drug interactions may be ruled out as an explanation for the high digoxin concentration. Digoxin concentrations, with maintenance therapy, should be drawn just prior to the administration of the next dose (trough concentration) or no sooner than 6 to 8 hours after the dose was administered. Her digoxin concentration in serum, however, was drawn 2.5 hours after her 9:00 a.m. dose and therefore does not yet reflect the concentration of digoxin at its myocardial target. To determine if digoxin is the primary cause of her GI symptoms and concomitant bradycardia, a repeat concentration should be drawn after 3:00 p.m. today to account for the distribution of digoxin to tissues. Changes to the medication regimen should be based on the correctly drawn concentration.

concentrations are used to determine the need for rescue therapy with leucovorin to minimize methotrexate toxicity.

Although samples for drug concentration measurements may be preferred at certain times during a dosing interval, visits to physician offices often do not coincide with desired times for blood draws. One is then faced with the matter of how to interpret a concentration that is drawn at a time that happens to be more convenient to the patient's appointment. The most critical pieces of information to obtain in this situation are (1) when the last drug dose was taken, (2) adherence, (3) timing of the sample relative to the last dose, and (4) the expected time of peak concentration. Some drugs are available as a wide variety of formulations (solutions, suspensions, immediate-release, and sustained-release or extended-release dosage forms), and the package insert may be the best source of information for the expected peak time. Once again, drugs with relatively long half-lives given as sustained-release or slowly absorbed products in divided doses will have the flattest concentration-versus-time profiles, and concentrations drawn anytime during the interval are going to be similar. However, immediate-release drugs with short half-lives given less frequently will show more fluctuation. Knowing the expected peak time for the formulation in question is especially important for drugs that show more fluctuation during that interval. In that case, one can at least judge if the reported concentration is closer to a peak, an average (if midway between the peak and trough), or a trough.

# USE OF CONCENTRATIONS FOR DOSAGE ADJUSTMENT

A chronic intermittent dosage regimen has three components: the dose rate, the dosing interval, and the dose. For the dosage regimen of 240 mg every 8 hours, the dose is 240 mg, the interval is 8 hours, and the dose rate can be expressed as 720 mg/day or 30 mg/hr. The degree of fluctuation between doses is highly influenced by the dosing interval. Dose rate is influenced by both the dose and interval; therefore, any change in the dose or interval will be associated with the corresponding change in the dose rate.

## Dosage Adjustments for Linear Behavior

If a drug is known to have first-order bioavailability and elimination behavior after the administration of therapeutic doses, one can use simple proportionality to make an adjustment in the daily dose:

- If average concentrations are being monitored or estimated, one can predict that the average, steady-state drug concentration will increase in proportion to the increase in total daily dose, regardless of any changes made to the dosing interval.

- If trough concentrations are monitored and the dosing interval is held constant, the trough concentration will increase in proportion to the increase in daily dose.

- If trough concentrations are monitored for a drug that exhibits considerable fluctuation during the dosing interval and both the dose and dosing interval will be adjusted, the trough concentration will not be as easy to predict at a new steady state and is beyond the scope of this chapter. If the

trough concentration can be used to estimate the $C_{ss,avg}$, as described previously, the $C_{ss,avg}$ can be predicted to change in proportion to the change in daily dose.

Sampling after a dosage regimen adjustment, if appropriate, should not be done until a new steady state has been reached. For a drug with first-order behavior, this should take the same time (three half-lives at a minimum) that it did after initiation of therapy with this drug.

## Dosage Adjustments for Drugs with Nonlinear Behavior

All drugs show nonlinear elimination behavior if sufficiently high doses are given. Some drugs, however, show pronounced nonlinear (Michaelis-Menten) elimination behavior after doses that produce therapeutic drug concentrations. This means that an increase in the dose of the drug results in a greater-than-proportional increase in the drug concentration. Phenytoin is an example of a drug with this behavior. Theophylline and procainamide also show some degree of nonlinear behavior but only at the higher end of their therapeutic ranges and not enough to require special dosing methods.

Methods have been described to permit predictions of the effect of dose increases for phenytoin using population averages or actual measurements of the parameters that define nonlinearity, namely $V_{max}$ (maximum rate of metabolism) and $K_m$ (the "Michaelis constant"), but they are beyond the scope of this chapter.[49] The most important rule to remember for dosage adjustments of drugs such as phenytoin is to be conservative; small increases in the dose produce unpredictably large increases in the serum drug concentration. It must also be noted that the half-life of a drug like phenytoin is progressively prolonged at higher concentrations. Increases in the dose require a longer period of time to reach a steady state as compared with when the drug was first initiated.

Population pharmacokinetic or Bayesian dosage adjustment methods, which involve the use of statistical probabilities, are preferred by many for computerized individualization of therapy and can be used for drugs with both linear and nonlinear behavior.[47,50]

# PROTEIN BINDING, ACTIVE METABOLITES, AND OTHER CONSIDERATIONS

## Altered Serum Binding

Total (unbound plus protein-bound) drug concentrations measured in blood, serum, or plasma are most frequently used for therapeutic drug monitoring, despite the fact that unbound drug concentrations are more closely correlated to drug effect.[35] While total concentrations are easier to measure, it should be noted the ratio of unbound to total drug concentration in serum is usually constant within and between individuals. For some drugs, however, the relationship between unbound and total drug concentration is extremely variable among patients, or it may be altered by disease or drug interactions. For drugs that undergo concentration-dependent serum binding, the relationship between unbound and total concentration varies within patients. In these situations, total drug concentration does not reflect the same concentration of activity as with normal binding and must be cautiously interpreted because the usual therapeutic range does not apply (**Minicase 3**).

The direct measurement of unbound drug concentration would seem to be appropriate in these situations. Drugs for which total concentration monitoring is routinely performed (but for which unbound concentration monitoring has been proposed) include carbamazepine, phenytoin, and VPA. Of these, correlations between unbound drug concentration and response have been weakly established for carbamazepine but more firmly established for phenytoin.[35,51,52]

Unbound drug concentration measurements involve an extra step prior to analysis—separation of the unbound from the bound drug. If unbound drug concentration measurements are unavailable, too costly, or considered impractical, the following alternative approaches to interpreting total drug concentrations in situations of altered serum protein binding may be used:

- **Use of equations to normalize the measured total concentration.** Sheiner and Tozer were the first to propose equations that can be used to convert a measured total concentration of drug (phenytoin in this case) to an approximation of what the total concentration would be if the patient had normal binding.[53] Equations to normalize PHT concentrations have been used for patients with hypoalbuminemia, impaired renal function, and concurrent VPA therapy.[54-56] Once the total concentration has been normalized, it may be compared with the conventional therapeutic range. It must be noted that this normalization method may not be a reliable substitute for the measurement of the unbound phenytoin concentration, particularly when clinical presentation does not correlate with the obtained drug concentration.

- **Normalization of the measured total concentration using literature estimates of the abnormal unbound drug fraction.** An alternative method for normalizing the total concentration can be used if reasonable estimates of the abnormal and normal unbound reactions of the drug can be ascertained (ie, from the literature). The normalized total concentration ($C_{normalized}$) can be estimated as

$$C_{normalized} = C_{measured} \times \frac{\text{abnormal unbound fraction}}{\text{normal unbound fraction}}$$

## MINICASE 3

## Value of Unbound Antiepileptic Drug Serum Concentrations

Trevor L., a 26-year-old White man, is discharged after a long inpatient admission following a high-speed vehicle accident, which led to significant brain swelling secondary to a traumatic brain injury. Consequently, he exhibited clinical findings of seizure activity while admitted and it was recommended he be discharged on phenytoin 200 mg TID. Today (4 weeks after discharge) is his follow-up appointment with the neurology department. The patient reveals to the neurologist that he has been experiencing ataxia and dizziness. The neurology resident is concerned about antiepileptic drug toxicity, namely, phenytoin toxicity, and orders a phenytoin total serum concentration, along with a complete metabolic panel as part of routine monitoring.

Results: Phenytoin: 16 mg/L (reference range 10 to 20 mg/L)
Albumin: 1.8 g/dL
Serum creatinine: 0.98 mg/dL

The neurology resident is perplexed given the phenytoin concentration is within therapeutic range and calls the hospital clinical pharmacist to discuss it further.

QUESTION: How is the total concentrations of phenytoin misleading in this case? What further recommendations should the pharmacist provide the resident to determine whether the symptoms the patient is experiencing are related to antiseizure therapy toxicity?

DISCUSSION: Assessing the patient's symptoms solely on the total phenytoin concentrations can be misleading and can lead to seeking alternative explanations for the patient's symptoms, thereby delaying necessary life-saving medication dose adjustments.

Phenytoin binds primarily to albumin in plasma. The patient has significant hypoalbuminemia; therefore, interpreting the phenytoin concentrations using total phenytoin only can be misleading and it is expected that the unbound concentration is likely higher than the therapeutic range of unbound concentration of 1 to 2 mg/L. Several approaches can be followed in a situation like this to assist with assessing the patient's clinical findings: (1) ordering an unbound phenytoin concentration, (2) calculating the unbound phenytoin concentration, or (3) using special equations to convert the phenytoin concentration to what it would be if the patient had normal serum protein binding. One specialized equation is commonly called the Winter-Tozer equation. This equation normalizes phenytoin concentration in patients with hypoalbuminemia.

Corrected phenytoin concentration is as follows:

(measured phenytoin)/(X * albumin + 0.1)

where *X* in this patient's case is 0.25 for low albumin in patients with head trauma.

Corrected phenytoin concentration is as follows:

(16 mg/L)/(0.25*1.8 g/dL + 0.1) = 29 mg/L

The corrected phenytoin concentration reveals a supratherapeutic concentration that is likely contributing to the patient's current symptoms and complaints.

where $C_{measured}$ is the measured total concentration reported by the laboratory.

- **Predictive linear regression equations.** Some studies have reported the ability to predict unbound drug concentrations in the presence of displacing drugs if the total concentrations of both drugs are known. This has been done to predict unbound concentrations of phenytoin and carbamazepine, both in the presence of VPA.[55,56] These unbound drug concentrations should be compared with corresponding therapeutic ranges of unbound drug, which can be estimated for any drug if the normal unbound fraction and the usual therapeutic range of total concentrations are known.

- **Use of saliva as a substitute for unbound drug concentration.** Saliva may be a reasonable alternative so long as studies have shown a strong correlation between unbound concentrations in serum and concentrations in saliva. The concentration of drug in saliva may not be equal to the concentration in serum ultrafiltrate; therefore, the laboratory should have determined a reliable conversion factor for this. The calculated unbound concentration may then be compared with the estimated therapeutic range for unbound concentrations as described previously. Saliva concentrations may also be used as a predictor of total drug concentrations, particularly for some of the AEDs.[57]

- **Active metabolites**—Interpretation of parent drug concentration alone, for drugs with active metabolites that are present to varying extents, is difficult at best. Active metabolites may contribute to therapeutic response, toxicity, or both. Because metabolites likely have different pharmacokinetic characteristics, they are affected differently than the parent drug under different physiologic and pathologic conditions. For drugs such as primidone (metabolized to phenobarbital) and procainamide (metabolized to *N*-acetylprocainamide [NAPA]), the laboratory typically reports both the parent drug and the metabolite as well as a therapeutic range for both. Although a therapeutic range for the sum of procainamide and NAPA may be reported by some laboratories, this practice is discouraged because the parent drug and metabolites have different types of pharmacologic activities.

- **Enantiomeric pairs.** Some drugs exist as an equal mixture (racemic mixture) of enantiomers, which are chemically identical but are mirror images of each other. Because they can interact differently with receptors, they may have different pharmacodynamic and pharmacokinetic properties. The relative proportions of the enantiomers can differ widely among and within patients. Thus, a given concentration of the summed enantiomers (what is routinely measured using achiral methods) can represent different activities.[31]

Table 5-3 provides relevant information about protein binding, active metabolites, and other influences on serum concentration interpretation for drugs discussed in the Applications sections that follow.

# APPLICATIONS

## Analgesic Drugs
### Acetaminophen

***Therapeutic range and clinical considerations.*** Acetaminophen is the first-line treatment for patients with osteoarthritis and mild-to-moderate chronic pain.[58,59] Additionally, acetaminophen is a commonly used antipyretic agent.[60] Acetaminophen serum concentrations should be monitored only when a suspected or confirmed overdose is a concern or in patients taking long-term acetaminophen with concomitant liver dysfunction.[61] Antipyretic activity is expected to occur at serum concentrations of 4 to 18 mg/L; analgesic activity is expected to occur at serum concentrations of 10 mg/L.[62] Historically, 4,000 mg/day has long been considered a safe therapeutic dose in normal patients.[63-65]

***Sample timing.*** Acetaminophen serum concentrations should be drawn at least 4 hours after suspected acute ingestion to ensure drug absorption; the Rumack–Matthew nomogram should be referenced to determine treatment decisions.[66] In the case of IV formulation overdose, reliable guidelines related to monitoring and management have not been established.

***Protein binding, active metabolites, and other considerations.*** Acetaminophen is 10% to 25% bound to protein at therapeutic concentrations and 8% to 43% at supratherapeutic concentrations.[60]

## Bronchodilators
### Aminophylline and Theophylline

***Therapeutic range and clinical considerations.*** Although aminophylline and theophylline are rarely used in practice, serum concentration monitoring may be necessary because of variable pharmacokinetics. These agents are not recommended for the treatment of asthma exacerbations according to the Global Initiative for Asthma 2020 guidelines due to efficacy and safety concerns.[67] The 2020 Global Initiative for Chronic Obstructive Lung Disease guidelines recommend using a more effective therapy of inhaled long-acting bronchodilators over theophylline when possible. In the management of chronic obstructive pulmonary disease exacerbations, IV theophylline is not recommended due to significant side effects. Peak concentrations of 5 to 20 mg/L are targeted with concentrations >20 mg/L being associated with adverse events.[68,69] There is an 85% probability of adverse effects with concentrations above 25 mg/L; concentrations above 30 to 40 mg/L are associated with dangerous adverse events.[70] Many patients do not tolerate theophylline; adverse effects typically experienced by adults include nausea, vomiting, diarrhea, irritability, and insomnia at concentrations above 15 mg/L; supraventricular tachycardia, hypotension, and ventricular arrhythmias at concentrations above 40 mg/L; and seizures, brain damage, and even death at higher concentrations.[71]

Theophylline is also indicated for treatment of neonatal apnea, although caffeine is preferred.[72] The therapeutic range of theophylline in neonates is generally considered to be 5 to 10 mg/L but may be as low as 3 mg/L or as high as 14 mg/L.[73-76] Adverse effects in neonates include lack of weight gain, sleeplessness, irritability, diuresis, dehydration, hyperreflexia, jitteriness, and serious cardiovascular and neurologic events.[70] Tachycardia has been reported in neonates with concentrations as low as 13 mg/L.[77]

In summary, there is considerable overlap of therapeutic and toxic effects within the usual therapeutic ranges reported for theophylline in neonates, children, and adults. Indications for theophylline monitoring include therapeutic confirmation of effective concentrations after initiation of therapy or a dosage regimen adjustment, anticipated drug–drug interactions, change in smoking habits, and changes in health status that might affect the metabolism of theophylline.

*Sample timing.* Concentrations should be measured 30 minutes after the end of the infusion if an aminophylline loading dose is given; continuous infusion monitoring should include monitoring serum concentrations at one half-life after the start of the infusion and at every 12 or 24 hours after the start of the infusion.[78] The half-life of theophylline can range anywhere from 20 to 30 hours in premature infants to 3 to 5 hours in children or adult smokers to as long as 50 hours in nonsmoking adults with severe heart failure or liver disease.[68,73] Steady state is reached in 24 hours for the average patient, with an elimination half-life of 8 hours, but requires a much longer elimination time for patients with heart failure or liver disease. The time to steady state in premature neonates may be as long as 9 days.[74]

The fluctuation of theophylline concentrations within a steady-state dosing interval can be quite variable, depending not only on the frequency of administration but also on the type of formulation, half-life, and whether the dose was taken with a meal.[70,71] Trough concentrations of theophylline are most reproducible and should be used for monitoring. Comparisons of trough concentrations from visit to visit can be facilitated if samples are obtained at the same time of day on each visit due to the diurnal variations in the rate of theophylline absorption.[70]

*Use of concentrations for dosage adjustment.* Theophylline is usually assumed to undergo first-order elimination, but some of its metabolic pathways are nonlinear at concentrations at the higher end of the therapeutic range. The clearance of theophylline decreases by 20% as daily doses are increased from 210 mg to 1,260 mg.[70] For IV formulations, concentrations should be checked every 24 hours to determine if dose adjustment is warranted; for oral formulations, intervals of 6 to 12 months are recommended once the daily dose has been stabilized.[68,79]

*Protein binding, active metabolites, and other considerations.* Theophylline is 35% bound to serum proteins in neonates and 40% to 50% in adults; therefore, significant alterations in serum protein binding are unlikely.[79] Theophylline is metabolized to the active metabolite caffeine, which is of minor consequence in adults. Caffeine concentrations in the serum of neonates, however, are approximately 30% of theophylline concentrations and contribute to treatment of neonatal apnea, which may account for the slightly lower therapeutic range of theophylline in neonates as compared with adults.[80]

## Caffeine

*Therapeutic range and clinical considerations.* Caffeine is indicated for neonatal apnea (apnea of prematurity) and is recommended over theophylline because it can be given once daily (due to a longer half-life), has a wider therapeutic index, and does not require drug concentration monitoring. [72,80] Concentrations as low as 5 mg/L may be effective, but most pediatric textbooks consider 10 mg/L to be the lower limit of the therapeutic range; an acceptable reference range is 8 to 14 mg/L.[76,81,82] Toxicity may occur at concentrations >20 mg/L, and serious toxicity is associated with serum concentrations above 50 mg/L. Signs of toxicity include jitteriness, vomiting, irritability, tremor of the extremities, tachypnea, and tonic-clonic movements. Serum concentration measurements of caffeine may not be routinely necessary for apnea of prematurity in neonates.[80,83] However, neonates who do not respond as expected or in whom there is recurrence of apnea after a favorable response may benefit.

*Sample timing.* The half-life of caffeine in preterm infants at birth ranges from 40 to 230 hours.[81,82] Thus, a loading dose is always administered to attain effective concentrations as soon as possible. The long half-life means that caffeine concentrations will not fluctuate much during the interval, even when caffeine is administered once daily. Sampling in the postdistribution phase is recommended, which is at least 2 hours after the dose.

Baseline concentrations of caffeine must be obtained prior to the first caffeine dose in the following situations: (1) if the infant had been previously treated with theophylline because caffeine is a metabolite of theophylline and (2) if the infant was born to a mother who consumed caffeine prior to delivery. Reductions in the usual caffeine dose are necessary if predose caffeine concentrations are present.

*Use of concentrations for dosage adjustment.* No data suggest that caffeine undergoes nonlinear elimination. Thus, dosage adjustments by proportionality are acceptable. Dosage adjustments for caffeine are complicated by the fact that a true steady state is not reached for at least 4 days, so any adjustments should be conservative.

*Protein binding, active metabolites, and other considerations.* Caffeine is only 31% bound to serum proteins and has no active metabolites.[81]

## Antiepileptic Drugs

Antiepileptic drugs (AEDs) have clearly defined therapeutic ranges for the indication of seizures, unless otherwise stated; however, concentrations associated with toxicity would apply across all indications. Because AEDs are used as prophylaxis for seizures that may not occur frequently, it is particularly important that effective serum concentrations of these drugs be ensured early in therapy. Although AEDs are often only used for prophylaxis, they provide a unique challenge because seizures occur irregularly and unpredictably to be able to correlate clinically with therapeutic drug monitoring. Indications for monitoring AEDs include (1) documentation of an effective steady-state concentration after initiation of therapy, (2) after dosage regimen adjustments, (3) after adding a drug that has potential for interaction, (4) changes in disease state or physiologic status that may affect the pharmacokinetics of the drug, (5) within hours of a seizure recurrence, (6) after an unexplained change in seizure frequency (7) suspected dose-related drug toxicity, and (8) suspected nonadherence.[14,84,85]

## Carbamazepine

***Therapeutic range and clinical considerations.*** Carbamazepine is indicated for the prevention of partial seizures and generalized tonic-clonic seizures as well as the treatment of pain associated with trigeminal neuralgia.[73,86] Extended-release formulations have been approved for the prevention and treatment of acute manic or mixed episodes in patients with bipolar I disorder.[87] Most textbooks report a therapeutic range of 4 to 12 mg/L. Concentrations above 12 mg/L are most often associated with nausea and vomiting, unsteadiness, blurred vision, drowsiness, dizziness, and headaches in patients taking carbamazepine alone.[39] Patients taking other AEDs, such as primidone, phenobarbital, VPA, or phenytoin, may show similar adverse effects at carbamazepine concentrations as low as 9 mg/L. Additionally, some central nervous system (CNS) effects such as drowsiness, dizziness, or headaches can be seen at concentrations >8 mg/L.[88] Many clinicians target the lower end of the therapeutic range (4 to 8 mg/L) to avoid adverse effects seen at concentrations of 11 to 15 mg/L (somnolence, nystagmus, ataxia) or toxicities at 15 to 25 mg/L of agitation, hallucinations, and chorea.[85,86] Toxicity is expected at concentrations >20 mg/L; serious adverse reactions are seen at concentrations >50 mg/L.[89,90]

Carbamazepine 10,11-epoxide is an active metabolite that can be present in concentrations containing 12% to 25% carbamazepine, but it is not routinely monitored along with the parent drug. A suggested therapeutic range for this metabolite, used at some research centers, is 0.4 to 4 mg/L; toxicity is expected at concentrations >9 mg/L.[73,91]

In addition to the usual indications for monitoring, it is important to monitor carbamazepine concentrations if the patient is switched to another formulation (eg, generic) because bioavailability may vary between formulations.[85]

***Sample timing.*** If a loading dose is administered, concentrations can be taken 2 hours after administration of the suspension formulation to ensure therapeutic concentrations have been achieved.[92] Because carbamazepine induces its own metabolism, it is recommended that initial doses of carbamazepine be relatively low and gradually increased over a 3- to 4-week period.[39] For maximal induction or deinduction to occur, 2 to 3 weeks may be required after the maximum dose has been attained. Thus, a total of 6 to 7 weeks may be required for a true steady state to be reached after initiation of therapy. After any dose changes or addition/discontinuation of enzyme-inducing or inhibiting drugs, 2 to 3 weeks is required to reach a new steady state.[73] It is recommended that during dose titration, carbamazepine concentrations be measured at weekly intervals. After reaching the maintenance dose, blood concentrations can be less frequently monitored at 3- to 6-month intervals.[92]

A trough concentration is generally preferred. The absorption of immediate-release carbamazepine tablets from the GI tract is relatively slow and erratic, reaching a peak between 3 and 8 hours after a dose.[93] Extended-release formulations are even more slowly absorbed. If carbamazepine is administered every 6 or 8 hours, serum concentrations during the dosing interval remain fairly flat, and all concentrations will be fairly representative of a trough concentration. Less frequent dosing results in more fluctuation, in which case the time of the concentration relative to the last dose should be documented for appropriate interpretation. Use of the extended-release formulation of carbamazepine minimizes fluctuations caused by diurnal variations.[94] Nevertheless, it is recommended that samples on repeated visits always be obtained at the same time of the day for purposes of comparison.[85]

***Use of concentrations for dosage adjustment.*** Carbamazepine exhibits nonlinear behavior due to autoinduction, which can lead to an increase in drug elimination.[95] An additional 10% to 20% should be added or subtracted for a dose increase or dose decrease, respectively, to account for the autoinduction previously described.[96] After the autoinduction period, if the dose is adjusted without a change in the interval, a concentration drawn at the same time within the interval increases in proportion to the increase in dose.

***Protein binding, active metabolites, and other considerations.*** The absorption of carbamazepine is variable after oral ingestion and is formulation dependent.[95] In most patients, carbamazepine is 70% to 80% bound to serum proteins, including albumin and α-1-acid glycoprotein (AAG).[97] In some patients, however, unbound percentages as low as 10% have been reported. Measurements of unbound carbamazepine concentrations are not generally recommended or necessary. Total concentrations should be carefully interpreted in situations of suspected altered protein binding. Decreased binding might be anticipated in uremia, liver disease, hypoalbuminemia, or hyperbilirubinemia.[73] Increased binding might be rarely expected in cases of physiologic trauma due to elevated AAG concentrations. Because VPA has been shown to displace carbamazepine from albumin, an equation was proposed to predict unbound carbamazepine concentrations in this situation.[56] Correlations between saliva and unbound carbamazepine concentrations are strong.[98] Thus, saliva sampling might be considered in situations of suspected alterations in carbamazepine binding.[99]

Drug–drug interactions that are expected to result in a higher proportion of active 10,11-epoxide metabolite relative to the parent drug (eg, concurrent phenytoin, phenobarbital, or VPA) may alter the activity associated with a given carbamazepine concentration. It is suggested that a lower therapeutic range of 4 to 8 mg/L be used when those drugs are given concurrently.[14] Carbamazepine-10, 11-epoxide is 50% protein bound.[100]

## Phenobarbital/Primidone

Primidone and phenobarbital are both used for the management of generalized tonic-clonic and partial seizures.[73] Phenobarbital is also used for febrile seizures in neonates and infants, while primidone is used for treatment of essential tremor.[85,101] Although primidone has activity of its own, most clinicians believe that phenobarbital—a metabolite of primidone—is predominantly responsible for primidone's therapeutic effects.

***Therapeutic ranges and clinical considerations.*** The therapeutic range of phenobarbital for treatment of tonic-clonic, febrile, and hypoxic ischemic seizures is generally regarded as 10 to 40 mg/L, while concentrations as high as 70 mg/L may be required for refractory status epilepticus.[85,101] Eighty-four percent of patients are likely to respond with concentrations between 10 and 40 mg/L.[101] Management of partial seizures generally requires higher phenobarbital concentrations than management of bilateral tonic-clonic seizures.[14] Concentrations of phenobarbital are almost always reported when primidone concentrations are ordered; site-specific laboratory protocols should be followed. The therapeutic range of primidone reported by most laboratories is 5 to 12 mg/L.[14,85] Fifteen percent to 20% of a primidone dose is metabolized to the active phenobarbital; the side effects of primidone are mostly related to phenobarbital.[73] CNS side effects such as sedation and ataxia generally occur in chronically treated patients at phenobarbital concentrations between 35 and 80 mg/L. Stupor and coma have been reported at phenobarbital concentrations above 65 mg/L.[93] Clinicians should consider drawing concentrations when nonadherence or toxicity is suspected if the patient is experiencing lack of efficacy, in patients with severe liver or kidney disease (including dialysis), and when interacting medications are initiated or discontinued.[102]

*Sample timing.* The half-life of phenobarbital is the rate-limiting step for determining the time to reach steady state after primidone administration. The half-life of phenobarbital averages 5 days for neonates and 4 days for adults.[101] Because phenobarbital or primidone dosage may be initiated gradually, steady state is not attained until 2 to 3 weeks after full dosage has been implemented. Because of phenobarbital's long half-life, concentrations obtained anytime during the day would provide reasonable estimates of a trough concentration. Ideally, concentrations should be obtained from visit to visit at similar times of the day.[101] If IV phenobarbital is administered, serum concentrations should be drawn at least 1 hour postinfusion.[103]

*Use of concentrations for dosage adjustment.* Phenobarbital and primidone exhibit linear elimination behavior; thus, a change in the dose of either drug will result in a proportional change in average steady-state serum concentrations.[93,101]

*Protein binding, active metabolites, and other considerations.* Phenobarbital is approximately 50% bound to serum proteins (albumin) in adults; primidone is not bound to serum proteins.[85,104] Thus, total concentrations of both drugs are reliable indicators of the active, unbound concentrations of these drugs. Although primidone has an active metabolite, phenylethylmalonamide, its contribution to activity is unlikely to be significant. Clearance of phenobarbital can increase or decrease depending on many patient-specific factors, including age (decreases in neonates and elderly patients), severe liver or kidney disease (decreases), interacting medications (increases or decreases), urine pH (increases), and malnutrition (increases).[105-111] Salivary phenobarbital concentrations correlate well with both plasma total and free phenobarbital concentrations, making salivary concentrations a useful alternative in therapeutic drug monitoring.[95]

## Phenytoin and Fosphenytoin

*Therapeutic range.* Phenytoin is primarily used for treatment of generalized tonic-clonic and complex partial seizures.[112] It may also be used in the treatment of trigeminal neuralgia and seizure prophylaxis after neurosurgery.[73,112] Studies have shown that serum concentrations of phenytoin between 10 and 20 mg/L result in maximum protection from primary or secondary generalized tonic-clonic seizures in most adult patients with normal protein binding. Ten percent of patients with controlled seizures have phenytoin concentrations <3 mg/L; 50% have concentrations <7 mg/L; and 90% have concentrations <15 mg/L. Concentrations at the lower end of the range are effective for bilateral seizures, while higher concentrations appear to be necessary for partial seizures.[14] The therapeutic range of total concentrations in infants is lower (6 to 11 mg/L) due to lower serum protein binding. Concentration-related side effects include nystagmus; CNS depression (ataxia, inability to concentrate, confusion, and drowsiness); and changes in mental status, coma, or seizures at concentrations >40 mg/L.[85] Although mild side effects may be observed at concentrations as low as 5 mg/L, there have been cases in which concentrations as high as 50 mg/L have been required for effective treatment without negative consequences.[113]

Some clinicians have proposed that monitoring of phenytoin be limited to unbound concentrations, particularly in patients who are critically ill or likely to have unusual protein binding.[52,114,115] Unbound phenytoin concentrations are more predictive of clinical toxicity than are total phenytoin concentrations in these individuals.[116] The therapeutic range of unbound phenytoin concentrations is presumed to be 1 to 2 mg/L for laboratories that determine the unbound phenytoin fraction at 25°C, and 1.5 to 3 mg/L if done at 37°C.[116]

Fosphenytoin is the IV prodrug of phenytoin; fosphenytoin pharmacokinetics and related monitoring are based on phenytoin calculations.[117-119]

*Sample timing.* The time required to attain steady state after initiation of phenytoin therapy is difficult to predict because of phenytoin's nonlinear elimination behavior. Although the $T_{50\%}$ is approximately 24 hours (considering the average population $V_{max}$ and $K_m$ values when concentrations are between 10 and 20 mg/L), there can be extreme variations in these population values. Half-lives between 6 and 60 hours have been reported in adults.[85] Thus, a steady state might not be attained for as long as 3 weeks. Some clinicians advise that samples be obtained prior to steady state (after 3 to 4 days) to make sure that concentrations are not climbing too rapidly.[112] Equations have been developed to predict the time required to reach a steady state once $V_{max}$ and $K_m$ values are known.[49] It is important to recognize that the time required to reach a steady state in a given patient is longer each time the dose is further increased.

Most clinicians advise that trough phenytoin concentrations be monitored.[85] Phenytoin is quite slowly absorbed, so that the concentration versus time profile is fairly flat. This is especially true when oral phenytoin is administered two or three times per day. In this case, a serum phenytoin sample drawn any time during the dosage interval is likely to be close to a trough concentration. The greatest fluctuation would be seen for the more quickly absorbed products (chewable tablets and suspension) in children (who have a higher clearance of phenytoin) given once daily. In this case, it is particularly important to document the time of sample relative to the dose to identify if the concentration is closer to a peak, a trough, or a $C_{ss,avg}$.

*Use of concentrations for dosage adjustment.* Phenytoin exhibits pronounced nonlinear behavior after therapeutic doses. Thus, increases in dose will produce greater-than-proportional increases in the average serum concentration during the dosing interval. Several methods, described elsewhere, use population and patient-specific $V_{max}$ and $K_m$ values to predict the most appropriate dose adjustment.[49] The clinician must be vigilant to limit phenytoin daily dose increases to less than 30 to 60 mg of sodium phenytoin and less than 25 to 50 mg of the chewable tablets.

***Protein binding, active metabolites, and other considerations.*** The metabolites of phenytoin have insignificant activity. Phenytoin binds primarily to albumin in plasma, and the normal unbound fraction of drug in plasma of adults is 0.1.[85,112] Lower serum binding of phenytoin is observed in neonates and infants and in patients with hypoalbuminemia, liver disease, nephrotic syndrome, end-stage renal disease (ESRD), pregnancy, cystic fibrosis, burns, trauma, malnourishment, acquired immunodeficiency syndrome (AIDS), and advanced age.[73,120] Concurrent drugs (VPA and salicylates) are known to displace phenytoin.[73] Therefore, a total concentration of phenytoin that is within the range of 10 to 20 mg/L in these patients might represent an unbound concentration that is higher than the therapeutic range of unbound concentrations of 1 to 2 mg/L. A total concentration of phenytoin in this situation can be misleading. Several approaches can be used in these situations: (1) an unbound phenytoin concentration can be ordered, if available; (2) the patient's unbound phenytoin concentration can be calculated by estimating the unbound fraction in the patient (using the literature) and multiplying that by the patient's measured phenytoin concentration (the resulting unbound concentration should then be compared with 1 to 2 mg/L); or (3) special equations may be used to convert the phenytoin concentration to what it would be if the patient had normal serum protein binding.

The following equation, commonly called the Winter-Tozer equation, was developed to normalize phenytoin concentrations in patients with hypoalbuminemia and renal failure and has been revised for use in various patient populations[73,112,121-123]:

$$\text{normalized PHT concentration} = \frac{\text{measured PHT concentration}}{(X \times \text{albumin concentration, g/dL}) + 0.1}$$

The value "X" is 0.25 for elderly patients or patients with head trauma with low albumin and creatinine clearances ≥25 mL/min; 0.2 for patients with normal or low albumin who are receiving dialysis; and 0.29 for neurocritical care. Additionally, a coefficient of 0.275 has been proposed as having more broad applicability to a variety of patients.[124] Total concentrations of phenytoin in patients with creatinine clearance values between 10 and 25 mL/min cannot be as accurately normalized; the clinical status of such patients should be carefully considered because total concentrations can be misleading. The Winter-Tozer equation for normalizing phenytoin concentrations has been tested by groups of investigators in different groups of patients with mixed reviews; it is emphasized that it should be used only as a guide.

Known to increase the unbound fraction of phenytoin in serum, VPA also has been variably reported to inhibit the metabolism of phenytoin.[125] These two occurrences together could mean that a concentration within the range of 10 to 20 mg/L is associated with adverse effects and an unbound phenytoin concentration of 2 mg/L. If unbound phenytoin concentrations

are not available, the following equations—modified from their original form—may be useful to normalize the phenytoin concentration if the concentration of VPA in that same sample has been measured.[54,112] Notably, some controversy remains regarding which equation provides better accuracy and may be dependent on the laboratory method used to obtain the total phenytoin concentration; therefore, clinical judgement should be used when determining which method is most appropriate for a particular situation.[54,126]

Haidukewych equation[55]:

$$\text{Corrected free PHT} = \big(0.095 + (0.001 * \text{VPA})\big) * \big(\text{Total PHT}\big)$$

May equation[56]:

$$\text{Corrected free PHT} = \big(0.0792 + (0.000636 * \text{VPA})\big) \\ * \big(\text{Total PHT}\big)$$

Salivary concentrations of phenytoin are strongly predictive of unbound phenytoin concentrations and have the added advantage of being noninvasive and thus an option for children and elderly patients.[57]

### Valproic Acid

***Therapeutic range.*** In addition to partial and generalized tonic-clonic and myoclonic seizures, VPA is used for management of absence seizures and for a variety of other conditions, including prophylaxis against migraine headaches and bipolar disorder.[85] Most laboratories use 50 to 100 mg/L as the therapeutic range for trough total VPA concentrations in the treatment of epilepsy; concentrations of 50 to 125 mg/L are considered therapeutic in the treatment of mania.[127] Some patients with epilepsy are effectively treated at lower concentrations, and others may require trough concentrations as high as 120 mg/L.[128] Concentrations at the upper end of the therapeutic range appear to be necessary for treatment of complex partial seizures.[128] The same therapeutic range has been used for patients with migraines or bipolar disorder, although the value of routine serum concentration monitoring for bipolar disorder has been questioned.[129,130] The following concentration-related side effects may be seen: ataxia, sedation, lethargy, and fatigue at concentrations >75 mg/L; tremor at concentrations >100 mg/L; and stupor and coma at concentrations >175 mg/L.[128] The therapeutic range of total VPA concentrations is confounded by the nonlinear serum protein binding of this drug, which might explain some of the variable response among and within patients at a given total serum concentration.[73]

***Sample timing.*** The half-life of VPA ranges between 7 and 18 hours in children and adults and 17 and 40 hours in infants.[85] Thus, as long as 5 days may be required to attain a steady state. The pattern of change in VPA concentrations varies from interval to interval during the day because of considerable diurnal variation.[85,128] It is, therefore, recommended that samples always be obtained prior to the morning dose as the trough concentration has been shown to be most consistent from day to day.[128] Considerable fluctuation within the interval is seen with the immediate-release capsule and syrup, which are rapidly absorbed. The enteric-coated, delayed-release tablet formulation of VPA displays a shift to the right with respect to its concentration-versus-time profile, such that the lowest concentration during the interval may not be observed until 4 to 6 hours into the next dosing interval.[93] It is important to know, however, that concentrations during the interval after administration of the enteric-coated tablet show considerable fluctuation. The extended-release formulations, if given in divided doses, provide less fluctuation in concentrations, and samples may be drawn at any time.

***Use of concentrations for dosage adjustment.*** The metabolism of unbound VPA is linear following therapeutic doses. Thus, unbound VPA concentrations increase in proportion to increases in dose.[83,93] Because VPA shows nonlinear, saturable protein binding in serum over the therapeutic range, total concentrations increase less than proportionally. This is important to keep in mind when interpreting total VPA concentrations.

***Protein binding, active metabolites, and other considerations.*** VPA is 90% to 95% bound to albumin and lipoproteins in serum. The unbound fraction of VPA shows considerable interpatient variability. It is increased in neonates, in conditions in adults associated with hypoalbuminemia (eg, liver disease, nephrotic syndrome, cystic fibrosis, burns, trauma, malnutrition, and advanced age), and as a result of displacement by endogenous substances (eg, bilirubin, free fatty acids, and uremic substances in ESRD) and other drugs (eg, salicylates).[73,130,131] The increase in the unbound fraction of VPA during labor is believed to be the result of displacement by higher concentrations of free fatty acids.[132] Intrapatient variability in the unbound fraction exists because of nonlinear binding. The unbound fraction of VPA is fairly constant at lower concentrations but progressively increases as total concentrations rise >75 mg/L.[85] Thus, total concentrations do not reflect unbound concentrations at the upper end of the therapeutic range. A therapeutic range for unbound VPA concentrations can only be approximated. Assuming unbound fractions of 0.05 to 0.1 and a therapeutic range of total VPA concentrations of 50 to 100 mg/L, an unbound therapeutic range of 2.5 to 10 mg/L can be deduced.

### Other Antiepileptic Drugs

Routine serum concentration monitoring is not recommended for most AEDs.[133,134] The following drugs' serum concentrations would only be monitored if toxicity or nonadherence was suspected:

- **Clobazam.** The therapeutic range and subsequently the correlation of serum concentrations and efficacy of clobazam are not fully established. de Leon and colleagues suggest that a concentration-to-dose ratio may be more appropriate for monitoring clobazam; however, at this time therapeutic drug monitoring is not routinely used.[135]

- **Ethosuximide.** The therapeutic range for ethosuximide is generally considered to be 40 to 100 mg/L.[136] Eighty percent of patients achieve partial control within that range, and 60% are seizure free. Some patients require concentrations up to 150 mg/L.[73] Side effects are usually seen at concentrations >70 mg/L and include drowsiness, fatigue, ataxia, and lethargy.[73] Ethosuximide does not require as much monitoring as some of the other antiepileptics, but it is important to ensure effective concentrations after initiation of therapy or a change in dosage regimen. The half-life of ethosuximide

is quite long—60 hours in adults and 30 hours in children.[93] Thus, it is advised to wait as long as 1 week to 12 days before obtaining ethosuximide concentrations for monitoring purposes.[14,136] Although it is generally advised that trough concentrations be obtained, concentrations drawn any time during the dosing interval should be acceptable because there will be little fluctuation if ethosuximide is given in divided doses. Peak concentrations of ethosuximide administered as a capsule are attained in 3 to 7 hours.[93,136] Ethosuximide is negligibly bound to serum proteins and its metabolites have insignificant activity. Although ethosuximide is administered as a racemic mixture, the enantiomers have the same pharmacokinetic properties. Thus, measurement of the summed enantiomers is acceptable.[137]

- **Felbamate.** It displays excellent bioavailability and is metabolized to multiple inactive metabolites. There is notable interindividual variation in felbamate's metabolism.[84] The therapeutic range of felbamate is considered to be between 30 and 60 mg/L. Dose decreases of up to 50% should be considered in patients with renal dysfunction.[138] Clinically, this medication is reserved to refractory treatment due to its side effect profile and increased incidence of aplastic anemia and acute liver failure.[138] Monitoring felbamate concentrations does not predict toxicity. Felbamate takes 3 to 5 days to reach steady-state concentration, and serum concentrations should not be drawn before this time. Felbamate is 22% to 25% bound to albumin and has no active metabolites. Felbamate decreases the concentration of carbamazepine and increases the concentration of carbamazepine 10, 11-epoxide, phenobarbital, phenytoin, and VPA when administered with these agents; a 20% to 25% dose reduction of aforementioned agents should be considered if it is initiated concomitantly with felbamate.[139-145] Simultaneously, coadministration of carbamazepine, phenobarbital, and phenytoin decreases felbamate concentrations, and VPA does not have a significant effect on felbamate concentrations.[138]

- **Gabapentin.** Although a great candidate for therapeutic drug monitoring because of wide intrapatient variability, in large part due to changes in concentration/dose ratio with age and changes in half-life related to renal impairment, it has limited clinical use.[143] Therapeutic drug monitoring is most useful in certain patient populations, including in patients with renal impairment or in those for whom adherence is questionable.[84,95] The therapeutic range of gabapentin is 2 to 20 mg/L; the toxic range is ≥25 mg/L. Gabapentin is mainly renally cleared; therefore, dose adjustments are necessary in renal impairment.[146] Steady state is achieved within 24 to 48 hours.[147,148] Gabapentin is minimally bound to protein (<3%) and is eliminated 99% unchanged (1% is excreted as the *N*-methyl metabolite).[149] It is recommended that serum concentrations of concomitant antiepileptic therapies be monitored if given with gabapentin.[150] Linear behavior is seen at doses up to 1,800 mg/day, however nonlinear behavior is reported at higher doses because of saturable intestinal absorption.

- **Lacosamide.** Due to a predictable pharmacokinetics profile and no clear correlations between therapeutic concentrations and efficacy or toxicity, therapeutic drug monitoring is not routinely recommended or needed.

- **Lamotrigine.** The considerable pharmacokinetic variability among patients taking lamotrigine, due in part to significant drug–drug interactions, makes it a good candidate for therapeutic drug monitoring.[133,151] The therapeutic range of lamotrigine is 2.5 to 15 mg/L.[26,135,152] It has been suggested that concomitant therapy with other antiepileptics may alter the response to lamotrigine or its side-effect profile.[151] The half-life of lamotrigine can range from 15 to 30 hours on monotherapy.[133] Thus, one should wait at least 1 week before obtaining samples after initiating or adjusting lamotrigine therapy.[151] This drug exhibits linear pharmacokinetics; therefore, dose rate adjustments result in proportional changes in average serum concentrations. Because it is only 55% bound to serum proteins, measurements of unbound lamotrigine concentrations in serum are not necessary.

- **Levetiracetam.** Serum concentration monitoring of levetiracetam is more important in pregnant women and in infants and children because of the higher clearance in these patients.[26,153] Furthermore, levetiracetam levels have been shown to be affected by weight and medication coadministration.[154] Routine monitoring of levetiracetam is not required for most patient populations due to the predictable dose response. The half-life ranges from 6 to 8 hours in adults, and a steady state should be attained within 1 week.[135] Serum concentrations between 5 and 45 mcg/mL are considered to be therapeutic.[155] Serum protein binding of levetiracetam is <10%, eliminating the need for measurement of unbound levetiracetam concentrations.[135] Ideally, serum concentrations should be drawn in the morning as a trough concentration due to diurinal variation in concentrations

- **Oxcarbazepine.** The pharmacologic effect of oxcarbazepine is primarily related to serum concentrations of its active monohydroxy metabolite, licarbazepine. A therapeutic range of licarbazepine is 12 to 35 mg/L.[156] The elimination half-life of licarbazepine is variable, ranging from 7 to 20 hours, and is prolonged in renal impairment. The serum protein binding of licarbazepine is low at 40%.

- **Pentobarbital.** As a sedative hypnotic, therapeutic effects of pentobarbital are seen at 1 to 5 mg/L; toxicity occurs at concentrations >10 mg/L. Pentobarbital is 45% to 70% bound to protein and is primarily eliminated via the kidneys. Therapeutic concentrations have not been established for antiepileptic purposes.[157]

- **Pregabalin.** Pregabalin is approved as adjunctive treatment for partial onset seizures and for the treatment of fibromyalgia or diabetic, spinal cord injury-related, and postherpetic neuralgia. It has excellent bioavailability estimated at 98% and poor protein binding with very few drug interactions.[158] It is primarily eliminated via the kidneys and, therefore, requires dose adjustment in patients with kidney dysfunction. There are no known significant active metabolites.[159] Pregabalin reaches a steady state concentration at 24 to 48 hours.[147,148] The therapeutic range has been defined as 3 to 8 mg/L.[160,161]

- **Tiagabine.** Tiagabine shows pronounced interpatient pharmacokinetic variability due to strong protein binding and hepatic metabolism.[162] Trough concentrations between 20 and 100 mcg/L are associated with improved seizure control, but there is wide variation in response at any given total concentration.[26,133,134] This could, in part, be due to variable serum binding (96% bound in serum on average). Salicylate, naproxen, and VPA have been shown to displace tiagabine from serum proteins.[133,134] Tiagabine half-life ranges from 5 to 13 hours and may be even shorter in the presence of enzyme-inducing drugs.[134,153] Tiagabine shows linear elimination behavior after therapeutic doses.

- **Topiramate.** Topiramate concentrations are particularly influenced by interactions with other drugs, with concentrations as much as 2-fold lower when enzyme-inducing drugs are administered concurrently.[163] The half-life ranges from 18 to 23 hours, and it has linear elimination behavior.[133,134,151] Topiramate is <40% bound to serum proteins but shows saturable binding to red blood cells, thus suggesting that whole blood might be a preferable specimen for monitoring.[134,151] Effective serum concentrations are generally reported to be between 2 and 25 mg/L.[164] No active metabolites have been identified. Routine therapeutic drug monitoring is only recommended in patients with hepatic or renal impairment.[162] Saliva concentrations have a strong correlation with serum and may be a viable option for monitoring chronic therapy.[165]

- **Zonisamide.** The pharmacokinetics of zonisamide are variable among patients and also highly influenced by interactions with other drugs.[133] Zonisamide is approximately 40% bound to serum albumin, and, like topiramate, shows saturable binding to red blood cells, suggesting that whole blood monitoring might be preferable.[135,151] The half-life is 50 to 70 hours but may be as short as 25 hours when enzyme inducers are coadministered.[135] Some reports suggest nonlinear behavior at higher doses. The serum concentration range associated with response is 10 to 38 mg/L; cognitive dysfunction is reported at concentrations >30 mg/L.[26,135,151] No active metabolites have been identified.[135]

## Antimicrobials

### Aminoglycosides

*Therapeutic ranges.* Aminoglycosides have been used for decades to treat infections caused by multidrug-resistant microorganisms. Most commonly used IV aminoglycosides today include amikacin, gentamicin, and tobramycin.[48] They are bactericidal and their efficacy is depends highly on peak concentration after an infusion.[166] Optimal bactericidal activity occurs when the peak:minimum inhibitory concentration (MIC) ratio is between 8:1 and 10:1.[167-169] They also exhibit a postantibiotic effect (PAE) in which bacterial killing continues even after the serum concentration falls below the MIC.[73] The concentration-dependent killing and PAE of aminoglycosides explain why extended-interval, or once-daily (pulse), dosing is shown to be safe and effective in many patients. Studies have shown improved peak concentrations of aminoglycosides after extended-interval dosing of aminoglycosides when compared with multiple daily dosing regimens (ie, thrice-daily dosing). Additionally, lower trough concentrations have been reported at the end of the dosing interval compared with multiple daily dosing regimens, reducing the risk of drug accumulation.[170] As a result, extended-interval aminoglycosides have been associated with improvement in efficacy and decreased nephrotoxicity.[171-174] Nephrotoxicity and ototoxicity are the most frequently reported adverse effects of aminoglycosides. Ototoxicity is associated with a prolonged course of treatment (for >7 to 10 days) with peaks above 12 to 14 mg/L for gentamicin and tobramycin and 35 to 40 mg/L for amikacin.[73] One study noted there was not a significant difference in the incidence of ototoxicity between once-daily and multiple-daily dosing aminoglycosides.[170] Patients with trough concentrations above 2 to 3 mg/L (gentamicin and tobramycin) or 10 mg/L (amikacin) for >5 to 7 days are predisposed to increased risk of nephrotoxicity.[73] The risk of nephrotoxicity is even further increased when aminoglycosides are given concomitantly with other nephrotoxic agents.

Therapeutic ranges for peaks and troughs are reported for the aminoglycosides and pertain only to dosing approaches that involve multiple doses during the day. For gentamicin and tobramycin, peaks between 6 and 10 mg/L and troughs between 0.5 and 2 mg/L are recommended.[175] The approximately 4-fold higher MIC for amikacin explains why peaks between 20 and 30 mg/L and troughs between 1 and 8 mg/L are recommended.[175] There is no therapeutic range when the extended-interval dosing method is used; doses are given to attain peaks that are approximately 8- to 10-fold the MIC, and troughs are intended to be nondetectable within 4 hours of administration of the next dose.[166,175]

There has been some concern over the years that aminoglycosides are overmonitored. Uncomplicated patients who have normal renal function, do not have life-threatening infections, and will be treated for <5 days may not need to have serum aminoglycoside concentrations measured.[176] At the other extreme, dosage individualization using serum concentrations of aminoglycosides is necessary in patients who are expected to be on prolonged treatment courses (≥5 days) or in whom unusual pharmacokinetic parameters are expected.[173-180]

***Sample timing.*** For extended-interval dosing patients with normal renal function, a steady state is never reached because each dose is washed out prior to the next dose. The method developed by Nicolau et al (the Hartford nomogram) requires that a single blood sample be obtained between 6 and 14 hours after the end of the first infusion.[167,181] This sample is referred to as a random sample, but the time of the collection must be documented. The concentration is used with a nomogram to determine if a different dosing interval should be used.[48,167] Concentrations that are too high according to the Hartford nomogram indicate that the drug is not being cleared as well as originally predicted, suggesting the need for a longer dosing interval. For traditional dosing, it is important to wait until a steady state is reached before obtaining serum concentrations. The half-lives of the aminoglycosides are 1.5 to 3 hours for adults with normal renal function but as long as 72 hours in patients with severe renal impairment.[73] A conservative rule of thumb is that steady state is reached after the third or fourth dose.[48] Some patients may have blood samples drawn immediately after the first dose ("off the load") to determine their

pharmacokinetic parameters for purposes of dosage regimen individualization. These would most likely be patients who are anticipated to have unpredictable or changing pharmacokinetic parameters, such as those in a critical care unit, and who require immediate effective treatment because of life-threatening infections.

Two blood samples are sufficient for purposes of individualizing traditional aminoglycoside dosing therapy and provide reasonable estimates of aminoglycoside pharmacokinetic parameters.[182] It is crucial that the times of the sample collections be accurately recorded.[48,166] The two samples should be spaced sufficiently apart from each other so that an accurate determination of the log-linear slope can be made to determine the elimination rate constant. The first sample, sometimes referred to as the measured peak, should be drawn no earlier than 1 hour after the end of a 30-minute infusion.[182-185] However, it is usually drawn within 30 minutes prior to the start of infusion of the next dose (assumed to be the trough).[48,164,176] Once the elimination rate constant has been calculated using these two concentrations, the true peak and true trough can be calculated and their values compared with desired target peaks and troughs.

***Use of concentrations for dosage adjustment.*** Various extended-interval dosing methods are used to take advantage of the concentration-related killing and PAE of aminoglycosides.[176] The original Hartford method involves giving a milligram-per-kilogram dose that is administered to attain a peak concentration that is approximately 10 times the MIC. Then a sample is obtained between 6 and 14 hours after the end of the infusion and compared with a nomogram, which indicates the appropriate maintenance dosing interval—usually 24, 36, or 48 hours.[167]

Serum concentrations of aminoglycosides obtained during traditional dosing are used to determine an individual patient's pharmacokinetic parameters as well as the true peak and true trough to compare these to desired target concentrations. Equations that account for time of drug infusion are used to determine an appropriate dosing interval and dose.[185] Other dosage adjustment methods include nomograms and population pharmacokinetic (Bayesian) methods.[177,185]

***Protein binding, active metabolites, and other considerations.*** Aminoglycosides are <10% bound to serum proteins, and unbound concentrations will always reflect total concentrations in the serum.[175] The metabolites of the aminoglycosides are inactive.

### Vancomycin

***Therapeutic range and clinical considerations.*** Vancomycin is a glycopeptide antibiotic that is used intravenously to treat gram-positive organisms, including those resistant to other antibiotics (ie, methicillin-resistant *Staphylococcus aureus* [MRSA]).[48,73] The emergence of vancomycin-resistant enterococci, vancomycin-resistant *S aureus*, vancomycin-intermediate *S aureus* (VISA), and heteroresistant VISA has led to the need to optimize and restrict vancomycin use. Major toxicities associated with vancomycin are nephrotoxicity and ototoxicity. Another adverse effect known as red man syndrome (intense flushing, tachycardia, and hypotension) is a histamine-related reaction associated with rapid infusion.[73,186]

Although some institutions may monitor both peaks and troughs of vancomycin, this practice has been questioned because of a lack of standardization in associating timing of sample draw and peak concentration. In contrast to aminoglycosides, the most important pharmacodynamic parameter of vancomycin when used against *S aureus* isolates is 24-hour AUC to MIC, with a target of 400 to 600 mg × h/L. Historically, due to ease of use and practicality, trough concentrations served as surrogates for the AUC/MIC target, with troughs of 15 to 20 mg/L recommended for infections caused by *S aureus* isolates with MICs ≤1.[187] Although this traditional trough-based monitoring recommendation has been widely practiced in recent years, benefits for maintaining higher troughs are not well supported, and more recent evidence has emerged noting that trough concentrations may not correlate well with AUC values—risking either overexposure (and increased risk of associated toxicities) or underexposure (and increased risk of emergence of antimicrobial resistance). Therefore, new guidelines recommend that in patients with suspected or confirmed MRSA infections that individualized AUC/MIC ratio of 400 to 600 mg × h/L is targeted using AUC-guided dosing and monitoring, which can be accomplished by either two-point kinetics or through the use of Bayesian software programs (preferred method). There remains a gap in available evidence on the most appropriate AUC/MIC ratio target for non-MRSA infections, which the recent guidelines have not addressed. Therefore, the use of the aforementioned targets for non-MRSA infections should be extrapolated with caution if opted to be used in these scenarios.[187]

*Sample timing.* The half-life of vancomycin is 7 to 9 hours in adults with normal renal function and 120 to 140 hours in patients with renal failure. A shorter half-life of 3 to 4 hours has been noted in certain patient populations (ie, obesity, burn victims).[73,188] For AUC-guided dosing and monitoring, either a two-point kinetic or Bayesian software approach can be followed. With two-point kinetics, it is recommended that once steady state is achieved, one concentration be obtained at the postdistribution phase (peak concentration at 1 to 2 hours after infusion) and a second concentration at the end of the dosing interval (trough). If Bayesian software is used, one or two vancomycin concentrations (with one of the concentrations being a trough) should be obtained to help estimate the AUC although a two-concentration approach is preferred. The latter approach does not require steady-state concentration to be reached first, thereby allowing for early AUC target assessment. Of note, a trough concentration may be appropriate to estimate the AUC using the Bayesian approach in certain patient populations.[187] For traditional (historical) concentration monitoring, samples should be obtained as troughs within 30 minutes to 1 hour of the start of the next infusion.

*Use of concentrations for dosage adjustment.* Because of the increased risk of nephrotoxicity in patients with serious MRSA infections, a trough-only based monitoring approach, targeting troughs of 15 to 20 mg/L, is no longer recommended and an AUC-monitoring approach is advocated instead. Of note, the aforementioned recommendation is only for serious MRSA infections. Whether a traditional trough-only monitoring versus an AUC-guided dosing and monitoring approach

is best for other infections has not been determined. Besides serious MRSA infections, monitoring is recommended for patients at high risk for nephrotoxicity, patients with unstable renal function, and patients receiving extended courses of vancomycin therapy (ie, >3 days). Vancomycin elimination is linear, and an increase in the dose (without a change in the dosing interval) can be expected to provide a proportional change in the trough serum concentration. It must be cautioned that vancomycin has a pronounced distribution phase, making the standardization of any peak sample to be especially important. More sophisticated prediction methods for dosing adjustments must be used if the dosing interval is adjusted with or without a change in dose.

Many methods have been proposed for vancomycin dosage regimen adjustments.[73,78,188,189] A relatively simple method, proposed by Ambrose and Winter, permits the use of a single trough concentration (drawn within 1 hour of the start of the next infusion) along with an assumption of the population distribution volume to predict the necessary pharmacokinetic parameters needed for individualization.[186] Once those parameters are determined, equations that account for drug infusion can be used to target desired peak and trough vancomycin concentrations. For AUC-guided dosing, monitoring of AUC exposure is recommended in obesity and patients with changing renal function. More frequent monitoring may be needed in patients exhibiting hemodynamic instability.

***Protein binding, active metabolites, and other considerations.*** Vancomycin is 30% to 55% bound to serum proteins in adults with normal renal function. The binding is lower (19%) in patients with ESRD.[189] With binding this low, total concentrations of vancomycin provide reliable reflection of the unbound concentrations in serum. Vancomycin metabolites are inactive and thus do not contribute to antibacterial effect or toxicity.

## β-Lactams

***Therapeutic range and clinical considerations.*** The β-lactam antibiotics demonstrate time-dependent bactericidal killing with efficacy related to the percentage of the dosing interval that free drug concentration remains above the MIC (fT>MIC). Studies have shown that the killing potential of β-lactams is maximized at concentrations that are three to four times the MIC, with higher concentrations providing little, if any, additional benefit.[190] Therefore, it is important to optimize exposure of β-lactams by increasing dosing frequency or infusion duration. Generally, fT>MIC of 40%, 50%, and 50% to 70% is required for the bactericidal killing potential of carbapenems, penicillins, and cephalosporins, respectively.[191] As demonstrated by an increase in $V_d$ and changes in antibiotic clearance (either increased or decreased), β-lactam antibiotic pharmacokinetics may be altered in critically ill patients. Additionally, obesity can similarly alter antibiotic pharmacokinetic parameters. As a result, standard doses of antibiotics may be suboptimal, leading to inadequate concentrations and even toxicities in some situations.[192] Roberts and colleagues noted that one-fifth of critically ill patients did not achieve a pharmacokinetic/pharmacodynamic target of 50% fT>MIC when standard antibiotic doses were used.[193] Historically, therapeutic drug monitoring of β-lactam was not undertaken because these agents lack a narrow therapeutic window and toxicity that would necessitate monitoring. As the incidence of multidrug-resistant microorganisms continues to increase, dosing optimization of currently available antibiotics is more important than ever and provides a potential role for β-lactam therapeutic drug monitoring, especially in the critically ill patient population and other patients with known pharmacokinetic variability.[190,194]

## Antifungal Agents

### Flucytosine (5-FC)

***Therapeutic range and clinical considerations.*** Flucytosine is a synthetic antifungal agent used in combination with amphotericin B for treatment of select systemic fungal infections (ie, cryptococcal meningitis).[195] In vivo and animal studies have noted that time above MIC is the most important pharmacodynamic parameter related to outcome with flucytosine therapy.[196] Flucytosine has significant interpatient pharmacokinetic variability. Although no exact target range for serum concentrations of flucytosine has been established, most clinicians agree that peak serum concentrations (2 hours postdose) of flucytosine should be kept below 100 mg/L to avoid dose-related hepatotoxicity, bone marrow suppression, and GI disturbances.[166,197,198] Additionally, concentrations should not fall below a trough concentration of <20 to 40 mg/L to avoid the development of resistance.[166,197-199] Hepatotoxicity and bone marrow suppression are usually reversible with discontinuation. Indications for monitoring flucytosine include avoidance of toxicity—particularly in patients with impaired renal function or those receiving concomitant amphotericin B—and avoidance of development of resistance due to sustained low concentrations.[167,195-197]

***Sample timing.*** Flucytosine is minimally protein bound (2% to 4%) and undergoes minimal hepatic metabolism. It is primarily (90%) excreted in the urine as unchanged drug, with an elimination half-life of 4 to 5 hours in patients with normal renal function and upwards of 250 hours in ESRD.[196,197,200] Maximum serum concentration is reached within 1 to 2 hours after an oral dose at steady state in patients with normal renal function.[199] Therefore, a 2-hour postdose concentration of flucytosine should be obtained after three to five doses have been administered, noting that steady state may not be reached for approximately 10 days in patients with renal failure.[195,196] Trough concentrations, if indicated, should be drawn within 30 minutes of the next dose.

***Use of concentrations for dosage adjustment.*** Because there are no reports of nonlinear elimination behavior, a given increase in dose should produce a proportional increase in serum flucytosine concentration. Therapeutic drug monitoring is considered standard of care for the use of flucytosine and it is recommended that serum concentrations be obtained at 72 hours after therapy initiation, when there are concerns with adherence, or if there are signs of drug-related toxicities.[199]

### Azole Antifungals

***Therapeutic ranges and clinical considerations.*** The incidence of fungal infections has been on the rise as the number of patients at risk has increased (eg, patients receiving immunosuppressive therapy). Azole antifungal agents are used to treat several different fungal infections, including invasive candidiasis, aspergillosis, and mucormycosis. The primary reason for monitoring azole antifungal drugs is to ensure efficacy and safety as they have demonstrated wide interpatient pharmacokinetic variability. Suboptimal azole antifungal concentrations have been associated with treatment failure and fungal breakthrough, whereas high concentrations have been related to toxicities (eg, hepatotoxicity).

***Itraconazole.*** Itraconazole concentrations are known to be relatively low in patients with AIDS or acute leukemia, most likely due to malabsorption and concurrent administration of enzyme-inducing drugs.[201] Additionally, absorption of the oral capsule formulation greatly depends on the gastric pH; itraconazole capsule formulation demonstrates improved absorption in an acidic environment. This necessitates the administration of the oral capsule with a full meal or acidic beverage (eg, cola). Conversely, the oral liquid solution's absorption is improved when not taken with food.[196] The newest formulation of itraconazole uses SUper-Bio-Available technology, which enhances the bioavailability of poorly soluble drugs, thereby increasing the relative bioavailability of itraconazole to 173% and involves less interpatient variability in plasma concentrations.[202,203] Itraconazole displays nonlinear pharmacokinetics. It undergoes significant first-pass metabolism into several metabolites—most importantly, hydroxy-itraconazole—with levels approximately double those of itraconazole. Although some isolates of yeasts and mold are more susceptible to hydroxy-itraconazole or itraconazole, they have comparable in vitro antifungal activity.[202] It has been noted that mortality and breakthrough infections are more common with itraconazole trough concentrations <0.5 mg/L and toxicity with concentrations >3 mg/L. Efficacy has been associated with itraconazole concentrations of 0.5 to 1 mg/L. Itraconazole accumulates slowly and reaches concentrations of 0.5 to 1 mg/L after 1 to 2 weeks. Due to slow accumulation, a loading dose is recommended to assist with reaching therapeutic concentrations sooner, namely in serious fungal infections. Additionally, itraconazole inhibits CYP3A4, leading to a number of significant drug interactions.[204] Due to interpatient and absorption variability based on the administered formulation, some consider the serum concentration monitoring of itraconazole to be essential in patients with life-threatening fungal infections.[205] Measuring itraconazole concentrations is recommended to ensure adequate absorption, monitor the need for dosage changes (eg, when interacting medications are added or discontinued), and assess adherence to therapy. Because of a long elimination half-life (34 to 42 hours after multiple doses), the concentration of itraconazole can be drawn at any time during a dosing interval once steady state is reached (at approximately 2 weeks).[206,207]

***Voriconazole.*** Voriconazole is a first-line treatment option for invasive aspergillosis and other invasive fungal infections. It exhibits nonlinear pharmacokinetics (Michaelis-Menten) related to saturable clearance mechanisms. This leads to greatly variable and unpredictable changes in drug exposure secondary to dosage adjustments and interpatient pharmacokinetic variability.[196,202] The most important pharmacodynamic parameter is AUC/MIC with a value of >25 associated with clinical efficacy in infections due to *Candida* and *Aspergillus* spp. Voriconazole has excellent bioavailability; however, it is metabolized by several significant CYP450 enzymes (ie, CYP2C9, CYP3A4, and CYP2C19). These enzymes may have significant interpatient variability due to enzyme polymorphism and, therefore, lead to varying voriconazole concentrations.[196] Suboptimal voriconazole concentrations have been associated with suboptimal response and treatment failure. Additionally, elevated voriconazole concentrations have been correlated with toxicities, which include hepatotoxicity, visual disturbances, and hallucinations. Based on available data, voriconazole concentrations between 1 mg/L and 4 to 6 mg/L are recommended to increase efficacy and decrease risk of toxicity. A trough concentration (eg, end of 12-hour dosing interval) should be drawn within the first week of therapy initiation or dosage adjustment.[196,204,208,209]

***Posaconazole.*** Posaconazole is indicated for the treatment of several invasive fungal infections, including mucormycosis. Posaconazole is available as an oral suspension, delayed-release tablet, and IV solution.[210] The oral formulations (oral suspension and delayed-release tablet) are not interchangeable because of noted pharmacokinetic differences. The oral formulations are influenced by food intake. Additionally, the oral suspension is influenced by gastric pH. It is recommended that the oral suspension be given with a high-fat meal to enhance bioavailability (by 2.6 to 4 times).[204,208] Similar to previously mentioned azole antifungals, posaconazole demonstrates large interpatient variability in its pharmacokinetic parameters. An exposure-toxicity relationship is still unknown for posaconazole.[196,202,208,209] Because of the prolonged half-life of posaconazole (26 to 35 hours), steady state is not reached until the end of first week of therapy, and serum concentrations can be measured at any time during the interval at that point.[204,208] Greater clinical response to posaconazole has been related to higher drug concentration exposure. Although a recommended trough concentration has not been defined, some have suggested a trough of >0.7 mg/L or >0.9 mcg/mL for prophylaxis, and a trough of >1 mg/L for primary therapy and >1.25 mg/L for salvage therapy or >1.8 mg/L in treatment of invasive fungal infections.[202,204]

***Fluconazole.*** Therapeutic drug monitoring of fluconazole is not required due to predictable concentrations based on currently available data. Additionally, it is less affected by drug–drug interactions. Of note, an AUC/MIC ratio >25 to 50 is related to improved clinical outcomes.[196,202,205]

***Isavuconazole.*** Although most patients achieve concentrations >1 mg/L with standard recommended doses, therapeutic drug monitoring of isavuconazole is not recommended at this time because of lack of efficacy or toxicity thresholds in the treatment of invasive aspergillosis or mucormycosis.[202,211]

## Antimycobacterials

Drugs that are FDA-approved and considered first line as part of an initial four-drug regimen are isoniazid, rifampin, pyrazinamide, and either ethambutol or streptomycin. Of these, isoniazid and rifampin are the most important based on their relatively high potency and favorable side-effect profiles. Second-line

agents that are more toxic must be used if drug resistance emerges and include ethionamide, cycloserine, capreomycin, para-aminosalicylic acid, and dapsone.[212]

The practice of therapeutic drug monitoring for antituberculosis drugs varies among experts. It is used to provide insight into drug dosing and dose adjustments. Scenarios in which therapeutic drug monitoring may be beneficial include poor response despite therapy adherence and drug-susceptible regimens, severe GI abnormalities in which absorption may be questioned, and drug–drug interactions.[213] Low concentrations of isoniazid and rifampin have been associated with slow disease response, relapse, and emergence of drug resistance.[214] In fact, poor treatment outcomes have been related to low tuberculosis (TB) drug exposure, noting an estimated 9-fold increase in treatment failure.[215] As a result, it is essential that adequate concentrations of these antimycobacterial drugs be present in serum for effective treatment and avoidance of negative consequences. This does not always occur, even in patients in whom adherence has been documented.[212] Lower-than-expected concentrations of antimycobacterial drugs have been reported in patients with diabetes and in individuals with HIV infections, which in some cases was associated with malabsorption.[216-218] There is also considerable potential for drug–drug interactions among the antimycobacterial drugs, given the effects of rifampin, isoniazid, and the fluoroquinolones in either inducing or inhibiting cytochrome P450 isozymes.[219] Drugs used to treat patients with HIV may also contribute to additional drug–drug interaction concerns.

A study in patients without HIV who are infected with TB who were not responding to treatment as expected showed that 29% to 68% of them had serum antimycobacterial drug concentrations below target ranges.[220] In another study, a small percentage of nonresponding patients all showed suboptimal concentrations of rifampin.[221] After dosage adjustments were made, all patients responded to treatment. The authors recommended that low serum rifampin concentrations be suspected in patients who do not respond after 3 months of supervised drug administration or earlier in patients with HIV infection, malnutrition, known GI or malabsorptive disease, or hepatic or renal disease.

Most TB drugs display AUC/MIC as the most important pharmacodynamic parameter; however, the relationship between dose or serum concentrations and toxicity is not well established (exceptions include pyrazinamide, ethambutol, and cycloserine). Several TB drugs display significant interpatient variability, necessitating therapeutic drug monitoring of these agents to avoid potential associated treatment failure, relapse, and toxicity.[222]

Specialized laboratories have been developed that offer sensitive and specific assays for serum concentrations for the most commonly used antimycobacterial drugs.[212] As more specific information about the efficacy of therapeutic drug monitoring of these drugs becomes available, more laboratories and services of this type will likely be available.[223]

## Antiretrovirals
### *Therapeutic Ranges and Clinical Considerations*

Overall, there is a paucity of published literature correlating clinical outcomes in adults infected with HIV and drug concentrations. Significant interpatient variability exists in regard to pharmacokinetics of antiretroviral drugs. Therapeutic concentration ranges, therefore, have not been established for most antiretrovirals.[224,225] Furthermore, antiretroviral regimens are administered as fixed doses; therefore, dose adjustments, as seen with other drug classes requiring therapeutic drug monitoring, may not be feasible or useful.[226] Although routine monitoring of antiretroviral agents is not recommended, there are some scenarios in which therapeutic drug monitoring should be considered. These situations include instances in which significant drug–drug or drug–food interactions may lead to reduced efficacy or toxicities; physiologic and anatomic changes (eg, GI) that may impair drug absorption or metabolism; pregnancy in which women do not achieve virologic clearance; and cases in which treatment-experienced patients have developed virologic failure.[227] There is some evidence that favors limited serum concentration monitoring of drugs used in the treatment of HIV-1 infection, in particular, the PIs and the non-nucleoside reverse-transcriptase inhibitors (NNRTIs).[228,229] These drugs, particularly the PIs, show marked interpatient variability in their pharmacokinetics, and their serum concentrations correlate with virologic response and failure.[230,231] A substudy of the randomized, prospective clinical trial AIDS Therapy Evaluation in the Netherlands showed that patients who underwent serum drug concentration monitoring for antiretroviral drugs had a significantly higher likelihood of virological response as compared with those who did not undergo monitoring.[230] Of note, the study was conducted in antiretroviral-naive patients. The same results have not been shown in subsets of antiretroviral-experienced patient populations. Assays for drug concentrations are available commercially for some antiretrovirals although there is a lag time in results being reported.[226,227]

Minimum concentration ($C_{min}$) is the proposed target concentration parameter.[229] Minimum effective concentrations have been determined for the most common PIs based on in vitro determinations of drug concentrations (corrected for serum binding) required for 50% or 90% inhibition of replication in a patient's virus isolate ($IC_{50}$ or $IC_{90}$). Attention has turned more recently, however, to the use of a new parameter that may be a better predictor of response. The inhibitory quotient (IQ) is the ratio of the trough plasma concentration to the $IC_{50}$ or $IC_{90}$.[230] A high IQ indicates more drug is present in the patient than is needed for a virologic response, whereas a low IQ indicates inadequate drug concentrations or a resistant virus. Recent studies show the virologic response may be better related to IQ than to trough concentrations alone.[230] Future studies may focus on the definition of therapeutic ranges of IQ rather than minimum concentrations.

Some clinicians advocate the monitoring of PI and NNRTIs in all patients upon the initiation of therapy to ensure adequate concentrations; others reserve the use for selected situations, including patients with renal or liver disease, pregnant patients, children, patients at risk for drug interactions, and patients with suspected toxicity.[230,232]

## Sample Timing

Half-lives of NNRTIs average 25 to 50 hours, and steady state is reached after a week in most patients.[233] However, a steady state is reached within 2 days for the PIs, which have half-lives ranging from 2 to 12 hours.[233] Predose samples are recommended as the minimum effective concentrations, and IQs are based on the lowest drug concentration during the dosing interval. There may be logistical problems with this timing, however, in cases in which the drug is administered once daily in the evening. Some drugs, such as nelfinavir, exhibit a lag in their absorption, such that the lowest concentration actually occurs about an hour after administration of the next dose.

## Use of Concentrations for Dosage Adjustment

Dosage adjustments of antiretroviral drugs, for the most part, should result in proportional changes in the trough serum drug concentration, provided the dosing interval is not altered. As mentioned previously, antiretroviral doses are fixed; therefore, there is no guidance on dose adjustment based on available drug concentrations. Reports showing serum drug concentrations to be unpredictable after dosage adjustments in some patients suggest that nonadherence with antiretroviral regimens is a major concern.[231] Serum concentrations of amprenavir, lopinavir, nelfinavir, and saquinavir may be difficult to maintain above their minimum effective concentrations because of rapid clearances and large first-pass effects. Rather than increasing their dose, ritonavir, a potent inhibitor of CYP3A4-mediated metabolism in the gut wall and liver, may be coadministered as a pharmacoenhancer. This results in decreased GI enzyme metabolism of the PI, higher trough concentrations, and, in most cases, prolonged elimination half-lives.[234]

## Protein Binding, Active Metabolites, and Other Considerations

The serum protein binding of nevirapine and indinavir is 50% to 60%, whereas the protein binding of the other antiretrovirals is >90%.[242,245] Albumin and AAG are the primary binding proteins for these drugs in serum.[232] As would be expected, there is considerable variability in the unbound fraction of these drugs in serum. In addition, AAG concentrations are elevated in patients with HIV-1 infection and can return to normal with treatment. Thus, the same total concentration of the drug would be expected to reflect a lower concentration of response early in treatment as compared with later. Clearly, total concentrations of the PIs and NNRTIs should be cautiously interpreted if unusual serum binding is anticipated, but no clear guidelines are yet available. Only nelfinavir has a metabolite that is known to be active.[230] Although studies indicate the measurement of the metabolite is probably not crucial, there is likely to be considerable variability among and within patients in the presence of this metabolite.

# Cardiac Drugs

## Digoxin

***Therapeutic range and clinical considerations.*** Since the advent of therapeutic drug monitoring, there has been a dramatic reduction in digoxin toxicity.[236] Routine monitoring is not necessary unless digoxin toxicity is expected, the patient has declining renal function, there is a suspected change in pharmacokinetics due to changing condition, or there is an initiation of concomitant interacting medications.[237] Additionally, patients with electrolyte abnormalities (eg, hypokalemia, hypomagnesemia, and hypercalcemia), hypothyroidism, myocardial ischemia, and acidotic states are at higher risk of toxicity. Patients with hyperthyroidism are believed to be more resistant to digoxin.[30]

Digoxin's inotropic effect is the basis for its use for the management of heart failure, while its chronotropic effects are the basis for the management of atrial arrhythmias, such as atrial fibrillation and atrial flutter. The commonly reported therapeutic range is 0.5 to 2 mcg/L in adults and 1 to 2.6 mcg/L in neonates.[76,235,237] The lower end of the range (0.5 to 1 mcg/L) is generally used for treatment of heart failure.[238] Results of the Digitalis Investigation Group trial found in a post hoc analysis that concentrations of 0.5 to 0.8 mcg/L in men with heart failure (left ventricular ejection fraction <46%) reduced hospitalizations.[239] Dosing strategies for patients with heart failure have been established based on kidney function, age >70 years, ideal body weight, and height.[240-242] Higher serum digoxin concentrations may be required for treatment of atrial arrhythmias (0.8 to 1.5 mcg/L), with concentrations up to 2 mcg/L previously showing benefit in some patients.[73] More recent studies have shown an increased mortality in patients treated with digoxin with a serum concentration of >1.2 mcg/L; however, as noted previously, routine monitoring is not indicated.

Fifty percent of patients with serum digoxin concentrations >2 mcg/L show some form of digoxin toxicity; toxicity may be experienced at lower concentrations, and management should be based on symptoms.[73,243] Symptoms of toxicity include muscle weakness; GI reports (anorexia, nausea, vomiting, abdominal pain, and constipation); CNS effects (headache, insomnia, confusion, vertigo, and changes in color vision); and serious cardiovascular effects (second- or third-degree atrioventricular bradycardia, premature ventricular contractions, and ventricular tachycardia) (**Table 5-4**).[73,237]

***Sample timing.*** The average digoxin half-life in adults with normal renal function is approximately 2 days; at least 7 days are recommended to attain a steady state.[237] In the case of treatment of digoxin overdose with digoxin-immune Fab fragments (a fragment of an antibody that is very specific for digoxin), blood samples for serum digoxin measurements should not be obtained sooner than 10 days after administration of the fragments.[235,237]

Samples drawn during the absorption and distribution phases after administration of digoxin cannot be appropriately

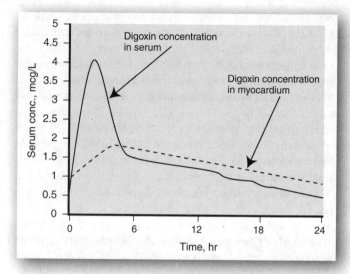

**FIGURE 5-5.** Simulated plot showing concentrations of digoxin in serum (microgram/liter) and concentrations in myocardial tissue (units not provided) after a dose of digoxin at steady state. Tissue concentrations do not parallel concentrations in serum until at least 6 hours after the dose.

interpreted by comparison with the usual therapeutic range. Digoxin concentrations in blood do not reflect the more important concentrations in myocardial tissue until at least 6 hours after the dose (some say at least 12 hours).[237,245,246] Therefore, blood samples should be drawn anytime between 6 hours after the dose and right before the next dose (**Figure 5-5**). Ideally, blood samples would be drawn as a trough concentration just prior to the next dose.

Inappropriate timing of samples for digoxin is problematic. One study revealed that 55% of the samples submitted to the laboratory for digoxin analysis lacked clinical value because of inappropriate timing.[247] In another study, standardization of digoxin administration and blood sampling times resulted in a dramatic reduction in inappropriately timed samples (ie, timed at 5:00 p.m. for digoxin administration and timed at 7:00 a.m. for blood sampling).[248] Another recommendation is that the laboratory immediately contact the clinician if digoxin concentrations are >3.5 mcg/L.[237] If it is confirmed that the sample was drawn too early after the dose, another sample should be requested. If monitoring is considered at the initiation of therapy, serum concentrations should be drawn within 12 to 24 hours of the loading dose; if no loading dose is administered, clinicians should wait 3 to 5 days after therapy initiation to evaluate concentrations.[249] It should be noted that concentrations drawn after administering a loading dose can assist in ensuring adequate concentrations are achieved; however, they cannot guide maintenance dosing.

***Use of concentrations for dose adjustment.*** Because of the linear elimination behavior of digoxin, a given increase in the daily digoxin dose produces a proportional increase in the serum concentration at that time during the dosing interval. To determine steady-state concentrations after dose adjustments, obtain a serum concentration 5 to 7 days after any dose change,

## TABLE 5-4. Digoxin Toxicities[245]

| Cardiac effects | • Arrhythmias <br> • Sinus bradycardia |
|---|---|
| CNS/GI effects | • Anorexia, nausea, vomiting, abdominal pain <br> • Visual disturbances: halos, photophobia, color perception dysfunction (red-green or yellow green), scotomata <br> • Fatigue, weakness, dizziness, headache, confusion, delirium, psychosis |

and periodically thereafter, particularly in instances of potential change in pharmacokinetics, as detailed previously. In patients with ESRD, steady state may not be obtained for 15 to 20 days.[249]

***Protein binding, active metabolites, and other considerations.*** Digoxin is only 20% to 30% bound to serum proteins.[29] Therefore, total concentrations in serum will reflect the pharmacologically active unbound concentration. The biologic activity of digoxin metabolites is modest compared with the parent drug, and variable presence of metabolites should not affect the interpretation of a digoxin serum concentration.

## Other Cardiac Drugs

***Amiodarone.*** Amiodarone is used for the treatment of life-threatening recurrent ventricular arrhythmias that do not respond to adequate doses of other antiarrhythmics and is commonly used in the management of recurrent atrial fibrillation/flutter. The primary metabolite, desethylamiodarone (DEA), has similar electrophysiologic properties as amiodarone and accumulates at concentrations similar to or higher than the parent drug, especially in patients with renal failure.[235] Concentrations of amiodarone and desethylamiodarone demonstrate linear pharmacokinetics with increasing doses of amiodarone.[250] The concentration versus effect relationship for amiodarone is poorly defined; some say that serum concentrations between 0.5 and 2.5 mg/L are associated with effectiveness with minimal toxicity.[235] The occurrence of toxicity has been reported at plasma concentrations >2.5 mg/L.[251-253] Laboratories that measure serum amiodarone concentrations report only the parent drug, despite high concentrations of the active metabolite. In general, therapeutic drug monitoring of amiodarone is of limited benefit because activity of the drug is mostly associated with concentrations in the tissue.[246] Serum concentrations might be most useful in cases of suspected nonadherence or toxicity.

***Lidocaine.*** Lidocaine is a type 1B antiarrhythmic used as second-line therapy for the acute treatment for ventricular tachycardia and fibrillation with modern use primarily as off-label for pain. The therapeutic range is generally considered to be 1.5 to 5 mg/L with concentrations >6 mg/L considered to be toxic.[73,238,255] Minor side effects—drowsiness, dizziness, euphoria, and paresthesias—may be observed at serum concentrations >3 mg/L. More serious side effects observed at concentrations >6 mg/L include muscle twitching, confusion, agitation, and psychoses, whereas cardiovascular depression, atrioventricular block, hypotension, seizures, and coma may be observed at concentrations >8 mg/L.[73,237,255] Lidocaine concentrations are not monitored as commonly with short-term use because its effect (abolishment of the electrocardiogram-monitored arrhythmia or pain relief) is easy to directly observe and is generally not indicated when used for pain management given administration is generally limited to single doses. Electrocardiogram monitoring may be indicated and is typically part of institutional protocols. Indications for drug concentration monitoring should be restricted to situations in which the expected response is not evident or when decreased hepatic clearance is suspected or anticipated: liver disease, heart failure, advanced age, severe trauma, and concurrent drugs such as β-adrenergic blockers, fluvoxamine, or cimetidine.[235,237,254]

Additionally, serum concentrations should be monitored in the case of extended use, although infusion duration beyond 6 hours is not recommended.[256] The half-life of lidocaine ranges from 1.5 hours to as long as 5 hours in patients with liver disease; thus, steady state may not be attained for 18 to 24 hours.[73,255] Because lidocaine is administered as a continuous infusion, there are no fluctuations in concentrations, and blood lidocaine serum concentrations can be drawn anytime once steady state is reached. Adjustments of lidocaine infusion rate should result in a proportional increase in lidocaine serum concentration. The unbound percentage of lidocaine is normally 30% but can range from 10% to 40% due to variations in AAG concentrations.[73,237] The combination of higher total concentrations of lidocaine during prolonged infusions and a lower unbound fraction mean that unbound lidocaine concentrations during prolonged infusions are probably therapeutic.[257] The monoethylglycinexylidide metabolite of lidocaine has 80% to 90% of the antiarrhythmic potency of lidocaine, and its concentration accumulates in renal failure.[73,254]

***Mexiletine.*** Several early studies with mexiletine have established a linear association with serum concentrations and toxicity. Currently, the clinically used therapeutic range is 0.8 to 2 mcg/mL; however, it should be noted the establishment of this therapeutic range was in the prophylaxis of ventricular tachycardia after myocardial infarction, not in the treatment of ventricular tachycardia, which is the most common use.[258-260] Despite the potential benefit of therapeutic drug monitoring for mexiletine in some patient populations, specifically those with hepatic dysfunction, serum concentrations are not widely used and when they are used, they do not often result in a change to therapy.

***Procainamide.*** Although the oral formulation is no longer available in the United States, the IV form of procainamide is used for patients with atrial fibrillation or flutter who require cardioversion.[261,262] The therapeutic range of procainamide is complicated by the presence of an active metabolite, NAPA, which has different electrophysiologic properties than the parent drug. Procainamide is a type 1A antiarrhythmic, whereas NAPA is a type III antiarrhythmic.[73,235,237] The enzyme that acetylates procainamide is bimodally distributed, such that patients are either slow or fast acetylators. In addition, NAPA depends more on the kidneys for elimination than procainamide.[247,263] Most patients respond when serum procainamide concentrations are between 4 and 8 mg/L; some patients receive additional benefit with concentrations up to 12 mg/L.[261] There have been reports of patients requiring concentrations between 15 and 20 mg/L without adverse effects.[261] Serum concentrations of NAPA associated with efficacy are reported to be as low as 5 mg/L and as high as 30 mg/L. Most clinicians consider toxic NAPA concentrations to be >30 to 40 mg/L.[237] Some clinicians feel that NAPA does not need to be monitored except in patients with renal impairment.[261] Most laboratories automatically measure both procainamide and NAPA concentrations in the same sample. The practice of summing the two concentrations and comparing it to a therapeutic range for summed procainamide and NAPA (often reported as 10 to 30 mg/L) is to be discouraged.[73,237,261] To do this validly, the molar units of the two chemicals would need to be used.[238] The best practice is to independently compare each chemical to its own reference range.[73,237,265] Side effects to procainamide and NAPA are similar. Anorexia, nausea, vomiting, diarrhea, weakness, and hypotension may be seen with procainamide concentrations >8 mg/L, although concentrations >12 mg/L may be associated with more serious adverse effects: heart block, ventricular conduction disturbances, new ventricular arrhythmias, and even cardiac arrest.[73] Indications for procainamide and NAPA serum concentration monitoring include recurrence of arrhythmias that were previously controlled, suspected toxicity or overdose, anticipated pharmacokinetic alterations caused by drug–drug interactions (including amiodarone, cimetidine, ethanol, ofloxacin, quinidine, ranitidine, and trimethoprim), and disease state changes (renal failure or heart failure, in particular).[73,237,261,263] The half-life of procainamide in adults without renal impairment or heart failure ranges from 2.5 hours (fast acetylator) to 5 hours (slow acetylator).[73,237] The half-life of NAPA is longer, averaging 6 hours in patients with normal renal function and 30 hours or longer in patients with renal impairment.[73,261] Thus, a steady state of both chemicals is not observed until at least 18 hours in patients with good renal function or as long as 4 days in renal impairment. The lower clearance of procainamide at higher doses has been attributed to nonlinear hepatic clearance.[264] The clinician should be aware that increases in infusion rate may produce somewhat greater-than-proportional increases in serum procainamide concentration in some patients, particularly those with serum concentrations at the upper end of the therapeutic range. Procainamide is only 10% to 20% bound to serum proteins.[235,238] Thus, total procainamide and NAPA concentrations always reflect the pharmacologically active unbound concentrations of these drugs.

**Quinidine.** The therapeutic range of quinidine for treatment of severe malaria due to *Plasmodium falciparum* is reported as 3 to 6 mg/L.[265] When used in combination with verapamil for prevention of atrial fibrillation, the therapeutic range of quinidine is reported to be 2 to 6 mg/L, although use of quinidine is not strongly recommended due to a 3-fold increased risk of cardiac death when compared with other antiarrhythmic agents.[265-268] Common side effects are anorexia, nausea, and diarrhea; more serious side effects include cinchonism, hypotension, and ventricular arrhythmias.[73,237] Torsades de pointes is more likely to occur at lower concentrations of the therapeutic range, thus complicating the interpretation of quinidine concentrations.[235] Indications for monitoring of quinidine concentrations include therapeutic confirmation, suspected toxicity, recurrence of arrhythmias, drug–drug interactions, suspected nonadherence, and changes in formulation.[73,237,268] The half-life of quinidine is reported to range from 4 to 8 hours in adults and up to 10 hours in patients with liver disease. Steady state should be attained within 2 or 3 days in patients with normal hepatic function, and most clinicians agree that samples should be drawn as a trough within 1 hour of the next dose.[73,235,237,268] Quinidine is a weak base that is normally between 70% and 80% bound to albumin and AAG.[237] The unbound fraction of quinidine was shown to be decreased in patients with atrial fibrillation or atrial flutter, and the unbound quinidine concentration was shown to correlate better with

electrocardiogram interval changes than total quinidine.[269,270] A total quinidine concentration that is >5 mg/L could be therapeutic with respect to unbound quinidine concentration. The dihydroquinidine impurity may be present in amounts that are between 10% and 15% of the labeled amount of quinidine and is believed to have similar electrophysiologic properties as quinidine.[237] The 3-hydroxyquinidine metabolite has activity that is less than the parent (anywhere between 20% and 80% have been reported), is less highly bound to serum proteins, and demonstrates accumulation with chronic treatment.[263,271]

## Cytotoxic Drugs

Although cytotoxic drugs have some characteristics that make them ideal candidates for therapeutic drug monitoring (narrow therapeutic indices and variable pharmacokinetics), they have many more characteristics that make therapeutic drug monitoring difficult or unsuitable.[272,273] They lack a simple, immediate indication of pharmacologic effect to aid definition of a therapeutic range (the ultimate outcome of cure could be years). They are given in combination with other cytotoxic drugs, such that concentration versus effect relationships for any single drug is difficult to isolate. They are used to treat cancer, which is a highly heterogeneous group of diseases, each possibly having its own concentration-versus-effect relationships. In summary, cytotoxic drugs are not routinely monitored because they need more clearly defined therapeutic ranges. If ranges are established, they are usually more helpful to avoid toxicity than to define zones for efficacy.

### Methotrexate

*Therapeutic range.* Methotrexate is the only antimetabolite drug for which serum concentrations are routinely monitored.[272] It acts by blocking the conversion of intracellular folate to reduced folate cofactors necessary for cell replication. Although cancer cells are more susceptible to the toxic effects of methotrexate, healthy host cells are also affected by prolonged exposure to methotrexate. It is for this reason that leucovorin, a folate analogue that prevents further cell damage, is administered following high-dose methotrexate treatments.[272] Measurements of serum methotrexate concentrations at critical times after high-dose methotrexate regimens are imperative to guide the amount and duration of leucovorin rescue treatments, thus preventing methotrexate toxicity. Institution of protocols for methotrexate serum concentration monitoring for this purpose has resulted in dramatic reductions in high-dose methotrexate-related toxicity and mortality.[274]

Although it is known that methotrexate concentrations must be sufficiently high to prevent relapse of the malignancy, the specific range of concentrations related to efficacy has been difficult to define.[274] However, the relationship between methotrexate concentrations and toxicity has been much more clearly defined. Prolonged high concentrations of methotrexate can lead to nephrotoxicity, myelosuppression, GI mucositis, and liver cirrhosis.[272,274] Serum concentration monitoring is not generally indicated when relatively low doses of methotrexate are given for chronic diseases such as rheumatoid arthritis, asthma, and psoriasis and maintenance for certain cancers.

*Sample timing.* The timing of samples for determination of methotrexate concentrations depends highly on the administration schedule. As one example of such a protocol, a methotrexate dose may be administered by IV infusion over 36 hours followed by a regimen of leucovorin doses administered over the next 72 hours.[275] Additional or larger leucovorin doses might be given depending on the methotrexate concentrations in samples drawn at various times after the start of the methotrexate infusion. It is important that methotrexate concentrations continue to be monitored until they are below the critical concentrations (usually between 0.05 μM/L and 0.1 μM/L).[272,275]

*Use of concentrations for dosage adjustment.* Methotrexate dose adjustments and leucovorin doses are based on institution-specific protocols.

*Protein binding, active metabolites, and other considerations.* Methotrexate binding to albumin in serum ranges from 20% to 57%.[272] Although studies have shown the unbound fraction of methotrexate to be increased by concomitant administration of nonsteroidal anti-inflammatory drugs, salicylate, sulfonamides, and probenecid, the implications for interpretation of methotrexate concentrations are probably negligible.[275] The methotrexate metabolite, 7-hydroxymethotrexate, has only one-one hundredth the activity of methotrexate but may cause nephrotoxicity due to precipitation in the renal tubules.[274]

### Other Cytotoxic Drugs

Petros and Evans provide an excellent summary of cytotoxic drugs and the types of measurements that have been used to predict their toxicity and response.[274] Correlations between the response or toxicity and serum concentration or AUC versus time curve for total drug have been shown for busulfan, carboplatin, cisplatin, cyclophosphamide, docetaxel, etoposide, 5-fluorouracil, irinotecan, paclitaxel, teniposide, topotecan, and vincristine.[274,276,277] The strong correlation between busulfan AUC and bone marrow transplant outcome led the FDA to include instructions for AUC monitoring in the package insert for IV busulfan. Unbound AUC values for etoposide and teniposide, which demonstrate concentration-dependent binding, correlate more strongly with toxicity than corresponding total plasma AUC values.[278] Systemic drug clearance has been predictive of response/toxicity for amsacrine, fluorouracil, methotrexate, and teniposide.[274,279] Steady-state average serum concentrations or concentrations at designated postdose times have also been predictive of response/toxicity for cisplatin, etoposide, and methotrexate.[274] Finally, concentrations of cytosine-arabinoside metabolite in leukemic blasts and concentrations of mercaptopurine metabolite in red blood cells have been predictive of response or toxicity for these drugs. Correlations between systemic exposure and response/toxicity for cyclophosphamide, carmustine, and thiotepa have also been reported.[280] Toxicity of doxorubicin has been found to be associated with peak plasma concentrations.[281] Although most studies up to this point have focused on the use of cytotoxic drug concentration measurements to minimize toxicity, future studies will increasingly focus on the use of drug concentrations to maximize efficacy.

## Immunosuppressant Drugs

Immunosuppressant drugs are used for a variety of indications, including prevention of rejection in organ transplant or treatment of autoimmune diseases. Therapeutic drug monitoring is widely used to ensure adequate doses are attained and to avoid toxicity. Although this chapter discusses commonly used therapeutic ranges, individualized targets may be used based upon patient-specific factors, time from transplant, or institutional protocols.

### Cyclosporine

*Therapeutic range and clinical considerations.* Cyclosporine is a potent cyclic polypeptide used for prevention of organ rejection in patients who have received kidney, liver, bone marrow, or heart transplants.[282] It is also used for the management of psoriasis, rheumatoid arthritis, and other autoimmune diseases. The therapeutic range of cyclosporine depends highly on the specimen (whole blood or serum/plasma) and assay. Whole blood is preferred given that cyclosporine binds to erythrocytes and lipoproteins. Most transplant centers use whole blood with one of the more specific assays—high-performance liquid chromatography or immunoassays that use monoclonal antibodies (monoclonal radioimmunoassay or monoclonal fluorescence polarization immunoassay).[73,283,284] The commonly cited therapeutic range for whole blood troughs using one of these specific methods is 100 to 500 mcg/L.[73,285] Troughs at the higher end of this range may be desired initially after transplantation and in patients at high risk for rejection.[285] The therapeutic range also depends on the specific organ transplantation procedure and the stage of treatment after surgery (higher concentrations during induction and lower concentrations during maintenance to minimize side effects) as well as comedications.[73,284-287] Thus, it is important that the therapeutic range guidelines established by each center be used. Although most centers still use single-trough concentrations to adjust cyclosporine doses, the area under the blood concentration versus time curve is believed to be a more sensitive predictor of clinical outcome.[287] Studies that have investigated the use of single cyclosporine concentrations measured 2 hours after the dose as a surrogate for the AUC value suggest a better clinical outcome as compared with the use of single-trough concentrations.[283,288,289]

Cyclosporine has a narrow therapeutic index and extremely variable pharmacokinetics among and within patients. The implications of ineffective therapy and adverse reactions are serious. Thus, it is imperative that cyclosporine concentrations be monitored in all patients starting immediately after transplant surgery. The primary side effects associated with high cyclosporine blood concentrations are nephrotoxicity, neurotoxicity, hypertension, hyperlipidemia, hirsutism, and gingival hyperplasia.[73,285,287] Blood cyclosporine concentrations should also be monitored when there is a dosage adjustment, signs of rejection or adverse reactions, suspected nonadherence, or the initiation or discontinuation of drugs known to induce or inhibit cyclosporine metabolism.[285,287]

*Sample timing.* Monitoring is often done immediately after surgery before a steady state is reached. Initially, concentrations may be obtained daily or every other day, then every 3 to 5 days, and then monthly. Changes in dose or initiation or discontinuation of potential enzyme inducers or inhibitors require resampling once a new steady state is reached. The half-life of cyclosporine ranges from 5 to 27 hours and depends on the particular formulation. Thus, every 3 to 5 days is generally adequate in most patients for attainment of a new steady state. Most centers continue to sample predose (trough) cyclosporine concentrations, while some are using 2-hour postdose concentrations, which appear to more closely predict total exposure to cyclosporine as measured by AUC.[283,289] Multiple samples to determine the AUC are generally unnecessary.

**Use of concentrations for dosage adjustment.** In most cases, simple proportionality may be used for dosage adjustments. Trough or 2-hour postdose concentrations will change in proportion to the change in dose so long as the dosing interval remains the same.

**Protein binding, active metabolites, and other considerations.** Cyclosporine is 90% bound to albumin and lipoproteins in blood.[286] Unbound fractions in blood vary widely among patients and are weakly correlated to lipoprotein concentrations in blood.[286] For example, lower unbound fractions of cyclosporine have been reported in patients with hypercholesterolemia.[287] Lindholm and Henricsson reported a significant drop in the unbound fraction of cyclosporine in plasma immediately prior to acute rejection episodes.[290] An association between low cholesterol concentrations (and presumably high unbound fractions of cyclosporine) and increased incidence of neurotoxicity has also been reported.[287] These studies suggest that efforts to maintain all patients within a certain range of total concentrations may be misleading. Routine monitoring of unbound cyclosporine concentrations is not yet feasible, given the many technical difficulties with this measurement. Instead, the clinician should cautiously interpret total concentrations of cyclosporine in situations in which altered protein binding of cyclosporine has been reported.

## Other Immunosuppressant Drugs

**Everolimus.** Everolimus is an mTOR (mammalian target of rapamycin) kinase inhibitor that is used in the treatment of many oncologic conditions, in patients with liver and renal transplants, and in a treatment of subependymal giant cell astrocytoma (SEGA).[291] Everolimus is primarily metabolized through CYP3A4 and has six known weak metabolites. The half-life is approximately 30 hours, and bioavailability decreases with high-fat meals.[291,292] Whole blood concentrations should be in the range of 3 to 8 mcg/L for liver and renal transplant patients; 5 to 15 mcg/L is the reference range in patients with SEGA. In patients with liver or renal transplant, trough concentrations should be drawn 4 to 5 days after therapy initiation, dose adjustments, or discontinuation of interacting medications. In patients with SEGA, concentrations should be monitored approximately 2 weeks after initiation or dose adjustment; when interacting medications are initiated, discontinued, or changed; with changes in everolimus formulation; or with changes in liver function. When a maintenance dose has been attained, trough concentrations should be monitored every 6 to 12 months. More frequent monitoring of 3 to 6 months is suggested if a patient's body surface area is fluctuating. Everolimus is 74% protein-bound.[291]

**Mycophenolic acid.** Mycophenolate mofetil, the prodrug of mycophenolic acid, is often used in combination with cyclosporine or tacrolimus with or without corticosteroids in patients who have received transplant and may be used alone in patients with various autoimmune diseases.[287] Although troughs of mycophenolic acid may be monitored (plasma concentrations between 2.5 and 4 mg/L are targeted with good success), AUC values appear to be better predictors of postoperative efficacy (avoidance of acute rejection).[289,293,294] Reliable measurements of AUC may be determined with as few as three samples (trough, 30 minutes postdose, and 120 minutes postdose) with a desired target AUC range of 30 to 60 mg × hr/L.[293] The half-life of mycophenolic acid is approximately 17 hours. Thus, a new steady state is attained approximately 3 days after a dose change or the addition/discontinuation of drugs that affect the metabolism of mycophenolic acid. Mycophenolic acid is 98% bound to plasma proteins, and the unbound fraction is greatly influenced by changes in albumin concentration, displacement by metabolites, renal failure, and hyperbilirubinemia.[283,293] Several groups of investigators suggest that unbound mycophenolic acid concentrations should be monitored when altered binding is suspected.[287,293-296] There is evidence that unbound mycophenolic acid concentration may be a better predictor of adverse effects than total concentration.[295,297]

**Sirolimus.** Sirolimus is a macrolide antibiotic with potent immunosuppressant activity. When used in combination with cyclosporine and corticosteroids, trough blood concentrations of 5 to 15 mcg/L are generally targeted.[285] With whole blood sampling, therapeutic concentrations measure 10 to 15 mcg/L with concomitant calcineurin inhibitors, and higher ranges of 15 to 25 mcg/L are targeted without calcineurin inhibitors.[298] It has a relatively long half-life (62 hours), and a new steady state is not attained in many patients until at least 6 days after dose adjustments or the addition or discontinuation of interacting drugs.[285] At present, trough concentrations are used for monitoring because they correlate well with AUC.[283]

**Tacrolimus.** Tacrolimus is a macrolide antibiotic with immunosuppressant activity and is generally used in combination with other immunosuppressant drugs. Trough blood concentrations of tacrolimus as high as 20 mcg/L are targeted during initial treatment and gradually decrease to between 5 and 10 mcg/L during maintenance therapy, often after 12 months, and are generally determined by indication and institution-specific protocols.[289] Toxicities to tacrolimus are similar to those with cyclosporine, including nephrotoxicity and neurotoxicity.[285,299] The unpredictable and variable extent of tacrolimus bioavailability (5% to 67%) contributes to the need for monitoring of this drug.[299] The advent of a once-daily extended-release formulation produced with advanced drug-delivery systems can enhance bioavailability and maintain stable serum concentrations over 24 hours.[300] Differences in pharmacogenomics (related to the CYP3A4*22 allele) have been associated with altered pharmacokinetics.[301] Monitoring should always be done after changes in dose or initiation/discontinuation of enzyme-inducing or inhibiting agents. The half-life of tacrolimus ranges from 4 to 41 hours for both immediate- and extended-release formulations, and a new steady state is attained after approximately 3 to 5 days.[285,287] Although trough concentrations are still the method of choice for monitoring, a second concentration might be needed if Bayesian approaches to dosage individualization are used.[289,302] Some evidence suggests the window for obtaining a blood sample for those patients receiving the extended-release formulation may be wider (±3 hours of the dose), which may allow more flexibility and reduce waste from improperly timed concentrations.[300] Tacrolimus exhibits linear elimination behavior; thus, an increase in the daily dose is expected to result in a proportional increase in the steady-state trough concentration. Tacrolimus is 75% to 99% bound to plasma proteins (albumin, α-1-glycoprotein, lipoproteins and globulins).[287,299] Reports of lower unbound serum concentrations of tacrolimus during episodes of rejection lead one to be cautious with interpretation of total tacrolimus concentrations in patients with suspected alterations in protein binding.[297]

## Psychotropics

### Tricyclic Antidepressants (Amitriptyline, Nortriptyline, Imipramine, Desipramine)

*Therapeutic ranges.* Although tricyclic antidepressants (TCAs) continue to be used for the treatment of depression, their use has significantly declined in favor of newer antidepressants.[303] The therapeutic ranges of amitriptyline, imipramine, desipramine, and nortriptyline are well defined for depression; however, they are not routinely used for other off-label indications, such as sleep or pain.[25,304,305] Desipramine and nortriptyline are also active metabolites of imipramine and amitriptyline, respectively.

When imipramine is administered, combined serum concentrations of imipramine and desipramine that are considered therapeutic but not toxic are between 180 and 350 mcg/L.[304,305] Combined concentrations above 500 mcg/L are extremely toxic.[305] When desipramine is administered, concentrations between 115 and 250 mcg/L are frequently associated with therapeutic effect.[304,305] When amitriptyline is administered, combined serum concentrations of amitriptyline and nortriptyline should be between 120 and 250 mcg/L.[304] Combined concentrations above 450 mcg/L are not likely to produce an additional response and are associated with cardiotoxicity and anticholinergic delirium.[305] The therapeutic range of nortriptyline is the most firmly established of these four drugs; target serum concentrations after nortriptyline administration are between 50 and 150 mcg/L.[304-306]

The most common side effects of the TCAs are anticholinergic in nature.[304] Toxicities seen at higher concentrations include cardiac conduction disturbances, seizures, and coma.[304] For all of the TCAs, these toxic effects occur at serum concentrations that are approximately five times those needed for antidepressant efficacy.[11] Indications for monitoring include suspected nonadherence or inadequate response, suspected toxicity, and suspected unusual or altered pharmacokinetics (seen in children and elderly persons and with drug interactions).

The TCAs in general are highly bound to serum proteins.[303] Thus, one would expect unbound TCA serum concentrations to be much better predictors of response than total concentrations, particularly in populations suspected to have unusually high or low serum binding. Until now, studies that have attempted to examine this have not been able to clarify relationships between response and total serum concentrations based on variable protein binding. The TCAs are extensively metabolized and undergo significant first-pass metabolism. Although the primary active metabolites have been identified and are separately measured, other active metabolites can accumulate in some circumstances and affect the response at a given parent drug concentration.[307]

### Other Antidepressants: Selective Serotonin Reuptake Inhibitor, Serotonin Norepinephrine Reuptake Inhibitor, Monoamine Oxidase Inhibitors

Assays have been developed to document the serum concentrations observed following the administration of other cyclic antidepressants as well as the selective serotonin reuptake inhibitors, serotonin and norepinephrine reuptake inhibitors, and norepinephrine reuptake inhibitors.[11,308,309-313] Although reference ranges have been established, there does not appear to be any compelling reason for routine monitoring of these drugs given their relatively wide therapeutic indices and more favorable side effect profiles. Because 50% of patients not achieving optimal relief from symptoms of depression, some clinicians advocate the use of serum concentration monitoring in patients who do not initially respond to identify nonadherence or unusually low serum concentrations.[11,25,307,314]

### Lithium

*Therapeutic range.* Lithium is a monovalent cation used for the treatment of bipolar disorder and the manic phase of affective disorders, and it is somewhat effective in the treatment of refractory depression.[314] The concentration units for lithium are expressed as milliequivalent/liter, which is the same as millimole/liter. Although the overall therapeutic range for treatment of bipolar disorder is commonly cited as 0.5 to 1.2 mEq/L, there appear to be two distinct ranges used in practice, depending on the stage of therapy.[26,305] For acute management of manic episodes, the therapeutic range of 0.8 to 1.2 mEq/L is desired, going up to 1.5 mEq/L if necessary.[73,315,316] For maintenance treatment, the therapeutic range of 0.6 to 1 mEq/L or 1 to 1.2 mEq/L is usually recommended.[73,310,315,317] In elderly patients, target therapeutic concentrations are as low as 0.2 mEq/L.[318] Serum concentrations >1.5 mEq/L are associated with fine tremors of the extremities, GI disturbances, muscle weakness, fatigue, polyuria, and polydipsia. Concentrations >2.5 mEq/L are associated with coarse tremors, confusion, delirium, slurred speech, and vomiting. Concentrations >2.5 to 3.5 mEq/L are associated with seizures, coma, and death.[304] It is important to point out that the values for the therapeutic ranges are based on samples obtained at a specific time during the day—just before the morning dose and at least 12 hours after the evening dose for patients on a BID or TID regimen.[315,319]

Most clinicians require that every patient taking lithium be regularly monitored, which is cost effective considering the potential avoidance of toxicity.[73,306] Specific indications for lithium concentration monitoring include evaluation of nonadherence, suspicion of toxicity, confirmation of the concentration associated with efficacy, and any situation in which altered pharmacokinetics of the drug is anticipated (drug–drug interactions, pregnancy, children, geriatric patients, and fluid and electrolyte imbalance). Despite the strong indication for lithium monitoring in all patients, 37% of lithium users on Medicaid did not have serum drug concentrations monitored.[320]

***Sample timing.*** The half-life of lithium ranges from 18 to 24 hours, and steady state is reached within a week of therapy.[315] However, 2 to 3 weeks of treatment may be required after that before the full response to the drug can be assessed.[315] When initiating lithium therapy, it is recommended that serum concentrations be measured every 2 to 3 days (before a steady state is reached) to ensure that concentrations do not exceed 1.2 mEq/L during that time.[73] Because of the extreme variability of serum lithium concentrations during the absorption and distribution periods, the current standard of practice is to draw all samples for lithium serum concentration determination 12 hours after the evening dose, regardless of whether a twice- or thrice-daily dosing schedule is used. For example, the time for blood sampling for a patient on a 9 a.m./3 p.m./9 p.m. schedule would be right before the 9 a.m. dose.[73] The timing of blood samples for a patient taking once-daily lithium is less clear given the greater degree of serum lithium concentration fluctuation with this dosing method.[315]

***Use of concentrations for dosage adjustment.*** Lithium exhibits linear elimination behavior, and proportionality can be assumed when dosage adjustments are made. The assumption of linearity is the basis for several dosing methods that are used for initiating lithium therapy in patients. The Cooper method involves drawing a sample for lithium analysis 24 hours after a first dose of 600 mg.[44] The resulting concentration, believed to provide a reflection of the drug's half-life, is used with a nomogram that indicates the optimal maintenance regimen. The Perry method requires that two concentrations be drawn during the postabsorption, postdistribution phase after a first dose of lithium.[45] These two concentrations are used to determine the first-order elimination rate constant, which can then be used to determine the expected extent of lithium accumulation in the patient. The maintenance regimen required to attain a desired target lithium concentration in that patient can then be determined. Population-pharmacokinetic, dosing-initiation methods (Bayesian) can also be used.[73]

***Protein binding, active metabolites, and other considerations.*** Lithium is not bound to serum proteins, nor is it metabolized.

***Antipsychotics.*** The existence of well-defined therapeutic ranges for most antipsychotic drugs remains controversial.[321-323] There is growing interest in therapeutic drug monitoring of antipsychotics and several drugs have more established therapeutic drug monitoring guidance.[25,324-326] The AGNP-TDM Expert Consensus Guidelines: Therapeutic Drug Monitoring in Psychiatry make several recommendations for serum drug concentration monitoring for several antipsychotics, including haloperidol, perphenazine, fluphenazine, amisulpride, clozapine, olanzapine, and risperidone. The focus of therapeutic drug monitoring for antipsychotics is for the prevention of adverse effects, especially extrapyramidal effects during dose titration for effect with an emphasis on quality of life rather than a concern for toxicity.[25] Additional considerations include assessment of adherence or lack of response at maximal doses.

Clozapine would be the only exception because toxicity can be seen at the upper end of the therapeutic range and the incidence of seizures with clozapine directly correlates with plasma concentrations.[25,327] Although there is a range of interpatient variability related to clozapine pharmacokinetics, Rajkumar and colleagues found that in patients with treatment-resistant schizophrenia, increasing doses of clozapine, caffeine intake, and VPA administration were most closely associated with serum clozapine concentrations.[325] Reference ranges for other antipsychotic drugs are primarily based on average serum concentrations observed during chronic therapy.[306,310] One difficulty in establishing clear therapeutic range guidelines and subsequent dose adjustments is that chronicity of illness and duration of antipsychotic drug exposure can shift the therapeutic range; separate therapeutic ranges may need to be developed depending on duration of illness. Furthermore, many medications are used for various psychotic indications in which dosing ranges and therapeutic concentrations may differ.

# FUTURE OF THERAPEUTIC DRUG MONITORING

Drug assays are rapidly improving with regard to specificity, sensitivity, speed, and convenience. Methods that separate drug enantiomers may help to elucidate therapeutic ranges for compounds administered as racemic mixtures.[328] Capillary electrophoresis-based assays will be increasingly used in clinical laboratories because of their low cost, specificity, use for small sample volumes, and speed.[329] Methods for measurement of drugs in hair samples are being proposed for assessment of long-term drug adherence.[330] Implanted amperometric biosensors, currently used for glucose monitoring, may be useful for continuous monitoring of drug concentrations.[331] Subcutaneous microdialysis probes may also be useful for continuous drug monitoring, particularly because they monitor pharmacologically active unbound drug concentrations.[332] Point-of-care assay methods, currently used in private physician offices, group practices, clinics, and emergency departments, could eventually be used in community pharmacies in the future.[333,334]

Therapeutic drug monitoring of the near future may also involve determination of genotypes, characterization of proteins produced in particular diseases (proteomics), and analysis of drug metabolite profiles (metabonomics).[335,336] Pharmacogenomics and related sciences may help to identify those subsets of patients who will be nonresponders or toxic responders and help to determine appropriate initial doses and patients who will benefit most from therapeutic drug monitoring. Such testing would not require special sample timing, might be possible using noninvasive methods (eg, hair, saliva, and buccal swabs), and would need to be done only once because the results would apply over a lifetime. This type of testing may help patients receive the best drug for the indication and rapid individualization of drug dosage to achieve desired target concentrations.[32,33,335,337] The addition of this testing will likely result in an increased demand for new types of tests from clinical laboratories currently involved in routine therapeutic drug monitoring.

There is a movement to change the terminology and practice of therapeutic drug monitoring to target concentration strategy, concentration intervention, and therapeutic drug management.[46,338] Critics of the therapeutic drug monitoring terminology claim that it suggests a passive process that is concerned only with after-the-fact monitoring to ensure that concentrations are within a range without proper regard to evaluating the response to the drug in an individual patient.[338] Target concentration intervention is essentially a new name for a process that has been used by clinical pharmacokinetics services for years and involves the following steps: (1) choosing a target concentration (usually within the commonly accepted therapeutic range) for a patient; (2) initiating therapy to attain that target concentration using best-guess population pharmacokinetic parameters; (3) fully evaluating the response at the resulting steady-state concentration; and (4) adjusting the regimen as needed using pharmacokinetic parameters that have been further refined by use of the drug concentration measurement(s).

The desire for positive clinical responses with new biologic agents, such as monoclonal antibodies, warrants further investigation as patients seek individualized and expensive treatment options. Studies do not currently recommend routine monitoring, but clinicians should be aware of further development in this area.[339,340] Methods to improve the therapeutic drug monitoring process itself are needed. Every effort should be made to focus on patients who are most likely to benefit from therapeutic drug monitoring, and minimize the time and money spent on monitoring that provides no value.[8] The biggest problems with the process continue to be lack of education, communication, and documentation.[5,23] Approaches to changing clinician behavior with regard to appropriate sampling and interpretation include educational sessions, the formation of formal therapeutic drug monitoring services, multidisciplinary quality improvement efforts, and the computerization of requests for drug concentration measurement samples.[341] Pharmacists will continue to play a pivotal role in the education of licensed independent practitioners and others involved in the therapeutic drug monitoring process. Future studies that evaluate the effect of therapeutic drug monitoring on patient outcomes will likely use quality management approaches.[342]

## LEARNING POINTS

1. *A female patient who was diagnosed with complex partial seizures was initiated on VPA, 750 mg/day. She returns to the clinic after 4 weeks and reports that she has not had any seizures since taking the VPA. There are no signs or symptoms consistent with VPA toxicity. Why should a serum VPA concentration be measured in this patient?*

   ANSWER: Given the endpoint of therapy is the absence of something (seizures in this case), there is no way to ensure that the patient is taking enough VPA. Some types of seizures occur infrequently, and it is possible that the patient's serum VPA concentration is low and she simply has not had a seizure yet. It is important to ensure that the concentration is within the therapeutic range of 50 to 100 mg/L (for patients with normal serum

albumin concentrations) before assuming the patient is adequately protected from future seizure activity.

2. *A 24-year-old female patient with hypoalbuminemia has been initiated on phenytoin for treatment of generalized tonic-clonic seizures. A serum phenytoin concentration is measured and reported as 16 mg/L. The patient reports that she has not experienced any seizures since starting the phenytoin, but she has noticed weakness and blurry vision since then. Nystagmus is observed on physical exam. The laboratory reports a serum albumin concentration of 2.5 g/dL (normal is 3.5 to 5 g/dL). How do you interpret the phenytoin concentration?*

   ANSWER: The target therapeutic range for phenytoin concentrations is reported as 10 to 20 mg/L. This range, however, assumes an albumin concentration that is within the normal range. A patient with abnormally low albumin concentrations is likely to show toxicity when phenytoin concentrations are between 10 and 20 mg/L. Due to the low albumin concentrations, the unbound concentration of phenytoin is high. Therefore, it is likely in this case that the dose of phenytoin is too high, thus accounting for the ataxia and nystagmus. A phenytoin concentration at the low end of the usual therapeutic range (or even below) would be a more appropriate goal. Furthermore, the use of free, or unbound, phenytoin concentrations to establish correlation may be of benefit.

3. *A 60-year-old male patient with normal renal function was initiated on oral digoxin 0.25 mg every morning for treatment of supraventricular arrhythmias. He returns to his primary care physician 1 month later for an 8 a.m. appointment. A blood sample, drawn at 8:30 a.m., reveals a digoxin serum concentration of 2.9 mcg/L. There are no signs or symptoms of digoxin toxicity. On further inquiry, the patient reveals that he took his digoxin dose at 7:30 a.m. that morning. A repeat sample drawn right before the next digoxin dose is 1.2 mcg/L. What is the reasoning for the discrepancy in the two reported digoxin concentrations?*

   ANSWER: This discrepancy illustrates the importance of blood sample timing relative to the intake of the last drug dose. The initial serum digoxin concentration in this case is above the upper limit generally defined for patients with atrial arrhythmias (1.2 mcg/L) and might lead to the conclusion that the daily digoxin dose is excessively high. However, the sample should have been drawn sometime between 6 hours after the dose and right before the next dose, allowing adequate time for digoxin in blood to have equilibrated with digoxin in myocardial tissue. Significant resources are wasted by inappropriate timing of blood samples for digoxin measurements, and incomplete documentation of dose or blood sample timing.

4. *A 35-year-old male patient with a history of lymphoma is admitted due to MRSA bacteremia and is receiving IV vancomycin therapy (dosed at 1,750 mg [18 mg/kg] IV every 8 hours). His renal function is normal and he is currently hemodynamically stable. A vancomycin concentration 7.5 hours after initial dose is drawn from his central line and reveals a concentration of 52 mg/L. The clinical*

*pharmacy specialist decides to hold the next dose and orders a repeat concentration (a total of 16 hours after dose), which reveals a concentration of <2 mg/L. What is/are reason(s) for the initial elevated vancomycin concentration?*

**ANSWER:** Appropriateness of drawn concentrations is key in the interpretation of concentrations. There are several reasons why a concentration may not make sense. Dosed appropriately, it is expected that the vancomycin concentration in this patient would be lower than what was observed, namely given the dose is appropriate for this younger patient with normal renal function and who does not have any signs of impending hemodynamic instability. One possible explanation for the higher-than-expected concentration is the fact that the sample was drawn from the central line. Some reports note falsely elevated concentrations when drawn from central lines, and therefore the recommendation is to draw drug concentration samples using peripheral sites instead. Additionally, it is possible that the sample was drawn from a line that was not flushed prior to sample withdrawal. Finally, there could be patient-specific factors that can contribute to the higher-than-expected concentrations or concomitant use of nephrotoxic agents.

5.  *A 47-year-old male patient with a history of bipolar I and recent new diagnosis of reduced ejection fraction heart failure presents to the emergency department with new-onset diarrhea, ataxia, confusion, and polyuria. His home medications include carvedilol 6.25 mg BID, lisinopril 2.5 mg daily, furosemide 20 mg daily, and lithium ER 300 mg BID. The physician orders a lithium concentration, which results as 2.1 mEq/L. What is/are the reason(s) for the patient's elevated lithium concentration?*

**ANSWER:** The patient had a recent addition of a diuretic (furosemide) and angiotensin-converting enzyme inhibitor (lisinopril), which can increase lithium concentrations through the reduced elimination of lithium. This case highlights the importance of drug interactions on serum concentrations of certain medications, which should be reviewed during the prescribing and dispensing process to ensure proper monitoring and adjustment.

# ACKNOWLEDGMENTS

The authors would like to acknowledge the contributions of Dr. Jaclyn A. Boyle and Dr. Janis J. MacKichan, who helped author this chapter in previous editions of this textbook.

# REFERENCES

1.  Evans WE. General principles of clinical pharmacokinetics. In: Burton ME, Shaw LM, Schentag JJ, et al, eds. *Applied Pharmacokinetics and Pharmacodynamics: Principles of Therapeutic Drug Monitoring.* 4th ed. Baltimore, MD: Lippincott Williams & Wilkins; 2006:3-7.

2.  Marshall EK. Experimental basis of chemotherapy in the treatment of bacterial infections. *Bull N Y Acad Med.* 1940;16(12):723-731.PubMed

3.  Shannon JA. The study of antimalarials and antimalarial activity in the human malarias. *Harvey Lect.* 1945-1946;41:43-89.PubMed

4.  Koch-Weser J. Drug therapy: serum drug concentrations as therapeutic guides. *N Engl J Med.* 1972;287(5):227-231.PubMed

5.  Carroll DJ, Austin GE, Stajich GV, et al. Effect of education on the appropriateness of serum drug concentration determination. *Ther Drug Monit.* 1992;14(1):81-84.PubMed

6.  Mason GD, Winter ME. Appropriateness of sampling times for therapeutic drug monitoring. *Am J Hosp Pharm.* 1984;41(9):1796-1801. PubMed

7.  Travers EM. Misuse of therapeutic drug monitoring: an analysis of causes and methods for improvement. *Clin Lab Med.* 1987;7(2):453-472.PubMed

8.  Ensom MH, Davis GA, Cropp CD, Ensom RJ. Clinical pharmacokinetics in the 21st century. Does the evidence support definitive outcomes? *Clin Pharmacokinet.* 1998;34(4):265-279.PubMed

9.  Touw DJ, Neef C, Thomson AH, Vinks AA. Cost-effectiveness of therapeutic drug monitoring: a systematic review. *Ther Drug Monit.* 2005;27(1):10-17.PubMed

10. Walson PD. Therapeutic drug monitoring in special populations. *Clin Chem.* 1998;44(2):415-419.PubMed

11. Burke MJ, Preskorn SH. Therapeutic drug monitoring of antidepressants: cost implications and relevance to clinical practice. *Clin Pharmacokinet.* 1999;37(2):147-165.PubMed

12. Patsalos PN, Berry DJ, Bourgeois BFD, et al. Antiepileptic drugs: best practice guidelines for therapeutic drug monitoring: a position paper by the subcommission on therapeutic drug monitoring, ILAE Commission on Therapeutic Strategies. *Epilepsia.* 2008;49(7):1239-1276.PubMed

13. Bates DW. Improving the use of therapeutic drug monitoring. *Ther Drug Monit.* 1998;20(5):550-555.PubMed

14. Eadie MJ. Therapeutic drug monitoring: antiepileptic drugs. *Br J Clin Pharmacol.* 2001;52(suppl 1):11S-20S.PubMed

15. Robinson JD, Taylor WJ. Interpretation of serum drug concentrations. In: Taylor WJ, and Caviness MHD, eds. *A Textbook for the Application of Therapeutic Drug Monitoring.* Irving, TX: Abbott Laboratories, Diagnostics Division; 1986:31-45.

16. Traub SL. Interpretation of serum drug concentrations. In: Traub SL, ed. *Basic Skills in Interpreting Laboratory Data.* 2nd ed. Bethesda, MD: American Society of Health-System Pharmacists; 1996:61-92.

17. Nierenberg DW. Measuring drug levels in the office: rationale, possible advantages, and potential problems. *Med Clin North Am.* 1987;71(4): 653-664.PubMed

18. Blecka LJ, Jackson GJ. Immunoassays in therapeutic drug monitoring. *Clin Lab Med.* 1987;7(2):357-370.PubMed

19. Taylor AT. Office therapeutic drug monitoring. *Prim Care.* 1986;13(4):743-760.PubMed

20. Tachi T, Hase T, Okamoto Y, et al. A clinical trial for therapeutic drug monitoring using microchip-based fluorescence polarization immunoassay. *Anal Bioanal Chem.* 2011;401(7):2301-2305.PubMed

21. D'Angio RG, Stevenson JG, Lively BT, Morgan JE. Therapeutic drug monitoring: improved performance through educational intervention. *Ther Drug Monit.* 1990;12(2):173-181.PubMed

22. Sieradzan R, Fuller AV. A multidisciplinary approach to enhance documentation of antibiotic serum sampling. *Hosp Pharm.* 1995;30(10):872-877.PubMed

23. Warner A. Setting standards of practice in therapeutic drug monitoring and clinical toxicology: a North American view. *Ther Drug Monit.* 2000;22(1):93-97.PubMed

24. Murphy JE. Introduction. In: Murphy JE, ed. *Clinical Pharmacokinetics.* 5th ed. Bethesda, MD: American Society of Health-System Pharmacists; 2012:xxix-xxxvii.

25. Hiemke C, Baumann P, Bergemann N, et al. AGNP consensus guidelines for therapeutic drug monitoring in psychiatry: update 2011. *Pharmacopsychiatry.* 2011;44:195-235.

26. Johannessen SIJ, Landmark CJ. Value of therapeutic drug monitoring in epilepsy. *Expert Rev Neurother.* 2008;8(6):929-939.PubMed

27. U.S. Food and Drug Administration. *Guidance for industry: exposure-response relationships. Study design, data analysis, and regulatory applications: 2003.* Silver Spring, MD: U.S. Department of Health & Human Services; 2003.

28. Reed MD, Blumer JL. Therapeutic drug monitoring in the pediatric intensive care unit. *Pediatr Clin North Am.* 1994;41(6):1227-1243.PubMed

29. Schentag JJ, Bang AJ, Kozinski-Tober JL. Digoxin. In: Burton ME, Shaw LM, Schentag JJ, et al, eds. *Applied Pharmacokinetics and Pharmacodynamics: Principles of Therapeutic Drug Monitoring.* 4th ed. Baltimore, MD: Lippincott Williams & Wilkins; 2006:410-439.

30. Lima JJ, Wenzke SC, Boudoulas H, Schaal SF. Antiarrhythmic activity and unbound concentrations of disopyramide enantiomers in patients. *Ther Drug Monit.* 1990;12(1):23-28.PubMed

31. Ensom MH, Chang TK, Patel P. Pharmacogenetics: the therapeutic drug monitoring of the future? *Clin Pharmacokinet.* 2001;40(11):783-802. PubMed

32. McLeod HL, Evans WE. Pharmacogenomics: unlocking the human genome for better drug therapy. *Annu Rev Pharmacol Toxicol.* 2001;41:101-121.PubMed

33. MacKichan JJ, Lee M. Factors contributing to drug-induced diseases. In: Tisdale JE, Miller DA, eds. *Drug-Induced Diseases: Prevention, Detection and Management.* Bethesda, MD: American Society of Health-System Pharmacists; 2010:23-30.

34. Hesse LM, He P, Krishnaswamy S, et al. Pharmacogenetic determinants of interindividual variability in bupropion hydroxylation by cytochrome P450 2B6 in human liver microsomes. *Pharmacogenetics.* 2004;14(4): 225-238.PubMed

35. MacKichan JJ. Influence of protein binding and use of unbound (free) drug concentrations. In: Burton ME, Shaw LM, Schentag JJ, et al, eds. *Applied Pharmacokinetics and Pharmacodynamics: Principles of Therapeutic Drug Monitoring.* 4th ed. Baltimore, MD: Lippincott Williams & Wilkins; 2006:82-120.

36. Traugott KA, Maxwell PR, Green K, et al. Effects of therapeutic drug monitoring criteria in a computerized prescriber-order-entry system on the appropriateness of vancomycin level orders. *Am J Health Syst Pharm.* 2011;68(4):347-352.PubMed

37. Bruguerolle B. Chronopharmacokinetics: current status. *Clin Pharmacokinet.* 1998;35(2):83-94.PubMed

38. Baraldo M. The influence of circadian rhythms on the kinetics of drugs in humans. *Expert Opin Drug Metab Toxicol.* 2008;4(2):175-192.PubMed

39. MacKichan JJ, Kutt H. Carbamazepine. In: Taylor WJ, and Finn AL, eds. *Individualizing Drug Therapy: Practical Applications of Drug Monitoring.* New York, NY: Gross, Townsend Frank Inc; 1981:1-25.

40. Bauer LA. Carbamazepine. In: Bauer LA. eds. Applied clinical pharmacokinetics. 3rd ed. http://accesspharmacy.mhmedical.com/. Accessed Jul 1, 2015.

41. Schäffler L, Bourgeois BF, Lüders HO. Rapid reversibility of autoinduction of carbamazepine metabolism after temporary discontinuation. *Epilepsia.* 1994;35(1):195-198.PubMed

42. Rodvold KA, Paloucek FP, Zell M. Accuracy of 11 methods for predicting theophylline dose. *Clin Pharm.* 1986;5(5):403-408.PubMed

43. Slattery JT, Gibaldi M, Koup JR. Prediction of maintenance dose required to attain a desired drug concentration at steady-state from a single determination of concentration after an initial dose. *Clin Pharmacokinet.* 1980;5(4):377-385.PubMed

44. Browne JL, Perry PJ, Alexander B, et al. Pharmacokinetic protocol for predicting plasma nortriptyline levels. *J Clin Psychopharmacol.* 1983;3(6):351-356.PubMed

45. Cooper TB, Simpson GM. The 24-hour lithium level as a prognosticator of dosage requirements: a 2-year follow-up study. *Am J Psychiatry.* 1976;133(4):440-443.PubMed

46. Perry PJ, Alexander B, Dunner FJ, et al. Pharmacokinetic protocol for predicting serum lithium levels. *J Clin Psychopharmacol.* 1982;2(2): 114-118.PubMed

47. Neely M, Jelliffe R. Practical, individualized dosing: 21st century therapeutics and the clinical pharmacometrician. *J Clin Pharmacol.* 2010;50(7):842-847.PubMed

48. Hammett-Stabler CA, Johns T. Laboratory guidelines for monitoring of antimicrobial drugs. *Clin Chem.* 1998;44(5):1129-1140.PubMed

49. Winter ME, Tozer TN. Phenytoin. In: Burton ME, Shaw LM, Schentag JJ, et al, eds. *Applied Pharmacokinetics and Pharmacodynamics: Principles of Therapeutic Drug Monitoring.* 4th ed. Baltimore, MD: Lippincott Williams & Wilkins; 2006:463-490.

50. Jelliffe RW, Schumitzky A, Van Guilder M, et al. Individualizing drug dosage regimens: roles of population pharmacokinetic and dynamic models, Bayesian fitting, and adaptive control. *Ther Drug Monit.* 1993;15(5):380-393.PubMed

51. Chan K, Beran RG. Value of therapeutic drug level monitoring and unbound (free) levels. *Seizure.* 2008;17(6):572-575.PubMed

52. Burt M, Anderson DC, Kloss J, Apple FS. Evidence-based implementation of free phenytoin therapeutic drug monitoring. *Clin Chem.* 2000;46(8 Pt 1): 1132-1135.PubMed

53. Sheiner LB, Tozer TN, Winter ME. Clinical pharmacokinetics: the use of plasma concentrations of drugs. In: Melmon KL, Morelli HF, eds. *Clinical Pharmacology: Basic Principles in Therapeutics.* New York, NY: MacMillan; 1978:71-109.

54. Kerrick JM, Wolff DL, Graves NM. Predicting unbound phenytoin concentrations in patients receiving valproic acid: a comparison of two prediction methods. *Ann Pharmacother.* 1995;29(5):470-474.PubMed

55. Haidukewych D, Rodin EA, Zielinski JJ. Derivation and evaluation of an equation for prediction of free phenytoin concentration in patients co-medicated with valproic acid. *Ther Drug Monit.* 1989;11(2):134-139. PubMed

56. May TW, Rambeck B, Nothbaum N. Nomogram for the prediction of unbound phenytoin concentrations in patients on a combined treatment of phenytoin and valproic acid. *Eur Neurol.* 1991;31(1):57-60.PubMed

57. Patsalos PN, Berry DJ. Therapeutic drug monitoring of antiepileptic drugs by use of saliva. *Ther Drug Monit.* 2013;35(1):4-29.PubMed

58. Felson DT. Osteoarthritis. In: Longo DL, Fauci AS, Kasper DL, et al., eds. Harrison's Principles of Internal Medicine. 18th ed. http:// accesspharmacy.mhmedical.com/. Accessed June 29, 2015.

59. Whelton A. Appropriate analgesia: an evidence-based evaluation of the role of acetaminophen in pain management. *Am J Ther.* 2005;12:43-45.

60. *Tylenol oral (acetaminophen oral) prescribing information.* Skillman, NJ: McNeil Consumer Healthcare; 2010.

61. Acetaminophen. In: *Lexicomp Online* [online database]. Hudson, OH: Lexi-Comp. https://www.wolterskluwer.com/en/solutions/lexicomp. Accessed August 13, 2015.

62. Wilson JT, Brown RD, Bocchini JA Jr, Kearns GL. Efficacy, disposition and pharmacodynamics of aspirin, acetaminophen and choline salicylate in young febrile children. *Ther Drug Monit.* 1982;4(2):147-180.PubMed

63. Ahlers SJGM, Van Gulik L, Van Dongen EPA, et al. Aminotransferase levels in relation to short-term use of acetaminophen four grams daily in postoperative cardiothoracic patients in the intensive care unit. *Anaesth Intensive Care.* 2011;39(6):1056-1063.PubMed

64. Watkins PB, Kaplowitz N, Slattery JT, et al. Aminotransferase elevations in healthy adults receiving 4 grams of acetaminophen daily: a randomized controlled trial. *JAMA.* 2006;296(1):87-93.PubMed

65. Krenzelok EP, Royal MA. Confusion: acetaminophen dosing changes based on NO evidence in adults. *Drugs R D.* 2012;12(2):45-48.PubMed

66. Rumack BH. Acetaminophen hepatotoxicity: the first 35 years. *J Toxicol Clin Toxicol.* 2002;40(1):3-20.PubMed

67. Global Initiative for Asthma (GINA). GINA report: global strategy for asthma management and prevention. https://ginasthma.org/wp-content /uploads/2020/06/GINA-2020-report_20_06_04-1-wms.pdf. Accessed Aug 22, 2020.

68. Aminophylline. In: *Lexicomp Online* [online database]. Hudson, OH: Lexi-Comp. https://www.wolterskluwer.com/en/solutions/lexicomp. Accessed October 16, 2020.

69. Global Initiative for Chronic Obstructive Lung Disease. Global strategy for the diagnosis, management, and prevention of chronic obstructive pulmonary disease: 2020 report. https://goldcopd.org/wp-content /uploads/2019/12/GOLD-2020-FINAL-ver1.2-03-Dec19_WMV.pdf. Accessed Aug 23, 2020.

70. Edwards DJ, Zarowitz BJ, Slaughter RL. Theophylline. In: Evans WE, Schentag JJ, Jusko WJ, eds. *Applied Pharmacokinetics: Principles of Therapeutic Drug Monitoring.* 3rd ed. Vancouver, WA: Applied Therapeutics Inc; 1992:1-38.

71. Murphy JE, Winter ME. Theophylline. In: Winter ME, ed. *Basic Clinical Pharmacokinetics.* 5th ed. Baltimore, MD: Lippincott Williams & Wilkins; 1020:403-441.

72. Scanlon JE, Chin KC, Morgan ME, et al. Caffeine or theophylline for neonatal apnoea? *Arch Dis Child.* 1992;67(4 Spec No):425-428.PubMed

73. Bauer LA. *Applied Clinical Pharmacokinetics.* 2nd ed. New York, NY: McGraw-Hill; 2008.

74. Murphy JE, Phan H. Theophylline. In: Murphy JE, ed. *Clinical Pharmacokinetics.* 5th ed. Bethesda, MD: American Society of Health System Pharmacists; 2012:315-325.

75. Juarez-Olguin H, Flores-Perez J, Perez-Guille G, et al. Therapeutic monitoring of theophylline in newborns with apnea. *P&T.* 2004;29: 322-324.

76. Koren G. Therapeutic drug monitoring principles in the neonate. National Academy of Clinical Biochemistry. *Clin Chem.* 1997;43(1): 222-227.PubMed

77. Aranda JV, Chemtob S, Laudignon N, Sasyniuk BI. Pharmacologic effects of theophylline in the newborn. *J Allergy Clin Immunol.* 1986; 78(4 Pt 2):773-780.PubMed

78. Aminophylline. In: *Lexicomp Online.* [online database]. Hudson, OH: Lexi-Comp. https://www.wolterskluwer.com/en/solutions/lexicomp. Accessed Sep 13, 2015.

79. Theophylline. In: *Lexicomp Online.* [online database]. Hudson, OH: Lexi-Comp. https://www.wolterskluwer.com/en/solutions/lexicomp. Accessed Oct 16, 2020.

80. Eichenwald EC. Apnea of Prematurity. *Pediatrics.* 2016;137(1).PubMed

81. de Wildt SN, Kerkvliet KT, Wezenberg MG, et al. Use of saliva in therapeutic drug monitoring of caffeine in preterm infants. *Ther Drug Monit.* 2001;23(3):250-254.PubMed

82. Caffeine. In: *Lexicomp Online.* [online database]. Hudson, OH: Lexi-Comp. https://www.wolterskluwer.com/en/solutions/lexicomp. Accessed May 3, 2017.

83. Natarajan G, Botica ML, Thomas R, Aranda JV. Therapeutic drug monitoring for caffeine in preterm neonates: an unnecessary exercise? *Pediatrics.* 2007;119(5):936-940.PubMed

84. McMillin GA, Krasowski MD. Therapeutic Drug Monitoring of Newer Antiepileptic Drugs. In: Clarke W, ed. *Clinical Challenges in Therapeutic Drug Monitoring: Special Populations, Physiological Conditions and Pharmacogenomics.* Amsterdam, Netherlands: Elsevier; 2016:101-134.

85. Warner A, Privitera M, Bates D. Standards of laboratory practice: antiepileptic drug monitoring. *Clin Chem.* 1998;44(5):1085-1095.PubMed

86. Van Tyle JH, Winter ME. Carbamazepine. In: Winter ME, ed. *Basic Clinical Pharmacokinetics.* 5th ed. Baltimore, MD: Lippincott Williams & Wilkins; 2010:182-197.

87. McEvoy GK, Snow ED, eds. *AHFS Drug Information.* Bethesda, MD: American Society of Health-System Pharmacists; 2012:2266-2273.

88. Bialer M, Levy RH, Perucca E. Does carbamazepine have a narrow therapeutic plasma concentration range? *Ther Drug Monit.* 1998;20(1):56-59.PubMed

89. Schulz M, Iwersen-Bergmann S, Andresen H, Schmoldt A. Therapeutic and toxic blood concentrations of nearly 1,000 drugs and other xenobiotics. *Crit Care.* 2012;16(4):R136.PubMed

90. Hiemke C, Baumann P, Bergemann N, et al. AGNP consensus guidelines for therapeutic drug monitoring in psychiatry: update 2011. *Pharmacopsychiatry.* 2011;44:195-235.

91. Shorvon SD. *Handbook of Epilepsy Treatment.* 3rd ed. Oxford: Wiley-Blackwell; 2010:436.

92. Cohen H. Carbamazepine. In: Cohen H, ed. *Casebook in Clinical Pharmacokinetics and Drug Dosing.* New York, NY: McGraw-Hill; 2015:57-63.

93. Garnett WR, Anderson GD, Collins RJ. Antiepileptic drugs. In: Burton ME, Shaw LM, Schentag JJ, et al, eds. *Applied Pharmacokinetics and Pharmacodynamics: Principles of Therapeutic Drug Monitoring.* 4th ed. Baltimore, MD: Lippincott Williams & Wilkins; 2006:491-511.

94. Bonneton J, Iliadis A, Genton P, et al. Steady state pharmacokinetics of conventional versus controlled-release carbamazepine in patients with epilepsy. *Epilepsy Res.* 1993;14(3):257-263.PubMed

95. Patsalos PN, Spencer EP, Berry DJ. Therapeutic drug monitoring of antiepileptic drugs in epilepsy: A 2018 update. *Ther Drug Monit.* 2018;40(5):526-548.PubMed

96. Bauer LA. Carbamazepine. In: Bauer LA, ed. *Applied Clinical Pharmacokinetics.* 3rd ed. http://accesspharmacy.mhmedical.com/. Accessed Jul 2, 2015.

97. MacKichan JJ, Zola EM. Determinants of carbamazepine and carbamazepine 10,11-epoxide binding to serum protein, albumin and alpha 1-acid glycoprotein. *Br J Clin Pharmacol.* 1984;18(4):487-493. PubMed

98. MacKichan JJ, Duffner PK, Cohen ME. Salivary concentrations and plasma protein binding of carbamazepine and carbamazepine 10,11-epoxide in epileptic patients. *Br J Clin Pharmacol.* 1981;12(1):31-37.PubMed

99. Chee KY, Lee D, Byron D, et al. A simple collection method for saliva in children: potential for home monitoring of carbamazepine therapy. *Br J Clin Pharmacol.* 1993;35(3):311-313.PubMed

100. Levy RH, Kerr BM. Clinical pharmacokinetics of carbamazepine. *J Clin Psychiatry.* 1988;49(suppl):58-62.PubMed

101. Tallian KB, Anderson DM. Phenobarbital. In: Murphy JE, ed. *Clinical Pharmacokinetics.* 5th ed. Bethesda, MD: American Society of Health-System Pharmacists; 2012:263-272.

102. Glauser TA, Pippenger CE. Controversies in blood-level monitoring: Reexamining its role in the treatment of epilepsy. *Epilepsia.* 2000; 41(suppl 8):S6-15.

103. Cohen H. Phenobarbital and primidone. In: Cohen H, ed. *Casebook in Clinical Pharmacokinetics and Drug Dosing.* New York, NY: McGraw-Hill; 2015:153-166.

104. Eadie MJ. Therapeutic drug monitoring: antiepileptic drugs. *Br J Clin Pharmacol.* 1998;46(3):185-193.PubMed

105. Hvidberg EF, Dam M. Clinical pharmacokinetics of anticonvulsants. *Clin Pharmacokinet.* 1976;1(3):161-188.PubMed

106. Nelson E, Powell JR, Conrad K, et al. Phenobarbital pharmacokinetics and bioavailability in adults. *J Clin Pharmacol.* 1982;22(2-3):141-148.PubMed

107. Alvin J, McHorse T, Hoyumpa A, et al. The effect of liver disease in man on the disposition of phenobarbital. *J Pharmacol Exp Ther.* 1975;192(1):224-235.PubMed

108. Lous P. Elimination of barbiturates. In: Johansen SH, ed. *Barbiturate Poisoning and Tetanus.* Boston, MA: Little Brown; 1966.

109. Asconapé JJ, Penry JK. Use of antiepileptic drugs in the presence of liver and kidney diseases: a review. *Epilepsia.* 1982;23(suppl 1):S65-S79.PubMed

110. Waddell WJ, Butler TC. The distribution and excretion of phenobarbital. *J Clin Invest.* 1957;36(8):1217-1226.PubMed

111. Anderson GD. Phenobarbital and other barbiturates: Chemistry, biotransformation, and pharmacokinetics. In: Levy RH, Mattson RH, Meldrum BS, et al, eds. *Antiepileptic Drugs.* New York, NY: Raven Press; 2002:496-503.

112. Winter ME. Phenytoin and fosphenytoin. In: Murphy JE, ed. *Clinical Pharmacokinetics.* 5th ed. Bethesda, MD: American Society of Health-System Pharmacists; 2012:273-287.

113. Kozer E, Parvez S, Minassian BA, et al. How high can we go with phenytoin? *Ther Drug Monit.* 2002;24(3):386-389.PubMed

114. Banh HL, Burton ME, Sperling MR. Interpatient and intrapatient variability in phenytoin protein binding. *Ther Drug Monit.* 2002;24(3):379-385.PubMed

115. Brodtkorb E, Reimers A. Seizure control and pharmacokinetics of antiepileptic drugs in pregnant women with epilepsy. *Seizure.* 2008;17(2):160-165.PubMed

116. von Winckelmann SL, Spriet I, Willems L. Therapeutic drug monitoring of phenytoin in critically ill patients. *Pharmacotherapy*. 2008;28(11): 1391-1400.PubMed

117. Phenytoin. In: *Lexicomp Online*. [online database]. Hudson, OH: Lexi-Comp. https://www.wolterskluwer.com/en/solutions/lexicomp. Accessed Aug 16, 2015.

118. Browne TR. Fosphenytoin (Cerebyx). *Clin Neuropharmacol*. 1997;20(1):1-12.PubMed

119. In: Cohen H. Phenytoin and fosphenytoin. Cohen H, ed. *Casebook in Clinical Pharmacokinetics and Drug Dosing*. New York, NY: McGraw-Hill; 2015:167-181.

120. Toler SM, Wilkerson MA, Porter WH, et al. Severe phenytoin intoxication as a result of altered protein binding in AIDS. *DICP*. 1990;24(7-8):698-700.PubMed

121. Anderson GD, Pak C, Doane KW, et al. Revised Winter-Tozer equation for normalized phenytoin concentrations in trauma and elderly patients with hypoalbuminemia. *Ann Pharmacother*. 1997;31(3):279-284. PubMed

122. Kane SP, Bress AP, Tesoro EP. Characterization of unbound phenytoin concentrations in neurointensive care unit patients using a revised Winter-Tozer equation. *Ann Pharmacother*. 2013;47(5):628-636. PubMed

123. Soriano VV, Tesoro EP, Kane SP. Characterization of free phenytoin concentrations in end-stage renal disease using the Winter-Tozer equation. *Ann Pharmacother*. 2017;51(8):669-674.PubMed

124. Cheng W, Kiang TK, Bring P, Ensom MH. Predictive performance of the Winter-Tozer and derivative equations for estimating free phenytoin concentration. *Can J Hosp Pharm*. 2016;69(4):269-279.PubMed

125. MacKichan JJ. Protein binding drug displacement interactions fact or fiction? *Clin Pharmacokinet*. 1989;16(2):65-73.PubMed

126. May TW, Rambeck B, Jürges U, et al. Comparison of total and free phenytoin serum concentrations measured by high-performance liquid chromatography and standard TDx assay: implications for the prediction of free phenytoin serum concentrations. *Ther Drug Monit*. 1998;20(6):619-623.PubMed

127. Valproic acid and derivatives. In: *Lexicomp Online*. [online database]. Hudson, OH: Lexi-Comp. https://www.wolterskluwer.com/en/solutions /lexicomp. Accessed Sep 14, 2015.

128. Gidal BE. Valproic acid. In: Murphy JE, ed. *Clinical Pharmacokinetics*. 5th ed. Bethesda, MD: American Society of Health-System Pharmacists; 2012:327-336.

129. Haymond J, Ensom MH. Does valproic acid warrant therapeutic drug monitoring in bipolar affective disorder? *Ther Drug Monit*. 2010;32(1): 19-29.PubMed

130. Ueshima S, Aiba T, Ishikawa N, et al. Poor applicability of estimation method for adults to calculate unbound serum concentrations of valproic acid in epileptic neonates and infants. *J Clin Pharm Ther*. 2009;34(4):415-422.PubMed

131. Dasgupta A, Volk A. Displacement of valproic acid and carbamazepine from protein binding in normal and uremic sera by tolmetin, ibuprofen, and naproxen: presence of inhibitor in uremic serum that blocks valproic acid-naproxen interactions. *Ther Drug Monit*. 1996;18(3): 284-287.PubMed

132. Bardy AH, Hiilesmaa VK, Teramo K, Neuvonen PJ. Protein binding of antiepileptic drugs during pregnancy, labor, and puerperium. *Ther Drug Monit*. 1990;12(1):40-46.PubMed

133. Johannessen SI, Tomson T. Pharmacokinetic variability of newer antiepileptic drugs: when is monitoring needed? *Clin Pharmacokinet*. 2006;45(11):1061-1075.PubMed

134. Garnett WR, Bainbridge JL, Egeberg MD, et al. Newer antiepileptic drugs. In: Murphy JE, ed. *Clinical Pharmacokinetics*. 5th ed. Bethesda, MD: American Society of Health-System Pharmacists; 2012:135-157.

135. de Leon J, Spina E, Diaz FJ. Clobazam therapeutic drug monitoring: a comprehensive review of the literature with proposals to improve future studies. *Ther Drug Monit*. 2013;35(1):30-47.PubMed

136. Garnett WR, Bainbridge JL, Johnson SL. Ethosuximide. In: Murphy JE, ed. *Clinical P.harmacokinetics*. 5th ed. Bethesda, MD: American Society of Health-System Pharmacists; 2012:197-201.

137. Villén T, Bertilsson L, Sjöqvist F. Nonstereoselective disposition of ethosuximide in humans. *Ther Drug Monit*. 1990;12(5):514-516.PubMed

138. Felbatol [package insert]. Somerset, NJ: MED Pharmaceuticals; 2008.

139 Felbamate. In: *Lexicomp Online*. [online database]. Hudson, OH: Lexi-Comp. https://www.wolterskluwer.com/en/solutions/lexicomp. Accessed Aug 29, 2020.

140. Hooper WDD, Franklin ME, Glue P, et al. Effect of felbamate on valproic acid disposition in healthy volunteers: inhibition of beta-oxidation. *Epilepsia*. 1996;37(1):91-97.PubMed

141. Reidenberg P, Glue P, Banfield CR, et al. Effects of felbamate on the pharmacokinetics of phenobarbital. *Clin Pharmacol Ther*. 1995;58(3): 279-287.PubMed

142. Sachdeo R, Wagner ML, Sachdeo S, et al. Coadministration of phenytoin and felbamate: evidence of additional phenytoin dose-reduction requirements based on pharmacokinetics and tolerability with increasing doses of felbamate. *Epilepsia*. 1999;40(8):1122-1128.PubMed

143. Armijo JA, Pena MA, Adín J, Vega-Gil N. Association between patient age and gabapentin serum concentration-to-dose ratio: a preliminary multivariate analysis. *Ther Drug Monit*. 2004;26(6): 633-637.PubMed

144. Wagner ML, Remmel RP, Graves NM, Leppik IE. Effect of felbamate on carbamazepine and its major metabolites. *Clin Pharmacol Ther*. 1993;53(5):536-543.PubMed

145. Albani F, Theodore WH, Washington P, et al. Effect of felbamate on plasma levels of carbamazepine and its metabolites. *Epilepsia*. 1991;32(1):130-132.PubMed

146. Neurontin [package insert]. New York: Parke-Davis Division of Pfizer; 2010.

147. Gidal BE, Radulovic LL, Kruger S, et al. Inter- and intra-subject variability in gabapentin absorption and absolute bioavailability. *Epilepsy Res*. 2000;40(2-3):123-127.PubMed

148, Alvey C, Bockbrader H, Gonyea-Polski S, et al. *An oral, rising, single- and multiple-dose, tolerance and pharmacokinetic study of pregabalin (CI-1008) capsules in healthy volunteers*. New York: Pfizer; 2000.

149. Bockbrader HN, Wesche D, Miller R, et al. A comparison of the pharmacokinetics and pharmacodynamics of pregabalin and gabapentin. *Clin Pharmacokinet*. 2010;49(10):661-669.PubMed

150. Gabapentin. In: *Lexicomp Online*. [online database]. Hudson, OH: Lexi-Comp. https://www.wolterskluwer.com/en/solutions/lexicomp. Accessed Aug 15, 2015.

151. Perucca E. Is there a role for therapeutic drug monitoring of new anticonvulsants? *Clin Pharmacokinet*. 2000;38(3):191-204.PubMed

152. Chong E, Dupuis LL. Therapeutic drug monitoring of lamotrigine. *Ann Pharmacother*. 2002;36(5):917-920.PubMed

153. Tomson T, Battino D. Pharmacokinetics and therapeutic drug monitoring of newer antiepileptic drugs during pregnancy and the puerperium. *Clin Pharmacokinet*. 2007;46(3):209-219.PubMed

154. Gupta V, Gupta K, Singh G, Kaushal S. An analytical study to correlate serum levels of levetiracetam with clinical course in patients with epilepsy. *J Neurosci Rural Pract*. 2016;7(suppl 1):S31-S36.PubMed

155. Keppra IV [package insert]. Smyrna, GA: UBC; 2010.

156. Trileptal [package insert]. East Hanover, NJ: Novartis Pharmaceuticals; 2011.

157. Pentobarbital. In: *Lexicomp Online*. [online database]. Hudson, OH: Lexi-Comp. https://www.wolterskluwer.com/en/solutions/lexicomp. Accessed Aug 15, 2015.

158. Ben-Menachem E. Pregabalin pharmacology and its relevance to clinical practice. *Epilepsia*. 2004;45(suppl 6):13-18.PubMed

159. Pregabalin. In: *Lexicomp Online*. [online database]. Hudson, OH: Lexi-Comp. https://www.wolterskluwer.com/en/solutions/lexicomp. Accessed Aug 15, 2015.

160. Patsalos PN, Berry DJ, Bourgeois BFD, et al. Antiepileptic drugs: best practice guidelines for therapeutic drug monitoring: a position paper by the subcommission on therapeutic drug monitoring, ILAE Commission on Therapeutic Strategies. *Epilepsia.* 2008;49(7):1239-1276.PubMed

161. Lyrica [package insert]. New York: Pfizer; 2009.

162. Jacob S, Nair AB. An updated overview on therapeutic drug monitoring of recent antiepileptic drugs. *Drugs R D.* 2016;16(4):303-316.PubMed

163. Contin M, Riva R, Albani F, et al. Topiramate therapeutic monitoring in patients with epilepsy: effect of concomitant antiepileptic drugs. *Ther Drug Monit.* 2002;24(3):332-337.PubMed

164. Topamax [package insert]. Titusville, NJ: Ortho-McNeil-Janssen Pharmaceuticals; 2009.

165. Miles MV, Tang PH, Glauser TA, et al. Topiramate concentration in saliva: an alternative to serum monitoring. *Pediatr Neurol.* 2003;29(2):143-147.PubMed

166. Begg EJ, Barclay ML, Kirkpatrick CM. The therapeutic monitoring of antimicrobial agents. *Br J Clin Pharmacol.* 2001;52(suppl 1):35S-43S. PubMed

167. Nicolau DP, Freeman CD, Belliveau PP, et al. Experience with a once-daily aminoglycoside program administered to 2,184 adult patients. *Antimicrob Agents Chemother.* 1995;39(3):650-655.PubMed

168. Maglio D, Nightingale CH, Nicolau DP. Extended interval aminoglycoside dosing: from concept to clinic. *Int J Antimicrob Agents.* 2002;19(4):341-348.PubMed

169. Moore RD, Lietman PS, Smith CR. Clinical response to aminoglycoside therapy: importance of the ratio of peak concentration to minimal inhibitory concentration. *J Infect Dis.* 1987;155(1):93-99.PubMed

170. Stankowicz MS, Ibrahim J, Brown DL. Once-daily aminoglycoside dosing: an update on current literature. *Am J Health Syst Pharm.* 2015;72(16):1357-1364.PubMed

171. van Lent-Evers NA, Mathôt RA, Geus WP, et al. Impact of goal-oriented and model-based clinical pharmacokinetic dosing of aminoglycosides on clinical outcome: a cost-effectiveness analysis. *Ther Drug Monit.* 1999;21(1):63-73.PubMed

172. Barclay ML, Kirkpatrick CM, Begg EJ. Once daily aminoglycoside therapy. Is it less toxic than multiple daily doses and how should it be monitored? *Clin Pharmacokinet.* 1999;36(2):89-98.PubMed

173. Bartal C, Danon A, Schlaeffer F, et al. Pharmacokinetic dosing of aminoglycosides: a controlled trial. *Am J Med.* 2003;114(3):194-198. PubMed

174. Streetman DS, Nafziger AN, Destache CJ, Bertino AS Jr. Individualized pharmacokinetic monitoring results in less aminoglycoside-associated nephrotoxicity and fewer associated costs. *Pharmacotherapy.* 2001;21(4):443-451.PubMed

175. Schentag JJ, Meagher AK, Jelliffe RW. Aminoglycosides. In: Burton ME, Shaw LM, Schentag JJ, et al, eds. *Applied Pharmacokinetics and Pharmacodynamics: Principles of Therapeutic Drug Monitoring.* 4th ed. Baltimore, MD: Lippincott Williams & Wilkins; 2006:285-327.

176. Murphy JE, Matthias KR. Aminoglycosides. In: Murphy JE, ed. *Clinical Pharmacokinetics.* 5th ed. Bethesda, MD: American Society of Health-System Pharmacists; 2012:91-118.

177. Petejova N, Zahalkova J, Duricova J, et al. Gentamicin pharmacokinetics during continuous venovenous hemofiltration in critically ill septic patients. *J Chemother.* 2012;24(2):107-112.PubMed

178. Boyer A, Gruson D, Bouchet S, et al. Aminoglycosides in septic shock: an overview, with specific consideration given to their nephrotoxic risk. *Drug Saf.* 2013;36(4):217-230.PubMed

179. Mueller EW, Boucher BA. The use of extended-interval aminoglycoside dosing strategies for the treatment of moderate-to-severe infections encountered in critically ill surgical patients. *Surg Infect (Larchmt).* 2009;10(6):563-570.PubMed

180. Prins JM, Weverling GJ, de Blok K, et al. Validation and nephrotoxicity of a simplified once-daily aminoglycoside dosing schedule and guidelines for monitoring therapy. *Antimicrob Agents Chemother.* 1996;40(11):2494-2499.PubMed

181. Wallace AW, Jones M, Bertino JS Jr. Evaluation of four once-daily aminoglycoside dosing nomograms. *Pharmacotherapy.* 2002;22(9): 1077-1083.PubMed

182. Begg EJ, Barclay ML, Duffull SB. A suggested approach to once-daily aminoglycoside dosing. *Br J Clin Pharmacol.* 1995;39(6):605-609. PubMed

183. Beringer P, Winter ME. Aminoglycoside antibiotics. In: Winter ME, ed. *Basic Clinical Pharmacokinetics.* 5th ed. Baltimore, MD: Lippincott Williams & Wilkins; 2010:134-181.

184. Botha FJ, van der Bijl P, Seifart HI, Parkin DP. Fluctuation of the volume of distribution of amikacin and its effect on once-daily dosage and clearance in a seriously ill patient. *Intensive Care Med.* 1996;22(5): 443-446.PubMed

185. Tod MM, Padoin C, Petitjean O. Individualising aminoglycoside dosage regimens after therapeutic drug monitoring: simple or complex pharmacokinetic methods? *Clin Pharmacokinet.* 2001;40(11):803-814. PubMed

186. Ambrose PJ, Winter ME. Vancomycin. In: Winter ME, ed. *Basic Clinical Pharmacokinetics.* 5th ed. Baltimore, MD: Lippincott Williams & Wilkins; 2010:459-487.

187. Rybak MJ, Le J, Louise TP, et al. Therapeutic monitoring of vancomycin for serious methicillin-resistant staphylococcus aureus infections: a revised consensus guideline and review by the American Society of Health-System Pharmacists, the Infectious Diseases Society of America, The Pediatric Infectious Diseases Society, and the Society of Infectious Disease Pharmacists. Clinical Infect Dis 2020 Jul 13. Online ahead of print, Sept 12, 2020, https://pubmed.ncbi.nlm.nih.gov/32658968/.

188. Matzke GR, McGory RW, Halstenson CE, Keane WF. Pharmacokinetics of vancomycin in patients with various degrees of renal function. *Antimicrob Agents Chemother.* 1984;25(4):433-437.PubMed

189. Moise-Broder PA. Vancomycin. In: Burton ME, Shaw LM, Schentag JJ, et al, eds. *Applied Pharmacokinetics and Pharmacodynamics: Principles of Therapeutic Drug Monitoring.* 4th ed. Baltimore, MD: Lippincott Williams & Wilkins; 2006:328-340.

190. Huttner A, Harbarth S, Hope WW, et al. Therapeutic drug monitoring of the β-lactam antibiotics: what is the evidence and which patients should we be using it for? *J Antimicrob Chemother.* 2015;70(12):3178-3183. PubMed

191. Cohen H. Continuous and intermittent infusion beta-lactam antibiotics. In: Cohen H, ed. *Casebook in Clinical Pharmacokinetics and Drug Dosing.* New York, NY: McGraw-Hill; 2015:31-41.

192. Hites M, Taccone FS, Wolff F, et al. Case-control study of drug monitoring of β-lactams in obese critically ill patients. *Antimicrob Agents Chemother.* 2013;57(2):708-715.PubMed

193. Roberts JA, Paul SK, Akova M, et al. DALI: defining antibiotic levels in intensive care unit patients: are current β-lactam antibiotic doses sufficient for critically ill patients? *Clin Infect Dis.* 2014;58(8):1072-1083. PubMed

194. Cusumano JA, Klinker KP, Huttner A, et al. Towards precision medicine: therapeutic drug monitoring-guided dosing of vancomycin and β-lactam antibiotics to maximize effectiveness and minimize toxicity. *Am J Health Syst Pharm.* 2020;77(14):1104-1112.PubMed

195. Petersen D, Demertzis S, Freund M, et al. Individualization of 5-fluorocytosine therapy. *Chemotherapy.* 1994;40(3):149-156.PubMed

196. Goodwin ML, Drew RH. Antifungal serum concentration monitoring: an update. *J Antimicrob Chemother.* 2008;61(1):17-25.PubMed

197. Vermes A, Guchelaar HJ, Dankert J. Flucytosine: a review of its pharmacology, clinical indications, pharmacokinetics, toxicity and drug interactions. *J Antimicrob Chemother.* 2000;46(2):171-179.PubMed

198. Summers KK, Hardin TC, Gore SJ, Graybill JR. Therapeutic drug monitoring of systemic antifungal therapy. *J Antimicrob Chemother.* 1997;40(6):753-764.PubMed

199. Stott KE, Hope WW. Therapeutic drug monitoring for invasive mould infections and disease: pharmacokinetic and pharmacodynamic considerations. *J Antimicrob Chemother* 2017;72(suppl ): i12-i18.

200. Flucytosine. In: *Lexicomp Online*. [online database]. Hudson, OH: Lexi-Comp. https://www.wolterskluwer.com/en/solutions/lexicomp. Accessed Aug 13, 2015.

201. Al-Rawithi S, Hussein R, Al-Moshen I, Raines D. Expedient microdetermination of itraconazole and hydroxyitraconazole in plasma by high-performance liquid chromatography with fluorescence detection. *Ther Drug Monit*. 2001;23(4):445-448.PubMed

202. John J, Loo A, Mazur S, Walsh TJ. Therapeutic drug monitoring of systemic antifungal agents: a pragmatic approach for adult and pediatric patients. *Expert Opin Drug Metab Toxicol*. 2019;15(11):881-895.PubMed

203. Mayne Pharma. SUBA Bioavailability technology. www.maynepharma.com/innovation/specialty-technologies/suba-bioavailability-technology. Accessed Aug 28, 2020.

204. Ashbee HR, Barnes RA, Johnson EM, et al. Therapeutic drug monitoring (TDM) of antifungal agents: guidelines from the British Society for Medical Mycology. *J Antimicrob Chemother*. 2014;69(5):1162-1176. PubMed

205. British Society for Antimicrobial Chemotherapy Working Party. Laboratory monitoring of antifungal chemotherapy. *Lancet*. 1991;337(8757):1577-1580.PubMed

206. Wheat LJ, Freifeld AG, Kleiman MB, et al. Clinical practice guidelines for the management of patients with histoplasmosis: 2007 update by the Infectious Diseases Society of America. *Clin Infect Dis*. 2007;45(7): 807-825.PubMed

207. Itraconazole. In: *Lexicomp Online*. [online database]. Hudson, OH: Lexi-Comp. https://www.wolterskluwer.com/en/solutions/lexicomp. Accessed Aug 20, 2015.

208. Cohen H. Extended-spectrum triazole antifungals: posaconazole and voriconazole. In: Cohen H, ed. *Casebook in Clinical Pharmacokinetics and Drug Dosing*. New York, NY: McGraw-Hill; 2015:183-193.

209. Patterson TF, Thompson GR 3rd, Denning DW, et al. Practice guidelines for the diagnosis and management of aspergillosis: 2016 update by the Infectious Diseases Society of America. *Clin Infect Dis*. 2016;63(4): e1-e60.PubMed

210. Posaconazole. In: *Lexicomp Online*. [online database]. Hudson, OH: Lexi-Comp. https://www.wolterskluwer.com/en/solutions/lexicomp. Accessed Aug 20, 2015.

211. Isavuconazole. In: *Lexicomp Online*. [online database]. Hudson, OH: Lexi-Comp. https://www.wolterskluwer.com/en/solutions/lexicomp. Accessed Aug 28, 2020.

212. Peloquin CA. Therapeutic drug monitoring in the treatment of tuberculosis. *Drugs*. 2002;62(15):2169-2183.PubMed

213. Nahid P, Dorman SE, Alipanah N, et al. Official American Thoracic Society/Centers for Disease Control and Prevention/Infectious Diseases Society of America clinical practice guidelines: treatment of drug-susceptible tuberculosis. *Clin Infect Dis*. 2016;63(7):e147-e195. PubMed

214. Babalik A, Babalik A, Mannix S, et al. Therapeutic drug monitoring in the treatment of active tuberculosis. *Can Respir J*. 2011;18(4):225-229. PubMed

215. van der Burgt EPM, Sturkenboom MGG, Bolhuis MS, et al. End TB with precision treatment! *Eur Respir J*. 2016;47(2):680-682.PubMed

216. Holland DP, Hamilton CD, Weintrob AC, et al. Therapeutic drug monitoring of antimycobacterial drugs in patients with both tuberculosis and advanced human immunodeficiency virus infection. *Pharmacotherapy*. 2009;29(5):503-510.PubMed

217. Sahai J, Gallicano K, Swick L, et al. Reduced plasma concentrations of antituberculosis drugs in patients with HIV infection. *Ann Intern Med*. 1997;127(4):289-293.PubMed

218. Heysell SK, Moore JL, Keller SJ, Houpt ER. Therapeutic drug monitoring for slow response to tuberculosis treatment in a state control program, Virginia, USA. *Emerg Infect Dis*. 2010;16(10): 1546-1553.PubMed

219. Yew WW. Clinically significant interactions with drugs used in the treatment of tuberculosis. *Drug Saf*. 2002;25(2):111-133.PubMed

220. Kimerling ME, Phillips P, Patterson P, et al. Low serum antimycobacterial drug levels in non-HIV-infected tuberculosis patients. *Chest*. 1998;113(5):1178-1183.PubMed

221. Mehta JB, Shantaveerapa H, Byrd RP Jr, et al. Utility of rifampin blood levels in the treatment and follow-up of active pulmonary tuberculosis in patients who were slow to respond to routine directly observed therapy. *Chest*. 2001;120(5):1520-1524.PubMed

222. Alsultan A, Peloquin CA. Therapeutic drug monitoring in the treatment of tuberculosis: an update. *Drugs*. 2014;74(8):839-854.PubMed

223. Yew WW. Therapeutic drug monitoring in antituberculosis chemotherapy: clinical perspectives. *Clin Chim Acta*. 2001;313(1-2): 31-36.PubMed

224. Bierman WF, van Agtmael MA, Nijhuis M, et al. HIV monotherapy with ritonavir-boosted protease inhibitors: a systematic review. *AIDS*. 2009;23(3):279-291.PubMed

225. Arribas JR, Clumeck N, Nelson M, et al. The MONET trial: week 144 analysis of the efficacy of darunavir/ritonavir (DRV/r) monotherapy versus DRV/r plus two nucleoside reverse transcriptase inhibitors, for patients with viral load < 50 HIV-1 RNA copies/mL at baseline. *HIV Med*. 2012;13(7):398-405.PubMed

226. Marzinke MA. Therapeutic drug monitoring of antiretrovirals. In: Clarke W, ed. *Clinical Challenges in Therapeutic Drug Monitoring: Special Populations, Physiological Conditions and Pharmacogenomics*. Amsterdam, Netherlands: Elsevier; 2016:135-163.

227. Guidelines for the use of antiretroviral agents in HIV-1 infected adults and adolescents. https://aidsinfo.nih.gov/contentfiles/lvguidelines/adultandadolescentgl.pdf. Accessed Aug 28, 2020.

228. Pretorius E, Klinker H, Rosenkranz B. The role of therapeutic drug monitoring in the management of patients with human immunodeficiency virus infection. *Ther Drug Monit*. 2011;33(3): 265-274.PubMed

229. Panel on Antiretroviral Guidelines for Adults and Adolescents. *Guidelines for the use of antiretrovirals in HIV-1-infected adults and adolescents*. Washington, DC: Department of Health and Human Services; 2011:1-67.

230. Rayner CR, Dooley JM, Nation RL. Antivirals for HIV. In: Burton ME, Shaw LM, Schentag JJ, et al, eds. *Applied Pharmacokinetics and Pharmacodynamics: Principles of Therapeutic Drug Monitoring*. 4th ed. Baltimore, MD: Lippincott Williams & Wilkins; 2006:354-409.

231. Back DJ, Khoo SH, Gibbons SE, Merry C. The role of therapeutic drug monitoring in treatment of HIV infection. *Br J Clin Pharmacol*. 2001;52(suppl 1):89S-96S.PubMed

232. Khoo SH, Gibbons SE, Back DJ. Therapeutic drug monitoring as a tool in treating HIV infection. *AIDS*. 2001;15(suppl 5):S171-S181.PubMed

233. Dasgupta A, Okhuysen PC. Pharmacokinetic and other drug interactions in patients with AIDS. *Ther Drug Monit*. 2001;23(6): 591-605.PubMed

234. Moyle GJ, Back D. Principles and practice of HIV-protease inhibitor pharmacoenhancement. *HIV Med*. 2001;2(2):105-113.PubMed

235. Campbell TJ, Williams KM. Therapeutic drug monitoring: antiarrhythmic drugs. *Br J Clin Pharmacol*. 2001;52(suppl 1):21S-34S. PubMed

236. Parker RB, Nappi JM, Cavallari LH. Chronic heart failure. In: DiPiro JT, Talbert RL, Yee GC, et al, eds. *Pharmacotherapy: A Pathophysiologic Approach*. 9th ed. http://accesspharmacy.mhmedical.com/. Accessed Jun 29, 2015.

237. Valdes R Jr, Jortani SA, Gheorghiade M. Standards of laboratory practice: cardiac drug monitoring. *Clin Chem*. 1998;44(5):1096-1109. PubMed

238. Yancy CW, Jessup M, Bozkurt B, et al. 2017 ACC/AHA/HFSA Focused Update of the 2013 ACCF/AHA Guideline for the Management of Heart Failure: A Report of the American College of Cardiology/American Heart Association Task Force on Clinical Practice Guidelines and the Heart Failure Society of America. *J Am Coll Cardiol*. 2017;70(6):776-803. PubMed

239. Rathore SS, Curtis JP, Wang Y, et al. Association of serum digoxin concentration and outcomes in patients with heart failure. *JAMA.* 2003;289(7):871-878.PubMed

240. Bauman JL, DiDomenico RJ, Viana M, Fitch M. A method of determining the dose of digoxin for heart failure in the modern era. *Arch Intern Med.* 2006;166(22):2539-2545.PubMed

241. Eichhorn EJ, Gheorghiade M. Digoxin. *Prog Cardiovasc Dis.* 2002;44(4):251-266.PubMed

242. Gheorghiade M, van Veldhuisen DJ, Colucci WS. Contemporary use of digoxin in the management of cardiovascular disorders. *Circulation.* 2006;113(21):2556-2564.PubMed

243. Schentag J, Bang A, Kozinski-Tober J. Digoxin. In: Burton M, Shaw L, Schentag J, Evans W, eds. *Applied Pharmacokinetics and Pharmacodynamics.* 4th ed. Baltimore, MD: Lippincott Williams & Wilkins; 2006:411-439.

244. Eichhorn EJ, Gheorghiade M. Digoxin. *Prog Cardiovasc Dis.* 2002;44(4):251-266.PubMed

245. Boro MS, Winter ME. Digoxin. In: Winter ME, ed. *Basic Clinical Pharmacokinetics.* 5th ed. Baltimore, MD: Lippincott Williams & Wilkins; 2010:198-239.

246. Page RL. Digoxin. In: Murphy JE, ed. *Clinical Pharmacokinetics.* 5th ed. Bethesda, MD: American Society of Health-System Pharmacists; 2012:185-195.

247. Bernard DW, Bowman RL, Grimm FA, et al. Nighttime dosing assures postdistribution sampling for therapeutic drug monitoring of digoxin. *Clin Chem.* 1996;42(1):45-49.PubMed

248. Matzuk MM, Shlomchik M, Shaw LM. Making digoxin therapeutic drug monitoring more effective. *Ther Drug Monit.* 1991;13(3):215-219. PubMed

249. Digoxin. In: *Lexicomp Online.* [online database]. Hudson, OH: Lexi-Comp. https://www.wolterskluwer.com/en/solutions/lexicomp. Accessed Aug 13, 2015.

250. Rotmensch HH, Belhassen B, Swanson BN, et al. Steady-state serum amiodarone concentrations: relationships with antiarrhythmic efficacy and toxicity. *Ann Intern Med.* 1984;101(4):462-469.PubMed

251. Singh BN, Vaughan Williams EM. The effect of amiodarone, a new anti-anginal drug, on cardiac muscle. *Br J Pharmacol.* 1970;39(4):657-667.PubMed

252. Mahmarian JJ, Smart FW, Moyé LA, et al. Exploring the minimal dose of amiodarone with antiarrhythmic and hemodynamic activity. *Am J Cardiol.* 1994;74(7):681-686.PubMed

253. Pollak PT. Clinical organ toxicity of antiarrhythmic compounds: ocular and pulmonary manifestations. *Am J Cardiol.* 1999;84(9A):37R-45R. PubMed

254. Nolan PE, Trujillo TC. Lidocaine. In: Murphy JE, ed. *Clinical Pharmacokinetics.* 5th ed. Bethesda, MD: American Society of Health-System Pharmacists; 2012:229-242.

255. Ohara KY, Winter ME. Lidocaine. In: Winter ME, ed. *Basic Clinical Pharmacokinetics.* 5th ed. Baltimore, MD: Lippincott Williams & Wilkins; 2010:277-293.

256. Cohen H. Lidocaine. In: *Casebook in Clinical Pharmacokinetics and Drug Dosing.* New York, NY: McGraw-Hill; 2015:97-102.

257. Bauer LA, Brown T, Gibaldi M, et al. Influence of long-term infusions on lidocaine kinetics. *Clin Pharmacol Ther.* 1982;31(4):433-437.PubMed

258. Ohashi K, Ebihara A, Hashimoto T, et al. Pharmacokinetics and the antiarrhythmic effect of mexiletine in patients with chronic ventricular arrhythmias. *Arzneimittelforschung.* 1984;34(4):503-507.PubMed

259. Talbot RG, Nimmo J, Julian DG, et al. Treatment of ventricular arrhythmias with mexiletine (Kö 1173). *Lancet.* 1973;2(7826):399-404. PubMed

260. Nei SD, Danelich IM, Lose JM, et al. Therapeutic drug monitoring of mexiletine at a large academic medical center. *SAGE Open Med.* 2016;4:2050312116670659.

261. Page RL, Murphy JE. Procainamide. In: Murphy JE, ed. *Clinical Pharmacokinetics.* 5th ed. Bethesda, MD: American Society of Health-System Pharmacists; 2012:289-298.

262. Cohen H. Procainamide. Cohen H, ed. *Casebook in Clinical Pharmacokinetics and Drug Dosing.* New York: McGraw-Hill; 2015: 195-202.

263. Brown JE, Shand DG. Therapeutic drug monitoring of antiarrhythmic agents. *Clin Pharmacokinet.* 1982;7(2):125-148.PubMed

264. Coyle JD, Lima JJ. Procainamide. In: Evans WE, Schentag JJ, Jusko WJ, eds. *Applied Pharmacokinetics: Principles of Therapeutic Drug Monitoring.* 3rd ed. Vancouver, WA: Applied Therapeutics; 1992:22.1-22.33.

265. Griffith KS, Lewis LS, Mali S, Parise ME. Treatment of malaria in the United States: a systematic review. *JAMA.* 2007;297(20):2264-2277.PubMed

266. Nolan PE, Trujillo TC, Yeaman CM. Quinidine. Murphy JE, ed. *Clinical Pharmacokinetics.* 5th ed. Bethesda, MD: American Society of Health-System Pharmacists; 2012:299-313.

267. Cardiac Arrhythmia Suppression Trial (CAST) Investigators. Preliminary report: effect of encainide and flecainide on mortality in a randomized trial of arrhythmia suppression after myocardial infarction. *N Engl J Med.* 1989;321(6):406-412.PubMed

268. Morganroth J, Goin JE. Quinidine-related mortality in the short-to-medium-term treatment of ventricular arrhythmias. A meta-analysis. *Circulation.* 1991;84(5):1977-1983.PubMed

269. McCollam PL, Crouch MA, Watson JE. Altered protein binding of quinidine in patients with atrial fibrillation and flutter. *Pharmacotherapy.* 1997;17(4):753-759.PubMed

270. Ochs HR, Grube E, Greenblatt DJ, et al. Intravenous quinidine: pharmacokinetic properties and effects on left ventricular performance in humans. *Am Heart J.* 1980;99(4):468-475.PubMed

271. Holford NHG, Coates PE, Guentert TW, et al. The effects of quinidine and its metabolites on the EKG and systolic time intervals: Concentration-effect relationships. *Br J Pharmacol.* 1981;11:187-195.PubMed

272. Lennard L. Therapeutic drug monitoring of cytotoxic drugs. *Br J Clin Pharmacol.* 2001;52(suppl 1):75S-87S.PubMed

273. Hon YY, Evans WE. Making TDM work to optimize cancer chemotherapy: a multidisciplinary team approach. *Clin Chem.* 1998;44(2):388-400.PubMed

274. Petros WP, Evans WE. Anticancer agents. In: Burton ME, Shaw LM, Schentag JJ, et al, eds. *Applied Pharmacokinetics and Pharmacodynamics: Principles of Therapeutic Drug Monitoring.* 4th ed. Baltimore, MD: Lippincott Williams & Wilkins; 2006:617-636.

275. Yuen CW, Winter ME. Methotrexate. In: Winter ME, ed. *Basic Clinical Pharmacokinetics.* 5th ed. Baltimore, MD: Lippincott Williams & Wilkins; 2010:304-325.

276. McCune JS, Gibbs JP, Slattery JT. Plasma concentration monitoring of busulfan: does it improve clinical outcome? *Clin Pharmacokinet.* 2000;39(2):155-165.PubMed

277. Tabak A, Hoffer E, Rowe JM, Krivoy N. Monitoring of busulfan area under the curve: estimation by a single measurement. *Ther Drug Monit.* 2001;23(5):526-528.PubMed

278. Sparreboom A, Nooter K, Loos WJ, Verweij J. The (ir)relevance of plasma protein binding of anticancer drugs. *Neth J Med.* 2001;59(4):196-207.PubMed

279. Gusella M, Ferrazzi E, Ferrari M, Padrini R. New limited sampling strategy for determining 5-fluorouracil area under the concentration-time curve after rapid intravenous bolus. *Ther Drug Monit.* 2002;24(3):425-431.PubMed

280. Petros WP, Colvin OM. Metabolic jeopardy with high-dose cyclophosphamide?–not so fast. *Clin Cancer Res.* 1999;5(4):723-724. PubMed

281. Zalupski M, Metch B, Balcerzak S, et al. Phase III comparison of doxorubicin and dacarbazine given by bolus versus infusion in patients with soft-tissue sarcomas: a Southwest Oncology Group study. *J Natl Cancer Inst.* 1991;83(13):926-932.PubMed

282. Cyclosporine. In: *Lexicomp Online*. [online database]. Hudson, OH: Lexi-Comp. https://www.wolterskluwer.com/en/solutions/lexicomp. Accessed Aug 13, 2015.

283. Holt DW, Armstrong VW, Griesmacher A, et al. International Federation of Clinical Chemistry/International Association of Therapeutic Drug Monitoring and Clinical Toxicology working group on immunosuppressive drug monitoring. *Ther Drug Monit*. 2002;24(1):59-67.PubMed

284. Oellerich M, Armstrong VW, Kahan B, et al. Lake Louise Consensus Conference on cyclosporin monitoring in organ transplantation: report of the consensus panel. *Ther Drug Monit*. 1995;17(6):642-654.PubMed

285. Formea CM, Karlix JL. Antirejection agents. In: Murphy JE, ed. *Clinical Pharmacokinetics*. 5th ed. Bethesda, MD: American Society of Health-System Pharmacists; 2012:159-166.

286. Johnston A, Holt DW. Cyclosporine. In: Burton ME, Shaw LM, Schentag JJ, et al, eds. *Applied Pharmacokinetics and Pharmacodynamics: Principles of Therapeutic Drug Monitoring*. 4th ed. Baltimore, MD: Lippincott Williams & Wilkins; 2006:512-528.

287. Wong SH. Therapeutic drug monitoring for immunosuppressants. *Clin Chim Acta*. 2001;313(1-2):241-253.PubMed

288. Quan DJ, Winter ME. Immunosuppressants: cyclosporine, tacrolimus, and sirolimus. In: Winter ME, ed. *Basic Clinical Pharmacokinetics*. 5th ed. Baltimore, MD: Lippincott Williams & Wilkins; 2010:250-276.

289. Johnston A, Holt DW. Immunosuppressant drugs: the role of therapeutic drug monitoring. *Br J Clin Pharmacol*. 2001;52(suppl 1):61S-73S. PubMed

290. Lindholm A, Henricsson S. Intra- and interindividual variability in the free fraction of cyclosporine in plasma in recipients of renal transplants. *Ther Drug Monit*. 1989;11(6):623-630.PubMed

291. Everolimus. In: *Lexicomp Online*. [online database]. Hudson, OH: Lexi-Comp. https://www.wolterskluwer.com/en/solutions/lexicomp. Accessed Sep 7, 2015.

292. Kovarik JM, Hartmann S, Figueiredo J, et al. Effect of food on everolimus absorption: quantification in healthy subjects and a confirmatory screening in patients with renal transplants. *Pharmacotherapy*. 2002;22(2):154-159.PubMed

293. Nawrocki A, Korecka M, Solari S, et al. Mycophenolic acid. In: Burton ME, Shaw LM, Schentag JJ, et al, eds. *Applied Pharmacokinetics and Pharmacodynamics: Principles of Therapeutic Drug Monitoring*. 4th ed. Baltimore, MD: Lippincott Williams & Wilkins; 2006:563-594.

294. Kuypers DRJ, Le Meur Y, Cantarovich M, et al. Consensus report on therapeutic drug monitoring of mycophenolic acid in solid organ transplantation. *Clin J Am Soc Nephrol*. 2010;5(2):341-358.PubMed

295. Weber LT, Shipkova M, Armstrong VW, et al. The pharmacokinetic-pharmacodynamic relationship for total and free mycophenolic acid in pediatric renal transplant recipients: a report of the German study group on mycophenolate mofetil therapy. *J Am Soc Nephrol*. 2002;13(3):759-768.PubMed

296. Ensom MH, Partovi N, Decarie D, et al. Pharmacokinetics and protein binding of mycophenolic acid in stable lung transplant recipients. *Ther Drug Monit*. 2002;24(2):310-314.PubMed

297. Dasgupta A. Usefulness of monitoring free (unbound) concentrations of therapeutic drugs in patient management. *Clin Chim Acta*. 2007;377 (1-2):1-13.PubMed

298. Schonder KS, Johnson HJ. Solid-organ transplantation. In: DiPiro JT, Talbert RL, Yee GC et al., eds. Pharmacotherapy: A Pathophysiologic Approach. http://accesspharmacy.mhmedical.com. Accessed Jun 29, 2015.

299. Christians U, Pokaiyavanichkul T, Chan L. Tacrolimus. In: Burton ME, Shaw LM, Schentag JJ, et al, eds. *Applied Pharmacokinetics and Pharmacodynamics: Principles of Therapeutic Drug Monitoring*. 4th ed. Baltimore, MD: Lippincott Williams & Wilkins; 2006:529-562.

300. Philosophe B, Leca N, West-Thielke PM, et al. Evaluation of flexible tacrolimus drug concentration monitoring approach in patients receiving extended-release once-daily tacrolimus tablets. *J Clin Pharmacol*. 2018;58(7):891-896.PubMed

301. Elens L, Capron A, van Schaik RH, et al. Impact of CYP3A4*22 allele on tacrolimus pharmacokinetics in early period after renal transplantation: toward updated genotype-based dosage guidelines. *Ther Drug Monit*. 2013;35(5):608-616.PubMed

302. Macchi-Andanson M, Charpiat B, Jelliffe RW, et al. Failure of traditional trough levels to predict tacrolimus concentrations. *Ther Drug Monit*. 2001;23(2):129-133.PubMed

303. DeVane CL. Cyclic antidepressants. In: Burton ME, Shaw LM, Schentag JJ, et al, eds. *Applied Pharmacokinetics and Pharmacodynamics: Principles of Therapeutic Drug Monitoring*. 4th ed. Baltimore, MD: Lippincott Williams & Wilkins; 2006:781-797.

304. Linder MW, Keck PE Jr. Standards of laboratory practice: antidepressant drug monitoring. *Clin Chem*. 1998;44(5):1073-1084.PubMed

305. Finley PR. Antidepressants. Murphy JE, ed. *Clinical Pharmacokinetics*. 5th ed. Bethesda, MD: American Society of Health-System Pharmacists; 2012:119-134.

306. Mitchell PB. Therapeutic drug monitoring of psychotropic medications. *Br J Clin Pharmacol*. 2001;52(suppl 1):45S-54S.PubMed

307. Lieberman JA, Cooper TB, Suckow RF, et al. Tricyclic antidepressant and metabolite levels in chronic renal failure. *Clin Pharmacol Ther*. 1985;37(3):301-307.PubMed

308. Fiaturi N, Greenblatt DJ. Therapeutic drug monitoring of antidepressants. *Handb Exp Pharmacol*. 2019;250:115-133.PubMed

309. Rasmussen BB, Brøsen K. Is therapeutic drug monitoring a case for optimizing clinical outcome and avoiding interactions of the selective serotonin reuptake inhibitors? *Ther Drug Monit*. 2000;22(2):143-154. PubMed

310. Ghibellini G, Carson SW. Lithium. In: Murphy JE, ed. *Clinical Pharmacokinetics*. 5th ed. Bethesda, MD: American Society of Health-System Pharmacists; 2012:243-262.

311. Burke MD. Principles of therapeutic drug monitoring. *Postgrad Med*. 1981;70(1):57-63.PubMed

312. Leucht S, Steimer W, Kreuz S, et al. Doxepin plasma concentrations: is there really a therapeutic range? *J Clin Psychopharmacol*. 2001;21(4):432-439.PubMed

313. DeVane CL. Metabolism and pharmacokinetics of selective serotonin reuptake inhibitors. *Cell Mol Neurobiol*. 1999;19(4):443-466. PubMed

314. McEvoy GK, Snow ED, eds. *AHFS Drug Information*. Bethesda, MD: American Society of Health-System Pharmacists; 2012:2662-2671.

315. Finley PR, Winter ME. Lithium. Winter ME, ed. *Basic Clinical Pharmacokinetics*. 5th ed. Baltimore, MD: Lippincott Williams & Wilkins; 2010:294-303.

316. American Psychiatric Association. Practice guideline for the treatment of patients with schizophrenia. *Am J Psychiat*. 2004;161 (suppl 2):1-56.

317. Cohen H. Lithium. Cohen H, ed. *Casebook in Clinical Pharmacokinetics and Drug Dosing*. New York: McGraw-Hill; 2015:103-108.

318. Shulman KI, Herrmann N. The nature and management of mania in old age. *Psychiatr Clin North Am*. 1999;22(3):649-665, ix.PubMed

319. Bettinger TL, Crismon ML. Lithium. In: Burton ME, Shaw LM, Schentag JJ, et al, eds. *Applied Pharmacokinetics and Pharmacodynamics: Principles of Therapeutic Drug Monitoring*. 4th ed. Baltimore: Lippincott Williams & Wilkins; 2006:798-812.

320. Marcus SC, Olfson M, Pincus HA, et al. Therapeutic drug monitoring of mood stabilizers in Medicaid patients with bipolar disorder. *Am J Psychiatry*. 1999;156(7):1014-1018.PubMed

321. Eilers R. Therapeutic drug monitoring for the treatment of psychiatric disorders. Clinical use and cost effectiveness. *Clin Pharmacokinet*. 1995;29(6):442-450.PubMed

322. Perel JM, Jann MW. Antipsychotics. In: Burton ME, Shaw LM, Schentag JJ, et al, eds. *Applied Pharmacokinetics and Pharmacodynamics: Principles of Therapeutic Drug Monitoring*. 4th ed. Baltimore, MD: Lippincott Williams & Wilkins; 2006:813-838.

323. Mauri MC, Volonteri LS, Colasanti A, et al. Clinical pharmacokinetics of atypical antipsychotics: a critical review of the relationship between plasma concentrations and clinical response. *Clin Pharmacokinet.* 2007;46(5):359-388.PubMed

324. Nielsen J, Damkier P, Lublin H, Taylor D. Optimizing clozapine treatment. *Acta Psychiatr Scand.* 2011;123(6):411-422.PubMed

325. Rajkumar AP, Poonkuzhali B, Kuruvilla A, et al. Clinical predictors of serum clozapine levels in patients with treatment-resistant schizophrenia. *Int Clin Psychopharmacol.* 2013;28(1):50-56.PubMed

326. Haloperidol. In: *Lexicomp Online.* [online database]. Hudson, OH: Lexi-Comp. https://www.wolterskluwer.com/en/solutions/lexicomp. Accessed Aug 19, 2015.

327. Remington G, Agid O, Foussias G, et al. Clozapine and therapeutic drug monitoring: is there sufficient evidence for an upper threshold? *Psychopharmacology (Berl).* 2013;225(3):505-518.PubMed

328. Williams ML, Wainer IW. Role of chiral chromatography in therapeutic drug monitoring and in clinical and forensic toxicology. *Ther Drug Monit.* 2002;24(2):290-296.PubMed

329. Thormann W, Theurillat R, Wind M, Kuldvee R. Therapeutic drug monitoring of antiepileptics by capillary electrophoresis. Characterization of assays via analysis of quality control sera containing 14 analytes. *J Chromatogr A.* 2001;924(1-2):429-437.PubMed

330. Williams J, Patsalos PN, Mei Z, et al. Relation between dosage of carbamazepine and concentration in hair and plasma samples from a compliant inpatient epileptic population. *Ther Drug Monit.* 2001;23(1):15-20.PubMed

331. Wang J. Amperometric biosensors for clinical and therapeutic drug monitoring: a review. *J Pharm Biomed Anal.* 1999;19(1-2):47-53.PubMed

332. Ståhle L, Alm C, Ekquist B, et al. Monitoring free extracellular valproic acid by microdialysis in epileptic patients. *Ther Drug Monit.* 1996;18(1):14-18.PubMed

333. Campbell M. Community-based therapeutic drug monitoring. Useful development or unnecessary distraction? *Clin Pharmacokinet.* 1995;28(4):271-274.PubMed

334. Hawksworth GM, Chrystyn H. Therapeutic drug and biochemical monitoring in a community pharmacy: Part 1. *Int J Pharm Pract.* 1995;3:133-138.

335. Nebert DW, Vesell ES. Can personalized drug therapy be achieved? A closer look at pharmaco-metabonomics. *Trends Pharmacol Sci.* 2006;27(11):580-586.PubMed

336. Ferraldeschi R, Newman WG. Pharmacogenetics and pharmacogenomics: a clinical reality. *Ann Clin Biochem.* 2011;48(Pt 5):410-417.PubMed

337. Innocenti F, Ratain MJ. Update on pharmacogenetics in cancer chemotherapy. *Eur J Cancer.* 2002;38(5):639-644.PubMed

338. Holford NH. Target concentration intervention: beyond Y2K. *Br J Clin Pharmacol.* 2001;52(suppl 1):55S-59S.PubMed

339. Oude Munnink TH, Henstra MJ, Segerink LI, et al. Therapeutic drug monitoring of monoclonal antibodies in inflammatory and malignant disease: Translating TNF-α experience to oncology. *Clin Pharmacol Ther.* 2016;99(4):419-431.PubMed

340. Gotta V, Widmer N, Decosterd LA, et al. Clinical usefulness of therapeutic concentration monitoring for imatinib dosage individualization: results from a randomized controlled trial. *Cancer Chemother Pharmacol.* 2014;74(6):1307-1319.PubMed

341. Bates DW, Soldin SJ, Rainey PM, Micelli JN. Strategies for physician education in therapeutic drug monitoring. *Clin Chem.* 1998;44(2):401-407.PubMed

342. Schumacher GE, Barr JT. Total testing process applied to therapeutic drug monitoring: impact on patients' outcomes and economics. *Clin Chem.* 1998;44(2):370-374.PubMed

## BIBLIOGRAPHY

Bauer LA. *Applied Clinical Pharmacokinetics.* 2nd ed. New York, NY: McGraw-Hill; 2008.

Burton ME, Shaw LM, Schentag JJ, et al, eds. *Applied Pharmacokinetics and Pharmacodynamics: Principles of Therapeutic Drug Monitoring.* 4th ed. Baltimore, MD: Lippincott Williams & Wilkins; 2006.

Cohen H. *Casebook in Clinical Pharmacokinetics and Drug Dosing.* New York, NY: McGraw-Hill; 2015.

Murphy JE, ed. *Clinical Pharmacokinetics.* 5th ed. Bethesda, MD: American Society of Health-System Pharmacists; 2012.

Taylor WJ, Caviness MHD, eds. *A Textbook for the Application of Therapeutic Drug Monitoring.* Irving, TX: Abbott Laboratories, Diagnostics Division; 1986.

Winter ME, ed. *Basic Clinical Pharmacokinetics.* 5th ed. Baltimore, MD: Lippincott Williams & Wilkins; 2010.

# 6

# Pharmacogenetics and Molecular Testing

## *Jason H. Karnes and Laura B. Ramsey*

## OBJECTIVES

*After completing this chapter, the reader should be able to*

- Define pharmacogenetics
- Differentiate germline and somatic mutations
- Describe the use of molecular testing in pharmacogenetics/pharmacogenomics as tools for personalizing therapy
- Describe the difference between empirical pharmacotherapy and genotype-guided pharmacotherapy
- Describe how pharmacogenetics can enhance therapeutic drug monitoring
- Assess the utility of genotype in addition to other patient-specific factors for specific medications in the provision of pharmaceutical care
- Discuss the role of laboratory medicine in pharmacogenetics in terms of turnaround time, interpretative reporting, and assay performance

## PHARMACOGENETICS

As early as the 1950s, the heritable nature of drug response was noted for agents such as succinylcholine, isoniazid, and primaquine.[1-3] Later, twin studies confirmed this heritability by showing that the half-lives of some drugs were tightly correlated in monozygotic twins and had little correlation in dizygotic twins.[4] Since that time, the fields of pharmacogenetics and pharmacogenomics have taken off, and the genetic basis for variability in drug metabolism, transport, and pharmacodynamic effect is increasingly being appreciated. In fact, pharmacogenetic and molecular tests are routinely used in therapeutic areas such as hematology/oncology and infectious disease, and their usefulness is being explored in every major therapeutic drug class.[5,6]

Pharmacogenetics/pharmacogenomics is the translational science of correlating interindividual genetic variation with variability in drug response, including both drug efficacy and safety (**Table 6-1**). Historically and practically, the terms *pharmacogenetics* and *pharmacogenomics* have been used interchangeably (as in this chapter). However, definitions may vary depending on the context. For example, pharmacogenetics can be seen as the study of variants in a handful of candidate genes. On the contrary, because of our expanding technological ability to simultaneously investigate millions of variants across the human genome using genome-wide genotyping arrays or high-throughput sequencing, pharmacogenomics may refer to genome-wide investigation of drug response variability.

Pharmacogenetics seeks to avoid adverse drug reactions and improve clinical efficacy, providing personalized medicine to patients, much the same way therapeutic drug monitoring by serum drug concentrations customizes certain medication regimens for individual patients. One goal of pharmacogenetics is to refine the current empirical approach to drug therapy management so that it is less "trial-and-error" in nature. There are often many drug classes available to treat a given condition and several drugs within each of those classes that a clinician may opt to use. This large armamentarium of drug therapy choices can lead to an inefficient, time-consuming management strategy in which the therapeutic decision is based on little more than clinician preference. Another goal of pharmacogenetics is to provide the appropriate dose to individual patients so that the "one dose fits all" strategy is avoided. Incorporating the results of genetic tests along with nongenetic factors (eg, age, sex, smoking status, kidney and liver function, drug–drug interactions) into pharmacotherapy decision making may help streamline this process such that the likelihood for response is maximized while the chance of toxicity is minimized.[7,8]

Understanding the results of molecular tests that are used in the application of pharmacogenetics is of critical importance to healthcare providers if this form of personalized medicine is going to improve patient care. Many institutions are attempting to implement preemptive genotyping so that results will be in the electronic medical record before a particular drug with a clinically actionable genetic test is prescribed. Furthermore, direct-to-consumer genetic tests are already available to patients, regardless of whether significant published evidence is available supporting that the test improves clinical care. Despite the great promise of personalized medicine, the field is changing rapidly, and exactly how and when tests should be applied clinically is still very much a work in progress. Therefore, this chapter focuses on

DOI 10.37573/9781585286423.006

**TABLE 6-1.** Key Terms Related to Genomics and Pharmacogenomics

| KEY TERMS | DEFINITION |
|---|---|
| Allele | A variant form of a gene or locus; an individual inherits two alleles for each gene or locus, one from each parent |
| Diplotype | The combination of two haplotypes or star alleles in a single individual |
| Gene | The basic physical unit of inheritance that is passed from parents to offspring and contains the information needed to specify traits |
| Genotype | The combination of alleles in an individual at a particular locus |
| Germline variant | Heritable DNA variant occurring in gametes and present in all nucleated cells |
| Haplotype | Combination of genetic variants inherited together on a single chromosome |
| Pharmacogenetics/Pharmacogenomics | The translational science of correlating interindividual genetic variation with variability in drug response, including both drug efficacy and safety |
| Phenotype | The observable characteristics or traits of an organism that are produced by the interaction of the genotype and the environment |
| Preemptive PGx test | PGx test done before a medication order or adverse reaction |
| Reactive PGx test | PGx test done after a medication order or adverse reaction |
| Somatic variant | DNA variant occurring in nongermline cells (not heritable) and occurring during the lifespan of an individual |
| Single nucleotide polymorphism (SNP) | Variation at a single position in a DNA sequence among individuals |
| Star allele | Combination of genetic variants inherited together, defined by PharmVar |

PGx = pharmacogenetic.

pharmacogenetic laboratory tests that are used commonly in clinical practice or are most likely to be incorporated into clinical practice in the near future.

While some organizations, such as the National Academy of Clinical Biochemistry (NACB), have established practice guidelines for the application of pharmacogenetics, clinical guidance for pharmacogenetic tests is often provided in disease-specific guidelines on a case-by-case basis.[9-11] The U.S. Food and Drug Administration (FDA) has released both a Table of Pharmacogenetic Associations (https://www.fda.gov/medical-devices/precision-medicine/table-pharmacogenetic-associations) and a Table of Pharmacogenomic Biomarkers in Drug Labeling (https://www.fda.gov/drugs/science-and-research-drugs/table-pharmacogenomic-biomarkers-drug-labeling). Clinical pharmacology groups such as the Clinical Pharmacogenetics Implementation Consortium (CPIC) have published practice guidelines for specific drug/gene pairs with clinical importance as data become available (**Table 6-2**; https://cpicpgx.org/guidelines).[12] CPIC guidelines are regularly updated, and the CPIC website should be checked for the most up-to-date information. CPIC guidelines have been endorsed by several professional societies, including the Association for Molecular Pathology, the American Society for Clinical Pharmacology and Therapeutics, and American Society of Health-System Pharmacists, and provide a concise summary of clinical recommendations and supporting evidence for pharmacogenetic tests.

An important consideration for CPIC guidelines is that they do not give recommendations on when to administer a pharmacogenetic test but give recommendations for clinical interventions in the event that a test result is already known. Taken together, guidelines from these organizations and others will likely be useful in bringing together the fields of laboratory medicine and clinical pharmacology in the application of pharmacogenetics.

## Pharmacogenetic Testing Versus Disease Genetic Testing

Laboratory testing for pharmacogenetic and genetic polymorphisms yields the same general types of results (ie, a patient's genotype[s] or diplotype[s]). However, the target populations and the use of test results for pharmacogenetic testing versus disease genetic testing may be quite different. Clinically used pharmacogenetic tests provide information that may aid in selection or dosing of medications. Therefore, individuals receiving pharmacogenetic tests typically are candidates for a particular therapeutic agent, which may or may not be administered. Individuals receiving disease genetic tests, on the other hand, are likely considered at risk for developing or suspected of having a particular disease or condition without regard to drug treatment. Because no drug exposure is necessary to consider a patient a risk and the presence or risk of disease may not be modifiable, implications of disease genetic tests are generally more severe.

**TABLE 6-2.** Drugs with Actionable Dosing/Patient Selection Guidelines Based on Germline Variation According to the CPIC[a]

| DRUG(S) | GENE(S) | CPIC GUIDELINE RECOMMENDATIONS SUMMARY |
|---|---|---|
| Abacavir | HLA-B | Alternative agent in carriers of HLA-B*57:01[113] |
| Allopurinol | HLA-B | Alternative agent in carriers of HLA-B*58:01[118] |
| Aminoglycosides | MT-RNR1 | Drug: aminoglycosides*, Gene: MT-RNR1, summary: Avoid aminoglycosides in patients susceptible to aminoglycoside-induced hearing loss based on MT-RNR1 genotype.[130] |
| Atazanavir | UGT1A1 | Alternative agent in UGT1A1 poor metabolizers[64] |
| Atomoxetine | CYP2D6 | Modified dosing based on CYP2D6 metabolizer status[27] |
| Carbamazepine Oxcarbazepine | HLA-B HLA-A | Alternative agent in carriers of HLA-B*15:02 and HLA-A*31:01[118] |
| Clopidogrel | CYP2C19 | Alternative agent in CYP2C19 poor and intermediate metabolizers[31] |
| Codeine | CYP2D6 | Alternative agent in CYP2D6 ultrarapid and poor metabolizers[23] |
| Efavirenz | CYP2B6 | Decreased dose in CYP2B6 intermediate and poor metabolizers[47] |
| Fluorouracil Capecitabine Tegafur | DPYD | Reduced dose in DPYD intermediate metabolizers and avoid agent in DPYD poor metabolizers[61] |
| Ivacaftor | CFTR | Use only with specific CFTR genotypes[125] |
| NSAIDs[b] | CYP2C9 | Reduced dose or alternative drug depending on CYP2C9 metabolizer status and specific NSAID[44] |
| Ondansetron Tropisetron | CYP2D6 | Alternative agent in CYP2D6 ultrarapid metabolizers[25] |
| Phenytoin | CYP2C9 HLA-B | Reduced dose in CYP2C9 intermediate and poor metabolizers; alternative agent in carriers of HLA-B*15:02[43] |
| Peginterferon alfa-2a Peginterferon alfa-2b Ribavirin | IFNL3 | Consider alternative agent in patients with unfavorable response genotype for IFNL3[126] |
| Proton pump inhibitors | CYP2C19 | Drug: proton pump inhibitors*, Gene: CYP2C19, summary: Increased dose for CYP2C19 rapid and ultrarapid metabolizers, reduced dose for chronic therapy in poor and intermediate metabolizers.[131] |
| Rasburicase | G6PD | Contraindicated for deficient WHO class II or III G6PD variants[66] |
| Simvastatin | SLCO1B1 | Decreased dose or alternative agent in low or intermediate SLCO1B1 function[127] |
| SSRIs[c] | CYP2D6 | Reduced dose or alternative drug depending on CYP2D6 metabolizer status and specific SSRI[29] |
|  | CYP2C19 | Reduced dose or alternative drug depending on CYP2C19 metabolizer status and specific SSRI[29] |
| Tacrolimus | CYP3A5 | Increased dose for CYP3A5 normal and intermediate metabolizers[46] |
| Tamoxifen | CYP2D6 | Alternative agent in CYP2D6 poor and some intermediate metabolizers[26] |
| Mercaptopurine Azathioprine Thioguanine | TPMT NUDT15 | Reduced dose for TPMT and/or NUDT15 intermediate or poor metabolizers depending on patient's condition[128] |

(continued)

**TABLE 6-2.** Drugs with Actionable Dosing/Patient Selection Guidelines Based on Germline Variation According to the CPIC[a], cont'd

| DRUG(S) | GENE(S) | CPIC GUIDELINE RECOMMENDATIONS SUMMARY |
|---|---|---|
| Tricyclic antidepressants[d] | CYP2D6 | Decreased dose or alternative agent depending on CYP2D6 and CYP2C19 metabolizer status and specific tricyclic antidepressant[28] |
| | CYP2C19 | Decreased dose or alternative agent depending on CYP2C19 metabolizer status and specific tricyclic antidepressant[28] |
| Volatile anesthetic agents[e] Succinylcholine | RYR1 CACNA1S | Alternative agent in patients susceptible to malignant hyperthermia based on RYR1 and CACNA1S genotypes[129] |
| Voriconazole | CYP2C19 | Alternative agent in CYP2C19 ultrarapid, rapid, and poor metabolizers; dose decrease for poor metabolizers in pediatric patients[39] |
| Warfarin | CYP2C9 VKORC1 CYP4F2 | Use of warfarin dosing algorithms with CYP2C9, VKORC1, and CYP4F2 polymorphisms depending on patient race[40] |

NSAID = nonsteroidal anti-inflammatory drug.
[a]Based on a table from https://cpicpgx.org/guidelines, which is regularly updated; not necessarily an all-inclusive list.
[b]Guidance for NSAIDs includes celecoxib, flurbiprofen, lornoxicam, ibuprofen, meloxicam, piroxicam, and tenoxicam.
[c]Guidance for SSRIs includes citalopram, escitalopram, fluvoxamine, paroxetine, and sertraline.
[d]Guidance for tricyclic antidepressants includes amitriptyline, clomipramine, desipramine, doxepin, imipramine, nortriptyline, and trimipramine.
[e]Guidance for volatile anesthetic agents include desflurane, enflurane, halothane, isoflurane, methoxyflurane, sevoflurane, and succinylcholine.
[*]Guidance for aminoglycosides includes amikacin, gentamicin, kanamycin, paromomycin, plazomicin, streptomycin, tobramycin.
[*]Guidance for proton pump inhibitors includes omeprazole, lansoprazole, pantoprazole, and dexlansoprazole

Historically, pharmacogenetic testing has been considered to have fewer ethical issues surrounding it than disease genetic testing.[13] However, while this is still generally considered to be the case, the risks of pharmacogenetic testing also have been outlined and a framework created to ensure appropriate delivery of pharmacogenetic information in the healthcare system.[14] This framework outlines three major considerations regarding whether a particular pharmacogenetic test raises ethical issues: whether the genetic variant is inherited or acquired, whether the goal of testing is to address a specific clinical question or to provide information for future clinical care, and whether the test reveals ancillary clinical information (eg, disease risk).[14]

## Pharmacogenetics and Personalized/Precision Medicine

Pharmacogenetics offers one piece to the puzzle of personalized or precision medicine. Personalized medicine seeks to tailor medical therapy to individual characteristics of patients. It can include genomic information, as in pharmacogenetics, or any other molecular analyses (eg, metabolomics, proteomics) in combination with commonly used clinical parameters such as age, weight, and renal function. Personalized medicine may also tailor therapy based on characteristics of tumors or pathogens. This chapter focuses on pharmacogenetic testing of patient DNA as a means of providing personalized medicine.

## Resources for Pharmacogenetics

The National Institutes of Health (NIH) has supported several pharmacogenetic resources. The Pharmacogenomics Knowledgebase (PharmGKB) collects, curates, and disseminates knowledge about clinically actionable gene–drug associations and genotype–phenotype relationships. This includes prescribing recommendations written by CPIC, the Dutch Pharmacogenetics Working Group, the Canadian Pharmacogenomics Network for Drug Safety, and American, Canadian, European, Swiss, and Japanese medication labels with pharmacogenomic information (**Table 6-3**). PharmGKB curates pathways of pharmacokinetics and pharmacodynamics. They catalog publications detailing the effects of individual variants in each gene, summarize gene–drug pairs, and give each gene–drug pair a strength of evidence rating. The PharmGKB website includes all the CPIC guideline recommendations, allowing the user to select a diplotype to get the CPIC recommendations for a specific drug. Some clinicians use this tool when they have a pharmacogenetic test that does not use CPIC's recommendations or come with an interpretation. CPIC's website contains all the guidelines published and assigns levels of evidence of gene–drug pairs nominated for guidelines. The guidelines are all peer reviewed and published as open access. Each guideline contains a large supplemental file with population frequencies of the alleles, diplotypes, and phenotypes as well as a rating of each publication reviewed during the guideline development (Table 6-3).

The combinations of specific polymorphisms on a single chromosome or haplotypes leading to these phenotypes are typically described using star (*) nomenclature as defined by the Pharmacogene Variation Consortium (Pharmvar; https://www.pharmvar.org).[15] The combination of haplotypes is referred to as a diplotype, such that each patient inherits two star alleles for a given gene (eg, CYP2C9*1/*1). For most genes, the *1 genotype is

**TABLE 6-3.** Commonly Used Online Resources for Pharmacogenomic Information

| RESOURCE | ACRONYM/ABBREVIATION | WEBSITE |
|---|---|---|
| Clinical Pharmacogenetic Implementation Consortium | CPIC | cpicpgx.org |
| Canadian Pharmacogenomics Network for Drug Safety | CPNDS | cpnds.ubc.ca |
| Database of Single Nucleotide Polymorphisms | dbSNP | ncbi.nlm.nih.gov/snp |
| Electronic Medical Records and Genomics Network | eMERGE | emerge-network.org |
| Implementing GeNomics In pracTicE | IGNITE | gmkb.org |
| Pharmacogenomics Research Network | PGRN | pgrn.org |
| Pharmacogenomics Knowledgebase | PharmGKB | pharmgkb.org |
| Pharmacogene Variation Consortium | PharmVar | pharmvar.org |
| Ubiquitous Pharmacogenomics | U-PGx | upgx.eu |

considered the common or normal, fully functioning form of the gene. It is important to note that the *1 allele is reported if all other alleles tested for are absent, but this is not usually accurate. If gene sequencing has not been performed and rare loss-of-function alleles have not been interrogated, a *1/*1 genotype may erroneously be reported. The Association for Molecular Pathology PGx Working Group has defined minimal alleles to test prior to designating *1 for CYP2C19, CYP2D6, CYP2C9, and VKORC1.[16,17,18] Star alleles contain one or more variants and can confer no function, decreased function, normal function, or increased function based on the functional consequences of the variant for the gene's protein product. The terms for allele function and phenotype are standardized by CPIC.[19] In PharmVar, the variants defining each star allele for each gene are annotated, with the function and references to the reports describing the function.[15]

Three large networks are studying pharmacogenetic implementation and incorporation into electronic medical records. The Electronic Medical Records and Genomics (eMERGE) Network combines DNA biorepositories with electronic medical record (EMR) systems for large scale, high-throughput genetic research in support of implementing genomic medicine (Table 6-3). This network has implemented pharmacogenetic testing and incorporation into EMRs. The Implementing GeNomics In pracTicE (IGNITE) Pragmatic Clinical Trials Network is dedicated to supporting the implementation of genomics in healthcare, with trials implementing pharmacogenetics in the treatment of depression and pain. The Ubiquitous Pharmacogenomics Consortium (U-PGx) is investigating whether pre-emptive genotyping of an entire panel of important pharmacogenetic markers is cost-effective and results in a better outcome for patients across several European countries.

## DRUG DISPOSITION-RELATED MOLECULAR TESTS

Pharmacokinetics is concerned with the fate of drugs or other substances once administered and studies the rate and extent of absorption, distribution, metabolism, and excretion. A great deal of interpatient variability exists in the pharmacokinetics of many drugs and a common source of interpatient variability occurs in drug metabolism. Drug disposition reactions can be divided into phase I, phase II, and phase III reactions. Phase I reactions typically involve processes such as oxidation, reduction, and hydrolysis of compounds and are typified by hepatic cytochrome P450 (CYP) drug metabolism. Phase II reactions include conjugation or synthetic reactions such as glucuronidation, sulfation, methylation, acetylation, and others. The purpose of phase II metabolism is to make compounds more water-soluble and facilitate excretion. Finally, phase III reactions are characterized by transport protein-mediated cellular efflux of drugs, usually at the level of the gut, liver, kidney, and highly sequestered tissues. While genetic variability occurs in each of the previously listed phases of drug disposition, many examples of actionable pharmacogenetic associations are found in phase I metabolism. For example, genes encoding many phase I enzymes (eg, CYP2C9, CYP2D6, CYP2C19) contain common genetic variation with a high impact on enzymatic function. When a drug is primarily metabolized through one of these enzymes, such variation has a large impact on drug concentration and thus drug response. Fewer phase II/III genes have actionable variants (eg, UGT1A1, NAT2, ABCB1).

## Cytochrome P450 System

Although many of the genes encoding CYP enzymes are highly polymorphic, CYP2D6, CYP2C9, and CYP2C19 have genetic variation (polymorphisms), which can describe fairly predictable distributions of drug concentrations, making them clinically relevant for some pharmacogenetic tests. Metabolizer status can be described as normal, intermediate, poor, rapid, or ultrarapid based on the presence or absence of gene variations.[19] This genotype–phenotype relationship could help identify poor metabolizers likely to experience side effects (or therapeutic failure in the case of prodrugs requiring activation) to usual doses of CYP450-metabolized drugs or ultrarapid metabolizers more prone to therapeutic failure (or toxicity in the case of prodrugs). With knowledge of genotype, drug doses in these individuals with altered metabolism could then be increased or decreased as appropriate or alternative drugs may be chosen. This ability of genotype to predict drug metabolizing phenotype may be especially important for drugs with narrow therapeutic indices and less important for wide therapeutic index drugs.[20]

## CYP2D6

The *CYP2D6* gene contains more than 120 alleles, which can lead to a normal function, reduced function, or no function. Increased *CYP2D6* function is also observed when there are multiple copies of the gene present. The most common no-function alleles are *3 (rs35742686), *4 (rs1065852, rs3892097, and rs1135840), *5 (gene deletion), and *6 (rs5030655). These single nucleotide polymorphism (SNP) reference numbers (rs numbers) are curated reference numbers for specific variants established by the National Center for Biotechnology Information (NCBI) SNP database (Database of Single Nucleotide Polymorphisms [dbSNP] at www.ncbi.nlm.nih.gov/snp). Multiple copies of the gene are designated by the allele number, the letter x, the the number of copies detected (e.g., *1x2). Due to the number of *CYP2D6* alleles and their disparate functional consequences, the conversion of diplotypes to standardized and clinically interpretable metabolizer phenotypes becomes particularly important.[19,21,22] An activity score system has been devised in which a numeric value is given to each allele, scores are summed for both alleles, and the resulting numeric value is converted into a CYP2D6 metabolizer phenotype. Each functional group is assigned an activity value ranging from 0 to 1 (eg, 0 for no function, 0.5 for decreased function, and 1 for normal function). If multiple copies of the *CYP2D6* gene are detected, the activity score is multiplied by the number of copies of each allele present. Therefore, a normal metabolizer with an activity score of 1.5 will have less enzymatic activity than a normal metabolizer with an activity score of 2. CYP2D6 metabolizer phenotypes include CYP2D6 ultrarapid metabolizer (activity score >2.25), normal metabolizer (activity score is 1.25 to 2.25), intermediate metabolizer (activity score is 0.25 to 1), and poor metabolizer (activity score is 0). CYP2D6 poor metabolizers are more common among individuals of European ancestry and CYP2D6 ultrarapid metabolizers are more common in individuals with Oceania and Near East ancestry.[23]

One of the most reproducible associations between *CYP2D6* genotype and a drug response occurs with codeine. Codeine is a prodrug requiring metabolism by CYP2D6 into its active form morphine for analgesic effect. Therefore, those individuals who are *CYP2D6* poor metabolizers are at risk for therapeutic failure and those who are ultrarapid metabolizers are at risk for toxicity. Alternative analgesic therapy is recommended in both groups of patients (**Minicase 1**).[23,24] In addition to codeine, several guidelines have been published with recommendations for *CYP2D6* genetic testing interpretation and suggested clinical action for the test results. These include guidelines for *CYP2D6* genotype and use of ondansetron/tropisetron, atomoxetine, and tamoxifen.[25-27] Additional guidelines are also available for use of *CYP2D6* genotype in combination with other CYP enzyme pharmacogenetic test results for tricyclic antidepressants and selective serotonin reuptake inhibitors (SSRIs).[28,29]

## CYP2C19

The *CYP2C19* gene contains more than 35 alleles leading to normal, decreased, no, or increased function. The most common no-function alleles are *2 (rs4244285) and *3 (rs4986893), which account for 85% of no function alleles in white and black individuals and 99% of no function alleles in Asians. The other decreased or no function alleles, *4 (rs28399504), *5 (rs56337013), *6 (rs72552267), *7 (rs72558186), *8 (rs41291556), and *10 (rs6413438) are less common. The *17 (rs12248560) allele is an increased function allele and has a frequency of 3% to 20% depending on ethnicity.[30,31] The Association for Molecular Pathology has determined the minimum set of alleles for testing in *CYP2C19* are *2, *3, and *17 based on their relatively high frequencies and functional consequences for the CYP2C19 enzyme.[32] Thus, guidelines typically reserve clinical recommendations for these alleles, and pharmacogenetic testing platforms often interrogate only these three *CYP2C19* loci.

One of the most extensively studied associations between *CYP2C19* polymorphisms and a drug response is with clopidogrel. Clopidogrel is a prodrug requiring activation by two CYP450-dependent steps, both of which involve CYP2C19. Individuals carrying no function *CYP2C19* alleles have been shown to have lower active metabolite concentrations, reduced inhibition of platelet aggregation, and increased risk of adverse cardiovascular outcomes when treated with clopidogrel at standard doses compared with those without reduced function alleles.[33-38] The FDA has updated the clopidogrel label to indicate that alternative treatment or treatment strategies be considered in individuals with two no function *CYP2C19* alleles. Guidelines have been published with treatment recommendations for clopidogrel based on *CYP2C19* genotype (**Minicase 2**).[30,31] Other guidelines use *CYP2C19* genotype for drug selection and dosing, including guidelines for voriconazole, tricyclic antidepressants, and SSRIs.[28,29,39]

## CYP2C9

*CYP2C9* contains more than 60 alleles, more than 30 of which are known to lead to decreased or no function.[40] The most common variants in white individuals in *CYP2C9* are the *2 (rs1799853) and *3 (rs1057910) alleles, whereas the *5 (rs28371686), *6 (rs9332131), *8 (rs7900194), and *11 (rs28371685) alleles are more prevalent in black persons. The *2 allele has a frequency of approximately 13% in white persons, 0% in Asians, and 3% in black persons. The *3 allele has a frequency of approximately 7% in white persons, 4% in Asians, and 2% in black persons. The Association for Molecular Pathology has determined the minimum set of alleles for testing in *CYP2C9* are *2, *3, *5, *6, *8, and *11.[41] One of the most well-documented associations with *CYP2C9* is with warfarin dose requirements (**Figure 6-1**; discussed in detail later).[40,42] Warfarin is a particularly interesting example because CPIC recommendations for pharmacogenetics are different based on a patient's age and self-reported race. These race-based recommendations for warfarin pharmacogenetics underscore the importance of patient race and its influence on the probability that a patient carries specific polymorphisms in relevant pharmacogenetic genes, which can have

## MINICASE 1

# Codeine Pharmacogenetics

J.P. is a 30-year-old woman who had a caesarean section and delivered a healthy baby boy 12 days ago. She was given codeine in the hospital for pain control and was given a codeine prescription upon discharge. She presents with her baby to the emergency department because her baby has been exhibiting extreme sleepiness, poor feeding, and trouble breathing. She is genotyped and found to be CYP2D6*1/*1X2.

QUESTION: Which gene(s) impact response to codeine?

DISCUSSION: Codeine is a prodrug that is activated to morphine by CYP2D6. Other genes that may impact codeine metabolism and response include UGT2B7, which is involved in the formation of morphine-6-glucuronide, the ABCB1 transporter gene, and the opioid receptor μ1 gene OPRM1.

QUESTION: Genotypes for CYP2D6 are represented by what four phenotypes?

DISCUSSION: (1) Normal (also known as *extensive*) metabolizers. This phenotype achieves the expected concentrations of morphine. (2) Intermediate metabolizer. This phenotype has intermediate enzyme activity and reduced morphine formation. (3) Poor metabolizers. This phenotype lacks CYP2D6 enzyme activity and has greatly reduced morphine formation, leading to insufficient pain relief when given codeine. (4) Ultrarapid metabolizers. This phenotype has increased enzyme activity and increased morphine formation, leading to an increased risk of toxicity.

QUESTION: What is an activity score, and which score goes with each phenotype from the previous question?

DISCUSSION: Activity score is used in addition to the traditional drug metabolizer phenotypes because of the large number of alleles present in CYP2D6 and the wide range of enzyme activity, even within phenotypic groups. To determine an activity score, the combination of alleles is used to determine diplotype. Each functional group is then assigned an activity value ranging from 0 to 1 (eg, 0 for no function, 0.5 for decreased function, and 1 for normal function). If multiple copies of the CYP2D6 gene are detected, the activity score is multiplied by the number of copies of each allele present. Therefore, a normal metabolizer with an activity score of 1.5 will have less enzyme activity than a normal metabolizer with an activity score of 2.

- Normal metabolizers: activity score is 1.25 to 2.25.
- Intermediate metabolizer: activity score is 0.25 to 1.
- Poor metabolizers: activity score is 0.
- Ultrarapid metabolizers: activity score is >2.25.

QUESTION: What do you suspect is going on with this patient's baby, and what treatment management decisions would you recommend based on her genotype?

DISCUSSION: Per the CPIC guidelines, this genotype is an ultrarapid metabolizer with increased enzyme activity (~1% to 2% of patients). CYP2D6 ultrarapid metabolizers treated with codeine have rapid intoxication, even with low doses, due to the increased formation of morphine. Codeine is excreted into the breastmilk; therefore, suspect that the baby is receiving toxic levels of morphine. Codeine should be avoided in ultrarapid metabolizers and alternative analgesics should be considered.

QUESTION: What analgesics are not impacted by CYP2D6? What other medications might variants in this gene affect?

DISCUSSION: Analgesics not impacted by CYP2D6 include morphine and nonopioids. Tramadol, hydrocodone, and, to a lesser extent, oxycodone all have metabolism impacted by CYP2D6.

dramatically different frequencies between race groups. Other guidelines are available to support the use of CYP2C9 genetic testing to guide treatment with nonsteroidal antiinflammatory drugs and phenytoin.[43,44]

## CYP3A5

CYP3A5 has predictable associations between polymorphisms and expression of CYP3A5 enzyme. The CYP3A5*3 allele is associated with slower metabolism compared with *1 and tacrolimus pharmacokinetics; patients carrying the *1 allele (CYP3A5 expressers) have significantly lower trough (predose) concentrations of tacrolimus for a given dose than nonexpressers. Approximately 10% to 20% of white persons, 85% of black persons, 60% of Hispanic persons, and 50% of East Asians are considered CYP3A5 expressers.[45] Consequently, these individuals may require dose modifications of CYP3A5-metabolized drugs, as normal doses are based on nonexpressers. CYP3A5 genetic variants have been implicated in variable drug responses for many drugs, including statins, antiepileptics, calcineurin

inhibitors, and tacrolimus. However, dosing guidelines based on genotype exist only for tacrolimus (**Minicase 3**).[46]

## Other CYP450s

Similar to CYP2C9, polymorphisms in the gene CYP4F2 have been associated with warfarin dose requirements.[40] However, the impact of CYP4F2 variation is not due to CYP4F2-mediated warfarin metabolism but to CYP4F2-mediated metabolism of reduced vitamin K, which affects a patient's ability to produce functioning clotting factors and thus a patient's stable warfarin dose (discussed in detail in the following section). A relatively recent example of CYP enzyme pharmacogenetics is CYP2B6. This enzyme is highly polymorphic with more than 35 known variant alleles.[47] Different race groups have substantial differences in the frequencies of CYP2B6 alleles, which include decreased function (eg, CYP2B6*6 and *9), no function (eg, CYP2B6*18), and increased function (eg, CYP2B6*4) alleles. These alleles can be used to guide dosing of efavirenz, a nonnucleoside reverse transcriptase inhibitor used to treat individuals with human

## MINICASE 2

# Cardiovascular Pharmacogenetics

J.K. is a 58-year-old 109 kg (240 lbs), 1.7 m (5'7"), white man who was admitted to the emergency department after experiencing an episode of sustained, substernal chest pain. He is diagnosed with an ST elevation myocardial infarction and sent immediately for coronary angiography and subsequent percutaneous coronary intervention. The patient is started on clopidogrel 75 mg daily, aspirin 325 mg daily, and metoprolol succinate 25 mg daily in addition to his current medication list. You are consulted for pharmacogenomics of clopidogrel and simvastatin.

Allergies: no known drug allergies

Past medical history: uncontrolled hypertension, hyperlipidemia, type 2 diabetes

Vital signs: blood pressure 155/92 mm Hg, pulse 55 beats/min, respiration rate 17 breaths/min, temperature 98.9°F

Medications prior to admission: lisinopril 20 mg daily, glipizide XL 10 mg daily, simvastatin 40 mg daily, omeprazole 20 mg daily

Pharmacogenetic test results: *CYP2D6 \*3/\*3* (poor metabolizer); *CYP2C19\*2/\*3* (poor metabolizer); *SLCO1B1 \*1a/\*1a* (normal function); *VKORC1-1639 G/A; CYP2C9\*1/\*3 (CYP2C9\*5, \*6, \*8, \*11* not tested); *CYP4F2 \*1/\*1*

QUESTION: Based on this patient's clinical and genotype information, what recommendations do you have for antiplatelet therapy (ie, clopidogrel treatment)?

DISCUSSION: According to CPIC guidelines, clinical recommendations for clopidogrel will depend on *CYP2C19* genotype results. If he is an ultrarapid (*CYP2C19\*17* carrier) or normal metabolizer (*\*1/\*1*), then he would be considered to have an adequate response to clopidogrel. If he is an intermediate metabolizer (*\*2* or *\*3* carrier) or poor metabolizer (*\*2/\*2, \*2/\*3, \*3/\*3*), then a switch to an alternative antiplatelet, such as prasugrel or ticagrelor, could be considered. Because this patient is a poor metabolizer, antiplatelet treatment with clopidogrel should be avoided and either prasugrel or ticagrelor should be started to avoid an inadequate antiplatelet treatment and a resulting stent thrombosis.

QUESTION: If this patient had a *CYP2C19\*1/\*17* genotype, what would be the best long-term antiplatelet therapy for him?

DISCUSSION: Because the *CYP2C19\*1/\*17* diplotype would indicate that he is an ultrarapid metabolizer, J.K.'s functional copies of CYP2C19 would result in efficient production of the active clopidogrel metabolite. So, clopidogrel is an effective option for J.K. to prevent stent thrombosis.

QUESTION: Does this patient's statin therapy need to be changed?

DISCUSSION: According to CPIC guidelines, minimization of rhabdomyolysis risk with simvastatin should be directed by *SLCO1B1* rs4149056 genotype. The patient's diplotype is *SLCO1B1 \*1a/\*1a*, indicating that his genotype is rs4149056 TT. The TT genotype indicates a normal risk for muscle toxicity with the drug. The treatment does not need to be changed unless additional cholesterol lowering is needed, in which case simvastatin should be switched to an alternative such as a higher potency statin. This is because simvastatin 80 mg is not recommended by the FDA due to increased incidence of rhabdomyolysis.

QUESTION: Before discharge, this patient develops atrial fibrillation. If warfarin is used for anticoagulation (baseline INR is 1.01 and target INR is 2.5), what initial dose of warfarin would you use?

DISCUSSION: Because the patient is white, the CPIC guidelines recommend use of a pharmacogenetic algorithm that includes *VKORC1-1639G>A* and *CYP2C9\*2* and *\*3* variants. Additional variants such as *CYP2C9\*5, \*6, \*8, \*11* can be included in the dosing algorithm or used to decrease the warfarin dose by 15% to 30% in variant carriers. The *CYP4F2\*3* allele can also be included in the dosing algorithm or used to increase warfarin dose 5% to 10%.

J.K.'s genotype results, discussed previously, are *VKORC1-1639 G/A, CYP2C9\*1/\*3,* and *CYP4F2 \*1/\*1,* but the *CYP2C9\*5, \*6, \*8, \*11* alleles have not been tested. If the patient reported African ancestry, then no genotype-guided algorithm should be used. Because the patient is white, then a dosing algorithm can be used, several of which are found at WarfarinDosing.org (http://warfarindosing.org /Source/Home.aspx). Using J.K.'s information on WarfarinDosing .org, a 3.4 mg/day therapeutic dose according to the Gauge algorithm and 4.1 mg/day according to the International Warfarin Pharmacogenetics Consortium algorithm are recommended. These therapeutic doses may be rounded to the nearest mg dose that is clinically available. INR monitoring should still be performed as per clinical recommendations. A starting dose of 5 mg is not recommended given genomic data are available.

immunodeficiency virus (HIV) infection. Although many other CYP enzymes are involved in drug metabolism, many do not have a marked impact on drug metabolism. *CYP3A4* contains more than 30 reported polymorphisms, but this variation is either rare or does not have major functional consequences for enzyme function. *CYP3A4* polymorphisms thereby result in a unimodal distribution of drug clearance, likely due to phenotypic variation influenced by food or other environmental factors. Thus, they are not typically used in the clinical setting.

Unlike *CYP2D6, CYP2C19,* or *CYP2C9,* only a small number of rare variations cause loss of CYP3A4 activity.[48]

## Solute Carrier Organic Anion Transporter Family Member 1B1

Solute carrier organic anion transporter family member 1B1 (*SLCO1B1*) encodes a transporter in the liver that facilitates the uptake of many endogenous compounds and drugs,

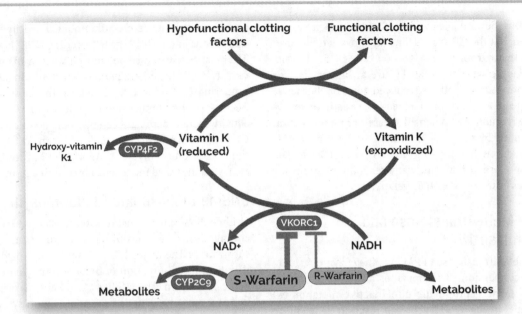

**FIGURE 6-1.** Visual representation of genes involved in warfarin metabolism and warfarin mechanism of action. Warfarin is administered via a racemic mixture of the *R*- and *S*-stereoisomers. The *S*-warfarin is markedly more potent than the *R*-warfarin and is metabolized predominantly by *CYP2C9*. Warfarin's mechanism of action involves inhibiting vitamin K epoxide reductase, encoded by *VKORC1*, and this limits the availability of reduced vitamin K, leading to decreased formation of functionally active clotting factors. *CYP4F2* functionally removes vitamin K from the vitamin K cycle by metabolizing reduced vitamin K to hydroxyl-vitamin K1.

## MINICASE 3

### Immunosuppressant Pharmacogenetics

D.L. is a 2-year-old African American girl who has renal dysplasia and recently received a kidney transplant. After the transplant, she was started on the usual dose of 0.1 mg/kg of tacrolimus twice a day. After a tacrolimus trough concentration was low, her dose was doubled. Two days later, a trough concentration was high. Her trough concentrations continued to vacillate above and below the target range as the dose was adjusted several times. After a dose of 0.3 mg/kg, D.L. suffered a seizure. The tacrolimus was held, and she developed acute kidney injury and rejection. *CYP3A5* testing was ordered at this time, with a genotype result of *1/*3 (expresser). In addition, azathioprine was started due to mycophenolic acid–related diarrhea. She became neutropenic, so TPMT phenotyping was ordered. (The TPMT phenotyping assay detects the TPMT enzyme activity in red blood cells.) After the results came back as TPMT normal metabolizer, the pharmacogenetics team was consulted, and it was discovered she had a blood transfusion prior to the TPMT phenotyping sample being drawn. The *TPMT* genotype test was ordered, resulting in a *1/*3A intermediate metabolizer. She developed a fever and was started on fluconazole. She was subsequently trialed on tacrolimus again, and the dose was adjusted due to the drug–drug interaction between fluconazole and tacrolimus.

QUESTION: Which pharmacogene(s) influence tacrolimus and azathioprine?

DISCUSSION: Up to 50% of the interpatient variability in tacrolimus pharmacokinetics is explained by variants in *CYP3A5*. This patient is an expresser and likely needs a higher-than-standard starting dose of tacrolimus. Myelosuppression related to azathioprine is influenced by *TPMT* and *NUDT15*. This patient is a TPMT intermediate metabolizer and may require reduced doses of thiopurines.

QUESTION: Why were the TPMT phenotyping and genotyping inconsistent?

DISCUSSION: The TPMT phenotype is testing with an assay for the enzyme's activity in red blood cells. Given the patient had a blood transfusion recently, the enzyme activity was for the transfused red blood cells, indicating normal activity. However, the genotyping was subsequently performed on the patient's white blood cells, where the genotype indicated she was an intermediate metabolizer.

QUESTION: What contributed to the seizures this patient experienced?

DISCUSSION: In a *CYP3A5* expresser, the tacrolimus trough concentrations are lower than expected. When the dose is increased, the trough concentration increases, as does the maximal concentration. This patient likely experienced a seizure because of the high maximal concentration of tacrolimus. The clinical team was comfortable initiating tacrolimus again when fluconazole was also part of the medication regimen because it inhibits CYP3A4, which slows the metabolism of tacrolimus, and lower doses are needed to receive the same exposure and trough concentrations. Some studies have demonstrated an association with the *CYP3A4*22* allele and tacrolimus pharmacokinetics; however, it is not included in the CPIC guideline.

including statins. Several alleles with decreased function have been described, but the CPIC guideline for simvastatin focuses on the alleles that harbor the rs4149056 C allele (*5, *15, *46, and *47).[49] People with these alleles are at higher risk for simvastatin-induced myopathy, so reduced doses or alternative lipid-lowering agents are recommended (pravastatin or rosuvastatin).[50] The frequency of having decreased or poor function varies significantly by race group, from 6% in Africans to 43% in Europeans. Although other drugs are substrates of SLCO1B1/OATP1B1, there are not currently any recommendations for adjusting doses based on *SLCO1B1* genotype.

## Thiopurine Methyltransferase and Nudix Hydrolase 15

Thiopurine methyltransferase (TPMT) is the enzyme responsible for the conversion of thiopurines azathioprine, thioguanine, and 6-mercaptopurine into inactive metabolites. Genetic variants in the *TPMT* gene can result in deficient or absent TPMT activity, leading to severe hematologic adverse effects with azathioprine or 6-mercaptopurine (6-MP) treatment. The most common variants in *TPMT* are referred to as *TPMT*\*2 (rs1800460), \*3A (rs1800460 and rs1142345), and \*3C (rs1142345). Individuals with one copy of a variant allele make up approximately 10% of the white population and require dose reductions of approximately 50%.[51,52] Individuals with two no-function alleles require dose reductions of thiopurines like 6-MP on the magnitude of 90% to avoid hematologic toxicity.

More recently, variants in nudix hydrolase 15 (*NUDT15*) were discovered to influence thiopurine tolerability in patients with leukemia and inflammatory bowel disease.[53,54] This enzyme inactivates thioguanine nucleotides; reduced or absent function is associated with more active metabolites of thiopurines. The \*2 and \*3 alleles confer no enzymatic function, resulting in high concentrations of active metabolites and an increased risk for myelosuppression. CPIC recommends reduced dosing in carriers of these alleles.[55] These alleles are most common in Asians and Hispanics, in whom *TPMT* no function alleles are less common.

Thiopurines are used in the treatment of childhood acute lymphoblastic leukemia and rheumatoid arthritis, the prevention of renal allograft rejection, and the management of inflammatory bowel disease. The FDA-approved drug label for mercaptopurine states that patients with severe myelosuppression should be evaluated for TPMT or NUDT15 deficiency while taking the drug and that patients with homozygous TPMT or NUDT15 deficiency require substantial dose reductions.[56] Many major academic medical centers routinely perform *TPMT* genotyping or activity testing prior to thiopurine dosing for leukemia, although the frequency of testing is lower in other specialties (eg, gastroenterology and rheumatology).[57]

## Dihydropyrimidine Dehydrogenase

Dihydropyrimidine dehydrogenase (DPD) metabolizes fluoropyrimidine agents (5-fluorouracil, capecitabine, and tegafur) commonly used in the treatment of solid organ tumors. In the mid-1980s, it was recognized that deficiencies in DPD were heritable and associated with severe 5-fluorouracil toxicity.[58,59] Many polymorphisms in the *DPYD* gene, encoding DPD, have been found. The most widely studied polymorphism is in an intron, IVS14 +1 G>A (*DPYD*\*2A, rs3918290), which results in a splicing defect rendering *DPYD* inactive, have been the most widely studied. Because of the number and complexity of *DPYD* variants, an activity score system has been implemented similar to *CYP2D6*. CPIC guidelines have been published with dosing recommendations based on genotype.[60,61] As with TPMT testing, DPD deficiency can be tested for genetically or with enzymatic testing.[62,63]

## Uridine Diphosphate Glucuronosyltransferase

Uridine diphosphate glucuronosyltransferases mediate phase II conjugation of glucuronic acid of drugs and endogenous substrates.[64] The major UGT1A subfamily enzyme, UGT1A1, is critical for elimination of bilirubin, the main byproduct of heme catabolism. The *UGT1A1*\*28 allele was originally identified as a causative genetic variant of Gilbert syndrome, a form of mild unconjugated hyperbilirubinemia.[65] Since then, multiple *UGT1A1* alleles have been identified that reduce the transcription of *UGT1A1*, making patients more susceptible to drugs that inhibit UGT1A1-mediated glucuronidation of bilirubin. Such drugs include atazanavir, which is a protease inhibitor used to treat HIV. To avoid hyperbilirubinemia associated with atazanavir, guidelines recommend avoiding atazanavir in UGT1A1 poor metabolizers. It is important to note that while *UGT1A1* (and *G6PD* described later) have guidelines to support clinical intervention based on pharmacogenetic testing, these enzymes have no direct role in the metabolism of their associated drugs. In these cases, drug therapy increases the risk for adverse reactions; therefore, guidelines recommend that these drugs be avoided in persons with enzymatic deficiencies.[64,66]

## Glucose-6-Phosphate Dehydrogenase

Glucose-6-phosphate dehydrogenase (G6PD) is an enzyme that produces reduced nicotinamide adenine dinucleotide phosphate (NADPH) from NADPH.[66,67] G6PD is particularly important in erythrocytes because in these cells G6PD is one of the only available sources of NADPH, which is required to protect erythrocytes from oxidative stress. Individuals who are deficient in G6PD have erythrocytes with a much-reduced capacity for NADPH production and a compromised ability to handle oxidative stress. G6PD-deficient individuals are more susceptible to hemolytic anemia resulting from drug-induced lysis from drugs such as rasburicase, which is used to treat hyperuricemia. Multiple polymorphisms in *G6PD* are known to cause G6PD deficiency, and a World Health Organization (WHO) class system is available to classify individuals who are G6PD deficient.[67] Accordingly, a guideline is available to guide the use of *G6PD* genotyping results to avoid rasburicase in G6PD deficient individuals. An interesting aspect of *G6PD* genotyping is that the gene is present on the X chromosome; thus, WHO classifications are primarily based on assessments in males, who have only one copy of the gene. Tests for G6PD deficiency can thereby result in incidental disease findings, including diagnosis of Klinefelter's syndrome, a rare genetic disease in male patients who have an extra X chromosome.

## Determination of Clinical Significance

When deciding whether drug metabolism polymorphisms might be clinically significant for particular drugs, it is helpful to consider three main factors. First, is the drug metabolism enzyme of interest an important route of elimination for the drug in question? If not, even functional polymorphisms in this gene may not have a great impact on the pharmacokinetics of the drug. Second, does the medication of interest have a narrow therapeutic index or steep exposure/response relationship? If not, changes in plasma concentrations may not be great enough to influence the dose-response relationship. Third, are other therapeutic alternatives available to the medication in question? If so, these alternatives may have other routes of metabolism that are not polymorphic, and the variability in pharmacokinetics could be avoided altogether. Determination of clinical significance for pharmacodynamic and immune-related genes requires different considerations, such as whether alternative agents are available and the associated risks (or cost) of alternative agents.

# DRUG TARGET–RELATED MOLECULAR TESTS

## Germline Variation and Genotype-Guided Therapy

Although pharmacokinetics is concerned with absorption, distribution, metabolism, and excretion, pharmacodynamics is concerned with drug effects on target molecules, tissues, and physiologic processes. This section discusses examples of how variation in genes that encode drug targets can affect drug disposition. There are illustrative examples in cardiology, oncology, infectious diseases, and others in which consideration of genetic variation affecting pharmacodynamics may improve drug therapy. This section focuses on germline mutations, which are heritable mutations present in all nucleated cells, rather than somatic mutations, which occur during the lifespan of an individual and are typically associated with cancer. Warfarin is the main example discussed and includes both pharmacokinetic and pharmacodynamic genes that can be used to improve dose prediction. The next section focuses on illustrative examples of drug-target related molecular tests for somatic mutations in oncology.

### Warfarin Pharmacogenetics

Warfarin is one of the most commonly prescribed anticoagulants for the treatment and prevention of thrombosis. Warfarin has a narrow therapeutic range (as measured by the international normalized ratio [INR]) below which thrombosis risk is increased and above which bleeding risk is increased. Although patient-specific factors such as age, sex, race, and diet partially explain variability in warfarin response, these factors do not reliably predict the likelihood of efficacy or bleeding risk. As such, investigators have studied the role of genetic variants in an enzyme responsible for warfarin's metabolism (CYP2C9) and vitamin K epoxide reductase complex subunit 1 (VKORC1) on warfarin responses (Figure 6-1). These studies have investigated the impact of genetic and nongenetic factors on endpoints related to INR, bleeding, and clinical efficacy.

VKORC1 catalyzes the conversion of vitamin K-epoxide to vitamin K, which is the rate-limiting step in vitamin K recycling.[68] Warfarin exerts its anticoagulant effect through inhibition of VKORC1, which in turn limits availability of reduced vitamin K, leading to decreased formation of functionally active clotting factors.[40] Pharmacogenetic studies have interrogated VKORC1 polymorphisms and determined that a common variant upstream of VKORC1 (c.-1639G>A, rs9923231) is significantly associated with warfarin sensitivity, and patients with one or two c.-1639G>A alleles require progressively lower warfarin doses than –1639G/G homozygotes. CYP2C9 is the major metabolic route for the more potent warfarin enantiomer S-warfarin. The CYP2C9*1 allele is associated with full metabolic capacity, while the well-studied *2 (rs1799853) and *3 (rs1057910) alleles are associated with decreased metabolic activity, diminished warfarin clearance, and lower warfarin dose requirements.[69-74] By extension, these variant carriers exhibit longer than normal time to achieve target INR and are at increased risk for bleeding.[75] Another CYP enzyme, CYP4F2, plays no direct role in the metabolism of warfarin, but CYP4F2 polymorphisms affect stable warfarin dose because CYP4F2 removes reduced vitamin K from the vitamin K cycle. Taken together, CYP2C9, CYP4F2, and VKORC1 polymorphisms, when considered with clinical correlates of warfarin dose, explain approximately 50% of the variability in warfarin dose requirements.[76,77] Dosing algorithms, including pharmacogenetic variation and clinical information, are continually being developed and tested, and the FDA updated the warfarin label with estimated doses by genotype.[78-80] Guidelines also have been published with recommendations for clinical interpretation of warfarin pharmacogenetics data.[40,80]

The CYP2C9*2 and *3 variants are common in individuals with European ancestry and were preferentially incorporated into genotype-guided warfarin dosing algorithms due in part to the fact that most of the evidence was generated in individuals with European ancestry.[81] Other CYP2C9 variants are associated with warfarin dose requirements in African Americans include CYP2C9*5, CYP2C9*6, CYP2C9*8, and CYP2C9*11.).[82-84] Another SNP in the CYP2C cluster of genes, rs12777823, has also been observed to have an important impact on warfarin dose in African Americans.[85] Early warfarin dosing guidelines did not differentiate recommendations based on race, but subsequent guidelines advise against the use of warfarin dosing algorithms in African Americans if CYP2C9*5, *6, *8, *11 have not been interrogated. For patients who do not report West African ancestry, CPIC guidelines recommend the use of a pharmacogenetic algorithm that includes VKORC1-1639G>A and CYP2C9*2 and *3 variants.[86] The additional variants CYP2C9*5, *6, *8, *11 can be included in the dosing algorithm or used to decrease the warfarin dose by 15% to 30% in variant carriers. The CYP4F2*3 allele can also be included in the dosing algorithm or used to increase warfarin dose 5% to 10%. Warfarin pharmacogenetics have been complicated by contradictory prospective clinical trials assessing pharmacogenetic-guided versus traditional dosing.[87-90] The U.S.-based study was called Clarification of Optimal Anticoagulation Through Genetics (COAG),[88] and the two European studies were called European Pharmacogenetics of Anticoagulant Therapy.[89,90] All of the studies had the same primary endpoint: time in the therapeutic range. To briefly summarize the trials' findings related to the primary outcome, pharmacogenetic-guided dosing was superior to empirical dosing; however, pharmacogenetic-guided dosing was not superior to a clinical dosing algorithm.[87-90] Further complicating the issue is that in COAG, African Americans fared significantly worse with a pharmacogenetic dosing algorithm compared with the clinical algorithm.[88] The pharmacogenetic algorithm used in these studies did not include variants that are associated with warfarin dose requirements in African Americans (CYP2C9*5, CYP2C9*6, CYP2C9*8, CYP2C9*11, and rs12777823).[82-84] The exclusion of these variants from the algorithm may have overestimated the dose in African American study subjects.[82] Although time in the therapeutic range (primary endpoint) did not differ between the groups, major bleeding was more common in the clinically guided dosing arm of the COAG trial compared with the genotype-guided dosing arm (HR 0.36; 95% CI 0.15-0.86; $P$ = .021).[88] Other randomized controlled trials have since been published that support implementation of genotype-guided warfarin dosing, including the Genetic Informatics Trial conducted primarily in white persons.[91,92]

## Tumor Molecular Testing to Guide Therapy Choices

In oncology, the advances in genomic technologies and the realization that many tumors can be subdivided in molecular subsets defined by specific genomic alterations have fueled the development of therapeutic agents targeting these molecular alterations. Therefore, genomic testing to identify patients to be considered for a specific therapy based on the patient's tumor molecular classification (and germline variation, for some drugs) is becoming the standard of care. Also, in addition to germline (inherited) variations, tumor cells also can exhibit acquired (somatic) variations only present in the tumor tissue. This adds a layer of complexity to molecular testing, involving the acquisition and processing of tumor tissue with adequate quality and quantity to accommodate the test of interest.

It is important to keep in mind that the biological understanding of the molecular landscape of tumors is constantly evolving, as are the genomic technologies used to assess molecular alterations in tumor samples, circulating tumor cells or cell-free tumor DNA. This section deals with two illustrative examples of molecular alterations in tumors at the gene and protein level used to guide therapy: (1) the epidermal growth factor receptor tyrosine kinase inhibitors (EGFR TKIs) erlotinib, gefitinib, and afatinib in EGFR mutation-positive non–small-cell lung cancer (NSCLC); and (2) the serine/threonine-protein kinase B-raf (BRAF) inhibitors vemurafenib and dabrafenib in BRAF mutation-positive melanoma.

### Epidermal Growth Factor Receptor Mutation-Positive Non–Small-Cell Lung Cancer and Epidermal Growth Factor Receptor Tyrosine Kinase Inhibitors

Epidermal growth factor receptor aberrant signaling is associated with development and prognosis of certain cancers. EGFR mutation-positive NSCLC depends on EGFR signaling for proliferation and survival. Therefore, EGFR therapeutic inhibition results in blockage of important processes in the pathogenesis of lung cancers.[93]

In NSCLC, the presence of certain EGFR-activating mutations in the tumor (mostly in exons 18 to 21 of the EGFR gene) defines a molecular subset of lung cancer associated with increased sensitivity to EGFR TKIs such as erlotinib, gefitinib, and afatinib in the metastatic setting. The best documented EGFR TKI-sensitizing mutations are exon 19 deletions and L858R in exon 21, representing approximately 90% of reported EGFR mutations in NSCLC. The remaining 10% of EGFR mutations represent a heterogeneous, less common, and less characterized group of mutations. EGFR mutations are most common in East Asians (35% versus 10% in white persons), female never-smokers, and patients with adenocarcinoma histology.[94,95] In a 2004 landmark study, Lynch and colleagues identified mutations in the EGFR gene in tumors of patients with NSCLC who were responsive to gefitinib.[96] Sensitivity and specificity were 89% and 100%, respectively; positive and negative predictive values were 100% and 88%. Since this publication, several clinical trials have prospectively tested the impact of EGFR mutations on clinical response to EGFR TKIs among patients with lung cancer. Results from these studies have underscored the importance of tumor molecular profiling, and EGFR mutation testing is currently a standard procedure in guiding therapy choices for advanced NSCLC.[97-99] First-generation (gefitinib, erlotinib) and second-generation (afatinib) EGFR TKIs are FDA approved for the first-line treatment of patients with metastatic NSCLC whose tumors have EGFR exon 19 deletions or exon 21 (L858R) substitution mutations as detected by an FDA-approved test. These drugs were approved in conjunction with polymerase chain reaction (PCR)-based companion diagnostic tests designed to detect defined EGFR mutations in patients considered for therapy with any of these drugs.

### BRAF Mutation-Positive Melanoma and BRAF Pathway Inhibitors

The presence of certain BRAF mutations defines a molecular subset of melanoma especially sensitive to inhibition by BRAF inhibitors as single agents or in combination with MEK inhibitors. Vemurafenib and dabrafenib are BRAF inhibitors indicated for the treatment of patients with unresectable or metastatic melanoma with BRAF V600E mutation as detected by an FDA-approved test. Mutated BRAF proteins often have elevated kinase activity leading to aberrant activation of survival and antiapoptotic signaling pathways in the tumor cells.[100] Approximately 40% to 60% of cutaneous melanomas are positive for BRAF V600 mutations. Among these, the V600E mutations constitute 80% to 90% of reported V600 BRAF mutations, but other less common BRAF mutations, such as V600K and V600D, also occur. Their role in conferring sensitivity to BRAF inhibitors, however, is not as well documented.[101]

As with other therapeutic agents targeting specific tumor molecular alterations, vemurafenib and dabrafenib also were developed along with PCR-based companion diagnostic tests designed to identify specific BRAF V600 mutations.[102] Currently,

BRAF inhibitors are not indicated for patients with wild-type *BRAF* melanoma because of the potential of paradoxical activation of the mitogen-activated protein kinase pathway and tumor promotion in certain cellular contexts, which highlights the importance of understanding test performance for determining therapy eligibility and the consequences of false-positive and false-negative results.[103]

## Resistance to Targeted Therapy

Only a percentage of patients respond to targeted therapies, and despite initial clinical benefit, responders often develop resistance. Elucidating underlying mechanisms of primary or acquired resistance at a molecular level is an intense area of research in oncology. For example, somatic point mutations in the *KRAS* gene, most commonly found in codons 12 and 13, have been strongly associated with primary resistance to the anti-EGFR monoclonal antibodies panitumumab and cetuximab in colorectal cancer. K-ras is downstream of EGFR signaling, so activating mutations in *KRAS* bypass the EGFR inhibition. Therefore, these antibodies are not indicated for colorectal cancer patients with tumors positive for these mutations. Of note, different *KRAS* mutations may not predict to the same extent resistance to anti-EGFR antibodies.[104] Point mutations, gene amplifications, changes in protein expression, and activation of alternate pathways are among the mechanisms implicated in resistance.[105] Molecular assays to identify these alterations and evaluate their clinical significance are in different stages of development. This is illustrated by osimertinib, which is a third-generation irreversible EGFR TKI first approved in conjunction with a PCR-based companion diagnostic assay for patients with metastatic *EGFR* T790M mutation-positive NSCLC who have progressed on or after EGFR TKI therapy. The *EGFR* T790M second-site mutation accounts for approximately 50% of the reported cases of acquired resistance to the reversible EGFR TKIs erlotinib and gefitinib. It was subsequently approved as first-line therapy for metastatic NSCLC to anticipate and avoid the development of the *EGFR* T790M mutation. Many other mechanisms of resistance to EGFR TKIs involving different molecular alterations have been reported in NSCLC.[106]

# IMMUNE-RELATED ADVERSE REACTIONS AND MOLECULAR TESTS

Variants in immune-related genes are increasingly being associated with drug-induced adverse events. In particular, human leukocyte antigen (HLA) screening has emerged as a preventive strategy for immune-mediated adverse drug reactions (IM-ADRs). *HLA* alleles are highly polymorphic and, within the genome-wide association study catalogue, more phenotype associations have been identified in the HLA region than any other region of the genome.[107,108] Immune response is modulated by the HLA system, and amino acid sequences of each HLA molecule determine peptide binding and antigen presentation to T-lymphocytes.[109] Variation in HLA is critical to prevent

allograft rejection and plays a key role in determining susceptibility to infection and autoimmune disease.

One of the earliest examples of HLA-associated IM-ADRs was with abacavir hypersensitivity reaction (HSR), for which a strong association was observed with *HLA-B\*57:01*.[110,111] Immune-mediated hypersensitivity reactions occur in 5% to 8% of patients treated with abacavir, usually within the first 6 weeks of treatment. The presence of at least one *HLA-B\*57:01* allele is necessary for the HSR reaction to occur, although the *HLA-B\*57:01* allele is not sufficient to predict HSR. Prospective randomized-controlled trials demonstrated that screening for the *HLA-B\*5701* allele eliminated immunologically confirmed hypersensitivity reactions with a negative predictive value of 100% and a positive predictive value of 47.9%.[111] Current HIV treatment guidelines recommend screening for *HLA-B\*5701* before initiation of an abacavir-containing treatment regimen.[10,112,113]

Subsequently, *HLA-B\*15:02* and *HLA-A\*31:01* were observed to be strongly associated with carbamazepine-induced Stevens-Johnson syndrome,[114-116] which is a severe, cutaneous immune-mediated reaction to several classes of drugs, including antiepileptics, antibiotics, and antivirals. *HLA-B\*15:02* has also been associated with IM-ADRs to other anticonvulsants, including oxcarbazepine, phenytoin, and lamotrigine.[107] Similarly, IM-ADRs caused by allopurinol, a drug used to treat gout and hyperuricemia, are associated with *HLA-B\*58:01*.[117]

Multiple guidelines are available that support the use of *HLA* allelic information to guide drug selection (Table 6-2). In these guidelines, if a patient carries an associated *HLA* allele, then the recommendation is to avoid that agent.[43,113,118,119] This is true whether the patient carries one or two copies of the *HLA* allele. Importantly, no dose adjustments are recommended based on *HLA* alleles given these alleles have no role in the metabolism or pharmacologic action of these drugs. In most cases, these alleles have a high negative predictive value (usually near 100%) but low positive predictive value for the IM-ADR. This indicates that the *HLA* allele is generally necessary to elicit the reaction in the presence of the drug, but drug treatment and the presence of an *HLA* allele are not deterministic for the IM-ADR. Furthermore, allele frequencies vary dramatically by race. In the case of *HLA-B\*15:02* and *HLA-B\*57:01*, carriage of these alleles is essentially nonexistent in many African populations but is as high as 20% in some Asian populations. This implies that the use of *HLA* screening to prevent IM-ADRs may only be cost-effective in populations that have increased frequencies of the associated *HLA* alleles.

## GENOTYPING PLATFORMS

Many commercial genetic tests are available for pharmacogenetic-related genes or gene panels. The AmpliChip (Roche Molecular Diagnostics, Basel, Switzerland) microarray is one such example that is FDA-cleared. It provides analysis for *CYP2D6* and *CYP2C19* genotypes to predict enzymatic activities. The assay tests for up to 33 *CYP2D6* alleles, including gene duplications and three *CYP2C19* variants, and includes software to predict the drug metabolism phenotype based on the combination of alleles present (eg, normal, intermediate, poor, and ultrarapid metabolizers). Luminex xTAG CYP2D6 Kit (Luminex Corporation, Austin, TX) is another FDA-cleared test that tests for 15 *CYP2D6* alleles as well as gene duplications. Because commercially available genetic testing options change frequently, we do not discuss all available tests. However, the Genetic Testing Registry provides a central location for voluntary submission of genetic test information by providers (www .ncbi.nlm.nih.gov/gtr/). Most pharmacogenomic testing panels are ordered by a provider rather than a patient, and many have not received FDA approval because they are considered laboratory-developed tests. The first and only pharmacogenetic test given FDA authorization for direct-to-consumer testing (rather than being ordered by a provider) is provided by 23andMe (Sunnyvale, CA).

Pharmacogenetic genotyping assays do have two limitations with which the clinician should be familiar: (1) New alleles that alter function are constantly being discovered, so there are patients who will not be perfectly assigned to a phenotype group or could be inappropriately assigned the *1/*1 genotype by default because these alleles are untested. (2) Because genotyping does not directly measure metabolic activity or drug concentrations, the effect of drug interactions on the drug metabolizing phenotype is not captured by the test. In other words, a person may genotypically be a normal metabolizer but phenotypically be a poor metabolizer because the person is taking a drug that inhibits the particular CYP450 enzyme. This limitation highlights the importance of proper patient-specific interpretation of CYP genotyping results in clinical practice.

To accommodate the growing number of genetic variants of (potential) clinical significance, clinical testing is moving from single variants to multiplexed panels that can simultaneously interrogate a limited number of variants (polymorphisms and hotspot mutations). Next-generation sequencing (NGS) technologies, although not yet implemented in routine practice, provide even more comprehensive genomic analysis, including genome copy number changes and structural rearrangements, which are not captured by multiplexed panels. NGS technologies can perform whole-genome sequencing, targeted sequencing, including whole-exome sequencing, transcriptome analysis, and epigenetic profiling. NGS-based approaches have been used to uncover underlying disease biology and to identify markers influencing response to therapies. In the context of clinical oncology, high-throughput gene sequencing has the potential to change patient care from diagnosis to disease management. However, the integration and accurate biological interpretation of the large genomic data generated by these platforms are still major challenges for clinical implementation.[120-122]

The cost of pharmacogenetic testing varies depending on the number of alleles being tested. Although multigene arrays are more cost-effective than genotyping individual SNPs, they currently do not have current procedural terminology codes for reimbursement; thus, genotyping for clinical care is often done as individual tests.[123] The turnaround time also varies, but it is usually 24 to 96 hours. In institutions in which the clinical laboratory is onsite, turnaround could be as fast as 4 hours depending on the assay. Generally, genotyping results that are to be used in the clinical care of patients need to be generated from certified laboratories (such as those approved or certified by the Clinical Laboratory Improvements Amendments [CLIA] or the College of Pathologists [CAP]). Germline variation is stable throughout a person's lifetime; therefore, in general, it only needs to be done once. However, it is important to note which alleles are tested because additional alleles may have been discovered, which will require additional testing to gain information on those alleles.

## Clinical Implementation of Pharmacogenomics

Perhaps the biggest barrier to the application of pharmacogenetics is the inability to apply genotype results. This application would require integration into the electronic health record and adequate clinical decision support to guide practitioners in the use of pharmacogenetic data. In this regard, the pharmacogenetics testing process could be interdisciplinary, involving physicians, translational scientists, clinical pharmacists, and others. Additionally, accreditation standards such as those put forth by The Joint Commission, CLIA, CAP and others will have to be addressed when formally incorporating pharmacogenetic testing into institution-based practice. Multiple medical centers, including primarily large academic medical centers, have addressed many of these issues and are implementing pharmacogenomics in clinical care. Developing this infrastructure is a key component of some NIH-supported resources such as eMERGE and IGNITE.

As mentioned elsewhere in the chapter, organizations, including the NACB and CPIC, are working in a multidisciplinary fashion to address issues related to pharmacogenetic test methodology, standardization and quality control/assurance of tests, selection of appropriate test panels, reporting and interpretation of results, and other issues related to testing applied in clinical practice.[9,12,19,22,124] Although expansive in scope, the NACB guidelines specifically highlight the role of the clinical laboratory in the development of genotyping strategies that maximize test performance (ie, sensitivity and specificity) for clinical application. Furthermore, guideline recommendations developed the following criteria for a pharmacogenetic test to be clinically useful: (1) *analytical reliability* (consistent measurement of the genotype/allele tested); (2) *operational implementation* (operational characteristics should not be beyond the complexity level certified by CLIA for reference laboratories); (3) *clinical predictive power* (specificity and sensitivity consistent with other diagnostics in use); and (4) *compatibility with therapeutic management* (interpretation of genotype results should inform clinical decision-making). Interestingly, model examples outlined by the guidelines for drugs in which pharmacogenetics can be implemented include warfarin (*CYP2C9* and *VKORC1*) and irinotecan (*UGT1A1*). CPIC has taken the approach of publishing clinical practice guidelines for specific drug/gene pairs as enough data becomes available to warrant clinical action based on genotype. A sample of drug/gene pairs that contain pharmacogenetic information, which can inform dosing or patient selection, is shown in Table 6-2.

## SUMMARY

Pharmacogenetics is currently being used most widely in hematology/oncology as well as infectious disease and holds the promise of improving patient care by adding another dimension to therapeutic drug monitoring in other diseases. As the evidence for pharmacogenetic relationships increases and the cost of genotyping decreases, the use of genetic information will likely be applied to chronic drug therapy for agents with narrow therapeutic indices, with critical pathways of metabolism and bioactivation, and with severe adverse drug reactions. The field of pharmacogenetics is evolving rapidly. Consequently, specific information regarding molecular tests and labeling information is likely to constantly change. Basic skills in interpreting genetic information will serve as an important foundation for laboratory medicine and drug therapy as more clinical applications of pharmacogenetics emerge.

For pharmacogenetics to translate to practice, the research and clinical communities jointly must create a meaningful level of evidence in support of pharmacogenetics-enhanced, therapeutic decision-making. Because of their unique training and position in the healthcare sector, pharmacists can foresee the forefront of pharmacogenetics research and application. Pharmacists will likely be called upon to synthesize evidence-based practices for incorporating genetic information into treatment algorithms. Once a genetic biomarker is validated (eg, thiopurine pharmacogenetics), clinicians (including pharmacists) will be responsible for the appropriate use and interpretation of the genetic test. The pharmacist's drug and disease expertise, coupled with an understanding of pharmacogenetic principles, may lead to a revolutionary treatment paradigm with enhanced patient outcome as the ultimate goal.

## LEARNING POINTS

### 1. What types of genes could impact drug response?

**ANSWER:** Genes that influence the pharmacokinetics (eg, drug metabolism enzymes or drug transporters) and pharmacodynamics (eg, drug targets) of a drug or immune response to a drug could impact drug response. Genetic variation that impacts pharmacogenetics could be germline (ie, host DNA) or somatic (eg, tumor DNA).

### 2. How might pharmacogenomics enhance therapeutic drug monitoring and management?

**ANSWER:** Traditional patient-specific factors such as age, sex, renal function, hepatic function, and body weight are frequently used to determine the appropriateness of a particular drug or dose for an individual. However, these factors only partially account for the likelihood of efficacy or toxicity. As our knowledge of how genetic variability impacts drug response is solidified, we can begin to incorporate pharmacogenetic information into algorithms for optimizing pharmacotherapy for individual patients and move toward personalized medicine.

### 3. Who is likely to be involved in incorporating pharmacogenomics into clinical decision-making?

**ANSWER:** The incorporation of pharmacogenomics requires an interdisciplinary team of healthcare providers with knowledge of the specific pharmacological properties of individual drugs, molecular biology, genetics, laboratory medicine, clinical medicine, genetic counseling, and economics. In addition, patients and consumers will likely be active participants and drivers of the use of genetic tests in clinical practice.

## ACKNOWLEDGMENTS

The authors would like to acknowledge the contributions of Dr. Amber L. Beitelshees and Dr. Rosane Charlab, who authored this chapter in previous editions of this textbook. The authors would also like to acknowledge Ms. Hayley Patterson for her graphic design assistance and administrative assistance with this chapter.

## REFERENCES

1. Evans DA, Manley KA, Mckusick VA. Genetic control of isoniazid metabolism in man. *BMJ*. 1960;2(5197):485-491.PubMed

2. Hughes HB, Biehl JP, Jones AP, Schmidt LH. Metabolism of isoniazid in man as related to the occurrence of peripheral neuritis. *Am Rev Tuberc*. 1954;70(2):266-273.PubMed

3. Alving AS, Carson PE, Flanagan CL, Ickes CE. Enzymatic deficiency in primaquine-sensitive erythrocytes. *Science*. 1956;124(3220):484-485. PubMed

4. Vesell ES, Page JG. Genetic control of the phenobarbital-induced shortening of plasma antipyrine half-lives in man. *J Clin Invest*. 1969;48(12):2202-2209. PubMed

5. Volpi S, Bult CJ, Chisholm RL, et al. Research directions in the clinical implementation of pharmacogenomics: an overview of us programs and projects. *Clin Pharmacol Ther*. 2018;103(5):778-786.PubMed

6. Zineh I, Pebanco GD, Aquilante CL, et al. Discordance between availability of pharmacogenetics studies and pharmacogenetics-based prescribing information for the top 200 drugs. *Ann Pharmacother*. 2006;40(4):639-644.PubMed

7. Zineh I, Johnson JA. Pharmacogenetics of chronic cardiovascular drugs: applications and implications. *Expert Opin Pharmacother*. 2006;7(11): 1417-1427.PubMed

8. Jameson JL, Longo DL. Precision medicine: personalized, problematic, and promising. *N Engl J Med*. 2015;372(23):2229-2234.PubMed

9. Laboratory analysis and application of pharmacogenetics to clinical practice. Https://www.Aacc.Org/science-and-research/practice -guidelines/pharmacogenetics Accessed Feb 22, 2016.

10. Aberg JA, Gallant JE, Ghanem KG, et al. Primary care guidelines for the management of persons infected with HIV: 2013 update by the HIV Medicine Association of the Infectious Diseases Society of America. *Clin Infect Dis*. 2014;58(1):e1-e34.PubMed

11. Wright RS, Anderson JL, Adams CD, et al. 2011 ACCF/AHA focused update incorporated into the ACC/AHA 2007 guidelines for the management of patients with unstable angina/non-ST-elevation myocardial infarction: a report of the American College Of Cardiology Foundation/American Heart Association Task Force on practice guidelines developed in collaboration with the American academy Of Family Physicians, Society For Cardiovascular Angiography And Interventions, and The Society Of Thoracic Surgeons. *J Am Coll Cardiol*. 2011;57(19):e215-e367.PubMed

12. Relling MV, Klein TE. Cpic: Clinical pharmacogenetics implementation consortium of the pharmacogenomics research network. *Clin Pharmacol Ther*. 2011;89(3):464-467.PubMed

13. Roses AD. Pharmacogenetics and the practice of medicine. *Nature*. 2000;405(6788):857-865.PubMed

14. Haga SB, Burke W. Pharmacogenetic testing: not as simple as it seems. *Genet Med*. 2008;10(6):391-395.PubMed

15. Gaedigk A, Whirl-Carrillo M, Pratt VM, et al. Pharmvar and the landscape of pharmacogenetic resources. *Clin Pharmacol Ther*. 2020;107(1):43-46.PubMed

16. Pratt VM, Cavallari LH, Del Tredici AL, et al. Recommendations for clinical warfarin genotyping allele selection: a report of The Association For Molecular *Pathology* and The College Of American Pathologists. *J Mol Diagn*. 2020;22(7):847-859.PubMed

17. Pratt VM, Cavallari LH, Del Tredici AL, et al. Recommendations for clinical cyp2c9 genotyping allele selection: A joint recommendation of the association for molecular pathology and College of American Pathologists. *J Mol Diagn*. 2019;21(5):746-755.PubMed

18. Pratt VM, Cavallari LH, Del Tredici AL, et al. *J Mol Diagn*. 2021 Sep;23(9):1047-1064. Epub 2021 Jun 10.PubMed

19. Caudle KE, Dunnenberger HM, Freimuth RR, et al. Standardizing terms for clinical pharmacogenetic test results: consensus terms from the Clinical Pharmacogenetics Implementation Consortium (CPIC). *Genet Med*. 2017;19(2):215-223.PubMed

20. Zineh I, Beitelshees AL, Gaedigk A, et al. Pharmacokinetics and CYP2D6 genotypes do not predict metoprolol adverse events or efficacy in hypertension. *Clin Pharmacol Ther*. 2004;76(6):536-544.PubMed

21. Gaedigk A, Sangkuhl K, Whirl-Carrillo M, et al. Prediction of CYP2D6 phenotype from genotype across world populations. *Genet Med*. 2017;19(1):69-76.PubMed

22. Caudle KE, Sangkuhl K, Whirl-Carrillo M, et al. Standardizing cyp2d6 genotype to phenotype translation: Consensus recommendations from the Clinical Pharmacogenetics Implementation Consortium and Dutch Pharmacogenetics Working Group. *Clin Transl Sci*. 2020;13(1):116-124. PubMed

23. Crews KR, Gaedigk A, Dunnenberger HM, et al. Clinical Pharmacogenetics Implementation Consortium guidelines for cytochrome P450 2D6 genotype and codeine therapy: 2014 update. *Clin Pharmacol Ther*. 2014;95(4):376-382.PubMed

24. Crews KR, Gaedigk A, Dunnenberger HM, et al. Clinical Pharmacogenetics Implementation Consortium (CPIC) guidelines for codeine therapy in the context of cytochrome P450 2D6 (CYP2D6) genotype. *Clin Pharmacol Ther*. 2012;91(2):321-326.PubMed

25. Bell GC, Caudle KE, Whirl-Carrillo M, et al. Clinical Pharmacogenetics Implementation Consortium (CPIC) guideline for CYP2D6 genotype and use of ondansetron and tropisetron. *Clin Pharmacol Ther*. 2017;102(2):213-218.PubMed

26. Goetz MP, Sangkuhl K, Guchelaar HJ, et al. Clinical pharmacogenetics implementation consortium (CPIC) guideline for CYP2D6 and tamoxifen therapy. *Clin Pharmacol Ther*. 2018;103(5):770-777.PubMed

27. Brown JT, Bishop JR, Sangkuhl K, et al. Clinical pharmacogenetics implementation consortium guideline for cytochrome p450 (CYP)2D6 genotype and atomoxetine therapy. *Clin Pharmacol Ther*. 2019;106(1): 94-102.PubMed

28. Hicks JK, Sangkuhl K, Swen JJ, et al. Clinical pharmacogenetics implementation consortium guideline (CPIC) for CYP2D6 and CYP2C19 genotypes and dosing of tricyclic antidepressants: 2016 update. *Clin Pharmacol Ther*. 2017;102(1):37-44.PubMed

29. Hicks JK, Bishop JR, Sangkuhl K, et al. Clinical pharmacogenetics implementation consortium (CPIC) guideline for cyp2d6 and cyp2c19 genotypes and dosing of selective serotonin reuptake inhibitors. *Clin Pharmacol Ther*. 2015;98(2):127-134.PubMed

30. Scott SA, Sangkuhl K, Gardner EE, et al. Clinical Pharmacogenetics Implementation Consortium guidelines for cytochrome P450-2C19 (CYP2C19) genotype and clopidogrel therapy. *Clin Pharmacol Ther*. 2011;90(2):328-332.PubMed

31. Scott SA, Sangkuhl K, Stein CM, et al. Clinical Pharmacogenetics Implementation Consortium guidelines for CYP2C19 genotype and clopidogrel therapy: 2013 update. *Clin Pharmacol Ther*. 2013;94(3): 317-323.PubMed

32. Pratt VM, Del Tredici AL, Hachad H, et al. Recommendations for clinical CYP2C19 genotyping allele selection: A report of the association for molecular pathology. *J Mol Diagn*. 2018;20(3):269-276.PubMed

33. Umemura K, Furuta T, Kondo K. The common gene variants of CYP2C19 affect pharmacokinetics and pharmacodynamics in an active metabolite of clopidogrel in healthy subjects. *J Thromb Haemost*. 2008;6(8): 1439-1441.PubMed

34. Shuldiner AR, O'Connell JR, Bliden KP, et al. Association of cytochrome P450 2C19 genotype with the antiplatelet effect and clinical efficacy of clopidogrel therapy. *JAMA*. 2009;302(8):849-857.PubMed

35. Hulot JS, Collet JP, Cayla G, et al. CYP2C19 but not PON1 genetic variants influence clopidogrel pharmacokinetics, pharmacodynamics, and clinical efficacy in post-myocardial infarction patients. *Circ Cardiovasc Interv*. 2011;4(5):422-428.PubMed

36. Mega JL, Close SL, Wiviott SD, et al. Cytochrome p-450 polymorphisms and response to clopidogrel. *N Engl J Med*. 2009;360(4):354-362.PubMed

37. Mega JL, Simon T, Collet JP, et al. Reduced-function CYP2C19 genotype and risk of adverse clinical outcomes among patients treated with clopidogrel predominantly for PCI: a meta-analysis. *JAMA*. 2010;304(16):1821-1830.PubMed

38. Cavallari LH, Lee CR, Beitelshees AL, et al. Multisite investigation of outcomes with implementation of cyp2c19 genotype-guided antiplatelet therapy after percutaneous coronary intervention. *JACC Cardiovasc Interv*. 2018;11(2):181-191.PubMed

39. Moriyama B, Obeng AO, Barbarino J, et al. Clinical pharmacogenetics implementation consortium (CPIC) guidelines for cyp2c19 and voriconazole therapy. *Clin Pharmacol Ther*. 2017;102(1):45-51.PubMed

40. Johnson JA, Caudle KE, Gong L, et al. Clinical pharmacogenetics implementation consortium (CPIC) guideline for pharmacogenetics-guided warfarin dosing: 2017 update. *Clin Pharmacol Ther*. 2017;102(3):397-404.PubMed

41. Pratt VM, Cavallari LH, Del Tredici AL, et al. Recommendations for clinical warfarin genotyping allele selection: a report of the Association For Molecular *Pathology* and the College of American Pathologists. *J Mol Diagn*. 2020;22(7):847-859.PubMed

42. Beitelshees AL, Voora D, Lewis JP. Personalized antiplatelet and anticoagulation therapy: applications and significance of pharmacogenomics. *Pharm Genomics Pers Med*. 2015;8:43-61.PubMed

43. Caudle KE, Rettie AE, Whirl-Carrillo M, et al. Clinical pharmacogenetics implementation consortium guidelines for CYP2C9 and HLA-B genotypes and phenytoin dosing. *Clin Pharmacol Ther*. 2014;96(5):542-548.PubMed

44. Theken KN, Lee CR, Gong L, et al. Clinical pharmacogenetics implementation consortium guideline (CPIC) for cyp2c9 and nonsteroidal anti-inflammatory drugs. *Clin Pharmacol Ther*. 2020;108(2):191-200.PubMed

45. Xie HG, Wood AJ, Kim RB, et al. Genetic variability in CYP3A5 and its possible consequences. *Pharmacogenomics*. 2004;5(3):243-272.PubMed

46. Birdwell KA, Decker B, Barbarino JM, et al. Clinical pharmacogenetics implementation consortium (CPIC) guidelines for CYP3A5 genotype and tacrolimus dosing. *Clin Pharmacol Ther*. 2015;98(1):19-24.PubMed

47. Desta Z, Gammal RS, Gong L, et al. Clinical pharmacogenetics implementation consortium (CPIC) guideline for CYP2B6 and efavirenz-containing antiretroviral therapy. *Clin Pharmacol Ther*. 2019;106(4): 726-733.PubMed

48. Werk AN, Cascorbi I. Functional gene variants of CYP3A4. *Clin Pharmacol Ther*. 2014;96(3):340-348.PubMed

49. Ramsey LB, Johnson SG, Caudle KE, et al. The clinical pharmacogenetics implementation consortium guideline for SLCO1B1 and simvastatin-induced myopathy: 2014 update. *Clin Pharmacol Ther*. 2014;96(4): 423-428.PubMed

50. Link E, Parish S, Armitage J, et al. SLCO1B1 variants and statin-induced myopathy: a genomewide study. *N Engl J Med*. 2008;359(8):789-799. PubMed

51. Purinethol [package insert]. Research Triangle Park, NC: Glaxosmithkline; 2004.

52. Relling MV, Gardner EE, Sandborn WJ, et al. Clinical Pharmacogenetics Implementation Consortium guidelines for thiopurine methyltransferase genotype and thiopurine dosing. *Clin Pharmacol Ther*. 2011;89(3): 387-391.PubMed

53. Yang JJ, Landier W, Yang W, et al. Inherited NUDT15 variant is a genetic determinant of mercaptopurine intolerance in children with acute lymphoblastic leukemia. *J Clin Oncol*. 2015;33(11):1235-1242.PubMed

54. Yang SK, Hong M, Baek J, et al. A common missense variant in NUDT15 confers susceptibility to thiopurine-induced leukopenia. *Nat Genet*. 2014;46(9):1017-1020.PubMed

55. Relling MV, Schwab M, Whirl-Carrillo M, et al. Clinical Pharmacogenetics Implementation Consortium guideline for thiopurine dosing based on TPMT and NUDT15 genotypes: 2018 update. *Clin Pharmacol Ther*. 2019;105(5):1095-1105.PubMed

56. Purixan (mercaptopurine) oral suspension [package insert]. Franklin, TN: Rare Disease Therapeutics, Inc.; April 2020.

57. Fargher EA, Tricker K, Newman W, et al. Current use of pharmacogenetic testing: a national survey of thiopurine methyltransferase testing prior to azathioprine prescription. *J Clin Pharm Ther*. 2007;32(2):187-195. PubMed

58. Diasio RB, Beavers TL, Carpenter JT. Familial deficiency of dihydropyrimidine dehydrogenase. Biochemical basis for familial pyrimidinemia and severe 5-fluorouracil-induced toxicity. *J Clin Invest*. 1988;81(1):47-51.PubMed

59. Tuchman M, Stoeckeler JS, Kiang DT, et al. Familial pyrimidinemia and pyrimidinuria associated with severe fluorouracil toxicity. *N Engl J Med*. 1985;313(4):245-249.PubMed

60. Caudle KE, Thorn CF, Klein TE, et al. Clinical Pharmacogenetics Implementation Consortium guidelines for dihydropyrimidine dehydrogenase genotype and fluoropyrimidine dosing. *Clin Pharmacol Ther*. 2013;94(6):640-645.PubMed

61. Amstutz U, Henricks LM, Offer SM, et al. Clinical pharmacogenetics implementation consortium (CPIC) guideline for dihydropyrimidine dehydrogenase genotype and fluoropyrimidine dosing: 2017 update. *Clin Pharmacol Ther*. 2018;103(2):210-216.PubMed

62. Yen JL, McLeod HL. Should DPD analysis be required prior to prescribing fluoropyrimidines? *Eur J Cancer*. 2007;43(6):1011-1016. PubMed

63. Lee AM, Shi Q, Pavey E, et al. DPYD variants as predictors of 5-fluorouracil toxicity in adjuvant colon cancer treatment (NCCTG N0147). *J Natl Cancer Inst*. 2014;106(12):dju298.PubMed

64. Gammal RS, Court MH, Haidar CE, et al. Clinical pharmacogenetics implementation consortium (CPIC) guideline for ugt1a1 and atazanavir prescribing. *Clin Pharmacol Ther*. 2016;99(4):363-369.PubMed

65. Bosma PJ, Chowdhury JR, Bakker C, et al. The genetic basis of the reduced expression of bilirubin UDP-glucuronosyltransferase 1 in Gilbert's syndrome. *N Engl J Med*. 1995;333(18):1171-1175.PubMed

66. Relling MV, McDonagh EM, Chang T, et al. Clinical Pharmacogenetics Implementation Consortium (CPIC) guidelines for rasburicase therapy in the context of G6PD deficiency genotype. *Clin Pharmacol Ther*. 2014;96(2):169-174.PubMed

67. Minucci A, Moradkhani K, Hwang MJ, et al. Glucose-6-phosphate dehydrogenase (G6PD) mutations database: review of the "old" and update of the new mutations. *Blood Cells Mol Dis*. 2012;48(3):154-165. PubMed

68. Wajih N, Hutson SM, Owen J, Wallin R. Increased production of functional recombinant human clotting factor IX by baby hamster kidney cells engineered to overexpress VKORC1, the vitamin K 2,3-epoxide-reducing enzyme of the vitamin K cycle. *J Biol Chem*. 2005;280(36):31603-31607.PubMed

69. Daly AK, Day CP, Aithal GP. CYP2C9 polymorphism and warfarin dose requirements. *Br J Clin Pharmacol*. 2002;53(4):408-409.PubMed

70. Daly AK, Aithal GP. Genetic regulation of warfarin metabolism and response. *Semin Vasc Med*. 2003;3(3):231-238.PubMed

71. Furuya H, Fernandez-Salguero P, Gregory W, et al. Genetic polymorphism of CYP2C9 and its effect on warfarin maintenance dose requirement in patients undergoing anticoagulation therapy. *Pharmacogenetics*. 1995;5(6):389-392.PubMed

72. Lee CR, Goldstein JA, Pieper JA. Cytochrome P450 2C9 polymorphisms: a comprehensive review of the in-vitro and human data. *Pharmacogenetics*. 2002;12(3):251-263.PubMed

73. Takahashi H, Echizen H. Pharmacogenetics of warfarin elimination and its clinical implications. *Clin Pharmacokinet*. 2001;40(8):587-603.PubMed

74. Takahashi H, Kashima T, Nomizo Y, et al. Metabolism of warfarin enantiomers in Japanese patients with heart disease having different CYP2C9 and CYP2C19 genotypes. *Clin Pharmacol Ther*. 1998;63(5): 519-528.PubMed

75. Aithal GP, Day CP, Kesteven PJ, Daly AK. Association of polymorphisms in the cytochrome P450 CYP2C9 with warfarin dose requirement and risk of bleeding complications. *Lancet*. 1999;353(9154):717-719.PubMed

76. Sconce EA, Khan TI, Wynne HA, et al. The impact of CYP2C9 and VKORC1 genetic polymorphism and patient characteristics upon warfarin dose requirements: proposal for a new dosing regimen. *Blood*. 2005;106(7):2329-2333.PubMed

77. Wadelius M, Chen LY, Downes K, et al. Common VKORC1 and GGCX polymorphisms associated with warfarin dose. *Pharmacogenomics J*. 2005;5(4):262-270.PubMed

78. Klein TE, Altman RB, Eriksson N, et al. Estimation of the warfarin dose with clinical and pharmacogenetic data. *N Engl J Med*. 2009;360(8): 753-764.PubMed

79. Coumadin [package insert]. Princeton, NJ: Bristol-Myers Squibb; 2011.

80. Johnson JA, Gong L, Whirl-Carrillo M, et al. Clinical Pharmacogenetics Implementation Consortium Guidelines for CYP2C9 and VKORC1 genotypes and warfarin dosing. *Clin Pharmacol Ther*. 2011;90(4):625-629. PubMed

81. Kaye JB, Schultz LE, Steiner HE, et al. Pharmacotherapy. 2017 Sep;37(9): 1150-1163. Epub 2017 Sep 6.PubMed

82. Drozda K, Wong S, Patel SR, et al. Poor warfarin dose prediction with pharmacogenetic algorithms that exclude genotypes important for African Americans. *Pharmacogenet Genomics*. 2015;25(2):73-81.PubMed

83. Hernandez W, Aquino-Michaels K, Drozda K, et al. Novel single nucleotide polymorphism in CYP2C9 is associated with changes in warfarin clearance and CYP2C9 expression levels in African Americans. *Transl Res*. 2015;165(6):651-657.PubMed

84. Limdi NA, Brown TM, Yan Q, et al. Race influences warfarin dose changes associated with genetic factors. *Blood*. 2015;126(4):539-545. PubMed

85. Perera MA, Cavallari LH, Limdi NA, et al. Genetic variants associated with warfarin dose in African-American individuals: a genome-wide association study. *Lancet*. 2013;382(9894):790-796.PubMed

86. Johnson JA, Caudle KE, Gong L, et al. Clinical pharmacogenetics implementation consortium (CPIC) guideline for pharmacogenetics-guided warfarin dosing: 2017 update. *Clin Pharmacol Ther*. 2017;102(3):397-404.PubMed

87. Anderson JL, Horne BD, Stevens SM, et al. Randomized trial of genotype-guided versus standard warfarin dosing in patients initiating oral anticoagulation. *Circulation*. 2007;116(22):2563-2570.PubMed

88. Kimmel SE, French B, Kasner SE, et al. A pharmacogenetic versus a clinical algorithm for warfarin dosing. *N Engl J Med*. 2013;369(24): 2283-2293.PubMed

89. Pirmohamed M, Burnside G, Eriksson N, et al. A randomized trial of genotype-guided dosing of warfarin. *N Engl J Med*. 2013;369(24): 2294-2303.PubMed

90. Verhoef TI, Ragia G, de Boer A, et al. A randomized trial of genotype-guided dosing of acenocoumarol and phenprocoumon. *N Engl J Med*. 2013;369(24):2304-2312.PubMed

91. Gage BF, Bass AR, Lin H, et al. Effect of genotype-guided warfarin dosing on clinical events and anticoagulation control among patients undergoing hip or knee arthroplasty: the gift randomized clinical trial. *JAMA*. 2017;318(12):1115-1124.PubMed

92. Guo C, Kuang Y, Zhou H, et al. Genotype-guided dosing of warfarin in Chinese adults: a multicenter randomized clinical trial. *Circ Genom Precis Med*. 2020;13(4):e002602.PubMed

93. Sharma SV, Bell DW, Settleman J, Haber DA. Epidermal growth factor receptor mutations in lung cancer. *Nat Rev Cancer*. 2007;7(3):169-181. PubMed

94. Gately K, O'Flaherty J, Cappuzzo F, et al. The role of the molecular footprint of EGFR in tailoring treatment decisions in NSCLC. *J Clin Pathol*. 2012;65(1):1-7.PubMed

95. Oxnard GR, Arcila ME, Chmielecki J, et al. New strategies in overcoming acquired resistance to epidermal growth factor receptor tyrosine kinase inhibitors in lung cancer. *Clin Cancer Res*. 2011;17(17):5530-5537.PubMed

96. Lynch TJ, Bell DW, Sordella R, et al. Activating mutations in the epidermal growth factor receptor underlying responsiveness of non-small-cell lung cancer to gefitinib. *N Engl J Med*. 2004;350(21):2129-2139.PubMed

97. Pao W, Chmielecki J. Rational, biologically based treatment of EGFR-mutant non-small-cell lung cancer. *Nat Rev Cancer*. 2010;10(11): 760-774.PubMed

98. Tanner NT, Pastis NJ, Sherman C, et al. The role of molecular analyses in the era of personalized therapy for advanced NSCLC. *Lung Cancer*. 2012;76(2):131-137.PubMed

99. Pao W, Ladanyi M. Epidermal growth factor receptor mutation testing in lung cancer: searching for the ideal method. *Clin Cancer Res*. 2007;13(17):4954-4955.PubMed

100. Fecher LA, Cummings SD, Keefe MJ, Alani RM. Toward a molecular classification of melanoma. *J Clin Oncol*. 2007;25(12):1606-1620.PubMed

101. Holderfield M, Deuker MM, McCormick F, McMahon M. Targeting RAF kinases for cancer therapy: BRAF-mutated melanoma and beyond. *Nat Rev Cancer*. 2014;14(7):455-467.PubMed

102. Chapman PB, Hauschild A, Robert C, et al. Improved survival with vemurafenib in melanoma with BRAF V600E mutation. *N Engl J Med*. 2011;364(26):2507-2516.PubMed

103. Hatzivassiliou G, Song K, Yen I, et al. RAF inhibitors prime wild-type RAF to activate the MAPK pathway and enhance growth. *Nature*. 2010;464(7287):431-435.PubMed

104. Dienstmann R, Vilar E, Tabernero J. Molecular predictors of response to chemotherapy in colorectal cancer. *Cancer J*. 2011;17(2):114-126.PubMed

105. Sierra JR, Cepero V, Giordano S. Molecular mechanisms of acquired resistance to tyrosine kinase targeted therapy. *Mol Cancer*. 2010;9:75. PubMed

106. Sabnis AJ, Bivona TG. Principles of resistance to targeted cancer therapy: lessons from basic and translational cancer biology. *Trends Mol Med*. 2019;25(3):185-197.PubMed

107. Karnes JH, Miller MA, White KD, et al. Applications of immunopharmacogenomics: predicting, preventing, and understanding immune-mediated adverse drug reactions. *Annu Rev Pharmacol Toxicol*. 2019;59:463-486.PubMed

108. Robinson J, Halliwell JA, McWilliam H, et al. The IMGT/HLA database. *Nucleic Acids Res*. 2013;41(database issue):D1222-D1227.PubMed

109. Nepom GT, Erlich H. MHC class-II molecules and autoimmunity. *Annu Rev Immunol*. 1991;9:493-525.PubMed

110. Mallal S, Nolan D, Witt C, et al. Association between presence of HLA-B*5701, HLA-DR7, and HLA-DQ3 and hypersensitivity to HIV-1 reverse-transcriptase inhibitor abacavir. *Lancet*. 2002;359(9308):727-732. PubMed

111. Mallal S, Phillips E, Carosi G, et al. HLA-B*5701 screening for hypersensitivity to abacavir. *N Engl J Med*. 2008;358(6):568-579.PubMed

112. Department of Health and Human Services. Guidelines for the use of antiretroviral agents in HIV-1 infected adults and adolescents. http://www.aidsinfo.nih.gov/contentfiles/adultandadolescentgl.pdf. Accessed Mar 20, 2013.

113. Martin MA, Hoffman JM, Freimuth RR, et al. Clinical pharmacogenetics implementation consortium guidelines for HLA-b genotype and abacavir dosing: 2014 update. *Clin Pharmacol Ther*. 2014;95(5):499-500.PubMed

114. McCormack M, Alfirevic A, Bourgeois S, et al. HLA-A*3101 and carbamazepine-induced hypersensitivity reactions in Europeans. *N Engl J Med*. 2011;364(12):1134-1143.PubMed

115. Ozeki T, Mushiroda T, Yowang A, et al. Genome-wide association study identifies HLA-A*3101 allele as a genetic risk factor for carbamazepine-induced cutaneous adverse drug reactions in Japanese population. *Hum Mol Genet*. 2011;20(5):1034-1041.PubMed

116. Chung WH, Hung SI, Hong HS, et al. Medical genetics: a marker for Stevens-Johnson syndrome. *Nature*. 2004;428(6982):486.PubMed

117. Hung SI, Chung WH, Liou LB, et al. HLA-B*5801 allele as a genetic marker for severe cutaneous adverse reactions caused by allopurinol. *Proc Natl Acad Sci USA*. 2005;102(11):4134-4139.PubMed

118. Saito Y, Stamp LK, Caudle KE, et al. Clinical Pharmacogenetics Implementation Consortium (CPIC) guidelines for human leukocyte antigen B (HLA-B) genotype and allopurinol dosing: 2015 update. *Clin Pharmacol Ther*. 2016;99(1):36-37.PubMed

119. Phillips EJ, Sukasem C, Whirl-Carrillo M, et al. Clinical pharmacogenetics implementation consortium guideline for HLA genotype and use of carbamazepine and oxcarbazepine: 2017 update. *Clin Pharmacol Ther*. 2018;103(4):574-581.PubMed

120. Dienstmann R, Rodon J, Tabernero J. Biomarker-driven patient selection for early clinical trials. *Curr Opin Oncol*. 2013;25(3):305-312.PubMed

121. Xuan J, Yu Y, Qing T, et al. Next-generation sequencing in the clinic: promises and challenges. *Cancer Lett*. 2013;340(2):284-295.PubMed

122. Thomas A, Rajan A, Lopez-Chavez A, et al. From targets to targeted therapies and molecular profiling in non-small cell lung carcinoma. *Ann Oncol*. 2013;24(3):577-585.PubMed

123. Carlson B. Seeking a coding solution for molecular tests: managing the estimated 1,700 molecular tests now on the market is impossible without a unique CPT code for each test. What's at stake? The future of personalized medicine. *Biotechnol Healthc*. 2010;7(4):16-20.PubMed

124. Bank PCD, Caudle KE, Swen JJ, et al. Comparison of the guidelines of the clinical pharmacogenetics implementation consortium and the Dutch Pharmacogenetics Working Group. *Clin Pharmacol Ther*. 2018;103(4):599-618.PubMed

125. Clancy JP, Johnson SG, Yee SW, et al. Clinical Pharmacogenetics Implementation Consortium (CPIC) guidelines for ivacaftor therapy in the context of CFTR genotype. *Clin Pharmacol Ther*. 2014;95(6):592-597. PubMed

126. Muir AJ, Gong L, Johnson SG, et al. Clinical Pharmacogenetics Implementation Consortium (CPIC) guidelines for IFNL3 (IL28B) genotype and PEG interferon-α-based regimens. *Clin Pharmacol Ther*. 2014;95(2):141-146.PubMed

127. Wilke RA, Ramsey LB, Johnson SG, et al. The Clinical Pharmacogenomics Implementation Consortium: CPIC guideline for SLCO1B1 and simvastatin-induced myopathy. *Clin Pharmacol Ther*. 2012;92(1):112-117.PubMed

128. Relling MV, Gardner EE, Sandborn WJ, et al. Clinical Pharmacogenetics Implementation Consortium guidelines for thiopurine methyltransferase genotype and thiopurine dosing: 2013 update. *Clin Pharmacol Ther*. 2013;93(4):324-325.PubMed

129. Gonsalves SG, Dirksen RT, Sangkuhl K, et al. Clinical Pharmacogenetics Implementation Consortium (CPIC) guideline for the use of potent volatile anesthetic agents and succinylcholine in the context of RYR1 or CACNA1S genotypes. *Clin Pharmacol Ther*. 2019;105(6):1338-1344. PubMed

130. McDermott JH, Wolf J, Hoshitsuki K, et al. Clinical pharmacogenetics implementation consortium guideline for the use of aminoglycosides based on MT-RNR1 genotype. *Clin Pharmacol Ther*. 2021.PubMed

131. Lima JJ, Thomas CD, Barbarino J, et al. Clinical pharmacogenetics implementation consortium (CPIC) guideline for CYP2C19 and proton pump inhibitor dosing. *Clin Pharmacol Ther*. 2021;109:1417-1423. PubMed

# PART II

## SYSTEM DISORDERS AND DIAGNOSTIC TESTS

# 7 Cardiac Function and Related Tests

*Jessica DeAngelo and Jacqueline Finger*

## OBJECTIVES

*After completing this chapter, the reader should be able to*

- Explain the roles of the different biochemical markers in the diagnosis of acute coronary syndrome and heart failure
- Assess the presence and type of acute coronary syndrome in a patient case
- Assess the presence and type of heart failure in a patient case

The purpose of the heart is to pump blood throughout the body, delivering oxygen and nutrients to the tissues. The heart muscle has two basic properties: electrical and mechanical. Heart cells responsible for these properties are (1) pacemaker cells, or the "electrical power" of the heart; (2) electrical conducting cells, or the "hardwiring circuitry" of the heart; and (3) myocardial cells, or the contractile units of the heart. Disturbances in the electrical system result in rhythm disorders, also known as *arrhythmias* or *dysrhythmias*. The pumping action is accomplished by means of striated cardiac muscle, which largely composes the myocardium. Several cardiovascular diseases disrupt the mechanical function of the heart, including acute coronary syndrome (ACS), and heart failure.[1]

The management and potential complications of these disease states contribute greatly to the overall health of and cost incurred by society. Laboratory tests are essential for establishing the diagnosis and determining the prognosis of patients. Accurate and expeditious assessment of a patient presenting with symptoms suggestive of ACS guides individualized treatment to optimize a patient's short-term and long-term outcomes. Conversely, rapid exclusion of the diagnosis permits early discharge from the coronary care unit or hospital. Laboratory and other diagnostic tests used in evaluating a patient with possible ACS or heart failure are discussed in this chapter.

## CARDIAC PHYSIOLOGY

The heart consists of two pumping units that operate in parallel, one on the right side and the other on the left side. Each unit is composed of an upper chamber called the *atrium* and a lower chamber called the *ventricle*. The atrium receives blood into the heart and serves as a weak pump that helps move blood into the ventricle. The atrial contraction, or atrial kick, is responsible for 20% to 30% of ventricular filling. The right and left ventricles pump blood outside the heart and supply the primary force that propels blood through the pulmonary and peripheral circulation, respectively.[1]

The functional unit of the heart is comprised of a network of noncontractile cells that form the conduction system, which is responsible for originating and conducting action potentials from the atria to the ventricles. This leads to the excitation and contraction of the cardiac muscle, which is responsible for pumping blood to the other organs.[1]

The normal adult human heart contracts rhythmically at approximately 70 beats per minute. Each cardiac cycle is divided into a systolic and diastolic phase. During each cycle, blood from the systemic circulation is returned to the heart via the veins, and blood empties from the superior and inferior vena cavae into the right atrium.[1] During the diastolic phase, blood passively fills the right ventricle through the tricuspid valve with an active filling phase by atrial contraction just prior to end-diastole. During the systole phase, blood is then pumped from the right ventricle through the pulmonary artery to the lungs, where carbon dioxide is removed and the blood is oxygenated. From the lungs, blood returns to the heart via the pulmonary veins and empties into the left atrium.[1] Again, during diastole, blood empties from the left atrium through the mitral valve into the main pumping chamber, the left ventricle. With systole, the left ventricle contracts and blood is forcefully propelled into the peripheral circulation via the aorta. At rest, the normal heart pumps approximately

DOI 10.37573/9781585286423.007

4 to 6 L of blood per minute, known as cardiac output (CO). Maintaining normal CO depends on the heart rate (HR) and stroke volume (SV).[1]

$$CO \text{ (mL/min)} = HR \text{ (beats/min)} \times SV \text{ (mL/beat)}$$

The SV, defined as the volume of blood ejected during systole, is determined by intrinsic and extrinsic factors, including myocardial contractility, preload, and afterload. The coronary arteries, which supply the heart muscle, branch from the aorta just beyond the aortic valve and are filled with blood primarily during diastole. In the face of increased myocardial metabolic needs, the heart can increase coronary blood flow by vasodilation to meet myocardial oxygen demand.[1]

Decreased CO compromises tissue perfusion and, depending on severity and duration, may lead to significant acute and chronic complications. Several cardiac conditions lead to decreased CO, including hypertensive heart diseases, heart failure, valvular heart diseases, congenital heart diseases, diseases of the myocardium, conduction abnormalities, stable ischemic heart disease (SIHD), and ACS. This chapter focuses on the various tests used in the diagnosis and assessment of patients presenting with ACS and heart failure.

# ACUTE CORONARY SYNDROME

Acute coronary syndrome (ACS) is a medical emergency resulting from atherosclerotic plaque rupture in a coronary artery. This rupture results in an obstruction of the coronary lumen by a thrombus composed of platelet aggregates, fibrin, and entrapped blood cells. The obstruction caused by the thrombus leads to myocardial ischemia. When a coronary artery is occluded, the location, extent, rate, and duration of occlusion determine the severity of myocardial ischemia resulting in one of three types of ACS: unstable angina, non–ST-segment elevation myocardial infarction (NSTEMI), or ST-segment elevation myocardial infarction (STEMI).[2-4]

Complications of a myocardial infarction (MI) include cardiogenic shock, heart failure, ventricular and atrial arrhythmias, ventricular rupture or ventricular septal defect formation, cardiac tamponade, pericarditis, papillary muscle rupture, mitral regurgitation, and embolism. Initial assessment of the patient presenting with ACS may be confounded by the presence and severity of the previously described complications.[2-4]

Myocardial infarction can be recognized by clinical presentation, electrocardiography, elevated biochemical markers of myocardial necrosis, and imaging. Clinical presentation of all types of ACS is similar and does not distinguish among unstable angina, NSTEMI, and STEMI. Interpretation of a 12-lead electrocardiogram (ECG) and the presence of positive biomarkers of necrosis are used to differentiate between the different types of ACS. Positive biomarkers, such as cardiac-specific troponins, are suggestive of NSTEMI and STEMI. In the era of reperfusion therapy, diagnosing ACS accurately and without delay is crucial for risk stratification and appropriate, life-saving treatment implementation. This section describes the laboratory and diagnostic tests used in the diagnosis of ACS.[2-4]

# Laboratory Tests
## Cardiac-Specific Troponins

Infarction of myocardial cells disrupts membrane integrity, leaking intracellular macromolecules into the peripheral circulation, where they are detected. Several biochemical cardiac markers are used in the diagnosis and evaluation of ACS. The cardiac-specific troponins (cTn) have several attractive features and have gained acceptance as the biochemical markers of choice in the evaluation of patients with ACS.[5]

The role of cTn within the cardiac tissue is to modulate the contractile function of the muscle. Troponin is a protein complex consisting of three subunits: troponin C (TnC), troponin I (TnI), and troponin T (TnT). The three subunits are located along thin filaments of myofibrils, and they regulate $Ca^{+2}$-mediated interaction of actin and myosin necessary for the contraction of cardiac muscles. Troponin C binds $Ca^{+2}$, TnI inhibits interaction with myosin heads, and TnT attaches to tropomyosin on the thin filaments.[5] The TnC expressed by myocardial cells in cardiac and skeletal muscle is identical. In contrast, TnI and TnT isoforms are specific to cardiac myocytes. Monoclonal antibody-based immunoassays have been developed to detect cardiac-specific TnI (cTnI) and cardiac-specific TnT (cTnT).[5]

Cardiac-specific TnI and cTnT are highly specific and sensitive for myocardial injury.[6-8] In the case of myocardial injury, serum cTnI and cTnT levels begin to rise above the upper reference limit within 3 to 12 hours, peak in 24 hours (cTnI) or 12 hours to 2 days (cTnT), and return to normal in 5 to 10 days (cTnI) or 5 to 14 days (cTnT) (**Table 7-1**). Levels typically increase more than 20 times above the reference limit. The prolonged time course of elevation of cTnI and cTnT is useful for the late diagnosis of MI.[6-8]

Serial troponin levels should be obtained at presentation and 3 to 6 hours after onset of symptoms. A level of cTnT and cTnI that exceeds the decision level on at least one occasion during the first 24 hours after an index clinical ischemic event indicates MI. Most commercial immunoassays measure cTnI. A pattern that shows rising and falling troponin levels is required for the diagnosis of ACS. This is especially helpful in differentiating troponin elevation caused by MI from that caused by chronic conditions. Additional troponin levels should be obtained beyond 6 hours if the clinical index of suspicion for ACS is high.[9]

Cardiac troponins have been endorsed internationally as the standard biomarkers for the detection of myocardial injury, diagnosis of MI, and risk stratification in patients with suspected ACS.[3,4,9,10] Significant prognostic information may be inferred from troponin levels. In a study of patients presenting to the emergency department with chest pain, negative qualitative bedside testing of cTnI and cTnT was associated with low risk for death or MI within 30 days (event rates of 0.3 and 1.1, respectively).[11] Other large clinical trials have documented that elevated troponin levels are strong, independent predictors of mortality and serious adverse outcome 30 to 42 days after ACS.[12-16] Troponin levels should always be used in conjunction with other clinical findings. In one study, in-hospital mortality was as high as 12.7% in a troponin-negative subgroup of

**TABLE 7-1.** Biochemical Markers Used in the Diagnosis of ACS

| MARKER | MOLECULAR WEIGHT (Da) | RANGE OF TIME TO INITIAL ELEVATIONS | MEAN TIME TO PEAK ELEVATIONS (Nonthrombolysis) | TIME TO RETURN TO NORMAL RANGE |
|---|---|---|---|---|
| cTnI | 23,500 | 3–12 hr | 24 hr | 5–10 days |
| cTnT | 33,000 | 3–12 hr | 12 hr–2 days | 5–14 days |

*Source:* Adapted with permission from Adams JE 3rd, Bodor GS, Dávila-Román VG, et al. Cardiac troponin I. A marker with high specificity for cardiac injury. *Circulation.* 1993;88(1):101–106; Apple FS. Tissue specificity of cardiac troponin I, cardiac troponin T and creatine kinase-MB. *Clin Chim Acta.* 1999;284(2):151–159; Mair J, Morandell D, Genser N, et al. Equivalent early sensitivities of myoglobin, creatine kinase MB mass, creatine kinase isoform ratios, and cardiac troponins I and T for acute myocardial infarction. *Clin Chem.* 1995;41(9):1266–1272.

patients with ACS.[17] While cTn levels are most commonly elevated in ACS, it is important to note that there are other causes of detectable cTn (**Table 7-2**).[5] "See **Minicase 1** for an example of the use of these laboratory values to assess a patient presenting with ACS."

***High-sensitivity troponins.*** High-sensitivity troponin I (hsTnI) and troponin T (hsTnT) assays have been developed to increase the clinical sensitivity for detection of myocardial injury. High-sensitivity troponin assays detect concentrations of the same proteins that conventional sensitivity assays are aimed at detecting but in much lower concentrations. These assays have substantially lower limits of detection (in the picogram/milliliter range versus the current assays in the nanogram/milliliter range) as well as improved assay precision. To be classified as high-sensitivity assays, concentrations below the 99th percentile should be detectable above the assay's limit of detection for >50% of healthy individuals in the population of interest. High-sensitivity assays, by expert consensus, should have a coefficient of variance of <10% at the 99th percentile value in the population of interest.[18-21]

Studies suggest that high-sensitivity troponins provide enhanced diagnostic and prognostic accuracy. In one study, hsTnT was superior to TnT but equivalent to third-generation TnI for the diagnosis of MI, and hsTnT was the most likely assay to be elevated at baseline. The study also showed that change in troponin levels increase specificity but reduce sensitivity for the detection of acute MI.[22] Another study comparing hsTnI (Architect STAT hsTnI assay, Abbott Diagnostics Scarborough, Inc.) and cTnI (Architect STAT cTnI assay, Abbott Diagnostics Scarborough, Inc.) revealed that measurement at 3 hours after admission may help rule out MI. Troponin measured using either assay was superior to other biomarkers (including creatinine kinase [CK] and creatinine kinase-myocardial band [CK-MB]) in ruling in or ruling out MI. The sensitivity and negative predictive values of the hsTnI assay were higher than the cTnI assay at admission (82.3% and 94.7% versus 79.4% and 94%, respectively); however, the negative predictive value of both assays was 99.4% at 3 hours. For patients with detectable troponin on admission (using the 99th percentile diagnostic cutoff value) and a 250% increase in troponin level at 3 hours, the probability of MI was 95.8%.[23]

Although the use of high-sensitivity troponin assays has been longstanding in Europe, these assays have only been

**TABLE 7-2.** Causes of Detectable Serum Levels of Troponins in the Absence of Acute Coronary Syndrome

Aortic dissection

Bradycardia or tachycardia

Burns affecting >30% of body surface area

Cardiac contusion or trauma (cardiac surgery, ablation, pacing, implantable cardioverter-defibrillator shocks, cardioversion, endomyocardial biopsy)

Cardiomyopathy

Cardiotoxicity (doxorubicin, fluorouracil, trastuzumab)

Cardiopulmonary resuscitation

Coronary angioplasty or vasospasm

Critical illness (respiratory failure, sepsis)

Heart failure (chronic and acute decompensation)

Heart transplant rejection

Infiltrative disorders with cardiac involvement (amyloidosis, sarcoidosis)

Left ventricular hypertrophy

Myocarditis or pericarditis

Neurologic diseases, acute (cerebrovascular accident, subarachnoid hemorrhage)

Pulmonary embolism or severe pulmonary hypertension

Rhabdomyolysis with cardiac injury

Renal failure and hemodialysis

*Source:* Adapted with permission from Richards M, Nicholls MG, Espiner EA, et al. Comparison of B-type natriuretic peptides for assessment of cardiac function and prognosis in stable ischemic heart disease. *J Am Coll Cardiol.* 2006;47(1):52–60; Jernberg T, Stridsberg M, Venge P, Lindahl B. N-terminal pro brain natriuretic peptide on admission for early risk stratification of patients with chest pain and no ST-segment elevation. *J Am Coll Cardiol.* 2002;40(3):437–445; James SK, Lindahl B, Siegbahn A, et al. N-terminal pro-brain natriuretic peptide and other risk markers for the separate prediction of mortality and subsequent myocardial infarction in patients with unstable coronary artery disease: a Global Utilization of Strategies to Open occluded arteries (GUSTO)-IV substudy. *Circulation.* 2003;108(3):275–281.

## MINICASE 1

### Acute Coronary Syndrome

Ethan W., a 68-year-old man with history of hypertension, dyslipidemia, and type 2 diabetes, presents to the emergency department with reports of substernal chest discomfort that radiates to the left arm, shortness of breath, and palpitations for the past 4 hours. He appears in distress. His vital signs include BP 150/90 mm Hg, HR 130 beats/min, and RR 24 breaths/min. His jugular venous pressure (JVP) is normal, and his lungs are clear. Cardiac exam reveals tachycardia with no murmurs or rub appreciated. A benign abdominal exam, with no hepatojugular reflux and lower extremities, reveals no edema. Chest radiograph does not show any evidence of cardiomegaly or congestion. ECG reveals ST elevation in anterior leads. At presentation, cTnI is 9 ng/mL. The institution's diagnostic level is cTnI ≥0.3 ng/mL. BNP is 300 pg/mL. An echocardiogram reveals normal left ventricular size with an estimated ejection fraction of 50% and anterior wall motion akinesis.

QUESTION: What is the most likely assessment of this patient's presentation?

DISCUSSION: This patient is considered at high risk for cardiac events given his history of diabetes, hypertension, and dyslipidemia. Based on the ECG findings, along with the symptoms and the elevated troponin level at presentation, he is experiencing an acute anterior STEMI. In addition, the wall motion abnormality noted on echocardiography is consistent with MI. He is not showing evidence of heart failure on exam, and the chest radiograph reveals no evidence of congestion. Elevated BNP levels in ACS have been shown to be prognostic of a poor outcome, even in the absence of clinical evidence of heart failure.

recently approved for use in the United States. Several hsTnT and hsTnI assays are now available and being implemented in health systems across the United States. As the use of these newer tests becomes more widespread, it is important to recognize that there is variability in cutoff values, sensitivity, specificity, and clinical interpretation among the different available assays.[24]

### Cardiac Enzymes

#### Creatine kinase

*Normal range: male patients, 55 to 170 IU/L (0.92 to 2.84 μkat/L); female patients, 30 to 135 IU/L (0.5 to 2.25 μkat/L)*

#### Creatine kinase isoenzymes

*Normal range: CK-MB ≤6 ng/mL (≤6 mcg/L)*

*Creatine kinase* (CK) is an enzyme that stimulates the transfer of high-energy phosphate groups, and it is found in skeletal muscle, the myocardium, and the brain. Circulating serum CK is directly related to an individual's muscle mass.

Given the availability and characteristics of cardiac troponins, CK and CK-MB measurements are no longer useful for the diagnosis of ACS. However, CK-MB may still be used by some clinicians to estimate size of infarct.[4]

The enzyme CK is a dimer of two B monomers (CK-BB), two M monomers (CK-MM), or a hybrid of the two (CK-MB). The three isoenzymes are found in different sources: CK-BB is found in the brain, lungs, and intestinal tract; CK-MM is found primarily in skeletal and cardiac muscle; and CK-MB is found predominantly in the myocardium but also in skeletal muscle. Fractionation of total CK into three isoenzymes increases the diagnostic specificity of the test for MI.[25]

The CK-MB isoenzyme is most specific for myocardial tissue and has been used for the diagnosis of ACS. Serum CK-MB concentrations begin to rise 6 to 12 hours after the onset of symptoms, peak in 24 hours, and return to baseline in 2 to 3 days.[26,27] Other causes for elevated CK-MB levels include trauma, strenuous exercise, skeletal muscle injury, kidney failure, intramuscular injection, and exposure to toxins or drugs.[28]

## HEART FAILURE

Heart failure is a clinical syndrome in which the heart is unable to pump sufficient blood to meet the demands of the body. Heart failure is diagnosed based on history and physical examination. Although no specific test is used to diagnose heart failure, it is classified based on an indirect measurement of the contractility of the left ventricle, called *left ventricular ejection fraction* (LVEF). Heart failure is currently defined as either heart failure with reduced ejection fraction (HFrEF) or preserved ejection fraction (HFpEF). HFrEF occurs when the LVEF is ≤40%. HFrEF is also referred to as *systolic heart failure* because the underlying issue is related to poor ventricular contraction during systole. HFpEF occurs when the LVEF is ≥50%. HFpEF is also referred to as *diastolic heart failure* because the problem is related to impaired ventricular filling during diastole. Patients falling in an intermediate group with LVEF between 41% and 49% are classified as having HFpEF, borderline. Patients with current LVEF >40% and a history of HFrEF in the past are classified as having HFpEF, improved.[29]

Common etiologies for heart failure include coronary artery disease, valvular diseases, and hypertension. Signs and symptoms consistent with heart failure may be attributed to volume overload and congestion (eg, elevated jugular venous pressure,

## MINICASE 2

### Heart Failure

Ruth G. is a 76-year-old woman with a history of poorly controlled hypertension and coronary artery disease who presents to the emergency department with 2 weeks of progressive dyspnea on exertion and now shortness of breath at rest. She reports sleeping in a recliner for the last three nights to breathe more comfortably. She denies any chest discomfort and admits to smoking and medication nonadherence.

On examination, Ruth G. is unable to complete full sentences secondary to breathing difficulty. Her vital signs include blood pressure (BP) 190/105 mm Hg, heart rate (HR) 100 beats/min, and respiration rate (RR) 30 breaths/min. $O_2$ saturation is 86% on room air. Physical exam reveals elevated JVP at 18 cm $H_2O$. Lung exam reveals bibasilar dullness to percussion with diffuse crackles. Cardiac exam reveals a regular tachycardic rate; S1, S2, S3 with 2/6 holosystolic murmur at apex and laterally displaced point of maximal intensity. She has a positive hepatojugular reflux and 2+ pitting edema in the lower extremities, bilaterally. Chest radiographs reveal an enlarged cardiac silhouette with moderate bilateral effusions and cephalization of vasculature. Blood work results are significant: sodium 132 mmol/L, potassium 3.7 mmol/L, blood urea nitrogen 30 mg/dL, creatinine 1.5 mg/dL with an estimated

GFR 46 mL/min/1.73 $m^2$, troponin I level of 0.06 ng/mL (remained at same level with repeat measurements), and BNP level of 2,156 pg/mL. Echocardiogram reveals a dilated left ventricle with global hypokinesis and moderately depressed systolic function with an estimated ejection fraction of 38%.

QUESTION: How should this patient's findings and laboratory values be interpreted?

DISCUSSION: This patient has multiple risk factors for heart failure, including a history of coronary artery disease and poorly controlled hypertension. Her clinical presentation is compatible with acute decompensated heart failure with evidence of volume overload on physical exam (elevated JVP, positive hepatojugular reflux, 2+ lower extremity pitting edema). Her chest radiograph confirms findings of heart failure. Her BNP level is also significantly elevated and is indicative of heart failure. The low troponin level that did not rise is likely the result of a silent subendocardial ischemia given her poorly controlled hypertension and heart failure in the setting of a decreased creatinine clearance. The clinical presentation, BNP level, and LVEF of 38% measured by echocardiography—the findings—are all consistent with a diagnosis of heart failure with reduced ejection fraction (HFrEF).

---

peripheral edema, pulmonary congestion and edema, and dyspnea) and hypoperfusion (eg, tachycardia, cold extremities, cyanosis, and fatigue).[29]

## Laboratory Tests

### Natriuretic Peptides

*Natriuretic peptides* are naturally secreted hormones that are released by various cells in response to increased volume or pressure. Several natriuretic peptides have been identified with atrial natriuretic peptide and B-type natriuretic peptide (BNP) being cardiac-specific peptides. The two peptides are structurally similar and exert potent diuretic, natriuretic, and vascular smooth muscle-relaxing effects. A 28-amino acid (aa) peptide, atrial natriuretic peptide, is primarily secreted by the atrial myocytes in response to increased atrial wall tension. A 32-aa peptide, BNP, is primarily secreted by the left ventricular myocytes in response to volume overload and increased ventricular wall tension.[30]

The precursor for BNP is PreproBNP, a 134-aa peptide that is enzymatically cleaved into proBNP, a 108-aa peptide. The latter is then further cleaved into the biologically active C-terminal 32-aa BNP and the biologically inactive amino-terminal portion of the prohormone, *N*-terminal-proBNP (NT-proBNP). Plasma levels of both BNP and NT-proBNP are elevated in response to increased volume and ventricular myocyte stretch in patients with heart failure. Once released into the peripheral circulation, BNP is cleared by enzymatic degradation via

endopeptidase and natriuretic peptide receptor-mediated endocytosis, whereas NT-proBNP is cleared renally. The elimination half-life of BNP is significantly shorter than that of NT-proBNP (20 minutes versus 120 minutes, respectively).[30]

The quantitative measurements of BNP and NT-proBNP levels are indicated for the evaluation of patients suspected of having heart failure, assessment of the severity of heart failure, and risk stratification of patients with heart failure and ACS.[31] In conjunction with standard clinical assessment, BNP and NT-proBNP levels at the approved cutoff points are highly sensitive and specific for the diagnosis of acute heart failure and correlate well with the severity of heart failure symptoms as evaluated by the New York Heart Association Classification.[32,33] In addition, BNP and NT-proBNP are strong independent markers of clinical outcomes in patients with heart failure, IHD, and ACS, even in the absence of previous history of heart failure or objective evidence of left ventricular dysfunction during hospitalization.[34-40]

The value of serial BNP and NT-proBNP measurements to guide optimal heart failure therapy has been investigated. Several randomized trials of patients with chronic heart failure have compared standard heart failure therapy plus BNP or NT-proBNP-guided therapy to standard heart failure treatment alone.[41-46] A meta-analysis of these trials confirmed the findings that BNP-guided heart failure therapy reduces all-cause mortality in patients with chronic heart failure compared with usual clinical care in patients younger than 75 years but not in those older than 75 years of age. Mortality reduction might be attributable to the higher percentage of patients achieving target doses of angiotensin-converting enzyme inhibitors and β blockers—classes of agents shown to delay or halt progression of cardiac dysfunction and improve mortality in patients with heart failure.[47] A >30% reduction in BNP levels in response to heart failure treatment indicates a good prognosis.[48]

Several factors impact the BNP and NT-proBNP levels, including gender, age, renal function, and obesity. Plasma BNP and NT-proBNP levels in normal volunteers are higher in women and increase with age. In addition, renal insufficiency at an estimated glomerular filtration rate (GFR) <60 mL/min/1.73 m² may impact the interpretation of the measured natriuretic peptides. Significant correlation between NT-proBNP level and GFRs has been shown, more so than that between BNP level and GFRs. This is because renal clearance is the primary route of elimination of NT-proBNP, and the measured levels of the biomarker are elevated in patients with mild renal insufficiency. However, evaluation of patients with GFRs as low as 14.8 mL/min/1.73 m² revealed that the test continues to be valuable for the evaluation of the patient with dyspnea regardless of renal function.[51] Higher diagnostic cutoffs for different GFR ranges may be necessary for optimal interpretation in patients with renal insufficiency.

Plasma levels of BNP and NT-proBNP are reduced in obese patients, limiting the clinical interpretation of the tests in these patients. An inverse relationship between the levels of these markers and body mass index (BMI) is observed.[49,50] The exact mechanism for this is not known, but a BMI-related defect in natriuretic peptide secretion has been suggested.[51] In one study, NT-proBNP levels were found to be lower in obese patients presenting with dyspnea (with or without acute heart failure), but the test seemed to retain its diagnostic and prognostic capacity across all BMI categories.[52] Similarly in another study, in patients with advanced systolic heart failure, the test predicted worse symptoms, impaired hemodynamics, and higher mortality at all levels of BMI. Although BNP levels were relatively lower in overweight and obese patients, optimal BNP cutoff levels for prediction of death or urgent transplant in lean, overweight, and obese patients were reported to be 590 pg/mL, 471 pg/mL, and 342 pg/mL, respectively.[53] To increase the specificity of BNP

levels for heart failure in obese and lean patients, a diagnostic cutoff level of ≥54 pg/mL for severely obese patients and a cutoff level of ≥170 pg/mL in lean patients have been suggested.[54]

Despite the fact that BNP and NT-proBNP have no role in the diagnosis of ACS, they are powerful prognostic markers and predictors of mortality in these patients.[48,55-58] The use of BNP levels in the assessment of cardiotoxicity associated with anthracycline chemotherapy has also been studied.[59-62] Several studies have shown an improvement in early detection of chemotherapy-related cardiotoxicity when biomarkers such as BNP and hsTnI were used in addition to serial evaluation of LVEF. This could potentially translate to earlier intervention and improved outcome.[63,64]

### B-type natriuretic peptide

#### Diagnostic level: 100 pg/mL (100 ng/L)

The clinical diagnostic cutoff level for heart failure is a BNP level of >100 pg/mL. In addition to standard clinical evaluation, a BNP level of >100 pg/mL is associated with sensitivity and specificity of 90% for heart failure in a patient presenting with shortness of breath.[65] The test has a high negative predictive value in ruling out heart failure as a primary cause for the presentation. A BNP level of 100 to 500 pg/mL is suggestive, whereas a level >500 pg/mL is indicative of heart failure as the likely etiology of acute dyspnea (Table 7-3).[48]

A study investigating the prognostic value of BNP levels in patients with heart failure showed that the risk ratio of all-cause mortality and first morbid event (defined as death, sudden death with resuscitation, hospitalization for heart failure, or intravenous inotropic or vasodilator therapy for at least 4 hours) for patients with baseline BNP above the median level of 97 pg/mL was significantly higher than for patients with values below the median. Furthermore, the study revealed a significant quartile-dependent increase in mortality and first morbid event (baseline values for BNP in quartiles were <41, 41 to <97, 97 to <238, and ≥238 pg/mL). Patients with the greatest percent decrease in BNP from baseline to 4- and 12-month follow-up periods had the lowest morbidity and mortality, whereas patients with greatest percent increase in BNP had the highest morbidity and

**TABLE 7-3.** Interpretation of BNP and NT-proBNP Levels in Patients with Acute Dyspnea

|  | AGE | HEART FAILURE UNLIKELY | GRAY ZONE | HEART FAILURE LIKELY |
|---|---|---|---|---|
| BNP[a] | All | <100 pg/mL | 100–500 pg/mL | >500 pg/mL |
| NT-pro-BNP[b] | <50 yr | <300 pg/mL |  | >450 pg/mL |
|  | 50–75 yr |  |  | >900 pg/mL |
|  | >75 yr |  |  | >1,800 pg/mL |

[a]In patients with estimated GFR <60 mL/min/1.73 m² and BMI >35 kg/m², different decision limits must be used.
[b]In patients with estimated GFR <60 mL/min/1.73 m², different decision limits must be used.
*Source:* Adapted with permission from Thygesen K, Mair J, Mueller C, et al. Recommendations for the use of natriuretic peptides in acute cardiac care: a position statement from the Study Group on Biomarkers in Cardiology of the ESC Working Group on Acute Cardiac Care. *Eur Heart J.* 2012;33(16):2001–2006.

mortality. Another study showed that admission BNP and cardiac troponin levels are significant independent predictors of in-hospital mortality in patients with acutely decompensated heart failure. Patients with BNP levels ≥840 pg/mL and increased troponin levels were at particularly high risk for mortality.[66]

### N-terminal-proBNP

*Diagnostic level: 300 pg/mL (300 ng/L)*

*N*-terminal-proBNP (NT-proBNP) is a more stable form of BNP that correlates well with BNP in patients with heart failure, although its levels are typically higher than BNP levels. In addition, NT-proBNP levels are elevated in elderly persons and, accordingly, the clinical diagnostic cutoff level for heart failure is higher in older patients. An NT-proBNP level <300 pg/mL was optimal for ruling out acute heart failure, with a negative predictive value of 99%. For cut points of >450 pg/mL for patients younger than 50 years and >900 pg/mL for patients older than 50 years, NT-proBNP levels were highly sensitive and specific for the diagnosis of acute heart failure (Table 7-3).[33,48]

The angiotensin receptor neprilysin inhibitor (ARNI) drug combination contains the neprilysin inhibitor called sacubitril. By inhibiting neprilysin, the ARNI results in increased levels of natriuretic peptides.[67] Because BNP is a substrate for neprilysin, the ARNI leads to increased BNP levels. Note that NT-proBNP is not a substrate for neprilysin, so levels of NT-proBNP are not directly affected by the use of an ARNI.

### Other Biochemical Markers

Elevated cardiac troponin levels in patients with heart failure have been shown to be related to the severity of heart failure and worse outcomes.[68-70] In patients presenting with acute decompensated heart failure, routine measurement of troponin levels is recommended.[42] In addition to baseline troponin levels, serial troponin measurements may be useful in predicting outcomes.[71] In a recent study of patients hospitalized for acute heart failure, 60% of patients had detectable cTnT levels (>0.01 ng/mL or >0.01 mcg/L) levels and 34% had positive values (>0.03 ng/mL or >0.03 mcg/L) at baseline. Of the patients with negative troponin level at baseline, 21% had elevated cTnT levels by day 7. Positive troponin levels at baseline and conversion to detectable levels were associated with a poor prognosis.[72]

### Recommendations for Measurement of Biochemical Markers

Measurement of BNP or NT-proBNP is useful for (1) supporting clinical decision-making regarding the diagnosis of heart failure in ambulatory patients with dyspnea or in a patient with acutely decompensated heart failure, especially in the setting of clinical uncertainty and (2) establishing prognosis or disease severity in patients with chronic and acute decompensated heart failure. BNP/NT-proBNP–guided heart failure therapy can be useful to achieve optimal dosing in select patients with clinical euvolemia in the ambulatory care setting, but they are less well established in patients with acute decompensated heart failure. However, it is recommended to obtain a baseline BNP or NT-proBNP at the time of hospital admission for prognostic purposes. In addition, a predischarge BNP or NT-proBNP level may aid in determining postdischarge prognosis. Lastly, measuring cardiac troponins as biomarkers of myocardial injury is helpful for establishing prognosis and risk stratification in the ambulatory/outpatient and acute settings.[29,73]

## SUMMARY

The heart is a muscle that circulates blood first to the lungs for oxygenation and then throughout the vascular system to supply oxygen and nutrients to each cell in the body. Many conditions affect the heart's ability to function effectively, including SIHD, ACS, and heart failure. Various diagnostic laboratory tests and procedures can be employed to diagnose these conditions.

Gold standard evaluation for SIHD includes noninvasive testing, such as exercise or pharmacologic stress testing. The classic laboratory workup for ACS includes measurement of cardiac troponin level to evaluate for presence of cTnI or cTnT or the more recently approved hsTnI or hsTnT. Classic ECG changes, such as T-wave inversion, ST-segment depression or elevation, and Q-wave appearance, may also be present and are useful in evaluating patients who present with ACS. In addition to confirming an equivocal diagnosis, imaging techniques may localize and estimate the size of MIs. For diagnosis and assessment of heart failure, BNP or NT-proBNP measurement is considered the gold standard laboratory test. Determining LVEF via echocardiography is essential for differentiating systolic (reduced LVEF) from diastolic (preserved LVEF) heart failure so therapy may be targeted accordingly.

The clinician must be well informed of various tests used to diagnose and assess patients with SIHD, ACS, and heart failure. Knowledge of these tests and their clinical significance greatly impacts decisions regarding the implementation of appropriate medication management strategies and preventive measures.

## ACKNOWLEDGMENTS

The authors would like to acknowledge the contributions of Dr. Samir Y. Dahdal and Dr. Wafa Y. Dahdal, who authored this chapter in previous editions of this textbook.

## LEARNING POINTS

1. *Explain the function of cTn within cardiac tissue and its role in diagnosing ACS.*

   **ANSWER:** The role of cTn in cardiac myoctes is to modulate the contractile function of the muscle. When myocardial injury occurs, cTn levels may be detected in the serum. Presence of serum cTn above the upper reference limit is suggestive of an ACS event, specifically NSTEMI or STEMI.

2. *Discuss the release kinetics of cardiac specific troponins and recommendations for measurement of this laboratory test in patients presenting with chest pain.*

   **ANSWER:** cTnI and cTnT levels are detectable above the upper reference limit by 3 hours from the onset of symptoms. Mean time to peak elevation levels without reperfusion therapy is 24 hours for cTnI and 12 hours to 2 days for cTnT. Because of continuous release from injured myocytes, cTnI levels may remain elevated for 5 to 10 days after an MI versus 5 to 14 days for cTnT. Levels are obtained at initial presentation of patients with chest discomfort and repeated 3 to 6 hours later to confirm the diagnosis of MI.

3. **Describe the mechanism of action of the ARNI and its effect on serum BNP and NT-proBNP.**

   **ANSWER:** The ARNI contains the angiotensin receptor blocker drug called valsartan and the neprilysin inhibitor drug called sacubitril. Sacubitril inhibits the enzyme neprilysin, which is responsible for the breakdown of BNP. Because BNP is a substrate for neprilysin, the inhibition of neprilysin by the ARNI leads to increased BNP levels. In contrast, NT-proBNP is not a substrate of neprilysin, so its serum levels remain relatively unaffected by the ARNI.

4. **Define the use of BNP levels in the clinical assessment of patients presenting with heart failure.**

   **ANSWER:** The BNP levels are a good marker of left ventricular dysfunction and a strong marker to predict morbidity and mortality in patients with heart failure. In conjunction with the standard clinical assessment, BNP is used to establish or exclude the diagnosis of heart failure in patients presenting to the emergency department for evaluation of acute dyspnea. Serum BNP levels correlate with the clinical severity of heart failure as assessed by New York Heart Association classification.

# REFERENCES

1. Loscalzo J, Libby P, MacRae CA. Basic biology of the cardiovascular system. In: Jameson J, Fauci AS, Kasper DL, et al, eds. *Harrison's Principles of Internal Medicine.* 20th edition. New York, NY: McGraw-Hill; 2018: Chapter 232, 1-22.

2. Thygesen K, Alpert JS, Jaffe AS et al. Fourth universal definition of myocardial infarction. *Circulation.* 2018;138:e618-e651.

3. O'Gara PT, Kushner FG, Ascheim DD, et al. 2013 ACCF/AHA guideline for the management of ST-elevation myocardial infarction. *Circulation.* 2013;127(4):e362-e425.PubMed

4. Amsterdam EA, Wenger NK, Brindis RG, et al. 2014 AHA/ACC guideline for the management of patient with non-ST-elevation acute coronary syndromes. *Circulation.* 2014;130:e344-e426.PubMed

5. Garg P, Morris P, Fazlanie AL, et al. Cardiac biomarkers of acute coronary syndrome: from history to high-sensitivity cardiac troponin. *Intern Emerg Med.* 2017;12(2):147-155.PubMed

6. Adams JE 3rd, Bodor GS, Dávila-Román VG, et al. Cardiac troponin I: a marker with high specificity for cardiac injury. *Circulation.* 1993;88(1):101-106.PubMed

7. Apple FS. Tissue specificity of cardiac troponin I, cardiac troponin T and creatine kinase-MB. *Clin Chim Acta.* 1999;284(2):151-159.PubMed

8. Mair J, Morandell D, Genser N, et al. Equivalent early sensitivities of myoglobin, creatine kinase MB mass, creatine kinase isoform ratios, and cardiac troponins I and T for acute myocardial infarction. *Clin Chem.* 1995;41(9):1266-1272.PubMed

9. Thygesen K, Alpert JS, Jaffe AS, et al. Third universal definition of myocardial infarction. *J Am Coll Cardiol.* 2012;60(16):1581-1598.PubMed

10. Roffi M, Patrono C, Collet JP, et al. 2015 ESC Guidelines for the management of acute coronary syndromes in patients presenting without persistent ST-segment elevation: Task Force for the Management of Acute Coronary Syndromes in Patients Presenting without Persistent ST-Segment Elevation of the European Society of Cardiology (ESC). *Eur Heart J.* 2016;37(3):267-315.PubMed

11. Hamm CW, Goldmann BU, Heeschen C, et al. Emergency room triage of patients with acute chest pain by means of rapid testing for cardiac troponin T or troponin I. *N Engl J Med.* 1997;337(23):1648-1653.PubMed

12. Antman EM, Tanasijevic MJ, Thompson B, et al. Cardiac-specific troponin I levels to predict the risk of mortality in patients with acute coronary syndromes. *N Engl J Med.* 1996;335(18):1342-1349.PubMed

13. Ohman EM, Armstrong PW, Christenson RH, et al. Cardiac troponin T levels for risk stratification in acute myocardial ischemia. *N Engl J Med.* 1996;335(18):1333-1341.PubMed

14. Hamm CW, Braunwald E. A classification of unstable angina revisited. *Circulation.* 2000;102(1):118-122.PubMed

15. Kontos MC, de Lemos JA, Ou FS, et al. Troponin-positive, MB-negative patients with non-ST-elevation myocardial infarction: an undertreated but high-risk patient group. Results from the National Cardiovascular Data Registry Acute Coronary Treatment and Intervention Outcomes Network-Get With The Guidelines (NCDR ACTION-GWTG) Registry. *Am Heart J.* 2010;160(5):819-825.PubMed

16. James SK, Lindahl B, Siegbahn A, et al. N-terminal pro-brain natriuretic peptide and other risk markers for the separate prediction of mortality and subsequent myocardial infarction in patients with unstable coronary artery disease: a Global Utilization of Strategies to Open occluded arteries (GUSTO)-IV substudy. *Circulation.* 2003;108(3):275-281.PubMed

17. Steg PG, FitzGerald G, Fox KA. Risk stratification in non-ST-segment elevation acute coronary syndromes: troponin alone is not enough. *Am J Med.* 2009;122(2):107-108.PubMed

18. Jaffe AS, Apple FS, Morrow DA, et al. Being rational about (im)precision: a statement from the biochemistry subcommittee of the joint European Society of Cardiology/American College of Cardiology Foundation/American Heart Association/World Heart Federation Task Force for the definition of myocardial infarction. *Clin Chem.* 2010;56(6):941-943. PubMed

19. Apple FS, Collinson PO. Analytical characteristics of high-sensitivity cardiac troponin assays. *Clin Chem.* 2012;58(1):54-61.PubMed

20. Wu A, Collinson P, Jaffe A, Morrow D. High-sensitivity cardiac troponin assays: what analytical and clinical issues need to be addressed before introduction into clinical practice? Interview by Fred S. Apple. *Clin Chem.* 2010;56(6):886-891.PubMed

21. Sherwood MW, Kristin Newby L. High-sensitivity troponin assays: evidence, indications, and reasonable use. *J Am Heart Assoc.* 2014;3(1):e000403.PubMed

22. Aldous SJ, Florkowski CM, Crozier IG, et al. Comparison of high sensitivity and contemporary troponin assays for the early detection of acute myocardial infarction in the emergency department. *Ann Clin Biochem.* 2011;48(Pt 3):241-248.PubMed

23. Keller T, Zeller T, Ojeda F, et al. Serial changes in highly sensitive troponin I assay and early diagnosis of myocardial infarction. *JAMA.* 2011;306(24):2684-2693.PubMed

24. Januzzi JL Jr, Mahler SA, Christenson RH, et al. Recommendations for institutions transitioning to high-sensitivity troponin testing: JACC scientific expert panel. *J Am Coll Cardiol.* 2019;73(9):1059-1077.PubMed

25. Al-Hadi HA, Fox KA. Cardiac markers in the early diagnosis and management of patients with acute coronary syndrome. *Sultan Qaboos Univ Med J.* 2009;9(3):231-246.PubMed

26. Puleo PR, Guadagno PA, Roberts R, et al. Early diagnosis of acute myocardial infarction based on assay for subforms of creatine kinase-MB. *Circulation.* 1990;82(3):759-764.PubMed

27. Puleo PR, Meyer D, Wathen C, et al. Use of a rapid assay of subforms of creatine kinase MB to diagnose or rule out acute myocardial infarction. *N Engl J Med.* 1994;331(9):561-566.PubMed

28. Ay H, Arsava EM, Sanbas O. Creatinine kinase-MB elevation after stroke is not cardiac in origin. *Stroke.* 2002;33:286-289.PubMed

29. Yancy CW, Jessup M, Bozkurt B, et al. 2013 ACCF/AHA guideline for the management of heart failure: a report of the American College of Cardiology Foundation/American Heart Association Task Force on practice guidelines. *Circulation.* 2013;128(16):e240-e327.PubMed

30. Pandit K, Mukhopadhyay P, Ghosh S, Chowdhury S. Natriuretic peptides: diagnostic and therapeutic use. *Indian J Endocrinol Metab*. 2011;15(Suppl 4):S345-S353.

31. Tang WH, Francis GS, Morrow DA, et al. National Academy of Clinical Biochemistry Laboratory Medicine practice guidelines: clinical utilization of cardiac biomarker testing in heart failure. *Circulation*. 2007;116(5):e99-e109.PubMed

32. Maisel AS, Krishnaswamy P, Nowak RM, et al. Rapid measurement of B-type natriuretic peptide in the emergency diagnosis of heart failure. *N Engl J Med*. 2002;347(3):161-167.PubMed

33. Januzzi JL Jr, Camargo CA, Anwaruddin S, et al. The N-terminal Pro-BNP investigation of dyspnea in the emergency department (PRIDE) study. *Am J Cardiol*. 2005;95(8):948-954.PubMed

34. Berger R, Huelsman M, Strecker K, et al. B-type natriuretic peptide predicts sudden death in patients with chronic heart failure. *Circulation*. 2002;105(20):2392-2397.PubMed

35. Masson S, Latini R, Anand IS, et al. Direct comparison of B-type natriuretic peptide (BNP) and amino-terminal proBNP in a large population of patients with chronic and symptomatic heart failure: the Valsartan Heart Failure (Val-HeFT) data. *Clin Chem*. 2006;52(8):1528-1538.PubMed

36. Richards M, Nicholls MG, Espiner EA, et al. Comparison of B-type natriuretic peptides for assessment of cardiac function and prognosis in stable ischemic heart disease. *J Am Coll Cardiol*. 2006;47(1):52-60. PubMed

37. Jernberg T, Stridsberg M, Venge P, Lindahl B. N-terminal pro brain natriuretic peptide on admission for early risk stratification of patients with chest pain and no ST-segment elevation. *J Am Coll Cardiol*. 2002;40(3):437-445.PubMed

38. James SK, Lindahl B, Siegbahn A, et al. N-terminal pro-brain natriuretic peptide and other risk markers for the separate prediction of mortality and subsequent myocardial infarction in patients with unstable coronary artery disease: a Global Utilization of Strategies To Open occluded arteries (GUSTO)-IV substudy. *Circulation*. 2003;108(3):275-281. PubMed

39. Morrow DA, de Lemos JA, Sabatine MS, et al. Evaluation of B-type natriuretic peptide for risk assessment in unstable angina/non-ST-elevation myocardial infarction: B-type natriuretic peptide and prognosis in TACTICS-TIMI 18. *J Am Coll Cardiol*. 2003;41(8):1264-1272.PubMed

40. Galvani M, Ottani F, Oltrona L, et al. N-terminal pro-brain natriuretic peptide on admission has prognostic value across the whole spectrum of acute coronary syndromes. *Circulation*. 2004;110(2):128-134.PubMed

41. Balion CM, McKelvie RS, Reichert S, et al. Monitoring the response to pharmacologic therapy in patients with stable chronic heart failure: is BNP or NT-proBNP a useful assessment tool? *Clin Biochem*. 2008;41(4-5):266-276.PubMed

42. Troughton RW, Frampton CM, Yandle TG, et al. Treatment of heart failure guided by plasma aminoterminal brain natriuretic peptide (N-BNP) concentrations. *Lancet*. 2000;355(9210):1126-1130.PubMed

43. Jourdain P, Jondeau G, Funck F, et al. Plasma brain natriuretic peptide-guided therapy to improve outcome in heart failure: the STARS-BNP Multicenter Study. *J Am Coll Cardiol*. 2007;49(16):1733-1739.PubMed

44. Berger R, Moertl D, Peter S, et al. N-terminal pro-B-type natriuretic peptide-guided, intensive patient management in addition to multidisciplinary care in chronic heart failure a 3-arm, prospective, randomized pilot study. *J Am Coll Cardiol*. 2010;55(7):645-653.PubMed

45. Lainchbury JG, Troughton RW, Strangman KM, et al. N-terminal pro-B-type natriuretic peptide-guided treatment for chronic heart failure: results from the BATTLESCARRED (NT-proBNP-Assisted Treatment To Lessen Serial Cardiac Readmissions and Death) trial. *J Am Coll Cardiol*. 2009;55(1):53-60.PubMed

46. Pfisterer M, Buser P, Rickli H, et al. BNP-guided vs symptom-guided heart failure therapy: the Trial of Intensified vs Standard Medical Therapy in Elderly Patients With Congestive Heart Failure (TIME-CHF) randomized trial. *JAMA*. 2009;301(4):383-392.PubMed

47. Porapakkham P, Porapakkham P, Zimmet H, et al. B-type natriuretic peptide-guided heart failure therapy: a meta-analysis. *Arch Intern Med*. 2010;170(6):507-514.PubMed

48. Thygesen K, Mair J, Mueller C, et al. Recommendations for the use of natriuretic peptides in acute cardiac care: a position statement from the Study Group on Biomarkers in Cardiology of the ESC Working Group on Acute Cardiac Care. *Eur Heart J*. 2012;33(16):2001-2006. PubMed

49. Mehra MR, Uber PA, Park MH, et al. Obesity and suppressed B-type natriuretic peptide levels in heart failure. *J Am Coll Cardiol*. 2004;43(9):1590-1595.PubMed

50. McCord J, Mundy BJ, Hudson MP, et al. Relationship between obesity and B-type natriuretic peptide levels. *Arch Intern Med*. 2004;164(20):2247-2252.PubMed

51. Krauser DG, Lloyd-Jones DM, Chae CU, et al. Effect of body mass index on natriuretic peptide levels in patients with acute congestive heart failure: a ProBNP Investigation of Dyspnea in the Emergency Department (PRIDE) substudy. *Am Heart J*. 2005;149(4):744-750. PubMed

52. Bayes-Genis A, Lloyd-Jones DM, van Kimmenade RR, et al. Effect of body mass index on diagnostic and prognostic usefulness of amino-terminal pro-brain natriuretic peptide in patients with acute dyspnea. *Arch Intern Med*. 2007;167(4):400-407.PubMed

53. Horwich TB, Hamilton MA, Fonarow GC. B-type natriuretic peptide levels in obese patients with advanced heart failure. *J Am Coll Cardiol*. 2006;47(1):85-90.PubMed

54. Daniels LB, Clopton P, Bhalla V, et al. How obesity affects the cut-points for B-type natriuretic peptide in the diagnosis of acute heart failure: results from the Breathing Not Properly Multinational Study. *Am Heart J*. 2006;151(5):999-1005.PubMed

55. de Lemos JA, Morrow DA, Bentley JH, et al. The prognostic value of B-type natriuretic peptide in patients with acute coronary syndromes. *N Engl J Med*. 2001;345(14):1014-1021.PubMed

56. Morrow DA, de Lemos JA, Blazing MA, et al. Prognostic value of serial B-type natriuretic peptide testing during follow-up of patients with unstable coronary artery disease. *JAMA*. 2005;294(22):2866-2871. PubMed

57. Richards AM, Nicholls MG, Yandle TG, et al. Plasma N-terminal pro-brain natriuretic peptide and adrenomedullin: new neurohormonal predictors of left ventricular function and prognosis after myocardial infarction. *Circulation*. 1998;97(19):1921-1929.PubMed

58. James SK, Lindahl B, Siegbahn A, et al. N-terminal pro-brain natriuretic peptide and other risk markers for the separate prediction of mortality and subsequent myocardial infarction in patients with unstable coronary artery disease: a Global Utilization of Strategies To Open occluded arteries (GUSTO)-IV substudy. *Circulation*. 2003;108(3):275-281. PubMed

59. Poutanen T, Tikanoja T, Riikonen P, et al. Long-term prospective follow-up study of cardiac function after cardiotoxic therapy for malignancy in children. *J Clin Oncol*. 2003;21(12):2349-2356.PubMed

60. Vogelsang TW, Jensen RJ, Hesse B, Kjaer A. BNP cannot replace gated equilibrium radionuclide ventriculography in monitoring of anthracycline-induced cardiotoxicity. *Int J Cardiol*. 2008;124(2):193-197.PubMed

61. Feola M, Garrone O, Occelli M, et al. Cardiotoxicity after anthracycline chemotherapy in breast carcinoma: effects on left ventricular ejection fraction, troponin I and brain natriuretic peptide. *Int J Cardiol*. 2011;148(2):194-198.PubMed

62. Goel S, Simes RJ, Beith JM. Exploratory analysis of cardiac biomarkers in women with normal cardiac function receiving trastuzumab for breast cancer. *Asia Pac J Clin Oncol*. 2011;7(3):276-280.PubMed

63. Stevens P, Freehardt D, Estis J, et al. The utility of cardiac biomarkers during anthracycline chemotherapy for the detection of cardiac events: comparison left ventricular ejection fraction. *J Am Coll Cardiol*. 2014;63:12.

64. Pun SC, Nguyen A, Ades S, et al. Predictive value of high-sensitivity cardiac troponin T, troponin I, NT-ProBNP, and high-sensitivity CRP in the detection of myocardial injury following anthracycline-based chemotherapy. *J Am Coll Cardiol.* 2015;65:10.

65. Morrison LK, Harrison A, Krishnaswamy P, et al. Utility of a rapid B-natriuretic peptide assay in differentiating congestive heart failure from lung disease in patients presenting with dyspnea. *J Am Coll Cardiol.* 2002;39(2):202-209.PubMed

66. Anand IS, Fisher LD, Chiang YT, et al. Changes in brain natriuretic peptide and norepinephrine over time and mortality and morbidity in the Valsartan Heart Failure Trial (Val-HeFT). *Circulation.* 2003;107(9): 1278-1283.PubMed

67. Entresto (sacubitril/valsartan) [prescribing information]. East Hanover, NJ: Novartis; 2019.

68. Perna ER, Macín SM, Cimbaro Canella JP, et al. Minor myocardial damage detected by troponin T is a powerful predictor of long-term prognosis in patients with acute decompensated heart failure. *Int J Cardiol.* 2005;99(2):253-261.PubMed

69. Demir M, Kanadasi M, Akpinar O, et al. Cardiac troponin T as a prognostic marker in patients with heart failure: a 3-year outcome study. *Angiology.* 2007;58(5):603-609.PubMed

70. Latini R, Masson S, Anand IS, et al. Prognostic value of very low plasma concentrations of troponin T in patients with stable chronic heart failure. *Circulation.* 2007;116(11):1242-1249.PubMed

71. Miller WL, Hartman KA, Burritt MF, et al. Profiles of serial changes in cardiac troponin T concentrations and outcome in ambulatory patients with chronic heart failure. *J Am Coll Cardiol.* 2009;54(18):1715-1721. PubMed

72. O'Connor CM, Fiuzat M, Lombardi C, et al. Impact of serial troponin release on outcomes in patients with acute heart failure: analysis from the PROTECT pilot study. *Circ Heart Fail.* 2011;4(6):724-732.PubMed

73. Yancy CW, Jessup M, Bozkurt B, et al. 2017 ACC/AHA/HFSA Focused Update of the 2013 ACCF/AHA Guideline for the Management of Heart Failure: a Report of the American College of Cardiology/American Heart Association Task Force on Clinical Practice Guidelines and the Heart Failure Society of America. *Circulation.* 2017;136(6):e137-e161.PubMed

# 8

# Lipid Disorders

*Jill S. Borchert and Kathy E. Komperda*

DOI 10.37573/9781585286423.008

## OBJECTIVES

*After completing this chapter, the reader should be able to*

- List primary and secondary causes of dyslipidemia

- Outline the physiology of lipid metabolism

- Identify clinical manifestations of dyslipidemias

- Calculate low-density lipoprotein when provided with total cholesterol, high-density lipoprotein, and triglyceride values

- Given a case study, interpret laboratory results from a lipid profile and discuss how they should guide treatment choices

Dyslipidemia, or an abnormal serum lipid profile, is a major risk factor in the development of atherosclerotic cardiovascular disease (ASCVD).[1] Clinical manifestations of ASCVD include acute coronary syndrome (eg, myocardial infarction), angina, coronary revascularization (eg, percutaneous coronary intervention), peripheral arterial disease, stroke, and transient ischemic attack.[1] More than 121 million adults in the United States are affected by cardiovascular disease, with social determinants of health affecting the burden of disease.[2] Cardiovascular disease is a leading cause of death and primary and secondary preventative efforts are essential to decrease associated morbidity and mortality.

Management of cholesterol is one of seven factors identified by the American Heart Association (AHA) as critical to address to decrease ASCVD risk.[2] Healthy People 2020 targets have been identified, with 2030 goals in development. Efforts in the management of dyslipidemia have contributed to a decline in the prevalence of high total cholesterol (TC) and a decline in mean serum TC for adults meeting the Healthy People 2020 target for the proportion of adults with high TC (TC ≥240 mg/dL). Nonetheless, the Healthy People 2020 target for mean TC (177.9 mg/dL) has not been met overall or in any race/ethnicity subgroup. Further, approximately 30% of American adults have not been screened for dyslipidemia with a lipid panel. Practitioners are being asked to assess the lipid panel in an effort to decrease overall cardiovascular risk.

This chapter primarily covers the physiology of cholesterol and metabolism of triglycerides (TGs), their actions as part of lipoproteins, disorders of lipids and lipoproteins, and consequences of elevated lipid levels. The effects of diet, exercise, and drugs on these lipid values are also discussed. A detailed interpretation of test results and drug therapy with regard to cardiovascular risk is beyond the scope of this chapter, but references provide additional information.[1,3,4]

## PHYSIOLOGY OF LIPID METABOLISM

Lipids are an essential component of several biological processes. The major plasma lipids are cholesterol, TGs, and phospholipids. Cholesterol serves as a structural component of cell wall membranes and is a precursor for the synthesis of steroid hormones and bile acids.[5-7] TGs, the esterified form of glycerol and fatty acids, constitute the main form of lipid storage in humans and serve as a reservoir of fatty acids to be used as an energy source for the body.[7] Phospholipids are lipid molecules that contain a phosphate group. Like cholesterol, phospholipids become constituents of cell wall membranes. Both cholesterol and TGs are hydrophobic, while phospholipids are hydrophilic. Cholesterol and TGs are surrounded by proteins and phospholipids to form lipoproteins. These lipoproteins are more water soluble and can then be transported in the body. Because the laboratory measurement of plasma lipids is the sum of cholesterol and TGs circulating in the different lipoproteins, an understanding of the synthesis and metabolism of these lipoproteins is necessary for proper diagnosis and treatment of dyslipidemia in efforts to reduce overall cardiovascular risk.

Cholesterol and TGs can be absorbed from the diet (exogenous) or synthesized in the body (endogenous) (**Figure 8-1**).[6] Cholesterol is continuously undergoing synthesis, degradation, and recycling. Approximately one- to two-thirds of cholesterol consumed in the diet is absorbed; however, dietary cholesterol directly contributes relatively little to serum cholesterol levels. Instead, exogenous dietary intake

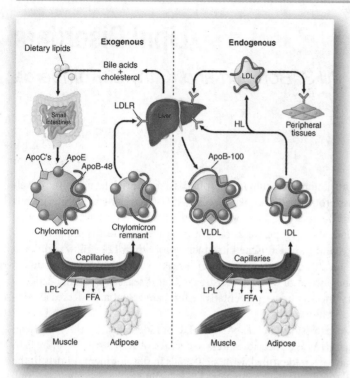

**FIGURE 8-1.** Lipid metabolism. Apo = apolipoprotein; FFA = free fatty acid; HL = hepatic lipase; IDL = intermediate-density lipoprotein; LDL = low-density lipoprotein; LDLR = low-density lipoprotein receptor; LPL = lipoprotein lipase; VLDL = very low-density lipoprotein. *Source*: Reprinted with permission from Jameson JL, Fauci AS, Kasper DL, et al, eds. *Harrison's Principles of Internal Medicine.* 20th ed. New York, NY: The McGraw-Hill Companies, Inc.; 2018.

of lipids and carbohydrates regulates endogenous synthesis of lipoproteins. Exogenous TGs are transported from the intestine to the systemic circulation via chylomicrons, which are predominantly TG-rich lipoproteins.[5,7] Endogenous production of cholesterol, TGs, and phospholipids primarily occurs in the liver and intestinal tract. Most serum cholesterol is created from cholesterol synthesis in the liver. Intestinal cholesterol absorption, hepatic cholesterol synthesis, and excretion of cholesterol and bile acids regulate serum cholesterol concentrations.[5-7] Most cholesterol synthesis occurs during the night.[8] The rate-limiting step in cholesterol synthesis is the conversion of hepatic hydroxymethylglutaryl-coenzyme A (HMG-CoA) to mevalonic acid.[5] This conversion is catalyzed by the enzyme HMG-CoA reductase.[5,6] An inhibitory feedback mechanism modulates cholesterol synthesis.[5] The presence of cholesterol in hepatic cells leads to decreased biosynthesis of cholesterol. Conversely, when hepatic cholesterol concentrations decrease, there is a resulting increase in hepatic cholesterol biosynthesis. However, the feedback inhibition mechanism is inadequate in preventing a rise in serum cholesterol levels in the presence of disorders of carbohydrate and lipid metabolism.[7]

Cholesterol, TGs, and phospholipid molecules complex with specialized proteins (apolipoproteins) to form lipoproteins, the transport form in which lipids are measured in the blood.[6,7] Because lipids are insoluble in aqueous plasma, they are formed into complexes with an outer hydrophilic coat of phospholipids and proteins and an inner core of fatty cholesterol and TGs. The apolipoproteins not only serve to support the formation of lipoproteins but also mediate binding to receptors and activate enzymes in lipoprotein metabolism. All lipoproteins contain phospholipids, TGs, and esterified and unesterified cholesterol in varying amounts. There are many ways to classify these lipoproteins; however, lipoproteins are classified most frequently by their density, size, and major apolipoprotein composition. **Table 8-1** summarizes the characteristics of the five major classes of lipoproteins.[6,7] The major apolipoproteins listed in Table 8-1 are a summary of the apolipoproteins involved in lipoprotein formation. Of note, atherogenic lipoproteins contain apolipoprotein B (apoB), while high-density lipoprotein (HDL) contains apoA. Another atherogenic lipoprotein is lipoprotein(a) [Lp(a)], which is associated with apo(a).[6]

All major lipoproteins play a role in cholesterol metabolism and transport in the body.[5,6] Chylomicrons, which are primarily TG rich, deliver TG from the gastrointestinal tract to the muscle and adipose tissue, where lipoprotein lipase (LPL) releases fatty acids and glycerol. After this process, the chylomicron is no longer TG rich and is now termed *chylomicron remnant*, which is delivered to the liver. The liver can export cholesterol and other TGs in the form of very low-density lipoproteins (VLDLs) into the circulation. Similar to chylomicrons, VLDLs are predominantly TG rich but have a higher cholesterol composition than chylomicrons (5 mg of TGs per 1 mg of cholesterol).[6] Once in circulation, VLDL undergoes the same hydrolyzation as chylomicrons via LPL.[5,6] This LPL activity then converts VLDL particles to intermediate-density lipoproteins (IDLs) and eventually low-density lipoproteins (LDLs). LDL typically carries the largest portion of cholesterol in the body. The liver degrades most circulating LDL; however, other tissues can take up a small portion of LDL that provides necessary cholesterol for cell membrane and steroid synthesis. LDL in general is considered atherogenic and has been a focus of dyslipidemia management. The last major lipoprotein is HDL and, unlike LDL, it is considered protection against atherosclerosis via a mechanism of reverse cholesterol transport (**Figure 8-2**). One role of HDL is to acquire excess cholesterol from degraded VLDL and the periphery. HDL undergoes an enzymatic reaction via lecithin cholesterol acyltransferase to become HDL cholesteryl ester and then is selectively taken up by the liver and targeted for excretion via bile. In addition, the cholesteryl ester transfer protein can transfer cholesteryl ester from HDL to the apoB-containing lipoproteins VLDL, IDL, and LDL, which then can be taken up by the liver more easily.

Elevated cholesterol is a known contributor to the development of atherosclerosis. Proper diagnosis and treatment of dyslipidemia can be an important preventative strategy. Numerous trials of effective treatment have demonstrated reductions in cardiovascular events, stroke, and total mortality in patients with ASCVD (secondary prevention) and in patients with asymptomatic dyslipidemia (primary prevention).[1]

**TABLE 8-1.** Characteristics of Lipoproteins

| LIPOPROTEIN | SIZE | DENSITY | MAJOR APOLIPOPROTEIN | ORIGIN | COMMENTS |
|---|---|---|---|---|---|
| Chylomicrons and chylomicron remnants | Largest | Least | ApoB-48 | Intestines | Primarily TGs |
| VLDL | ↑ | ↓ | ApoB-100 | Liver and intestines | Primarily TGs |
| IDL or remnants | | | ApoB-100 | Chylomicrons and VLDL | Transitional forms |
| LDL | | | ApoB-100 | End product of VLDL | Major carrier of cholesterol |
| HDL | Smallest | Most | ApoA-I | Intestines and liver | Removes cholesterol from atherosclerotic plaques in arteries |

*Source*: Adapted from Rader DJ, Kathiresan S. Disorders of lipoprotein metabolism. In: Jameson JL, Fauci AS, Kasper DL, et al, eds. *Harrison's Principles of Internal Medicine*. 20th ed. New York, NY: The McGraw-Hill Companies, Inc.; 2018:2889–2902; Freeman MW, Walford GA. Lipoprotein metabolism and the treatment of lipid disorders. In: Jameson JL, De Groot LJ, de Kretser DM, et al, eds. *Endocrinology: Adult and Pediatric*. 7th ed. Philadelphia, PA: W.B. Saunders Elsevier; 2016:715–736.

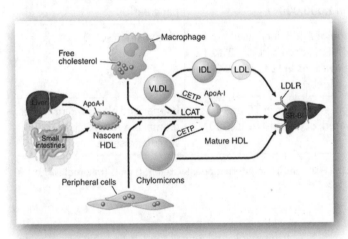

**FIGURE 8-2.** HDL metabolism and reverse cholesterol transport. Apo = apolipoprotein; CETP = cholesteryl ester transfer protein; HDL = high-density lipoprotein; IDL = intermediate-density lipoprotein; LCAT = lecithin-cholesterol acyltransferase; LDL = low-density lipoprotein; LDLR = low-density lipoprotein receptor; SR-BI = scavenger receptor class BI; VLDL = very low-density lipoprotein. *Source*: Reprinted with permission from Jameson JL, Fauci AS, Kasper DL, et al, eds. *Harrison's Principles of Internal Medicine*. 20th ed. New York, NY: The McGraw-Hill Companies, Inc.; 2018.

## Primary Lipid Disorders

*Dyslipidemias*, or abnormal concentrations of any lipoprotein type, are classified by etiology into primary or secondary disorders. Primary disorders are caused by genetic defects in the synthesis or metabolism of the lipoproteins. **Table 8-2** shows the characteristics of the major primary dyslipidemias.[3,6,9,10] Historically, familial dyslipidemias were categorized by the Fredrickson electrophoresis profile of lipoproteins. Currently, clinicians classify by the primary lipid parameter affected. Primary lipid disorders rarely occur alone, and it is unlikely for a genetic predisposition to be the sole cause of a lipid disorder. Clinically, other causes, such as diet or medications, should be considered and minimized in all patients.

## Secondary Lipid Disorders

*Secondary dyslipidemias* are disorders precipitated by other disease states, medications, or lifestyle (**Table 8-3**).[6,11-13] When a secondary cause is likely responsible for the lipid abnormality, treatment of the underlying cause should be strongly considered.

Common disease-related causes of dyslipidemia are diabetes and thyroid disorders. Patients with type 2 diabetes may present with elevated TG levels, decreased HDL cholesterol levels, and increased levels of small, dense LDL.[3,14] These abnormalities may persist despite adequate glycemic control, but optimization of glycemic control is still considered an important step. LDL cholesterol concentrations and, in some cases, TG levels increase in hypothyroidism.[6] In addition to these endocrine disorders, chronic kidney disease and liver disorders should be excluded. Alterations in lipid concentrations depend on the type of renal disorder present. For example, patients with chronic kidney disease present with elevations in TGs, whereas lipid profiles in patients with nephrotic syndrome are characterized by markedly elevated LDL cholesterol and TGs.[6,12,14] Different liver disorders also have varying effects on lipid profiles.[6] It is recommended that secondary causes be excluded by patient history, physical examination, and laboratory data. Laboratory tests such as fasting blood glucose, thyroid-stimulating hormone, serum creatinine, and urinalysis for proteinuria are useful to exclude common secondary causes of dyslipidemia.

In drug-induced dyslipidemia, changes are not always clinically significant, and withdrawal of the precipitating medication usually leads to a reversal of secondary dyslipidemia.

**TABLE 8-2.** Classification of Selected Primary Dyslipidemias

| PRIMARY LIPID ABNORMALITY | PRIMARY DYSLIPIDEMIA | SELECTED FEATURES[a] | CLINICAL MANIFESTATIONS |
|---|---|---|---|
| Increased LDL | Familial hypercholesterolemia | LDL receptor defect, LDL 200–500 in heterozygous, 500–800 in homozygous; prevalence 1 in 500 | Tendinous xanthomas, premature ASCVD |
| | Familial defective ApoB-100 | ApoB-100 mutation impairs LDL binding, LDL 200–400 in heterozygous, 500–800 in homozygous; prevalence 1 in 1,500 | Tendinous xanthomas, premature ASCVD |
| Increased TGs | Familial hypertriglyceridemia | Increases TG-rich VLDL particles, TGs >250; prevalence 5% | Often asymptomatic unless associated with metabolic syndrome |
| | Familial apoC-II deficiency | Autosomal recessive disorder; TGs >1,000; prevalence <1 in 1,000,000 | Eruptive xanthomas, hepatosplenomegaly, pancreatitis |
| | Lipoprotein lipase deficiency | Autosomal recessive disorder, mutation in lipoprotein lipase gene, TGs >1,000; prevalence 1 in 1,000,000 | Eruptive xanthomas, hepatosplenomegaly, pancreatitis |
| Increased TGs and cholesterol | Familial combined hyperlipidemia | Overproduction of ApoB, increased production of VLDL, occurs in 1%–2% of population, elevations in LDL, TGs, TC, but degree varies widely | Premature ASCVD |
| | Familial dysbetalipoproteinemia | ApoE mutation, elevations in TC and TGs similarly elevated; occurs in 1 in 10,000 | Palmar and plantar xanthomas, premature ASCVD, peripheral vascular disease |

[a]TGs, LDL, HDL, and TC in milligrams/deciliter. Conversion factor for LDL, HDL, and TC in International System (SI) units (millimoles/liter) is 0.02586. Conversion factor for TGs in SI units (millimoles/liter) is 0.01129.
*Source*: Adapted from References 3,6,9,10.

Nonetheless, when interpreting a lipid profile, it is important to evaluate how medication-related changes may have contributed to the profile. For example, antihypertensive agents are frequently administered to patients with cardiovascular risk. Nonselective beta-blocking agents, except carvedilol, which also has α 1-adrenergic receptor–blocking activity, may increase TG concentrations and reduce HDL cholesterol concentrations.[11] The effects on the lipid panel seem to be greater in individuals with high baseline TG concentrations. Thiazide diuretics increase TC, LDL cholesterol, and TG concentrations. Thiazide effects on the lipid panel are most pronounced with higher dosages; use of low doses is recommended. Although it is important to realize the effect of antihypertensive agents on the lipid profile, agents that adversely affect the lipid profile are not contraindicated in patients with dyslipidemia. Careful consideration of patient-specific factors is warranted.

Other drug classes have been implicated as sources of lipid abnormalities; however, effects on the lipid panel should not be considered a class effect for these medications. Atypical antipsychotics are known to cause lipid abnormalities, with olanzapine and clozapine possessing the greatest potential to increase LDL cholesterol, TC, and TG levels.[11] Other atypical antipsychotics,

such as aripiprazole and ziprasidone, have a low risk of metabolic effects. Similar variability has been seen among oral contraceptives, immunosuppressive drugs, and protease inhibitors. Various oral contraceptives affect lipoproteins differently. Combination oral contraceptives increase TG concentrations. Effects on LDL and HDL are variable, depending on oral contraceptive components. Oral contraceptives with second-generation progestins (eg, levonorgestrel) that have strong androgenic properties may increase TG and LDL cholesterol levels and decrease HDL cholesterol levels. However, combined oral contraceptives with third-generation progestins (eg, desogestrel) do not cause unfavorable effects on HDL and LDL cholesterol levels but may increase TGs. Immunosuppressive drugs such as cyclosporine, sirolimus, and corticosteroids adversely affect the lipid profile, but tacrolimus does not impact the lipid profile with the same magnitude, and mycophenolate mofetil has no effect.

Protease inhibitors are known to primarily cause an increase in TG levels but may also increase LDL.[13] Ritonavir-boosted lopinavir seems to have the greatest impact over ritonavir-boosted darunavir or atazanavir. Lipid abnormalities have also been identified with other antiretroviral therapies, including the nucleoside reverse transcriptase inhibitor abacavir, the nonnucleoside

**TABLE 8-3.** Secondary Causes of Dyslipidemia and Major Associated Changes in Lipoprotein Component

| MEDICAL OR DIET[a] | DRUG[a] |
|---|---|
| Acute hepatitis (↑TGs) | Alcohol (↑TGs) |
| Anorexia (↑LDL) | Anabolic steroids (↑LDL, ↓HDL) |
| Autoimmune disease (↑LDL, ↑TGs) | Atypical antipsychotics (↑TGs, ↓HDL) |
| Chronic kidney disease (↑LDL, ↑TGs) | Beta blockers (↑TGs, ↓HDL) |
| Cigarette use (↓HDL) | Combined contraceptives[b]: oral, vaginal ring (↑TGs) |
| Diabetes mellitus (↓HDL, ↑TGs) | Corticosteroids (↑LDL, ↑TGs) |
| Diet high in saturated or *trans* fats (↑LDL, ↑TGs) | Cyclosporine (↑LDL, ↑TGs) |
| Diet high in carbohydrates (↑TGs) | Estrogens, oral (↑TGs, ↑HDL, ↓LDL) |
| Glycogen storage disease (↑TGs) | Estrogen-receptor modulators (↓LDL, ↑TGs) |
| Hypothyroidism (↑LDL, ↑TGs) | Isotretinoin (↑LDL, ↓HDL, ↑TGs) |
| Liver failure (↓LDL, ↓TGs) | Progestins (↑LDL, ↓HDL, ↓TGs) |
| Metabolic syndrome (↑TGs) | Protease inhibitors (↑TGs) |
| Nephrotic syndrome (↑LDL, ↑TG) | Propofol (↑TGs) |
| Obesity (↓HDL, ↑TGs) | Sirolimus (↑LDL, ↑TGs) |
| Obstructive liver disease (↑LDL) | Thiazide diuretics (↑LDL, ↑TGs) |
| Polycystic ovary syndrome (↑LDL, ↑TGs) | |
| Pregnancy (↑LDL, ↑TGs) | |
| Sedentary lifestyle (↑TGs) | |

[a]↑ = increase; ↓ = decrease.
[b]Effect on HDL and LDL depends on specific components.
*Source:* Adapted from References 6,11–13.

reverse transcriptase inhibitor efavirenz, and the integrase inhibitor elvitegravir. Tenofovir disoproxil fumarate has been associated with improvements in the lipid profile, but switching to tenofovir alafenamide may increase lipids. Because drug-associated adverse effects on the lipid profile have not been directly correlated with increased risk for ASCVD, the importance of the efficacy, toxicity, and pill burden of the antiretroviral regimen is emphasized when considering a patient-centered treatment plan.

Lifestyle also may affect lipoprotein concentrations. Besides contributing to ASCVD risk, obesity and cigarette smoking cause a decrease in HDL cholesterol, and obesity further causes an increase in serum TGs.[6] Lifestyle modifications, including smoking cessation, physical activity, heart-healthy dietary patterns, and maintenance of a healthy weight, aid in reducing ASCVD risk and atherogenic lipid levels.[1,2,4] A diet that is high in saturated fats and *trans* fatty acids increases LDL cholesterol levels. A diet low in saturated fats with avoidance of *trans* fatty acids is recommended to reduce risk of ASCVD.[4] Low-carbohydrate diets favorably change TGs and HDL cholesterol, but they may increase LDL cholesterol levels and contribute to increased mortality if carbohydrates are replaced with animal-derived protein and fat. Light-to-moderate alcohol intake (one to two glasses of beer or wine or 1 to 2 oz of liquor per day) increases HDL.[6,15] The actual effect of alcohol consumption on TGs is variable.[3] It appears that light alcohol consumption may be associated with little to no change in TG levels. However, TG levels increase as alcohol consumption increases, particularly when excess alcohol is consumed with a diet high in saturated fat.

# LABORATORY TESTS FOR LIPIDS AND LIPOPROTEINS

Laboratory tests can be used to assess the concentrations of various lipids in the blood, making ASCVD risk assessment possible. Identification of patients at risk for ASCVD is a two-part process. First, a laboratory assessment of the lipid profile must occur. Second, an assessment of the overall ASCVD risk, including an assessment of additional cardiovascular risk factors, must occur. Multiple guidelines regarding dyslipidemia screening and management are available.[1,14] Some differences between the guidelines exist, and a detailed summary of the recommendations is beyond the scope of this chapter; however, key messages regarding lipid monitoring are discussed.

The American College of Cardiology (ACC) and the AHA published dyslipidemia guidelines (AHA/ACC guidelines) in 2018 with input and approval from several other professional organizations.[1] ASCVD risk assessment for primary prevention, including a lipid panel, is recommended every 4 to 6 years for any adult patient between 20 and 39 years old. This monitoring could be repeated more often if a clinician determines a patient's ASCVD risk has increased[14] or for adults between 40 and 75 years.[4] The standard lipid panel includes TC, TGs, HDL, and calculated LDL. This is only one component of the overall ASCVD risk assessment and should be done in conjunction with a review of information associated with established risk factors, such as age, diet, physical activity, weight, gender, blood pressure, diabetes, and smoking status.[1,4]

Screening recommendations differ for pediatric patients. The Expert Panel on Integrated Guidelines for Cardiovascular Health and Risk Reduction in Children and Adolescents recommends a fasting lipid panel for children between the ages of 2 and 8 years if a child has a positive family history for premature cardiovascular disease or has a parent with known dyslipidemia or if the child has cardiovascular risk factors, such as hypertension, diabetes, or elevated body mass index.[16] In addition, universal screening is recommended in all pediatric patients between 9 and 11 years. No routine screening is recommended during puberty because levels may fluctuate. Reference ranges and treatment strategies for pediatric patients differ from the adult population. A review of such pediatric recommendations is beyond the scope of this chapter.

Recent guidelines recommend that a fasting or nonfasting lipid panel can be used in ASCVD risk assessment.[1,16] The lipid panel was historically drawn as a fasting sample, requiring a 9- to 12-hour fast. However, eating causes clinically insignificant differences in TC and HDL levels.[17] Previous recommendations for fasting were based on the increase of TGs demonstrated with a fat tolerance test, which typically includes a much higher fat intake than average meals.[18,19] It has been estimated that compared with the fasting state, a nonfasting LDL cholesterol level is up to 10% lower and a nonfasting TG level is up to 20% higher.[20] These changes typically do not affect clinical decision-making. Allowing nonfasting lipid panels may increase screening rates, especially if the burden of obtaining the lipid panel under fasting conditions may delay and/or prevent lipid testing.[21] Exceptions to nonfasting measurement in which a fasting lipid panel is recommended are if TG measurement is the focus of the lab test or if TGs are >400 mg/dL in a nonfasting sample.[1]

Several laboratory factors may cause deviations in the lipid values obtained. Ideally, the patient should remain seated 5 minutes before phlebotomy, and tourniquet application should be limited to <1 minute to avoid hemoconcentration, which may cause falsely elevated lipid levels.[3,17] Plasma concentration lipid values are approximately 3% lower than those values associated with serum measurements.[3,17]

Patient-specific factors may also interfere with the lipid panel results. Recent weight changes, pregnancy, acute infection, trauma, and cardiovascular events may result in levels that are not representative of the patient's usual value.[17] For some of these circumstances (eg, pregnancy and acute infection), it may be beneficial to wait several weeks to months to obtain a lipid panel. For other circumstances, such as in the setting of acute coronary syndrome, a lipid panel should not be delayed. Measurement of plasma lipids in the setting of acute coronary syndrome usually provides LDL values that are lower than baseline 25 to 48 hours after an event.[22] A more recent study demonstrated that cholesterol levels remained relatively stable in the 4 days after an ACS event; however, no comparisons to pre-ACS levels were performed.[23] Despite the possible effect of cardiovascular events on lipid levels, the recommendations are to obtain a lipid panel, preferably within the first 24 hours after the event.[24,25]

Unlike most other laboratory values, "normal" ranges for lipid lab values are not determined by reference studies of normal subjects. Instead, values below a certain value (TC, LDL, and TGs) or values above a certain value (HDL) have been identified based on epidemiologic studies to determine ideal levels for decreasing cardiovascular disease risk.[26] Methods used to assay lipid panels vary among institutions. It is important to become familiar with the method of lipid profile measurement used by the laboratory that the clinician uses regularly.

## Total Cholesterol

For adults ≥20 years, total cholesterol levels are categorized in the following ways[27]:

desirable: <200 mg/dL (5.2 mmol/L)

borderline high: 200 to 239 mg/dL (5.2 to 6.2 mmol/L)

high: ≥240 mg/dL (6.2 mmol/L)

Current recommendations are to use the other components of the lipid panel (eg, LDL) instead of TC to guide patient-care decisions.[1] However, TC is still reported as part of a lipid panel, and the desirable levels included on laboratory reports are typically those from previous versions of cholesterol guidelines.[27]

## Triglycerides

For adults ≥20 years, TG levels are categorized in the following ways[12]:

normal: <150 mg/dL (1.7 mmol/L)

borderline high: 150 to 199 mg/dL (1.7 to 2.2 mmol/L)

high: 200 to 499 mg/dL (2.3 to 5.6 mmol/L)

very high: ≥500 mg/dL (5.6 mmol/L)

Disorders leading to hypertriglyceridemia involve dysregulation of chylomicrons and/or VLDL. Chylomicrons are typically only present postprandially, whereas VLDL, LDL, and HDL are present in the fasting state.[17] TGs in the form of chylomicrons appear in the plasma soon after eating and are typically eliminated within 6 to 9 hours after a meal. If chylomicrons persist 12 hours postprandially, this indicates an abnormal state. As previously discussed, an overnight fast is recommended if TGs are the focus of measurement or if TGs are >400 mg/dL on a nonfasting sample[1] because a high-fat meal (>50 g of fat) may provide a clinically significant 50% increase in TGs whereas a low-fat meal (<15 g of fat) does not.[3] If a nonfasting TG level is elevated, it is important to inquire about a patient's eating pattern to determine if retesting is valuable. Retesting in 2 to 4 weeks can be considered if a high-fat meal was ingested before the measurement.

Triglyceride classification varies slightly between sources,[1,3,12] but recommendations aimed at reducing complications of hypertriglyceridemia are consistent with a focus on lifestyle modifications and drug therapy, when necessary. The AHA/ACC guidelines classify fasting or nonfasting TGs of 175 to 499 mg/dL (2.0 to 5.6 mmol/L) as moderate hypertriglyceridemia and fasting TGs of 500 mg/dL (5.6 mmol/L) or higher as severe hypertriglyceridemia.[1] In moderate hypertriglyceridemia, VLDL is the primary carrier of excess TGs, whereas patients with severe hypertriglyceridemia often have both elevated VLDL and chylomicrons. Excess VLDL increases ASCVD risk, and chylomicrons contribute to the elevated risk of acute pancreatitis. Severe hypertriglyceridemia, especially concentrations ≥1,000 mg/dL or 11.3 mmol/L, may precipitate pancreatitis.[1,28] Before initiating drug therapy, underlying factors should be addressed, such as physical inactivity, poor diet, uncontrolled diabetes, and use of medications that increase TGs. In patients with severe hypertriglyceridemia, the goal of therapy is to reduce TGs <500 mg/dL (5.6 mmol/L).[28] Dietary modification includes an avoidance of *trans* fats and reduction in saturated fats without a concomitant increase in carbohydrates.[1,3] For patients with diabetes, glycemic control may help to lower TG concentrations. For very high TGs, the drugs of choice for lowering TGs are fibrates or omega-3 fatty acids.[1] An alternative approach to drug therapy for patients at lower risk for pancreatitis is to intensify statin therapy, which provides some reduction in TGs. Bile acid sequestrants should be avoided because these agents are known to increase TG concentrations (**Minicase 1**).

In addition to the risk of pancreatitis, extremely high concentrations of TGs—concentrations in excess of 2,000 mg/dL (22.6 mmol/L)—may also lead to eruptive cutaneous xanthomas on the elbows, knees, and buttocks.[26] Once TG concentrations are reduced, the xanthomas gradually disappear over the course of 1 to 3 months. Such extremely high TGs may also manifest as lipemia retinalis (a salmon-pink cast in the vascular bed of the retina) because TG particles scatter light in the blood, which is seen in the retinal vessels during an eye exam. The presence of such signs and symptoms warrants a detailed patient history and laboratory testing to ensure appropriate treatment.

Many patients with high TGs lead a sedentary lifestyle and are obese. Patients encountered in clinical practice with elevated TGs often have similar lipid and nonlipid risk factors of metabolic origin termed *metabolic syndrome*, which is associated with an increased ASCVD risk.[1,3] Metabolic syndrome is characterized by abdominal obesity, insulin resistance, hypertension, low HDL, and elevations in TGs. Metabolic syndrome is managed by correcting underlying causes, such as obesity, with lifestyle modifications and treating associated lipid risk factors.

Enzymatic methods for TG measurements are susceptible to interference by glycerol, which is normally present in serum.[17,26] Clinically significant increases in glycerol concentrations can occur in uncontrolled diabetes or after extremely vigorous physical exercise.[17] However, clinical laboratories incorporate means for correcting excess glycerol as part of the measurement process to provide accurate TG measurements.[17,26]

An excess of TGs in the blood can lead to errors in other laboratory measurements. Patients with severe hypertriglyceridemia may have lipemic samples, characterized by a milky appearance.[29] Although it does not affect laboratory TG measurement,

## MINICASE 1

## Hypertriglyceridemia

Felicia C., a 52-year-old woman, presents to the clinic to review lab results provided recently for routine screening. Her past medical history is significant for hypertension, bipolar disorder, and obesity. She has no premature family history of ASCVD. Daily medications include lisinopril 40 mg and olanzapine 15 mg. Her diet primarily consists of processed foods and significant amounts of carbohydrates. She denies any history of tobacco use but does report one to two glasses of wine most nights of the week. Physical activity is minimal beyond general daily activities. Felicia C. has no physical complaints. She is 5'6" and 220 lb. Lab results are as follows: TC, 242 mg/dL; TG, 594 mg/dL; HDL, 40 mg/dL; and direct LDL, 80 mg/dL. The labs were drawn at 9 a.m.

QUESTION: How should the lipid results be interpreted? What should be done next?

DISCUSSION: The first step should be to confirm with the patient if the lab specimens were obtained when the patient was fasting. TGs are affected by recent food intake, and the impact varies depending on the fat content of the meal. If a typical low-fat meal is ingested before lab measurements, then the effect is clinically insignificant. However, if the meal contains >50 g of fat, then the TG levels could be increased by as high as 50%.[3] If a patient fails to fast and the TG levels are >400 mg/dL upon screening, a repeat fasting lipid panel to confirm elevated TG levels should be ordered.[1] Felicia C. confirms the lipids were drawn in the fasting state. The LDL value in her lipid panel is a direct measurement. Lipid panels are often ordered to provide a calculated LDL with a reflex measurement of direct LDL if the TGs are >400 mg/dL because LDL can only be calculated with the Friedewald formula when TGs are <400 mg/dL.

Felicia C. has very high TGs, with a TG level >500 mg/dL; therefore, TG lowering is the initial therapeutic goal.[28] Very high TG levels, especially those >1,000 mg/dL, are associated with an increased risk of pancreatitis. Despite no symptoms or physical signs of pancreatitis, Felicia C. should take immediate steps to reduce her risk. To prevent acute pancreatitis, TGs should be lowered through lifestyle modifications, including dietary changes, alcohol avoidance, weight loss, and exercise. Dietary modifications include a reduction in saturated fat and avoidance of *trans* fat intake without an increase in carbohydrates.[3] Felicia C.'s current diet is high in saturated fat and carbohydrates, which is an established secondary cause of hypertriglyceridemia. Abstention from all alcohol intake is important to minimize the risk of pancreatitis. Of the atypical antipsychotics, olanzapine has a greater potential to contribute to increases in TGs than other agents, such as aripiprazole or ziprasidone. However, the risks and benefits of modifications in therapy must be carefully weighed, and any changes to her bipolar treatment should only occur in consultation with her mental health care provider for close monitoring. Hypertriglyceridemia is often present in patients who are obese and physically inactive. Because diabetes or metabolic syndrome is a common secondary cause of hypertriglyceridemia, a fasting glucose level should be obtained to determine if this is a factor in Felicia C.'s case. Further, a TG-lowering drug, such as a fibrate or omega-3 fatty acid, should be considered.[1] Bile acid sequestrants should be avoided because they may increase TGs. If Felicia C. experiences epigastric pain or vomiting, it may be prudent to check amylase and lipase levels and proceed with further evaluation for pancreatitis. Once TG levels have been lowered to <500 mg/dL, then attention can be turned to assessment of the lipid panel for ASCVD risk reduction.

it may cause interference in measurement of other laboratory tests such as alanine aminotransferase and aspartate aminotransferase, which depend on spectrophotometric methods for analysis. Most technologists and automated systems can identify lipemic samples, and processes can be used to remove lipemia. This produces a clear specimen and eliminates interferences in these assay methods.

## Low-Density Lipoprotein Cholesterol

For adults ≥20 years, LDL levels are categorized in the following ways[12]:

desirable: <100 mg/dL (2.6 mmol/L)

above desirable: 100 to 129 mg/dL (2.6 to 3.3 mmol/L)

borderline high: 130 to 159 mg/dL (3.4 to 4.1 mmol/L)

high: 160 to 189 mg/dL (4.1 to 4.9 mmol/L)

very high: ≥190 mg/dL (4.9 mmol/L)

Low-density lipoprotein cholesterol can be measured directly or estimated indirectly by a method determined by Friedewald.[30] The Friedewald formula subtracts the HDL and VLDL cholesterol from TC. The VLDL is estimated to be the TG level divided by five. Using the following formula (all in milligrams/deciliter), LDL may be estimated in patients with a TG concentration <400 mg/dL (4.5 mmol/L):

$$LDL = TC - HDL - (TGs/5)$$

If a patient's serum TG concentration exceeds 400 mg/dL (4.5 mmol/L), LDL cholesterol should not be calculated with this formula. A direct LDL measurement by laboratory would provide an LDL value. In patients with severe hypertriglyceridemia, TG-lowering therapy is often implemented to reduce pancreatitis risk. Once TG values have decreased to <400 mg/dL (4.5 mmol/L), a standard lipid panel provides LDL cholesterol data. Clinicians should be aware that other factors, such as low LDL levels (<70 mg/dL), especially when TGs are above normal, may also affect the reliability of the Friedewald equation and that calculation adjustments have been published.[1,31,32] AHA/ACC guidelines recommend initiating statin therapy in patients based on ASCVD risk.[1] Patients at high risk, including presence of clinical ASCVD or very high LDL levels (≥190 mg/dL or ≥4.9 mmol/L), would benefit from high-intensity statin therapy, with a goal LDL reduction of ≥50%. In patients between 40 and 75 years of age with diabetes, a moderate intensity statin with a goal LDL reduction of 30% to 49% is recommended. A high-intensity statin can be considered for select patients with diabetes with additional risk factors. For all other patients (ie, patients considered for primary prevention therapy without diabetes), an estimation of ASCVD risk is recommended via use of a risk calculator. Ten-year ASCVD risk calculations of 7.5% to 19.9% are classified as intermediate risk, whereas ≥20% are high risk. A patient's ASCVD risk calculation and the presence of risk-enhancing factors (eg, family history of premature ASCVD, chronic kidney disease, metabolic syndrome) can help guide the clinician–patient risk discussion on statin therapy. When risk discussion favors the initiation of statin therapy, a moderate intensity statin can be used in patients with an intermediate ASCVD risk calculation, whereas a high-intensity statin can be recommended in a patient with a high 10-year ASCVD risk (**Minicases 2 and 3**).

Lifestyle modifications aimed at lowering ASCVD risk are appropriate for all patients.[1] Detailed education should be provided to patients regarding the adoption of a low saturated fat diet that reduces the percent of calories from saturated fats and avoids *trans* fats.[4,33] Physical activity should also be encouraged, with a goal of at least 150 min/wk of moderate-intensity exercise. Improvements in diet and physical activity are imperative to aid in weight loss in overweight or obese patients. A weight loss of ≥5% has been associated with a significant improvement in LDL and TGs.[4] For patients at elevated ASCVD risk, lifestyle modifications with concurrent statin therapy should be recommended.[1]

## High-Density Lipoprotein Cholesterol

For adults ≥20 years, HDL levels are categorized in the following ways[12]:

low (men): <40 mg/dL (1.0 mmol/L)

low (women): <50 mg/dL (1.3 mmol/L)

Based on epidemiologic evidence, HDL acts as an antiatherogenic factor.[12] Whereas a high HDL concentration is associated with cardioprotection, low levels are associated with increased risk of ASCVD. The Framingham Study demonstrated that higher HDL levels are protective against cardiovascular risk, even in the setting of elevations in LDL.[34] HDL has several antiatherogenic properties, such as reverse cholesterol transport and antiplatelet activity; however, clinical studies aimed at raising HDL with medications have failed to demonstrate a decrease in cardiovascular risk.[12,34] Therefore, the mechanism of the association between low HDL and cardiovascular risk is not fully understood. It is possible that low HDL may be a marker of other atherogenic changes in the full lipid profile.

HDL cholesterol <40 mg/dL (1.0 mmol/L) in men or <50 mg/dL (1.3 mmol/L) in women is considered a risk factor of metabolic syndrome.[1] Most patients with low HDL levels have concomitant elevated TG levels.[6] In these patients, lifestyle therapy or drug therapy to decrease other atherosclerotic particles usually results in a desirable increase in HDL.[34] HDL is negatively correlated with TGs, smoking, and obesity and positively correlated with physical activity and smoking cessation. Women typically have higher HDL levels than men, likely due to the beneficial effects of estrogen.[6,34] Because of a lack of evidence, drug therapy decisions are not centered on raising HDL alone.[1]

## Non–High-Density Lipoprotein Cholesterol

For adults ≥20 years, non-HDL levels are categorized in the following ways[12]:

desirable: <130 mg/dL (3.4 mmol/L)

above desirable: 130 to 159 mg/dL (3.4 to 4.1 mmol/L)

borderline high: 160 to 189 mg/dL (4.1 to 4.9 mmol/L)

high: 190 to 219 mg/dL (4.9 to 5.7 mmol/L)

very high: ≥220 mg/dL (5.7 mmol/L)

Non-HDL cholesterol (TC–HDL) provides an estimate of the sum of cholesterol carried by atherogenic particles that

## MINICASE 2

### Primary Prevention

Julia K., a 46-year-old woman, presents to the clinic for a new patient consultation. She has been receiving care from a specialist (rheumatologist) but has not seen a primary care provider in many years. Her past medical history includes rheumatoid arthritis but no other chronic conditions; she is premenopausal and has an intrauterine device for pregnancy prevention. Her only medication is biweekly adalimumab, and she states the medication controls her symptoms well. She does not follow a specific diet but notes that she tries to limit her fast-food intake and eat a variety of fruits and vegetables. She walks at a moderate pace for 30 minutes three times a week. She denies any current tobacco use; she quit 10 years ago after smoking one pack per day for 10 years. She reports drinking one to two glasses of wine once a month. Her family history is notable, with a father who had a myocardial infarction at age 54. At her office visit, she has an unremarkable physical exam with a blood pressure reading of 112/74 mm Hg. She had a set of labs drawn the previous day that were nonfasting. The following laboratory results were obtained: TC, 270 mg/dL; HDL, 48 mg/dL; TG, 135 mg/dL; LDL, 195 mg/dL; and glucose, 102 mg/dL. Electrolyte, hematology, liver, renal, and thyroid tests are all normal. She is 5'6" and weighs 159 lb.

QUESTION: How should the lipid results be interpreted? Based on this interpretation, is medication therapy recommended?

DISCUSSION: Julia K. is asymptomatic and follows a reasonable lifestyle that includes a diet rich in fruits and vegetables, routine aerobic exercise, no tobacco use, and low alcohol intake.

Autoimmune disorders such as rheumatoid arthritis may be a secondary cause of dyslipidemia, and chronic inflammatory conditions may be a risk-enhancing factor for ASCVD.[1] She does not have type 2 diabetes or thyroid, renal, or liver disease. She has a family history of premature ASCVD, with her father having a clinical ASCVD event at an age <55 years.

Guidelines recommend checking a lipid panel in a fasting or nonfasting state because evidence suggests the variation between fasting and nonfasting results is clinically insignificant if labs are drawn after a standard meal.[1] Julia K.'s LDL is very high, her TC is high, her HDL is low, and her TGs are in normal range. The primary concern is the very high LDL because LDL ≥190 mg/dL highly suggests the presence of a primary lipid disorder. Patients with very high LDL cholesterol are known to be at an increased lifetime risk for ASCVD events because of their lifetime exposure to elevated atherogenic cholesterol. Julia K. would be considered high risk for ASCVD because of her very high LDL.

Julia K. should be encouraged to adhere to a low saturated fat diet that emphasizes reduced saturated fat and avoidance of *trans* fat and to maintain her physical activity. Because she is considered at high risk, high-intensity statin therapy is recommended. AHA/ACC guidelines recommend high-intensity statins for all adult patients with an LDL ≥190 mg/dL.[1] Once treatment is started, a repeat lipid panel could be ordered in 4 to 12 weeks to assess for adherence and percentage reduction in LDL.

---

contain apolipoprotein B (apoB) such as LDL, VLDL chylomicrons, and Lp(a).[1,12] For patients at very-high ASCVD risk (eg, multiple ASCVD events), non-HDL levels as well as LDL levels may guide when nonstatin therapies (eg, ezetimibe) are recommended.[1]

### Risk-Enhancing Factors

A number of risk-enhancing factors may be incorporated into patient-specific ASCVD risk assessment, including apoB, Lp(a), and high-sensitivity C reactive protein (hs-CRP).[1] ApoB and Lp(a) are lipid specific markers whereas hs-CRP is an inflammatory marker. Current AHA/ACC guidelines do not offer specific testing recommendations for these laboratory tests. However, guidelines do recommend considering these results, when available, as part of the clinician–patient risk discussion, especially for primary prevention in patients at either borderline or intermediate risk. Elevated levels of these markers imply higher ASCVD risk and support statin initiation for primary prevention or the intensification of statin therapy in patients with high-risk or very high-risk ASCVD. ApoB is a major component of all atherogenic lipoproteins; however, apoB levels have not demonstrated superiority over non-HDL levels in ASCVD risk prediction.[12] Thus, apoB is typically not measured because non-HDL is readily available with a standard lipid profile. Lp(a) is an atherogenic lipoprotein that can predict elevated ASCVD

risk independent of other atherogenic lipid values.[35] Lp(a) levels are stable throughout a patient's life and are not affected by diet, exercise, fasting status, or statins. There is concern about the lack of standardization of Lp(a) measurement in clinical laboratories, and results may be reported in either milligrams/deciliter or nanomoles/liter. There is no acceptable conversion factor between the two units, and the preference is for assays that are calibrated and report results in nanomoles/liter. Currently, no evidence exists that treatment directed at lowering Lp(a) provides any additional ASCVD risk reduction beyond guideline recommendations. Of the LDL-lowering drugs, proprotein convertase subtilisin/kexin type 9 (PCSK9) inhibitors have been shown to lower Lp(a). Finally, hs-CRP is an inflammatory marker that has been linked to excess ASCVD risk.[1,36] In a meta-analysis, elevated hs-CRP levels were linked to the risk of cardiovascular events, cerebrovascular events, and cardiovascular mortality.[37] Therefore, current AHA/ACC guidelines consider elevated hs-CRP levels as a risk enhancing factor to be incorporated into a patient's ASCVD risk assessment.[1] Currently, there are no clear recommendations on when these laboratory markers should be ordered, but elevated results can assist in identifying patients who benefit from statin initiation or intensification of LDL-lowering therapy.

When the ASCVD risk assessment, including a lipid panel, results in an uncertain statin therapy decision, the coronary

# MINICASE 3

## Secondary Prevention

James P., a 62-year-old man who is 5' 9" and weighs 260 lb, presents to the clinic after a positive stress test and is diagnosed with stable angina. He reported chest pain and shortness of breath with physical exertion that prompted the stress test. His past medical history is significant for obesity, hypertension treated with hydrochlorothiazide, and tobacco dependence. He does not have a history of diabetes or thyroid disorder. In addition to his hydrochlorothiazide, he is being prescribed metoprolol succinate, atorvastatin, and low-dose aspirin daily. He is hesitant to start these new medications and wonders if they are all necessary. He has never previously taken cholesterol-lowering medication. He does plan to quit smoking, has already purchased a nicotine replacement patch, and has set a quit date in the next week. His wife does most of the cooking and tries to prepare low-fat and low-salt meals, but he eats fast food for lunch most days of the week. He does not exercise routinely because exercise was limited by his chest pain but he would like to start walking regularly. His mother died of a stroke at age 62.

His blood pressure today at the clinic is 138/86 mm Hg, and his heart rate is 80 beats/min. Fasting lipid profile is as follows: TC, 212 mg/dL; TG, 160 mg/dL; LDL, 140 mg/dL; and HDL 40 mg/dL. Fasting glucose is 88 mg/dL; electrolyte, hematology, liver, renal, and thyroid test results are all normal.

QUESTION: How should the lipid profile be interpreted? Why should James P. receive a prescription for a lipid-lowering medication?

DISCUSSION: Even before this diagnosis, James P. was at risk for clinical ASCVD. At that time, he was an obese, male smoker—older than 45 years—with hypertension who lived a sedentary lifestyle and had some poor dietary habits. His mother died prematurely of ASCVD (female age <65 years).[1] James P. is obese, which may contribute to an increase in TGs and decrease in HDL cholesterol; he has no other evidence of disease-related secondary causes of dyslipidemia (eg, diabetes, hypothyroidism, obstructive liver disease, renal dysfunction). However, there are potential substance- or medication-related secondary causes of dyslipidemia in James P.'s case. Although hydrochlorothiazide may increase LDL cholesterol and TGs, the effect is most pronounced at higher doses.[11] Consideration of the lowest effective dose for blood pressure control would be valuable. He is a smoker but does have plans to quit in the immediate future. Smoking is associated with decreases in HDL cholesterol. James P.'s newly prescribed beta blocker may impact the lipid profile by causing decreases in HDL and increases in TGs. However, James P. should still start therapy with a beta blocker because the benefits of beta blockers in stable angina outweigh the impact on the lipid profile.

James P. should initiate therapy with a high-intensity statin (eg, atorvastatin 40 to 80 mg, rosuvastatin 20 mg). AHA/ACC recommendations are to initiate a high-intensity statin in all patients with clinical ASCVD, such as stable angina.[1] Lifestyle modifications are appropriate for James P., including weight loss, increasing physical activity, and a greater emphasis on reducing saturated fat and avoiding *trans* fat in the diet. His smoking cessation efforts should be supported and assessed periodically. A lipid panel and hepatic transaminases were performed recently, and no additional baseline laboratory tests are needed. After starting atorvastatin, the lipid profile should be repeated in 4 to 12 weeks to check for adherence and LDL response.

---

artery calcium (CAC) score is recommended by AHA/ACC guidelines.[1,38] This is not a laboratory test but a scan that can assist in guiding decisions of statin initiation in primary prevention. If the CAC score is zero, then patients can be considered lower risk and statin therapy can be delayed. However, in certain patients (ie, current smokers and patients with diabetes, premature ASCVD family history, or certain inflammatory conditions) ASCVD risk may still be elevated despite the zero CAC score. Because CAC scans do expose patients to radiation, it is recommended that these tests be ordered by clinicians who are knowledgeable in diagnostic radiology.

## Point-of-Care Testing Options

In addition to laboratory monitoring, point-of-care testing (POCT) options that range from at-home testing kits to healthcare practitioner–administered fingerstick tests are available.[39,40] Many at-home testing kits only provide TC results, providing limited results for an ASCVD risk assessment. Other over-the-counter testing kits provide results of the full lipid panel. At-home tests typically require a patient to apply blood to a card and mail the sample into a laboratory for processing. In addition to at-home testing methods, there are relatively inexpensive compact devices for POCT outside the laboratory that are waived from the Clinical Laboratory Improvement Amendments. These devices enable testing for TC, HDL, TGs, and calculated LDL.

One important consideration when evaluating POCT devices is awareness that some variability may be explained by the fact that different sample types are often compared. For example, a fingerstick provides a sample with capillary blood and a venous draw provides venous whole blood. No strong evidence supports that these two sample types give equivalent results.[17] The general conclusion is capillary blood samples provide lower lipid values than venous collection. Nevertheless, the POCT devices are accepted methods for screening for dyslipidemia and are frequently used at health fairs and other screening opportunities. In any POCT setting, quality control should be ensured to maintain accuracy of testing.

One of the benefits of POCT is that it involves the patient in the laboratory process. These visits become opportunities for the clinician to provide the patient with feedback on progress and reinforce the steps needed to reduce ASCVD risk. Because guidelines recommend a complete ASCVD risk assessment on all adult patients, it is important that patients still follow-up with

**TABLE 8-4.** Effects of Hypolipemic Medications

| DRUG CLASS | EFFECTS ON LIPOPROTEINS[a] | SAFETY LABORATORY PARAMETERS[a] |
|---|---|---|
| HMG-CoA reductase inhibitors (statins) | LDL: ↓ 18%–55%<br>HDL: ↑ 5%–15%<br>TG: ↓ 7%–30% | Creatine kinase[b]: ↑<br>Liver transaminases[b]: ↑ |
| Ezetimibe | LDL: ↓ 13%–20%<br>HDL: ↑ 3%–5%<br>TG: ↓ 5%–11% | Liver transaminases[b]: ↑ |
| Bile acid sequestrants | LDL: ↓ 15%–30%<br>HDL: ↑ 3%–5%<br>TG: ↑ 0%–10% | N/A |
| Niacin | LDL: ↓ 5%–25%<br>HDL: ↑ 15%–35%<br>TG: ↓ 20%–50% | Serum glucose[c]: ↑<br>Uric acid[c]: ↑<br>Liver transaminases[c]: ↑ |
| Fibrates | LDL: ↓ 5%–↑ 20%<br>HDL: ↑ 10%–20%<br>TG: ↓ 20%–50% | Creatine kinase[b]: ↑<br>Serum creatinine[c]: ↑ |
| Omega-3 fatty acids | LDL[d]: ↓ 6%–↑ 25%<br>HDL[d]: ↓ 5%–↑ 7%<br>TG: ↓ 19%–44% | N/A |
| PCSK9 inhibitors | LDL: ↓ 43%–64% | N/A |
| Bempedoic acid | LDL: ↓ 18%<br>HDL[e]: ↓ 6%<br>TG[e]: ↓ 2%–↑ 3% | Uric acid[c]: ↑<br>Serum creatinine[f]: ↑<br>BUN[f]: ↑<br>Liver transaminases[f]: ↑<br>Platelets[f]: ↑<br>Creatinine kinase[f]: ↑<br>Hemoglobin[f]: ↓<br>WBC[f]: ↓ |

BUN = blood urea nitrogen; WBC = white blood cell.
[a] ↑ = increase; ↓ = decrease.
[b] Routine monitoring of this lab test is not recommended with use of this drug therapy.
[c] Routine monitoring of this lab test is recommended with use of this drug therapy.
[d] Different omega-3 fatty acid products exhibit varying effects on LDL and HDL depending on whether product contains both dehydroepiandrosterone and eicosapentaenoic acid or eicosapentaenoic acid only.
[e] This information was not statistically analyzed in clinical trials but rather reported as exploratory endpoints.
[f] Due to lack of data, there are no current recommendations for or against routine monitoring of this lab test with use of this drug therapy.

a provider for a complete cardiovascular risk assessment because lipids are only one component of cardiovascular health.[4]

## EFFECTS OF HYPOLIPEMIC MEDICATIONS

Clinicians must be aware of how hypolipemic drugs can influence laboratory test results. The ultimate goal of drug therapy is to reduce ASCVD risk or, in the case of very high TGs alone, reduce the risk of pancreatitis. In general, HMG-CoA reductase inhibitors (statins), ezetimibe, bile acid sequestrants, PCSK9 inhibitors, and bempedoic acid are considered LDL-lowering

drug therapy. Fibrates and omega-3 fatty acids are considered drugs for lowering TGs. Niacin is an agent that has a favorable effect on multiple lipid parameters; however, it is no longer routinely recommended. Specific actions of the drugs and laboratory parameters used for monitoring safety are summarized in **Table 8-4**.[1,12,28,41-43]

## SUMMARY

The lipid panel consisting of TC, LDL cholesterol, HDL cholesterol, and TGs is an essential component of ASCVD risk assessment. Assessment of the lipid panel guides the identification of patients that may benefit from lifestyle modifications and/or drug therapy to reduce ASCVD risk. In the setting of hypertriglyceridemia, assessment of the lipid profile aids the clinician in identifying patients at risk for pancreatitis and assists with diagnostic, prognostic, and therapeutic decisions. For all patients with dyslipidemia, periodic measurement of the lipid profile is recommended to monitor progress and/or adherence.

## LEARNING POINTS

**1.    *Who should receive lipid testing?***

> **ANSWER:** The lipid panel, including TC, TGs, HDL, and LDL, is part of the ASCVD risk assessment that is recommended every 4 to 6 years for any adult patient between 20 and 39 years.[1] This monitoring could be repeated more often for adults between 40 and 75 years[4] or if a clinician determines that a patient's ASCVD risk has increased.[14] Screening is also recommended in all pediatric patients between 9 and 11 years.[16]

**2.    *Why is the measured LDL marked as calculated or direct?***

> **ANSWER:** LDL cholesterol concentrations can be estimated indirectly by a calculation method determined by Friedewald[1]: LDL = TC – HDL – (TGs/5). If a patient's serum TG concentration exceeds 400 mg/dL (4.5 mmol/L), LDL cholesterol cannot be calculated with this formula. Direct measurement of LDL is performed when the calculation would be inaccurate. Laboratory results typically indicate whether the LDL value is calculated or directly measured.

**3.    *If a lipid panel is drawn in the nonfasting state, are the results clinically usable?***

> **ANSWER:** Recent guidelines recommend that a fasting or nonfasting lipid panel can be used in ASCVD risk assessment.[1,19] The lipid panel was historically performed under fasting conditions after a 9- to 12-hour fast.[17] Recent literature suggests the change in lipid levels after a meal are less significant; however, meals with >50 g of fat may increase TGs substantially.[3,18-20] If TG measurement is the focus of the lab or if TGs are >400 mg/dL in a nonfasting sample, then a fasting lipid panel should be performed.[1]

## REFERENCES

1.   Grundy SM, Stone NJ, Bailey AL, et al. 2018 AHA/ACC/AACVPR/ AAPA/ABC/ACPM/ADA/AGS/APhA/ASPC/NLA/PCNA Guideline on the Management of Blood Cholesterol: a report of the American College of Cardiology/American Heart Association Task Force on Clinical Practice Guidelines. *J Am Coll Cardiol.* 2019;73(24):e285-e350.PubMed

2.   Virani SS, Alonso A, Benjamin EJ, et al. Heart disease and stroke statistics-2020 update: a report from the American Heart Association. *Circulation.* 2020;141(9):e139-e596.PubMed

3.   Miller M, Stone NJ, Ballantyne C, et al. Triglycerides and cardiovascular disease: a scientific statement from the American Heart Association. *Circulation.* 2011;123(20):2292-2333.PubMed

4.   Arnett DK, Blumenthal RS, Albert MA, et al. 2019 ACC/AHA guideline on the Primary Prevention of Cardiovascular Disease: a report of the American College of Cardiology/American Heart Association Task Force on Clinical Practice Guidelines. *Circulation.* 2019;140:e593-e646.

5.   Suchy F. Hepatobiliary function. In: Boron W, El B, eds. *Medical Physiology: A Cellular And Molecular Approach.* 2nd ed. Philadelphia, PA: W.B. Saunders; 2012:980-1007.

6.   Rader DJ, Kathiresan S. Disorders of lipoprotien metabolism. In: Jameson JL, Fauci AS, Kasper DL, et al, eds. *Harrison's Principles of Internal Medicine.* 20th ed. New York, NY: The McGraw-Hill Companies, Inc.; 2018:2889-2902.

7.   Freeman MW, Walford GA. Lipoprotein metabolism and the treatment of lipid disorders. In: Jameson JL, De Groot LJ, de Kretser DM, et al, eds. *Endocrinology: Adult and pediatric.* 7th ed. Philadelphia, PA: Saunders Elsevier; 2016:715-736.

8.   Jones PJ, Schoeller DA. Evidence for diurnal periodicity in human cholesterol synthesis. *J Lipid Res.* 1990;31(4):667-673.PubMed

9.   Civeria F, Pocovi M. Monogenic hypercholesterolemias. In: Garg A, ed. *Dyslipidemias: Pathophysiology, Evaluation and Management.* Totowa, NJ: Humana Press; 2015:177-203.

10.  Brahm A, Hegele RA. Primary hypertriglyceridemia. In: Garg A, ed. *Dyslipidemias: Pathophysiology, Evaluation and Management.* Totowa, NJ: Humana Press; 2015:205-220.

11.  Simha V. Drug-induced dyslipidemia. In: Garg A, ed. *Dyslipidemias: Pathophysiology, Evaluation and Management.* Totowa, NJ: Humana Press; 2015:267-286.

12.  Jacobson TA, Ito MK, Maki KC, et al. National lipid association recommendations for patient-centered management of dyslipidemia: part 1. Full report. *J Clin Lipidol.* 2015;9(2):129-169.PubMed

13.  Panel on Antiretroviral Guidelines for Adults and Adolescents. Guidelines for the Use of Antiretroviral Agents in Adults and Adolescents with HIV. Department of Health and Human Services. http://www .aidsinfo.nih.gov/ContentFiles/AdultandAdolescentGL.pdf. Accessed Jun 28, 2020.

14.  Jellinger PS, Handelsman Y, Rosenblit PD, et al. American Association of Clinical Endocrinologists and American College of Endocrinology guidelines for management of dyslipidemia and prevention of cardiovascular disease. *Endocr Pract.* 2017;23(suppl 2):1-87.PubMed

15.  Goldberg IJ, Mosca L, Piano MR, Fisher EA. AHA Science Advisory: wine and your heart: a science advisory for healthcare professionals from the Nutrition Committee, Council on Epidemiology and Prevention, and Council on Cardiovascular Nursing of the American Heart Association. *Circulation.* 2001;103(3):472-475.PubMed

16.  Expert Panel on Integrated Guidelines for Cardiovascular Health and Risk Reduction in Children and Adolescents. Expert panel on integrated guidelines for cardiovascular health and risk reduction in children and adolescents: summary report. *Pediatrics.* 2011;128(suppl 5):S213-S256. PubMed

17.  Chen X, Zhou L, Hussain MM. Lipids and dyslipoproteinemia. In: McPherson RA, Pincus MR, eds. *Henry's Clinical Diagnosis and Management by Laboratory methods.* 23rd ed. St. Louis, MO: Elsevier; 2017:221-243.

18.  Langsted A, Freiberg JJ, Nordestgaard BG. Fasting and nonfasting lipid levels: influence of normal food intake on lipids, lipoproteins, apolipoproteins, and cardiovascular risk prediction. *Circulation.* 2008;118(20):2047-2056.PubMed

19.  Nordestgaard BG, Langsted A, Mora S, et al. Fasting is not routinely required for determination of a lipid profile: clinical and laboratory implications including flagging at desirable concentration cut-points: a joint consensus statement from the European Atherosclerosis Society and European Federation of Clinical Chemistry and Laboratory Medicine. *Eur Heart J.* 2016;37(25):1944-1958.PubMed

20.  Sidhu D, Naugler C. Fasting time and lipid levels in a community-based population: a cross-sectional study. *Arch Intern Med.* 2012;172(22): 1707-1710.PubMed

21.  US Department of Veterans Affairs, US Department of Defense. VA/ DoD clinical practice guideline for the management of dyslipidemia for cardiovascular risk reduction. http://www.healthquality.va.gov/guidelines /CD/lipids. Accessed Jun 28, 2020.

22. Faulkner MA, Hilleman DE, Destache CJ, Mooss AN. Potential influence of timing of low-density lipoprotein cholesterol evaluation in patients with acute coronary syndrome. *Pharmacotherapy*. 2001;21(9):1055-1060. PubMed

23. Pitt B, Loscalzo J, Ycas J, Raichlen JS. Lipid levels after acute coronary syndromes. *J Am Coll Cardiol*. 2008;51(15):1440-1445.PubMed

24. O'Gara PT, Kushner FG, Ascheim DD, et al. 2013 ACCF/AHA guideline for the management of ST-elevation myocardial infarction: a report of the American College of Cardiology Foundation/American Heart Association Task Force on Practice Guidelines. *J Am Coll Cardiol*. 2013;61(4):e78-e140.PubMed

25. Amsterdam EA, Wenger NK, Brindis RG, et al. 2014 AHA/ACC Guideline for the Management of Patients with Non-ST-Elevation Acute Coronary Syndromes: a report of the American College of Cardiology/ American Heart Association Task Force on Practice Guidelines. *J Am Coll Cardiol*. 2014;64(24):e139-e228.PubMed

26. Devaraj S, Remaley AT. Lipids, lipoproteins, apolipoproteins, and other cardiac risk factors. In: Rifai N, Horvath AR, Wittwer CT, eds. *Tietz Fundamentals of Clinical Chemistry and Molecular Diagnostics*. 8th ed. St. Louis, MO: Elsevier; 2019:391-418.

27. Expert Panel on Detection, Evaluation, and Treatment of High Blood Cholesterol in Adults. Executive Summary of The Third Report of The National Cholesterol Education Program (NCEP) Expert Panel on Detection, Evaluation, And Treatment of High Blood Cholesterol In Adults (Adult Treatment Panel III). *JAMA*. 2001;285(19):2486-2497. PubMed

28. Skulas-Ray AC, Wilson PWF, Harris WS, et al. Omega-3 fatty acids for the management of hypertriglyceridemia: a science advisory from the American Heart Association. *Circulation*. 2019;140(12):e673-e691. PubMed

29. Nikolac N. Lipemia: causes, interference mechanisms, detection and management. *Biochem Med (Zagreb)*. 2014;24(1):57-67.PubMed

30. Friedewald WT, Levy RI, Fredrickson DS. Estimation of the concentration of low-density lipoprotein cholesterol in plasma, without use of the preparative ultracentrifuge. *Clin Chem*. 1972;18(6):499-502. PubMed

31. Martin SS, Blaha MJ, Elshazly MB, et al. Comparison of a novel method vs the Friedewald equation for estimating low-density lipoprotein cholesterol levels from the standard lipid profile. *JAMA*. 2013;310(19):2061-2068.PubMed

32. Martin SS, Blaha MJ, Elshazly MB, et al. Friedewald-estimated versus directly measured low-density lipoprotein cholesterol and treatment implications. *J Am Coll Cardiol*. 2013;62(8):732-739.PubMed

33. Eckel RH, Jakicic JM, Ard JD, et al. 2013 AHA/ACC guideline on lifestyle management to reduce cardiovascular risk: a report of the American College of Cardiology/American Heart Association Task Force on Practice Guidelines. *Circulation*. 2014;129(25 suppl 2):S76-S99.PubMed

34. Dhingra R, Vasan R. Lipoproteins and cardiovascular risk. In: Garg A, ed. *Dyslipidemias: Pathophysiology, Evaluation and Management*. Totowa, NJ: Humana Press; 2015:57-65.

35. Wilson DP, Jacobson TA, Jones PH, et al. Use of Lipoprotein(a) in clinical practice: a biomarker whose time has come. A scientific statement from the National Lipid Association. *J Clin Lipidol*. 2019;13(3):374-392. PubMed

36. Ridker PM, Danielson E, Fonseca FA, et al. Rosuvastatin to prevent vascular events in men and women with elevated C-reactive protein. *N Engl J Med*. 2008;359(21):2195-2207.PubMed

37. Kaptoge S, Di Angelantonio E, Lowe G, et al. C-reactive protein concentration and risk of coronary heart disease, stroke, and mortality: an individual participant meta-analysis. *Lancet*. 2010;375(9709):132-140. PubMed

38. Greenland P, Blaha MJ, Budoff MJ, et al. Coronary calcium score and cardiovascular risk. *J Am Coll Cardiol*. 2018;72(4):434-447.PubMed

39. Haggerty L, Tran D. Cholesterol point-of-care testing for community pharmacies: a review of the current literature. *J Pharm Pract*. 2017;30(4):451-458.PubMed

40. Scolaro KL, Stamm PL, Lloyd KB. Devices for ambulatory and home monitoring of blood pressure, lipids, coagulation, and weight management, part 1. *Am J Health Syst Pharm*. 2005;62(17):1802-1812. PubMed

41. Stone NJ, Robinson JG, Lichtenstein AH, et al. 2013 ACC/AHA guideline on the treatment of blood cholesterol to reduce atherosclerotic cardiovascular risk in adults: a report of the American College of Cardiology/American Heart Association Task Force on Practice Guidelines. *Circulation*. 2014;129(25 suppl 2):S1-S45.PubMed

42. Jun M, Perkovic V. Fibrates: risk, benefits and role in treating dyslipidemias. In: Garg A, ed. *Dyslipidemias: Pathophysiology, Evaluation and management*. Totowa, NJ: Humana Press; 2015:423-438.

43. Nexletol [package insert]. Ann Arbor, MI: Esperion Therapeutics, Inc.; 2020.

## QUICKVIEW | Triglycerides

| PARAMETER | DESCRIPTION | COMMENTS |
|---|---|---|
| **Common reference ranges** | | |
| Adults | Normal: <150 mg/dL (1.7 mmol/L)<br>Borderline high: 150–199 mg/dL (1.7–2.2 mmol/L)<br>High: 200–499 mg/dL (2.3–5.6 mmol/L)<br>Very high: ≥500 mg/dL (5.6 mmol/L) | SI conversion factor: 0.01129 (mmol/L) |
| Pediatrics | Acceptable:<br>  0–9 yr: <75 mg/dL (0.8 mmol/L)<br>  10–19 yr: <90 mg/dL (1.0 mmol/L)<br><br>Borderline high:<br>  0–9 yr: 75–99 mg/dL (0.8–1.1 mmol/L)<br>  10–19 yr: 90–129 mg/dL (1.0–1.5 mmol/L)<br><br>High:<br>  0–9 yr: ≥100 mg/dL (1.1 mmol/L)<br>  10–19 yr: ≥130 mg/dL (1.5 mmol/L) | |
| **Critical value** | 500 mg/dL (5.6 mmol/L) | High risk of pancreatitis |
| **Inherent activity?** | Intermediary for other active substances and stored energy in adipose tissue | Needed for formation of other lipids and fatty acids |
| **Location** | | |
| Production | Liver and intestines | From ingested food |
| Storage | Adipose tissue | |
| Secretion/excretion | None | |
| **Causes of abnormal values** | | |
| High | Excess carbohydrate intake<br>Genetic defects<br>Drugs<br>Alcohol | Tables 8-2 and 8-3<br>Associated with obesity, diabetes, and metabolic syndrome |
| Low | Hypolipidemics<br>Lifestyle modifications | Statins, niacin, fibrates, omega-3 fatty acids |
| **Signs and symptoms** | | |
| High level | Pancreatitis<br>Eruptive xanthomas<br>Lipemia retinalis | Increased risk of ASCVD |
| Low level | None | |
| **After event, time to…** | | |
| Initial elevation | Days to weeks | Single high-fat meal has major effect on TG concentration within 2 hr |
| Peak values | Days to weeks | Increases with aging |
| Normalization | Days to weeks | After diet changes or drug treatment is started |
| **Causes of spurious results** | Glycerol, recent high-fat meal, alcohol, lipid emulsion | |
| **Additional information** | TGs are not the primary target of therapy unless TGs ≥500 mg/dL (5.6 mmol/L) | |

## QUICKVIEW | Total Cholesterol

| PARAMETER | DESCRIPTION | COMMENTS |
|---|---|---|
| **Common reference ranges** | | |
| Adults | Desirable: <200 mg/dL (5.2 mmol/L) | SI conversion factor: 0.02586 (mmol/L) |
| | Borderline high: 200–239 mg/dL (5.2–6.2 mmol/L) | |
| | High: ≥240 mg/dL (6.2 mmol/L) | |
| Pediatrics | Acceptable: <170 mg/dL (4.4 mmol/L) | |
| | Borderline high: 170–199 mg/dL (4.4–5.1 mmol/L) | |
| | High: ≥200 mg/dL (5.2 mmol/L) | |
| **Critical value** | Not acutely critical | Depends on risk factors, LDL, TGs, and HDL |
| **Inherent activity?** | Intermediary for other active substances | Needed for cell wall, steroid, and bile acid production |
| **Location** | | |
| Production | Liver and intestines | Ingested in diet |
| Storage | Lipoproteins | |
| Secretion/excretion | Excreted in bile | Also recycled to liver |
| **Causes of abnormal values** | | |
| High | Diet high in saturated fats and *trans* fats | Tables 8–2 and 8–3 |
| | Genetic defects | |
| | Drugs | |
| Low | Hyperthyroidism | |
| | Liver disease | Statins, ezetimibe, niacin, fibrates, bile acid sequestrants, PCSK9 inhibitors, bempedoic acid |
| | Hypolipidemics | |
| | Lifestyle modifications | |
| **Signs and symptoms** | | |
| High level | Tendon xanthomas | Increased risk of ASCVD |
| Low level | None | Usually considered sign of good health |
| **After event, time to…** | | |
| Initial elevation | Days to weeks | Single meal has little effect on TC concentration |
| Peak values | Days to weeks | Can increase with aging; does not change acutely |
| Normalization | Weeks to months | After diet changes or drugs |
| **Causes of spurious results** | Prolonged tourniquet application | Causes venous stasis (increase 5%–10%) |
| **Additional information** | Not applicable | |

## QUICKVIEW | LDL Cholesterol

| PARAMETER | DESCRIPTION | COMMENTS |
|---|---|---|
| **Common reference ranges** | | |
| Adults | Desirable: <100 mg/dL (2.6 mmol/L) | SI conversion factor: 0.02586 (mmol/L) |
| | Above desirable: 100–129 mg/dL (2.6–3.3 mmol/L) | |
| | Borderline high: 130–159 mg/dL (3.4–4.1 mmol/L) | |
| | High: 160–189 mg/dL (4.1–4.9 mmol/L) | |
| | Very high: ≥190 mg/dL (4.9 mmol/L) | |
| Pediatrics | Acceptable: <110 mg/dL (2.8 mmol/L) | |
| | Borderline high: 110–129 mg/dL (2.8–3.3 mmol/L) | |
| | High: ≥130 mg/dL (3.4 mmol/L) | |
| **Critical value** | Not acutely critical | Depends on risk factors and ASCVD history |
| **Inherent activity?** | Intermediary for other active substances | Needed for cell wall, steroid, and bile acid production |
| **Location** | | |
| Production | Liver and intestines | Ingested in diet |
| Storage | Lipoproteins | |
| Secretion/excretion | Excreted to bile | Also recycled to liver |
| **Causes of abnormal values** | | |
| High | Diet high in saturated fats and *trans* fats, genetic defects, hypothyroidism, nephrotic syndrome | Tables 8-2 and 8-3 |
| Low | Drugs, hyperthyroidism, liver disease, hypolipidemics, lifestyle modifications | Table 8-3<br>Statins, ezetimibe, niacin, bile acid sequestrants, PCSK9 inhibitors, bempedoic acid |
| **Signs and symptoms** | | |
| High level | Atherosclerotic vascular disease, tendon xanthomas | Clinical ASCVD |
| Low level | None | Usually considered sign of good health |
| **After event, time to…** | | |
| Initial elevation | Days to weeks | Single meal has little effect on LDL cholesterol concentration |
| Peak values | Days to weeks | Can increase with aging; does not change acutely |
| Normalization | Weeks to months | After diet changes or medications |
| **Causes of spurious results** | Acute coronary syndrome | LDL levels decline within a few hours of event and may remain low for several weeks |
| **Additional information** | LDL may be a target of therapy<br>Indirect methods are typically used to calculate LDL cholesterol, with the most common being the Friedewald equation: LDL = TC – HDL – (TGs/5)<br>This equation cannot be used if TGs >400 mg/dL (4.5 mmol/L) and LDL would need to be directly measured | |

*Source*: Adapted from References 1,12,28,41–43.

# 9 Endocrine Disorders

*Eva Vivian*

DOI 10.37573/9781585286423.009

## OBJECTIVES

*After completing this chapter, the reader should be able to*

- Describe the use of glycated hemoglobin, fasting plasma glucose, and oral glucose tolerance tests as diagnostic tools for type 1 and type 2 diabetes mellitus

- Explain the major differences between laboratory values found in patients with diabetic ketoacidosis and those in a hyperosmolar hyperglycemic state

- Describe the actions of thyroxine, triiodothyronine, and thyroid-stimulating hormone and the feedback mechanisms regulating them

- Given a case description including thyroid function test results, identify the type of thyroid disorder and describe how tests are used to monitor and adjust related therapy

- Describe the relationship between urine osmolality, serum osmolality, and antidiuretic hormone as they relate to diabetes insipidus

- Describe the laboratory tests used to diagnose Addison disease and Cushing syndrome

The endocrine system consists of hormones that serve as regulators, which stimulate or inhibit a biological response to maintain homeostasis within the body. Endocrine disorders often result from a deficiency or an excess of a hormone, leading to an imbalance in physiologic functions of the body. Usually, negative feedback mechanisms regulate hormone concentrations (**Figure 9-1**). Therefore, laboratory assessment of an endocrine disorder is based on the concentrations of a plasma hormone and integrity of the feedback mechanism regulating that hormone. In this chapter, the relationship between a hormone (insulin) and a target substrate (glucose) serves as an example of these concepts. Evaluations of the functions of the thyroid and adrenal glands are also described. The relationships between vasopressin (antidiuretic hormone [ADH]) and serum and urine osmolality are used to demonstrate the basis for the water deprivation test in diagnosing diabetes insipidus.

## GLUCOSE HOMEOSTASIS

Glucose serves as the fuel for most cellular functions and is necessary to sustain life. Carbohydrates ingested from a meal are metabolized in the body into glucose. Glucose is absorbed from the gastrointestinal (GI) tract into the bloodstream, where it is used in skeletal muscle and the brain for energy. Excess glucose is stored in the liver in the form of glycogen (glycogenesis) and is converted in adipose tissue to fats and triglycerides (lipogenesis). Insulin, which is produced, stored, and released from β cells of the pancreas, facilitates these anabolic processes. The liver, skeletal muscle, brain, and adipose tissue are the main tissues affected by insulin. To induce glucose uptake, insulin must bind to specific cell-surface receptors. Most secreted insulin is taken up by the liver, while the remainder is metabolized by the kidneys.

In the fasting state, insulin levels decrease, resulting in an increase in glycogen breakdown by the liver (glycogenolysis) and an increase in the conversion of free fatty acids to ketone bodies (lipolysis).[1] When glucose concentrations fall below 70 mg/dL, an event known as *hypoglycemia* occurs, resulting in the release of glucagon by the pancreatic α cell. Glucagon stimulates the formation of glucose in the liver (gluconeogenesis) and glycogenolysis. Glucagon also facilitates the breakdown of stored triglycerides in adipose tissue into fatty acids (lipolysis), which can be used for energy in the liver and skeletal muscle. In addition to glucagon secretion, hypoglycemia leads to secretion of counterregulatory hormones such as epinephrine, cortisol, and growth hormone. Epinephrine release in response to hypoglycemia results in neurogenic symptoms such as sweating, palpitations, tremulousness, anxiety, and hunger. Glucagon and, to a lesser degree, epinephrine promote an immediate breakdown of glycogen and the synthesis of glucose by the liver. Cortisol increases glucose levels by stimulating gluconeogenesis. Growth hormone inhibits the uptake of glucose by tissues when glucose levels fall below 70 mg/dL.[1]

In individuals without diabetes, once plasma glucose concentrations exceed 180 mg/dL (the renal threshold), renal glucose reabsorption is saturated and glucose starts to appear in the urine. In individuals with hyperglycemia, large amounts of glucose may be excreted into the urine. However, in diabetes mellitus (DM), the renal glucose threshold may increase up to 240 mg/dL, causing reabsorption of more glucose, which further contributes to hyperglycemia.[1]

In summary, glucose concentrations are affected by any factor that can influence glucose production or utilization, glucose absorption from the GI tract, glycogen catabolism, or insulin production or secretion. Fasting suppresses the rate of insulin secretion, and eating generally increases insulin secretion.

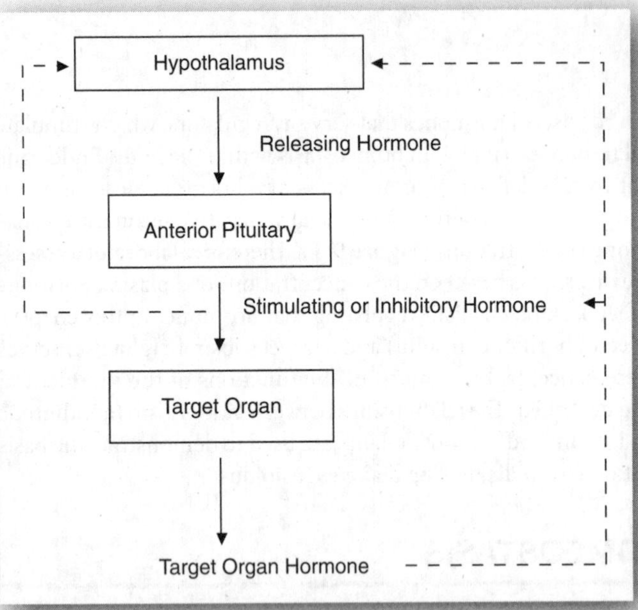

**FIGURE 9-1.** The hypothalamus may secrete a releasing hormone in response to low levels of stimulating, inhibitory, or target organ hormone. This releasing hormone causes the release of a stimulating or inhibitory hormone that, in turn, controls the release of target organ hormone.

Increased insulin secretion lowers serum glucose concentrations, whereas decreased secretion raises glucose concentrations.[1]

# DIABETES MELLITUS

The three most commonly encountered types of DM are as follows:

1. Type 1 DM, formally known as insulin-dependent DM
2. Type 2 DM, formerly known as adult-onset or noninsulin-dependent DM[2]
3. Gestational DM (GDM)

Type 1 DM is characterized by a lack of endogenous insulin, a predisposition to ketoacidosis, and abrupt onset. Some patients present with ketoacidosis after experiencing polyuria, polyphagia, and polydipsia for several days. Typically, this type of DM is diagnosed in children and adolescents but may also occur at a later age. In contrast, patients with type 2 DM do not normally depend on exogenous insulin to sustain life and are not usually ketosis prone, but they are usually obese and >40 years old. There is an alarming increase in the number of children and adolescents diagnosed with type 2 DM. Although there is a genetic predisposition to the development of type 2 DM, environmental factors such as high-fat diet and sedentary lifestyle contribute to the disorder. Patients with type 2 DM are both insulin deficient and insulin resistant (**Table 9-1**).[1]

Many patients with type 2 DM are asymptomatic, so diagnosis often depends on laboratory studies. Concentrations of ketone bodies in the blood and urine are typically low or absent, even in the presence of hyperglycemia. This finding is common because the lack of insulin is not severe enough to lead to abnormalities in lipolysis and significant ketosis or acidosis.

Because of the chronicity of asymptomatic type 2 DM, many patients with type 2 DM present with evidence of microvascular

**TABLE 9-1.** General Characteristics of Type 1 and Type 2 Diabetes Mellitus

| CHARACTERISTICS | TYPE 1 | TYPE 2 |
|---|---|---|
| Usual age of onset | Childhood or adolescence | >40 yr old |
| Rapidity of onset | Abrupt | Gradual |
| Family studies | Increased prevalence of type 1 DM | Increased prevalence of type 2 DM |
| Body weight | Unusually thin | Obesity is common |
| Islet cell antibodies and pancreatic cell-mediated immunity | Yes | No |
| Ketosis | Possible | Unlikely; if present, associated with severe stress or infection |
| Insulin | Markedly diminished early in disease or totally absent | Levels may be low, normal, or high (indicating insulin resistance) |
| Symptoms | Polyuria, polydipsia, polyphagia, weight loss | May be asymptomatic; polyuria, polydipsia, polyphagia may be present |

*Source*: Adapted from American Diabetes Association. Classification and diagnosis of diabetes: standards of medical care in diabetes: 2021. *Diabetes Care* 2021;44(suppl 1):S152S33.

complications (neuropathy, nephropathy, and retinopathy) and macrovascular complications (coronary artery, cerebral vascular, and peripheral arterial disease) at the time of diagnosis. Type 2 DM is often discovered incidentally during glucose screening sponsored by hospitals and other healthcare institutions.[1]

Gestational DM, a third type of glucose intolerance, develops during the third trimester of pregnancy. Patients with GDM have a 30% to 50% chance of developing type 2 DM later in life.[2] Women with diabetes who become pregnant or women diagnosed with diabetes early in pregnancy are not included in this category.

## Diagnostic Laboratory Tests

### C-Peptide

Categories of C-peptide values are as follows:
- Fasting range: 0.78 to 1.89 ng/mL (0.26 to 0.62 nmol/L)
- Range 1 hour after a glucose load: 5 to 12 ng/mL
- During a glucose tolerance test: 1.66 to 3.97 nmol/L

Insulin is synthesized in the β cells of the islets of Langerhans as the precursor, proinsulin. Proinsulin is cleaved to form C-peptide and insulin, which are both secreted in equimolar amounts into the portal circulation. By measuring the levels of C-peptide, the level of insulin can also be calculated. C-peptide levels are also used to evaluate residual β-cell function. High levels of C-peptide generally indicate high levels of endogenous insulin production, which may be a response to high levels of blood glucose caused by glucose intake and insulin resistance. Also, high levels of C-peptide also are seen with insulinomas (insulin-producing tumors) and may be seen with hypokalemia, pregnancy, Cushing syndrome, and renal failure. Low levels of C-peptide are associated with low levels of insulin production, which can occur when insufficient insulin is produced due to a decrease in the number of functional insulin-producing β cells associated with type 1 DM or long-term type 2 DM or with suppression tests that involve substances such as somatostatin.[3]

A C-peptide test can be performed to distinguish between type 1 and type 2 DM. A patient with type 1 DM has a low level of insulin and C-peptide. A patient with newly diagnosed type 2 DM typically has a normal or high level of C-peptide. When a patient has newly diagnosed type 1 or type 2 DM, C-peptide can be used to help determine how much insulin the patient's pancreas is still producing. With type 2 DM, the test may be ordered to monitor the status of β-cell function and insulin production over time and determine if insulin injections may be required.

A C-peptide test may differentiate the cause of hypoglycemia, such as excessive use of medicine to treat diabetes or a noncancerous growth (tumor) in the pancreas (insulinoma). Because man-made (synthetic) insulin does not have C-peptide, a person with a low blood sugar level from taking too much insulin has a low C-peptide level but a high level of insulin. Insulinomas are the most common cause of hypoglycemia resulting from endogenous hyperinsulinism. A person with an insulinoma has a high level of C-peptide in the blood when the he or she has a high level of insulin.

Although they are produced at the same rate, C-peptide and insulin leave the body by different routes. Insulin is processed and eliminated by the liver and kidneys, whereas C-peptide is removed primarily by the kidneys. The half-life of C-peptide is 30 minutes as compared with the half-life of insulin, which is 5 minutes. Thus, there is usually about five times as much C-peptide in the bloodstream as endogenous insulin.[3]

### Diabetes-Related Autoantibody Testing

*Diabetes-related (islet) autoantibody testing* is used to distinguish between autoimmune type 1 DM and type 2 DM, allowing for early initiation of the most appropriate treatment, which may minimize disease complications. The four most commonly used autoantibody tests are islet cell cytoplasmic autoantibodies (ICA), glutamic acid decarboxylase autoantibodies (GADA), insulinoma-associated-2 autoantibodies (IA-2A), and insulin autoantibodies (IAA). Of these, ICA and GADA, which are autoantibodies directed against islet cell proteins or β-cell antigen, are present in 70% to 80% of adult patients with type 1 DM. IA-2A autoantibodies are present in approximately 60% of adult patients with type 1 DM. The majority of people, 95% or more, with new-onset type 1 DM will have at least one islet autoantibody.[2] Some people who have type 1 DM will never develop detectable amounts of islet autoantibodies, but this is rare.

The autoantibodies seen in children are often different than those seen in adults. IAA is usually the first marker to appear in young children. As the disease evolves, IAA may disappear and ICA, GADA, and IA-2A become more important. Approximately 50% of children with new-onset type 1 DM will be IAA positive.

A combination of these autoantibodies may be ordered when a person is newly diagnosed with diabetes and the healthcare provider wants to distinguish between type 1 and type 2 DM. In addition, these tests may be used when the diagnosis is unclear in persons with diabetes who have been diagnosed as type 2 DM, but who have great difficulty in controlling their glucose levels with oral medications. If ICA, GADA, and IA-2A are present in a person with symptoms of DM, the diagnosis of type 1 DM is confirmed. Likewise, if IAA is present in a child with DM who is not insulin-treated, type 1 DM is the cause. If no diabetes-related autoantibodies are present, then it is unlikely that the diabetes is type 1 DM.[2]

Latent autoimmune diabetes in adults (LADA) is a slow-progressing form of autoimmune diabetes. Patients may present with characteristics of both type 1 and type 2 DM.[4,5] The clinical features of type 1 diabetes seen in LADA include a lower body mass index (BMI) compared with what is typical in type 2 DM and autoimmunity against one or more of the following antibodies: ICA, autoantibodies to glutamic acid decarboxylase (GAD), IA-2, and IAA[6,7] The characteristics of type 2 DM that may present in LADA include older age at onset and insulin resistance or deficiency. Characteristics of LADA tend to include an intermediate level of β-cell dysfunction between those in type 1 and type 2 DM, faster decline of C-peptide compared with type 2 DM, and a level of insulin resistance that is comparable to type 1 DM.[8] β-cell decline is variable in LADA, as measured by C-peptide levels.[8,9]

## Laboratory Tests to Assess Glucose Control

The two most common methods used for evaluating glucose homeostasis are the fasting plasma glucose (FPG) and glycated hemoglobin (A1c) tests. The oral glucose tolerance test (OGTT) is most commonly used to diagnosis GDM.[2]

With all blood tests, proper collection and storage of the sample and performance of the procedure are important. Improper collection and storage of samples for glucose determinations can lead to false results and interpretations. After collection, red blood cells (RBCs) and white blood cells (WBCs) continue to metabolize glucose in the sample tube. This process occurs unless (1) the RBCs can be separated from the serum using serum separator tubes or (2) the metabolism is inhibited using sodium fluoride–containing (gray-top) tubes or refrigeration of the specimen. Without such precautions, the glucose concentration drops by 5 to 10 mg/dL (0.3 to 0.6 mmol/L) per hour, and the measured glucose level does not reflect the patient's FPG at collection time. In vitro, metabolic loss of glucose is hastened in samples of patients with leukocytosis or leukemia.[10-15]

### Fasting Plasma Glucose and Two-Hour Postprandial Glucose

The categories of FPG values are as follows:

- FPG <100 mg/dL (5.6 mmol/L) represents normal fasting glucose
- FPG ≥100 (5.6 mmol/L) and <126 mg/dL (7 mmol/L) represents *prediabetes* (previously termed *impaired fasting glucose*)
- FPG ≥126 mg/dL (7 mmol/L) represents provisional diagnosis of diabetes (the diagnosis must be confirmed as described in **Table 9-2**)[2]

An FPG concentration measures the ability of endogenous or exogenous insulin to prevent fasting hyperglycemia by regulating glucose anabolism and catabolism. FPG may be used to monitor therapy in patients being treated for glucose abnormalities. For this test, the patient maintains his or her usual diet, and the assay is performed on awakening (before breakfast).

This timing allows for an 8-hour fast. An FPG >126 mg/dL (>7 mmol/L), in abnormal test results from the same sample or in two separate test samples, is diagnostic for DM. If the initial single test is an abnormal FPG result, either the same or a different test can be taken on a different day to confirm the diagnosis for DM.

Testing in asymptomatic people should be considered in adults of any age who are overweight or obese (BMI ≥25 kg/m² or ≥23 kg/m² for individuals of Asian-Pacific descent) with one or more risk factors[2]:

- First-degree relative with diabetes
- High-risk ethnic groups (eg, high-risk ethnic groups: Hispanic, African American, Native American, South or East Asian, or Pacific Island descent)
- History of cardiovascular disease
- Hypertension (≥140/90 mm Hg or on therapy for hypertension)
- High-density lipoprotein cholesterol level of 35 mg/dL (0.90 mmol/L) and/or a triglyceride level of 250 mg/dL (2.82 mmol/L)
- Women with polycystic ovary syndrome
- Physical inactivity• A1c ≥5.7%, impaired glucose tolerance, or elevated fasting glucose on a previous testing (should be tested annually)
- Polycystic ovary syndrome
- Other clinical conditions associated with insulin resistance (eg, severe obesity, acanthosis nigricans)

Patients with prediabetes (A1C ≥5.7% [39 mmol/mol], impaired glucose tolerance [IGT]; impaired fasting glucose [IFG]) should be tested yearly. Women who were diagnosed with GDM should have lifelong testing at least every 3 years. Individuals without these risk factors should be screened no later than 45 years of age. If results are normal, testing should be repeated at a minimum of 3-year intervals, with consideration of more frequent testing depending on initial results and risk

**TABLE 9-2.** Diagnosis of DM Based on Fasting Plasma Glucose Concentration, Oral Glucose Tolerance Test, or Glycosylated Hemoglobin

| LEVEL OF GLUCOSE TOLERANCE | | VENOUS PLASMA GLUCOSE AFTER 75-g OGTT[a] (mg/dL) | | |
| --- | --- | --- | --- | --- |
| | FPG | 30, 60, or 90 min | 2 hr | A1c |
| "Normal" | <100 | NA | <140 | <5.7% |
| Prediabetes | 100–125 | NA | 140–199 | 5.7%–6.4% |
| DM | ≥126 | NA | >200 | ≥6.5% |
| GDM | >92 | >180 (1 hr) | >153 | |

NA = not applicable.
[a]Multiply number by 0.056 to convert glucose to International System (SI) units (mmol/L).
*Source*: Adapted from American Diabetes Association. Classification and diagnosis of diabetes: standards of medical care in diabetes-2021. *Diabetes Care* 2021;44(suppl 1):S152S33.

status. The American Diabetes Association (ADA) also recommends that individuals from high-risk groups aged >30 years be screened for DM every 3 years.[2]

### Oral Glucose Tolerance Test

The categories for the 75-g OGTT are as follows:

- 2-hour postload glucose (PG), <140 mg/dL (7.8 mmol/L) represents normal glucose tolerance
- 2-hour PG 140 to 199 mg/dL (7.8 to 11 mmol/L) represents prediabetes (previously termed *impaired glucose tolerance*)
- 2-hour PG ≥200 mg/dL (≥11.1 mmol/L) represents provisional diagnosis of diabetes

The OGTT can be used to assess patients who have signs and symptoms of DM but whose FPG is normal or suggests prediabetes (<126 mg/dL or <7 mmol/L). The OGTT measures both the ability of the pancreas to secrete insulin following a glucose load and the body's response to insulin. Interpretation of the test is based on the plasma glucose concentrations drawn before and during the exam. This exam may also be used in diagnosing DM with onset during pregnancy if the disease threatens the health of the mother and fetus.

The OGTT is performed by giving a standard 75-g dose of an oral glucose solution over 5 minutes after an overnight fast. The pediatric dose is 1.75 g/kg up to a maximum of 75 g. Blood samples commonly are drawn before the glucose load and at 120 minutes after the glucose load. The samples should be collected into tubes containing sodium fluoride unless the assay will be performed immediately.[2] If the patient vomits the test dose, the exam is invalid and must be repeated.

Pregnant women with risk factors such as overweight or obese with a BMI >25; family history of type 2 DM; hypertension; hyperlipidemia; and high-risk ethnic groups (eg, Hispanic, African American, Native American, South or East Asian, or Pacific Island descent) should be screened at the first prenatal visit using standard diagnostic criteria for type 2 DM. Pregnant women not previously known to have DM or risk factors can be screened for GDM at 24 to 28 weeks' gestation. GDM diagnosis can be accomplished with either of two strategies:

1. The "one-step" 75-g OGTT
2. The older "two-step" approach with a 50-g (nonfasting) screen followed by a 100-g OGTT for women who screen positive

## One-Step Strategy

A 75-g OGTT is performed with plasma glucose measurement when the patient is fasting and at 1 and 2 hours.[2] The OGTT should be performed in the morning after an overnight fast of at least 8 hours. The diagnosis of GDM is made when any of the following plasma glucose values are met or exceeded:

- FPG ≥92 mg/dL (5.1 mmol/L)
- OGTT value at 1 hour ≥180 mg/dL (10 mmol/L)
- OGTT value at 2 hours ≥153 mg/dL[16] (8.5 mmol/L)

## Two-Step Strategy

Step 1: Perform a 50-g OGTT (nonfasting), with plasma glucose measurement at 1 hour. If the plasma glucose level measured 1 hour after the load is ≥130, 135, or 140 mg/dL (7.2, 7.5, or 7.8 mmol/L, respectively), proceed to a 100-g OGTT. Cutoff values of 130, 135, and 140 are all used clinically for screening. The lower values are more sensitive but less specific for GDM.

Step 2: The 100-g OGTT should be performed when the patient is fasting.[2] The diagnosis of GDM is made when at least two of the following four plasma glucose levels are met or exceeded (measured fasting and at 1, 2, and 3 hours during OGTT):

- Fasting: 95 mg/dL (5.3 mmol/L)
- 1 hour: 180 mg/dL (10.0 mmol/L)
- 2 hours: 155 mg/dL (8.6 mmol/L)
- 3 hours: 140 mg/dL (7.8 mmol/L)

### Glycated Hemoglobin

*Normal range: 4% to 5.6%*

*Glycated hemoglobin* (A1c), also known as *glycosylated A1c*, is a component of the hemoglobin molecule. During the 120-day lifespan of an RBC, glucose is irreversibly bound to the hemoglobin moieties in proportion to the average serum glucose. The process is called *glycosylation*. Measurement of A1c is, therefore, indicative of glucose control during the preceding 3 months. The entire hemoglobin A1 molecule—composed of A1a, A1b, and A1c—is not used because subfractions A1a and A1b are more susceptible to nonglucose adducts in the blood of patients with opiate addiction, lead poisoning, uremia, and alcoholism.[14] Because the test measures a component of hemoglobin, the specimen analyzed is RBC and not serum or plasma.

Results are not affected by daily fluctuations in the blood glucose concentration, and a fasting sample is not required. Results can reflect overall patient compliance to various treatment regimens. With most assays, 95% of a normal individual's hemoglobin is 4% to 5.6% glycated; a level of 5.7% to 6.4% indicates prediabetes, and a level of ≥6.5% indicates diabetes. An A1c ≥7% suggests less-than-ideal glucose control for most patients. Patients with A1c of ≥9% are considered to have poorly controlled glucose levels.[16]

For years, the A1c has been used to monitor glucose control in people already diagnosed with DM. Initially, it was not recommended for diagnosis because the test variability from laboratory to laboratory was too great for a diagnostic test. The A1c cut-point of ≥6.5% identifies one-third fewer cases of undiagnosed DM than a fasting glucose cut-point of ≥126 mg/dL. However, the lower sensitivity of the test at the cut-point is offset by the test's greater practicality, and wider use of this more convenient test may result in an increase in the number of diagnoses.[2]

A few situations confound interpretation of test results. False elevations in A1c may be noted with uremia, chronic alcohol intake, and hypertriglyceridemia.[16] Recent blood transfusion, use of drugs that stimulate erythropoiesis, and end-stage kidney disease may also compromise the accuracy of the A1C result.[2] Patients who have diseases with chronic or episodic hemolysis (eg, sickle cell disease and thalassemia) generally have spuriously low A1c concentrations caused by the predominance of young RBCs (which carry less A1c) in the circulation. In splenectomized patients and those with polycythemia, A1c is increased.

If these disorders are stable, the test still can be used, but values must be compared with the patient's previous results rather than published normal values. Both falsely elevated and falsely lowered measurements of A1c may also occur during pregnancy. Therefore, A1c should not be used to screen for GDM.[16]

The A1C test should be performed using a method that is certified by the NGSP (www.ngsp.org). Although point-of-care (POC) A1C assays may be NGSP certified and cleared by the U.S. Food and Drug Administration (FDA) for use in monitoring glycemic control in people with diabetes in both Clinical Laboratory Improvement Amendments (CLIA)-regulated and CLIA-waived settings, only those POC A1C assays that are also cleared by the FDA for use in the diagnosis of diabetes should be used for this purpose, and only in the clinical settings for which they are cleared. POC A1C assays may be more generally applied for the assessment of glycemic control in the clinic. Portable analyzers are available that can provide A1c results at the POC within 5 to 8 minutes.[16] The ADA recommends A1c testing one to two times a year for patients with good glycemic control and quarterly in patients with poor control or whose therapy has changed.[2]

### Fructosamine

*Normal range: 170 to 285 µmol/L*

*Fructosamine* is a general term that is applied to any glycosylated protein. Unlike the A1c test, only glycosylated proteins in the serum or plasma (eg, albumin)—not erythrocytes—are measured. In patients without diabetes, the unstable complex dissociates into glucose and protein. Therefore, only small quantities of fructosamine circulate. In patients with DM, higher glucose concentrations favor the generation of more stable glycation, and higher concentrations of fructosamine are found.

Fructosamine has no known inherent toxicological activity but can be used as a marker of medium-term glucose control. Fructosamine correlates with glucose control over 2 to 3 weeks based on the half-lives of albumin (14 to 20 days) and other serum proteins (2.5 to 23 days). As a result, high-fructosamine concentrations may alert caregivers to deteriorating glycemic control earlier than increases in A1c.

Falsely elevated results may occur for the following reasons:

- Serum (not whole blood) hemoglobin concentrations are >100 mg/dL (normally <15 mg/dL)
- Serum bilirubin is >4 mg/dL
- Serum ascorbic acid is >5 mg/dL[17]

Methyldopa and calcium dobesilate (the latter is used outside the United States to minimize myocardial damage after an acute infarction) may also cause falsely elevated results. Serum fructosamine concentrations are lower in obese patients with DM as compared with lean patients with DM.[18] Falsely low fructosamine levels can be observed in patients with low serum protein or albumin levels. Some clinicians advocate the use of fructosamine concentrations as a monitoring tool for short-term changes in glycemic control (eg, GDM, recent addition of medication). A fructosamine test can be used as an alternative test in cases in which the A1C may be unreliable, such as blood loss or hemolytic anemia, sickle cell anemia, or other hemoglobin variants. The hemoglobin A1c test is also less reliable and the fructosamine test may be preferred.[18]

### Urine Glucose

*Normal range: negative*

Glucose "spills" into the urine when the serum glucose concentration exceeds the renal threshold for glucose reabsorption (normally 180 mg/dL). However, a poor correlation exists between urine glucose and concurrent serum glucose concentrations. This poor correlation occurs because urine is "produced" hours before it is tested unless the inconvenient double-void method (urine is collected 30 minutes after emptying of the bladder) is used. Furthermore, the renal threshold varies among patients and tends to increase in diabetes over time, especially if renal function is declining. Urine testing gradually has been replaced by convenient fingerstick blood sugar testing. Urine glucose testing should be recommended only if a patient is unable or unwilling to perform blood glucose monitoring.[19]

### Self-Monitoring Tests for Blood Glucose

*Blood glucose meters* and *reagent test strips* are commercially available so that patients may perform blood glucose monitoring at home. These systems are also used in hospitals, where healthcare providers rely on quick results for determining insulin requirements. The meters currently marketed are lightweight, relatively inexpensive, accurate, and user friendly.[20]

The first generation of self-monitoring blood glucose (SMBG) meters relied on a photometric analysis that was based on a dye-related reaction. This method, also termed *reflectance photometry, light reflectance,* or *enzyme photometry*, involves a chemical reaction between capillary blood and a chemical on the strip that produces a change in color. The amount of color reflected from the strip is measured photometrically. The reflected color is directly related to the amount of glucose in the blood. The darker color the test strip, the higher the glucose concentration. The disadvantages of this method are that the test strip has to be developed after a precise interval (after the blood is washed away), a large sample size of blood (>12 µL) is required, and the meter requires frequent calibration.[21]

Most SMBG meters today utilize an electrochemical or enzyme electrode process, which determines glucose levels by measuring an electrical charge produced by the glucose-reagent reaction. These second-generation glucose meters can further be subdivided according to the electrochemical principle used: amperometry or colorimetry.[21]

*Amperometry* biosensor technology requires a large sample size (4 to 10 µL). Amperometric technology measures only a small percentage of the glucose and uses a multiplier to convert it to a numerical value. Therefore, blood glucose readings may be affected by environmental temperature, hematocrit (Hct), medications, and other factors. Also, small samples may result in inaccurate readings because of a weak signal being generated.[22]

The *colorimetry* method involves converting the glucose sample into an electrochemical charge, which is then captured for measurement. An advantage of this system is that a small amount of blood (eg, 0.3 mL) is enough to determine the blood glucose level. The colorimetry method is not influenced by changes in temperature and Hct levels. These monitors can use blood samples extracted from the arm and thigh, too. At these alternative sites, there are fewer capillaries and nerve endings, allowing for a less painful needle stick. Some examples of second-generation glucometers that use the colorimetry method include Nova Max Plus, OneTouch Verio, and FreeStyle Lite. A chart that lists the current glucose meters and their features can be found at http://main.diabetes.org/dforg/pdfs/2020/2020-cg-blood-glucose-meters.pdf.[22]

Although new SMBG meters report results as plasma values, older meters may report results as whole blood values, which are approximately 10% to 15% lower than plasma values. The ADA recommends whole blood fasting readings of 80 to 130 mg/dL (4.4 to 6.7 mmol/L) and postprandial readings of <180 mg/dL.[2]

***Special features of glucose meters.*** Blood glucose testing can be challenging for adults with poor vision or limited dexterity and children with small hands. Patients should try several meters by checking their ease of use with the lancing device and lancets, test strips, packaging, and meter features before committing to one. Many meters like the Glucocard Shine Express, Advocate Redi-Code Plus Speaking Meter, and For a Test N'GO Advance Voice offer an audio function that is available in several different languages. Individuals with visual impairment may benefit from larger display screen, screen backlight, or test strip port light. Examples of meters that offer a screen backlight include the FreeStyle Lite, Presto, Presto Pro, OneTouch Ultra 2, and Contour Next Link USB.[22]

Some children are more comfortable monitoring their blood glucose than others. Some children may like glucometers that come in bright or "cool" colors. Many "auto-code" or "no-code" meters, which do not require manually programming the meter to recognize a specific group of test strips, are ideal choices for children who are learning how to monitor their blood glucose levels. Parents should select a meter that requires a small blood sample size.

Most meters hold from 100 to 450 test results, although a few save over 1,000. This makes it easier to track blood glucose control over time. Many meters on the market have computer-download capabilities through a USB connection.[22]

Generally, blood glucose concentrations determined by these methods are clinically useful estimates of corresponding plasma glucose concentrations measured by the laboratory. Therefore, at-home blood glucose monitoring is preferred to urine testing.[22] At-home blood testing clarifies the relationship between symptomatology and blood glucose concentrations. The best meter for a patient is an individual decision. Patients should be encouraged to try different brands of meters to find the device with which they are most comfortable.[20]

The use of *continuous glucose monitoring* (CGM) is recognized as the standard of care for individuals with type 1 diabetes and a subset of those with type 2 diabetes requiring insulin therapy.[23] CGM provides readings every few minutes throughout the day. This method allows patients and providers an opportunity to observe trends in glucose levels throughout the day and make the appropriate adjustments to medication, meal, or exercise regimens. A small, sterile, disposable glucose-sensing device called a *sensor* is inserted into the subcutaneous tissue. This sensor measures the change in glucose levels in interstitial fluid and sends the information to a reader that can store from 3 to 90 days of data. Real-time CGM systems include Dexcom G5 and Dexcom G6 sensors (manufactured by Dexcom); Eversense CGM System (manufactured by Senseonics) and Guardian Connect CGM System (manufactured by Medtronic Diabetes). Monitors are typically calibrated daily by entering at least two blood glucose readings obtained at different times using a standard blood glucose meter. The monitors have an alert system to warn patients if their blood glucose level is dangerously low or high. The monitor may be part of an insulin pump or a separate device that can be carried in a pocket or purse. Smartphone apps are also used in conjunction with CGMs. The FreeStyle Libre Flash Glucose Monitoring System and FreeStyle Libre 2 System (Abbott Diabetes Care) are the only intermittently scanned system currently available. After the sensor is inserted, there is a 12-hour warm-up time, and no initial or daily calibration is required during the 14-day wear period. Unlike with the real-time CGM system, the patient has to purposely scan the sensor to obtain changes in glucose levels.[23,24]

Quality control, which consists of control solution testing, calibration, and system maintenance, is a necessary component of accurate glucose testing. Control solutions can be purchased to assess the accuracy of the test strip. Control solutions should be used every time a new container of test strips is opened, when the blood glucose meter is mishandled or dropped, or whenever the accuracy of the results is questioned. The technique of verifying accuracy operates the same way that the patient analyzes a drop of blood. A few meters require manual calibration prior to use, but most have an automatic calibration mode for ease of use. In photometric meters, the blood sample intended for the strip may come in contact with the meter and soil the optic window resulting in inaccurate results.[21] Pharmacists should guide patients through the instructions for cleaning the meter that is usually provided by the manufacturer.[20]

***Factors affecting glucose readings.*** User error is the most common reason for inaccurate results. Some of the most common errors include not putting enough blood on the reagent portion of the strip. Patients should be asked periodically to demonstrate how they operate the meter.[25]

Environmental factors such as temperature, humidity, altitude, and light may influence the accuracy of glucose readings. Exposing glucometers to extremes of temperature can alter battery life and performance. Therefore, glucometers should be stored at room temperature to ensure accuracy (most will function at temperatures between 50°F and 104°F). Temperature changes and humidity may decrease the shelf life of test strips, resulting in inaccurate test results. Test strips should not be stored in areas of high humidity, such as a bathroom, or in areas with notable temperature changes, such as the car. Individuals should check the expiration date of the test strips. Because test strips are costly, patients are often tempted to use expired strips, which result in inaccurate readings.[26,27] Most test strips expire within 90 to 180 days after being opened.

At higher altitudes, changes in oxygen content and temperature alter glucose testing results. Results of studies evaluating the accuracy of glucometers at altitudes >10,000 feet have revealed major alterations in blood glucose levels. These changes are attributed to variations in metabolic rate, hydration, diet, physical exercise, Hct, and temperature associated with higher altitudes. Patients should be educated on how to use glucometers at high altitudes. Changes in light exposure can also alter results with photometric glucometers.[26] Additional variables such as hypotension, hypoxia, high triglyceride concentrations, and various drugs can alter readings; each patient should be evaluated for the presence of such variables and medication-related effects.[25-27]

***Accuracy of glucose readings.*** The FDA requires 95% of all meter test results to be within 20% of the actual blood glucose level for results ≥75 mg/dL (4.2 mmol/L). An actual blood glucose that is 100 mg/dL (5.6 mmol/L) could show on a meter as being between 80 and 120 mg/dL (4.4 to 6.7 mmol/L) and still be considered accurate. The FDA is currently reviewing more stringent standards that will require 98% of meter test results to be within 15% of the actual blood glucose level for results ≥75 mg/dL (4.2 mmol/L). For example, an actual blood glucose result of 100 mg/dL (5.6 mmol/L) could potentially show on a meter as any value between 85 and 115 mg/dL (4.7 to 6.4 mmol/L) and meet the standard.[28]

The guidelines for results in the hypoglycemic range, defined as a blood glucose level <72mg/dL (4.2 mmol/L), stipulate that 98% of test results must be within ±15 mg/dL of the actual blood glucose level. Therefore, if an actual blood glucose level is 60 mg/dL, the guidance says the reading would need to be between 45 and 75 mg/dL (2.5 to 4.2 mmol/L) to meet accuracy standards.[28,29]

The FDA guidance also recommends that meter boxes and test strip vials include easy-to-understand accuracy data—both on the outside of the package and on the insert inside. The FDA does not regularly monitor blood glucose meters or strips once they enter the commercial market. This means some companies may not maintain the same level of quality and accuracy as when the products were initially approved.[28,29]

***Frequency of glucose monitoring.*** Glucose monitoring requirements may vary based on the pharmacologic therapy administered. It is generally unnecessary in patients who manage their diabetes with diet alone or who take oral medications that do not cause hypoglycemia. Patients taking insulin injections twice a day should check blood glucose levels at least twice a day. Patients on intensive insulin therapy should monitor blood glucose levels three to four times a day. Patients on insulin pumps need monitoring four to six times a day to determine the effectiveness of the basal and bolus doses. In general, premeal glucose measurements are needed to monitor the effectiveness of the basal insulin dose (eg, glargine or detemir) dose. Two-hour postprandial glucose (PPG) readings are needed to monitor rapid-acting insulins (eg, lispro, glulisine, aspart, and Afrezza inhaled). Oral blood glucose–lowering agents, such as metformin, thiazolidinediones, sitagliptin, and glipizide, are evaluated using 2-hour postprandial readings. Pregnancy requires frequent monitoring of blood glucose levels four to six times a day to ensure tight control. Premeal testing is required during acute illness to determine the need for supplemental insulin.[30-37]

# Diagnosis of Hyperglycemia

The diagnosis of patients with *hyperglycemia* commonly falls into one of three categories: (1) DM or prediabetes, (2) diabetic ketoacidosis (DKA), and (3) hyperosmolar hyperglycemia state (HHS).[2]

## Diabetes Mellitus or Prediabetes

***Goals of therapy.*** Once DM is diagnosed, the clinician needs to establish a therapeutic goal with respect to glucose control. The ADA recommends that an A1C goal for many nonpregnant adults of <7% (53 mmol/mol) is appropriate. On the basis of provider judgment and patient preference, achieving lower A1C levels (eg, <6.5%) may be acceptable if it can be achieved safely without significant hypoglycemia or other adverse effects of treatment. Less stringent A1C goals (eg, <8% [64 mmol/mol]) may be appropriate for patients with a history of severe hypoglycemia, limited life expectancy, advanced microvascular or macrovascular complications, extensive comorbid conditions, or long-standing diabetes in whom the goal is difficult to achieve despite diabetes self-management education, appropriate glucose monitoring, and effective doses of multiple glucose-lowering agents, including insulin.

## Diabetic Ketoacidosis

Insulin deficiency can result in impaired glucose use by peripheral tissues and the liver. Prolonged insulin deficiency results in protein breakdown and increased glucose production (gluconeogenesis) by the liver and an increased release of counterregulatory hormones such as glucagon, catecholamines (eg, epinephrine and norepinephrine), cortisol, and growth hormones. In the face of lipolysis, free fatty acids are converted by the liver to ketone bodies (β-hydroxybutyric acid and acetoacetic acid), which can result in metabolic acidosis. DKA, which occurs most commonly in patients with type 1 DM, is initiated by insulin deficiency (**Minicase 1**). The most common causes of DKA include the following[38]:

- Infections, illness, and emotional stress
- Nonadherence or inadequate insulin dosage
- Undiagnosed type 1 DM
- Unknown or no precipitating event

Clinically, patients with DKA typically present with dehydration, lethargy, acetone-smelling breath, abdominal pain, tachycardia, orthostatic hypotension, tachypnea, and, occasionally, mild hypothermia and lethargy or coma. Because of a patient's tendency toward low body temperatures, fever strongly suggests infection as a precipitant of DKA. DKA is typically associated with a high glucose concentration. This concentration is typically >250 mg/dL or 13.9 mmol/L; however, in the setting of sodium-glucose cotransporter-2 (SGLT2) inhibitors use and other uncommon conditions, the blood glucose can be in the normal range (euglycemic DKA).[39]

# MINICASE 1

## Diabetic Ketoacidosis

Rena M. is a 40-year-old woman with a 2-year history of type 2 DM. She presents to the ED with a pH of 7.25, $HCO_3$ of 9, and blood glucose of 180 mg/dL. Her husband brought her to the ED after finding her "out of it" when attempting to wake her. She was vomiting and unable to eat over the last 24 hours, and she experienced labored breathing, fever, chills, and unusual fatigue.

Approximately 1 year ago, her provider started her on Janumet (sitagliptin–metformin, 50 mg/1,000 mg) at breakfast and dinner. At her most recent clinic appointment 1 month ago, her laboratory results indicated that her HbA1c has dropped from 9.2 to 7.8 since starting sitagliptin–metformin. Her doctor decided to add dapagliflozin 10 mg to her regimen to obtain an HbA1c below 7%. Rena M. also takes atorvastatin 40 mg at bedtime for elevated cholesterol and lisinopril 10 mg daily and hydrochlorothiazide 25 mg daily for hypertension. She has tolerated all of her medications and adheres to the indicated daily schedule. Physical examination reveals a lethargic woman with vital signs including BP 116/68 mm Hg (which dropped to 95/50 when standing); HR 105 beats/min; respiratory rate (RR) 30 breaths/min (deep and regular); and an oral temperature 101.4°F (38.6°C). Her skin turgor is poor, her mucous membranes are dry, and she is disoriented and confused. Her laboratory results are as follows:

- Sodium, 142 mEq/L (136 to 142 mEq/L)
- Potassium, 5 mEq/L (3.8 to 5 mEq/L)
- Chloride, 99 mEq/L (95 to 103 mEq/L)
- BUN, 28 mg/dL (8 to 23 mg/dL)
- SCr, 1.8 mg/dL (0.6 to 1.2 mg/dL)
- Phosphorus, 2.7 mg/dL (2.3 to 4.7 mg/dL)
- Amylase, 200 International Units/L (30 to 220 International Units/L)
- pH, 7.25 (7.38 to 7.44)
- Bicarbonate, 9 mEq/L (21 to 28 mEq/L)
- Hct, 52% (36% to 45%)
- WBC count, 16 × $10^3$ cells/mm³ (4.8 to 10.8 × $10^3$ cells/mm³)
- Calcium, 9 mg/dL (9.2 to 11 mg/dL)
- Glucose, 180 mg/dL (70 to 110 mg/dL)
- Ketones, 3+ at 1:8 serum dilution (normal = 0)
- Osmolality, 304 mOsm/kg (280 to 295 mOsm/kg)
- Triglycerides, 174 mg/dL (10 to 150 mg/dL)
- Lipase, 1.4 units/mL (<1.5 units/mL)
- Magnesium, 2 mEq/L (1.3 to 2.1 mEq/L)

A urine screen with Multistix indicates a large (160 mg/dL) amount of ketones (the highest designation on the strip).

QUESTION: Based on clinical and laboratory findings, what is the most likely diagnosis for this patient? What precipitated this metabolic disorder? Can an interpretation of any results be influenced by her acidosis or hyperglycemia? Are there potential medication interferences with any laboratory tests?

DISCUSSION: The patient has type 2 DM and presents with DKA, which is less commonly observed in patients with type 2 DM compared with type 1 DM. Since 2014, the FDA has received many reports of DKA in patients treated with SGLT2 inhibitors. The FDA reports that DKA case presentations associated with SGLT2 inhibitors are atypical in that glucose levels can be normal or mildly elevated, whereas patients with a typical DKA presentation (type 1 DM or type 2 DM) typically have glucose levels >300 mg/dL. This patient has a fever, which suggest a potential infection. She should be examined for infection by obtaining a urinalysis and blood culture. The cause of preserved euglycemia could be greater urinary loss of glucose triggered by counterregulatory hormones, hepatic glucose production observed during a fasting state, or the SGLT2 inhibitor. A key physiologic determinant is the quantity of food she ingested before development of DKA. That is, when patients are well fed, their liver contains large amounts of glycogen, which primes the liver to produce glucose and suppress ketogenesis. However, when patients have been vomiting and unable to eat, the liver is depleted of glycogen and primed to produce ketones. Thus, patients such as Rena M. with euglycemic ketoacidosis are usually in the fasting state before they become ill.

Clinically, Rena M. presents with typical signs of ketoacidosis, which include difficulty breathing, nausea, vomiting, abdominal pain, confusion, and unusual fatigue and sleepiness. Her decreased skin turgor, dry mucous membranes, tachycardia (HR 105 beats/min), and orthostatic hypotension are consistent with dehydration, a common condition in patients with DKA. Her breathing is rapid and deep. Although she is not comatose, she is lethargic, confused, and disoriented. Chemically, she probably has a total body deficit of sodium and potassium despite serum concentration results within normal limits.

The decreased intravascular volume associated with DKA causes hemoconcentration on electrolytes. Therefore, these values do not reflect total body stores, and the clinician can expect them to decline rapidly if unsupplemented fluids are infused. Although her phosphorus concentration is in the normal range (lower end), it likely will decrease after rehydration and insulin. Serial electrolyte testing should be done every 3 to 4 hours during the first 24 hours.

Serial glucose, ketones, and acid-base measurements, typical of DKA, should show gradual improvement with proper therapy. Potassium balance is altered in patients with DKA because of combined urinary and GI losses. Although total potassium is depleted, the serum potassium concentration may be high, normal, or low, depending on the degree of acidosis. Her metabolic acidosis has resulted in an extracellular shifting of potassium, causing an elevated serum potassium concentration. Potassium supplementation may be withheld for the first hour or until serum levels begin to drop. Potassium replacement should begin when potassium levels reach normal. Low serum potassium in the face of pronounced acidosis suggests severe potassium depletion that requires early, aggressive therapy to prevent life-threatening hypokalemia during treatment.

Decreased intravascular volume has led to a hemoconcentrated Hct and BUN, which is also elevated by decreased renal perfusion (prerenal azotemia), although intrinsic renal causes should be considered if SCr is also elevated. Fortunately, as is probably the case with this patient, high SCr may be an artifact caused by the

*Continued*

## MINICASE 1 (cont'd)

influence of ketone bodies on the assay. If so, SCr concentrations should decline with ketone concentrations.

She may be exhibiting leukocytosis unrelated to infection, but no lab data were provided in the case to actually rule out infection. Her estimated plasma osmolarity based on the osmolarity estimation

formula would be $(2 \times 142) + (180/18) + (28/2.8) = 304$ mOsm/L, which is approximately equal to the actual measured laboratory result.

The serum ketone results still would have to be interpreted as real and significant, given all of the other signs and symptoms. A urine screen also indicated the presence of ketones.

---

DKA is also characterized by low venous bicarbonate (0 to 15 mEq/L), a decreased arterial pH (<7.0 to 7.2), and the presence of an anion gap (>12) (see Chapter 13 for more information on anion gap). Glucose spilling in the urine can lead to osmotic diuresis, resulting in hypotonic fluid losses, dehydration, and electrolyte loss. Sodium and potassium concentrations may be low, normal, or high on initial presentation. Sodium concentrations are reflective of the amount of total body water and sodium lost and replaced. In the presence of hyperglycemia, sodium concentrations may be decreased because of the movement of water from the intracellular space to the extracellular space. The potassium level reflects a balance between the amount of potassium lost in the urine and insulin deficiency, which causes higher concentrations of serum potassium as potassium shifts from intracellular spaces to extracellular fluid. Hypertonicity and acidosis can cause potassium to move from the intracellular space to the extracellular space, resulting in elevated potassium levels. Patients with low or normal potassium levels on presentation should be placed on intravenous (IV) potassium replacement and monitored closely because DKA and its subsequent treatment can result in a low serum potassium and total body potassium levels that may place the patient at risk for cardiac dysrhythmia.[38,39]

The phosphate level is usually normal or slightly elevated but may decrease during treatment and should be monitored.[38] Creatinine and blood urea nitrogen (BUN) are usually elevated due to dehydration with an increased BUN to Scr ratio. These levels usually return to normal after rehydration unless there was preexisting renal insufficiency. Hemoglobin, Hct, and total protein levels are mildly elevated due to decreased plasma volume and dehydration. Amylase levels may be increased due to increased secretion by the salivary glands. Liver function tests are usually elevated but return to normal in 3 to 4 weeks.

Serum osmolality is typically elevated at 300 to 320 mOsm/kg (normally, 280 to 295 mOsm/kg). Serum osmolarity (milliosmoles/liter), which is practically equivalent to osmolality (milliosmoles/kilogram), can be estimated using the following formula:

$$\text{serum osmolarity (mOsm/L)} = (2'\text{sodium}) + \text{glucose}/18 + \text{BUN}/2.8$$

where *glucose* and *BUN* units are expressed as milligrams/deciliter.

***Blood and urine ketones.*** Ketones are present in the blood and urine of patients with DKA, as the name of this disorder implies. Formation of ketone bodies results from fat metabolism. Three

principal ketone bodies include acetoacetate, acetone, and β-hydroxybutyrate, which is the predominant ketone in the blood of patients with DKA.[38] DKA can be prevented if patients are educated about detection of hyperglycemia and ketonuria. It is recommended that all patients with DM test their urine for ketones during acute illness or stress when blood glucose levels are consistently >250 mg/dL (14 mmol/L), during pregnancy, or when any symptoms of ketoacidosis—such as nausea, vomiting, or abdominal pain—are present.[40]

All of the commercially available urine testing methods are based on the reaction of acetoacetic acid with sodium nitroprusside (nitroferricyanide) in a strongly basic medium. The colors range from beige or buff-pink for a "negative" reading to pink and pink-purple for a "positive" reading (Acetest, Ketostix, Laboratorystix, and Multistix). These nitroprusside-based (nitroferricyanide) assays do not detect β-hydroxybutyric acid and are 15 to 20 times more sensitive to acetoacetate than to acetone. In a few situations (eg, severe hypovolemia, hypotension, low partial pressure of oxygen [$pO_2$], and alcoholism) where β-hydroxybutyrate predominates, assessment of ketones may be falsely low. As DKA resolves, β-hydroxybutyric acid is converted to acetoacetate, the assay-reactive ketone body. Therefore, a stronger reaction may be encountered in laboratory results. However, this reaction does not necessarily mean a worsening of the ketoacidotic state.[41]

Clinicians must keep in mind that ketonuria may also result from starvation, high-fat diets, fever, and anesthesia, but these conditions are not associated with hyperglycemia. Levodopa, mesna, acetylcysteine (irrigation), methyldopa, phenazopyridine, pyrazinamide, valproic acid, captopril, and high-dose aspirin may cause false-positive results with urine ketone tests.[42-44] The influence of these drugs on serum ketone tests has not been studied extensively. If the ketone concentration is increased, a typical series of dipstick results includes the following results:

1. Negative
2. Trace (5 mg/dL)
3. Small (15 mg/dL)
4. Moderate (40 mg/dL)
5. Large (80 mg/dL)
6. Very large (160 mg/dL)

False-negative readings have been reported when test strips have been exposed to air for an extended period of time or when urine specimens have been highly acidic, such as after large intakes of ascorbic acid.[40] Urine ketone tests should not be used for diagnosing or monitoring the treatment of DKA. Acetoacetic and β-hydroxybutyric acids concentrations in urine greatly exceed blood concentrations. Therefore, the presence of ketone bodies in urine cannot be used to diagnose DKA. Conversely, during recovery from ketoacidosis, ketone bodies may be detected in urine long after blood concentrations have fallen.[43,45] In addition, urine testing only provides an estimate of blood ketone levels 2 to 4 hours before testing and depends on the person being able to pass urine.[40,41]

Blood β-ketone testing can provide a patient with an early warning of impending DKA.[45,46] While blood β-ketone testing is routinely conducted in a medical setting, patients may also use an at-home kit to test for ketones in blood. While instructions may vary, kits will include some kind of device for the patient to prick their finger (similar to blood glucose testing). The brands of meters currently marketed are CareTouch, Keto-Mojo, Nova Max Plus, and Precision Xtra. All of these meters can also be used to measure blood glucose levels. Patients should purchase the glucose strips made for their meter to use this feature. In addition, each meter can be tested against control. A β-hydroxybutyric acid level <0.6 mmol/L is considered normal. Patients with levels between 0.6 and 1 mmol/L should take additional insulin and increase their fluid intake to flush out the ketones. Patients should contact their physician if levels are between 1 and 3 mmol/L. Patients should be advised to report to the emergency department (ED) immediately if their levels are >3 mmol/L.[46]

### Hyperosmolar Hyperglycemia State

*Hyperosmolar hyperglycemia state* (HHS) is a condition that occurs most frequently in elderly patients with type 2 DM, and it is usually precipitated by stress or illness when such patients do not drink enough to keep up with osmotic diuresis. Patients usually present with severe hyperglycemia (glucose concentrations >600 mg/dL or >33.3 mmol/L); decreased mentation (eg, lethargy, confusion, dehydration); neurologic manifestations (eg, seizures and hemisensory deficits); and an absence of ketosis. Insulin deficiency is not as severe in HHS as in DKA. Therefore, lipolysis, which is necessary for the formation of ketone bodies, does not occur (**Minicase 2**). The absence of ketosis results in significantly milder GI symptoms than patients with DKA. Therefore, patients often fail to seek medical attention. Patients with HHS tend to have much higher blood glucose concentrations than in DKA and are usually more dehydrated on presentation than patients with DKA due to impairment in the thirst mechanism, which results in prolonged diuresis and dehydration.[46-48]

In some cases, patients are taking medications that cause glucose intolerance (eg, diuretics, steroids, and phenytoin). Stroke and infection are disease-related predisposing factors. Initially, electrolytes are within normal ranges, but BUN routinely is elevated. Serum osmolalities characteristically are higher than those in DKA—in the range of 320 to 400 mOsm/kg. Serum electrolytes (eg, magnesium, phosphorus, and calcium) are typically abnormal and should be monitored until they return to normal range.[47,48]

## Hypoglycemia

*Hypoglycemia* is defined as a blood glucose level of 70 mg/dL (3.9 mmol/L) or lower.

- Level 1 (mild) hypoglycemia: blood glucose is <70 mg/dL but ≥54 mg/dL.
- Level 2 (moderate) hypoglycemia: Blood glucose is <54 mg/dL.
- Level 3 (severe) hypoglycemia: A person is unable to function because of mental or physical changes. They need help from another person. In this case, blood glucose is often <40 mg/dL.

The classification of hypoglycemia is based on an individual's ability to self-treat. Mild hypoglycemia is characterized by symptoms such as sweating, trembling, shaking, rapid heartbeat, heavy breathing, and difficulty concentrating. The symptoms associated with mild hypoglycemia vary in severity and do not imply that the symptoms experienced by the individual are minor or easily tolerated. Although patients may experience profuse sweating, dizziness, and lack of coordination, they still may be able to self-treat. These symptoms resolve after consuming readily absorbable carbohydrates (eg, fruit juice, milk, or hard candy).[16,49]

## Other Laboratory Tests Used in the Management of Diabetes Mellitus

The 2021 ADA standards recommend urinalysis for detection of proteinuria should be obtained in patients with DM on a yearly basis.[50] This should begin at the time of diagnosis in patients with type 2 DM and 5 years after diagnosis in patients with type 1 DM.[50] A quantitative test for urine protein should follow a positive result on urinalysis. If urinalysis is negative for proteinuria, testing for increased albumin excretion (previously termed *microalbuminuria*) should be obtained. Increased albumin excretion indicates glomerular damage and is predictive of clinical nephropathy.[50]

Three methods are available to screen for increased albumin excretion. One method is measurement of the urine albumin to creatinine ratio in a spot urine sample. This method is convenient in the clinical setting because it requires only one urine sample. A morning sample is preferred to take into account the diurnal variation of albumin excretion. A second method is a 24-hour urine collection for determination of albumin excretion. This method may be tedious and accuracy relies on proper collection techniques. An advantage of this method is that renal function can simultaneously be quantified. A third alternative method to the 24-hour collection is a timed urine collection for albumin. Moderately increased albuminuria is defined as a urinary albumin excretion of 30 to 299 mcg/mL on a spot urine sample, 30 to 299 mg/24 hr on a 24-hour urine collection, or 20 to 199 mcg/min on a timed urine collection. Transient rises in albumin excretion can be associated with exercise, hyperglycemia, hypertension, urinary tract infection, heart failure, and fever. Therefore, if any of these conditions are present, they may result in false-positive results on screening tests. Variability exists in the excretion of albumin; thus, moderately increased albuminuria must be confirmed in two repeated tests in a 3- to 6-month period. Two of three positive screening tests for moderately increased albuminuria confirm the diagnosis.[50]

# MINICASE 2

## Hyperosmolar Hyperglycemia State Secondary to Uncontrolled Type 2 Diabetes Mellitus

Jimmy C. is a 63-year-old African American man with a 19-year history of type 2 DM, hypertension, and dyslipidemia. He lives alone. His medication list includes metformin 1,000 mg BID, simvastatin 20 mg daily at bedtime, lisinopril 20 mg daily, hydrochlorothiazide 25 mg daily, and ASA 325 mg daily. He monitors his blood glucose once a day, and his results have ranged from 215 to 400 mg/dL. His fasting blood glucose has averaged 200 mg/dL over the last week. He reports frequent urination throughout the day and night, which has increased over the last 6 days. He denies any nausea or vomiting but states he has not had much of an appetite lately. His daughter accompanies him to the doctor's office because she thinks he has not been his usual self lately.

The physical examination reveals a disoriented and confused man with vital signs including BP 120/60 mm Hg (which decreased to 100/60 when standing); HR 100 beats/min; RR 20 breaths/min (deep and regular); and oral temperature 101.4°F (38.6°C). His skin turgor is poor, and his mucous membranes are dry. His laboratory results are as follows:

- Sodium, 139 mEq/L (136 to 142 mEq/L)
- Potassium, 4.6 mEq/L (3.8 to 5 mEq/L)
- Chloride, 102 mEq/L (95 to 103 mEq/L)
- BUN, 50 mg/dL (8 to 23 mg/dL)
- SCr, 1.2 mg/dL (0.6 to 1.2 mg/dL)
- Phosphorus, 2.7 mg/dL (2.3 to 4.7 mg/dL)
- pH, 7.38 (7.36 to 7.44)
- Bicarbonate, 26 mEq/L (21 to 28 mEq/L)
- Hct, 39% (42% to 50%)
- WBC count, $9.4 \times 10^3$ cells/mm³ (4.8 to 10.8 × 10³ cells/mm³)
- Calcium, 9 mg/dL (9.2 to 11 mg/dL)
- Glucose, 715 mg/dL (70 to 110 mg/dL)
- Ketones, 0 (normal = 0)
- Osmolality, 335 mOsm/kg (280 to 295 mOsm/kg)
- Triglycerides, 174 mg/dL (10 to 150 mg/dL)
- Lipase, 1.4 units/mL (<1.5 units/mL)
- Magnesium, 2 mEq/L (1.3 to 2.1 mEq/L)
- Hemoglobin A1c, 9.5 (4% to 5.6%)

QUESTION: Based on the subjective and objective data provided, what is the most likely diagnosis for this patient? What signs and symptoms support the diagnosis? What could have precipitated this disorder?

DISCUSSION: Jimmy C. is older than 60 years. HHS occurs most frequently in patients older than 60 years. He reports symptoms for more than 5 days. He has decreased skin turgor, dry mucous membranes, tachycardia (HR 100 beats/min), and orthostatic hypotension (a fall of systolic BP 20 mm Hg after 1 minute of standing), which are consistent with dehydration. He is lethargic, confused, and disoriented. Patients with HHS are generally more dehydrated than patients with DKA; therefore, mentation changes are more commonly seen in patients with HHS than in DKA. Elderly persons often have an impaired thirst mechanism that increases the risk of HHS. Jimmy C.'s plasma glucose level is >600 mg/dL; bicarbonate concentration is normal; and pH is normal. Negative ketone bodies <2+ in 1:1 dilution confirms the diagnosis of HHS (and not DKA, in which ketones are present in the blood and urine of patients). Insulin deficiency is less profound in HHS; therefore, lipolysis resulting in the production of ketone bodies does not occur. His plasma osmolarity can be estimated using a formula:

$$pOsm = (2 \times serum\ sodium) + glucose/18 + BUN/2.8$$

The estimated osmolality is $(2 \times 139) + (715/18) + 50/2.8 = 335$ mOsm/kg, which is the same as the actual laboratory value. Massive fluid loss due to prolonged osmotic diuresis secondary to hyperglycemia may have precipitated the onset of HHS.

The patient should be given IV fluids for hydration because of the mental status changes. An IV insulin drip should also be administered. Although his sodium and potassium are within normal limits, the presence of orthostatic hypotension is consistent with decreased intravascular volume, causing hemoconcentration of sodium and potassium. These levels may decline when the patient is rehydrated with fluids. Potassium replacement is required. Phosphorus is also within normal limits but may decrease after rehydration and insulin. Decreased intravascular volume has led to hemoconcentration of Hct and BUN, which is also elevated because of decreased renal perfusion (prerenal azotemia), although intrinsic renal causes should be considered if SCr is also elevated.

Given the patient's symptoms and diagnosis of HHS, metformin in combination with a once-daily injection of long-acting insulin administered at breakfast or bedtime is a reasonable option because he did not obtain glycemic control on oral agent(s). Metformin can be continued if glomerular filtration rate >30 mL/min/1.73m² and long-acting insulin can be administered at bedtime.

Based on results of landmark studies, the ADA recommends angiotension-converting enzyme (ACE) inhibitors or angiotension receptor blockers (ARBs) for the treatment of both moderately increased albuminuria (previously termed *microalbumuria* and defined as a urinary albumin excretion 30 to 299 mg/day) and severely increased albuminuria (previously termed *macroalbuminuria* and defined as a urinary albumin excretion >300 mg/day). If one class is not tolerated, the other should be substituted.

The leading cause of death in patients with DM is cardiovascular disease. Control of hypertension and dyslipidemia is necessary to decrease the risk of macrovascular complications. Under the new American College of Cardiology and American Heart Association lipid guidelines, patients should be placed on statin medications based on risk stratification and treated with varying intensity statin dosing regimens.[51,52]

Patients with DM and hypertension should be treated with pharmacologic therapy regimen that includes either an ACE inhibitor or an ARB.[50] Although ARBs have been shown to delay the progression of nephropathy in patients with type 2 DM, hypertension, moderately increased albuminuria, and renal insufficiency, ACE inhibitors are the initial agents of choice in patients with type 1 DM with hypertension and any degree of albuminuria. Thiazide diuretics, β-blockers, or calcium channel blockers should be used as an add-on agent to further decrease BP (blood pressure). Avoidance of nephrotoxic drugs and use of SGLT2i therapy is also recommended.[50]

# THYROID

## Anatomy and Physiology

The *thyroid* gland is a butterfly-shaped organ composed of two connecting lobes that span the width of the trachea. The thyroid produces the hormones thyroxine ($T_4$) and triiodothyronine ($T_3$). Approximately 80 and 30 mcg of $T_4$ and $T_3$, respectively, are produced daily in normal adults. Although $T_4$ is produced solely by the thyroid gland, only about 20% to 25% of $T_3$ is directly secreted by this gland. Approximately 80% of $T_3$ is formed by hepatic and renal deiodination of $T_4$.[53]

$T_4$ has a longer half-life than $T_3$, approximately 7 days versus 1 day, respectively. At the cellular level, however, $T_3$ is three to four times more active physiologically than $T_4$.[49] When the conversion of $T_4$ to $T_3$ is impaired, a stereoisomer of $T_3$, known as *reverse* $T_3$, is produced; reverse $T_3$ has no known biological effect.

Thyroid hormones have many biological effects, both at the molecular level and on specific organ systems. These hormones stimulate the basal metabolic rate and can affect protein, carbohydrate, and lipid metabolism. They are also essential for normal growth and development. Thyroid hormones act to do the following tasks:

- Stimulate neural and skeletal development during fetal life
- Stimulate oxygen consumption at rest
- Stimulate bone turnover by increasing bone formation and resorption
- Promote conversion of carotene to vitamin A
- Promote chronotropic and inotropic effects on the heart
- Increase number of catecholamine receptors in heart muscle cells
- Increase basal body temperature
- Increase production of RBCs
- Increase metabolism and clearance of steroid hormones
- Alter metabolism of carbohydrates, fats, and protein
- Control normal hypoxic and hypercapnic respiratory drives

The synthesis of thyroid hormones depends on iodine and the amino acid tyrosine. The thyroid gland, using an energy-requiring process, transports dietary iodide ($I^-$) from the circulation into the thyroid follicular cell. Iodide is oxidized to iodine ($I_2$), and then combined with tyrosyl residues within the thyroglobulin molecule to form thyroid hormones (iodothyronine). Thus, thyroid hormones are formed and stored within the thyroglobulin protein for release into the circulation.[54,55]

Both $T_4$ and $T_3$ circulate in human serum bound to three proteins: thyroxine-binding globulin (TBG); transthyretin, previously known as *thyroid-binding prealbumin*; and albumin. Of the three proteins, 80% of $T_4$ and $T_3$ is bound to TBG. Only 0.02% of $T_4$ and 0.2% of $T_3$ circulate unbound, free to diffuse into tissues. The "free" fraction is the physiologically active component. Total and free hormones exist in an equilibrium state in which the protein-bound fraction serves as a reservoir for making the free fraction available to tissues.[55]

Thyroid hormone secretion is regulated by a feedback mechanism involving the hypothalamus, anterior pituitary, and thyroid gland itself (**Figure 9-2**). The release of $T_4$ and $T_3$ from the thyroid gland is regulated by *thyrotropin*, also called *thyroid stimulating hormone* (TSH), which is secreted by the anterior pituitary. The intrathyroidal iodine concentration also influences thyroid gland activity, and TSH secretion primarily is regulated by a dual negative feedback mechanism:

Thyrotropin-releasing hormone (TRH), or protirelin, is released by the hypothalamus, which stimulates the synthesis and release of TSH from the pituitary gland. Basal TSH concentrations in persons with normal thyroid function are 0.3 to 5 milliunits/L. The inverse relationship between TSH and free $T_4$ is logarithmic. A 50% decrease in free $T_4$ concentrations leads to a 50-fold increase in TSH concentrations and vice versa.[49] Unbound $T_4$ and $T_3$ (mainly the concentration of intracellular $T_3$ in the pituitary) directly inhibit pituitary TSH secretion. Consequently, increased concentrations of free thyroid hormones cause decreased TSH secretion, and decreased concentrations of $T_4$ and $T_3$ cause increased TSH secretion.[55]

Prolonged exposure to cold and acute psychosis may activate the hypothalamic-pituitary-thyroid axis, whereas severe stress may inhibit it. Although TRH stimulates pituitary TSH release, somatostatin, corticosteroids, and dopamine inhibit it. Small amounts of iodide are needed for $T_4$ and $T_3$ production, but large amounts inhibit their production and release. Evidence from the most sensitive assays suggests that no physiologically relevant change in serum TSH concentrations occurs in relation to age.[54]

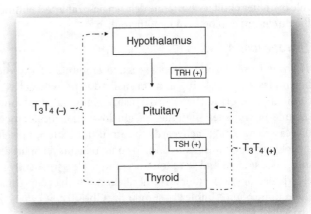

**FIGURE 9-2.** The hypothalamic-pituitary-thyroid axis.

## Thyroid Disorders

Patients with a normally functioning thyroid gland are said to be in a *euthyroid* state. When this state is disrupted, thyroid disease may result, which occurs four times more often in women than in men. Thyroid disease may occur at any age but peaks between the third and sixth decades of life. A family history of this disease often is present, especially for autoimmune thyroid diseases. Diseases of the thyroid usually involve an alteration in the quantity or quality of thyroid hormone secretion and may manifest as *hypothyroidism* or *hyperthyroidism*. In addition to the signs and symptoms discussed next, thyroid disease may produce an enlargement of the thyroid gland known as *goiter*.[51]

### Hypothyroidism

*Hypothyroidism* results from a deficiency of thyroid hormone production, causing the body metabolism to slow down. This condition affects about 2% of women and 0.2% of men, and the incidence increases with age. Symptoms include lethargy; constipation; dry, coarse skin and hair; paresthesias and slowed deep tendon reflexes; facial puffiness; cold intolerance; decreased sweating; impaired memory, confusion, and dementia; slow speech and motor activity; and anemia and growth retardation in children. Interestingly, these typical signs and symptoms have been observed in as little as 25% of elderly hypothyroid patients.[57]

Hypothyroidism is usually caused by one of three mechanisms. Primary hypothyroidism is a failure of the thyroid to produce thyroid hormone; secondary hypothyroidism is failure of the anterior pituitary to secrete TSH; and tertiary hypothyroidism is failure of the hypothalamus to produce TRH. The classification is commonly referred to as primary (problem originating within the thyroid gland) or secondary (disease originating from the pituitary or hypothalamus).

Most patients with symptomatic primary hypothyroidism have TSH concentrations >20 milliunits/L. Patients with mild signs or symptoms (usually not the reason for the visit to the doctor) have TSH values of 10 to 20 milliunits/L. Patients with secondary and tertiary hypothyroidism may have a low or normal TSH. In such patients, other pituitary hormones (eg, adrenocorticotropic hormone [ACTH], antidiuretic hormone [ADH], prolactin, growth hormone, and luteinizing hormone/follicle-stimulating hormone [LH/FSH]) should be measured to rule out other pituitary hormone deficiencies. **Table 9-3** outlines the numerous etiologies of hypothyroidism.[57]

### Thyrotoxicosis

*Thyrotoxicosis* results when excessive amounts of thyroid hormones are circulating and is usually due to hyperactivity of the thyroid gland (hyperthyroidism). Signs and symptoms include nervousness; fatigue; weight loss; heat intolerance; increased sweating; tachycardia or atrial fibrillation; muscle atrophy; warm, moist skin; and, in some patients, exophthalmos.[58] These signs and symptoms occur much less frequently in elderly persons, except for atrial fibrillation, which occurs three times more often.[59] **Table 9-4** summarizes the specific causes of hyperthyroidism.

## TABLE 9-3. Classification of Hypothyroidism by Etiology

**Primary**

Iodine deficiency

Excessive iodide intake (eg, kelp and contrast dyes)

Thyroid ablation: surgical removal of the thyroid, post $^{131}$I (radioactive iodine $^{131}$I) treatment of thyrotoxicosis, radiation of neoplasm

Hashimoto (autoimmune) thyroiditis

Subacute thyroiditis

Genetic abnormalities of thyroid hormone synthesis

Medications: propylthiouracil, methimazole, thiocyanate, lithium, amiodarone, alfa-interferon, some antineoplastic agents (ipilimumab, bexarotene, sunitinib, nivolumab)

Food: excessive intake of goitrogenic foods (eg, cabbage and turnips)

**Secondary**

Hypopituitarism: adenoma, ablative therapy, pituitary destruction, sarcoidosis hypothalamic dysfunction

**Other**

Abnormalities of $T_4$ receptor

$T_4$ = thyroxine.
*Source*: Adapted from Cryer PE. Hypoglycemia: pathophysiology, diagnosis and treatment. New York: Oxford University Press; 1997; Grundy SM, Stone NJ, Bailey AL, et al. 2018 AHA/ACC/AACVPR/AAPA/ABC/ACPM/ADA/AGS/APhA/ASPC/NLA/PCNA Guideline on the Management of Blood Cholesterol: a report of the American College of Cardiology/American Heart Association Task Force on Clinical Practice Guidelines. *Circulation*. 2019;139(25):e1082–e1143.

## Nonthyroid Laboratory Tests in Patients with Thyroid Disease

Thyroid disease may present with a wide range of signs, symptoms, and abnormal laboratory results. **Table 9-5** lists nonthyroid laboratory tests that may indicate a thyroid disorder. The influence on these tests reflects the widespread effects of thyroid hormones on peripheral tissues. Findings from these tests cannot be used alone to diagnose a thyroid disorder. However, they may support a diagnosis of thyroid dysfunction when used with specific thyroid function tests and the patient's presenting signs and symptoms.[60]

## Thyroid Function Tests

Tests more specific for thyroid status or function can be categorized as those that (1) measure the concentration of products secreted by the thyroid gland, (2) evaluate the integrity of the hypothalamic-pituitary-thyroid axis, (3) assess intrinsic thyroid gland function, and (4) detect antibodies to thyroid tissue.[60]

**TABLE 9-4.** Classification of Hyperthyroidism by Etiology

Overproduction of thyroid hormone

    Graves disease[a]

    TSH-secreting pituitary adenomas

    Hydatidiform moles/choriocarcinomas[b]

    Multinodular goiter

"Leaking" thyroid hormone due to thyroid destruction

    Lymphocytic thyroiditis

    Granulomatous thyroiditis

    Subacute thyroiditis

    Radiation

Medications: thyroid-replacement drugs (excessive), amiodarone, iodinated radiocontrast agents, iodine excess, kelp[c]

Ovarian teratomas with thyroid elements

Metastatic thyroid carcinoma

[a]Most frequent cause. The mechanism is production of thyroid-stimulating antibodies; usually associated with diffuse goiter and ophthalmopathy.
[b]Tumor production of chorionic gonadotropin, which stimulates the thyroid.
[c]Patients at risk for hyperthyroidism from these agents usually have some degree of thyroid autonomy.
*Source*: Adapted from Cryer PE. *Hypoglycemia: Pathophysiology, Diagnosis and Treatment*. New York: Oxford University Press; 1997; American Diabetes Association. Cardiovascular disease and risk management: standards of medical care in diabetes: 2020. *Diabetes Care*. 2020;43(suppl 1):S111–S134.

Tests that directly or indirectly measure the concentrations of $T_4$ and $T_3$ include the following:

- Free $T_4$
- Total serum $T_4$
- Serum $T_3$ resin uptake
- Free $T_4$ index
- Total serum $T_3$

Test results that are higher than normal are consistent with hyperthyroidism, whereas test results that are lower than normal indicate hypothyroidism.

The integrity of the hypothalamic-pituitary-thyroid axis is assessed by measuring TSH and TRH. A radioactive iodine uptake test assesses intrinsic thyroid gland function, and an antithyroid antibodies test detects antibodies to thyroid tissue.

### Free $T_4$

*Normal range: 0.9 to 2.3 ng/dL (11.6 to 29.6 pmol/L)*

This test measures the unbound $T_4$ in the serum and is the most accurate reflection of thyrometabolic status (**Tables 9-6**

**TABLE 9-5.** Nonthyroid Laboratory Tests Consistent with Thyroid Disorders

| HYPOTHYROIDISM | HYPERTHYROIDISM |
|---|---|
| Decreased | |
|   Hgb/Hct[a] | Granulocytes |
|   Serum glucose | Serum cholesterol |
|   Serum sodium | Serum triglycerides |
|   Urinary excretion of 17-hydroxysteroids | |
|   Urinary excretion of 17-ketosteroids | |
| Increased | |
|   AST/SGOT | Alkaline phosphatase |
|   Capillary fragility | Lymphocytes |
|   Cerebrospinal fluid protein | Serum ferritin |
|   LDH | Urinary calcium excretion |
|   $pCO_2$ | |
|   Serum carotene | |
|   Serum cholesterol | |
|   CPK | |
|   Serum prolactin | |
|   Serum triglycerides | |

AST = aspartate aminotransferase; CPK = serum creatine phosphokinase; Hgb = hemoglobin; LDH = lactate dehydrogenase; $pCO_2$ = partial pressure of carbon dioxide; SGOT = serum glutamic-oxaloacetic transaminase.
[a]Associated with normocytic and macrocytic anemias.
*Source*: Adapted from Grundy SM, Stone NJ, Bailey AL, et al. 2018 AHA/ACC/AACVPR/AAPA/ABC/ACPM/ADA/AGS/APhA/ASPC/NLA/PCNA Guideline on the Management of Blood Cholesterol: a report of the American College of Cardiology/American Heart Association Task Force on Clinical Practice Guidelines. *Circulation*. 2019;139(25):e1082–e1143; American Diabetes Association. Cardiovascular disease and risk management: standards of medical care in diabetes: 2020. *Diabetes Care*. 2020;43(suppl 1):S111–S134.

and **9-7**). Several methods are available to determine free $T_4$ concentrations. Some methods perform well only in otherwise healthy hypothyroid and hyperthyroid patients and in euthyroid patients with mild abnormalities of TBG. However, in patients with severe alterations of $T_4$ binding to carrier proteins (eg, severe nonthyroidal illness), only the direct equilibrium dialysis method maintains accuracy (Table 9-7).[61]

### Total Serum $T_4$

*Normal range: 5.5 to 12.5 mcg/dL (71 to 161 nmol/L)*

In most patients, the *total serum* $T_4$ level is a sensitive test for the functional status of the thyroid gland. It is high in 90% of

**TABLE 9-6.** Free T$_4$ and TSH in Thyroidal and Nonthyroidal Disorders

| DIAGNOSIS | FREE T$_4$ INDEX OR DIRECT EQUILIBRIUM DIALYSIS FREE T$_4$ | TSH (milliunits/L) |
|---|---|---|
| Hypothyroidism | | |
| Primary Normal | ↓ | ↑ |
| On dopamine or glucocorticoids | ↓ | ↓ |
| Secondary or tertiary: functional hypopituitarism | ↓ | ↓ |
| Recent thyroid supplement withdrawal | ↓ | <0.1 |
| Recently treated hyperthyroidism | ↓ | <0.1 |
| Hyperthyroidism | ↑ | <0.1[a] |
| With severe nonthyroidal illness | ↓/WNL/↑[b] | <0.1[a] |
| Euthyroid states | WNL | WNL |
| Low total T$_4$ of nonthyroidal illness | ↓/WNL/↑[c] | WNL/↑ |
| After T$_3$ therapy | ↓ | WNL/↓ |
| After T$_4$ therapy | WNL | WNL |
| High total T$_4$ of nonthyroidal illness | ↑ | WNL/↑ |
| High total T$_4$ from amiodarone or iodinated contrast media | ↑ | ↑ |
| Decreased T$_4$-binding proteins | ↑/WNL[d] | WNL |

↑ = increased; ↓ = decreased; T$_3$ = triiodothyronine; T$_4$ = thyroxine; WNL = within normal limits.
[a]Usually absent TSH response to TRH; also may be normal with hyperthyroidism from TSH-secreting tumors.
[b]Normal or low using free T$_4$ index estimation; increased using the direct equilibrium dialysis free T$_4$ assay.
[c]Decreased using free T$_4$ index estimation; normal to high using the direct equilibrium dialysis free T$_4$ assay.
[d]Decreased using free T$_4$ index estimation; normal using the direct equilibrium dialysis free T$_4$ assay.
*Source*: Adapted from Jenklass J, Talbert RL. Thyroid disorders. In: DiPiro JT, Talbert RL, Yee GC, eds. *Pharmacotherapy: A Pathophysiologic Approach.* 9th ed. New York, NY: McGraw-Hill; 2014:1191–1216; Mokshagundam S, Barzel US. Thyroid disease in the elderly. *J Am Geriatr Soc.* 1993;41(12):1361–1369.

patients with hyperthyroidism and low in 85% of patients with hypothyroidism. This test measures both bound and free T$_4$ and is, therefore, influenced by any alteration in the concentration or binding affinity of thyroid-binding protein.[56]

Conditions that increase or decrease thyroid-binding protein result in an increased or decreased total serum T$_4$, respectively, but do not affect the amount of metabolically active free T$_4$ in the circulation. Therefore, thyrometabolic status may not always be truly represented by the results. **Table 9-8** lists factors that alter thyroid-binding protein.[61]

***Increased total serum T4.*** An increased total serum T$_4$ may indicate hyperthyroidism, elevated concentrations of thyroid-binding proteins (as seen in pregnancy or in women receiving oral contraceptive therapy), or nonthyroid illness. Total serum T$_4$ elevations have been noted in patients, particularly elderly persons, with relatively minor illnesses. These transient elevations may be due to increased TSH secretion stimulated by a low T$_3$ concentration. Similarly, up to 20% of all patients admitted to psychiatric hospitals have had transient total serum T$_4$ elevations on admission.[61] Thus, the differential diagnosis for a patient with this elevation must include nonthyroid illness versus hyperthyroidism if other signs and symptoms of thyroid disease are absent or inconsistent.[61]

***Decreased total serum T4.*** A decreased total serum T$_4$ may indicate hypothyroidism, decreased concentrations of thyroid-binding proteins, or *nonthyroid illness* (also called *euthyroid sick syndrome*). Nonthyroid illness may lower the total serum T$_4$ concentration with no change in thyrometabolic status. Typically in this syndrome, total serum T$_4$ is decreased (or normal), total serum T$_3$ is decreased, reverse T$_3$ is increased, and TSH is decreased (or normal). Neoplastic disease, DM, burns, trauma, liver disease, renal failure, prolonged infections, and cardiovascular disease are nonthyroid illnesses that can lower total serum T$_4$ concentrations.[61]

Several mechanisms probably contribute to this low T$_4$ state. Diminished T$_4$ in nonthyroid illness may be due to low TBG concentrations caused by protease cleavage at inflammatory sites during acute inflammatory illness. In some, but not all, patients with chronic illness, a desialylated form of TBG is synthesized by the liver, which has one-tenth the binding capacity of that of normal TBG. This results in a fall in the circulating levels of total thyroid hormone as a consequence of the diminished thyroid hormone-binding capacity. In addition, peripheral deiodination of T$_4$ to T$_3$ is impaired because of diminished activity of type I deiodinase enzyme. Diminished enzyme activity accounts for decreased deiodination of T$_4$ to T$_3$ and an increase in the production of reverse T$_3$.[60,61]

In general, a correlation exists between the degree of total serum T$_4$ depression and the prognosis of the illness (ie, the lower the total serum T$_4$, the poorer the disease outcome). Because severely ill patients may appear to be hypothyroid, it is important to differentiate between patients with serious nonthyroid illnesses and those who are truly hypothyroid.[61] After recovery from a nonthyroid illness, thyroid function test result abnormalities should be completely reversible.

**TABLE 9-7.** Performance and Availability of Free $T_4$ Methods

| ASSAY | % OF EUTHYROID PATIENTS WITH SEVERE TBG DEPRESSION OR SEVERE NONTHYROIDAL ILLNESS IN WHICH ASSAY UNDERESTIMATES FREE $T_4$ | COMMENTS |
|---|---|---|
| Free $T_4$ index[a] or single-step | 50%–80% | Available in most clinical laboratory tests |
| Immunoextraction or RIA[b] | 10%–30% | Available in some clinical laboratory tests |
| Direct equilibrium dialysis[c] | 0%–5% | Available in reference laboratory tests and large medical center laboratory tests; gold standard |
| Ultrafiltration[d] | 0%–5% | Available only in research laboratory tests |

[a]Corrects total $T_4$ values using an assessment of $T_4$-binding proteins.
[b]Uses a $T_4$ analog or two-step-back titration with solid-phase $T_4$ antibody but does not use membranes to separate free from bound hormone.
[c]Uses minimally diluted serum that separates free $T_4$ from bound $T_4$ using a semipermeable membrane.
[d]May be underestimated in 25% of patients on dopamine. A decreased direct equilibrium dialysis free $T_4$ with an elevated TSH is diagnostic of primary hypothyroidism, even in patients with severely depressed TBG. Conversely, an increased direct equilibrium dialysis free $T_4$ with a TSH of <0.10 milliunit/L is consistent with nonpituitary hyperthyroidism.[53] Decreased direct equilibrium dialysis free $T_4$ with normal or decreased TSH concentrations may be seen in patients on $T_3$ therapy (Table 9-8). Although free $T_4$ assays are becoming widely available (Table 9-12), most clinicians initially rely on the traditional total serum $T_4$ measurement by RIA.
*Source*: Adapted from Walsh JP. Managing thyroid disease in general practice. *Med J Aust*. 2016;205(4):179–184; Kaptein EM. Clinical application of free thyroxine determinations. *Clin Lab Med*. 1993;13:653–672.

**TABLE 9-8.** Factors Altering Thyroid-Binding Protein

| FACTORS THAT INCREASE THYROID-BINDING PROTEIN | FACTORS THAT DECREASE THYROID-BINDING PROTEIN |
|---|---|
| Acute infectious hepatitis | Acromegaly |
| Acute intermittent porphyria | Androgen therapy |
| Chronic active hepatitis | L-asparaginase |
| Clofibrate | Cirrhosis |
| Estrogen-containing oral contraceptives | Danazol |
| Estrogen-producing tumors | Salsalate |
| Estrogen therapy | Genetic deficiency of TBG |
| 5-fluorouracil | Glucocorticoid therapy (high dose) |
| Genetic excess of total binding protein | Furosemide (high dose) |
| Heroin | Hypoproteinemia |
| Methadone maintenance | Malnutrition |
| Perphenazine | Nephrotic syndrome |
| Pregnancy | Phenytoin |
| Tamoxifen | Salicylates |
| | Testosterone-producing tumors |

*Source*: Adapted from Walsh JP. Managing thyroid disease in general practice. *Med J Aust*. 2016;205(4):179–184; Mokshagundam S, Barzel US. Thyroid disease in the elderly. *J Am Geriatr Soc*. 1993; 41(12):1361–1369; Klee GG, Hay ID. Role of thyrotropin measurements in the diagnosis and management of thyroid disease. (review). *Clin Lab Med*. 1993;13(3):673–682.

*Drugs causing true alterations in total serum thyroxine.* Medications can cause a true alteration in total serum $T_4$ and a corresponding change in free $T_4$ concentrations (**Tables 9-9 and 9-10**).[62] In such cases, the total serum $T_4$ (and free $T_4$) result remains a true reflection of thyrometabolic status. High-dose salicylates and phenytoin also may lower total serum $T_4$ significantly via decreased protein binding in vivo. Salicylates inhibit binding of $T_4$ and $T_3$ to TBG. An initial increase in serum free $T_4$ is followed by return of free $T_4$ to normal levels with sustained therapeutic serum salicylate concentrations, although total $T_4$ levels may decrease by as much as 30%. Phenytoin displaces $T_4$ and $T_3$ from serum binding proteins, resulting in an initial increase in free $T_4$ and $T_3$ and a decrease in total $T_4$ levels.[62,63]

Iodides may also *increase* thyroid function. A previously euthyroid patient may develop thyrotoxicosis from exposure to increased quantities of iodine. Supplemental iodine causes autonomously functioning thyroid tissue to produce and secrete thyroid hormones, leading to a significant increase in $T_4$ and $T_3$ concentrations. This phenomenon commonly occurs during therapeutic iodine replacement in patients who live in areas of endemic iodine deficiency.

Similarly, patients with underlying goiter who live in iodine-sufficient areas may develop hyperthyroidism when given pharmacological doses of iodide. The heavily iodinated antiarrhythmic medication amiodarone may induce hyperthyroidism (1% to 5% of patients) as well as hypothyroidism (6% to 10% of patients).[64] Propylthiouracil and methimazole are used in patients with hyperthyroidism to decrease hormone concentrations. Both $T_4$ and $T_3$ concentrations decrease more rapidly with methimazole than propylthiouracil.[65]

### Serum $T_3$ Resin Uptake

*Normal range: 25% to 38%*

Although rarely used, the *serum $T_3$ resin uptake* test indirectly estimates the number of binding sites on thyroid-binding

**TABLE 9-9.** Medications That Cause a True Alteration in Total Serum $T_4$ and Free $T_4$ Measurements[a]

| MECHANISM | INCREASE TOTAL SERUM $T_4$ AND FREE $T_4$ | DECREASE TOTAL SERUM $T_4$ AND FREE $T_4$ |
|---|---|---|
| Interference in central regulation of TSH secretion at hypothalamic-pituitary level | Amphetamines | Glucocorticoids (acutely) Octreotide Dobutamine Dopamine |
| Interference with thyroid hormone synthesis or release from thyroid gland | Amiodarone,[b] lithium[b] | Aminoglutethimide, amiodarone,[b] 6-mercaptopurine, sulfonamides Iodides[b] Thionamides Lithium[b] |
| Altered thyroid hormone metabolism | Amiodarone, iopanoic acid, ipodate, propranolol (high dose) | Phenobarbital Carbamazepine Rifampin Phenytoin |
| Inhibition of GI absorption of exogenous thyroid hormone | | Antacids, orlistat cholestyramine, colestipol, iron, sodium polystyrene sulfonate, soybean flour (infant formulas), sucralfate Omeprazole lansoprazole |

[a]In true alterations, the concentration change is not due to assay interference or alteration in thyroid-binding proteins. As noted in Table 9-10, iodides can significantly alter thyroid status. They have the potential to inhibit thyroid hormone release and impair the organification of iodine. In healthy individuals, this effect lasts only 1 to 2 weeks. However, individuals with subclinical hypothyroid disease may develop clinical hypothyroidism after treatment with iodides. Iodide-induced hypothyroidism has also been noted in patients with cystic fibrosis and emphysema.[57]
[b]May increase or decrease total serum $T_4$ and free $T_4$.
*Source:* Compiled, in part, from references 55,57,58.

**TABLE 9-10.** Iodine-Containing Compounds That May Influence Thyroid Status

Oral radiopaque agents
  Diatrizoate
  Iocetamic acid
  Iopanoic acid
  Ipodate
  Tyropanoate

Expectorants
  Iodinated glycerol[a]
  Potassium iodide solution
  SSKI

Parenteral radiopaque agents
  Diatrizoate meglumine
  Iodamide meglumine
  Iopamidol
  Iothalamate meglumine
  Metrizamide

Miscellaneous compounds
Amiodarone
Kelp-containing nutritional supplements

SSKI = supersaturated potassium iodide.
[a]No longer available; most products reformulated with guaifenesin.
*Source:* Compiled, in part, from references 58 and 59.

protein occupied by $T_3$. This result is also referred to as the *thyroid hormone-binding ratio.* The $T_3$ resin uptake is usually low when the concentration of thyroid-binding proteins is high.[60]

In this test, radiolabeled $T_3$ is added to a specimen that contains endogenous hormone. An aliquot of this mixture is then added to a resin that competes with endogenous thyroid-binding proteins for the free hormone. Radiolabeled $T_3$ binds to any free endogenous thyroid-binding protein; at the saturation point, the remainder binds to the resin. The amount of thyroid-binding protein can be estimated from the amount of radiolabeled $T_3$ taken up by the resin. The $T_3$ resin uptake result is expressed as a percentage of the total radiolabeled $T_3$ that binds to the resin. The $T_3$ resin uptake can verify the clinical significance of measured total serum $T_4$ and $T_3$ concentrations because it is an indicator of thyroid-binding protein-induced alterations of these measurements; however, it is rarely used in contemporary practice because of the availability of the free T4 test.[60]

Elevated $T_3$ resin uptake concentrations are consistent with hyperthyroidism, whereas decreased concentrations are consistent with hypothyroidism. However, this test is never used alone for diagnosis. The $T_3$ resin uptake is low in hypothyroidism because of the increased availability of binding sites on the TBG. However, in nonthyroidal illnesses with a low $T_4$, the $T_3$ resin uptake is elevated. Therefore, the test may be used to differentiate between true hypothyroidism and a low $T_4$ state caused by nonthyroid illness.[60]

All of the disease states and medications listed in **Table 9-11** can influence thyroid-binding protein and, consequently, alter $T_3$

resin uptake results. Radioactive substances taken by the patient also interfere with this test. In practice, the T$_3$ resin uptake test is used only to calculate the free T$_4$ index.[61,62]

### Free T$_4$ Index

*Normal range: 1 to 4 units*

The *free T$_4$ index* is the product of total serum T$_4$ multiplied by the percentage of T$_3$ resin uptake:

$$\text{free T}_4 \text{ index} = \text{total serum T}_4(\text{mcg/dL}) \times \text{T}_3 \text{ resin uptake (\%)}$$

The free T$_4$ index adjusts for the effects of alterations in thyroid-binding protein on the total serum T$_4$ assay. The index is high in hyperthyroidism and low in hypothyroidism. Patients taking phenytoin or salicylates have low total serum T$_4$ and high T$_3$ resin uptake with a normal free T$_4$ index. Pregnant patients have high total serum T$_4$ and low T$_3$ resin uptake with a normal free T$_4$ index. Patients taking therapeutic doses of levothyroxine may have a high free T$_4$ index because total serum T$_4$ and T$_3$ resin uptake are high. In addition to affecting total serum T$_4$ and free T$_4$, propranolol and nadolol block the conversion of T$_4$ to T$_3$, which may cause mild elevations in the free T$_4$ index.[60]

### Total Serum T$_3$

*Normal range: 80 to 200 ng/dL (1.2 to 3.1 nmol/L)*

Using radioimmunoassay (RIA), highly active thyroid hormone T$_3$ is measured. Like T$_4$, almost all of T$_3$ is protein bound. Therefore, any alteration in thyroid-binding protein influences this measurement. As with the total serum T$_4$ test, changes in thyroid-binding protein increase or decrease total serum T$_3$ but do not affect the metabolically active free T$_3$ in the circulation. Therefore, the patient's thyrometabolic status remains unchanged.[60]

Total serum T$_3$ is primarily used as an indicator of hyperthyroidism (**Minicase 3**). This measurement is usually made to detect T$_3$ toxicosis when T$_3$, but not T$_4$, is elevated. Generally, the serum T$_3$ assay is not a reliable indicator of hypothyroidism because of the lack of reliability of the assay in the low to normal range. Drugs that affect T$_4$ concentrations have a corresponding effect on T$_3$ concentrations. Additionally, propranolol, propylthiouracil, and glucocorticoids inhibit the peripheral conversion of T$_4$ to T$_3$ and cause decreased T$_3$ concentration (T$_4$ usually stays normal).[60]

Total serum T$_3$ concentrations can be low in euthyroid patients with conditions (eg, malnutrition, cirrhosis, and uremia) in which the conversion of T$_4$ to T$_3$ is suppressed. T$_3$ is low in only half of hypothyroid patients because these patients tend to produce relatively more T$_3$ than T$_4$. A patient with a normal total serum T$_4$, a low T$_3$, and a patient with high reverse T$_3$ has euthyroid sick syndrome.[60]

### Thyroid-Stimulating Hormone

*Normal range: 0.5 to 5.0 milliunits/L*

*Thyroid stimulating hormone* (TSH) is a glycoprotein with two subunits: α and β. The α subunit is similar to those of

**TABLE 9-11.** Test Results Seen in Common Thyroid Disorders and Drug Effects on Test Results

| DISEASE | TOTAL SERUM T$_4$ | TOTAL SERUM T$_3$ | T$_3$ RESIN UPTAKE | FREE T$_4$ INDEX | RAIU | TSH | COMMENT |
|---|---|---|---|---|---|---|---|
| Hypothyroidism | ↓ | ↓ | ↓ | ↓ | ↓ | ↑/↓ [a] | |
| Hyperthyroidism | ↑ | ↑ | ↑ | ↑ | ↑ | ↓ | |
| T$_3$ thyrotoxicosis | No change | ↑ | No change | No change | No change | ↓ | T$_3$ resin uptake may be slightly increased |
| Euthyroid sick | No change/↓ | ↓ | ↑ | Variable | No change | No change syndrome | |
| Corticosteroids | ↓ | No change/↓ | ↑ | No change | ↓ | No change/↓ | |
| Phenytoin/aspirin | ↓ | ↓ | ↑ | No change | ↓ | No change | Large salicylate dose |
| Radiopaque media | No change/↑ | No change/↓ | No change | No change/↑ | ↓ | No change | |

↑ = increased; ↓ = decreased; RAIU = radioactive iodine uptake test.
[a]Increased TSH diagnostic of primary hypothyroidism. TSH is decreased in secondary and tertiary types.
*Source*: Adapted from Surks MI, Sievert R. Drugs and thyroid function. *N Engl J Med.* 1995;333(25):1688–1694; Kaptein EM. Clinical application of free thyroxine determinations. *Clin Lab Med.* 1993;13(3):653–672.

## MINICASE 3

### A Patient with Hyperthyroidism

A 35-year-old nurse complains of nervousness, mood swings, weakness, and palpitations with exertion for the past 6 months. Recently, she noticed excessive sweating and wanted to sleep with fewer blankets than her husband. Menstrual periods had been regular, but there was less bleeding. She has lost 20 lb over the last 6 months despite eating twice as much as she did 1 year ago. Her HR is 92 beats/min and BP is 150/90 mm Hg. She appears anxious. She has smooth, warm, moist skin; she has a fine tremor; and she cannot rise from a deep knee bend without aid. Upon physical exam, her thyroid contains three nodules—two on the right and one on the left with a total gland size of 60 g (three times normal size). All nodules are of firm consistency, and there is no lymphadenopathy.

- Sodium, 145 mEq/L (136 to 142 mEq/L)
- Potassium, 4 mEq/L (3.8 to 5 mEq/L)
- Chloride, 101 mEq/L (95 to 103 mEq/L)
- Carbon dioxide, 26 mEq/L (21 to 28 mEq/L)
- BUN, 10 mg/dL (8 to 23 mg/dL)
- SCr, 0.8 mg/dL (0.6 to 1.2 mg/dL)
- Hemoglobin, 12 g/dL (12 to 16 g/dL)
- Hct, 36% (36% to 45%)
- RBC count, 3.5 M/mm$^3$ (4 to 5.2 M/mm$^3$)

- Antithyroid antibodies, 1:200
- Mean cell (corpuscular) volume, 104 mm$^3$ (80 to 100 mm$^3$)
- WBC count, 16 × 10$^3$ cells/mm$^3$ (4.8 to 10.8 × 10$^3$ cells/mm$^3$)
- Calcium, 9 mg/dL (9.2 to 11 mg/dL)
- Glucose, 96 mg/dL (70 to 110 mg/dL)
- Free T$_4$, 4.6 ng/dL (0.9 to 2.3 ng/dL)
- T$_3$, 250 ng/dL (80 to 200 ng/dL)
- TSH, 0.3 microunits/mL (0.5 to 5 microunits/mL)

QUESTION: How should these results be interpreted? Are confirmatory tests needed?

DISCUSSION: This patient presents with many of the clinical features of hyperthyroidism, including rapid heart rate, weight loss, and heat intolerance. Her thyroid gland is visibly enlarged (goiter). She also has elevated BP and complains of nervousness, sweating, and hand tremors. The diagnosis of hyperthyroidism can be confirmed by her laboratory results of a high T4 and a below-normal TSH value. She has a toxic multinodular goiter that should be treated with radioactive iodine or surgery with antithyroid drug and iodine pretreatment.

other hormones secreted from the anterior pituitary: follicle-stimulating hormone, human chorionic gonadotropin (hCG), and luteinizing hormone. The β subunit of TSH is unique and renders its specific physiologic properties.[61,62]

Although the older "first-generation" TSH assays have been useful in diagnosing primary hypothyroidism, they have not been useful in diagnosing hyperthyroidism. Almost all patients with symptomatic primary hypothyroidism have TSH concentrations >20 milliunits/L; those with mild signs or symptoms have TSH values of 10 to 20 milliunits/L. Often, TSH concentrations become elevated before T$_4$ concentrations decline. All assays can accurately measure high concentrations of TSH.[61,66]

The first-generation TSH assays, however, cannot distinguish low-normal from abnormally low values because their lower limit of detection is 1 milliunit/L, whereas the lower limit of basal TSH is 0.2 to 0.3 milliunits/L in most euthyroid persons. This distinction can usually be ascertained with the second-generation assays, which can accurately measure TSH concentrations as low as 0.05 milliunits/L. Occasionally, some euthyroid patients have levels of 0.05 to 0.5 milliunits/L. Therefore, supersensitive, third- and fourth-generation assays have been developed; they can detect TSH concentrations as low as 0.005 milliunits/L and 0.004 milliunits/L, respectively. Although third-generation assays are usually not required to make or confirm this diagnosis, they provide a wider margin of tolerance so that discrimination at 0.1 milliunit/L can be ensured even when the assay is not performing optimally. Concentrations

<0.05 milliunits/L are almost always diagnostic of primary hyperthyroidism in patients <70 years.[61]

*Use in therapy.* In patients with primary hypothyroidism, TSH concentrations are also used to adjust the dosage of thyroid hormone replacement therapy. In addition to achieving a clinical euthyroid state, typically the goal should be to lower TSH into the midnormal range (**Minicase 4**). The exception is in patients with recently diagnosed papillary or follicular thyroid cancer, where the goal TSH level may be in the 0.1 to 0.2 milliunits/L range. Although TSH concentrations reflect long-term thyroid status, serum T$_4$ concentrations reflect acute changes. Patients with long-standing hypothyroidism often notice an improvement in well-being two to three weeks after starting therapy. Significant improvements in heart rate (HR), weight, and puffiness are seen early in therapy, but hoarseness, anemia, and skin/hair changes may take many months to resolve.[66]

Unless undesirable changes in signs or symptoms occur, it is rational to wait at least 6 to 8 weeks after starting or changing therapy to repeat TSH and T$_4$ concentrations to refine dosing.[56] The hypothalamic-pituitary-axis requires this time to respond fully to changes in circulating thyroid hormone concentrations. For example, noncompliant patients with hypothyroidism who wait to take their thyroid hormone replacement therapy until days before their appointment may have elevated TSH concentrations despite a normal T$_4$ concentration.[61]

Patients with thyroid cancer are often treated with TSH suppressive therapy, usually levothyroxine. The therapeutic

## MINICASE 4

## A Case of Possible Hypothyroidism

Diane G. is a 45-year-old homemaker who presents to clinic complaining of progressive weight gain of 20 lb in 1 year, fatigue, postural dizziness, loss of memory, slow speech, deepening of her voice, dry skin, constipation, and cold intolerance. Her HR is 58 beats/min, and her BP is 110/70 mm Hg. Her physical exam is normal, except for a mildly enlarged thyroid gland, pallor, and diminished tendon reflexes. She denies taking any medications or changing her diet. Diane G.'s chemistry results are as follows:

- Sodium, 130 mEq/L (136 to 142 mEq/L)
- Potassium, 3.8 mEq/L (3.8 to 5 mEq/L)
- Carbon dioxide, 28 mEq/L (21 to 28 mEq/L)
- Calcium, 9.5 mg/dL (9.2 to 11 mg/dL)
- Magnesium, 2 mEq/L (1.3 to 2.1 mEq/L)
- Glucose, 80 mg/dL (70 to 110 mg/dL)
- BUN, 20 mg/dL (8 to 23 mg/dL)
- SCr, 1.1 mg/dL (0.6 to 1.2 mg/dL)
- Cholesterol, 255 mg/dL (<200 mg/dL)

The cholesterol concentration is elevated since a screening 6 months ago. A test for mononucleosis is negative. Hct is low at 36% (36% to 45%)—close to her usual. Her total serum $T_4$ is 3.8 mcg/dL (5.5 to 12.5 mcg/dL), her $T_3$ resin uptake is 15% (25% to 38%), her free $T_4$ index is 1.0 (1 to 4), and her TSH is 65 milliunits/L (0.3 to 5 milliunits/L).

QUESTION: How should these results be interpreted?

DISCUSSION: Clinically, all of the history and physical findings point to hypothyroidism. The pallor and weakness are also consistent with anemia, but an Hct of 35% is unlikely to cause such significant symptoms. Her cholesterol recently became elevated, consistent with primary hypothyroidism.[93] Both the total serum $T_4$ and $T_3$ resin uptake are low and TSH level is high.

QUESTION: Does this information help to elucidate the diagnosis?

DISCUSSION: An elevated TSH confirms primary hypothyroidism. Diane G. is started on levothyroxine 0.2 mg/day, and her TSH is 6 milliunits/L 3 weeks later. Clinically, she improves but is not fully back to normal. Six weeks after starting therapy, she complains of jitteriness, palpitations, and increased sweating. Her TSH is <0.3 milliunit/L. Her physician lowers the dose of levothyroxine to 0.1 mg/day, and she becomes asymptomatic after about 2 weeks. Eight weeks later, her TSH is 1.5 milliunits/L, and she remains asymptomatic. Her cholesterol is 200 mg/dL, sodium is 138 mEq/L, and Hct is 40%.

QUESTION: Which test(s) should be used to determine proper dosing of levothyroxine? How long after a dosage change should clinicians wait before repeating the test(s)?

DISCUSSION: Although total serum $T_4$, $T_3$ resin uptake, and free $T_4$ index can be used to monitor and adjust doses of thyroid supplements in patients with a hypothyroid disorder, the highly sensitive TSH test is most reliable. Chemically, the goal is to achieve a TSH in the normal range, as was ultimately achieved in this patient (TSH of 1.5 milliunits/L).

The TSH is the standard for adjusting thyroid replacement therapy. The 0.2-mg levothyroxine dose is excessive for this patient, as evidenced by her "hyperthyroid" symptoms and the fully suppressed TSH. Eight weeks later, after $T_4$ steady state has been reached on the 0.1-mg/day dose and after the hypothalamic-pituitary-thyroid axis reached homeostasis, TSH is within the desired range. Her cholesterol, sodium, and Hct also normalized when she became euthyroid.

endpoint is a basal TSH concentration of about 0.1 milliunit/L. Some clinicians suggest more complete suppression with TSH concentrations <0.005 milliunit/L, whereas others think that it leads to toxic effects of overreplacement (eg, accelerated bone loss, new onset atrial fibrillation).[61,66]

*Potential misinterpretation and drug interference.* Some TSH assays may yield falsely elevated results whenever hCG concentrations are high (eg, pregnancy) due to the similarity in structure of these two proteins. Most patients who have secondary or tertiary hypothyroidism have low or normal TSH concentrations. In patients with nonthyroid illness, TSH may be suppressed by factors other than thyroid hyperfunction. As mentioned previously, the TSH concentration typically is normal in patients with euthyroid sick syndrome.[62,66]

Thyroid function tests are known to be altered in depressed patients. With the advent of the third-generation TSH assays, it was hoped that TSH concentrations could help to determine various types of depression and response to therapies. Unfortunately, TSH has not proven useful in this way.[66] Because

endogenous dopamine inhibits the stimulatory effects of TRH, any drug with dopaminergic activity can inhibit TSH secretion. Therefore, levodopa, glucocorticoids, bromocriptine, and dopamine are likely to lower TSH results. The converse is also true—dopamine antagonists (metoclopramide) may increase TSH concentrations.[62,63]

### Radioactive Iodine Uptake Test

This test is used to detect the ability of the thyroid gland to trap and concentrate iodine and, thereby, produce thyroid hormone. In other words, this test assesses the intrinsic function of the thyroid gland. This test is not specific, and its reference range must be adjusted to the local population. Therefore, its use is declining. In patients with a normal thyroid gland, 12% to 20% of the radioactive iodine is absorbed by the gland after 6 hours and 5% to 25% is absorbed after 24 hours. The radioactive iodine uptake test is an indirect measure of thyroid gland activity and should not be used as a basic screening test of thyroid function. This test is most useful in distinguishing causes of hyperthyroidism, including that caused by subacute thyroiditis, which results in an absent or reduced uptake of iodine.[56]

A high radioactive iodine uptake is noted with the following conditions[51]:

- Thyrotoxicosis
- Iodine deficiency
- Postthyroiditis
- Withdrawal rebound after thyroid hormone or antithyroid drug therapy

A low test result occurs in the following persons[51]:

- Individuals with acute thyroiditis
- Euthyroid patients who ingest iodine-containing products
- Patients on exogenous thyroid hormone therapy
- Patients who are taking antithyroid drugs such as propylthiouracil
- Individuals with hypothyroidism

The radioactive iodine uptake test is affected by the body's store of iodine. Therefore, the patient should be carefully questioned about the use of iodine-containing products before the test. This test is contraindicated during pregnancy.

### Antithyroid Antibodies

*Normal range: varies with antibody*

Antibodies that "attack" various thyroid tissue components can be detected in the serum of patients with autoimmune disorders such as Hashimoto thyroiditis and Graves disease. Thyroid microsomal antibody is found in 95% of patients with Hashimoto thyroiditis, 55% of patients with Graves disease, and 10% of adults without thyroid disease. In patients who have nodular goiters, high-antibody titers strongly suggest Hashimoto thyroiditis as opposed to cancer. In Graves disease, hyperthyroidism is caused by antibodies, which activate TSH receptors. In chronic autoimmune thyroiditis, hypothyroidism may be caused by antibodies competitively binding to TSH receptors, thereby blocking TSH from eliciting a response.[66]

Results are reported as titers. Titers in excess of 1:100 are significant and usually can be detected even during remission. Antibodies (>1:10) to thyroglobulin are present in 60% to 70% of adults with active Hashimoto thyroiditis but typically are not detected during remission. Titers above 1:1,000 are found only in Hashimoto thyroiditis or Graves disease (25% to 10%, respectively). Lower titers may be seen in 4% of the normal population, although the frequency increases with the age in female patients. The thyroid microsomal antibody and thyroglobulin antibody serological tests may be elevated or positive in patients with nonthyroidal autoimmune disease.

Anti-TSH receptor antibodies are present in virtually all patients with Graves disease, but the test is usually not necessary for diagnosis. These antibodies mostly stimulate TSH receptors (eg, thyroid-stimulating immunoglobulin) but also may compete with TSH and inhibit TSH stimulation of the thyroid gland. High titers allow a confirmation of Graves disease in asymptomatic patients, such as those whose only manifestation is exophthalmos.[66,67]

## Laboratory Diagnosis of Hypothalamic-Pituitary-Thyroid Axis Dysfunction

The laboratory diagnosis of primary hypothyroidism can be made with a low free $T_4$ index and an elevated TSH concentration. The presence of a low free $T_4$ index and a normal or low serum TSH concentration indicates secondary or tertiary hypothyroidism or nonthyroid illness. In such patients, the $T_3$ resin uptake may differentiate between hypothyroidism and a low $T_4$ state due to nonthyroid illness. An elevated reverse $T_3$ concentration also suggests nonthyroid illness. $T_3$ is of limited usefulness in diagnosing hypothyroidism because it may be normal in up to one-third of patients with hypothyroidism.[55,61] With the availability of ultrasensitive TSH assays, many clinicians begin their evaluations with this test.

The total serum $T_4$ and free $T_4$ or free $T_4$ indexes are commonly used and are increased in almost all patients with hyperthyroidism. Usually, both $T_3$ and $T_4$ are elevated. However, a few (<5%) patients with hyperthyroidism exhibit normal $T_4$ with elevated $T_3$ ($T_3$ toxicosis). Second-line tests such as antithyroid antibody serologies are necessary to diagnose autoimmune thyroid disorders.[66]

## ADRENAL DISORDERS

The adrenal glands are located extraperitoneally at the upper poles of each kidney. The adrenal medulla, which makes up 10% of the adrenal gland, secretes catecholamines (eg, epinephrine and norepinephrine). The adrenal cortex, which comprises 90% of the adrenal gland, is divided into three areas.

1. The outer layer of the adrenal gland, known as the *zona glomerulosa*, makes up 15% of the adrenal gland and is responsible for production of aldosterone, a mineralocorticoid that regulates electrolyte and volume homeostasis.

2. The *zona fasciculata*, located in the center of the adrenal gland, occupies 60% of the gland and is responsible for glucocorticoid production. Cortisol, a principal end product of glucocorticoid production, regulates fat, carbohydrate, and protein metabolism. Glucocorticoids maintain the body's homeostasis by regulating bodily functions involved in stress as well as normal activities.

3. The *zona reticularis* makes up 25% of the adrenal gland and secretes mostly inactive androgen precursors that undergo peripheral conversion to adrenal androgens, such as dehydroepiandrosterone (DHEA), DHEA sulfate (DHEA-S), and androstenedione (the precursor to testosterone). These hormones influence the development of the reproductive system.[68,69]

## Cushing Syndrome

*Cushing syndrome*, first described 70 years ago, is the result of excessive concentrations of cortisol. It is an extremely rare disease in children, with a peak in adults in the third or fourth decade. In most cases, hypercortisolism is the result of overproduction of cortisol by the adrenal glands due to an ACTH-secreting pituitary tumor. Long-term use of glucocorticoids, the most common cause of Cushing's disease, and adrenal tumors can result in hypercortisolism.

Patients with hypercortisolism generally present with facial plethora (moon face) as a result of atrophy of the skin and underlying tissue. A common sign of hypercortisolism is fat accumulation in the dorsocervical area often referred to as "buffalo hump." Other cardinal signs and symptoms include hypertension, osteopenia, glucose intolerance, myopathy, bruising, back pain, proximal muscle weakness, and depression. Hyperpigmentation is present in patients with ACTH-secreting pituitary tumors. Hair loss, acne, and oligomenorrhea are also the result of superfluous cortical secretion.[70]

## Diagnostic Tests

It is important to rule out iatrogenic Cushing's syndrome when there is long-term steroid therapy and assess pretest probability of Cushing's syndrome based on relatively specific signs stated previously (**Minicase 5**).

In healthy individuals, the level of serum cortisol reaches a peak in the morning around 7 a.m. to 9 a.m. (5 to 23 mcg/dL) and reaches the lowest level between bedtime and 2 a.m. (usually <5 ug/dL).

One of the first signs of Cushing's syndrome is the loss of this diurnal variation. Accordingly, the three first-line biochemical screening tests recommended for the diagnosis of endogenous hypercortisolism are to prove that the patients has lost this normal secretion of cortisol, and thus it is recommended that patients are screened with these tests. The following tests are used to identify patients with Cushing syndrome: 24-hour urine-free cortisol (UFC), midnight plasma cortisol, and the low-dose dexamethasone suppression test (DST) using 1 mg for the overnight test or 0.5 mg every 6 hours for the 2-day study. The most frequently used test to identify patients with hypercortisolism is the 24-hour UFC test, which measures free

## MINICASE 5

## Steroid-Induced Hypercortisolism

Teresa S. is a 35-year-old woman with a past medical history of type 2 diabetes that was diagnosed in her late 20s. She has been taking metformin 1,000 mg twice a day regularly since her diagnosis. Teresa S. was diagnosed with rheumatoid arthritis 6 months ago and started on regular treatment with prednisolone 30 mg daily. She reports to her primary care provider for general muscle weakness and low back pain. She has been having low back pain for a little over 4 months. The general muscle weakness has been getting progressively worse over the past month and is beginning to concern her. Teresa S. also reports having trouble making it through her Zumba class on Tuesdays and Thursdays. She says that lately she has little interest in her regular activities and has been experiencing fatigue without physical exertion. Lastly, Teresa S. reports having irregular menstrual cycles for the past 2 years accompanied by unexplained weight gain in her abdomen.

Physical exam reveals purple/pink stretch marks on arms, abdomen, and thighs. The patient has multiple cuts and bruises on her arms and hands, with an explanation of having thin skin. The patient is obese with noticeable fatty deposits in the upper back and midsection. Her BP is 154/76 mm Hg, and her heart rate is 74 beats/min.

The patient would like to have little to no back pain. She also would like to be able to increase her strength and endurance to resume her normal Zumba classes twice a week. Goals for her blood test results are as follows:

- Sodium, 142 mEq/L (136 to 142 mEq/L)
- Potassium, 3.3 mEq/L (3.8 to 5 mEq/L)
- Chloride, 99 mEq/L (95 to 103 mEq/L)
- BUN, 28 mg/dL (8 to 23 mg/dL)
- SCr, 1.8 mg/dL (0.6 to 1.2 mg/dL)
- Hct, 40% (36% to 45%)
- WBC count, 6.2 × $10^3$ cells/mm$^3$ (4.8 to 10.8 × $10^3$ cells/mm$^3$)

- Calcium, 10 mg/dL (9.2 to 11 mg/dL)
- Glucose, 180 mg/dL (70 to 110 mg/dL)
- Ketones, 0 at 1:8 serum dilution (normal = 0)
- Osmolality, 285 mOsm/kg (280 to 295 mOsm/kg)
- Triglycerides, 207 mg/dL (10 to 150 mg/dL)
- Lipase, 1.0 units/mL (<1.5 units/mL)
- Magnesium, 1.7 mEq/L (1.3 to 2.1 mEq/L)
- Hemoglobin A1c, 6.1 (4% to 5.6%)
- 8 a.m. Cortisol, 33.4 mcg/dL

QUESTION: Based on the subjective and objective data provided, what is the most likely diagnosis for this patient? What signs and symptoms support the diagnosis? What could have precipitated this disorder?

DISCUSSION: The patient complained of unusual fatigue, back pain, headaches, irregular menstrual cycles, generalized weakness, and a recent lack of interest in her normal hobbies/activities. Teresa S.'s reports are accompanied by objective findings of elevated BP, proximal weakness, purple/pink stretch marks, multiple bruises, and noticeable fatty deposits.

The diagnosis of hypercortisolism due to the chronic use of prednisolone is supported by her lab results of an elevated 8 a.m. serum cortisol of 33.4 mcg/dL, potassium level of 3.3 mmol/L, elevated fasting blood glucose level 180 mg/dL, and serum triglyceride levels of 207 mg/dL. Based on subjective and objective evidence, the patient is diagnosed as having Cushing syndrome caused by the chronic use of prednisolone. The prednisolone dose is tapered, alternative treatment options for rheumatoid arthritis are considered, and the serum cortisol level is measured after 3 months during a follow-up appointment. BP and cholesterol levels will be rechecked at the follow-up appointment.

cortisol levels and creatinine in a urine sample that is collected over a 24-hour period. Laboratory tests in adults with Cushing syndrome include the following results:

1.  24-hour UFC at least three times above normal
2.  Midnight plasma cortisol 5 mcg/dL (138 mmol/L) or more
3.  Low-dose DST plasma cortisol exceeds 2 mcg/dL (50 nmol/L) when drawn between 8:00 a.m. and 9:00 a.m. [71]

Of the suppression tests, the overnight DST, is the least laborious test to perform. The patient is given 1 mg of dexamethasone at 11:00 p.m. A plasma cortisol levels is obtained at 8:00 a.m. the next morning. Patients with Cushing syndrome have high cortisol concentrations (>5 mcg/dL or >138 nmol/L) because of an inability to suppress the negative-feedback mechanism of the hypothalamic-pituitary-adrenal axis.[63,64]

Once hypercortisolism is confirmed, one of the following tests should be performed to identify the source of hypersecretion, which could include the pituitary gland, adrenal gland, or production from an ectopic site. Such tests include high-dose DST; plasma ACTH via immunoradiometric assay (IRMA) or RIA; adrenal vein catheterization; metyrapone stimulation test; adrenal, chest, or abdominal computed tomography; corticotropin-releasing hormone (CRH) stimulation test; inferior petrosal sinus sampling; and pituitary magnetic resonance imaging. Other possible tests and procedures include insulin-induced hypoglycemia, somatostatin receptor scintigraphy, desmopressin stimulation test, naloxone CRH stimulation test, loperamide test, hexarelin stimulation test, and radionuclide imaging. Additional tests should be performed to confirm the diagnosis because other factors (eg, starvation, topical steroid application, and acute stress) influence the results of the previously mentioned tests.[69,70]

Plasma ACTH concentrations can be measured by RIA procedures. Interpretation of the results is as follows:

*   ACTH levels <10 pg/mL indicate an ACTH-independent adrenal source, such as an adrenal tumor or long-term use of steroids
*   ACTH levels between 5 and 10 pg/mL should be followed by a CRH test
*   ACTH levels >10 pg/mL indicate an ACTH-dependent syndrome

The CRH test can be employed to determine if the source of hypercortisolism is pituitary or ectopic (extrapituitary). Baseline ACTH and CRH levels are obtained. Then, ACTH and cortisol levels are measured 15 to 30 and 45 to 60 minutes after the administration of a 100-mcg IV dose of CRH. A 50% increase from baseline in ACTH levels indicates an ACTH-dependent syndrome.[70]

### Adrenal Insufficiency (Addison Disease)

*Adrenal insufficiency (Addison disease* or *primary adrenal insufficiency)* is the result of an autoimmune destruction of all regions of the adrenal cortex. Tuberculosis, fungal infections, acquired immunodeficiency syndrome, metastatic cancer, and lymphomas can also precipitate adrenal insufficiency. Adrenal insufficiency results in deficiencies in cortisol, aldosterone, and androgens. Patients usually present with weakness, weight loss,

increased pigmentation, hypotension, GI symptoms, postural dizziness, and vertigo.

Secondary adrenal insufficiency can result from the use of high doses or extended duration of use of exogenous steroids, which suppress the hypothalamic-pituitary axis, resulting in a decrease in the release of ACTH. Patients with secondary adrenal insufficiency maintain normal aldosterone levels and do not exhibit signs of hyperpigmentation.[71,72]

***Diagnostic tests.*** Measurement and interpretation of plasma corticotropin (ACTH) levels are recommended to distinguish between primary adrenal insufficiency and secondary adrenal insufficiency. A high normal or elevated ACTH concentration is consistent with primary adrenal insufficiency, whereas a low normal or undetectable level suggests secondary adrenal insufficiency.

The cosyntropin stimulation test is used to diagnose patients with low cortisol levels. Patients receive 250 mcg of synthetic ACTH or cosyntropin intravenously or intramuscularly. Serum cortisol levels are drawn at the time of injection and 30 minutes and 1 hour after injection. Cortisol levels >18 to 20 mcg/dL (497 to 552 nmol/L) indicate an adequate response from the adrenal gland, thus ruling out adrenal insufficiency. The cosyntropin stimulation test results may be normal in patients with secondary adrenal insufficiency or mild primary adrenal insufficiency due to the high dose of corticotropin given. Therefore, many endocrinologists recommend that higher cutoff values (≥22 to 25 mcg/dL or 607 to 690 nmol/L) be used. To distinguish primary from secondary adrenal insufficiency, ACTH, renin, and aldosterone levels are measured.[71,72]

# DIABETES INSIPIDUS

*Diabetes insipidus* is a syndrome in which the body's inability to conserve water manifests as excretion of large volumes of dilute urine. This section explores related pathophysiology, types of diabetes insipidus, and interpretation of test results to evaluate this disorder.[73]

## Physiology

Normally, serum osmolality is maintained around 285 mOsm/kg and is determined by the amounts of sodium, chloride, bicarbonate, glucose, and urea in the serum. The excretion of these solutes along with water is a primary factor in determining urine volume and concentration. In turn, the amount of water excreted by the kidneys is determined by renal function and ADH (vasopressin). ADH reduces renal elimination of water and produces concentrated urine.

ADH is synthesized in the hypothalamus and stored in the posterior pituitary gland. This hormone is released into the circulation after physiologic stimulation, such as an increase in serum osmolality or blood volume detected by the osmoregulatory centers in the hypothalamus.[73,74] Congestive heart failure lowers the osmotic threshold for ADH release, whereas nausea—but not vomiting—strongly stimulates ADH. In general, α-adrenergic agonists stimulate ADH release, whereas β-adrenergic agonists inhibit release and acts on the distal renal tubule and the collecting duct to cause water reabsorption. Chlorpropamide potentiates the effect of ADH on renal concentrating ability. When ADH is lacking or the renal tubules do not respond to the hormone, polyuria ensues. If the polyuria is severe enough, a diagnosis of diabetes insipidus is considered.[73,74]

## Clinical Diagnosis

Diabetes insipidus should be differentiated from other causes of polyuria, such as osmotic diuresis (eg, hyperglycemia, mannitol, and contrast media), renal tubular acidosis, diuretic therapy, and psychogenic polydipsia. Patients usually excrete 16 to 24 L of dilute urine in 24 hours. The urine specific gravity is <1.005 and urine osmolality <300 mOsm/kg.[73] As long as the thirst mechanism is intact and a patient can drink, no electrolyte problems result. However, if a patient is unable to replace fluids lost through excessive urine output, he or she can develop dehydration and hypernatremia.

Although diabetes insipidus is usually caused by a defect in the pituitary secretion (neurogenic, also called *central*) or renal activity (nephrogenic) of ADH, it can also be caused by a defect in thirst (dipsogenic) or psychological function (psychogenic), with resultant excessive intake of water. If left untreated, diabetes insipidus can lead to significant morbidity and mortality; therefore, the underlying cause should be sought to ensure proper diagnosis and therapy. The specific type of diabetes insipidus often can be identified by the clinical setting. If the diagnosis is equivocal, a therapeutic trial with an antidiuretic drug or measurement of plasma ADH is necessary (**Table 9-12**).[74]

### Central Diabetes Insipidus

*Central diabetes insipidus* (ADH deficiency) may be the result of any disruption in the pituitary-hypothalamic regulation of ADH. Patients often present with a sudden onset of polyuria (in the absence of hyperglycemia) and preference for iced drinks. Tumors or metastases in or around the pituitary or hypothalamus, head trauma, neurosurgery, genetic abnormalities, Guillain-Barré syndrome, meningitis, encephalitis, toxoplasmosis, cytomegalovirus, tuberculosis, and aneurysms are some of the known causes. In addition, phenytoin and alcohol inhibit ADH release from the pituitary. In response to deficient secretion of ADH and subsequent hyperosmolality of the plasma, thirst is stimulated. The absence of effective ADH results in polyuria.[73]

### Nephrogenic Diabetes Insipidus

In *nephrogenic diabetes insipidus* (ADH resistance), the secretion of ADH is normal, but the renal tubules do not respond to ADH.[75] In the kidney, the actions of ADH on its type-2 receptor (V2R) induce increased water reabsorption in addition to polyphosphorylation and membrane targeting of the water channel aquaporin-2. Mutations in the V2R have been found to be associated with nephrogenic diabetes insipidus. Causes of nephrogenic diabetes insipidus include chronic renal failure, pyelonephritis, hypokalemia, hypercalciuria, malnutrition, genetic defects, and sickle cell disease. Additionally, lithium toxicity, colchicine, glyburide, demeclocycline, cidofovir, and methoxyflurane occasionally cause this disorder.[74]

### Diabetes Insipidus of Pregnancy

A transient diabetes insipidus, originally thought to be a form of nephrogenic diabetes insipidus, may develop during late pregnancy from excessive vasopressinase (ADHase) activity. This kind of diabetes insipidus is associated with preeclampsia with liver involvement. Because vasopressinase does not metabolize desmopressin acetate, this is the treatment of choice.[76]

***Laboratory diagnosis.*** Some clinicians avoid dehydration testing and rely on measuring plasma ADH concentrations to distinguish central from nephrogenic diabetes insipidus. In otherwise healthy adults, the average basal plasma ADH concentration is 1.3 to 4 pg/mL (1.2 to 3.7 pmol/L). Based on medical history, symptoms, and signs, an elevated basal plasma ADH level almost always indicates nephrogenic diabetes insipidus. If the basal plasma ADH concentration is low (<1 pg/mL) or immeasurable, the result is inconclusive and a dehydration test should be done.

The theory behind the water deprivation test is that in normal individuals, dehydration stimulates ADH release and the urine becomes concentrated. An injection of vasopressin at this point

**TABLE 9-12.** Differential Diagnosis of Diabetes Insipidus Based on Water Deprivation Test

| DIAGNOSIS | URINE SPECIFIC GRAVITY | AVERAGE URINE OSMOLALITY (mOsm/kg) | PLATEAU URINE OSMOLALITY (mOsm/kg) | AVERAGE SERUM OSMOLALITY (mOsm/kg) | CHANGE IN URINE OSMOLALITY AFTER VASOPRESSIN |
|---|---|---|---|---|---|
| Normal individuals | >1.015 | 300–800 | <1,600 | 280–295 | Little change |
| Central diabetes insipidus | <1.010 | <300 | <300 | Normal or increased | Increases |
| Nephrogenic diabetes insipidus | <1.010 | <300 | <300 | Normal or increased | Little change |

*Source*: Sowers JR, Zieve FJ. Clinical disorders of vasopression. In: Lavin N, ed. *Manual of Endocrinology and metabolism*. Boston, MA: Little, Brown; 1986-65-74. Young DS. *Effects of Drugs on Clinical Laboratory Tests*. 3rd ed. Washington, DC: American Association for Clinical Chemistry Press; 1990.

does not further concentrate the urine. In contrast, the urine of patients with central diabetes insipidus is not maximally concentrated after fluid deprivation but will be after vasopressin injection.[77]

To perform the test, patients are deprived of fluid intake (up to 18 hours) until the urine osmolality of three consecutive samples varies by no more than 30 mOsm/kg. Urine osmolality and specific gravity are measured hourly. At this time, 5 units of aqueous vasopressin is administered subcutaneously, and urine osmolality is measured 1 hour later. Plasma osmolality is measured before the test, when urine osmolality has stabilized, and after vasopressin has been administered.

In healthy individuals, fluid deprivation for 8 to 12 hours results in normal serum osmolality and a urine osmolality of 800 mOsm/kg. The urine osmolality plateaus after 16 to 18 hours. Patients with central diabetes insipidus have an immediate rise in urine osmolality to 600 mOsm/kg, with a corresponding decrease in urine output with vasopressin injection. Patients with nephrogenic diabetes insipidus are unable to increase urine osmolality above 300 mOsm/kg because vasopressin injection has little effect.[77]

In addition to being inconvenient and expensive, dehydration procedures are reliable only if the diabetes insipidus is severe enough that—even with induced dehydration—the urine still cannot be concentrated.

Accurate interpretation requires consideration of potential confounding factors. If the laboratory cannot ensure accurate and precise plasma (not serum) osmolality measurements, plasma sodium should be used. Patients should be observed for nonosmotic stimuli, such as vasovagal reactions, that may affect ADH release. Lastly, if the patient has previously received ADH therapy, ADH antibodies may cause false-positive results suggestive of nephrogenic diabetes insipidus.[74,75]

## SUMMARY

Endocrine disorders typically result from a deficiency or excess of a hormone. Laboratory tests that measure the actual hormone, precursors, or metabolites can help to elucidate whether and why a hormonal or metabolic imbalance exists. Tests used to assess thyroid, adrenal, glucose, and water homeostasis or receptors have been discussed.

The FPG and the 2-hour PPG concentration tests are the most commonly performed tests for evaluation of glucose homeostasis. Glycated hemoglobin assesses average glucose control over the previous 2 to 3 months, whereas fructosamine assesses average control over the previous 2 to 3 weeks.

DKA and hyperosmolar nonketotic hyperglycemia are the most severe disorders along the continuum of glucose intolerance. Extreme hyperglycemia (600 to 2,000 mg/dL) with insignificant ketonemia/acidosis is consistent with hyperosmolar nonketotic hyperglycemia, whereas less severe or even absent hyperglycemia with ketonemia and acidosis is characteristic of DKA (350 to 650 mg/dL). Hyperglycemia with ketonemia and acidosis is characteristic of DKA.

Thyroid tests can be divided into those that (1) measure the concentration of products secreted by the thyroid gland ($T_3$ and $T_4$);

(2) evaluate the integrity of the hypothalamic-pituitary-thyroid axis (TSH and TRH); (3) assess intrinsic thyroid gland function (radioactive iodine uptake test); and (4) detect antibodies to thyroid tissue (thyroid microsomal antibody). Although TSH concentrations are usually undetectable or <0.3 milliunit/L in patients with hyperthyroidism, $T_4$ concentrations are usually high in patients with overt hyperthyroidism. The TSH concentrations are low or undetectable in patients with hypothyroidism from hypothalamic or pituitary insufficiency and in patients with nonthyroidal illness. In contrast, TSH concentrations are high and $T_4$ concentrations are low in patients with primary hypothyroidism.

Glucocorticoids maintain the body's homeostasis by regulating bodily functions involved in stress and normal activities. Sex hormone precursors are all produced in the adrenal glands. Cushing syndrome is the result of excessive cortisol in the body. Addison disease occurs when there is a deficiency in cortisol production.

Diabetes insipidus is a syndrome in which the body's inability to conserve water manifests as excretion of large volumes of dilute urine. It most often is caused by a defect in the secretion (neurogenic, also called *central*) or renal activity (nephrogenic) of ADH. Urine and plasma osmolality are key tests. With the advent of high-performance assays, the use of plasma vasopressin concentrations to distinguish central from nephrogenic types may obviate the need for provocative iatrogenic dehydration testing procedures.

## LEARNING POINTS

1. *Which patients with diabetes benefit from self-monitoring of blood glucose and how can different test results (premeal, postmeal, and fasting) be used in diabetes management?*

ANSWER: The ADA recommends self-monitoring of blood glucose for all people with diabetes who use insulin.[78] Self-monitoring provides information that patients can use to adjust insulin doses, physical activity, and carbohydrate intake in response to high or low glucose levels. The goal of self-monitoring of blood glucose is to prevent hypoglycemia while maintaining blood glucose levels as close to normal as possible. Most people with type 1 DM must use self-monitoring of blood glucose to achieve this goal. Although patients with type 2 DM receiving insulin therapy benefit from self-monitoring of blood glucose, the benefit of self-monitoring of blood glucose for individuals with type 2 DM who do not use insulin is not firmly established.[78] The ADA states that self-monitoring of blood glucose may be desirable in patients treated with sulfonylureas or other drugs that increase the risk of hypoglycemia.[78] The frequency and timing of self-monitoring of blood glucose vary based on several factors, including an individual's glycemic goals, the current level of glucose control, and the treatment regimen. The ADA recommends self-monitoring of blood glucose three or more times per day for most individuals who have type 1 DM and seven-point testing for pregnant women who use insulin.[74] More frequent testing (four to six times per day) may be needed to monitor pump therapy.[79,80] In patients with type 1 DM, self-monitoring of blood glucose is most commonly recommended four times a day: before meals and at bedtime. A periodic 2:00 a.m. test is recommended to monitor for nighttime hypoglycemia. These measurements are used to adjust insulin doses and attain the fasting glucose goal. However, there is evidence that blood glucose measurements taken after lunch, after dinner, and at bedtime have the highest correlation to A1c values.[79,80] When premeal or fasting goals are reached but A1c values are not optimal, self-monitoring of blood glucose 2 hours after meals can provide guidance for further adjustment of insulin regimens. Postmeal measurements are also used to evaluate the effects of rapid-acting insulins (eg, lispro, aspart), which are injected just before meals. Patients with type 2 DM who use multiple daily injections of insulin should generally test as often as patients with type 1 (at least three times per day). Patients on once-daily insulin and oral medications may also benefit from testing before meals and at bedtime when therapy is initiated or if control is poor.[81,82]

**2. What factors should a pharmacist consider when helping a patient select an SMBG meter?**

**ANSWER:** Meters offer a variety of features that should be considered in the selection process. The key features are meter size; the amount of blood required for each test; ease of use; speed of testing; cleaning and calibration requirements; alternate site testing capability; meter and test strip cost; language choice; and the capability to store readings, average readings over time, and download data. Patient factors to consider include lifestyle (where they will be testing, importance of portability, and speed), preferences (importance of small sample size or alternate site capability), dexterity (whether they can they operate the meter), visual acuity, and insurance coverage.[83]

**3. What are some of the advantages of CGM?**

**ANSWER:** Continuous glucose monitoring can provide a near-continuous readout of interstitial glucose concentration, which adequately reflects blood glucose concentration and can help to identify trends and patterns in glucose control with only a single needle stick to place the sensor. In addition, in the case of real-time CGM, monitors can be programmed to alarm for either high or low glucose values, thus allowing the patient to treat for these abnormal values and potentially reduce the risks associated with hypoglycemia or hyperglycemia as well as diminish patient fear of such an occurrence.[23,24]

**4. What factors may affect the accuracy of an A1c result?**

**ANSWER:** False elevations in A1c may be noted with uremia, chronic alcohol intake, and hypertriglyceridemia. Patients who have diseases with chronic or episodic hemolysis (eg, sickle cell disease and thalassemia) generally have spuriously low A1c concentrations caused by the predominance of young RBCs (which carry less A1c) in the circulation. In splenectomized patients and those with polycythemia, A1c is increased. If these disorders are stable, the test still can be used, but values must be compared with the patient's previous results rather than published normal values. Both falsely elevated and falsely lowered measurements of A1c may also occur during pregnancy. Therefore, it should not be used to screen for GDM.[10,12,15]

**5. Which laboratory tests are recommended in the initial evaluation of thyroid disorders?**

**ANSWER:** The principal laboratory tests recommended in the initial evaluation of a suspected thyroid disorder are the sensitive TSH and the free $T_4$ levels. Free $T_4$ is the most accurate reflection of thyrometabolic status. The free $T_4$ is the most reliable diagnostic test for the evaluation of hypothyroidism and hyperthyroidism when thyroid hormone–binding abnormalities exist. If a direct measure of the free $T_4$ level is not available, the estimated free $T_4$ index can provide comparable information. Total serum $T_4$ is still the standard initial screening test to assess thyroid function because of its wide availability and quick turnaround time. In most patients, the total serum $T_4$ level is a sensitive test to evaluate the function of the thyroid gland. This test measures both bound and free $T_4$ and is, therefore, less reliable than the free $T_4$ or free $T_4$ index when alterations in TBG or nonthyroidal illnesses exist. The serum TSH is the most sensitive test to evaluate decreased thyroid function. TSH secreted by the pituitary is elevated in early or subclinical hypothyroidism (when thyroid hormone levels appear normal) or when thyroid hormone replacement therapy is inadequate.[56,60]

# REFERENCES

1. Skyler JS, Bakris GL, Bonifacio E, et al. Differentiation of diabetes by pathophysiology, natural history, and prognosis. *Diabetes*. 2017;66(2):241-255. doi:10.2337/db16-0806

2. American Diabetes Association. Classification and diagnosis of diabetes: Standards of medical care in diabetes-2021. *Diabetes Care*. 2021;44 (Suppl. 1):S152S33.

3. Sacks DB, Arnold M, Bakris GL, et al. Guidelines and recommendations for laboratory analysis in the diagnosis and management of diabetes mellitus. *Clin Chem*. 2011;57:e1-e47.

4. Lutgens M, Meijer M, Peeters B, et al. Easily obtainable clinical features increase the diagnostic accuracy for latent autoimmune diabetes in adults: an evidence-based report. *Prim Care Diabetes*. 2008;2:207211.

5. Appel SJ, Wadas TM, Rosenthal RS, Ovalle F. Latent autoimmune diabetes of adulthood (LADA): an often misdiagnosed type of diabetes mellitus. *J Am Acad Nurse Pract*. 2009 Mar;21(3):156-159. doi: 10.1111/j.1745-7599.2009.00399.x

6. Naik RG, Brooks-Worrell BM, Palmer JP. Latent autoimmune diabetes in adults. *J Clin Endocrinol Metab*. 2009 Dec;94(12):4635-4644. doi: 10.1210/jc.2009-1120

7. Pipi E, Marketou M, Tsirogianni A. Distinct clinical and laboratory characteristics of latent autoimmune diabetes in adults in relation to type 1 and type 2 diabetes mellitus. *World J Diabetes* 2014;5:505-510.

8. Fourlanos S, Dotta F, Greebuam CJ, et al. Latent autoimmune diabetes in adults (LADA) should be less latent. *Diabetologia*. 2005;48:2206-2212.

9. Hawa M, Buchan AP, Ola T, et al. LADA and CARDS: a prospective study of clinical outcome in established adult-onset autoimmune diabetes. *Diabetes Care*. 2014;37:1643-1649.

10. Goldstein DE, Little RR, Wiedmeyer HM, et al. Glycated hemoglobin: methodologies and clinical applications. *Clin Chem*. 1986;32(suppl 10):B64-B70.

11. Yarrison G, Allen L, King N, et al. Lipemic interference in Beckman Diatrac hemoglobin A1c procedure removed. *Clin Chem*. 1993;39:2351-2352.

12. Goldstein DE, Parker M, England JD, et al. Clinical application of glycosylated hemoglobin measurements. *Diabetes*. 1982;31(suppl 3):70-78.

13. American Diabetes Association. Resource guide 2003: glycohemoglobin tests diabetes forecast. Alexandria, VA: American Diabetes Association; 2003;(suppl 1):67.

14. The International Expert Committee. International Expert Committee report on the role of the A1C assay in the diagnosis of diabetes. *Diabetes Care*. 2009;32:1327-1334.

15. Tahara Y, Shima K. Kinetics of HbA1c, glycated albumin, and fructosamine and analysis of their weight functions against preceding plasma glucose level. *Diabetes Care*. 1995;18:440-447.

16. American Diabetes Association. Glycemic targets: Standards of medical care in diabetes 2021. *Diabetes Care*. 2021;44(Suppl. 1):S73-S84.

17. Masharani U, German MS. Pancreatic hormones and diabetes mellitus. Gardner DG, Shoback D, eds. *Greenspan's Basic and Clinical Endocrinology*. 10th ed. New York, NY: McGraw-Hill Education; 2018. 628.

18. Vasista P, Tziaferi V, Greening J, et al. G472(P) Glycosylated haemoglobin (HbA1c): Is it a reliable measure of glycaemic control in all patients with type 1 diabetes mellitus? *Archives of Disease in Childhood*. 2016;101:A281.

19. Riley RS, McPherson RA. Basic examination of urine. In: McPherson RA, Pincus MR, eds. *Henry's Clinical Diagnosis and Management by Laboratory Methods*. 23rd ed. St Louis, MO: Elsevier; 2017:chap 28.

20. Holland, K. Choosing a glucose meter. https://www.healthline.com/health/type-2-diabetes/choosing-glucose-meter (assessed 2021 November 11).

21. Yoo EH, Lee SY. Glucose biosensors: an overview of use in clinical practice. *Sensors (Basel)*. 2010;10(5):4558-4576. doi:10.3390/s100504558

22. Diabetes Forecast [online]. 2020 consumer guide: http://main.diabetes.org/dforg/pdfs/2020/2020-cg-blood-glucose-meters.pdf (accessed 2021 November 11).

23. Fonseca VA, Grunberger G, Anhalt H, et al. Consensus Conference Writing Committee. Continuous glucose monitoring: a consensus conference of the American Association of Clinical Endocrinologists and American College of Endocrinology. *Endocr Pract*. 2016;22:1008-1021.

24. Diabetes Forecast [online]. 2020 consumer guide: continuous glucose monitors. http://main.diabetes.org/dforg/pdfs/2020/2020-cg-continuous-glucose-monitors.pdf?utm_source=Offline&utm_medium=Print&utm_content=cgms&utm_campaign=DF&s_src=vanity&s_subsrc=cgms (accessed 2020 May 19).

25. Ginsberg BH. Factors affecting blood glucose monitoring: sources of errors in measurement. *J Diabetes Sci Technol*. 2009;3:903-913.

26. Sylvester AC, Price CP, Burrin JM. Investigation of the potential for interference with whole blood glucose strips. *Ann Clin Biochem*. 1994;31:94-96.

27. Tonyushkina K, Nichols JH. Glucose meters: a review of technical challenges to obtaining accurate results. *J Diabetes Sci Technol*. 2009;3:971-980.

28. US Food and Drug Administration. Blood glucose monitoring test systems for prescription point-of-care use: draft guidance for industry and food and drug administration staff (November 2018). http://www.fda.gov/downloads/MedicalDevices/DeviceRegulationandGuidance/GuidanceDocuments/UCM380325.pdf (accessed 2020 June 24).

29. US Food and Drug Administration. Self-monitoring blood glucose test systems for over-the-counter use: draft guidance for industry and Food and Drug Administration staff (October 2016). http://www.fda.gov/downloads/MedicalDevices/DeviceRegulationandGuidance/GuidanceDocuments/UCM380327.pdf (accessed 2020 June 24).

30. McGeoch G, Derry S, Moore RA. Self-monitoring of blood glucose in type 2 diabetes mellitus: what is the evidence? *Diabetes Metab Res Rev*. 2007;23:423-440.

31. Benjamin EM. Self-monitoring of blood glucose: the basics. *Clin Diabetes*. 2002;20:45-47.

32. Banerji MA. The foundation of diabetes self-management: glucose monitoring. *Diabetes Educ*. 2007;33(suppl 4):87S-90S.

33. Sacks DB, Arnold M, Bakris GL, et al. Guidelines and recommendations for laboratory analysis in the diagnosis and management of diabetes mellitus. *Diabetes Care*. 2011;34:e61-69.

34. Avignon A, Radauceanu A, Monnier L. Nonfasting plasma glucose is a better marker of diabetic control than fasting plasma glucose. *Diabetes Care*. 1997;20:1822-1826.

35. Bell DS, Ovalle F, Shadmany S. Postprandial rather than preprandial glucose levels should be used for adjustment of rapid-acting insulins. *Endocr Pract*. 2000;6:477-478.

36. Daudek CD, Derr RL, Kalyani RR. Assessing glycemia in diabetes using self-monitoring blood glucose and hemoglobin A1c. *JAMA*. 2006;295:1688-1697.

37. Austin MM, Haas L, Johnson T, et al. Self-monitoring of blood glucose: benefits and utilization. *The Diabetes Educator*. 2006;328:35-47.

38. Maletkovic J, Drexler A. Diabetic ketoacidosis and hyperglycemic hyperosmolar state. *Endocrinol Metab Clin North Am*. 2013;42(4):677-95. doi: 10.1016/j.ecl.2013.07.001.

39. Musso Giovanni, Saba Francesca, Cassader Maurizio, et al. Diabetic ketoacidosis with SGLT2 inhibitors. *BMJ*. 2020;371:m4147.

40. Corwell B, Knight B, Olivieri L, Willis GC. Current diagnosis and treatment of hyperglycemic emergencies. *Emerg Med Clin North Am*. 2014 May;32(2):437-452. doi: 10.1016/j.emc.2014.01.004.

41. Mitchell R, Thomas SD, Langlois NE. How sensitive and specific is urinalysis 'dipstick' testing for detection of hyperglycaemia and ketosis? An audit of findings from coronial autopsies. *Pathology*. 2013;45(6):587-590. doi:10.1097/PAT.0b013e3283650b93

42. Goren MP, Pratt CB. False-positive ketone tests: a bedside measure of urinary mesna. *Cancer Chemother Pharmacol*. 1990;25:371-372.

43. Savage MW, Dhatariya KK, Kilvert A, et al. Joint British Diabetes Societies guideline for the management of diabetic ketoacidosis. *Diabet. Med*. 2011;28:508-515. doi: 10.1111/j.1464-5491.2011.03246.x

44. Graham P, Naidoo D. False-positive Ketostix in a diabetic on antihypertensive therapy. *Clin Chem*. 1987;33:1490.

45. Gosmanov AR, Gosmanova EO, Kitabchi AE. Hyperglycemic Crises: Diabetic Ketoacidosis and Hyperglycemic Hyperosmolar State. In: Feingold KR, Anawalt B, Boyce A, et al., eds. *Endotext*. South Dartmouth (MA): MDText.com, Inc.; May 9, 2021.

46. Fayfman M, Pasquel FJ, Umpierrez GE. Management of hyperglycemic crises: Diabetic ketoacidosis and hyperglycemic hyperosmolar state. *Med Clin North Am*. 2017 May;101(3):587-606. doi: 10.1016/j.mcna.2016.12.011. PMID: 28372715; PMCID: PMC6535398

47. Matz R. Hyperosmolar nonacidotic diabetes (HNAD). In: Porte D Jr, Sherwin RS, eds. *Diabetes mellitus: theory and practice*. 5th ed. Amsterdam, Netherlands: Elsevier; 1997:845-860.

48. Burge MD, Hardy KJ, Schade DS. Short-term fasting is a mechanism for the development of euglycemic ketoacidosis during periods of insulin deficiency. *J Clin Endocrinol Metab*. 1993;76:1192-1198.

49. Iqbal A, Heller S. Managing hypoglycaemia. *Best Pract Res Clin Endocrinol Metab*. 2016;30(3):413-430. doi:10.1016/j.beem.2016.06.004

50. American Diabetes Association. Microvascular complications and foot care: Standards of Medical Care in Diabetes 2021. *Diabetes Care*. 2021;44(Suppl. 1):S151-S167.

51. Grundy SM, Stone NJ, Bailey AL, et al. 2018 AHA/ACC/AACVPR/AAPA/ABC/ACPM/ADA/AGS/APhA/ASPC/NLA/PCNA guideline on the management of blood cholesterol: a report of the American College of Cardiology/American Heart Association Task Force on Clinical Practice Guidelines. *Circulation*. 2019;139:e1082-e1143. DOI: 10.1161/CIR.0000000000000625

52. American Diabetes Association. Cardiovascular disease and risk management: Standards of Medical Care in Diabetes 2021. *Diabetes Care*. 2021;44(Suppl.1):S125-S150.

53. Walsh JP. Managing thyroid disease in general practice. *Med J Aust*. 2016;205(4):179-184. doi:10.5694/mja16.00545

54. Jenklass J, Talbert RL. Thyroid disorders. In: DiPiro JT, Talbert RL, Yee GC, eds. Pharmacotherapy: a pathophysiologic approach. 9th ed. New York: McGraw-Hill; 2014:1191-1216.

55. Ingbar SH, Woeber KA. The thyroid gland. In: Williams RH, ed. Textbook of endocrinology. 6th ed. Philadelphia: WB Saunders; 1981:117-248.

56. Hershman JM. Hypothyroidism and hyperthyroidism. In: Lavin N, ed. Manual of endocrinology and metabolism. Boston: Little Brown; 1986:365-378.

57. Garber JR, Cobin RH, Gharib H, et al. for the American Association of Clinical Endocrinologists and American Thyroid Association Taskforce on Hypothyroidism in Adults. Clinical practice guidelines for hypothyroidism in adults: cosponsored by the American Association of Clinical Endocrinologists and the American Thyroid Association. *Endocr Pract.* 2012;18:988-1028.

58. Bahn RS, Burch HB, Cooper DS, et al.for the American Thyroid Association and American Association of Clinical Endocrinologists. Hyperthyroidism and other causes of thyrotoxicosis: management guidelines of the American Thyroid Association and American Association of Clinical Endocrinologists. *Endocr Pract.* 2011;17:456-520.

59. Mokshagundam S, Barzel US. Thyroid disease in the elderly. *J Am Geriatr Soc.* 1993;41:1361-1369.

60. Becker DV, Bigos ST, Gaitan E, et al. Optimal use of blood tests for assessment of thyroid function. *JAMA.* 1993;269:2736-2737.

61. Spencer CA. Thyroid profiling for the 1990s: free $T_4$ estimate or sensitive TSH measurement. *J Clin Immunoassay.* 1989;12:82-85.

62. Singer PA. Thyroid function tests and effects of drugs on thyroid function. In: Lavin N, ed. Manual of endocrinology and metabolism. Boston, MA: Little Brown; 1986:341-354.

63. Surks MI, Sievert R. Drugs and thyroid function. *N Engl J Med.* 1995;333:1688-1694.

64. Khanderia U, Jaffe CA, Theisen V. Amiodarone-induced thyroid dysfunction. *Clin Pharm.* 1993;12:774-779.

65. Okamura K, Ikenoue H, Shiroozu A, et al. Reevaluation of the effects of methylmercaptoimidazole and propylthiouracil in patients with Graves' hyperthyroidism. *J Clin Endocrinol Metab.* 1987;65:719-723.

66. Hinkle J, Cheever K. Brunner & Suddarth's Handbook of Laboratory and Diagnostic Tests. 2nd Ed, Kindle. Philadelphia: Wolters Kluwer Health, Lippincott Williams & Wilkins; c2014. Thyroid-Stimulating Hormone, Serum; p. 484.

67. Nelson JC, Wilcox RB, Pandin MR. Dependence of free thyroxine estimates obtained with equilibrium tracer dialysis on the concentration of thyroxine-binding globulin. *Clin Chem.* 1992;38:1294-1300.

68. Michalakis K, Ilias I. Medical management of adrenal disease: a narrative review. *Endocr Regul.* 2009 Jul;43(3):127-135. PMID: 19817507

69. Fitzgerald PA. Pituitary disorders. In: Fitzgerald PA, ed. Handbook of clinical endocrinology. Greenbrae, CA: Jones Medical Publications; 1986:22-29.

70. Lacroix A, Feelders RA, Stratakis CA, Nieman LK. Cushing's syndrome. *Lancet.* 2015;386:913-927.

71. Dorin RI, Qualls Cr, Crapo LM. Diagnosis of adrenal insufficiency. *Ann Intern Med.* 2003;139:194-204.

72. Arlt W, Allolio B. Adrenal insufficiency. *Lancet.* 2003;361:1881-1893.

73. Lightman SL. Molecular insights into diabetes insipidus. *N Engl J Med.* 1993;328:1562-1563.

74. Bichet DG. Nephrogenic diabetes insipidus. *Adv Chronic Kidney Dis.* 2006 Apr;13(2):96-104.

75. Olesen ET, Rützler MR, Moeller HB, Praetorius HA, Fenton RA. Vasopressin-independent targeting of aquaporin-2 by selective E-prostanoid receptor agonists alleviates nephrogenic diabetes insipidus. *Proc Natl Acad Sci U S A.* 2011 Aug 2;108(31):12949-12954. doi: 10.1073/pnas.1104691108

76. Krege J, Katz VL, Bowes WA Jr. Transient diabetes insipidus of pregnancy. *Obstet Gynecol Surv.* 1989;44:789-795.

77. Sowers JR, Zieve FJ. Clinical disorders of vasopressin. In: Lavin N, ed. Manual of endocrinology and metabolism. Boston, MA: Little Brown; 1986:65-74.

78. American Diabetes Association. Diabetes technology: Standards of Medical Care in Diabetes 2021. *Diabetes Care.* 2021;44(Suppl. 1):S85-S99.

79. Benjamin EM. Self-monitoring of blood glucose: the basics. *Clinical Diabetes.* 2002;20:45-47.

80. Banerji MA. The foundation of diabetes self-management: glucose monitoring. *The Diabetes Educator.* 2007;87S-90S.

81. Bell D, Ovalle F, Shadmany S. Postprandial rather than preprandial glucose levels should be used for adjustment of rapid-acting insulins. *Endocr Pract.* 2000;6:477-478.

82. Austin MM, Haas L, Johnson T, et al. Self-monitoring of blood glucose: benefits and utilization. *Diabetes Educ.* 2006;32835-32847.

83. Mensing C. Helping patients choose the right glucose meter. *Nurse Pract.* 2004;29:43-45.

## QUICKVIEW | Total Serum $T_3$

| PARAMETER | DESCRIPTION | COMMENTS |
|---|---|---|
| **Common reference ranges** | | |
| Adults and children | 80–200 ng/dL | Affected by TBG changes |
| | (1.2–3.1 nmol/L) | SI conversion factor = 0.0154 (nmol/L) |
| **Critical value** | Not established | Extremely high or low values should be reported quickly |
| **Natural substance?** | Yes | Only 0.2% of $T_3$ is unbound |
| **Inherent activity?** | Only free portion | Total assumed to correlate with free $T_3$ activity |
| **Location** | | |
| Production and storage | 20%–25% secreted by thyroid gland, remainder produced by conversion of $T_4$ to $T_3$ | Bound mostly to thyroglobulin |
| Secretion/excretion | From thyroid, liver, and kidneys to blood | |
| **Major causes of...** | | |
| **High results** | Hyperthyroidism | Not truly a cause but a reflection of high result |
| | $T_4$ and $T_3$ supplements | |
| | Other causes | |
| Associated signs and symptoms | Signs and symptoms of hyperthyroidism | Nervousness, weight loss, heat intolerance, tachycardia, diaphoresis |
| **Low results** | Hypothyroidism | Not truly a cause but a reflection of low result |
| | Other causes | |
| | Propranolol | |
| | Propylthiouracil | |
| | Glucocorticoids | |
| Associated signs and symptoms | Signs and symptoms of hypothyroidism | Lethargy, constipation, dry skin, cold intolerance, slow speech, confusion |
| **After insult, time to...** | | |
| Initial elevation or depression | Weeks to months | Increases within hours in acute $T_4$ or $T_3$ overdose |
| Peak values | Weeks to months | Increases within hours in acute $T_4$ or $T_3$ overdose |
| Normalization | Usually same time as onset | Assumes insult removed or effectively treated |
| **Drugs often monitored with test** | $T_4$ and $T_3$ | Other drugs |
| **Causes of spurious results** | Increased or decreased TBG leads to falsely increased or decreased total serum $T_3$, respectively; nonthyroidal illness leads to falsely increased or decreased total serum $T_3$ | |

## QUICKVIEW | Total Serum T$_4$

| PARAMETER | DESCRIPTION | COMMENTS |
|---|---|---|
| **Common reference ranges** | | |
| Adults and children | 5.5–12.5 mcg/dL (71–161 nmol/L) | Affected by TBG changes with nonthyroidal illness |
| | | SI conversion factor = 12.87 (nmol/L) |
| Newborn/3–5 days | 11–23/9–18 mcg/dL | Affected by TBG changes with nonthyroidal illness |
| **Critical value** | Not established | Extremely high or low values should be reported quickly, especially in newborns |
| **Natural substance?** | Yes | Only 0.02% of T$_4$ is unbound |
| **Inherent activity?** | Only free portion | Total assumed to correlate with free T$_4$ activity |
| **Location** | | |
| Production and storage | Thyroid gland | Bound mostly to thyroglobulin |
| Secretion/excretion | From thyroid to blood | About 33% converted to T$_3$ outside thyroid |
| **Major causes of...** | | |
| **High results** | Hyperthyroidism | Not truly a cause but a reflection of high result |
| | T$_4$ supplements | |
| | Other causes (Tables 9-6 and 9-8) | |
| Associated signs and symptoms | Signs and symptoms of hyperthyroidism | Nervousness, weight loss, heat intolerance, tachycardia, diaphoresis |
| **Low results** | Hypothyroidism | Not truly a cause but a reflection of low result |
| | Other causes (Tables 9-5 and 9-8) | |
| | Signs and symptoms of hyperthyroidism | Lethargy, constipation, dry skin, cold intolerance, slow speech, confusion |
| **After insult, time to...** | | |
| Initial elevation or depression | Weeks to months | Increases within hours in acute T$_4$ overdose |
| Peak values | Weeks to months | Increases within hours in acute T$_4$ overdose |
| Normalization | Usually same time as onset | Assumes insult removed or effectively treated |
| **Drugs often monitored with test** | T$_4$ | Other drugs |
| **Causes of spurious results** | Increased or decreased TBG leads to falsely increased or decreased total serum T$_4$, respectively; nonthyroidal illness leads to falsely increased or decreased total serum T$_4$ | |

## QUICKVIEW | Free T$_4$

| PARAMETER | DESCRIPTION | COMMENTS |
|---|---|---|
| **Common reference ranges** | | |
| Adults and children | 0.9–2.3 ng/dL (11.6–29.6 pmol/L) | Higher in infants <1 mo; direct equilibrium dialysis assay not affected by TBG changes or severe nonthyroidal illness<br>SI conversion factor = 12.87 (pmol/L) |
| **Critical value** | Not established | Extremely high or low values should be reported quickly |
| **Natural substance?** | Yes | Only 0.02% of T$_4$ is unbound |
| **Inherent activity?** | Probably | Some influence on basal metabolic rate; T$_3$ most active |
| **Location** | | |
| Production and storage | Thyroid gland | Bound mostly to thyroglobulin |
| Secretion/excretion | From thyroid to blood | 33% converted to T$_3$ outside thyroid |
| **Major causes of…** | | |
| **High results** | Hyperthyroidism | Not truly a cause but a reflection of high result |
| | T$_4$ supplements | |
| | Other causes (Table 9-8) | |
| Associated signs and symptoms | Signs and symptoms of hyperthyroidism | Nervousness, weight loss, heat intolerance, tachycardia, diaphoresis |
| **Low results** | Hypothyroidism | Not truly a cause but a reflection of low result |
| | Other causes (Table 9-8) | |
| Associated signs and symptoms | Signs and symptoms of hypothyroidism | Lethargy, constipation, dry skin, cold intolerance, slow speech, confusion |
| **After insult, time to…** | | |
| Initial elevation or depression | Weeks to months | Increases within hours in acute T$_4$ overdose |
| Peak values | Weeks to months | Increases within hours in acute T$_4$ overdose |
| Normalization | Usually same time as onset | Assumes insult removed or effectively treated |
| **Drugs often monitored with test** | T$_4$ | Other drugs |
| **Causes of spurious results** | Rare with direct equilibrium dialysis assay (Table 9-9) | Decreased direct equilibrium dialysis assay for free T$_4$ with decreased or normal TSH may occur in patients |

## QUICKVIEW | TSH

| PARAMETER | DESCRIPTION | COMMENTS |
|---|---|---|
| **Common reference ranges** | | |
| Adults and children | 0.5–5.0 milliunits/L | |
| **Critical value** | Not established | Extremely high or low values should be reported quickly |
| **Natural substance?** | Yes | |
| **Inherent activity?** | Yes | Stimulates thyroid to secrete hormone |
| **Location** | | |
| Production and storage | Anterior pituitary | |
| Secretion/excretion | Unknown | |
| **Major causes of...** | | |
| **High results** | Primary hypothyroidism Antithyroid drugs<br><br>Other causes (Table 9-6) | Causes of primary hypothyroidism |
| Associated signs and symptoms | Signs and symptoms of hypothyroidism | Lethargy, constipation, dry skin, cold intolerance, slow speech, confusion |
| **Low results** | Primary hyperthyroidism | Must be $\leq 0.05$ milliunit/L for definitive diagnosis of (primary hyperthyroidism); may be decreased or normal in secondary or tertiary hypothyroidism |
| | Other causes (Tables 9-5 and 9-8) | |
| Associated signs and symptoms | Signs and symptoms of hyperthyroidism | Nervousness, weight loss, heat intolerance, HR increase, diaphoresis |
| **After insult, time to...** | | |
| Initial elevation or depression | Weeks to months | Decreases within hours in acute $T_4$ overdose |
| Peak values | Weeks to months | Decreases within hours in acute $T_4$ overdose |
| Normalization | Usually same time as onset | Assumes insult removed or effectively treated |
| **Drugs often monitored with test** | $T_4$ and $T_3$ | Also antithyroid drugs (methimazole and propylthiouracil) |
| **Causes of spurious results** | Increased TSH: dopamine antagonists | Metoclopramide and domperidone |
| | Decreased TSH: dopamine agonists | Dopamine, bromocriptine, levodopa, glucocorticoids |
| | Above TSH measurements are accurate here | These drugs decrease TSH, but the change is not reflective of primary hypothyroidism or hyperthyroidism; therefore, the results are not truly spurious |

## QUICKVIEW | Plasma Glucose

| PARAMETER | DESCRIPTION | COMMENTS |
|---|---|---|
| **Common reference ranges** | | |
| Adults | Adult fasting: <100 mg/dL (5.6 mmol/L)<br>Adult 2-hr postprandial: <140 mg/dL (7.8 mmol/L)<br>Full-term infant normal: 20–90 mg/dL (1.11–5 mmol/L) | Multiply by 0.056 for SI units (mmol/L) |
| Critical value | Adult fasting, no previous history: >126 mg/dL (7 mmol/L)<br>Anytime: <50 mg/dL (<2.8 mmol/L) | In known patient with diabetes, increased glucose is not an immediate concern unless patient is symptomatic; an increased glucose is not critical if serial levels are decreasing over time |
| Natural substance? | Yes | Always present in blood |
| Inherent activity? | Yes | Major source of energy for cellular metabolism |
| **Location** | | |
| Production | Liver and muscle | Dietary intake |
| Storage | Liver and muscle | As glycogen |
| Secretion/excretion | Mostly metabolized for energy | Levels >180 mg/dL (10 mmol/L) spill into urine |
| **Major causes of...** | | |
| High results | Type 1 and 2 DM<br>Drugs (Table 9-2)<br>Excess intake | |
| Associated signs and symptoms | Polyuria, polydipsia, polyphagia, weakness | Long term: damage to kidneys, retina, neurons, and vessels |
| Low results | Insulin secretion/dose excessive relative to diet<br>Sulfonylureas or other hypoglycemic agents<br>Insulinomas | Most common in patients with diabetes |
| Associated signs and symptoms | Hunger, sweating, weakness, trembling, headache, confusion, seizures, coma | From neuroglycopenia and adrenergic discharge |
| **After insult, time to...** | | |
| Initial elevation | Type 1 DM: months to elevation<br>Type 2 DM: years to elevation<br>After insulin: minutes to decrease<br>After meal: 15–30 min to elevation<br>After epinephrine or glucagon: minutes<br>After steroids and growth hormone: hours | |
| Normalization | After insulin: minutes | Depends on insulin type |
| | After exercise: minutes to hours | Depends on intensity and duration |
| Drugs often monitored with test | Insulin, sulfonylureas, biguanides (eg, metformin), thiazolidinediones, or other hypoglycemic agents | Also, diazoxide, L-asparaginase, total parenteral nutrition |
| Causes of spurious results | High-dose vitamin C, acetaminophen | With some glucometers |
| | Metronidazole | With some automated assays |

## QUICKVIEW | A1c

| PARAMETER | DESCRIPTION | COMMENTS |
|---|---|---|
| **Common reference ranges** | | |
| Adults and children | 4%–5.6% | Fasting not required; represents average glucose levels past 8 wk |
| **Critical value** | Not applicable | Reflects long-term glycemic control; >9% suggests poor control |
| **Natural substance?** | Yes | Subunit of Hgb |
| **Inherent activity?** | Yes | Oxygen carrier; also carries glucose |
| **Location** | | |
| Production | Bone marrow | In newborns in liver and spleen |
| Storage | Not stored | Circulates in blood |
| Secretion/excretion | Older cell removed by spleen | Converted to bilirubin |
| **Major causes of…** | | |
| **High results** | DM | Any cause of prolonged hyperglycemia |
| | Chronic hyperglycemia | |
| Signs and symptoms | Signs and symptoms of diabetes | |
| **Low results** | | |
| Associated signs and symptoms | Not clinically useful | |
| **After insult, time to…** | | |
| Initial elevation | 2–4 mo | Initial insult is chronic hyperglycemia |
| Normalization | 2–4 mo | Assumes sudden and persistent euglycemia |
| **Drugs often monitored with test** | biguanides (eg, metformin), sulfonylureas (eg, glimepiride), meglitinides (eg, repaglinide), thiazolidinediones (eg, pioglitazone), dipeptidyl peptidase IV inhibitors (eg, sitagliptin), and α-glucosidase inhibitors (eg, acarbose), insulin (eg, glargine) | Also diet and exercise |
| **Causes of spurious results** | High results: alcoholism, uremia, increased triglycerides, hypertriglyceridemia, hemolysis, polycythemia | Also seen in pregnant and splenectomized patients |
| | Low results: sickle cell anemia, thalassemia | |

# 10

# Renal Function and Related Tests

*Kimmy T. Nguyen*

## OBJECTIVES

*After completing this chapter, the reader should be able to*

- Describe clinical situations in which blood urea nitrogen and serum creatinine are elevated

- Discuss the evolving role of cystatin C in estimating glomerular filtration rate

- Recognize the limitations in the usefulness of the serum creatinine concentration in estimating kidney function

- Explain the clinical use of the Cockcroft-Gault equation, the Modification of Diet in Renal Disease equation, and the Chronic Kidney Disease Epidemiology Collaboration equation to assess kidney function

- Determine creatinine clearance given a patient's 24-hour urine creatinine excretion and serum creatinine

- Estimate creatinine clearance given a patient's height, weight, sex, age, and serum creatinine and identify limitations of the methods for estimation of kidney function

- Recognize the classification of chronic kidney disease, glomerular filtration rate categories, and albuminuria as predictors of disease

- Discuss the various components assessed by macroscopic, microscopic, and chemical analysis of the urine

- Describe the role of commonly obtained urinary electrolytes and the fractional excretion of sodium in the diagnostic process

Through the excretion of water and solutes, the kidneys are largely responsible for maintaining homeostasis within the body. They also function in the activation and synthesis of many substances that affect blood pressure (BP), mineral metabolism, and red blood cell (RBC) production. The purpose of this chapter is to provide insight into the interpretation of laboratory tests in the assessment of kidney function as well as provide an overview of the interpretation of a urinalysis.

## KIDNEY PHYSIOLOGY

The functional unit of the kidneys is the nephron, and each healthy kidney contains approximately 1 million nephrons. The major components of the nephron include the glomerulus, proximal tubule, loop of Henle, distal tubule, and collecting duct. Afferent arterioles deliver blood to the glomerulus, where it undergoes filtration. Molecular weight and electrical charge affect filtration through glomerular capillary pores. Substances with a molecular weight of <7,000 Da freely cross the filtration barrier. In contrast, plasma proteins, such as albumin (MW 66,000 Da), have particularly low levels of filterability due to their size. As molecular weight increases, the ability to undergo filtration decreases. Most drugs are small enough to be freely filtered at the glomerulus, with the exception of large proteins and drugs bound to plasma proteins. Electrical charge affects macromolecule filtration because the filtration barrier contains fixed polyanions. As a result, negatively charged macromolecules are restricted by the filtration barrier, leading to a lesser extent of filtration compared with positively charged or neutral macromolecules. When there is a loss of negative ionic charge in the filtration barrier from diseases that affect the glomerulus, negatively charged macromolecules, such as albumin, are able to undergo filtration and lead to albuminuria. Smaller molecules, such as mineral anions, are not hindered by the filtration barrier and are freely filtered.[1] Additionally, a drug's volume of distribution ($V_D$) plays a role in clearance. Drugs with a high $V_D$ are unlikely to be significantly removed by the kidneys because there are higher concentrations in the extravascular tissue than in the vascular compartment.[2]

The proximal tubule reabsorbs large quantities of water. As water is reabsorbed back into the blood, sodium passively follows. Other solutes primarily reabsorbed in the proximal tubule include glucose, amino acids, phosphate, uric acid, chloride, bicarbonate, urea, hydrogen, calcium, and magnesium. Water, sodium, calcium, chloride, and magnesium are further reabsorbed in the loop of Henle. The distal tubule regulates the amount of sodium, potassium, bicarbonate, phosphate, and hydrogen that is excreted, and the collecting duct regulates the amount of water in the urine through the action of antidiuretic hormone (ADH), which facilitates water reabsorption.[1]

Substances can enter the nephron from the peritubular blood or interstitial space via secretion. Additionally, substances may be reabsorbed from the distal tubule back into the systemic circulation via the peritubular vasculature. Tubular secretion occurs via three primary pathways in the proximal tubule: the organic acid transport system, the organic cation transport system, and the organic anion transport system.[3] Although each system is somewhat specific for anions and cations, some drugs, such as probenecid, are secreted by both pathways. Creatinine enters the tubule primarily

DOI 10.37573/9781585286423.010

by filtration through the glomerulus. However, a small amount of creatinine is also secreted by the organic cation transport system into the proximal tubule. This becomes important when using renal clearance of creatinine to estimate kidney function.[1]

The rate of renal blood flow (RBF) is 1 L/min, which represents ~20% of cardiac output. The direct relationship between renal plasma flow (RPF) and RBF and hematocrit (Hct) is described by the following equation[4]:

$$RPF = RBF \times (1 - Hct) \qquad (1)$$

The normal value for RPF is ~625 mL/min.[4] Of the plasma that reaches the glomerulus, ~20% is filtered and enters the proximal tubule, providing the glomerular filtration rate (GFR). A normal GFR is ~125 mL/min. The GFR is often used as a measure of the degree of kidney excretory function. In the absence of kidney disease, the kidneys filter ~180 L of fluid each day; of this amount, they only excrete ~1.5 L as urine. This amount varies widely depending on fluid intake. Regardless, more than 99% of the initial glomerular filtrate is reabsorbed into the bloodstream. Many solutes, such as creatinine, and many renally eliminated drugs are concentrated in the urine.[1]

# DEFINITION AND CLASSIFICATION OF CHRONIC KIDNEY DISEASE

The classification of *chronic kidney disease* (CKD) is based on the nature or cause of the abnormality (structure, function), the GFR category (g1 through g5), and the albuminuria category (a1 through a3). The prognostic categories can be found at www.kdigo.org.[5] CKD has been defined as GFR <60 mL/min/1.73 m² for longer than 3 months.[5] The use of estimating equations (eGFR) or the measurement of GFR rather than using serum creatinine (SCr) or cystatin C alone can provide the basis for the classification of kidney function. Additionally, markers of kidney damage are used for prognosis of risk, and examples include albuminuria (albumin excretion rate >30 mg/24 h, albumin-to-creatinine [ACR] ratio 30 mg/g), structural (eg, polycystic kidney disease, hydronephrosis, renal artery stenosis), or functional anomalies (eg, urinary sediment such as casts or renal tubular disorders). Risk is categorized as low risk (no markers of kidney disease), moderately increased risk, high risk, and very high risk.[5] This information is useful to guide therapy and further monitor CKD complications.

# ASSESSMENT OF KIDNEY FUNCTION

Classification of kidney disease and dosing of medications depend on an accurate and reliable method of assessing kidney function.[5] Direct measurement of GFR using markers, such as inulin and iothalamate, is the most accurate assessment of kidney function. However, use is not routine in clinical practice because of cost and practical concerns. Measurements of timed 24-hour urine creatinine (UCr) collections are difficult by design, flawed by collection errors, and used only when determination of GFR, and more specifically creatinine clearance (CrCl), are vital and estimating equations are not reliable. Widespread availability of

eGFR strengthens its use in determining renal function in pharmacokinetic studies for drug dosing.[6,7] However, CrCl, as calculated through equations such as Cockcroft-Gault, is a widely accepted surrogate of GFR and may still be used to assess renal function. Serum concentrations of cystatin C, an endogenous polypeptide, have been evaluated as an alternative method to predict GFR in children and adults.[8-10]

Estimated GFR was initially validated using the Modification of Diet in Renal Disease (MDRD) equation and was used to stage and monitor CKD.[11-15] However, the 2009 CKD Epidemiology Collaboration (CKD-EPI) equation, or an alternative creatinine-based GFR estimating equation with superior accuracy to the CKD-EPI equation, is currently recommended to estimate GFR.[5] It is important to note that the MDRD is still used to estimate GFR in many laboratories, and values >60 mL/min may simply be reported as GFR >60 when this equation is used.[16] In 2010, the U.S. Food and Drug Administration (FDA) Guidance to Industry draft revision proposed that both eGFR and CrCl be incorporated into package insert dosage recommendations for patients with decreased renal function.[17] The use of eGFR to adjust medication doses has become commonplace, with more clinical laboratories reporting eGFR values and pharmacokinetic data referencing both eGFR and CrCl for new medications. It is important to note that use of different equations leads to variation in kidney function estimates, and renal dosing decisions require clinical judgment.

## Exogenous Markers
### Inulin Clearance

*Inulin* is a polysaccharide starch, an inert carbohydrate, with a molecular weight of 5,000 Da.[1] Inulin is not bound to plasma proteins and is freely filtered through the glomerulus and into the urine without undergoing metabolism, secretion, or reabsorption. As a result, inulin is an ideal marker for measuring GFR in adults and older children.[18] Neonates and younger children may present logistical problems in obtaining accurate urine flow rates.[14] However, the expensive and cumbersome nature of multiple timed urine collection makes this approach largely impractical.

## I-Iothalamate and Iohexol Clearance

Urinary clearance of *I-iothalamate* and *iohexol* allows measurement of GFR. Unlike I-iothalamate, iohexol is nonionic and does not undergo active secretion or absorption.[19] The test involves injection of the radioactive exogenous marker, repeated blood sampling, and timed urine collection.[20] The invasiveness and associated costs prohibit widespread application. As with inulin, the need for intravenous administration and plasma sampling for these markers makes them impractical for routine use.

## Endogenous Markers
### Cystatin C

*Normal reference range[21]: 18–49 years: 0.63–1.03 mg/L; ≥50 years: 0.67–1.21 mg/L; 0–17 years: Reference values have not been established. Refer to eGFR.*

*Cystatin C* is a low-molecular weight polypeptide produced at a steady state by all nucleated cells. It is filtered by the glomerulus and removed from the bloodstream through degradation via the kidneys.[22] As a result, serum cystatin C concentrations are inversely proportional to GFR, and changes in serum concentrations may be an indirect reflection of GFR. It had been originally proposed that cystatin C may be more sensitive than SCr in tracking changes in kidney function because it is less affected by factors like race, age, and sex.[23] Combining SCr with cystatin C, age, sex, and race in estimating GFR has provided better results than equations based on a single filtration marker.[24] However, limited availability and cost of cystatin C make its use uncommon.

There is conflicting evidence regarding cystatin C in predicting different forms of acute kidney injury (AKI). Compared with creatinine, cystatin C was found to be a better predictor of contrast-induced AKI in patients with CKD.[25] Cystatin C was also found to be a useful marker for detecting acute renal failure up to 2 days earlier than SCr in critically ill patients.[26] However, previous studies have not captured the benefits of cystatin C to predict AKI in the settings of cardiopulmonary bypass and cardiothoracic surgery.[27,28]

Cystatin C concentrations have been used in equations for estimating GFR in pediatric patients.[8] The use of certified cystatin C concentrations in eGFR equations is evolving rapidly with the relatively recent certification of reference material.[29] The National Kidney Disease Education Program (NKDEP) recommends the use of cystatin C equations derived from data with the ERM-DA471/IFCC reference material that has been certified. Currently, it is recommended that inclusion of traceable cystatin C be used in eGFR equations rather than relying on the absolute value in the assessment of CKD.[5] Data also support the correlation of elevated cystatin C levels and cardiovascular disease mortality.[30] However, current data do not support implementation of cystatin c for the diagnosis of CKD in the primary care setting.[31]

### β-Trace Protein and β-2-Microglobulin

*Normal reference range[32]: men, 0.37-0.77 mg/L; women, 0.40 to 0.70 mg/L*

β-trace protein (BTP) and β-2-microglobulin (B2M) are low molecular weight proteins. Similar to cystatin C, BTP and B2M undergo glomerular filtration before reabsorption through the proximal tubule. BTP and B2M do not undergo urinary excretion under normal conditions, and elevated serum concentrations suggest renal impairment.[33] In contrast to creatinine, BTP and B2M appear less affected by age, sex, and race.[34] However, current data do not support the use of BTP and B2M because they do not provide significant prognostic information and are limited by assay availability, standards, and cost.[35]

### Serum creatinine

*Normal range: adults, 0.6 to 1.2 mg/dL (53 to 106 μmol/L); young children, 0.2 to 0.7 mg/dL (18 to 62 μmol/L)*

*Creatinine* and its precursor, creatine, are nonprotein, nitrogenous biochemicals of the blood. After synthesis in the liver, creatine diffuses into the bloodstream. Creatine is then taken up by muscle cells, where some of it is stored in a high-energy form called *creatine phosphate*. Creatine phosphate acts as a readily available source of phosphorus for regeneration of adenosine

triphosphate and is required for transforming chemical energy to muscle action.

Creatinine, which is produced in the muscle, is a spontaneous decomposition product of creatine and creatine phosphate. The daily production of creatinine is ~2% of total body creatine, which remains constant if muscle mass is not significantly changed. In normal patients at steady state, the rate of creatinine production equals its excretion. Therefore, SCr concentrations vary little from day to day in patients with healthy kidneys. Although there is an inverse relationship between SCr and kidney function, SCr should not be the sole basis for the evaluation of renal function.[14] Several issues should be considered when evaluating a patient's SCr. Some of the factors that affect SCr concentrations include muscle mass, sex, age, race, medications, method of laboratory analysis, and low-protein diets. Additionally, acute changes in a patient's GFR, such as in AKI, may not be initially manifested as an increase in SCr concentration because it takes time for new steady-state concentrations of SCr to be achieved. The time required to reach 95% of steady state in patients with 50%, 25%, and 10% of normal kidney function is about 1, 2, and 4 days, respectively. Steady-state concentrations of SCr become important because they are integral in clinical practice estimations of renal function.

An SCr concentration within the reference ranges as reported by clinical laboratories does not necessarily indicate normal kidney function. For example, an SCr concentration of 1.5 mg/dL in a 45-year-old man who weighs 150 lb and a 78-year-old woman who weighs 92 lb would correspond to different GFRs.

Clinicians can surmise that an increased SCr almost always reflects a decreased GFR in the absence of abnormalities in muscle mass or muscle breakdown (rhabdomyolysis), dietary protein intake, changes in hydration, and intense physical activity. The converse is not always true; a normal SCr does not necessarily imply a normal GFR. As part of the aging process, both muscle mass and renal function diminish. Decreasing amounts of creatinine coupled with a decrease in the kidney's ability to filter and excrete creatinine may result in an SCr that remains within normal limits. Thus, practitioners should not rely solely on SCr as an index of renal function.

Besides aging and alterations in muscle mass, some pathophysiological changes can affect the relationship between SCr and kidney function. For example, renal function may be overestimated based on SCr alone in patients with cirrhosis. In this patient population, the low SCr is due to a decreased hepatic synthesis of creatine, the precursor of creatinine. In patients with cirrhosis, it is prudent to perform a measured 24-hour CrCl. If a patient also has hyperbilirubinemia, assay interference by elevated bilirubin may also contribute to a low SCr.

***Laboratory measurement and reporting of serum creatinine.*** Historically, the laboratory methods used to measure SCr included the alkaline picrate method, inorganic enzymatic methods, and high-pressure liquid chromatography. The alkaline picrate assay (Jaffe) was the most commonly used method to measure SCr; however, interfering substances, such as noncreatinine chromogens, often led to underestimation of kidney function. Causes of falsely elevated SCr results included unusually large amounts of noncreatinine chromogens (eg, uric acid, glucose, fructose, acetone, acetoacetate, pyruvic acid, and ascorbic acid) in the serum. For example, an increase in glucose of 100 mg/dL (5.6 mmol/L) could falsely elevate SCr by 0.5 mg/dL (44 μmol/L) in some assays. Likewise, serum ketones high enough to spill into the urine may falsely increase SCr and UCr. In patients with diabetic ketoacidosis, a false elevation in SCr could prompt unnecessary evaluation for renal failure when presenting with ketoacidosis. Like ketones, high levels of acetoacetate may cause a falsely elevated SCr after a 48-hour fast or in patients with diabetic ketoacidosis Another endogenous substance, bilirubin, may falsely lower SCr results with both the alkaline picrate and enzymatic assays. At low GFRs, however, creatinine secretion overtakes the balancing effects of measuring noncreatinine chromogens, causing an overestimation of GFRs by as much as 50%.[36]

Reliable and accurate measurement and subsequent reporting of SCr concentrations is important. The MDRD and CKD-EPI equations use SCr concentrations as one of the variables to stage kidney damage based on the estimation of GFR. The Cockcroft-Gault equation, which depends greatly on the SCr concentration, has been used as the accepted methodology for drug dosing based on an estimation of CrCl.[37] The greater the imprecision of the assay, the less accurate the resultant GFR or CrCl estimations. The primary source of measurement errors includes systematic bias and interlaboratory, intralaboratory, and random variability in daily calibration of SCr values. Interlaboratory commutability is also problematic secondary to the variations in assay methodologies. A report from the Laboratory Working Group of the National Kidney Disease Program made recommendations to improve and standardize the measurement of SCr.[38,39] As of 2011, creatinine standardization is reported to be nationwide (in the United States), and calibration should be traceable to isotope dilution mass spectrometry (IDMS). Of note, SCr concentrations are lower than had been previously reported with older methods. This discrepancy may present a limiting factor in drug dosing for older medications when previous assays had yielded higher creatinine concentrations.

### Urea (Blood Urea Nitrogen)

*Normal range 8 to 23 mg/dL (2.9 to 8.2 mmol/L)*
*Blood urea nitrogen* (BUN) is the concentration of nitrogen (as urea) in the serum and not in RBCs, as the name implies. Although the renal clearance of urea can be measured, it cannot be used by itself to assess kidney function. Its serum concentration depends on urea production (which occurs in the liver), glomerular filtration, and tubular reabsorption. Therefore, clinicians must consider factors other than filtration when interpreting changes in BUN.

When viewed with other laboratory and clinical data, BUN can be used to assess or monitor hydration, renal function, protein tolerance, and catabolism in numerous clinical settings (**Table 10-1**).[40] Also, it is used to predict the risk of uremic syndrome in patients with severe renal failure. Concentrations above 100 mg/dL (35.7 mmol/L) are associated with this risk.

***Elevated blood urea nitrogen.*** Urea production is increased by a high-protein diet (including amino acid infusions), upper gastrointestinal (GI) bleeding, and the administration of

### TABLE 10-1. Common Causes of True BUN Elevations (Azotemia)

| Prerenal causes |
| --- |
| Decreased renal perfusion: dehydration, blood loss, shock, severe heart failure |

| Intrarenal (intrinsic) causes |
| --- |
| Acute kidney failure: nephrotoxic drugs, severe hypertension, glomerulonephritis, tubular necrosis |
| Chronic kidney dysfunction: pyelonephritis, diabetes, glomerulonephritis, renal tubular disease, amyloidosis, arteriosclerosis, collagen vascular disease, polycystic kidney disease, overuse of NSAIDs |

| Postrenal causes |
| --- |
| Obstruction of ureter, bladder neck, or urethra |

corticosteroids, tetracyclines, or any other drug with antianabolic effects. Usually, ~50% of the filtered urea is reabsorbed, but this amount is inversely related to the rate of urine flow in the tubules. In other words, the slower the urine flows, the more time the urea has to leave the tubule and reenter surrounding capillaries (reabsorption). Urea reabsorption tends to change in parallel with sodium, chloride, and water reabsorption. Because patients with volume depletion avidly reabsorb sodium, chloride, and water, larger amounts of urea are also absorbed.

Likewise, a patient with a pathologically low BP may develop diminished urine flow secondary to decreased RBF with a subsequently diminished GFR. Congestive heart failure and reduced RBF, despite increased intravascular volume, are common causes of elevated BUN. Types of renal failure that can cause an abnormally high BUN (also called *azotemia*) are listed in **Table 10-1**.

***Decreased blood urea nitrogen.*** In and of itself, a low BUN does not have pathophysiological consequences. BUN may be low in patients who are malnourished or have profound liver damage (due to an inability to synthesize urea). Intravascular fluid overload may initially dilute BUN and result in low concentrations. However, many causes of extravascular volume overload, which are associated with third spacing of fluids into tissues (eg, congestive heart failure, renal failure, and nephrotic syndrome), result in an increase in BUN because effective circulating volume is decreased.

***Blood urea nitrogen to serum creatinine ratio.*** Simultaneous BUN and SCr determinations are commonly made and can furnish valuable information to assess kidney function. This is particularly true for AKI. In AKI caused by volume depletion, both BUN and SCr are elevated. However, the BUN:SCr ratio is often >20:1. This observation is due to the differences in the renal handling of urea and creatinine. Recall that urea is reabsorbed with water, and under conditions of decreased renal perfusion, both urea and water reabsorption are increased. Because creatinine is not reabsorbed, it is not affected by increased water reabsorption. Thus, the concentrations of both substances may increase in this setting, but the BUN would be increased to a greater degree, leading to a BUN:SCr >20:1.

In summary, when acute changes in kidney function are observed and both BUN and SCr are greater than normal limits, BUN:SCr ratios >20:1 suggest prerenal causes of acute renal impairment (Table 10-1), whereas ratios from 10:1 to 20:1 suggest intrinsic kidney damage. Furthermore, a ratio >20:1 is not clinically important if both SCr and BUN are within normal limits (eg, SCr = 0.8 mg/dL and BUN = 20 mg/dL) (**Minicase 1**).

## Measurement of Creatinine Clearance

A complete 24-hour urine collection to measure CrCl is preferred over creatinine-based estimating equations in clinical situations of unstable SCr.[41] It important to note that if kidney function is unstable, measurement of CrCl by urine collection only reflects the function at the time of the measurement. The National Kidney Foundation indicates that these measured CrCls are not better than the estimates of CrCl provided through recommended equations.[5] However, a 24-hour timed urine measurement of CrCl may be useful in the following clinical situations: patients starting dialysis, patients with comorbid medical conditions, evaluation of patient dietary intake, patients with extremes in muscle mass, health enthusiasts taking creatine supplementation, vegetarians, patients with quadriplegia or paraplegia, and patients who have undergone amputation.[5]

### Interpreting Creatinine Clearance Values With Other Renal Parameters

As noted previously, the most common clinical uses for CrCl and SCr are as follows:

- Assessing kidney function in patients with CKD
- Monitoring the effects of drug therapy on slowing the progression of kidney disease
- Monitoring patients on nephrotoxic drugs
- Determining dosage adjustments for renally eliminated drugs

Because the relationship between SCr and CrCl is inverse and geometric as opposed to linear (**Figure 10-1**), significant declines in CrCl may occur before SCr rises above the normal range. For example, as CrCl slows, SCr rises little until there is a significant reduction in renal function. Therefore, SCr alone is not a sensitive indicator of early kidney dysfunction.

*Calculating creatinine clearance from a timed urine collection.* Although shorter collection periods (3 to 8 hours) appear to be adequate and may be more reliable, CrCl is routinely calculated using a 12-hour or 24-hour urine collection. Creatinine excretion is normally 20 to 28 mg/kg/24 h in men and 15 to 21 mg/kg/24 h in women. In children, normal excretion (mg/kg/24 h) should be approximately 15+ (0.5 × age), in which *age* is in years.

## MINICASE 1

## Estimating Equations for GFR

Marisela F., a 58-year-old woman (non–African American), arrives for routine follow-up after a recent diagnosis of type 2 diabetes mellitus. Her laboratory test results were as follows:

- Sodium, 138 mEq/L (136 to 145 mEq/L)
- Potassium, 4 mEq/L (3.5 to 5 mEq/L)
- Chloride, 102 mEq/L (96 to 106 mEq/L)
- Carbon dioxide, 25 mEq/L (24 to 30 mEq/L)
- Magnesium, 1.8 mEq/L (1.5 to 2.2 mEq/L)
- Glucose, 280 mg/dL (70 to 110 mg/dL)
- BUN, 19 mg/dL (8 to 20 mg/dL)
- SCr, 0.9 mg/dL (0.7 to 1.5 mg/dL)
- Urinary albumin: 1 mg
- Urinary creatinine: 18.5 g
- HbA1c, 11.4 (4% to 5.6%)

She is currently taking the following medications:

- Chlorthalidone 25 mg PO daily
- Metformin 1,000 mg PO twice daily

Her vital signs and information were as follows: height 5'5"; weight 125 lb; body mass index 20.8; BP 160/96 mm Hg; heart rate 94 beats/min; respiratory rate 18 beats/min; and temperature 101.6°F.

QUESTION: Which equation should be used to evaluate eGFR?

DISCUSSION: The CKD-EPI equation is preferred because it has greater accuracy compared with the MDRD equation. Using the 2009 CKD-EPI equation (12), the calculated eGFR for this patient is 71 mL/min/1.73 m² (stage G2). The MDRD equation is known to underestimate renal function for patients with an eGFR >60 mL/min/1.73 m², which may lead to falsely identifying patients with CKD. The CKD-EPI equation is more accurate when looking at an eGFR >60 mL/min/1.73 m².

QUESTION: How should the ACR be interpreted?

DISCUSSION: The ACR is 54 mg/g, which is elevated (≤30 mg/g). An elevated ACR may reflect damage to the glomerulus. However, the presence of fever, marked hyperglycemia as evidenced by the glucose and hemoglobin A1c, and elevated blood pressure may increase the ACR independently of kidney damage. Multiple abnormal readings are required to confirm albuminuria, and repeat testing is recommended.[5] If there was documentation of several abnormal ACR results over at least 3 months, the patient's albuminuria would be classified as category A2 (moderately increased) based on a finding of 54 mg/g.

QUESTION: How should the BUN:SCr ratio be interpreted?

DISCUSSION: The BUN:SCr ratio is >20:1. However, this ratio is not clinically significant because both the BUN and SCr are within normal limits. If one or both of the results were elevated, a BUN:SCr >20:1 would suggest a prerenal cause of acute renal impairment.

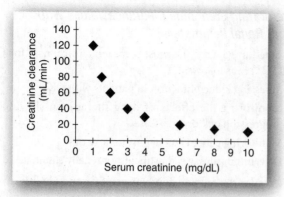

**FIGURE 10-1.** This plot represents the inverse relationship between SCr and CrCl. Relatively small changes in SCr at lower levels represent significant change in kidney function as assessed by CrCl.

Because its excretion remains relatively consistent within these ranges, UCr is often used as a check for completion of urine collection. In adults, some clinicians discount a urine sample if it contains <10 mg of creatinine/kg/24 h and assume that the collection was incomplete. However, 8.5 mg/kg/day might be a better cutoff, especially in critically ill elderly patients. UCr assays are affected by most of the same substances that affect SCr. To interfere significantly, however, the substance must appear in the urine in concentrations at least equal to those found in the blood.

Measured CrCl is calculated using the following formula:

$$CrCl\ (mL/min/1.73\,m^2) = [UCr \times V]/[Scr \times T] \times \frac{1.73}{BSA} \quad (2)$$

where *CrCl* is the CrCl in mL/min/1.73 m², *UCr* is urine creatinine concentration (mg/dL), *V* is volume of urine produced during the collection interval (mL), *SCr* is serum creatinine concentration (mg/dL), *T* is time of the collection interval (minutes), and *BSA* is body surface area (m²).

BSA can be estimated using the standard method of Dubois and Dubois[42]:

$$BSA\ (m^2) = 0.20247 \times height\ (m)^{0.725} \times weight\ (kg)^{0.425} \quad (3)$$

BSA also can be estimated using the following equations from Mosteller[43]:

$$BSA\ (m^2) = \sqrt{[height\ (cm) \times weight\ (kg)]/3{,}600} \quad (4)$$

$$BSA\ (m^2) = \sqrt{[height\ (in) \times weight\ (lb)]/3{,}131} \quad (5)$$

Adjustment of eGFR to a standard BSA (1.73 m²) allows direct comparison with normal CrCl ranges because such tables are in units of milliliters per minute per 1.73 m². The CrCl value adjusted for BSA is the number of milliliters cleared per minute for each 1.73 m² of the patient's BSA. Therefore, such adjustment in a large person (>1.73 m²) reduces the original nonadjusted clearance value because the assumption is that clearance would be lower if the patient were smaller. In practice, de-indexed values in which CrCl is in millimeters per minute should be used, and adjustment for body size is accomplished through a weight-based equation.

## Estimation of Creatinine Clearance

In practice, dosage recommendations for medications excreted through the kidneys have been traditionally based on the Cockcroft-Gault estimation of CrCl. With the implementation of standardized reporting of creatinine values, calculated CrCl values may be 5% to 20% higher and may not correlate with dosage guidelines based on renal dose adjustments on creatinine values from older assays.

***Cockcroft-Gault equation.*** This formula provides an estimation of CrCl.[37] The patient's age, body weight, and SCr concentration are necessary for the estimation. There is some controversy regarding which type of patient weight (total body weight [TBW], ideal body weight [IBW], adjusted body weight [ABW]) to use in the formula. Each weight affects the CrCl differently and may be preferred in certain situations over others. TBW may underestimate CrCl in underweight patients. In contrast, IBW was more accurate than TBW in normal weight patients. If TBW is less than IBW, use TBW to calculate CrCl. Lastly, ABW using a factor of 0.4 was found to be the least biased and most accurate method in patients who are obese because TBW overestimates the CrCl in this situation.[44]

Additional attempts to improve the Cockcroft-Gault equation include rounding the SCr when values are <1.0 mg/dL. By rounding the SCr to 1.0 mg/dL, the calculated CrCl is lower than the value given by using the actual SCr. A lower CrCl may lead to more conservative drug dosing. However, rounding of SCr has resulted in significant underestimation of CrCl.[45,46] The results of a meta-analysis suggest that actual SCr most closely estimates CrCl.[47] Based on the available data, rounding of SCr in elderly patients should be considered on a case-by-case basis because of limited evidence that this approach improves accuracy. Conflicting data exist for using lean body weight (LBW) to improve CrCl calculation in patients who are overweight, obese, or morbidly obese. Without clinical validation, both rounding of SCr and using lean body weight should be used cautiously.[46]

Additionally, this equation should be used cautiously in patients with unstable renal function. Instead, other methods, like cystatin C and the 6-variable MDRD equations, may provide more accurate results in critically ill patients with fluctuating renal function, but validation is lacking.[48]

$$CrCl\ (mL/min) = \frac{(140 - age) \times weight\ (kg)}{72 \times SCr\ (mg/dL)} \times 0.85\ (if\ female) \quad (6)$$

Body Weights Used with the Cockcroft-Gault Equation

| Weight (kg) | Calculation |
| --- | --- |
| TBW | Total body weight |
| IBW (male) | (2.3 x inches > 5 feet) + 50 kg |
| IBW (female) | (2.3 x inches > 5 feet) + 45.5 kg |
| ABW | IBW (kg) + 0.4 x (TBW (kg) – IBW (kg)) |

To illustrate the variations in CrCl based on different weights, consider a 50-year-old man with the following information: height 72" (182.88 cm); weight 115 kg; BMI 34.3; SCr 1.7 mg/dL.

The CrCl would be 84.6 mL/min with TBW, 57.1 mL/min using IBW, and 68.1 mL/min using ABW. These differences may affect diagnosis of CKD and renal dose adjustments for certain medications. Because the patient is obese, CrCl using TBW may overestimate the CrCl, whereas using ABW may provide a more accurate calculation.

**Estimation of Glomerular Filtration Rate–Modification of Diet in Renal Disease Equation.** The MDRD equation had been developed as a tool to identify patients at risk for complications arising from CKD.[14,49] (See **Table 10-2** for the stages of CKD.) Although the CKD-EPI equation is largely considered more accurate and less biased than the MDRD equation, some laboratories still use the MDRD equation for reporting eGFR. The MDRD equation provides an estimated GFR, which was developed using measured GFR I-iothalamate reference values in patients with CKD. The abbreviated MDRD equation has been reexpressed to include standardized SCr traceable to IDMS values.[11,39,50-52] Patients at age extremes may be particularly vulnerable to errors of estimated GFR.[9,13] In addition, results of the MDRD equation should be interpreted cautiously in patients with low muscle mass (eg, cachectic patients) or those with unstable renal function.

One well-known limitation identified with the MDRD equation is underestimation of renal function for patients with eGFR >60 mL/min/1.73 m[2,53] Because this study did not include patients with normal kidney function, the MDRD equation is considered particularly less accurate at higher GFRs.[54] This can lead to more patients being falsely identified with CKD. In these populations, the Kidney Disease: Improving Global Outcomes (KDIGO) working group recommends the measurement of cystatin C or direct measurement of CrCl when SCr concentration is less accurate.[5]

The original MDRD equation was also known as the 6-variable MDRD because it was based on six variables that included age, sex, ethnicity, SCr, urea, and albumin.[11] The

simplified 4-variable MDRD, shown below, uses four variables that include age, sex, ethnicity, and a revised calibration for SCr:

$$GFR\ (mL/min/1.73\ m^2) = 175 \times standardized\ SCr^{(-1.154)}$$
$$\times age^{(-0.203)} \times 1.212\ (if\ African\ American) \quad (7)$$
$$\times 0.742\ (if\ female)$$

## Estimation of Glomerular Filtration Rate–Chronic Kidney Disease Epidemiology Collaboration Creatinine Equation 2009

Introduced in 2009, the Chronic Kidney Disease Epidemiology Collaboration (CKD-EPI) equation is also based on standardized SCr, age, sex, and race. This equation performs with the same degree of accuracy as the MDRD equation for patients with eGFR <60 mL/min/1.73 m[2,55,56] However, it corrects the inadequacy of the MDRD equation, which leads to underestimations in patients with eGFR >60 mL/min/1.73 m[2]. Both the CKD-EPI and the MDRD equations account for age of the patient. Like all SCr-based equations, the Cockcroft-Gault, MDRD, and CKD-EPI equations succumb to the same inherent problems associated with this endogenous surrogate marker (ie, the formula should not be used in patients with unstable renal function). At the same SCr, younger patients who have more muscle mass have a higher GFR than older adults with low muscle mass. The usefulness of the CKD-EPI equation may be particularly evident in younger patients without kidney disease, younger patients with type 1 diabetes without microalbuminuria, or persons considering kidney donation with GFR rates approximating normal values. Additionally, data support its advantage over Cockcroft-Gault and MDRD in prognostic value in predicting cardiovascular mortality.[57] KDIGO currently recommends the CKD-EPI equation to estimate GFR.[5,55,56]:

$$GFR\ (mL/min/1.73\ m^2) = 141 \times min\ (S_c/\kappa,1)^{\alpha} \times$$
$$max\ (S_c/\kappa,1)^{-1.209} \times 0.993^{age} \times 1.018\ (if\ female) \times \quad (8)$$
$$1.159\ (if\ African\ American)$$

where $S_c$ = standardized SCr, $\kappa$ = 0.7 for women and 0.9 for men, $\alpha$ = −0.329 for women and −0.411 for men, *min* indicates the minimum of $S_c/\kappa$ or 1, and *max* indicates the maximum of $S_c/\kappa$ or 1.

## Cystatin C Equations

Recently, there has been calibration and standardization of traceable cystatin C concentrations to international reference standards. The 2012 NKF KDOQI Clinical Practice Guidelines for the Evaluation and Management of CKD recommend measuring cystatin C in adults with eGFR between 45 and 59 mL/min/1.73 m[2] who do not have confirmatory kidney damage.[5] The measurements of IDMS traceable cystatin C concentrations are not universally available in many community settings.

### *2012 Chronic Kidney Disease Epidemiology Collaboration Cystatin C Equation[5]:*

$$133 \times min\ (SCysC/0.8,1)^{-0.499} \times max\ (SCysC/0.8,1)^{-0.1328}$$
$$\times 0.996^{age} \times 0.932\ (if\ female) \quad (9)$$

**TABLE 10-2.** Chronic Kidney Disease Stages

| STAGE | GFR (ML/MIN/1.73 M²) | INTERPRETATION |
|---|---|---|
| 1* | >90 | Normal or high GFR |
| 2* | 60–89 | Mildly decreased |
| 3 | A 45–59 | Mildly to moderately decreased |
| | B 30–44 | Moderately to severely decreased |
| 4 | 15–29 | Significantly decreased |
| 5 | <15 | Kidney failure |

*In the absence of kidney damage, neither GFR category G1 nor G2 fulfil the criteria for CKD.
*Source*: Adapted with permission from Levey AS, Stevens PE, Bilous RW, et al. KDIGO 2012 Clinical practice guideline for the evaluation and management of chronic kidney disease. https://kdigo.org/guidelines/ckd-evaluation-and-management.

where SCysC is serum cystatin C (in mg/L), *min* indicates the minimum of SCysC/0.8 or 1, and *max* indicates the maximum of SCysC/0.8 or 1.

### *2012 Chronic Kidney Disease Epidemiology Collaboration Creatinine–Cystatin C Equation[5]:*

$$135 \times \min (SCr/k,1)^{\alpha} \times \max (SCr/k,1)^{-0.601} \times$$
$$\min (SCysC/0.8,1)^{-0.375} \times \max (SCysC/0.8,1)^{-0.711} \times$$
$$0.995^{age} \times (0.969 \text{ if female}) \times$$
$$(1.08 \text{ if African American}) \qquad (10)$$

where *SCr* is serum creatinine (in mg/dL), *SCysC* is serum cystatin C (in mg/L), *k* is 0.7 for women and 0.9 for men, α is −0.248 for women and −0.207 for men, *min(SCr/k, 1)* indicates the minimum of SCr/k or 1, *max(SCr/k, 1)* indicates the maximum of SCr/k or 1, *min(SCysC/0.8, 1)* indicates the minimum of SCysC/0.8 or 1, and *max(SCysC/0.8, 1)* indicates the maximum of SCysC/0.8 or 1.

***Clinical controversy: Cockcroft-Gault versus estimated glomerular filtration rate equations.*** The appropriate dosing of renally eliminated medications is necessary to prevent overdosage or underdosage. Overdosage of a medication can cause significant clinical consequences and contribute to poor patient outcomes. Similarly, underdosing medications can lead to therapeutic failures. In both scenarios, inappropriate medication dosing can lead to increased length of stay, higher healthcare costs, and preventable medication-related problems. The MDRD equation provides a more accurate estimation of kidney excretory function than the Cockcroft-Gault equation.[11,58,59] At this time, the optimal single best equation that can be used universally in all populations does not exist.

The usefulness of the MDRD equation in staging kidney disease is indisputable. Recently, manufacturers have provided some dosage guidance based on eGFR for patients with deteriorating kidney function. Recent studies support the agreement of the MDRD equation with measured GFR and FDA-assigned kidney function categories for medication dose adjustment.[60] The NKDEP in 2009 suggested the use of either the CrCl as estimated by Cockcroft-Gault or the eGFR for dosing medications in CKD for most patients.[61] However, this is controversial because most renal drug dosing is still based on CrCl. An important caveat that is often overlooked in the NKDEP recommendation is that the eGFR needs to be individualized in patients at the extremes in body size by multiplying the eGFR/1.73 m[2] by patient BSA to convert units to milliliters per minute:

$$\text{Individualized MDRD} = eGFR/1.73 \text{ m}^2 \times$$
$$\text{estimated BSA (m}^2) = eGFR \text{ for drug dosing} \qquad (11)$$

Alternatively, in patients who are considered to be high risk for adverse medication events, who are taking drugs that have a narrow therapeutic index, or in whom estimations of kidney function vary or are inaccurate, consider measuring CrCl or GFR using exogenous markers.[5] The Nephrology Practice and Research Network of the American College of Clinical Pharmacy

has suggested an algorithm for dosing medications eliminated by the kidneys using SCr-based equations.[62] Additionally, safety and efficacy considerations affect decisions regarding dosing of renally eliminated medications that include both patient factors (clinical condition, cachexia) and drug-specific properties (therapeutic index). In summary, individualized patient characteristics and the specific clinical situation necessitate medication dosing decisions based on benefits and risks rather them numbers purely derived from generalized equations.

## MEDICATION SAFETY

Pharmacists are responsible for optimizing the use of medications in their patients. Medications eliminated by the kidneys require caution in patients with acute kidney disease and CKD because the need for modifying the drug dose, extending the dosing interval, discontinuing use, and totally avoiding nephrotoxic drugs must be considered. Drug manufacturers provide drug information for use in patients with diminished renal function. Serum levels of medications that depend on renal elimination can be elevated, contributing to the increased likelihood of drug toxicity and subsequent adverse drug reactions. As mentioned, the use of eGFR estimating equations or direct measurements of CrCl, where appropriate, can provide important information for medication use and drug dosing. In situations in which SCr is not suitable, consider the use of a cystatin C equation (Equation 14).[5] Ensuring appropriate medication use and dosing in patients with acute kidney disease and CKD is one of the major contributions made by pharmacists. In acute kidney disease, temporarily hold administration of drugs that may contribute to or exacerbate kidney damage. **Table 10-3** identifies medication safety considerations for use in patients with acute or chronic kidney disease. However, specific medication recommendations from more than one reference should be reviewed before committing to dosing decisions (**Minicase 2**).

## URINALYSIS

*Urinalysis* is a commonly used clinical tool for the evaluation of various renal and nonrenal problems (eg, endocrine, metabolic, and genetic). A routine urinalysis is performed as a screening test during many hospital admissions and initial physician visits. It is also performed periodically in patients in nursing homes and other settings. The most common components of the urinalysis are discussed here.

An accurate interpretation of a urinalysis can be made only if the urine specimen is properly collected and handled. Techniques are fairly standardized and, keeping in mind that urine is normally sterile, aim to avoid contamination by normal flora of the external environment (mucous membranes of the vagina or uncircumcised penis or by microorganisms on the hands). Therefore, these areas are cleansed and physically kept away from the urine stream. During menses or heavy vaginal secretions, a fresh tampon should be inserted before cleansing.

A first-morning, midstream collection is customarily used as the specimen.[69] Once voided, the urine should be brought to the laboratory as soon as possible to prevent deterioration. If the sample is not refrigerated, bacteria multiply and use glucose (if present) as a food

**TABLE 10-3.** Medication Safety in Patients with CKD

| AGENTS | CAUTIONARY NOTES |
| --- | --- |
| **Antihypertensives/cardiac medications** | |
| RAAS antagonists (ACE-I, ARB, aldosterone antagonists, direct renin inhibitors) | • Avoid in people with suspected functional renal artery stenosis<br>• Start at lower dose in people with GFR <45 mL/min/1.73 m²<br>• Assess GFR and measure serum potassium within 1 wk of starting or following any dose escalation<br>• Temporarily suspend during intercurrent illness, planned IV radiocontrast administration, bowel preparation prior to colonoscopy, or before major surgery<br>• Do not routinely discontinue in people with GFR <30 mL/min/1.73 m² because they remain nephroprotective |
| β-blockers<br>Digoxin | • Reduce dose by 50% in people with GFR <30 mL/min/1.73 m²<br>• Reduce dose based on plasma concentrations |
| **Analgesics** | |
| NSAIDs | • Avoid in people with GFR <30 mL/min/1.73 m²<br>• Prolonged therapy is not recommended in people with GFR <60 mL/min/1.73 m²<br>• Should not be used in people taking lithium<br>• Avoid in people taking RAAS blocking agents |
| Opioids | • Reduce dose when GFR <60 mL/min/1.73 m²<br>• Use with caution in people with GFR <15 mL/min/1.73 m² |
| **Antimicrobials** | |
| Penicillin | • Risk of crystalluria when GFR <15 mL/min/1.73 m² with high doses<br>• Neurotoxicity with benzylpenicillin when GFR <15 mL/min/1.73 m² with high doses (maximum 6 g/day) |
| Aminoglycosides | • Reduce dose and increase dosage interval when GFR <60 mL/min/1.73 m²<br>• Monitor serum levels (trough and peak)<br>• Avoid concomitant ototoxic agents such as furosemide |
| Macrolides | • Reduce dose by 50% when GFR <30 mL/min/1.73 m² |
| Fluoroquinolones | • Reduce dose by 50% when GFR <15 mL/min/1.73 m² |
| Tetracyclines | • Reduce dose when GFR <45 mL/min/1.73 m²; can exacerbate uremia |
| Antifungals | • Avoid amphotericin unless no alternative when GFR <60 mL/min/1.73 m²<br>• Reduce maintenance dose of fluconazole by 50% when GFR <45 mL/min/1.73 m²<br>• Reduce dose of flucytosine when GFR <60 mL/min/1.73 m² |
| **Hypoglycemics** | |
| Sulfonylureas | • Avoid agents that are mainly renally excreted (eg, glyburide/glibenclamide)<br>• Other agents that are mainly metabolized in the liver may need reduced dose when GFR <30 mL/min/1.73 m² (eg, gliclazide, gliquidone) |
| Insulin | • Partly renally excreted and may need reduced dose when GFR <30 mL/min/1.73 m² |
| Metformin | • Suggest avoiding when GFR <30 mL/min/1.73 m² but consider risk–benefit if GFR is stable<br>• Review use when GFR <45 mL/min/1.73 m²<br>• Probably safe when GFR ≥45 mL/min/1.73 m²<br>• Suspend in people who become acutely unwell |
| GLP-1 RA[1] | • Renal dose adjustment required (exenatide, lixisenatide)<br>• Caution when initiating or increasing dose due to potential risk of AKI<br>• Benefit in slowing progression of diabetic kidney disease with liraglutide |

(continued)

## TABLE 10-3. Medication Safety in Patients with CKD, cont'd

| AGENTS | CAUTIONARY NOTES |
|---|---|
| SGLT2i[1] | • Renal dose adjustment required<br>• Benefit in slowing progression of diabetic kidney disease with canagliflozin, empagliflozin, dapagliflozin<br>• Talk about cutoffs with the four |
| **Lipid-lowering** | |
| Statins | • No increase in toxicity for simvastatin dosed at 20 mg per day or simvastatin 20 mg/ezetimide 10-mg combinations per day in people with GFR <30 mL/min/1.73 m² or on dialysis[83]<br>• Other trials of statins in people with GFR <15 mL/min/1.73 m² or on dialysis also showed no excess toxicity |
| Fenofibrate | • Increases SCr by ~0.13 mg/dL (12 μmol/L) |
| **Chemotherapeutic** | |
| Cisplatin | • Reduce dose when GFR <60 mL/min/1.73 m²<br>• Avoid when GFR <30 mL/min/1.73 m² |
| Melphalan | • Reduce dose when GFR <60 mL/min/1.73 m² |
| Methotrexate | • Reduce dose when GFR <60 mL/min/1.73 m²<br>• Avoid if possible when GFR <15 mL/min/1.73 m² |
| **Anticoagulants** | |
| Low-molecular-weight heparins | • Halve the dose when GFR <30 mL/min/1.73 m²<br>• Consider switch to conventional heparin or alternatively monitor plasma antifactor Xa in persons at high risk for bleeding |
| Warfarin | • Increased risk of bleeding when GFR <30 mL/min/1.73 m²<br>• Use lower doses and monitor closely when GFR <30 mL/min/1.73 m² |
| DOAC | • Edoxaban is not approved for patients with poor renal function (CrCl <30 mL/min) or upper range renal function (CrCl >95 mL/min)<br>• Renal dose adjustment needed at different CrCl levels based on each DOAC and specific indication due to lack of clinical trial data on safety or efficacy in patients with advanced CKD |
| **Miscellaneous** | |
| Lithium | • Nephrotoxic and may cause renal tubular dysfunction with prolonged use even at therapeutic levels<br>• Monitor GFR, electrolytes, and lithium levels monthly or more frequently if the dose changes or the patient is acutely unwell<br>• Avoid using concomitant NSAIDs<br>• Maintain hydration during intercurrent illness<br>• Risk–benefit of drug in specific situation must be weighed |
| Radiocontrast agents | • Use with caution in advanced renal disease<br>• Iodinated and ionic iodinated contrast media may cause acute renal failure as serious adverse effect<br>• Iodinated and ionic iodinated contrast media contraindicated in severe CKD (GFR <30 mL/min/1.73 m²) or in AKI |

ACE-I = angiotensin-converting enzyme inhibitor; ARB = angiotensin-receptor blocker; DOAC = direct oral anticoagulant; GLP-1 RA = glucagon-like peptide-1 receptor agonists; KDIGO = Kidney Disease: Improving Global Outcomes; RAAS = renin-angiotensin-aldosterone system.
Data as of January 2013.
*Source:* Reproduced with permission from KDIGO[5]; adapted from References 63–68.

# MINICASE 2

## Heart Failure

Elle K., an 83-year-old woman with a long history of congestive heart failure, is admitted to the hospital with reports of shortness of breath (she has been sleeping in her recliner and is unable to sleep in her bed despite using two pillows), a 15-lb weight gain, and fluid retention in her lower extremities. She also has anorexia, nausea, fatigue, and weakness. All have worsened over the past 2 weeks.

Physical examination reveals a frail (5'3", 78 kg) woman in moderate distress; heart rate 108 beats/min; BP 96/60 mm Hg; S3/S4 heart sounds; and +3 pitting edema bilateral lower extremities. Chest radiograph reveals bilateral pleural effusions. Past medical history is significant for hypertension, osteoarthritis of the knee, and atrial fibrillation.

Her current medications include the following:

- Lisinopril, 20 mg PO daily
- Metoprolol succinate, 100 mg PO daily
- Furosemide, 40 mg PO daily
- KCl, 10 mEq PO twice daily
- Ibuprofen, 400 mg PO four times daily PRN for knee pain

Laboratory test results are as follows:

- Sodium, 130 mEq/L (136 to 142 mEq/L)
- Potassium, 3.2 mEq/L (3.8 to 5 mEq/L)
- Chloride, 96 mEq/L (95 to 103 mEq/L)
- Carbon dioxide, 30 mEq/L (24 to 30 mEq/L or mmol/L)
- Magnesium, 1.6 mEq/L (1.3 to 2.1 mEq/L)
- Glucose, 78 mg/dL (70 to 110 mg/dL)
- Hgb, 11.5 g/dL (12.3 to 15.3 g/dL)
- BUN, 76 mg/dL (8 to 23 mg/dL)
- SCr, 2.5 mg/dL (0.6 to 1.2 mg/dL)
- BNP, 1,200 pg/mL (<100 pg/mL)
- Urinalysis, normal

Over the next 2 days, Elle K. receives aggressive diuretic therapy (intravenous [IV] furosemide 80 mg twice a day), and all electrolyte abnormalities were corrected. Her physical exam results were much improved, and she was no longer short of breath.

On the morning of day 4, her laboratory results were as follows:

- Sodium, 135 mEq/L
- Potassium, 3.2 mEq/L
- Chloride, 100 mEq/L
- Carbon dioxide, 34 mEq/L
- Magnesium, 1.4 mEq/L
- Glucose, 80 mg/dL
- Hgb, 11.4 g/dL
- BUN, 40 mg/dL
- SCr, 1.9 mg/dL
- BNP, 400 pg/mL

QUESTION: What type of renal dysfunction was this patient experiencing on admission to the hospital? What are the likely causes of her elevated BUN and SCr? Which formula would be best to estimate CrCl or eGFR?

DISCUSSION: This is a rather complex case because of the involvement of the kidneys in heart failure. Initially, the elevated BUN and SCr could be attributed to a prerenal state secondary to increased edema (hypervolemia) caused by worsening heart failure. This is supported by her clinical presentation (weight gain, symptoms of heart failure, chest X-ray, elevated BNP, and an elevated BUN:SCr ratio with a ratio of >20:1). A normal urinalysis would not reveal any cells that may indicate an intrinsic AKI (see Urinalysis section). Additionally, diuretics may increase BUN, which may complicate the picture, but the other evidence supports the diagnosis of prerenal azotemia. Assessment of kidney function on day 1 is difficult because the Cockcroft-Gault, MDRD, or CKD-EPI equation should not be used in patients with acute alterations in kidney function. In suspected cases of AKI and when there is a need to assess GFR, measurement of CrCl through collection of urine may be considered; however, this technique is associated with significant limitations in the setting of rapidly changing renal function.

QUESTION: What factors may have contributed to this patient's heart failure exacerbation?

DISCUSSION: She has several risk factors that can worsen heart failure. She has a history of hypertension and atrial fibrillation. If her osteoarthritis has worsened, she may have been using more ibuprofen more frequently and for an extended period of time. Additional risk factors that could also contribute to exacerbation of heart failure include nonadherence to medications (eg, furosemide) and noncompliance with fluid (2 L) and diet (2 g sodium/day) restriction recommendations.

QUESTION: What other electrolyte abnormalities have resulted?

DISCUSSION: Several electrolyte abnormalities were identified during initial presentation and subsequent laboratory analysis: increased BUN and SCr, increased serum bicarbonate, hypokalemia, hypomagnesemia, and hyponatremia. On admission, worsening heart failure resulted in decreased RBF. As with creatinine, there will be a reduction in BUN filtration at the glomerulus; however, urea is avidly reabsorbed in the proximal tubule (following sodium and water), resulting in an elevated ratio of BUN out of proportion to the creatinine (>20:1). This patient also presented initially with hypervolemic hyponatremia, most likely caused by worsening heart failure, diminished blood flow to the kidneys, peripheral edema, and subsequent weight gain. As she becomes euvolemic, the hyponatremia will gradually be corrected. After aggressive diuresis with IV furosemide, hypokalemia and hypomagnesemia require replacement therapy. Loop diuretics can also cause metabolic alkalosis (increased serum bicarbonate). Overaggressive diuresis can cause elevations in BUN and SCr without evidence of overt heart failure.

source. Subsequently, glucose concentrations decrease and ketones may evaporate with prolonged standing. Another problem is that formed elements (see Microscopic Analysis section) begin decomposing within 2 hours. With excessive exposure to light, bilirubin and urobilinogen are oxidized. Unlike other substances, however, protein is minimally affected by prolonged standing.

After a urine sample is collected, it may undergo three types of testing: macroscopic, microscopic, and chemical (dipstick).

## Macroscopic Analysis (General Appearance)

The color of normal urine varies greatly—from totally clear to dark yellow or amber—depending on the concentration of solutes. Color comes primarily from the pigments urochrome and urobilin. Fresh normal urine is not cloudy or hazy, but urine may become cloudy if urates (in an acid environment) or phosphates (in an alkaline environment) crystallize or precipitate out of solution. These salts become less soluble as the urine cools from body temperature.

Turbidity may also occur when large numbers of RBCs or white blood cells (WBCs) are present. An unusual amount of foam may be from protein or bile acids. **Table 10-4** lists causes of different urine colors. Some of the changes noted may be urine pH–dependent. In general, drug-induced changes in urine color are fairly rare. Drugs that cause or exacerbate any of the medical problems listed in Table 10-4 can also be considered indirect causes of discolored urine.

## Microscopic Analysis (Formed Elements)

Microscopic analysis typically involves the following steps[71]:

- Centrifuging the urine (12 mL) at 2,000 revolutions per minute for 5 minutes
- Pouring off all "loose" supernatant
- Mixing the sediment with the residual supernatant
- Examining the resulting suspension under 400 to 440× magnification (also described as high-power field)

**TABLE 10-4.** Potential Causes of Various Urine Coloring

| COLOR | CAUSE | POSSIBLE UNDERLYING ETIOLOGIES |
|---|---|---|
| Red to orange | Myoglobin | Crush injuries, electric shock, seizures, cocaine-induced muscle damage, rhabdomyolysis |
| | Hemoglobin/ erythrocytes | Hemolysis (malaria, drugs, strenuous exercise), menstrual contamination; kidney stones |
| | Porphyrins | Porphyria, lead poisoning, liver disease |
| | Drugs/chemicals | Drugs/chemicals causing previously mentioned diseases; as dyes: rifampin, isoniazid, riboflavin, sulfasalazine, warfarin, chlorpromazine, thioridazine, phenazopyridine, daunorubicin, doxorubicin, phenolphthalein, phenothiazines, senna, chlorzoxazone, hydroxocobalamin |
| | Food | Beets, rhubarb, blackberries, cold drink dyes, carrots |
| Blue to green | Biliverdin | Oxidation of bilirubin (poorly preserved specimen) |
| | Bacteria | *Pseudomonas* or *Proteus* in urinary tract infections (rare), particularly in urine drainage bags |
| | Drugs/chemicals | As dyes: amitriptyline, azuresin, methylene blue, Clorets abuse, Clinitest ingestion, mitoxantrone, triamterene, resorcinol, promethazine, cimetidine, amitriptyline, metoclopramide, indomethacin, and propofol |
| Brown to black | Myoglobin | Crush injuries, electric shock, seizures, cocaine-induced muscle damage, rhabdomyolysis |
| | Bile pigments | Hemolysis, bleed into tissues, liver disease |
| | Melanin | Melanoma (prolonged exposure to air) |
| | Methemoglobin | Methemoglobinemia from drugs, dyes |
| | Porphyrins | Porphyria and sickle cell crisis |
| | Drugs/chemicals | As dyes: cascara, chloroquine, clofazimine, emodin, senna; as chemicals: ferrous salts, methocarbamol, metronidazole, nitrofurantoin, sulfonamides, sorbitol, α-methyldopa, statins, L-dopa |

*Source*: Adapted from References 70–73.

Microscopic analysis can be done either routinely or selectively. In either case, one should look for the three "Cs"—cells, casts, and crystals.

## Cells

Theoretically, no cells should be seen during microscopic examination of urine. In practice, however, an occasional cell or two is found. These cells include microorganisms, RBCs, WBCs, and tubular epithelial cells.

**Microorganisms (normal range: zero to trace).** If bacteria are found in the urine sediment, contamination should be the first consideration. Of course, fungi, bacteria, and other single-cell organisms can be seen in patients with a urinary tract infection (UTI) or colonization. Even if ordered, some laboratories do not perform urine cultures unless there is significant bacteriuria. *Significant bacteriuria* may be defined as an initial positive dipstick screen for leukocyte esterase and nitrites (Chemical Analysis section). Likewise, some laboratories do not process cultures further (eg, identification, quantification, and susceptibility) if more than one or two different bacterial species are seen on initial plating. Additionally, some laboratories do not perform susceptibility testing if more than one organism (some more than two) is isolated or if <100,000 (some use 50,000 as the cutoff) colony-forming units (CFU) per milliliter per organism are measured with a midstream, clean-catch sample. The common cutoff for urine obtained through a catheter is <10,000 CFU/mL/organism. If multiple types of bacteria are present, contamination by flora from vaginal, rectal, hand, skin, or other body site is assumed.

**Red blood cells (erythrocytes) (normal range: one to three per high-power field).** Hematuria is the abnormal renal excretion of erythrocytes detected in two of three urine samples. A few RBCs are occasionally found in the urine of a healthy man or woman, particularly after exertion, trauma, or fever. If persistent, even small numbers (more than two to three per high-powered field) may reflect urinary tract pathology. Increased numbers of RBCs are seen (among others) in glomerulonephritis, infection (pyelonephritis), renal infarction or papillary necrosis, tumors, stones, and coagulopathies. In some of these disorders, hematuria may turn the urine pink or red (gross hematuria). If a specimen is not collected properly, vaginal blood may contaminate the urine.

**White blood cells (leukocytes) (normal range: zero to two per high-power field).** Potentially significant pyuria has been defined as three or more WBCs per high-power field of centrifuged urine sediment. Pyuria is usually associated with UTIs (upper or lower). However, inflammatory conditions (glomerulonephritis, interstitial nephritis) may also lead to this finding.[71,72]

**Epithelial cells (normal range: zero to one per high-power field).** Epithelial cells may be categorized as either squamous or nonsquamous. Squamous cells originate from the surfaces of external genitalia and the lower urinary tract. Presence of a large number of squamous epithelial cells usually suggests specimen contamination.[74,75]

**Tubular epithelial cells (normal range: zero or one per high-power field).** One epithelial cell per high-power field is often found in normal subjects. Cells originating from the renal tubules are small, oval, and mononuclear. Nonsquamous epithelial cells include transitional cells and renal tubular epithelial cells, and their presence indicates acute tubular necrosis, acute interstitial nephritis, and proliferative glomerulonephritis.[75] Their quantity increases dramatically when the tubules are damaged (eg, acute tubular necrosis) or when there is inflammation from interstitial nephritis or glomerulonephritis.[71]

## Casts

*Casts* are cylindrical masses of glycoproteins (eg, Tamm-Horsfall mucoprotein) that form in the tubules. Casts have relatively smooth and regular margins (as opposed to clumps of cells) because they conform to the shape of the tubular lumen. Under certain conditions, casts are released into the urine (called *cylindruria*). Even normal urine can contain a few clear casts. These formed elements are fragile and dissolve more quickly in warm, alkaline urine. Types include hyaline, cellular, granular, and waxy (broad); their causes are listed in **Table 10-5**.

**TABLE 10-5.** Causes of Various Types of Casts in Urine

| CAST | CAUSE |
|---|---|
| Red blood cell | Classically seen with acute glomerulonephritis; can be seen in patients who play contact sports and uncommonly with tubular interstitial disease |
| White blood cell | Classically seen with urinary tract infections and cystitis; also seen with glomerulonephritis and interstitial nephritis |
| Squamous epithelial cell | Nonspecific and may not be pathologic; seen with perineal or vaginal specimen contamination in females or foreskin contamination in males |
| Tubular epithelial cell | Nonspecific; acute tubular necrosis, glomerulonephritis, tubulointerstitial disease; also seen with cytomegalovirus infection and toxicity from salicylates and heavy metals, ethylene glycol |
| Hyaline | Nonspecific and may not be pathologic; seen with prerenal azotemia and strenuous exercise |
| Granular | Nonspecific but pathologic; may be seen in acute tubular necrosis; volume depletion, glomerulonephritis, tubulointerstitial disease |
| Waxy (broad) | Nonspecific but pathologic; may be seen with advanced or chronic renal failure |

Source: Adapted with permission from References 71,72,74.

**Hyaline casts.** Being clear, hyaline casts are difficult to observe under a microscope and are, by themselves, not indicative of disease. Hyaline casts can be seen in concentrated urine or with the use of diuretics.[72,75]

**Cellular casts.** In contrast to hyaline casts, cellular casts are seen with intrinsic renal disease. They form when leukocytes, RBCs, or renal tubular epithelial cells become entrapped in the gelatinous matrix forming in the tubule. Their clinical significance is the same as that of the cells themselves; unlike free cells, however, cells in casts originate from within the kidneys. The identification of a particular cast-type is often used to assist in diagnosis. WBC casts suggest intrarenal inflammation (eg, acute interstitial nephritis) or pyelonephritis. Epithelial cell casts suggest tubular destruction; they may also be noted in glomerulonephritis. RBC casts are seen in glomerulonephritis.[71,75]

**Granular and waxy casts.** Granular and waxy casts are older, degenerated forms of the other types. Granular (also called *muddy brown*) casts can be seen in many conditions, such as acute tubular necrosis, glomerulonephritis, and tubulointerstitial disease. Because waxy casts occur in many diseases, they do not offer much diagnostic information.[71,75]

### Crystals

The presence of *crystals* in the urine depends on urinary pH, the degree of saturation of the urine by the substance that is forming crystals, and the presence of other substances in the urine that may promote crystallization. Numerous types of crystals can be detected in the urine (**Figure 10-2**). Crystalluria, if differentiated by type, can help identify patients with certain local and systemic diseases. Cystine crystals occur with the condition cystinuria, and struvite (magnesium ammonium phosphate) crystals are seen with struvite stones. Calcium oxalate, calcium phosphate, and uric acid crystals are also suggestive of stones. Many crystals can be detected in otherwise healthy patients.[70,75]

## CHEMICAL ANALYSIS (SEMIQUANTITATIVE TESTS, URINE DIPSTICK TESTS)

For this discussion, biochemical analysis of urine includes protein; pH; specific gravity; bilirubin, bile, and urobilinogen; blood and hemoglobin; leukocyte esterase; nitrite; glucose; and ketones. These semiquantitative tests can be performed quickly using modern dipsticks containing one or more reagent-impregnated pads. When using these strips, the clinician must carefully apply the urine to the pads as instructed and wait the designated time before comparing pad colors to the color chart. Possible results associated with various colors are displayed in **Table 10-6**.

### Protein

*Normal range: zero to trace on dipstick or <200 mg/g (urine protein to creatinine ratio)*

The normal urinary proteins are albumin and low molecular weight serum globulins. However, albumin has a molecular weight of 66,000 Da and is typically restricted from passing through the glomerulus into the urine. The smaller serum globulins that are filtered in the nephron are generally reabsorbed in the proximal tubule. Therefore, healthy individuals excrete small amounts of protein in the urine (80 to <150 mg of protein per day). In the presence of kidney damage, larger quantities of protein may be excreted. Increased excretion of albumin is associated with diabetic nephropathy, glomerular disease, and uncontrolled hypertension. If low molecular globulins are detected, it is more likely a tubulointerstitial process. The term *proteinuria* is a general term that refers to the renal loss of protein (albumin and globulins). The term *albuminuria* specifically refers to the abnormal renal excretion of albumin. Clinical proteinuria is defined as the loss of >500 mg/day of protein urine. Patients with microalbuminuria are excreting relatively small, but still pathogenic, amounts (30 to 300 mg/day) of albumin. Common causes of proteinuria are listed in **Table 10-7**. It should be noted that proteinuria is sometimes intermittent and is not always pathologic (eg, after exercise and fever).

Because of difficulties with overnight and 24-hour collections, KDIGO recommends spot (untimed) urine testing. The ACR ratio is convenient and accounts for urine volume effects on protein concentration and standardizes the protein or albumin excretion to creatinine excretion. The ratio of protein (or albumin) to creatinine in an untimed urine sample is an accurate estimate of the total amount of protein (or albumin) excreted in the urine over 24 hours.[5] The current criteria for staging and prognosis of CKD recommends testing for albuminuria. The KDIGO working group recommends the urine ACR ratio as the preferred method to assess for kidney damage in addition to estimation of GFR. Like GFR, albuminuria should be assessed at least annually in patients with CKD and more frequently in high-risk populations in whom measurements may affect clinical decisions.[5]

Color indicator test strips (eg, Albustix, Multistix) used to detect and measure protein in the urine contain a buffer mixed with a dye (usually tetrabromophenol blue). In the absence of albumin, the buffer holds the pH at 3, maintaining a yellow color. If albumin is present, it reduces the activity coefficient of hydrogen ions (the pH rises), producing a blue color. Of note, these tests are fairly insensitive to the presence of low molecular globulins, including the Bence-Jones protein. Results can be affected by the urinary concentration. At both extremes of urinary concentrations, false-positive and false-negative results may occur. The potential for this can be easily assessed if specific gravity is measured concomitantly. Substances that cause abnormal urine color may affect the readability of the strips, including blood, bilirubin, phenazopyridine nitrofurantoin, and riboflavin.[78] Standard dipsticks do not detect microalbuminuria; however, newer dye-impregnated strips are available that can detect lower concentrations of albumin. The KIDIGO recommends confirming positive albuminuria test strips with quantitative laboratory measurements as a ratio to creatinine when possible.[5]

### pH

*Normal range: 4.6 to 8*

Sulfuric acid, resulting from the metabolism of sulfur-containing amino acids, is the primary acid generated by the

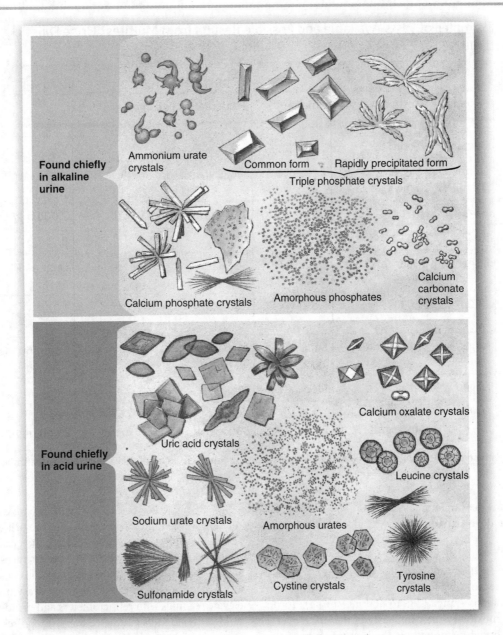

**FIGURE 10-2.** Inorganic elements that may be found in urinary sediment. Elements founds in alkaline urine are shown in the top half of the figure; those found in acidic urine are represented in the bottom half of the figure. *Source*: Reprinted with permission from Runge MS, Greganti MA. *Netter's Internal Medicine*. 2nd ed. Philadelphia, PA: Saunders; 2008:766. Copyright© 2008. Netter medical illustration used with permission of Elsevier. All rights reserved.

daily ingestion of food. The pH is usually estimated in 0.5-unit increments by use of test strips containing methyl red and bromthymol blue indicators. These strips undergo a series of color changes from orange to blue over a pH range of 5 to 8.5. Additionally, pH can be precisely measured with electronic pH meters. Normally, the kidneys can eliminate the acid load by excreting acid itself and sodium hydroxide ions. In fact, healthy persons can acidify urine to pH 4.5, although the average pH is around 6. Any pH close to the reference range can be interpreted as normal as long as it reflects the kidneys' attempts at regulating blood pH. Urinary pH can be affected by the various acid–base disorders. Determination of the urinary pH is often used in the setting of a UTI.[74,75] In general, acidic (versus neutral) urine deters bacterial colonization. Alkaline urine may be seen with either UTIs caused by urea-splitting bacteria, such as *Proteus mirabilis* (via ammonia production), or tubular defects causing decreased net tubular hydrogen ion secretion, as in renal tubular acidosis.

By their intended or unintended pharmacological actions, drugs can also cause true pH changes; they do not interfere with the reagents used to estimate urine pH. Drugs that induce diseases associated with pH changes are indirect causes. These and other causes of acidic and alkaline urine are listed in **Table 10-8**. Persistent pHs >7 are associated with calcium carbonate, calcium

**TABLE 10-6.** Examples of Tests Available and Possible Results from Multitest Urine Dipstick (Bayer Multistix 10 SG)

| TEST | RESULT | | | | | | |
|---|---|---|---|---|---|---|---|
| Leukocyte esterase | Negative | Trace | Small + | Moderate ++ | Large +++ | | |
| Nitrite | Negative | Positive | | | | | |
| Urobilinogen | Normal 0.2 mg/dL | Normal 1 mg/dL | 2 mg/dL | 4 mg/dL | 8 mg/dL | | |
| Protein | Negative | Trace | 30 mg/dL + | 100 mg/dL ++ | 300 mg/dL +++ | 2,000 mg/dL ++++ | |
| pH | 5 | 6 | 6.5 | 7 | 7.5 | 8 | 8.5 |
| Blood (Hgb) | Negative | Nonhemolyzed trace | Hemolyzed trace | Small + | Moderate ++ | Large +++ | |
| Specific gravity | 1.000 | 1.005 | 1.010 | 1.015 | 1.020 | 1.025 | 1.030 |
| Ketones | Negative | Trace 5 mg/dL | Small 15 mg/dL | Moderate 40 mg/dL | Large 80 mg/dL | Large 160 mg/dL | |
| Bilirubin | Negative | Small + | Moderate ++ | Large +++ | | | |
| Glucose | Negative | 1/10 g/dL (trace) 100 mg/dL | 1/4 g/dL 250 mg/dL | 1/2 g/dL 500 mg/dL | 1 g/dL 1,000 mg/dL | 2 g/dL 2,000 mg/dL | |

*Source*: Adapted with permission from Multistix (various) Reagent Strips [product information]. Elkhart, IN: Bayer HealthCare LLC; 2005.

phosphate, and magnesium–ammonium phosphate stones; pHs <5.5 are associated with cystine and uric acid stones.

## Specific Gravity

*Normal range: 1.016 to 1.022 (normal fluid intake)*
The kidneys are responsible for maintaining the blood's osmolality within a narrow range (285 to 300 mOsm/kg). To do so, the kidneys must vary the osmolality of the urine over a wide range. Although osmolality is the best measure of the kidneys' concentrating ability, determining osmolality is difficult. Fortunately, it correlates well with specific gravity when urine contains normal constituents. *Specific gravity* is the ratio of the weight of a given fluid to the weight of an equal volume of distilled water. Sodium, urea, sulfate, and phosphate contribute most to the specific gravity of urine. Because specific gravity is related to the weight (and not the number) of particles in solution, particles with a weight different from that of sodium chloride (the solute usually in the highest concentration there) can widen the disparity. Patients with normal kidney function can dilute urine to approximately 1.001 and concentrate urine to 1.035, which correlates to an osmolality of 50 to 1,000 mOsm/kg, respectively. A urinary specific gravity of 1.010 is considered isosthenuric; that is, the urinary osmolality is the same as plasma.[71,72,74]

Specific gravity can be measured by reagent strips (dipstick), a urinometer (hydrometer), or a refractometer. The reagent strips change color based on the $pK_a$ change of the strips in relation to the ionic concentration of the urine. The indicator substance on the strip changes color, which can be then correlated to the specific gravity. Specific gravity measured by reagent strips is not affected by high concentrations of substances such as glucose, protein, or radiographic contrast media, which may elevate readings with refractometers and urinometers. The urinometer is akin to a graduated buoy; it requires sufficient urine volume to float freely. The reading is adjusted according to the urine temperature. The refractometer uses the refractive index as a basis and needs only a few milliliters of urine and no temperature adjustment.[71,72,74]

Several conditions can affect specific gravity. In general, urinary specific gravity should be considered abnormal if it is the opposite (high versus low and vice versa) of that which should be produced based on the concurrent plasma osmolality. Patients who are volume depleted should present with a concentrated urine (specific gravity ≥1.020) as a normal compensatory mechanism. Patients with prerenal disease will likely have relatively concentrated urine, whereas patients with intrinsic damage to the renal tubules are more likely to produce urine, which is isosthenuric (the tubules are unable to dilute or concentrate the urine, so the urine is the same concentration as the filtrate). The urine of patients with diabetes insipidus has low values (<1.005) despite a relatively hypertonic plasma. On the other hand, patients with the syndrome of inappropriate syndrome

## TABLE 10-7. Causes of Proteins in Urine

Mild proteinuria (<0.5 g/day)

High blood pressure

Lower UTI

Fever

Renal tubular damage

Exercise

Moderate proteinuria (0.5–3 g/day)

Congestive heart failure

Chronic glomerulonephritis

Acute glomerulonephritis

Diabetic nephropathy

Pyelonephritis

Multiple myeloma

Preeclampsia of pregnancy

Rhabdomyolysis

Significant proteinuria (>3 g/day)

Glomerulonephritis

Amyloid

Chronic glomerulonephritis (severe)

Diabetic nephropathy

Lupus nephritis

Rhabdomyolysis

*Source*: Adapted with permission from Sacher RA, McPherson RA. Laboratory assessment of body fluids. *Widmann's Clinical Interpretation of Laboratory Tests*. 11th ed. Philadelphia, PA: FA Davis Company; 2000:924–1014; Bosch X, Poch E, Grau JM. Rhabdomyolysis and acute kidney injury. *N Engl J Med*. 2009;361(1):62–72.

of antidiuretic hormone (SIADH) have concentrated urine and relatively hypotonic serum.[71,72,74]

## Urobilinogen

*Normal range: 0.3 to 1 Ehrlich unit*

*Urobilinogen* (formed by bacterial conversion of conjugated bilirubin in the intestine) is normally present in urine and increases when the turnover of heme pigments is abnormally rapid, as in hemolytic anemia, congestive heart failure with liver congestion, cirrhosis, viral hepatitis, and drug-induced hepatotoxicity. Elevated urobilinogen may be premonitory of early hepatocellular injury, such as hepatitis, because it is evident in urine before serum bilirubin levels increase. Alkaline urine is also associated with increased urobilinogen concentrations caused by enhanced renal elimination. Urobilinogen may decrease (if previously elevated) in patients started on antibiotics (eg, neomycin, chloramphenicol, and tetracycline) that reduce the intestinal flora producing this substance. Urobilinogen is usually absent in total biliary obstruction because the substance cannot be formed. Increased urobilinogen in the absence of bilirubin in the urine suggests a hemolytic process.

## Bilirubin

*Normal range: negative*

A dark yellow or greenish-brown color generally suggests *bilirubin* in the urine (bilirubinuria). Most test strips rely on the reaction between bilirubin with a diazotized organic dye to yield a distinct color. Bilirubinuria may be seen in patients with intrahepatic cholestasis or obstruction of the bile duct (stones or tumor). False-negative results may occur in patients taking ascorbic acid.

## Blood and Hemoglobin

*Normal range: negative*

Dipsticks for blood depend on the oxidation of an indicator dye due to the peroxidase activity of hemoglobin. A dipstick test can detect as few as one to two RBCs per high-power field. Even small amounts of blood noted on dipstick require further investigation. It is important to note that in addition to hemoglobin, myoglobin can also catalyze this reaction so that a positive dipstick result for blood may indicate hematuria (blood), hemoglobinuria (free hemoglobin in urine), or myoglobinuria. Microscopic examination of the urine is needed to distinguish hematuria. The presence of ascorbic acid in the urine may lead to a false-negative result with these tests, which is usually associated with a fairly large oral intake of vitamin C.[72,74,78]

Hemoglobinuria suggests the presence of intravascular hemolysis or directed damage to the small blood vessels. The presence of myoglobin in the urine is highly suggestive of rhabdomyolysis, the acute destruction of muscle cells. With rhabdomyolysis, myoglobin is cleared rapidly by the kidneys and can be detected in the urine.[72]

The clinical distinction between hematuria, hemoglobinuria, and myoglobinuria is important because the clinical conditions that cause them are very different. The color of the urine is not specific; all three may lead to red or dark brown urine. As noted with dipsticks for blood, all three conditions lead to a positive test result. Microscopic analysis demonstrates many more erythrocytes with hematuria, but RBCs can be seen with hemoglobinuria and myoglobinuria. Erythrocytes may be few in hematuria because of lysis of the RBCs if the urine has a low specific gravity (<1.005).

## Leukocyte Esterase

*Normal range: negative to trace*

Many dipsticks can detect *leukocyte esterase*, give a semiquantitative estimate of pyuria (pus in the urine), and thus be considered an indirect test for UTIs. The presence of esterase activity correlates well with significant numbers of neutrophils (either present or lysed) in the urine. The leukocyte esterase test is important because the presence of actual neutrophils in the urine is not a specific indicator for UTI.[72,74]

**TABLE 10-8.** Factors Affecting Urine pH

| URINE PH AND FACTORS | CAUSES AND COMMENTS |
|---|---|
| **Alkaline** | |
| Postprandial | Specimens voided shortly after meals |
| Vegetarianism | Vegetables do not produce fixed acid residues |
| Alkalosis (metabolic or respiratory) | Hyperventilation, severe vomiting, GI suctioning |
| UTI | Some bacteria (eg, *Proteus*) split urea to ammonia, which is alkalinizing |
| Renal tubular acidosis | Impaired tubular acidification of urine and low bicarbonate and pH in blood |
| Drugs | Acetazolamide, bicarbonate salts, thiazides, citrate, and acetate salts |
| **Acidic** | |
| Drugs | Ammonium chloride, ascorbic acid (high dose), methenamine |
| Food | Cranberries, prunes, plums, fruit juices |
| Ketoacidosis | Diabetes mellitus, starvation, high fever |
| Metabolic acidosis | Increased ammonium excretion and cellular hypoxia with lactic acid production (shock) |
| Sleep | Mild respiratory acidosis |

*Source*: Adapted with permission from Sacher RA, McPherson RA. Laboratory assessment of body fluids. *Widmann's Clinical Interpretation of Laboratory Tests*. 11th ed. Philadelphia, PA: FA Davis Company; 2000:924–1014; McPherson RA, Ben-Ezra J, Zhao S. Basic examination of urine. In: McPherson RA, Pincus MR, eds. *Henry's Clinical Diagnosis and Management by Laboratory Methods*. 21st ed. Philadelphia, PA: Saunders Elsevier; 2007:393–425.

## Nitrite

*Normal range: negative*

The presence of *nitrite* in the urine is another indirect indicator of a UTI. Many organisms, such as *Escherichia coli, Klebsiella, Enterobacter, Proteus, Staphylococcus*, and *Pseudomonas*, are able to reduce nitrate to nitrite; thus, a positive urine test result would suggest a UTI. If nitrite-positive, a culture of the urine should be obtained. A first-morning urine specimen is preferred because an incubation period is necessary for bacteria to convert urinary nitrate to nitrite. A positive test result is suggestive of a UTI, but a negative test result cannot rule out a UTI (ie, the test is specific but not highly sensitive). False-positive test results may be caused by strips that are exposed to air. False-negative results occur with infections caused by non–nitrite-producing organisms (*Enterococcus*).[72,74]

## Glucose and Ketones

*Normal range: none*

Although glucose is filtered in the glomerulus, it is almost completely reabsorbed in the proximal tubule so that glucose is generally absent in the urine. However, at glucose concentrations >180 mg/dL, the capacity to reabsorb glucose is exceeded and glycosuria occurs. Glucose in the urine is suggestive of diabetes mellitus although other less common conditions can cause glycosuria.

Additionally, certain medications may cause intentional glycosuria through their mechanism of action. One notable example includes the sodium-glucose cotransporter 2 inhibitor (SGLT2i) drug class, which is indicated primarily for type 2 diabetes mellitus but is supported by an increasing body of evidence for use in heart failure with reduced ejection fraction.[79] SGLT2i are proteins located on the proximal convoluted tubule that are responsible for ~90% of filtered glucose reabsorption. SGLT2i prevent glucose reabsorption and facilitate excretion in the urine, resulting in intended glycosuria.[80,81] As a result of various factors that affect or cause glycosuria, use of urinary glucose to screen and monitor for diabetes is no longer a standard of care.[72,74,75]

Ketones in the urine typically indicate a derangement of carbohydrate metabolism resulting in use of fatty acids as an energy source. Ketonuria in association with glucose in the urine is suggestive of uncontrolled type 1 diabetes mellitus. Ketonuria can also occur with pregnancy, carbohydrate-free diets, and starvation. Aspirin has been reported to cause a false-negative ketone test result, whereas levodopa and phenazopyridine may cause false-positive ketone results (**Minicase 3**).[72,74,75]

## Urinary Electrolytes

Like most laboratory tests, *urinary electrolytes* are rarely definitive for any diagnosis. They can confirm suspicions of a particular medical problem from the history, physical examination, and

## MINICASE 3

### Glycosuria/Ketonuria

Mason L. is a 20-year-old man who presents to an urgent care facility with reports of fatigue and nausea. He notes losing 10 lb despite experiencing increased appetite and thirst over the past 3 months. He describes increased frequency of urination but denies any pain or burning sensations upon voiding.

| URINALYSIS | RESULT | REFERENCE STANDARD/RANGES |
|---|---|---|
| Color | Yellow | Yellow |
| Specific gravity | 1.020 | 1.016–1.022 |
| Ketones | 5+ | Negative |
| Glucose | 4+ | Negative |
| pH | 5 | 4.6–8 |
| Blood | Negative | Negative |
| Protein | Negative | Negative |
| Nitrite | Negative | Negative |
| Leukocyte esterase | Negative | Negative-trace |
| Bacteria | 0 | 0-trace |
| WBC | 0 | 0-2/HPF |
| RBC | 1/HPF | 1-3/HPF |
| Epithelial cells | 0 | 0-1/HPF |

QUESTION: What condition is suggested by the patient's presentation and urinalysis results?

DISCUSSION: The patient requires further evaluation for type 1 diabetes mellitus and diabetic ketoacidosis. Glycosuria suggests diabetes mellitus because glucose is usually completely reabsorbed in the proximal tubule. Reports of polyphagia, polydipsia, and polyuria are hallmark characteristics of hyperglycemia. Type 1 diabetes mellitus is typically diagnosed in children, teens, and young adults. The presence of ketones suggests uncontrolled type 1 diabetes mellitus because of improper carbohydrate metabolism. The subsequent catabolism of fatty acids for energy leads to weight loss. Along with ketonuria, the patient's symptoms of fatigue and nausea prompt concerns for diabetic ketoacidosis.

---

other laboratory data. Along with the results of a urinalysis and serum electrolytes, urinary electrolyte tests allow the practitioner to rule in or out possible diseases of the differential diagnosis. These tests are relatively simple to perform and widely used in the clinical setting.

"Normal" values for urinary electrolytes are a bit of a misnomer because the kidneys should be retaining or excreting electrolytes based on intake and any endogenous production. Any concentration in the urine is normal if it favors a normal fluid and serum electrolyte status. A related test, the urinary fractional excretion of sodium ($\%FE_{Na}$), can assist with common diagnostic dilemmas involving the kidneys' ability to regulate electrolytes.

### Urinary Sodium and Potassium

The electrolyte that is most commonly measured in urine is sodium. Occasionally, it is useful to measure potassium and chloride. For these electrolytes, there is no conversion factor to International System (SI) units because milliequivalents per liter are equivalent to millimoles per liter.

### Sodium

*Normal range: varies widely*

Regulation of urinary excretion of sodium maintains an effective systemic circulating volume. For this reason, the urinary sodium concentration is often used to assess volume status in a patient. Less often, a 24-hour assessment of sodium excretion (via a urine collection) can be used to assess adherence to sodium restriction in a patient with hypertension and heart failure.[82,83] This is because the total urinary sodium excretion should equal the amount of sodium taken in through the diet. For example, a patient following a low-sodium diet should ingest <90 mEq (90 mmol) of sodium per day and would, therefore, have a 24-hour urine sodium <90 mEq (90 mmol) per day if the patient is following the diet accurately. Sodium and water balance is an extremely complex process, and only the most common disorders that may alter sodium and water balance (and hence urine sodium) are discussed here.

*Hyponatremia* is the most common electrolyte disorder seen in clinical practice, and it is most often observed in volume depletion (GI loss and diuretics) and in SIADH, which is not uncommon. In particular, SIADH can be seen in elderly patienets who are maintained on drugs known to cause excess secretion of ADH, such as selective serotonin reuptake inhibitors. Urine sodium concentrations of <20 mEq/L generally suggest volume depletion—the kidneys are responding to the low volume by reabsorbing sodium. In the case of SIADH, which is characterized by inappropriate retention of water in the distal tubule, the urine sodium is generally >20 to 40 mEq/L.

*Hypernatremia* is less common and occurs when there is limited access to free water because otherwise healthy adults become thirsty in the face of hypernatremia. Diabetes insipidus, which is characterized by a decreased production or response to ADH, is another cause of hypernatremia. With diabetes insipidus, the urine sodium concentration is low despite the presence of clinical euvolemia. This is due to dilution of the urinary sodium secondary to inappropriate loss of water in the urine.[83,84]

Urine sodium concentrations are also useful in the diagnosis of AKI. In the presence of prerenal azotemia, urine sodium concentrations are low because of the kidneys' attempt to maintain volume and blood flow to the kidneys. On the other hand, with acute tubular necrosis, the urinary sodium is generally >40 mEq/L because the damaged renal tubules are unable to reabsorb sodium and concentrate urine.[83] The fractional excretion of sodium ($FE_{Na}$) may be used to test the resorptive function of renal tubules. Diuretics can also interfere with the assessment of urinary sodium. Even with volume depletion, urinary sodium levels can be high due to the effect of the diuretic on renal sodium handling.[83]

**%$FE_{Na}$ test.** Although assessment of urine sodium concentrations is useful in determining volume status, concentration of sodium in the urine is affected by the degree of water reabsorption in the tubules. The $FE_{Na}$ is the percentage of sodium (fraction) that is filtered in the glomerulus that eventually is excreted in the urine and corrects for the amount of water in the filtrate. An $FE_{Na}$ can be estimated from a spot (random) urine sample with a concomitant serum sample. The calculation is as follows:

$$FE_{Na}(\%) = \left( \frac{U_{Na} \times S_{Cr}}{S_{Na} \times U_{Cr}} \right) \times 100 \qquad (12)$$

where $U_{Na}$ and $S_{Na}$ are urine and serum sodium in milliequivalents per liter or millimoles per liter and $U_{Cr}$ and $S_{Cr}$ are in milligrams per deciliter or micromoles per liter.

In the face of AKI, the $FE_{Na}$ can be useful to discriminate between a prerenal process (ie, volume depletion) and acute tubular necrosis. In the hypovolemic, prerenal state, the kidneys conserve sodium and the $FE_{Na}$ is <1%. With tubular damage, the $FE_{Na}$ generally is >2% to 3%. As with the assessment of urine sodium, the $FE_{Na}$ can be affected by diuretic therapy and may be somewhat high despite volume depletion.[82,83]

### Potassium

*Normal range: varies widely*

As is the case with sodium, urinary excretion of potassium varies based on dietary intake and other factors that may affect serum potassium concentrations. For patients with unexplained hypokalemia, urinary potassium may provide useful information. Concentrations >10 mEq/L in a hypokalemic patient usually mean that the kidneys are responsible for the loss. This may occur with potassium-wasting diuretics, high-dose sodium penicillin therapy (eg, ticarcillin/clavulanate and piperacillin/tazobactam), metabolic acidosis or alkalosis, and renal tubular acidosis. Concomitant hypokalemia and low urinary potassium (<10 mEq/L) suggest GI loss (including chronic laxative abuse) as the cause of low serum potassium. In the setting of hyperkalemia, assessment of urinary potassium concentrations is less useful. Hyperkalemia is often due to kidney failure (with or without drugs that affect potassium homeostasis), so potassium concentrations in the urine would be low.[83] A 24-hour urine potassium measurement or the transtubular potassium gradient (TTKG) may be used to differentiate between renal and nonrenal causes of potassium abnormalities. The TTKG measures potassium secretion by the distal nephron corrected for urine osmolality:

$$TTKG = (Ku/Ks) \times \left( S_{osm} / U_{osm} \right) \qquad (13)$$

where *Ku* and *Ks* are the concentrations of potassium in the urine and serum and $S_{osm}$ and $U_{osm}$ are the osmolarities of the serum and urine, respectively.[85,86] A TTKG value of <6 suggests a renal cause of hyperkalemia, whereas values >6 may indicate extrarenal causes of hyperkalemia, such as increased potassium intake, acidosis, or rhabdomyolysis.[87]

## SUMMARY

The kidneys play a major role in the regulation of fluids, electrolytes, and the acid–base balance. Kidney function is affected by the cardiovascular, pulmonary, endocrine, and central nervous systems. Therefore, abnormalities in these systems may be reflected in renal or urine tests. Urinalysis is useful as a mirror for organ systems that generate substances (eg, blood/biliary system and urobilinogen) ultimately eliminated in the urine. Urinalysis allows indirect examination without invasive procedures.

A rise in BUN without a simultaneous rise in SCr is not specific for kidney dysfunction. However, concomitant elevations in BUN and SCr almost always reflect some disturbance in the kidneys' ability to clear substances from the body. Renal functions should be estimated based on a patient's SCr and demographic characteristics using either the 2009 CKD-EPI or Cockcroft-Gault equation. These equations are a more reliable index of kidney function than SCr alone. Evolving evidence may show better estimation of GFR with creatinine–cystatin-C equations.[88] A thoughtful examination of urine (macroscopic, microscopic, and chemical) is an indispensable tool in identifying kidney and other pathologic processes that may be present in a patient.

## ACKNOWLEDGMENTS

The authors acknowledge the contributions of Dr. Dominick P. Trombetta, who authored this chapter in previous editions of this textbook.

# LEARNING POINTS

**1. *What is the relevance in knowing the eGFR?***

**ANSWER:** The importance is in the assessment of whether the GFR is stable or changing. Classification of kidney disease is based on estimates of GFR and ranges of albuminuria, and it identifies patients who need to be under the care of nephrologists. Also, changes in GFR may be reflective of worsening disease severity. Many medications are eliminated by renal excretion. Inappropriate use of nephrotoxic drugs or inappropriate dosing in patients with reduced renal function as evidenced by low eGFR may contribute to adverse drug reactions. The eGFR may assist the pharmacist in assessing medication use and determining dose and frequency adjustment. Lastly, staging may help identify appropriate screening for other conditions and comorbidities, such as anemia and mineral and bone disorder, and prepare patients for dialysis.

**2. *Which is better to use for drug dosing, the Cockcroft-Gault, MDRD, or CKD-EPI equation?***

**ANSWER:** Either the CrCl using Cockcroft-Gault equation or the eGFR multiplied by BSA may be used to calculate drug doses for most patients. In some cases, manufacturer labeling provides specific renal dose adjustments in terms of eGFR, such as for metformin and SGLT2 inhibitors; others use CrCl as calculated by Cockcroft-Gault equation. Consider measuring CrCl for patients who are considered at high risk (very young and very old patients), for patients receiving drugs that have a narrow therapeutic index, or for patients in whom estimations of kidney function vary or are likely to be inaccurate. This is especially important in assessing patients for kidney transplant.

**3. *What is the clinical significance of measuring albuminuria?***

**ANSWER:** Under normal conditions, a small amount of total body albumin is filtered by the kidneys. The filtered albumin and low molecular weight serum globulins are then generally reabsorbed in the proximal tubule, which means only small amounts are detected in the urine. The presence of albumin in the urine may suggest glomerular dysfunction, and albuminuria and GFR categories are used to classify CKD. Additionally, the category of albuminuria should be considered when assessing CKD prognosis. The ACR ratio is recommended to assess kidney damage in addition to the GFR. However, proteinuria may be intermittent and benign when caused by transient factors. As a result, evaluating other causes and arranging confirmatory testing may be recommended to distinguish between benign and pathologic albuminuria.

# REFERENCES

1. Eaton DC, Pooler J. *Vander's Renal Physiology.* 9th ed. New York, NY: McGraw-Hill; 2009.

2. Holford NHG. Pharmacokinetics and pharmacodynamics: rational dosing and the time course of drug action. In: Katzung BG, ed. *Basic and Clinical Pharmacology.* 14th ed. New York, NY: McGraw-Hill; 2018: Chapter 3, 41-55.

3. Dowling T. Evaluation of kidney. In: DiPiro JT, Yee GC, Posey L, et al, eds. *Pharmacotherapy: A Pathophysiologic Approach.* 11th ed. New York, NY: McGraw-Hill; 2020: Chapter 59 Evaluation of kidney function.

4. Barrett KE, Barman SM, Brooks HL, Yuan JXJ. *Ganong's Review of Medical Physiology.* 26th ed. New York, NY: McGraw-Hill; 2019.

5. Levey AS, Stevens PE, Bilous RW, et al. KDIGO 2012 Clinical practice guideline for the evaluation and management of chronic kidney disease. https://kdigo.org/wp-content/uploads/2017/02/KDIGO_2012_CKD_GL.pdf. Accessed Apr 18, 2020.

6. Hudson JQ, Nolin TD. Pragmatic use of kidney function estimates for drug dosing: the tide is turning. *Adv Chronic Kidney Dis.* 2018;25(1): 14-20.PubMed

7. Matzke GR, Aronoff GR, Atkinson AJ Jr, et al. Drug dosing consideration in patients with acute and chronic kidney disease-a clinical update from Kidney Disease: Improving Global Outcomes (KDIGO). *Kidney Int.* 2011;80(11):1122-1137.PubMed

8. Zappitelli M, Parvex P, Joseph L, et al. Derivation and validation of cystatin C-based prediction equations for GFR in children. *Am J Kidney Dis.* 2006;48(2):221-230.PubMed

9. Zappitelli M, Joseph L, Gupta IR, et al. Validation of child serum creatinine-based prediction equations for glomerular filtration rate. *Pediatr Nephrol.* 2007;22(2):272-281.PubMed

10. Shlipak MG, Mattes MD, Peralta CA. Update on cystatin C: incorporation into clinical practice. *Am J Kidney Dis.* 2013;62(3):595-603.PubMed

11. Levey AS, Coresh J, Greene T, et al. Using standardized serum creatinine values in the modification of diet in renal disease study equation for estimating glomerular filtration rate. *Ann Intern Med.* 2006;145(4): 247-254.PubMed

12. Brosius FC 3rd, Hostetter TH, Kelepouris E, et al. Detection of chronic kidney disease in patients with or at increased risk of cardiovascular disease: a science advisory from the American Heart Association Kidney And Cardiovascular Disease Council; the Councils on High Blood Pressure Research, Cardiovascular Disease in the Young, and Epidemiology and Prevention; and the Quality of Care and Outcomes Research Interdisciplinary Working Group: developed in collaboration with the National Kidney Foundation. *Circulation.* 2006;114(10): 1083-1087.PubMed

13. Lamb EJ, Webb MC, Simpson DE, et al. Estimation of glomerular filtration rate in older patients with chronic renal insufficiency: is the modification of diet in renal disease formula an improvement? *J Am Geriatr Soc.* 2003;51(7):1012-1017.PubMed

14. National Kidney Foundation. K/DOQI clinical practice guidelines for chronic kidney disease: evaluation, classification, and stratification. *Am J Kidney Dis.* 2002;39(2 suppl 1):S1-S266.PubMed

15. Counahan R, Chantler C, Ghazali S, et al. Estimation of glomerular filtration rate from plasma creatinine concentration in children. *Arch Dis Child.* 1976;51(11):875-878.PubMed

16. The Renal Association. About eGFR. https://renal.org/information-resources/the-uk-eckd-guide/about-egfr. Accessed Sep 24, 2020.

17. U.S. Food and Drug Administration. Guidance for industry: pharmacokinetics in patients with impaired renal function—study design, data analysis, and impact on doing and labeling, draft guidance. http://www.fda.gov/downloads/Drugs/GuidanceComplianceRegulatory Information/Guidances/ucm204959.pdf. Accessed Apr 18, 2020.

18. Inker LA, Levey AS. Assessment of glomerular filtration rate in acute and chronic settings. In: Gilbert SJ, Weiner DE, Gipson DS, et al., eds. *Primer on Kidney Diseases.* 6th ed. Philadelphia, PA: Elsevier Saunders; 2014: 26-32.

19. Delanaye P, Ebert N, Melsom T, et al. Iohexol plasma clearance for measuring glomerular filtration rate in clinical practice and research: a review. Part 1: How to measure glomerular filtration rate with iohexol? *Clin Kidney J.* 2016;9(5):682-699.PubMed

20. Papadakis MA, McPhee SJ, Rabow MW. *Current Medical Diagnosis and Treatment 2020.* 59th ed. New York, NY: McGraw-Hill; 2020.

21. Mayo Clinic, Mayo Clinical Laboratories. Cystatin C with estimated GFR serum. https://www.mayocliniclabs.com/test-catalog/Clinical+and+Inter pretive/35038. Accessed Apr 7, 2020.

22. Perkins BA, Nelson RG, Ostrander BE, et al. Detection of renal function decline in patients with diabetes and normal or elevated GFR by serial measurements of serum cystatin C concentration: results of a 4-year follow-up study. *J Am Soc Nephrol.* 2005;16(5):1404-1412. PubMed

23. Nicoll D, Lu CM, McPhee SJ. *Guide to Diagnostic Tests.* 7th ed. New York, NY: McGraw-Hill; 2017.

24. Stevens LA, Coresh J, Schmid CH, et al. Estimating GFR using serum cystatin C alone and in combination with serum creatinine: a pooled analysis of 3,418 individuals with CKD. *Am J Kidney Dis.* 2008;51(3):395-406.PubMed

25. Briguori C, Visconti G, Rivera NV, et al. Cystatin C and contrast-induced acute kidney injury. *Circulation.* 2010;121(19):2117-2122.PubMed

26. Herget-Rosenthal S, Marggraf G, Hüsing J, et al. Early detection of acute renal failure by serum cystatin C. *Kidney Int.* 2004;66(3):1115-1122. PubMed

27. Wald R, Liangos O, Perianayagam MC, et al. Plasma cystatin C and acute kidney injury after cardiopulmonary bypass. *Clin J Am Soc Nephrol.* 2010;5(8):1373-1379.PubMed

28. Koyner JL, Bennett MR, Worcester EM, et al. Urinary cystatin C as an early biomarker of acute kidney injury following adult cardiothoracic surgery. *Kidney Int.* 2008;74(8):1059-1069.PubMed

29. National Institute of Diabetes and Digestive and Kidney Diseases. Update on Cystatin C. https://www.niddk.nih.gov/health-information /professionals/clinical-tools-patient-management/kidney-disease /laboratory-evaluation/glomerular-filtration-rate/update-cystatin-c. Accessed May 5, 2020.

30. Menon V, Shlipak MG, Wang X, et al. Cystatin C as a risk factor for outcomes in chronic kidney disease. *Ann Intern Med.* 2007;147(1):19-27. PubMed

31. Shardlow A, McIntyre NJ, Fraser SDS, et al. The clinical utility and cost impact of cystatin C measurement in the diagnosis and management of chronic kidney disease: a primary care cohort study. *PLoS Med.* 2017;14(10):e1002400.PubMed

32. Donadio C, Bozzoli L. Urinary β-trace protein: a unique biomarker to screen early glomerular filtration rate impairment. *Medicine (Baltimore).* 2016;95(49):e5553.PubMed

33. DiPiro JT, Yee GC, Posey L, Haines ST, Nolin TD, Ellingrod V, eds. *Pharmacotherapy: A Pathophysiologic Approach,* 11th edition. New York, NY: McGraw-Hill; 2020.

34. Inker LA, Tighiouart H, Coresh J, et al. GFR estimation using β-trace protein and β2-microglobulin in CKD. *Am J Kidney Dis.* 2016;67(1):40-48.PubMed

35. Inker LA, Coresh J, Sang Y, et al. Filtration markers as predictors of esrd and mortality: individual participant data meta-analysis. *Clin J Am Soc Nephrol.* 2017;12(1):69-78.PubMed

36. Oh MS. Evaluation of renal function, water, electrolyte and acid-base. In: McPherson RA, Pincus MR, eds. *Henry's Clinical Diagnosis and Management by laboratory Methods.* 21st ed. Philadelphia, PA: Saunders Elsevier; 2007:147-169.

37. Cockcroft DW, Gault MH. Prediction of creatinine clearance from serum creatinine. *Nephron.* 1976;16(1):31-41.PubMed

38. Myers GL, Miller WG, Coresh J, et al. Recommendations for improving serum creatinine measurement: a report from the Laboratory Working Group of the National Kidney Disease Education Program. *Clin Chem.* 2006;52(1):5-18.PubMed

39. Wade WE, Spruill WJ. New serum creatinine assay standardization: implications for drug dosing. *Ann Pharmacother.* 2007;41(3):475-480. PubMed

40. Macedo E, Mehta RL. Clinical approach to the diagnosis of acute kidney injury. In: Gilbert SJ, Weiner DE, Gipson DS, et al., eds. *Primer on Kidney Diseases.* 6th ed. Philadelphia, PA: Elsevier Saunders; 2014:294-297.

41. National Institute of Diabetes and Digestive and Kidney Diseases. When not to use creatinine-based estimating equations. https://www.niddk.nih .gov/health-information/professionals/clinical-tools-patient-management /kidney-disease/identify-manage-patients/evaluate-ckd/estimate -glomerular-filtration-rate. Accessed May 7, 2020.

42. DuBois D, DuBois EF. A formula to estimate the approximate surface area if height and weight be known. *Arch Intern Med.* 1916;17:863-871.

43. Mosteller RD. Simplified calculation of body-surface area. *N Engl J Med.* 1987;317(17):1098.PubMed

44. Scappaticci GB, Regal RE. Cockcroft-Gault revisited: N\new deliverance on recommendations for use in cirrhosis. *World J Hepatol.* 2017;9(3):131-138.PubMed

45. Smythe M, Hoffman J, Kizy K, Dmuchowski C. Estimating creatinine clearance in elderly patients with low serum creatinine concentrations. *Am J Hosp Pharm.* 1994;51(2):198-204.PubMed

46. Winter MA, Guhr KN, Berg GM. Impact of various body weights and serum creatinine concentrations on the bias and accuracy of the Cockcroft-Gault equation. *Pharmacotherapy.* 2012;32(7):604-612. PubMed

47. Wilhelm SM, Kale-Pradhan PB. Estimating creatinine clearance: a meta-analysis. *Pharmacotherapy.* 2011;31(7):658-664.PubMed

48. Sunder S, Jayaraman R, Mahapatra HS, et al. Estimation of renal function in the intensive care unit: the covert concepts brought to light. *J Intensive Care.* 2014;2(1):31.PubMed

49. Levey AS, Bosch JP, Lewis JB, et al. A more accurate method to estimate glomerular filtration rate from serum creatinine: a new prediction equation. *Ann Intern Med.* 1999;130(6):461-470.PubMed

50. Verhave JC, Fesler P, Ribstein J, et al. Estimation of renal function in subjects with normal serum creatinine levels: influence of age and body mass index. *Am J Kidney Dis.* 2005;46(2):233-241.PubMed

51. Levey AS, Coresh J, Greene T, et al. Expressing the Modification of Diet in Renal Disease Study equation for estimating glomerular filtration rate with standardized serum creatinine values. *Clin Chem.* 2007;53(4):766-772.PubMed

52. National Kidney Disease Education Program. GFR MDRD Calculator for Adults (Conventional Units). https://www.niddk.nih.gov/health -information/professionals/clinical-tools-patient-management/kidney -disease/laboratory-evaluation/glomerular-filtration-rate-calculators /mdrd-adults-conventional-units. Accessed Apr 7, 2020.

53. National Kidney Foundation. Frequently asked questions about GFR estimates. https://www.kidney.org/sites/default/files/docs/12-10-4004 _abe_faqs_aboutgfrrev1b_singleb.pdf. Accessed Apr 7, 2020.

54. Klahr S, Levey AS, Beck GJ, et al. The effects of dietary protein restriction and blood-pressure control on the progression of chronic renal disease. *N Engl J Med.* 1994;330(13):877-884.PubMed

55. Levey AS, Stevens LA, Schmid CH, et al. A new equation to estimate glomerular filtration rate. *Ann Intern Med.* 2009;150(9):604-612.PubMed

56. Levey AS, Stevens LA. Estimating GFR using the CKD Epidemiology Collaboration (CKD-EPI) creatinine equation: more accurate GFR estimates, lower CKD prevalence estimates, and better risk predictions. *Am J Kidney Dis.* 2010;55(4):622-627.PubMed

57. Ferreira JP, Girerd N, Pellicori P, et al. Renal function estimation and Cockcroft-Gault formulas for predicting cardiovascular mortality in population-based, cardiovascular risk, heart failure and post-myocardial infarction cohorts: The Heart 'Omics' in AGEing (HOMAGE) and the high-risk myocardial infarction database initiatives. *BMC Med.* 2016;14(1):181.PubMed

58. Schwartz GJ, Work DF. Measurement and estimation of GFR in children and adolescents. *Clin J Am Soc Nephrol.* 2009;4(11):1832-1843.PubMed

59. Froissart M, Rossert J, Jacquot C, et al. Predictive performance of the modification of diet in renal disease and Cockcroft-Gault equations for estimating renal function. *J Am Soc Nephrol.* 2005;16(3):763-773.PubMed

60. Stevens LA, Nolin TD, Richardson MM, et al. Comparison of drug dosing recommendations based on measured GFR and kidney function estimating equations. *Am J Kidney Dis.* 2009;54(1):33-42.PubMed

61. National Kidney Disease Education Program. CKD and drug dosing: information for providers. https://www.niddk.nih.gov/health-information/professionals/advanced-search/ckd-drug-dosing-providers. Accessed Apr 7, 2020.

62. Nyman HA, Dowling TC, Hudson JQ, et al. Comparative evaluation of the Cockcroft-Gault Equation and the Modification of Diet in Renal Disease (MDRD) study equation for drug dosing: an opinion of the Nephrology Practice and Research Network of the American College of Clinical Pharmacy. *Pharmacotherapy*. 2011;31(11):1130-1144. PubMed

63. American Diabetes Association. Pharmacologic approaches to glycemic treatment: standards of medical care in diabetes: 2020. https://care.diabetesjournals.org/content/43/Supplement_1/S98. Accessed Sep 24, 2020.

64. Edoxaban [prescribing information]. Tokyo, Japan: Daiichi Sankyo Co.; 2015. https://www.accessdata.fda.gov/drugsatfda_docs/label/2015/206316lbl.pdf. Accessed Sep 24, 2020.

65. Cholografin meglumine [prescribing information]. Monroe Township, NJ: Bracco Diagnostics, Inc.; 2017. https://www.accessdata.fda.gov/drugsatfda_docs/label/2017/009321s030lbl.pdf. Accessed Sep 24, 2020.

66. Cholografin meglumine and diatrizoate sodium [prescribing information]. Raleigh, NC: Liebel-Flarsheim Company; 2017. https://www.accessdata.fda.gov/drugsatfda_docs/label/2017/019292s011lbl.pdf. Accessed Sep 24, 2020.

67. Iothalamate meglumine [prescribing information]. Raleigh, NC: Liebel-Flarsheim Company; 2017. https://www.accessdata.fda.gov/drugsatfda_docs/label/2017/013295s070lbl.pdf. Accessed Sep 24, 2020.

68. Ethiodized oil [prescribing information]. Bloomington, IN: Guerbet LLC; 2014. https://www.accessdata.fda.gov/drugsatfda_docs/label/2014/009190s024lbl.pdf. Accessed Sep 24, 2020.

69. Sacher RA, McPherson RA. Laboratory assessment of body fluids. In: *Widmann's Clinical Interpretation of Laboratory Tests*. 11th ed. Philadelphia, PA: FA Davis Company; 2000:924-1014.

70. Wallach J. Urine. In: *Interpretation of Diagnostic Tests*. 8th ed. Philadelphia, PA: Lippincott Williams & Wilkins; 2007:89-110.

71. Greenberg A. Urinalysis. In: Gilbert SJ, Weiner DE, Gipson DS, et al., eds. *Primer on Kidney Diseases*. 6th ed. Philadelphia, PA: Elsevier Saunders; 2014:33-41.

72. McPherson RA, Ben-Ezra J, Zhao S. Basic examination of urine. In: McPherson RA, Pincus MR, eds. *Henry's Clinical Diagnosis and Management by Laboratory Methods*. 21st ed. Philadelphia, PA: Saunders Elsevier; 2007:393-425.

73. Gill CB. Medscape reference. Drugs, diseases, and procedures: discoloration, urine. http://emedicine.medscape.com/article/2172371-overview. Accessed May 5, 2020.

74. Simerville JA, Maxted WC, Pahira JJ. Urinalysis: a comprehensive review. *Am Fam Physician*. 2005;71(6):1153-1162.PubMed

75. Wald R. Urinalysis in the diagnosis of renal disease. In: *UpToDate*. Waltham, MA: UpToDate; 2019: 1-53.

76. Multistix (various) Reagent Strips [product information]. Elkhart, IN: Bayer HealthCare LLC; 2005.

77. Bosch X, Poch E, Grau JM. Rhabdomyolysis and acute kidney injury [Erratum appears in *N Engl J Med*. 2011;19:364(20):1982]. *N Engl J Med*. 2009;361(1):62-72 PubMed

78. Jayne D, Yiu V. Hematuria and proteinuria. In: Gilbert SJ, Weiner DE, Gipson DS, et al., eds. *Primer on Kidney Diseases*. 6th ed. Philadelphia, PA: Elsevier Saunders; 2014:42-50.

79. U.S. Food and Drug Administration. FDA news release. FDA approves new treatment for a type of heart failure. May 2020. https://www.fda.gov/news-events/press-announcements/fda-approves-new-treatment-type-heart-failure. Accessed Sep 24, 2020.

80. Hsia DS, Grove O, Cefalu WT. An update on sodium-glucose co-transporter-2 inhibitors for the treatment of diabetes mellitus. *Curr Opin Endocrinol Diabetes Obes*. 2017;24(1):73-79.PubMed

81. Kalra S. Sodium glucose co-transporter-2 (SGLT2) inhibitors: a review of their basic and clinical pharmacology [Erratum appears in *Diabetes Ther*. 2015;6(1):95]. *Diabetes Ther*. 2014;5(2):355-366.PubMed

82. Kamel KS, Davids MR, Lin S-H, et al. Interpretation of electrolyte and acid-base parameters in blood and urine. In: *Brenner and Rector's The Kidney*. Philadelphia, PA: Elsevier; 2016:804-845.e2.

83. Rose BD. *Meaning and Application of Urine Chemistries. Clinical Physiology of Acid-Base and Electrolyte Disorders*. 5th ed. New York, NY: McGraw-Hill Inc; 2001:405-414.

84. Foote EF. Syndrome of inappropriate antidiuretic hormone secretion and diabetes insipidus. In: Tisdale JE, Miller DA, eds. *Drug-induced diseases*. Bethesda, MD: American Society of Health-System Pharmacists; 2005:611-624.

85. West ML, Marsden PA, Richardson RM, et al. New clinical approach to evaluate disorders of potassium excretion. *Miner Electrolyte Metab*. 1986;12(4):234-238.PubMed

86. Ethier JH, Kamel KS, Magner PO, et al. The transtubular potassium concentration in patients with hypokalemia and hyperkalemia. *Am J Kidney Dis*. 1990;15(4):309-315.PubMed

87. Choi MJ, Ziyadeh FN. The utility of the transtubular potassium gradient in the evaluation of hyperkalemia. *J Am Soc Nephrol*. 2008;19(3):424-426. PubMed

88. Inker LA, Schmid CH, Tighiouart H, et al. Estimating glomerular filtration rate from serum creatinine and cystatin C. *N Engl J Med*. 2012;367(1):20-29.PubMed

# QUICKVIEW | BUN

| PARAMETER | DESCRIPTION | COMMENTS |
|---|---|---|
| **Common reference range** | | |
| Adults<br>Children | 8–23 mg/dL (2.9–8.2 mmol/L)<br>5–18 mg/dL (1.8–6.4 mmol/L) | BUN represents concentration of nitrogen in serum |
| | | Usually measured with creatinine to assess renal function |
| | | A normal BUN:creatinine ratio is 6:1 to 20:1; if ratio is >20:1, it suggests prerenal etiology of renal failure; if ratio is 10–20:1, it suggests intrarenal etiology of renal failure |
| Critical value | 100 mg/dL (35.7 mmol/L) | Associated with uremic syndrome in patients with severe renal failure |
| Inherent activity | Extremely high BUN levels lead to uremia, which includes symptoms of nausea, vomiting, and other metabolic and endocrine abnormalities | |
| **Location** | | |
| Production | Urea is byproduct of hepatic protein metabolism; source of protein can be exogenous (eg, protein in diet) or endogenous (eg, breakdown of RBCs or muscle cells) | Urea is primary way that body eliminates excess nitrogen |
| Storage | Not applicable | |
| Secretion/excretion | Urea is 100% filtered by glomerulus and then undergoes proximal tubule reabsorption | Percentage that is reabsorbed by proximal tubule is inversely related to patient's intravascular volume; if intravascular volume is lower than normal, then percentage of BUN reabsorbed in proximal tubule is increased |
| **Causes of abnormal values** | | |
| High | Prerenal causes: dehydration, blood loss, shock, congestive heart failure, hypotension, increased protein catabolism (due to fever, infection, severe burns) | |
| | Intrarenal causes: acute or chronic renal failure due to any cause, glomerulonephritis, acute tubular necrosis, severe hypertension | |
| | Postrenal causes: obstruction of ureter, bladder neck, or urethra due to stones, enlarged prostate, or stricture, respectively | |
| | Nonrenal causes: excessive amino acid infusions, upper gastrointestinal tract bleeding | |
| | Drugs with antianabolic effects or protein catabolic effects: corticosteroids, tetracyclines | |
| | Drugs that contribute to prerenal or intrarenal failure: ACE inhibitor, acetaminophen, acyclovir, diuretics, aminoglycosides, antibiotics, angiotensin II receptor blockers, NSAIDs, radiographic contrast media | |

## QUICKVIEW | BUN (cont'd)

| PARAMETER | DESCRIPTION | COMMENTS |
|---|---|---|
| Low | Starving or malnourished patients with inadequate protein intake or patients with muscle-wasting disease | |
| | Excess intravascular volume (eg, congestive heart failure) or SIADH may dilute BUN and have low levels | |
| | Chloramphenicol, guanethidine, or streptomycin use | |
| **Signs and symptoms** | | |
| High level | Azotemia refers to elevated BUN, which occurs when GFR is 20%–35% of normal | |
| | Uremia refers to elevated BUN plus fluid and electrolyte, endocrine, neuromuscular, hematologic, or dermatologic, and metabolic abnormalities; it occurs when patient has overt renal failure and GFR is <20%–25% | |
| Low level | No symptoms | |
| **After event, time to....** | | |
| Initial elevation | Variable, depending on etiology of increase in BUN | |
| Peak values | Can exceed 100 mg/dL | |
| Normalization | If prerenal or postrenal etiology of renal failure is corrected, BUN will return to normal range quickly; however, if intrarenal etiology of renal failure results in permanent nephron injury, high levels of BUN may persist; in this case, when uremia develops, patient may be dialyzed, which will reduce BUN level | |
| **Causes of spurious results** | Avoid collecting blood specimens in tubes containing sodium fluoride, which inhibits urease | |

## QUICKVIEW | Creatinine

| PARAMETER | DESCRIPTION | COMMENTS |
|---|---|---|
| **Common reference range** | | |
| Adults<br>Children | 0.6–1.2 mg/dL (53–106 µmol/L)<br>0.2–0.7 mg/dL (18–62 µmol/L) | Usually measured with BUN to assess renal function<br><br>Normal range for SCr varies based on patient age, muscle mass of the patient, and gender; however, usually, normal range for adults applies to both men and women |
| Critical value | Variable based on age, race, muscle mass, low-protein diets, and medications | SCr should not be used alone as indicator of renal function; acute decrease in GFR may not be immediately manifested as increased SCr |
| Inherent activity | None | |
| **Location** | | |
| Production | Creatinine is produced in muscle; it is waste product of creatine and creatine phosphate | |
| Storage | Not applicable | |
| Secretion/excretion | 70%–80% of creatinine is filtered by glomerulus, and rest undergoes tubular secretion via the organic cation pathway | |
| **Causes of abnormal values** | | |
| High | Prerenal causes: dehydration, blood loss, shock, congestive heart failure, hypotension, increased intake of meat<br><br>Intrarenal causes: acute or chronic renal failure due to any cause, glomerulonephritis, acute tubular necrosis, severe hypertension<br><br>Postrenal causes: obstruction of ureter, bladder neck, or urethra due to stones, enlarged prostate, or stricture, respectively<br><br>Exposure to nephrotoxins (eg, aminoglycosides, vancomycin, loop diuretics, penicillinase- resistant penicillins) | |
| Low | Aging: older patients have less muscle mass; therefore, SCr may be lower than in younger patients<br><br>Malnourished patients have low muscle mass; therefore, SCr may be decreased | |
| **Signs and symptoms** | | |
| High level | If increased SCr is due to intrinsic renal disease, patients typically have other laboratory abnormalities; eg, when GFR is ~25 mL/min, increased serum phosphate, uric acid, potassium, and hydrogen ion result; when the GFR is <10 mL/min, increased sodium and chloride result | |

## QUICKVIEW | Creatinine (cont'd)

| PARAMETER | DESCRIPTION | COMMENTS |
|---|---|---|
| Low level | Signs and symptoms of underlying cause of low creatinine levels are evident (eg, malnourished patient appears cachectic) | |
| **After event, time to....** | | |
| Initial elevation | Variable, depending on etiology of increase in creatinine; eg, in acute renal failure, SCr often rises within 24–48 hr; after radiocontrast media exposure, SCr rises in 3–5 days; after ischemic renal failure, SCr increases in 7–10 days | |
| Peak values | Not applicable | |
| Normalization | If prerenal or postrenal etiology of renal failure is corrected, creatinine returns to normal range quickly; however, if intrarenal etiology of renal failure results in permanent nephron injury, high levels of creatinine may persist; after cause has been eliminated, increase in SCr may persist if patient had irreversible renal dysfunction or may persist for 7–14 days if patient had reversible renal dysfunction | |
| **Causes of spurious results** | Uric acid, glucose, fructose, acetone, acetoacetate, pyruvic acid, and ascorbic acid, cefoxitin, or flucytosine can cause false elevations in measured creatinine when using the alkaline picrate (Jaffe) assay; can lead to an underestimation of a patient's creatinine clearance | |
| | Bilirubin can falsely lower measured creatinine when using alkaline picrate assay or enzymatic assays; can lead to an overestimation of patient's creatinine clearance | |
| | Cimetidine, trimethoprim, pyrimethamine, dronedarone, or dapsone can compete through organic cation pathway for tubular secretin of creatinine; these drugs can cause false elevations in SCr | |
| | Hemolysis of blood sample can falsely increase creatinine measurement | |

# 11

# Electrolytes, Other Minerals, and Trace Elements

*Lingtak-Neander Chan and Jasmine S. Mangrum*

DOI 10.37573/9781585286423.011

## OBJECTIVES

*After completing this chapter, the reader should be able to*

- Describe the homeostatic mechanisms involved in sodium and water balance, hyponatremia, and hypernatremia

- Describe the physiology of intracellular and extracellular potassium regulation as well as the signs and symptoms of hypokalemia and hyperkalemia

- List common causes of serum chloride abnormalities

- List common conditions resulting in serum magnesium abnormalities and describe signs and symptoms of hypomagnesemia and hypermagnesemia

- Describe the metabolic and physiologic relationships among the metabolism of calcium, phosphate, parathyroid hormone, and vitamin D

- List common conditions resulting in serum calcium abnormalities and describe signs and symptoms of hypocalcemia and hypercalcemia

- List common conditions resulting in altered copper, zinc, manganese, selenium, and chromium homeostasis and describe the signs and symptoms associated with their clinical deficiencies

- Interpret the results of laboratory tests used to assess sodium, potassium, chloride, calcium, phosphate, magnesium, copper, zinc, manganese, selenium, and chromium (in the context of a clinical case description, including history and physical examination)

Serum or plasma electrolyte concentrations are among the most commonly used laboratory tests by clinicians in assessing a patient's health status, clinical conditions, and disease progression. The purpose of this chapter is to present the physiologic basis for the need to assess serum concentrations of common electrolytes and minerals. Interpretation of these laboratory results and the clinical significance of abnormal results are addressed.

Serum concentrations of sodium, potassium, chloride, and total carbon dioxide content (often referred to as *serum bicarbonate*) are among the most commonly monitored electrolytes in clinical practice. Magnesium, calcium, and phosphorus are also monitored, as determined by a patient's disease states and clinical indication. The homeostasis of calcium and phosphate is frequently discussed in the context of the endocrine system because of the effects of vitamin D and the parathyroid hormone (PTH) on the regulation of these minerals. Serum total carbon dioxide content, often measured in conjunction with electrolytes, is discussed in Chapter 13 because of its significance for the assessment of acid–base status. Listed in **Table 11-1** are the current dietary reference intake for electrolytes, minerals, and trace elements.

## ELECTROLYTES

The traditional units, International System (SI) units, and their conversion factors for electrolytes, minerals, and trace elements discussed in this chapter are listed in **Table 11-2**. Although the normal ranges of serum concentrations for each of the electrolytes are listed later, clinicians should always confirm with the institutional clinical laboratory department for their institutional reference range because of the variance introduced by equipment, analytical technique, and quality assurance data.

### Sodium

*Normal range: 135 to 145 mEq/L (135 to 145 mmol/L)*

Sodium is the most abundant cation in the extracellular fluid and is the major regulating factor for bodily fluid and water balance. Extracellular (ie, intravascular and interstitial) and intracellular sodium contents are closely affected by body fluid status. Thus, an accurate interpretation of serum sodium concentration must include an understanding of body water homeostasis and the interrelationship between the regulation of sodium and water.[1]

#### Physiology

Sodium is essential for maintaining the optimal transmembrane electric potential for action potential and neuromuscular functioning as well as regulating serum osmolality and water balance. Serum osmolality is an estimate of the water–solute ratio in the vascular fluid. It can be measured in the laboratory or estimated using the following equation:

$$\text{Estimated serum osmolality (mOsm/kg)} = (2 \times \text{serum[Na]}) + [\text{glucose, in mg/dL}]/18 + [\text{blood urea nitrogen, in mg/dL}]/2.8$$

**TABLE 11-1.** Recommended Dietary Reference Intake of Electrolytes and Minerals for Healthy Adults According to the Dietary Guidelines 2015 to 2020

| NUTRIENT | DIETARY REFERENCE INTAKE* | |
|---|---|---|
| | Men | Women |
| Sodium | Not to exceed 2,300 mg (100 mEq) | |
| Potassium | 4,700 mg (~120 mEq) | |
| Chloride | Varies with potassium and sodium intakes | |
| Magnesium | 19–30 years: 400 mg<br>≥31 years: 420 mg | 19–30 years: 310 mg<br>≥31 years: 320 mg |
| Calcium | 19–70 years: 1,000 mg<br>≥71 years: 1,200 mg | 19–50 years: 1,000 mg<br>≥51 years: 1,200 mg |
| Phosphorus | 700 mg | |
| Copper | 900 mcg | |
| Zinc | 11 mg | 8 mg |
| Manganese | 2.3 mg | 1.8 mg |
| Chromium† | 19–50 years: 35 mcg<br>≥51 years: 30 mcg | 19–50 years: 25 mcg<br>≥51 years: 20 mcg |

*According to the recommendations from 2015–2020 Dietary Guidelines for Americans. https://health.gov/our-work/food-nutrition/2015-2020-dietary-guidelines. Accessed July 30, 2020.
†Adequate intakes according to Institute of Medicine (U.S.) Food and Nutrition Board. Dietary reference intakes. Washington, DC: National Academies Press; 2001.

**TABLE 11-2.** Conversion Factors to SI Units

| NUTRIENT | TRADITIONAL UNITS | CONVERSION FACTORS TO SI UNITS | SI UNITS |
|---|---|---|---|
| Sodium | mEq/L | 1 | mmol/L |
| Potassium | mEq/L | 1 | mmol/L |
| Chloride | mEq/L | 1 | mmol/L |
| Magnesium | mEq/L | 0.5 | mmol/L |
| Calcium | mg/dL | 0.25 | mmol/L |
| Phosphorus | mg/dL | 0.3229 | mmol/L |
| Copper | mcg/dL | 0.1574 | µmol/L |
| Zinc | mcg/dL | 0.153 | µmol/L |
| Manganese | mcg/L | 18.2 | nmol/L |
| Chromium | mcg/L | 19.2 | nmol/L |

By strict definition, there is a difference between *osmolality*, which refers to the number of solute particles in 1 kg of solvent (expressed as mOsm/kg), and *osmolarity*, which describes the number of solute particles per 1 L of solvent (expressed as mOsm/L). Osmolality is generally used to describe serum and other physiologic solutions, whereas osmolarity is the term for intravenous (IV) solutions for infusion, such as IV fluids and parenteral nutrition solutions.

The normal range of serum osmolality is 285 to 295 mOsm/kg. The measured osmolality should not exceed the estimated value by more than 10 mOsm/kg. A difference of >10 mOsm/kg between the measured and estimate values is considered an increased osmolal gap, which may suggest the presence of other unmeasured solutes (eg, organic solvents, alcohol) and is useful to providing assessments in clinical toxicology. Decreased serum osmolality usually suggests a water excess, whereas increased serum osmolality suggests a water deficit. Although serum osmolality may be helpful in assessing water status, especially the intravascular volume, it should not be the primary and only parameter in assessing fluid status. Also, the results should be interpreted in the context of the ability of the solute to cross cellular membranes (eg, uremia causing hyperosmolality without relative intracellular depletion) and a patient's symptoms and signs of disease. **Figure 11-1** summarizes the interrelationship and regulation between water and sodium.

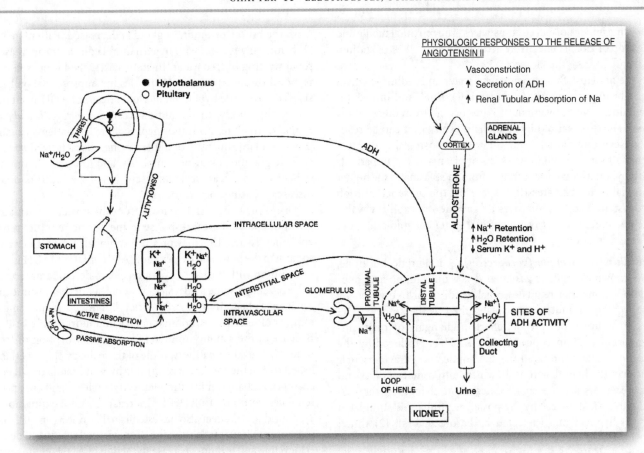

**FIGURE 11-1.** Homeostatic mechanisms involved in sodium, potassium, and water balance. Sodium is the principal cation in blood that contributes to serum osmolality and intravascular volume. When serum osmolality and intravascular volume are increased, baroreceptors in the carotid sinus, aortic arch, cardiac atria, hypothalamus, and juxtaglomerular apparatus in the kidney promote urinary loss of sodium and water. The synthesis and release of ADH are increased, which leads to increased water retention. In addition, elevated serum osmolality with increased serum sodium would suppress aldosterone release, which results in increased renal sodium excretion. In contrast, when serum osmolality is low due to excess intravascular water and decreased sodium, water passively moves from the bloodstream to interstitial spaces (resulting in edema) and into cells (in brain cells, this can cause brain swelling). In addition, low serum osmolality detected by hypothalamic osmoreceptors suppresses the release of ADH, resulting in decreased water reabsorption in the distal tubule, and stimulates the renin-angiotensin-aldosterone system (which enhances distal tubular reabsorption of sodium and potassium secretion). Serum osmolality also regulates the thirst response. When serum osmolality is high, hypothalamic osmoreceptors stimulate thirst so that the patient increases water intake. Together with increased ADH release, the body increases free water retention and eventually drives serum osmolality back within the normal range.

Changes in body water and total plasma volume can affect the serum sodium concentration. For example, as the result of changes in effective circulating volume, baroreceptors and osmoreceptors respond accordingly to restore an isovolemic state of the body. Baroreceptors are located in the carotid sinus, aortic arch, cardiac atria, hypothalamus, and juxtaglomerular apparatus in the kidney. An increase in plasma volume stimulates these receptors and promotes urinary loss of water and sodium. Osmoreceptors are present primarily in the hypothalamus. The three major effectors in response to the stimulation of the osmoreceptors include vasopressin or antidiuretic hormone

(ADH), the renin–angiotensin–aldosterone system, and natriuretic peptides. The resultant renal effects from these three distinct pathways collectively regulate the homeostasis of water and sodium.

The kidneys are the primary organ responsible for the retention and excretion of body sodium and water. The glomeruli receive and filter approximately 180 L of plasma fluid daily. On average, <2 L of water and between 0.1 and 40 g of sodium is excreted in the urine, depending on the fluid status and sodium intake of the individual. Although almost 100% of the serum sodium is filtered by the glomeruli, <1% is eventually excreted in the urine under normal circumstances. The proximal tubule and the loop of Henle collectively account for up to 90% of sodium reabsorbed from the kidneys.

The homeostatic mechanism for water and sodium involves equilibrium among intravascular, interstitial, and intracellular fluids.[2,3] Net movement of water occurs from areas of low osmolality to areas of high osmolality. This effect can be readily observed in patients with a low serum osmolality due to a deficit of serum sodium or excess of plasma water. In patients with hyponatremia, water moves from the plasma to the higher osmolality in the interstitial space. In the presence of high hydrostatic and oncotic pressure gaps across capillary walls, the net effect is excessive interstitial water accumulation and edema formation.[2,3]

*Antidiuretic hormone (vasopressin).* Antidiuretic hormone, also known as *arginine vasopressin*, is a nine amino acid peptide hormone that regulates renal handling of free water. By altering the amount of water reabsorbed by the kidney, ADH has an indirect, but pivotal, effect in changing or maintaining serum sodium concentration. ADH is produced by the magnocellular neurons in the supraoptic and paraventricular nuclei of the hypothalamus, in which both osmoreceptors and baroreceptors are present to detect fluid changes in the vasculature. ADH release by the posterior pituitary is stimulated by (1) hypovolemia (detected by baroreceptors); (2) thirst; (3) increased serum osmolality; and (4) angiotensin II. The plasma half-life of ADH is 10 to 20 minutes, and it is rapidly deactivated and eliminated by the liver, kidneys, and a plasma enzyme vasopressinase.

Antidiuretic hormone regulates urinary water loss by augmenting the permeability of the collecting tubules to increase the net reabsorption of water. Circulating serum ADH binds to type 2 vasopressin (V2) receptors starting at the thick ascending loop, which contributes to the corticomedullary gradient and mechanism of water retention. More importantly, ADH also binds to the V2 receptors in the collecting tubule and promotes the formation of a water channel, known as *aquaporin-2* (AQP2). AQP2 facilitates the reabsorption of water from the lumen back into the renal blood supply in the systemic circulation, causing a decrease in diuresis and net retention of water. However, if serum sodium is high but blood volume is normal (eg, normovolemia with hyperosmolality), the effect from the baroreceptors overrides the further release of ADH, thus preventing volume overload (ie, hypervolemia).[2]

The changes in plasma water content associated with ADH may alter serum osmolality and affect serum sodium concentration. In patients with the syndrome of inappropriate ADH (SIADH) secretion, an abnormally high quantity of ADH is present in the systemic circulation. This condition results in increased water reabsorption, which could cause a dilutional effect in serum sodium. In conjunction with increased free water intake, a low serum sodium concentration is commonly observed in these patients. Urine osmolality and urine electrolyte concentrations are often increased in SIADH because of decreased urinary excretion of free water associated with the increased effect of ADH. Conversely, in patients with central diabetes insipidus (DI), hypothalamic ADH synthesis or its release

from the posterior pituitary gland is decreased. Patients with DI commonly present with hypernatremia due to the increased renal wasting of free water. In some cases, the kidneys fail to respond to the circulating ADH despite appropriate synthesis ADH from the hypothalamus and release of ADH from the posterior pituitary. This condition is called *nephrogenic diabetes insipidus*. In either central or nephrogenic DI, patients usually produce a large quantity of diluted urine, characterized by low specific gravity, low urine osmolality, and low urine sodium.[2] (Chapter 10 offers an in-depth discussion of the effects of other diseases on urine composition.)

Drugs may alter ADH release from the posterior pituitary gland or the biological response to the hormone in the renal epithelial tissues. This may produce an imbalance of water and sodium in the body and exacerbate SIADH or DI.[4,5] SIADH is not uncommon with the use of cyclophosphamide, carbamazepine, oxcarbazepine, some analgesics, oxytocin, a number of anticancer agents, phenothiazines, some tricyclic antidepressants, and a number of selective serotonin reuptake inhibitors (**Table 11-3**).[6] Because of their ability to increase renal reabsorption of free water via the ADH pathway, some of these drugs play an established role in the treatment of chronic hypernatremia or DI. For example, carbamazepine stimulates ADH release and enhances renal cell response to ADH by increasing AQP2 expression.[7] This antidiuretic effect also has established its role as an off-label pharmacotherapeutic option for DI, however. In contrast, demeclocycline and lithium decrease the action of ADH on the renal epithelial water reabsorption mediated by aquaporin. They have been used off-label in the treatment of SIADH. Other drugs that decrease the release and impair the renal response to ADH also may precipitate DI (**Table 11-4**). Based on published data, lithium, foscarnet, and clozapine are the most commonly reported causes of drug-induced DI. In addition, conivaptan, a vasopressin receptor antagonist (V1A and V2 receptors), and tolvaptan, a selective V2 receptor antagonist, both modulate the renal handling of water by reducing renal water absorption and affect sodium homeostasis. These two drugs are approved by the U.S. Food and Drug Administration for the treatment of euvolemic and hypervolemic hyponatremia.

*Renin–angiotensin–aldosterone system.* Renin is a glycoprotein that catalyzes the conversion of angiotensinogen to angiotensin I, which is further converted to angiotensin II, primarily in the lungs. However, angiotensin II also can be formed locally in the kidneys. Angiotensin II, a potent vasoconstrictor, is important in maintaining optimal perfusion pressure to end organs, especially when plasma volume is decreased. In addition, it induces the release of aldosterone, ADH, and, to a lesser extent, cortisol.

Aldosterone is a hormone with potent mineralocorticoid activity. It affects the distal tubular reabsorption of sodium, which also contributes to plasma volume retention.[3] This hormone is released from the adrenal cortex. Besides angiotensin II, various dietary and neurohormonal factors, including low serum sodium, high serum potassium, and low blood volume, can stimulate its release. Aldosterone acts on renal sodium–potassium–adenosine triphosphate (Na-K-ATPase) to increase urinary excretion of potassium from the distal tubules

## TABLE 11-3. Medications That Can Cause Hyponatremia Based on Published Data

Drugs that alter sodium and water homeostasis
  Amiloride
  Indapamide
  Loop diuretics
  Thiazide diuretics
  Trimethoprim

Drugs that alter water homeostasis
  Stimulator of central ADH production or release
    Antidepressants:
      Monoamine oxidase inhibitors
      Selective serotonin reuptake inhibitors
      Tricyclic antidepressants (more common with amitriptyline, desipramine, protriptyline)
    Antiepileptic drugs
      Carbamazepine
      Oxcarbazepine
      Valproic acid
    Antipsychotic agents
      Phenothiazines (eg, thioridazine, trifluoperazine)
      Butyrophenones (eg, haloperidol)
    Antineoplastic agents
      Alkylating agents (cyclophosphamide, ifosfamide, melphalan)
      Platinum (cisplatin, carboplatin, oxaliplatin)
      Vinca alkaloids (more common with vinblastine and vincristine)
    Others: levamisole, methotrexate
      Cotrimoxazole (especially at high doses)
      Opioid analgesics
      3,4-methylenedioxymethylamphetamine (MDMA, known as Ecstasy)
Enhancers of ADH effect
  Antiepileptic drugs (primarily carbamazepine and lamotrigine)
  Antineoplastic agents (mostly cyclophosphamide)
  Nonsteroidal antiinflammatory drugs
Oral hypoglycemic agents
  Chlorpropamide
  Tolbutamide
Drugs with unclear mechanisms
  ACE inhibitors
  Bromocriptine
  Oxytocin
  Venlafaxine

## TABLE 11-4. Drugs That Can Cause Diabetes Insipidus by Decreasing Renal Response to ADH

Precipitant of Nephrogenic DI
  Amphotericin B
  Cidofovir
  Cimetidine
  Clozapine
  Colchicine
  Conivaptan
  Cyclophosphamide
  Demeclocycline
  Epirubicin
  Ethanol*
  Fluvoxamine
  Foscarnet
  Gentamicin
  Lithium
  Methicillin[†]
  Phenytoin* (uncommon at therapeutic doses)
  Propoxyphene[†]
  Tolvaptan
  Verapamil
  Vinblastine

*Likely also involves central effect by inhibiting ADH release.
[†]Currently no longer available in the United States although still available in some other countries.

in exchange for sodium reabsorption. Because of its effect on renal Na-K exchange, aldosterone has a profound effect on serum potassium, although its effect on serum sodium is relatively modest. As serum sodium increases, so does water reabsorption, which follows the osmotic gradient.[3] Renal arteriolar blood pressure (BP) then increases, which helps maintain the glomerular filtration rate (GFR). Ultimately, more water and sodium pass through the distal tubules, overriding the initial effect of aldosterone.[2,3]

*Natriuretic peptides.* Atrial natriuretic factor (ANF), also known as *atrial natriuretic peptide*, is a vasodilatory hormone synthesized and primarily released by the right atrium. It is secreted in response to plasma volume expansion as a result of increased atrial stretch. ANF inhibits the juxtaglomerular apparatus, zona glomerulosa cells of the adrenal gland, and the hypothalamus–posterior pituitary. As a result, a global downregulation of renin, aldosterone, and ADH, respectively, is achieved. ANF directly induces glomerular hyperfiltration and reduces sodium reabsorption in the collecting tubule. A net increase in sodium excretion is achieved. Therefore, ANF can decrease serum and total body sodium. Brain natriuretic peptide (BNP) is produced and secreted primarily by the ventricles in the brain, and to a much smaller extent, the atrium. Similar to atrial natriuretic peptide, BNP also regulates natriuretic, endocrine, and hemodynamic responses and may affect sodium homeostasis. An increase in blood volume or pressure, such as chronic heart failure (CHF) and hypertension, enhances BNP secretion, which induces a significant increase in natriuresis and to a lesser extent, urinary flow (ie, diuresis). Plasma BNP concentrations correlate with the magnitude of left ventricular heart failure and the clinical prognosis of patients with heart failure.

## Hyponatremia

*Hyponatremia* is defined as a serum sodium concentration <135 mEq/L (<135 mmol/L). Although it can be the direct result of sodium deficit, hyponatremia may also occur when total body fluid content is low (ie, volume depletion, dehydration), normal, or high (ie, fluid overload). Therefore, natremic status must be evaluated in concert with volume status to determine the nature of an underlying disorder. Fluid status should be assessed based on history of oral intake; vital signs; other supportive laboratory findings if available (eg, serum blood urea nitrogen [BUN]–serum creatinine [SCr] ratio, hematocrit to hemoglobin [Hgb] concentration ratio, or urine electrolyte assessment); recent changes in body weight; recent medical, surgical, and nutrition history; and findings from the physical examination. More important, a patient's renal function, hydration status, and fluid intake and output must be thoroughly evaluated and closely monitored.

Most patients with hyponatremia remain asymptomatic until serum sodium approaches 120 mEq/L. In most cases, hyponatremia can be effectively and safely managed with mild fluid restriction and the use of physiologic saline solution (eg, NaCl 0.9%). Infusion of hypertonic saline (eg, NaCl 3%) is usually not necessary unless serum sodium concentration is <120 mEq/L, altered mental status is present, or the patient is fluid restricted (eg, CHF, chronic renal failure). As with most electrolyte disorders, the chronicity of the imbalance is a major determinant of the severity of signs and symptoms. For example, hyponatremia in a patient with CHF secondary to chronic, progressive volume overload and decreased renal perfusion is less likely to be symptomatic than a patient who is hyponatremic due to rapid infusion of a hypotonic solution. The most commonly reported symptom associated with hyponatremia is altered mental status (**Table 11-5**). If serum sodium continues to fall, cerebral edema can worsen and intracranial pressure continue to rise. More severe symptoms such as seizure, coma, and, subsequently, death may result.[2-6]

The most common causes of hyponatremia can be broken down into two types: (1) sodium depletion in excess of total body water loss (eg, severe hypovolemia with true depletion of total body sodium); or (2) dilutional hyponatremia (ie, free water intake greater than water output with no change in sodium loss). Dilutional hyponatremia can be further categorized into five subtypes: (1) primary dilutional hyponatremia (eg, SIADH and renal failure); (2) neuroendocrine conditions (eg, adrenal insufficiency and myxedema); (3) psychiatric disorder (eg, psychogenic polydipsia); (4) osmotic hyponatremia (eg, severe hyperglycemia); and (5) thiazide diuretic-induced conditions.

## TABLE 11-5. Signs and Symptoms of Hyponatremia

Agitation

Anorexia

Apathy

Depressed deep tendon reflexes

Disorientation

Headache

Hypothermia

Lethargy

Muscle cramps

Nausea

Seizures

Vomiting

***Hyponatremia associated with total body sodium depletion.*** Hyponatremia associated with low total body sodium reflects a reduction in total body water, with an even larger reduction in total body sodium. This condition is primarily caused by depletion of extracellular fluid, which stimulates ADH release to increase renal water reabsorption, even at the expense of causing a transient hypoosmotic state. Some common causes include vomiting, diarrhea, intravascular fluid losses due to burn injury and pancreatitis, Addison disease, and certain forms of renal failure (eg, salt-wasting nephropathy).[2] This type of hyponatremia may also occur in patients treated too aggressively with diuretics who receive sodium-free solutions as replacement fluid.

***Hyponatremia associated with normal total body sodium.*** Also called *euvolemic* or *dilutional hyponatremia*, this condition refers to impaired free water excretion without alteration in sodium excretion. Etiologies include any mechanism that enhances ADH secretion or potentiates its action at the renal collecting tubules. This condition can occur as a result of glucocorticoid deficiency, severe hypothyroidism, and administration of water to a patient with impaired water excretion capacity.[2,5] SIADH is associated with excessive renal reabsorption of free water in the body due to continued ADH secretion, despite low serum osmolality. This results in hyponatremia and increased urinary sodium loss. Patients with SIADH produce concentrated urine with high urine osmolality (usually greater than serum osmolality) and urine sodium excretion (as reflected in a urine sodium concentration that is usually >20 mEq/L). They have normal renal, adrenal, and thyroid function and no evidence of volume abnormalities.[2,4,5]

Impaired ADH response can be precipitated by many factors, including medications. SIADH has been reported in patients with certain tumors, such as lung cancer, pancreatic carcinoma, thymoma, and lymphoma. ADH release from the parvicellular and magnocellular neurons may be stimulated by cytokines such as interleukin-1β, 2, 6, and tumor necrosis factor-α. Likewise, head trauma, subarachnoid hemorrhage, hydrocephalus, Guillain-Barré syndrome, pulmonary aspergillosis, and occasionally

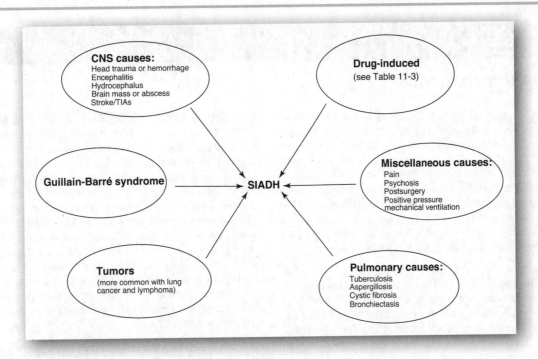

**FIGURE 11-2.** Etiologies of SIADH. TIA = transient ischemic attack.

tuberculosis may increase hypothalamic ADH production and release, leading to SIADH (**Figure 11-2**).

In some cases, hyponatremia may not be associated with a sodium deficit. This scenario is associated with normal or even slightly elevated total body sodium, which is distributed in a much larger volume of total body water. It is frequently observed in hypervolemic states with compromised renal function, such as CHF, cirrhosis, nephrotic syndrome, and chronic kidney disease (CKD). In these patients, renal handling of water and sodium is often impaired.[2,5]

The initial goal of therapy for most patients with hyponatremia, based on the most recent European and American consensus guidelines, is to raise the serum sodium concentration by 5 mEq/L.[8] Mild, asymptomatic hyponatremia (>125 mEq/L) can usually be safely managed with a sodium-containing oral rehydration solution or an increase in oral sodium intake, provided that the oral route is viable (ie, vomiting and diarrhea are controlled, evidence of functional gastrointestinal [GI] tract). IV sodium therapy is preferred in severe cases of hyponatremia or in patients with severe symptoms. In most cases, sodium chloride 0.9% is used, although the recent guidelines recommend using NaCl 3.0% in symptomatic patients.[8] If a hypertonic saline solution (eg, ≥NaCl 3.0%) is used, it must be infused via a central venous catheter because of its high osmolarity.

The initial goal for treating acute hyponatremia is to prevent further decline in serum sodium concentration, reverse or prevent neurologic symptoms, and avoid excessive correction of serum sodium in patients at risk for osmotic demyelination syndrome. In patients with sodium concentration >120 mEq/L with no or mild symptoms, acute correction of serum sodium concentration may not be warranted. In symptomatic patients with serum sodium concentration <120 mEq, increase serum

sodium by up to 4 to 6 mEq/L within 24 hours of baseline or until symptoms improve. The risk of osmotic demyelination syndrome has been reported after correction by 9 mEq/L per day.[8] Neurologic deficits would improve with this target rate of change in serum sodium concentration. The average rate of increase in serum sodium should not exceed 1 to 2 mEq/L/hr and a total of 9 mEq/L in any given 24-hour period. Excessive correction of serum sodium concentration during the course of treatment, and not just the first or second day, may result in osmotic demyelination syndrome. There is no evidence that the first day's correction should be greater than on other days. There is no evidence that correction of serum sodium by >10 mEq/L in 24 h or 18 mEq/L in 48 hours improves outcomes in patients with acute or chronic hyponatremia[8,9] (**Minicase 1**).

## TESTS FOR ASSESSING FLUID STATUS

### Fractional Excretion of Sodium

*Normal range: 1% to 2%*

In most cases, natremic disorders cannot be effectively managed without first optimizing the overall fluid status of the patient. Therefore, when a serum sodium value is abnormal, the clinician should first evaluate whether vascular volume is optimal. In addition to physical examinations and history, the *fractional excretion of sodium* ($FE_{Na}$) may help validate these findings, especially in patients whose physical examination results may be limited by other confounders (eg, use of antihypertensive drugs, CHF, or with acute renal failure). $FE_{Na}$ is most useful in the acute onset of oliguria in which a clinical history cannot be

## MINICASE 1

## A Case of Hyponatremia

Jessica F., a 24-year-old woman, presents to the emergency department with lower abdominal pain, fatigue, headache, and dizziness. She has had four episodes of vomiting and six episodes of diarrhea in the last 24 hours. She had salad at a salad bar for lunch the day before. About 2 hours after her lunch, she started to feel nauseated. The abdominal pain and vomiting started shortly thereafter, and the diarrhea started in the evening. She vomited her lunch, and her diarrhea was mostly watery without blood. She also experienced a headache this morning. She has not been eating for the last 24 hours and can tolerate only small sips of water.

Upon presentation, she looks pale with sunken eyes. She is alert and oriented to time, person, and place. Neurologic examination reveals no deficits. Her vital signs include BP 105/70 mm Hg in supine position (standing BP 90/65 mm Hg), heart rate (HR) 92 beats/min (standing 108 beats/min), and respiratory rate (RR) 20 breaths/min. She also has a temperature of 100.6°F. Blood work for serum electrolytes and complete blood count is ordered. Her electrolyte panel shows the following results:

- Sodium, 128 mEq/L
- Potassium, 3.3 mEq/L
- Chloride, 90 mEq/L
- $CO_2$ content, 21 mEq/L
- BUN, 28 mg/dL
- Creatinine, 1.05 mg/dL
- Glucose, 77 mg/dL

She has not taken any medication prior to this admission.

QUESTION: How would you interpret this patient's serum sodium concentration?

DISCUSSION: The patient's serum sodium concentration is lower than the normal range, suggesting hyponatremia. However, as mentioned previously, sodium disorder cannot be fully assessed without evaluating a person's fluid status. Based on the history, she had excessive fluid loss due to repeated episodes of vomiting and diarrhea. Fever also will increase insensible fluid loss. Therefore, her headache is likely caused by hypovolemia with hyponatremia. Her vital signs (orthostatic hypotension with reflex tachycardia) and the findings from physical exam support volume depletion. The laboratory results show an elevated BUN:SCr ratio of 28:1, which also is consistent with volume depletion. Increased loss of body fluids, especially from the GI tract, will lead to increased water and sodium loss. Her fluid intake has been limited and likely inadequate to replenish the continued sodium loss, which results in hyponatremia. She is likely experiencing hyponatremia associated with total sodium deficiency due to uncontrolled vomiting, diarrhea, and insufficient oral intake.

The onset of the patient's hyponatremia is likely acute because there are no other established factors that would lead to chronic hyponatremia (eg, use of diuretic drugs, selective serotonin reuptake inhibitors). Her symptoms of hyponatremia are mild as she shows no neurologic deficit. Her headache is likely associated with her volume depletion, mild hyponatremia, and possibly acid–base changes.

In summary, this patient has mild hyponatremia with hypovolemia. The cause seems to be from her acute illness—uncontrolled vomiting and diarrhea leading to increased water and sodium loss with insufficient sodium intake. She does not seem to experience major acute symptoms associated with hyponatremia at this point. The logical treatment approach for her involves controlling her nausea, diarrhea, and vomiting as well as treating hypovolemia with a sodium-containing fluid (eg, oral rehydration solution or IV NaCl 0.9%) and managing other electrolyte disturbances.

---

ascertained.[10] The value may be determined by the use of a random urine sample to determine renal handling of sodium. $FE_{Na}$, the measure of the percentage of filtered sodium excreted in the urine, can be calculated using the following equation:

$$FE_{Na} = 100 \times \frac{sodium_{urinary} \times creatinine_{plasma}}{sodium_{plasma} \times creatinine_{urinary}}$$

$$FE_{Na} = 100 \times [sodium\,(urine) \times creatinine\,(serum)] / [sodium\,(serum) \times creatinine\,(urine)]$$

Values >2% usually suggest that the kidneys are excreting a higher than normal fraction of the filtered sodium, implying likely renal tubular damage. Conversely, $FE_{Na}$ values <1% generally imply preservation of intravascular fluid through renal sodium retention, suggesting prerenal causes of renal dysfunction (eg, hypovolemia and cardiac failure). Because acute diuretic therapy can increase the $FE_{Na}$ to 20% or more, urine samples should be obtained at least 24 hours after diuretics have been discontinued.

## Blood Urea Nitrogen: Serum Creatinine Ratio

*Normal range: <20:1*

The *BUN:SCr ratio* can provide useful information to assess fluid status. When this ratio is higher than 20:1, contraction of plasma volume is usually present. While the terms dehydration and volume depletion are often used interchangeably, *dehydration* implies total body water depletion with most of which being intracellular, so the patient may or may not have hemodynamic compromise. On the other hand, *volume depletion* generally refers to a loss of plasma or intravascular volume, which tends to have a more profound cardiovascular effect.[11] As intravascular volume decreases, the rate of increase in serum urea is faster than that with SCr. Therefore, BUN increases by a larger magnitude than the SCr concentration in plasma volume depleted individuals, leading to a rise in the BUN:SCr ratio. However, it should be noted that BUN increases in the face of internal bleeding, CHF, renal failure, high dose corticosteroids, or high protein intake. Conversely, in patients with sarcopenia, low muscle mass, or low caloric intake, BUN concentration may remain low regardless of status of the plasma volume. If any of these conditions are present, additional signs and symptoms of volume depletion should be assessed along with the increased BUN:SCr ratio.

### Hypernatremia

*Hypernatremia* is defined as a serum sodium concentration >145 mEq/L (>145 mmol/L). By definition, all hypernatremic states lead to increased serum osmolality. There are four main causes of hypernatremia: inadequate water intake, extrarenal hypotonic fluid loss, renal concentrating defect, and excessive salt intake.[12] Depending on the etiology, hypernatremia may occur in the presence of high, normal, or low total body water content.[2,12]

The clinical manifestations of hypernatremia primarily involve the neurologic system. These manifestations are the consequence of dehydration, particularly in the brain. In adults, acute elevation in serum sodium >160 mEq/L (>160 mmol/L) may result in death. To assess the etiology of hypernatremia, it is important to evaluate (1) urine production, (2) sodium intake, and (3) renal solute concentrating ability, which reflects ADH activity. In most cases, history of presentation and urine analysis, including urine osmolality and urine sodium concentration, would help establish the cause of hypernatremia.[12]

***Hypernatremia associated with low total body water.*** This occurs when the loss of water exceeds the loss of sodium (ie, free water deficit).[3] The thirst mechanism generally increases water intake, but this adjustment is not always possible (eg, patients unable to tolerate oral intake or patients who are obtunded). This condition also may be iatrogenic when hypotonic fluid losses (eg, profuse sweating and diarrhea) are replaced with an excessive amount of salt-containing fluids, such as NaCl 0.9%. In these circumstances, fluid loss should be replaced with IV dextrose solutions or solutions with lower sodium content, such as NaCl 0.45%, which serve as a source of free water.[3,12] In patients with hypernatremia who present with high urine osmolality (>800 mOsm/kg, roughly equivalent to a specific gravity of 1.023) and low urine sodium concentrations (<10 mEq/L), these laboratory results reflect an intact renal concentrating mechanism. Signs and symptoms of dehydration should be carefully monitored. These include orthostatic hypotension, flat neck veins, tachycardia, poor skin turgor, and dry mucous membranes. In addition, the BUN:SCr ratio may be >20 secondary to dehydration.[2,11]

***Hypernatremia may be associated with normal total body water, also known as euvolemic hypernatremia.*** This condition refers to an increased loss of free water without concurrent sodium loss.[2,12,13] Because of water redistribution between the intracellular and extracellular fluid, no plasma volume contraction is usually evident unless water loss is substantial. In most cases, intravascular volume is further maintained by increased fluid intake. Etiologies include increased insensible water loss (eg, fever, extensive burns) and central and nephrogenic DI. It is worth noting that hypercalcemia, hypokalemia, acute tubular necrosis, amyloidosis, Sjögren's syndrome, sarcoidosis, and a number of medications can all independently precipitate nephrogenic DI. In evaluating a patient with hypernatremia, the clinician should carefully evaluate potential contribution by the existing pharmacotherapeutic agents and determine whether therapy should be modified. (Table 11-4).[13,14] Mild cases of DI can be safely and effectively managed by sufficient water intake. The removal of aggravating factors, if feasible, can further improve polyuria. If oral or enteral water intake in not adequate or tolerated, IV fluid administration with dextrose 5% is necessary for correcting hypernatremia and preventing hypovolemia. If the diagnosis of central DI is subsequently established, vasopressin or desmopressin, a synthetic analog of vasopressin, is a reasonable option for long-term maintenance therapy.

Hypernatremia also may be associated with increased total body water. This form of hypernatremia is the least common because sodium homeostasis is maintained indirectly through the control of water, and defects in the system usually affect total body water more than total body sodium.[3,13] Primary hyperaldosteronism and Cushing syndrome may cause total body water to increase. In other patients, high total body water usually results from exogenous administration of solutions containing large amounts of sodium (**Minicase 2**):

- Resuscitative efforts using large amount of sodium-containing solutions
- Inadvertent IV infusion of hypertonic saline solutions
- Inadvertent dialysis against high sodium-containing solutions
- Sea water, near drowning

## Potassium

*Normal range: 3.8 to 5.0 mEq/L (3.8 to 5.0 mmol/L)*
Potassium is the primary intracellular cation with an average intracellular fluid concentration of about 140 mEq/L (140 mmol/L). The major physiologic role of potassium is in the regulation of muscle and nerve excitability. It may also play important roles in the control of intracellular volume (similar to the ability of sodium in controlling extracellular volume), protein synthesis, enzymatic reactions, and carbohydrate metabolism.[14,15]

### Physiology

The most important aspect of potassium physiology is its effect on action potential, especially on muscle and nervous tissue excitability.[16,17] During periods of potassium imbalance, the cardiovascular system is of principal concern because of the life-threatening arrhythmias that may result from either high or low serum potassium concentrations. Cardiac muscle cells depend on their ability to change their electrical potentials, with accompanying potassium flux when exposed to the proper stimulus, to result in muscle contraction and nerve conduction.[16] One important aspect of potassium homeostasis is its distribution

## MINICASE 2

## A Case of Hypernatremia After Resection of Pituitary Tumor

Mrs. Lee, a 49-year-old woman with a recently diagnosed pituitary tumor, was admitted to the hospital 2 days ago for tumor resection. On postoperative day 2, she reports that she feels thirsty and a little dizzy. The nurse reports that she has been asking for water throughout the morning. She also has used the bathroom four times this morning.

Current vital signs: BP 108/80 mm Hg supine (standing BP 105/80 mm Hg); HR 84 to 90 beats/min; RR 10 to 14 breaths/min; $SpO_2$ (saturation of peripheral oxygen via pulse oximetry) 99% on room air; breathing comfortably. Intake (last 24 hours): five 8-oz glasses of water, 200 mL juice from breakfast, and two cups of hot tea.

Output: 3,130 mL of urine in the last 16 hours; weight: 63.7 kg today (64.2 kg yesterday; 64.7 kg before surgery).

Her laboratory results are as follows:

- Sodium, 155 mEq/L
- Potassium, 3.2 mEq/L
- Chloride, 101 mEq/L
- BUN, 18 mg/dL
- $CO_2$ content, 24 mEq/L
- Creatinine, 1.02 mg/dL
- Glucose, 72 mg/dL
- Urine osmolality, 105 mOsm/kg $H_2O$
- Urine specific gravity, 1.001

QUESTION: How would you interpret this patient's serum sodium concentration?

DISCUSSION: The patient's serum sodium concentration is elevated, suggesting hypernatremia. The next step is to assess her fluid status and determine the cause(s) of the disorder(s). Based on her history, the patient has an unusually high urine output (>3 L in 16 hours and frequent urination). Her urine osmolality and specific gravity show that she has diluted urine, which suggests that an excessive loss of free water likely has contributed to her hypernatremia. She is currently not volume depleted (based on her vital signs, BUN:SCr ratio) because she has been able to catch up with her urinary fluid loss with oral fluid intake due to thirst. Her weight change suggests that she is trending toward a mild fluid deficit. Thus, she can be described as having normovolemic hypernatremia.

The onset of her hypernatremia is likely acute because it occurred within 2 days after her surgery, and hyponatremia is more commonly seen after surgery because of elevated ADH releases. Her symptom of hypernatremia is limited to dizziness. Surgical procedures that could potentially affect pituitary gland function are a major risk factor for sodium disorders because the release and regulation of ADH may be affected. In this patient's case, the supraopticohypophyseal tract was likely affected during removal of the tumor, which precipitated the symptoms and signs that are currently observed. The elevated urine output with persistent thirst suggests that an ADH-related disorder, central DI, is likely present with a serious risk of altered sodium homeostasis. Her relatively normal vital signs were maintained by her ability to temporarily increase oral fluid intake. If the DI defect is not corrected, however, she will develop hypovolemia quickly. This is an acute medical problem, and the diagnosis should be established quickly with the help of several laboratory tests, such as urine sodium, serum sodium, and urine osmolality.

In summary, this patient has hypernatremia, which appears to be manifested by altered renal water/salt regulation based on the urine osmolality. Although her volume status appears normal at this point, she can quickly develop hypovolemia if she is unable to keep up with oral fluid intake. The cause of hypernatremia is likely related to the pituitary gland resection that caused central DI. The logical treatment approach for her involves free water provision to prevent free water deficit and treatment of DI. If her oral water intake is unable to match the urinary water loss, she will require concurrent IV fluid therapy to prevent severe hypovolemia.

---

equilibrium. In a 70-kg man, the total body potassium content is about 4,000 mEq. Of that amount, only a small fraction (about 60 mEq) is distributed in the extracellular fluid; the remainder resides within cells. The average daily Western diet contains 50 to 100 mEq of potassium, which is completely and passively absorbed in the upper GI tract. To enter cells, potassium must first pass through the extracellular compartment.

If the serum potassium concentration rises above 6 mEq/L (>6 mmol/L), symptomatic hyperkalemia is usually expected. Potassium homeostasis is altered by insulin, aldosterone, adrenergic responses, changes in acid–base balance, renal function, or GI and skin losses. These conditions can be modulated by various pathologic states as well as pharmacotherapy. Although potassium may affect different bodily functions, its effect on cardiac muscle is by far the most important clinical monitoring parameter.[15,16,18]

### Renal Homeostasis

When the serum potassium concentration is high, the body has two different mechanisms to restore potassium balance. A short-term solution is to shift the serum potassium into cells, whereas the other slower mechanism is renal elimination.[16] The kidneys are the primary organs involved in the control and elimination of potassium. Potassium is freely filtered at the glomeruli and almost completely reabsorbed before the filtrate reaches the collecting tubules. Only about 10% of the filtered potassium is secreted into the urine at the distal and collecting tubules. Virtually all the potassium recovered in urine is, therefore, regulated via tubular secretion rather than glomerular filtration.

In the distal tubule, potassium is secreted whereas sodium is reabsorbed. There are several mechanisms that can modulate this sodium–potassium exchange. Aldosterone plays an

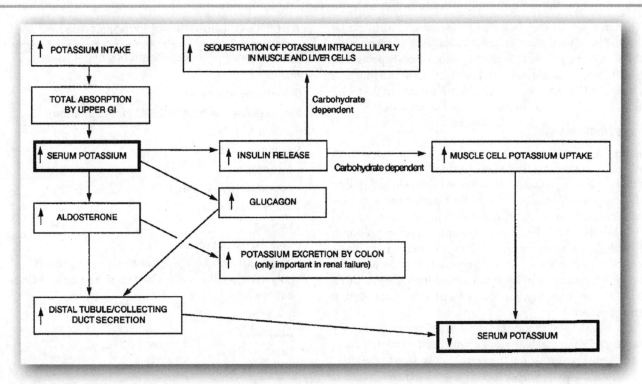

**FIGURE 11-3.** The acute homeostatic sequence of events in the body to maintain serum potassium within a narrow concentration range. An increased serum potassium triggers an increase in aldosterone secretion, which increases distal tubular potassium secretion. In patients with hyperkalemia and renal failure, aldosterone increases colonic potassium excretion. In patients with hyperkalemia and hyperglycemia, administration of insulin can shift potassium from the intravascular space into cells.

important role because it increases potassium secretion into the urine (**Figures 11-1** and **11-3**).[16] The hormone is secreted by the adrenal glands in response to high serum potassium concentrations. The delivery of large quantities of sodium and fluid to the distal tubules may also cause potassium secretion and its subsequent elimination, as seen in diuretic-induced hypokalemia. As the delivery of sodium and fluid is decreased, potassium secretion declines.

The presence of other anions in the distal tubules can increase renal potassium loss because the negatively charged anions attract positively charged potassium ions. This mechanism is responsible for hypokalemia caused by renal tubular acidosis and the administration large amount of sodium (eg, hypertonic saline solutions, or using sodium containing solution exclusively as vehicles for drugs).[16] Potassium secretion also is influenced by the potassium concentration in distal tubular cells. When the intracellular potassium concentration is high, such as during intravascular volume depletion, potassium secretion into the urine is increased. The modulation of renal potassium excretion by these mechanisms may take hours to correct a serum potassium concentration, even during drastic, acute changes. Extrarenal mechanisms, therefore, often play important roles in keeping the serum potassium concentration within the narrow acceptable range. Although the kidneys are the primary route of elimination, potassium secretion into the colon becomes important in patients with advanced renal failure.

### Acid–Base Homeostasis

Another potentially relevant factor influencing renal potassium secretion is serum pH. When arterial pH increases due to metabolic alkalosis, a compensatory efflux of hydrogen ions from the cells into the extracellular fluid (bloodstream) takes place with a concurrent influx of potassium ions into the cells to maintain an electropotential gradient.[17] During the early phase of metabolic alkalosis, the serum potassium concentration is transiently reduced because of a pH-dependent intracellular influx of serum potassium from the serum without altering the total body amount. Thus, although there is no immediate change in the amount of total body potassium, this movement of ions increases the cellular potassium content and results in hypokalemia. However, a shift in potassium and hydrogen ions also takes place in the renal distal tubular cells. In the presence of persistent alkalemia, renal potassium secretion into the urine is increased. Over time, the serum potassium concentration declines through increased renal loss, resulting in a reduced body store.

Metabolic acidosis has the opposite effect. Decreased pH results in an extracellular shift of potassium as a result of an intracellular shift of hydrogen ions, causing an elevated serum potassium concentration.[17] Because the intracellular potassium content of the distal tubular cell is decreased, secretion of potassium in the urine is diminished. Chronically, however, renal potassium loss gradually increases due to unknown mechanisms.

When a severe metabolic acid–base abnormality exists, adjustment of the measured serum potassium concentration may be necessary to more accurately estimate body potassium status when pH is normalized. For every 0.1 unit reduction in arterial pH from 7.40, roughly 0.6 mEq/L (range: 0.2 to 1.7 mEq/L) could be added to the serum potassium value.[17,19]

### Acute Homeostasis

Figure 11-3 summarizes the acute homeostatic mechanism involved in potassium distribution. During hyperkalemia, along with the release of aldosterone, increased glucagon and insulin release also contribute to reducing the serum potassium concentration. Glucagon stimulates potassium secretion into the distal tubules and collecting ducts whereas insulin promotes intracellular potassium uptake. Although insulin is not a major controlling factor in potassium homeostasis, it is useful for the emergency treatment of hyperkalemia. Administration of IV sodium bicarbonate may cause a transient intracellular shift of serum potassium.[14,16]

Pharmacological stimulation of β-2 adrenergic receptors may also affect the transcellular equilibrium of potassium. It leads to the movement of potassium from extracellular fluid to the intracellular fluid compartment. Therefore, β-2 adrenergic agonists (eg, albuterol) can be used short-term to treat certain hyperkalemic patients.[16,18]

### Hypokalemia

*Hypokalemia* is defined as a serum potassium concentration <3.5 mEq/L (<3.5 mmol/L).[16] To interpret the significance of low potassium values, clinicians should determine whether hypokalemia is caused by intracellular shifting of potassium (apparent deficit) or increased loss from the body (true deficit) (**Table 11-6**). Intracellular shifting occurs as a result of metabolic alkalosis, after administration of insulin, or giving large doses of β-2 adrenergic agonists (eg, continuous or hourly use of albuterol in patients in the intensive care unit (ICU) who are receiving mechanical ventilation). Increased elimination of potassium can occur in the kidneys or the GI tract. Other causes of hypokalemia include targeted temperature management, toxin exposure, refeeding syndrome, hyperaldosteronism, and Cushing syndrome. In children, several inherited disorders are associated with increased potassium wasting.[16,20,21]

### Drug-Associated Hypokalemia

***Amphotericin B.*** Proximal tubular damage can occur with amphotericin B therapy, resulting in renal tubular acidosis. Amphotericin B directly impairs the reabsorption of potassium, magnesium, and bicarbonate and leads to hypokalemia, hypomagnesemia, and metabolic acidosis. A concurrent deficiency in magnesium may affect the ability to restore potassium balance. Magnesium functions as a cofactor to maintain the sodium–potassium ATP pump activity and facilitates renal preservation of potassium. A patient with concurrent hypokalemia and hypomagnesemia does not respond to potassium replacement therapy effectively unless magnesium balance is restored first.[22,23] Lipid formulations of amphotericin B may still affect potassium homeostasis, although the magnitude may be less severe and the presentation is less acute.

## TABLE 11-6. Etiologies of Hypokalemia

Apparent deficit—intracellular shifting of potassium
  Alkalemia
  β-2 adrenergic stimulation
  Insulin (more common with IV bolus or infusion)
True deficit
  Decreased intake
    Alcoholism
    Potassium-free IV fluids
    Anorexia nervosa
    Bulimia
  Increased output (extrarenal)
    Potassium exchange resins or binders (eg, sodium polystyrene sulfonate, sodium zirconium cyclosilicate, patiromer)
    Vomiting
    Diarrhea
    Laxative abuse
    Intestinal fistulas
  Renal loss
    Corticosteroids, especially fludrocortisone and hydrocortisone
    Amphotericin B
    Loop and thiazide diuretics
    Hyperaldosteronism
    Cushing syndrome
    Licorice ingestion

***Diuretic.*** Non–potassium-sparing diuretic agents are drugs most commonly associated with renal potassium wasting. Although their mechanisms of natriuretic action differ, diuretic-induced hypokalemia is primarily caused by increased secretion of potassium at the distal sites in the nephron in response to an increased load of exchangeable sodium. Diuretics increase the distal urinary flow by inhibiting sodium reabsorption. This increased delivery of fluid and sodium in the distal segment of the nephron results in an increase in sodium reabsorption at that site. To maintain a neutral electrochemical gradient in the lumen, potassium is excreted as sodium is reabsorbed. Therefore, any inhibition of sodium absorption by diuretics proximal to or at the distal tubules can increase potassium loss. Renal potassium excretion is further enhanced when nonabsorbable anions are present in the urine.

Loop diuretics (eg, furosemide) or thiazides (eg, hydrochlorothiazide) are associated with hypokalemia and the effect is dose-dependent. Serum potassium concentrations should be monitored regularly, especially in patients receiving high doses of loop diuretics, to avoid the increased risk of cardiovascular events secondary to hypokalemia and other electrolyte imbalances. In addition, elderly patients with ischemic heart disease and patients receiving digoxin are more susceptible to the adverse consequences of hypokalemia. Other drugs commonly used in managing hypertension and other cardiac diseases such as spironolactone, triamterene, amiloride, eplerenone, angiotensin-converting enzyme (ACE) inhibitors, and angiotensin receptor antagonists are not expected to cause potassium loss due to their mode of action. On the contrary, they cause retention of potassium because of their effects related to aldosterone-dependent exchange sites in the collecting tubules.[24]

***Other causes.*** Conditions that cause hyperaldosteronism, either primary (eg, adrenal tumor) or secondary (eg, renovascular hypertension), can produce hypokalemia.[21] Cushing syndrome leads to increased circulation of mineralocorticoids such as aldosterone. Corticosteroids with strong mineralocorticoid activity (eg, fludrocortisone and hydrocortisone) also can cause hypokalemia. The hypokalemic effect of fludrocortisone is sometimes utilized to treat patients with chronic hyperkalemia.[25,26]

Gastrointestinal loss of potassium can be important. Aldosterone influences both renal and intestinal potassium handling.[17] A decrease in extracellular volume increases aldosterone secretion, which promotes renal and colonic potassium wasting. The potassium concentration in the GI fluid varies depending on the location of the GI tract, ranging from 5 mEq/L (bile, duodenum) to 30 mEq/L (colon). Therefore, profuse and uncontrolled diarrhea can result in potassium depletion. In contrast, upper GI secretion contains a much lower amount of potassium, and loss secondary to vomiting is unlikely to be significant. However, with severe vomiting, the resultant metabolic alkalosis may lead to hypokalemia due to intracellular shifting of potassium and enhanced urinary elimination. Finally, patients receiving potassium-free parenteral fluids can develop hypokalemia if not monitored properly.

***Clinical diagnosis.*** Signs and symptoms of hypokalemia involve many physiologic systems. Abnormalities in the cardiovascular system may result in serious consequences, including disturbances in cardiac rhythm. Hypokalemia-induced arrhythmias are of particular concern in patients receiving digoxin. Both digitalis glycosides and hypokalemia inhibit the sodium–potassium ATP pump in the cardiac cells. Together, they can deplete intracellular potassium, which may result in fatal arrhythmias. The signs and symptoms of hypokalemia are listed in **Table 11-7**.[1,20,21]

### Hyperkalemia

*Hyperkalemia* is generally defined as a serum potassium concentration >5.5 mEq/L (>5.5 mmol/L). As with hypokalemia, hyperkalemia may indicate a true or apparent potassium imbalance, although the signs and symptoms are indistinguishable.[16] To interpret a high serum potassium value, the clinician should determine whether hyperkalemia is due to apparent excess caused by extracellular shifting of potassium or true potassium excess in the body caused by increased intake with diminished excretion (**Table 11-8**).[14,16-18]

***Causes.*** Because renal excretion is the major route of potassium elimination, renal failure is the most common cause of hyperkalemia. However, potassium handling by the nephrons

## TABLE 11-7. Signs, Symptoms, and Effects of Hypokalemia on Various Organ Systems

Cardiovascular
  Decrease in T-wave amplitude
  Development of U waves
  Hypotension
  Increased risk of digoxin toxicity
  PR prolongation (with severe hypokalemia)
  Rhythm disturbances
  ST segment depression
  QRS widening (with severe hypokalemia)
Metabolic/endocrine (mostly serve as compensatory mechanisms)
  Decreased aldosterone release
  Decreased insulin release
  Decreased renal responsiveness to antidiuretic hormone
Neuromuscular
  Areflexia (with severe hypokalemia)
  Cramps
  Loss of smooth muscle function (ileus and urinary retention with severe hypokalemia)
  Weakness
Renal
  Inability to concentrate urine
  Nephropathy

is relatively well-preserved until the GFR falls to <10% of normal. Therefore, many patients with renal impairment can maintain a near normal, serum potassium concentration. They are still prone to developing hyperkalemia if excessive potassium is consumed and when renal function deteriorates.[16,17] It should also be noted that acid-base disorders can lead to changes in serum potassium concentration. For example, acidemia causes an efflux of intracellular potassium which may lead to hyperkalemia. The change is generally transient and serum potassium concentration would decline quickly with the correction of serum pH. However, if an excessive renal loss of serum potassium happens (eg, diuresis) during the transient period of potassium efflux, a total body potassium deficit may occur even after the normalization of serum pH.

Increased potassium intake rarely causes any problem in subjects in the absence of significant renal impairment. With normal renal function, increased potassium intake leads to increased renal excretion and redistribution to the intracellular space through the action of endogenous aldosterone and insulin, respectively. Interference with either mechanism may result in hyperkalemia. Decreased aldosterone secretion can occur with Addison disease or other defects affecting the hormone's adrenal output. Pathologic changes affecting the proximal or distal renal tubules also can lead to hyperkalemia.[16,17]

Use of potassium-sparing diuretics (eg, spironolactone) is a common cause of hyperkalemia, especially in patients with renal

## TABLE 11-8. Etiologies of Hyperkalemia

Extracellular shifting of potassium associated with acidemia

True excess

Increased release of intracellular potassium into bloodstream

Hemolysis

Tumor lysis syndrome

Rhabdomyolysis

Muscle crush injuries

Burns

Increased total body potassium

Increased potassium intake (eg, salt substitute, diet)

Decreased excretion or increased retention

Chronic or acute renal failure

Potassium-sparing diuretics

ACE inhibitors

Nonsteroidal antiinflammatory agents

Aldosterone receptor antagonists

Angiotensin II receptor antagonists

Unfractionated heparin

Trimethoprim (including drugs such as cotrimoxazole)

Deficiency of adrenal corticosteroids (especially mineralocorticoids)

Addison disease

Factious causes

Leukocytosis

Thrombocytosis

Hemolyzed specimen

---

function impairment. Concurrent use of potassium supplements (including potassium-rich salt substitutes) also increases the risk. Similar to hypokalemia, hyperkalemia can result from transcellular shifting of potassium. In the presence of severe acidemia, potassium shifts from the intracellular to the extracellular space, which may result in a clinically significant increase in the serum potassium concentration.[19]

**Clinical diagnosis.** The cardiovascular manifestations of hyperkalemia are of major concern. They include cardiac rhythm disturbances, bradycardia, hypotension, and, in severe cases, cardiac arrest. At times, muscle weakness may occur before these cardiac signs and symptoms. To appreciate the potent effect of potassium on the heart, one has to realize that potassium is the principal component of cardioplegic solutions commonly used to arrest the rhythm of the heart during cardiac surgeries.[14,16,18]

**Causes of spurious laboratory results.** Several conditions result in transient hyperkalemia, in which the high serum concentration reported is not expected to have significant

clinical sequelae. Erythrocytes also have high potassium content. When there is substantial hemolysis in the specimen collection tube, the red cells release potassium in quantities large enough to produce misleading results. Hemolysis may occur when a small needle is used for blood draw, when the tourniquet is too tight, or when the specimen stands too long or is mishandled. When a high serum potassium concentration is reported in a patient without pertinent signs and symptoms, the test needs to be repeated to rule out hemolysis. A similar phenomenon can occur when the specimen is allowed to clot (when nonheparinized tubes are used) because platelets and white cells are also rich in potassium.

Management of chronic hyperkalemia includes decreasing dietary intake of potassium, use of diuretics if feasible, and treatment of metabolic acidosis if present. If the cause is drug induced (eg, ACE inhibitors), the use of an alternative therapeutic agent should be considered. When changing to an alternative therapy is not an option (eg, tacrolimus in transplant patients), the addition of a chronic potassium-lowering agent, such as fludrocortisone or sodium-zirconium cyclosilicate, may be needed. For rapid correction of acute, symptomatic hyperkalemia, measures include correcting metabolic acidosis with IV sodium bicarbonate; administering IV dextrose and regular insulin or inhaled β-adrenergic agonists to shift potassium from the extracellular to the intracellular space; using high doses of loop diuretics to enhance renal excretion of potassium; administering patiromer, sodium zirconium cyclosilicate, or sodium polystyrene sulfonate to increase colonic elimination of potassium; and initiating dialysis in the most severe cases (**Minicase 3**).

## Chloride

*Normal range: 95 to 103 mEq/L (95 to 103 mmol/L)*

### Physiology

Chloride is the most abundant extracellular anion with a low intracellular concentration (about 4 mEq/L). Chloride is passively absorbed from the upper small intestine. In the distal ileum and large intestine, its absorption is coupled with bicarbonate ion secretion. Chloride excretion is primarily regulated by the renal proximal tubules, where it is exchanged for bicarbonate ions. Throughout the rest of the nephron, chloride passively follows sodium and water. In addition, the luminal and interstitial chloride-bicarbonate ($Cl/HCO_3$) exchangers in the collecting duct also contribute to the renal regulation of chloride.

Chloride is influenced by the extracellular fluid balance and acid–base balance.[19,20] Although homeostatic mechanisms do not directly regulate chloride, they indirectly regulate it through changes in sodium and bicarbonate. The physiologic role of chloride is primarily passive. It balances out positive charges in the extracellular fluid and, by passively following sodium, helps to maintain extracellular osmolality.

### Hypochloremia and Hyperchloremia

Serum chloride values are used as confirmatory tests to identify fluid balance and acid–base abnormalities.[27,28] Like sodium, a

## MINICASE 3

## A Case of Hyperkalemia

Raj P. a 68-year-old man, is admitted to the cardiology service for further examination of dyspnea and shortness of breath. His chief complaints include worsening of shortness of breath in the last 2 days, swelling of his legs, and the need for extra pillows before he can go to bed for the past week. He experiences worsening fatigue and dyspnea with ordinary activities.

He missed his furosemide doses for the past 2 to 3 days because it makes him go the bathroom a lot. He has been told that he needs furosemide for worsening shortness of breath. Otherwise, he takes his other medications consistently as instructed by his healthcare providers.

Past medical history includes congestive heart failure (ejection fraction of 31% checked 5.5 months ago), chronic atrial fibrillation, and type 2 diabetes mellitus. His home medications are as follows:

- Carvedilol, 12.5 mg PO q 12 hours
- Furosemide, 60 mg PO every morning and 20 mg every evening
- Glargine insulin, 30 units SC daily
- Lisinopril, 20 mg PO Twice daily
- Potassium chloride, 20 mEq PO daily
- Spironolactone, 12.5 mg PO daily
- Warfarin, 5 mg PO daily

Vital signs on admission: BP 110/78 mm Hg (baseline BP 118/82 mm Hg), HR 69 beats/min (baseline HR 68 beats/min), and weight 90 kg (4 weeks ago, clinic record; 80 kg upon clinic admission).

Raj's laboratory results are as follows:

- Brain natriuretic peptide (BNP), 532 pg/mL
- Sodium, 133 mEq/L
- Potassium, 5.7 mEq/L
- Chloride, 101 mEq/L
- $CO_2$ content, 22 mEq/L
- BUN, 37 mg/dL
- Creatinine, 2.1 mg/dL (baseline creatinine 1.5 mg/dL)
- Glucose, 72 mg/dL

Other tests include EKG and oxygen saturation 92% on room air.

QUESTION: How would you interpret this patient's serum potassium concentration?

DISCUSSION: His serum potassium concentration, at 5.7 mEq/L, is elevated. It is possible that his baseline potassium concentration is mildly elevated because there are several factors that would contribute to hyperkalemia: (1) he is taking a potassium supplement, (2) he is taking two drugs that can increase serum potassium (spironolactone and lisinopril), (3) he has renal insufficiency at baseline (creatinine 1.5 mg/dL). It is likely that his potassium concentration has increased more significantly in the last 2 days. His current state of hyperkalemia is likely exacerbated by two recent events: (1) nonadherence with furosemide in the last 3 days, which results in decreased renal potassium loss; and (2) worsening of heart failure (as suggested by increased BNP, weight gain of 10 kg, and increased leg swelling), which in turn decreases renal blood flow and results in worsening of acute renal failure (as suggested by an increased serum creatinine from 1.5 to 2.1 mg/dL).

The primary goal for managing hyperkalemia is to prevent/reverse cardiac symptoms. With a serum potassium of 5.7 mEq/L, there is a definite risk for arrhythmias. Therefore, a 12-lead EKG should be obtained. If EKG changes are present and consistent with hyperkalemia, interventions to decrease serum potassium concentration, such as IV insulin and dextrose or IV sodium bicarbonate, should be initiated right away. IV calcium (calcium gluconate 1 g) also should be administered to reduce the risk of arrhythmias. Note that IV calcium administration has no effect in removing serum potassium and should never be used alone in the management of symptomatic hyperkalemia. Regardless of the cardiac symptoms, his potassium supplement should be withheld. Because his blood pressure is not elevated, it also is reasonable to withhold spironolactone for now until the potassium concentration starts to decline.

In summary, this patient has hyperkalemia, most likely exacerbated by acute renal failure and continued use of a potassium supplement. Assessment of symptoms and signs of hyperkalemia should be performed as soon as possible.

change in the serum chloride concentration does not necessarily reflect a change in total body content. Rather, it indicates an alteration in fluid status and acid–base balance. One of the most common causes of hyperchloremia in hospitalized patients results from saline infusion.[29] Chloride has the added feature of being influenced by bicarbonate. Therefore, it would be expected to decrease to the same proportion as sodium when serum is diluted with fluid and increase to the same proportion as sodium during intravascular volume depletion. However, when a patient has been receiving continuous or frequent nasogastric suction, or has profuse vomiting, a greater loss of chloride than sodium can occur because gastric fluid contains 1.5 to 3 times more chloride than sodium. Gastric outlet obstruction, protracted vomiting, and self-induced vomiting also can lead to hypochloremia.

*Drug and IV fluid-associated causes.* Although drugs can influence serum chloride concentrations, they rarely do so directly. For example, although loop diuretics (eg, furosemide) and thiazide diuretics (eg, hydrochlorothiazide) inhibit chloride uptake at the loop of Henle and distal nephron, respectively, the hypochloremia that may result is due to the concurrent loss of sodium and contraction alkalosis.[30,31] Because chloride ions passively follow sodium ions, salt and water retention can transiently raise serum chloride concentrations. This effect occurs with corticosteroids and nonsteroidal antiinflammatory agents such as ibuprofen. Also, IV fluids or parenteral nutrition solutions with high chloride concentrations are associated with an increased risk of hyperchloremia. Replacing some of the cations with an acetate salt instead of a chloride salt (eg, potassium acetate instead of potassium chloride) can reduce this risk. The sources of chloride ions should be carefully monitored daily, especially among hospitalized patients receiving multiple IV drips and medications using a saline-based fluid as the vehicle.

***Acid–base status and other causes.*** Acid–base balance is partly regulated by renal production and excretion of bicarbonate ions. The proximal tubules are the primary regulators of bicarbonate. These proximal tubules cells exchange bicarbonate with chloride to maintain the intracellular electrochemical gradient. Renal excretion of chloride increases during metabolic alkalosis, resulting in a reduced serum chloride concentration.

The opposite situation also may be true: metabolic or respiratory acidosis results in an elevated serum chloride concentration. Hyperchloremic metabolic acidosis may occur when the kidneys are unable to conserve bicarbonate, as in interstitial renal disease (eg, obstruction, pyelonephritis, and analgesic nephropathy), GI bicarbonate loss from diarrhea, and acetazolamide-induced carbonic anhydrase inhibition.[31] One of the most common causes of hyperchloremia in hospitalized patients is excessive use of IV saline solution.[29] Falsely elevated chloride is rare but may occur with bromide toxicity due to an inability to distinguish between these two halogens by the laboratory's chemical analyzer. Because the signs and symptoms associated with hyperchloremia and hypochloremia are related to fluid status or a patient's acid–base status and its underlying causes, rather than to chloride itself, the reader is referred to discussions in Chapter 13.

# OTHER MINERALS

## Magnesium

*Normal range: 1.7 to 2.4 mg/dL (0.7 to 1 mmol/L) or 1.4 to 2 mEq/L*

### Physiology

Magnesium has a widespread physiologic role in maintaining neuromuscular functions and enzymatic functions. Magnesium acts as a cofactor for phosphorylation of ATPs from adenosine phosphates. Magnesium also is vital for binding macromolecules to organelles (eg, messenger ribonucleic acid to ribosomes).

The average adult body contains 21 to 29 g (1,750 to 2,400 mEq) of magnesium with the following distribution:

- Approximately 50% in bone (about 30% or less of this pool is slowly exchangeable with extracellular fluid)
- 20% in muscle
- Approximately 10% in nonmuscle soft tissues
- 1% to 2% in extracellular fluid (for plasma magnesium, about 50% is free; about 15% is complexed to anions; and 30% is bound to protein, primarily albumin)

Approximately 30% to 40% of the ingested magnesium is absorbed from the jejunum and ileum through transcellular and paracellular mechanisms. The regulation of oral magnesium absorption is by both passive diffusion down an electrochemical gradient and active transport process. TRPM6 is the transport protein that is highly expressed along the brush border membrane of the enterocytes and plays a key role in regulating the absorption of magnesium. The extent of magnesium absorption may be affected by dietary magnesium intake, calcium intake, vitamin D, and PTH. However, conflicting data are available, and the extent to which these parameters affect absorption is unresolved. Certain medications (eg, cyclosporine, tacrolimus, cisplatin, amphotericin B) can significantly increase renal magnesium loss, predisposing the patient to hypomagnesemia.[32,33]

Urinary magnesium accounts for one-third of the total daily magnesium output, whereas the other two-thirds are in the GI tract (eg, stool). Unbound serum magnesium is freely filtered at the glomerulus. All but 3% to 5% of filtered magnesium is normally reabsorbed (100 mg/day). In other words, 95% to 97% of the filtered magnesium is reabsorbed under normal physiology. Reabsorption is primarily through the ascending limb of the loop of Henle (50% to 60%). About 30% is reabsorbed in the proximal tubule and 7% from the distal tubule. This explains why loop diuretics have a profound effect on renal magnesium wasting. The drive of magnesium reabsorption is mediated by the charge difference generated by the sodium–potassium–chloride cotransport system in the lumen.

The regulation of magnesium is primarily driven by the serum magnesium concentration. Changes in serum magnesium concentrations have potent effects on renal reabsorption and stool losses. These effects are seen over 3 to 5 days and may persist for a long time. Hormonal regulation of magnesium seems to be much less critical for its homeostasis.

Factors affecting calcium homeostasis also affect magnesium homeostasis.[17,32] A decline in serum magnesium concentration stimulates the release of PTH, which increases serum magnesium by promoting its release from the bone store and enhancing renal reabsorption. Hyperaldosteronism causes increased magnesium renal excretion. Insulin by itself does not alter the serum magnesium concentration, but in a hyperglycemic state, insulin causes rapid intracellular uptake of glucose. This process causes an increase in the phosphorylation by sodium–potassium ATPase on the cell membrane. Because magnesium is used as a cofactor for sodium potassium ATPase, serum magnesium concentration declines, resulting in hypomagnesemia. Excretion of magnesium is influenced by serum calcium and phosphorus concentrations. Magnesium movement generally follows that of phosphorus (ie, if phosphorus declines, magnesium also declines) and is the opposite of calcium.[32,34,35] Other factors that increase magnesium reabsorption include acute metabolic acidosis, hyperthyroidism, and chronic alcohol use.

Magnesium also regulates neuromuscular function. Magnesium depletion results in neuromuscular weakness as the release of acetylcholine to motor endplates is enhanced by the presence of magnesium. Motor endplate sensitivity to acetylcholine also is affected. When serum magnesium decreases, acetylcholine release increases, resulting in increased muscle excitation, which may lead to increased deep tendon reflexes. Common symptoms associated with hypomagnesemia include weakness, muscle fasciculation with tremor, tetany, and increased deep tendon reflexes. In addition, vasodilation may occur by a direct effect on blood vessels and ganglionic blockade due to hypomagnesemia.

## Hypomagnesemia

*Hypomagnesemia* is loosely defined as a serum magnesium concentration <1.7 mg/dL (<0.7 mmol/L). The common causes of hypomagnesemia include renal wasting, chronic alcohol use, diabetes mellitus, protein-calorie malnutrition, refeeding syndrome, GI losses from chronic diarrhea or high ileostomy output, and postparathyroidectomy. Because serum magnesium deficiency can be offset by magnesium release from bone, muscle, and the heart, the serum value may not be a useful indicator of cellular depletion and complications (eg, arrhythmias). However, low serum magnesium usually indicates low cellular magnesium as long as the patient has a normal extracellular fluid volume.[34]

***Causes.*** Magnesium deficiency is more common than magnesium excess. Depletion usually results from excessive loss from the GI tract or kidneys (eg, use of loop diuretics). Magnesium depletion is not commonly the result of decreased intake because the kidneys can cease magnesium elimination in four to seven days to conserve the ion. However, with chronic alcohol consumption, deficiency can occur from a combination of poor intake, poor GI absorption (eg, vomiting or diarrhea), and increased renal elimination. Depletion also can occur from poor intestinal absorption (eg, small-bowel resection). Diarrhea can be a source of magnesium loss because diarrhea stools may contain as much as 14 mEq/L (7 mmol/L) of magnesium. Chronic use of proton-pump inhibitors also has been associated with hypomagnesemia.

Urinary magnesium loss may result from diuresis or tubular defects, such as the diuretic phase of acute tubular injuries. Some patients with hypoparathyroidism may exhibit low magnesium serum concentrations from renal loss and, possibly, decreased intestinal absorption. Other conditions associated with magnesium deficiency include hyperthyroidism, primary aldosteronism, diabetic ketoacidosis, and pancreatitis. Magnesium deficiency associated with these conditions may be particularly dangerous because often there are concurrent potassium and calcium deficiencies. Although loop diuretics lead to significant magnesium depletion, thiazide diuretics alone rarely cause hypomagnesemia, especially at lower doses (hydrochlorothiazide <50 mg/day). Furthermore, potassium-sparing diuretics (eg, spironolactone, triamterene, and amiloride) have some magnesium-sparing effect and, therefore, play a limited clinical role in preserving body magnesium and preventing hypomagnesemia.

***Clinical diagnosis.*** Magnesium affects the central nervous system (CNS). Magnesium depletion can cause personality changes, disorientation, convulsions, psychosis, stupor, and coma.[32,34] Severe hypomagnesemia may result in hypocalcemia due to intracellular cationic shifts. Many symptoms of magnesium deficiency result from concurrent hypocalcemia.

Perhaps the most important effects of magnesium imbalance are on the heart. Decreased magnesium in cardiac cells may manifest as a prolonged QT interval, which is associated with an increased risk of arrhythmias, especially torsades de pointes, which can be effectively treated by IV magnesium.[17,36,37] Moderately decreased concentrations can cause electrocardiogram (EKG) abnormalities similar to those observed with hypokalemia.

## Hypermagnesemia

*Hypermagnesemia* is defined as a serum magnesium concentration >2.4 mg/dL (>1 mmol/L).

***Causes.*** Besides magnesium overload (eg, overreplacement of magnesium, treatment for preeclampsia, and antacid/laxative overuse), the most important risk factor for hypermagnesemia is renal dysfunction, especially CKD. Rapid infusions of IV solutions containing large amounts of magnesium may result in transient hypermagnesemia.

***Clinical diagnosis.*** Serum magnesium concentrations <6 mg/dL (<2.5 mmol/L) rarely cause serious symptoms. Nonspecific symptoms, such as muscle weakness, decrease in deep tendon reflexes, or fatigue, may be present. As magnesium concentration rises above 6 mg/dL, more notable symptoms such as lethargy, mental confusion, and hypotension may be observed (**Table 11-9**).[35,38] In severe hypermagnesemia (12 mg/dL), life-threatening symptoms, including coma, paralysis, or cardiac arrest, can be observed and urgent therapy is indicated.

Treatment for severe or symptomatic hypermagnesemia may include IV calcium gluconate 1 to 2 g over 30 minutes to reverse the neuromuscular and cardiovascular blockade of magnesium. Increased renal elimination of magnesium can be achieved by forced diuresis with IV saline hydration and a loop diuretic agent. Hemodialysis should be reserved as a last resort.

## Calcium

*Normal range: 9.2 to 11 mg/dL (2.3 to 2.8 mmol/L) for adults*

**TABLE 11-9.** Signs and Symptoms of Hypermagnesemia

| SERUM MAGNESIUM CONCENTRATION | | MAJOR CLINICAL SIGNS AND SYMPTOMS |
|---|---|---|
| 6–8.5 mg/dL | 5–7 mEq/L | Bradycardia, flushing, sweating, sensation of warmth, fatigue, drowsiness |
| 8.5–12 mg/dL | 7–10 mEq/L | Hypotension, decreased deep tendon reflexes, altered mental status possible |
| >12 mg/dL | >10 mEq/L | Flaccid paralysis and increased PR and QRS intervals, severe mental confusion, coma, respiratory distress, and asystole |

## Physiology

Calcium plays an important role in the propagation of neuro-muscular activity, regulation of endocrine functions (eg, pancreatic insulin release and gastric hydrogen secretion), blood coagulation including platelet aggregation, and bone and tooth metabolism.[17,35,39]

The serum calcium concentration is closely regulated by complex interactions among PTH, serum phosphorus, vitamin D system, and the target organ (**Figure 11-4**). About one-third of the ingested calcium is actively absorbed from the proximal area of the small intestine, facilitated by 1,25-dihydroxycholecalciferol (1,25-DHCC or calcitriol, the most active form of vitamin D). Passive intestinal absorption is negligible with intake of <2 g/day. The average daily calcium intake is 2 to 2.5 g/day.

The normal adult body contains approximately 1,000 g of calcium, with only 0.5% found in the extracellular fluid; 99.5%

is integrated into bones. Therefore, the tissue concentration of calcium is small. Because bone is constantly remodeled by osteoblasts and osteoclasts, a small quantity of bone calcium is in equilibrium with extracellular fluid. Extracellular calcium exists in three forms:

1. Complexed to bicarbonate, citrates, and phosphates (6%)
2. Protein bound, mostly to albumin (40%)
3. Ionized or free fraction (54%)

***Intracellular calcium.*** The imbalance of body calcium results in disturbances in neuromuscular actions. Within the cells, calcium maintains a low concentration. The calcium that is attracted into the negatively charged cell is either actively effluxed out of the cells or sequestered by mitochondria or the endoplasmic reticulum. Such differences in concentrations allow calcium to be used for transmembrane signaling.

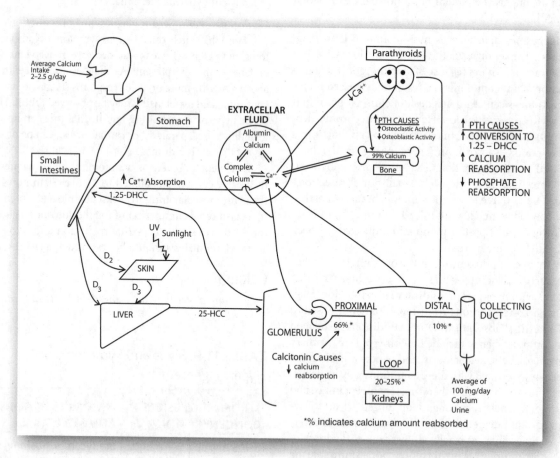

**FIGURE 11-4.** Calcium physiology: relationship with vitamin D, calcitonin, PTH, and albumin. The primary source of calcium is from diet. Absorption of calcium takes place in the small intestine. Vitamin D, more specifically calcitriol or 1,25-DHCC, has the most potent effect on intestinal extraction of calcium. Once absorbed, calcium is transported in the extracellular fluid by albumin to various organs. Bones serve as an important reservoir for calcium. When serum calcium concentration decreases, PTH release increases, and it stimulates osteoclast activity, which releases calcium into the plasma to maintain normocalcemia. Calcium also is excreted renally. Only about 10% of dietary calcium is normally lost in the urine. Although humans can synthesize a limited amount of vitamin D with optimal ultraviolet B exposure, most vitamin D comes from the diet, which many include ergocalciferol (vitamin D$_2$, primarily from plants) and cholecalciferol (vitamin D$_3$, primarily from animal sources). The endogenous vitamin D formed by the body is cholecalciferol (D$_3$).

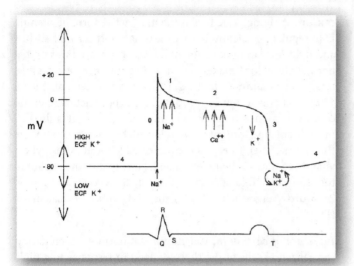

**FIGURE 11-5.** Cardiac intracellular potential and its relationship to the EKG.

In response to stimuli, calcium ions either enter a cell or are released from internal cellular stores where they interact with specific intracellular proteins to regulate cellular functions or metabolic processes.[17,39,40] Calcium enters cells through one of the three types of calcium channels: T (transient or fast), N (neuronal), and L (long-lasting or slow).

In the muscle, calcium is released from the intracellular sarcoplasmic reticulum. The released calcium binds to troponin and stops troponin from inhibiting the interaction of actin and myosin. This interaction results in muscle contraction. Conversely, muscle relaxation occurs when calcium is pumped back into the sarcoplasmic reticulum. In cardiac tissue, calcium becomes important during phase 2 of the action potential. During this phase, fast entry of sodium stops and calcium entry through the slow channels begins (**Figure 11-5**), resulting in contraction. During repolarization, calcium is actively pumped out of the cell.[17]

Calcium channel blockers (eg, nifedipine, diltiazem, and verapamil) inhibit the movement of calcium into muscle cells, thus decreasing the strength of contraction. They primarily affect the L-channels. The areas that are most sensitive to these effects appear to be the sinoatrial and atrioventricular nodes and vascular smooth muscles, which explains the hypotensive effects of nifedipine.

***Extracellular calcium.*** Complexed calcium usually accounts for <1 mg/dL (<0.25 mmol/L) of blood calcium. The calcium complex usually is formed with bicarbonate, citrate, or phosphate. In patients with CKD, calcium also may be bound with sulfate because of the decreased renal elimination of sulfate ions. Phosphorus plays an important role in calcium homeostasis. Under normal physiologic conditions, the product of total serum calcium concentration and serum phosphorus concentration (calcium–phosphate product) is relatively constant: an increase in one ion necessitates a corresponding decline in the other. In addition, many homeostatic mechanisms that control calcium also regulate phosphate. This relationship is particularly important in renal failure; the decreased phosphate excretion associated with CKD may ultimately lead to hypocalcemia, if hyperphosphatemia is untreated.[17,40]

Calcium also binds to serum proteins such as albumin (80%) and globulins (20%). Protein-bound calcium is in equilibrium with ionized calcium, which is affected by the serum anion concentration and blood pH. This equilibrium is important because ionized calcium is the physiologically active moiety. Alkalemia increases protein binding of calcium, resulting in a lower free fraction, whereas acidemia has the opposite effect. In patients with uncompensated respiratory or metabolic alkalosis, the signs and symptoms of hypocalcemia may become more pronounced due to increased binding. Conversely, signs and symptoms of hypercalcemia become more apparent in patients with uncompensated metabolic or respiratory acidosis. Therefore, total serum calcium concentration, which is commonly reported by clinical laboratories, is not as clinically significant as the quantity of available ionized calcium. In fact, it is the free calcium concentration that is closely regulated by the different homeostatic mechanisms.

Clinically, serum protein concentrations, especially albumin, have an important influence on regulating the amount of physiologically active calcium in the serum. The normal serum calcium range is 9.2 to 11 mg/dL (2.3 to 2.8 mmol/L) for a patient with a serum albumin of 4 g/dL. In normal healthy adults, only 40% to 50% of the total serum calcium is free from protein-binding and thus considered physiologically active. In patients with hypoalbuminemia (eg, due to acute illnesses, severe malnutrition), the free concentration of calcium is elevated despite a "normal" total serum calcium concentration. Therefore, it is a common practice either to measure ionized calcium or correct the total serum calcium concentration based on the measured albumin concentration. The following formula is commonly used in an attempt to "correct" total serum calcium concentration:

$$Ca_{corr} = ([4.0 - albumin] \times 0.8 \text{ mg/dL}) + Ca_{uncorr}$$

where $Ca corr$ is the corrected serum calcium concentration and $Ca uncorr$ is the uncorrected (or measured total) serum calcium concentration. For example, a clinician may be asked to write parenteral nutrition orders for an emaciated cancer patient with a GI obstruction. The serum albumin is 1.9 g/dL (19 g/L), and the total serum calcium concentration is 7.7 mg/dL (1.9 mmol/L). At first glance, one might consider the calcium to be low; however, with the reduced serum albumin concentration, more ionized calcium is available to cells.

$$Ca_{corr} = ([4.0 - 1.9] \times 0.8) + 7.7 = 9.4 \text{ mg/dL} (2.34 \text{ mmol/L})$$

The corrected serum calcium concentration is, thus, within the normal range. More importantly, the patient does not exhibit any signs and symptoms of hypocalcemia; thus, calcium supplementation is not indicated. In the presence of severe hypoalbuminemia, as in critically ill patients, an apparently low total serum calcium may in fact be sufficient or, in some instances, excessive.

Although this serum calcium correction method may be useful, the clinician must be aware of its limitations and potential for inaccuracy. The correction factor of 0.8 represents an average fraction of calcium bound to albumin under normal physiology. To have an accurate determination of the free concentration, a direct measurement of serum ionized calcium concentration is preferred (normal range: 4 to 4.8 mg/dL or 1 to 1.2 mmol/L). Ultimately, a patient's clinical presentation is the most important factor to determine if immediate treatment for a calcium disorder is indicated.

Although calcium absorption takes place throughout the entire small intestine, the proximal regions of the small intestine (jejunum and proximal ileum) are the most active and regulated areas. Calcium absorption from the human GI tract is mediated by two processes: (1) transcellular active transport, a saturable, vitamin D–responsive process mediated by specific calcium-binding proteins primarily in the upper GI tract, particularly in the distal duodenum and upper jejunum; and (2) paracellular process, a nonsaturable linear transfer via diffusion that occurs throughout the entire length of the intestine. Under normal physiology, the total calcium absorptive capacity is the highest in the ileum because of longer residence time. The rate of paracellular calcium absorption remains stable regardless of calcium intake. However, when dietary calcium intake is relatively limited, the efficiency of transcellular calcium transport becomes higher and accounts for a significant fraction of the absorbed calcium. Transcellular calcium transport is closely regulated by vitamin D, although other mechanisms also may be involved.[43,44] Specifically, 1,25-DHCC induces the intestinal expressions of transcellular calcium transporters through its binding with the vitamin D receptors in the intestinal epithelial cells.

**Effect of vitamin D.** A small amount of calcium is excreted daily into the GI tract through saliva, bile, and pancreatic and intestinal secretions. However, the primary route of elimination is filtration by the kidneys. Calcium is freely filtered at the glomeruli, where approximately 65% is reabsorbed at the proximal tubules under partial control by calcitonin and 1,25-DHCC. Roughly 25% is reabsorbed in the loop of Henle, and another 10% is reabsorbed at the distal tubules under the influence of PTH.[41,45]

Despite being classified as a vitamin, the physiologic functions of vitamin D more closely resemble a hormone. Vitamin D is important for the following functions:

- Intestinal absorption of calcium
- PTH-induced mobilization of calcium from bone
- Calcium reabsorption in the proximal renal tubules

Vitamin D is absorbed by the intestines in two forms, 7-dehydrocholesterol and cholecalciferol. 7-dehydrocholesterol is also converted into cholecalciferol in the skin by ultraviolet-B radiation from the sun. Hepatic and intestinal enzymes, including CYP27A1, CYP2J2, and CYP3A4, convert cholecalciferol to 25-hydroxycholecalciferol (25-HCC or calcidiol or calcifediol), which is then further converted by CYP27B1 in the kidneys to form 1,25-DHCC or calcitriol. This last conversion step is regulated by PTH and serum calcium concentration.[43,46] When PTH is increased during hypocalcemia, renal production of calcitriol increases, which increases intestinal absorption of calcium. Although calcitriol is the most active form of vitamin D in regulating calcium homeostasis, its short serum half-life and tight regulation of serum and tissue concentrations under normal physiology make it an inaccurate marker for assessing total body vitamin D status. Calcidiol has a serum half-life of 14 days, and its serum concentration does not fluctuate significantly in response to serum calcium concentration. It is also the main circulating form of vitamin D with high concentration in the plasma. Therefore, it is the preferred laboratory test when vitamin D status is being evaluated. Note that in most laboratories, the calcidiol assay measures the total concentration of 25-hydroxy-ergocalciferol (D2) and 25-hydroxycholecalciferol (D3).[47]

**Influence of calcitonin.** Calcitonin is a hormone secreted by specialized C cells of the thyroid gland in response to a high level of circulating ionized calcium. Calcitonin lowers serum calcium levels in part by inhibiting osteoclastic activity, thereby inhibiting bone resorption. It also decreases calcium reabsorption in the renal proximal tubules, resulting in increased renal calcium clearance. Calcitonin is used for the treatment of acute hypercalcemia; several different forms of the hormone are available.

**Influence of parathyroid hormone.** PTH is an important hormone involved in calcium homeostasis. It is secreted by the parathyroid glands, which are embedded in the thyroid, in direct response to low circulating ionized calcium. PTH closely regulates, and is regulated by, the vitamin D system to maintain serum ionized calcium concentration within a narrow range. Generally, PTH increases the serum calcium concentration and stimulates the enzymatic activity of CYP27B1 to promote renal conversion of calcidiol to calcitriol, which enhances intestinal calcium absorption. Elevated calcitriol concentration also serves as a potent suppressor of PTH synthesis via a negative feedback mechanism that is independent of the serum calcium concentration.[41,43] The normal reference range for serum PTH concentrations is 10 to 65 pg/mL (10 to 65 ng/L).

Tubular reabsorption of calcium and phosphate at the nephron is controlled by PTH; it increases renal reabsorption of calcium and decreases the reabsorption of phosphate, resulting in lower serum phosphorus and higher serum calcium concentrations. Perhaps the most important effect of PTH is on the bone. In the presence of PTH, osteoblastic activity is diminished and bone resorption processes of osteoclasts are increased. These effects increase serum ionized calcium, which feeds back to the parathyroid glands to decrease PTH output.

The suppressive effect of calcitriol on PTH secretion is used clinically in patients with CKD who have excessively high serum PTH concentrations caused by secondary hyperparathyroidism. PTH is a known uremic toxin, and its presence in supraphysiological concentrations has many adverse effects (eg, suppression of bone marrow erythropoiesis and increased osteoclastic bone resorption with replacement by fibrous tissue).[41] **Figure 11-6** depicts the relationship between serum PTH and serum calcium concentrations.

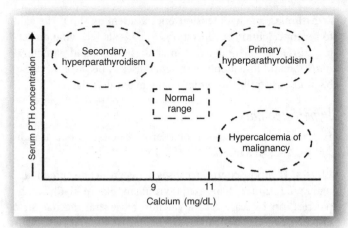

**FIGURE 11-6.** Interpretation of serum PTH concentrations with concomitant serum calcium concentrations.

**TABLE 11-10.** Common Etiologies of Hypocalcemia

| |
| --- |
| Decreased nutrient intake |
| Medications (see text) |
| Hyperphosphatemia |
| Hypoalbuminemia |
| Hypomagnesemia |
| Hypoparathyroidism |
| Acute pancreatitis |
| CKD |
| Secondary hyperparathyroidism |

**Abnormalities.** True abnormal serum concentrations of calcium may result from an abnormality in any of the previously mentioned mechanisms, such as

- Altered intestinal absorption
- Altered number or activity of osteoclast and osteoblast cells in bone
- Changes in renal reabsorption of calcium
- Calcium or phosphate IV infusions

Patients with CKD have increased serum phosphorus and decreased serum calcium concentrations as a result of the following factors that interact via a complex mechanism: decreased phosphate clearance by the kidneys, decreased renal production of calcitriol, and skeletal resistance to the calcemic action of PTH. This interaction is further complicated by the metabolic acidosis of renal failure, which can increase bone resorption to result in decreased bone integrity.

### Hypocalcemia

Hypocalcemia is defined as a total serum calcium concentration of <9.2 mg/dL (<2.3 mmol/L). The most common cause of hypocalcemia is low serum proteins. As discussed previously, decreased serum proteins leads to an increased free fraction of ionized calcium despite a mild reduction of total serum calcium concentration. If there is no other coexisting factor that could impair or alter calcium homeostasis, this should not be associated with a functional calcium deficit and clinical symptoms. Therefore, serum protein concentrations should always be taken into consideration when interpreting total serum calcium concentration. Even in the case of true, mild hypocalcemia, the patient may remain asymptomatic and often no treatment is required.

The most common causes of a true reduction in total serum calcium are disorders of vitamin D metabolism or impaired PTH production (**Table 11-10**). Osteomalacia (in adults) and rickets (in children) can result from severe deficiency in dietary calcium or vitamin D, diminished synthesis of vitamin $D_3$ from

insufficient sunlight exposure, or resistance of the intestinal wall to the action of vitamin D. The reduction in serum calcium leads to secondary hyperparathyroidism, which increases bone resorption. Over a long period of time, bones lose their structural integrity and become more susceptible to fracture. The diminished serum calcium concentration, if significant, may result in tetany. Other notable findings may include EKG changes (QT prolongation) and arrhythmias.

**Insufficient daily intake.** Although uncommon, diminished intake of calcium is an important cause of hypocalcemia, especially in patients receiving long-term parental nutrition solutions.[48,49]

**Medications.** Excessive use of certain drugs to lower serum calcium by either increasing bone deposition or decreasing renal reabsorption of calcium may lead to hypocalcemia. These drugs include calcitonin, corticosteroids, loop diuretics, pamidronate, alendronate, zoledronic acid, cinacalcet, and denosumab.[50]

Intravenous bicarbonate administration and hyperventilation can lead to alkalemia, resulting in decreased serum ionized calcium. This decrease is usually important only in patients who already have low total serum calcium concentrations. Drugs such as phenytoin, phenobarbital, carbamazepine, dexamethasone, and rifampin activate pregnane X receptor and thereby increase the metabolism of vitamin D. Over time, it may lead to mild hypocalcemia if chronic hypovitaminosis D is present. Calcium absorption may be impaired by aluminum-containing antacids.

Rapid IV administration of phosphate salts, especially at high doses, can also precipitate acute hypocalcemia. Phosphate can bind calcium ions and form an insoluble complex that can deposit into soft tissues and clog the microcirculation, causing metastatic calcification, hardening of normally pliable tissues, or blockage of capillary blood flow.[37,38] Soft-tissue deposition of the calcium–phosphate complex in lungs and blood vessels occurs when the serum solubility product of calcium times phosphorus is high. The product of total serum calcium and phosphorus concentrations (both expressed in milligrams/deciliter) is often calculated, especially in patients with CKD, to minimize the risk for tissue calcification. An increased risk of deposition is likely in patients with a calcium–phosphate product that exceeds 50 $mg^2/dL^2$ or in patients with alkalemia.

**Hypoparathyroidism.** Hypoparathyroidism can reduce serum calcium concentrations. The most common cause of hypoparathyroidism is thyroidectomy, in which the parathyroid glands are removed along with the thyroid glands. Because PTH is the major hormone regulating calcium balance, its absence significantly reduces serum calcium.[41]

**Secondary hyperparathyroidism.** Hypocalcemia is commonly seen in patients with secondary hyperparathyroidism resulting from CKD (Figure 11-6). The mechanism is complex and involves elevated serum phosphorus concentrations and reduced activation of vitamin D. PTH acts on bone to increase calcium and phosphate resorption. Because renal phosphate elimination is reduced because of renal failure, the serum phosphorus concentration is often high and depresses the serum calcium level. Because of the high phosphate concentrations in the intestinal lumen, dietary calcium is bound and absorption is impaired, while phosphate absorption continues.

**Metabolic acidosis.** Common in CKD, metabolic acidosis further enhances bone resorption. With prolonged severe hyperparathyroidism, excessive osteoclastic resorption of bones results in replacement of bone material with fibrous tissues. This condition is termed *osteitis fibrosa cystica.*[40] Such diminution of bone density may result in pathologic fractures. Although total serum calcium concentrations are low, patients may not show symptoms of hypocalcemia because the accompanying acidosis helps to maintain serum ionized calcium through the reduction in protein binding.

**Magnesium.** Similar to potassium, calcium balance is affected by magnesium homeostasis. Therefore, if a patient develops concurrent hypocalcemia and hypomagnesemia as a result of loop diuretic therapy, calcium replacement therapy may not be effective until magnesium balance is restored.

**Clinical diagnosis.** As with any electrolyte disorder, the severity of the clinical manifestations of hypocalcemia depends on the acuteness of onset. Hypocalcemia can, at times, be a medical emergency, with symptoms primarily in the neuromuscular system, including fatigue, depression, memory loss, hallucinations, and, in severe cases, seizures and tetany. The early signs of hypocalcemia are finger numbness, tingling and burning of extremities, and paresthesia. Mental instability and confusion may be seen in some patients as the primary manifestation.

Tetany is the hallmark of severe hypocalcemia. The mechanism of muscle fasciculation during tetany is the loss of the inhibitory effect of ionized calcium on muscle proteins. In extreme cases, this loss leads to increased neuromuscular excitability that can progress to laryngospasm and tonic-clonic seizures. Chvostek and Trousseau signs are hallmarks of hypocalcemia. The *Chvostek sign* is a unilateral spasm induced by a slight tap over the facial nerve. The *Trousseau sign* is a carpal spasm elicited when the upper arm is compressed by an inflated BP cuff.[48,49]

As hypocalcemia worsens, the cardiovascular system may be affected, as evidenced by myocardial failure, cardiac arrhythmias, and hypotension. Special attention should be paid to serum calcium concentrations in patients receiving diuretics, corticosteroids, digoxin, antacids, lithium, and parenteral nutrition and in patients with renal disease, because they may be more susceptible to symptomatic hypocalcemia.

## Hypercalcemia

*Hypercalcemia* indicates a total serum calcium concentration >11 mg/dL (>2.8 mmol/L).

**Causes.** The most common causes of hypercalcemia are malignancy and primary hyperparathyroidism (Figure 11-6). Malignancies can increase serum calcium by several mechanisms. Osteolytic metastases can arise from breast, lung, thyroid, kidney, or bladder cancer. These tumor cells invade bone and produce substances that directly dissolve bone matrix and mineral content. Some malignancies, such as multiple myeloma, can produce factors that stimulate osteoclast proliferation and activity. Another mechanism is the ectopic production of PTH or PTH-like substances by tumor cells, resulting in a pseudohyperparathyroid state.[50,51]

In primary hyperparathyroidism, inappropriate secretion of PTH from the parathyroid gland, usually due to an adenoma, increases serum calcium concentrations. The other major cause of hypercalcemia in hyperparathyroidism is the increased renal conversion of calcidiol to calcitriol. As the serum calcium concentration rises, the renal ability to reabsorb calcium may be exceeded, leading to an increased urinary calcium concentration and the subsequent formation of calcium–phosphate and calcium–oxalate renal stones. Typically, this condition results from parathyroid adenomas but also may be caused by primary parathyroid hyperplasia of chief cells or parathyroid carcinomas.[50]

Approximately 2% of patients treated with thiazide diuretics may develop hypercalcemia. Patients at risk are those with hyperparathyroidism. The mechanism appears to be multifactorial and includes enhanced renal reabsorption of calcium and decreased plasma volume.

The milk-alkali syndrome (Burnett syndrome), rarely observed today, is another drug-related cause of hypercalcemia.[52] This syndrome occurs from a chronic high intake of milk or calcium products combined with an absorbable antacid (eg, calcium carbonate, sodium bicarbonate, or magnesium hydroxide). This syndrome was more common in the past when milk or cream was used to treat gastric ulcers and before the advent of nonabsorbable antacids. Renal failure can occur as a result of calcium deposition in soft tissues.

Hypercalcemia also can result from the following conditions[2]:

- Excessive administration of IV calcium salts
- Chronic high-dose oral or enteral calcium supplements
- Chronic immobilization
- Paget disease
- Sarcoidosis
- Hyperthyroidism
- Acute adrenal insufficiency

- Lithium-induced renal calcium reabsorption
- Excessive intake of vitamin D, vitamin A, or thyroid hormone
- Drugs (eg, tamoxifen, teriparatide, androgenic hormones)

***Clinical diagnosis.*** Similar to hypocalcemia and other electrolyte disorders, the severity of the clinical manifestations of hypercalcemia depends on the acuteness of onset. Hypercalcemia can be a medical emergency, especially when serum concentrations rise above 14 mg/dL (>3.5 mmol/L). Symptoms associated with this condition often consist of vague GI complaints, such as nausea, vomiting, abdominal pain, dyspepsia, and anorexia. More severe GI complications include peptic ulcer disease, possibly due to increased gastrin release and acute pancreatitis.[50,51]

Severe hypercalcemic symptoms primarily involve the neuromuscular system (eg, lethargy, obtundation, psychosis, cerebellar ataxia, and, in severe cases, coma and death). However, EKG changes and spontaneous ventricular arrhythmias also may be seen. Hypercalcemia also may enhance the inotropic effects of digoxin, increasing the likelihood of cardiac arrhythmias.

Renal function may be affected by hypercalcemia through the ability of calcium to inhibit the adenyl cyclase–cyclic adenosine monophosphate system that mediates ADH effects on the collecting ducts. This inhibition results in diminished conservation of water by the kidneys. The renal effect is further compounded by diminished solute transport in the loop of Henle, leading to polyuria, nocturia, and polydipsia. Other chronic renal manifestations include nephrolithiasis, nephrocalcinosis, chronic interstitial nephritis, and renal tubular acidosis.

In addition, hypercalcemia can cause vasoconstriction of the renal vasculature, resulting in a decrease in renal blood flow and GFR. If hypercalcemia is allowed to progress, oliguric acute renal failure may ensue. In the presence of high calcium–phosphate product, soft-tissue calcification by the calcium–phosphate complex may occur. The signs and symptoms described previously are mostly seen in patients with severe hypercalcemia. With serum concentrations <13 mg/dL (3.2 mmol/L), most patients should be asymptomatic.

***Causes of spurious laboratory results.*** False hypercalcemia can occur if the tourniquet is left in place too long when the blood specimen is drawn. This results from increased plasma-protein pooling in the phlebotomized arm. Falsely elevated calcium should be suspected if serum albumin is >5 g/dL. **Table 11-11** contains the normal range values for tests related to calcium metabolism.

## Phosphate

*Normal range: 2.3 to 4.7 mg/dL (0.74 to 1.52 mmol/L) for adults*

Many of the factors that influence serum calcium concentrations also affect serum phosphorus, either directly or indirectly. Laboratory values for calcium and phosphorus should, therefore, be interpreted together. Because phosphate exists as several organic and inorganic moieties in the body, some clinical laboratories simply report the phosphate value as phosphorus.

**TABLE 11-11.** Normal Ranges for Tests Related to Calcium Metabolism in Adults

| LABORATORY PARAMETER | REFERENCE RANGE |
|---|---|
| Calcium (free) | 4.6–5.8 mg/dL |
| Calcium (total) | 9.2–11.0 mg/dL |
| Phosphorus | 2.3–4.7 mg/dL |
| PTH | 10–65 pg/mL |
| Urine calcium | <250 mg/day in men<br><200 mg/day in women |
| Urine phosphorus | 1 g/day (average) |

### Physiology

Phosphate is a major intracellular anion with several functions. It is important for intracellular metabolism of proteins, lipids, and carbohydrates, and it is a major component in phospholipid membranes, ribonucleic acids, nicotinamide diphosphate (an enzyme cofactor), cyclic adenine and guanine nucleotides (second messengers), and phosphoproteins. Another important function of phosphate is in the formation of high-energy bonds for the production of ATP, which is a source of energy for many cellular reactions. Phosphate is a component of 2,3-diphosphoglycerate (2,3-DPG), which regulates the release of oxygen from Hgb to tissues. In addition, phosphate has a regulatory role in the glycolysis and hydroxylation of cholecalciferol. It is also an important acid–base buffer.[17,40]

A balanced diet for adults usually contains 800 to 1,500 mg/day of phosphate. About two-thirds is actively absorbed from the small intestine. Some of the phosphate is absorbed passively with calcium, and some is absorbed under the influence of calcitriol, which also increases the intestinal absorption of calcium. However, phosphate is the first of the two to be absorbed.[42]

Phosphate absorption is diminished when a large amount of calcium or aluminum is present in the intestine due to the formation of insoluble phosphate compounds. Such large amounts of calcium and aluminum may result from the consumption of antacids. In fact, for patients with CKD who have high serum phosphorus concentrations, calcium- and aluminum-containing antacids may be given with meals as phosphate binders to reduce intestinal phosphate absorption.[42] It should be noted that due to concerns of detrimental accumulation of aluminum in the CNS as well as the ability to worsen anemia and bone disease, chronic use of aluminum-containing antacids should be avoided.

Phosphate is widely distributed in the body throughout the plasma, extracellular fluid, cell membrane structures, intracellular fluid, collagen, and bone. Bone contains 85% of the phosphate in the body. About 90% of serum phosphorus is filtered at the glomeruli, and most is actively reabsorbed at the proximal tubule. Some reabsorption also takes place in the loop of Henle, distal tubules, and possibly the collecting ducts.[17,40,53] The amount of renal phosphate excretion is, therefore, the amount filtered minus the amount reabsorbed. Increased urinary phosphate excretion can result from an increase in plasma volume and the action of PTH, which can block phosphate reabsorption throughout the nephron. In contrast, vitamin $D_3$ and its metabolites can directly stimulate proximal tubular phosphate reabsorption. In all, 90% of eliminated phosphate is excreted renally, while the remainder is secreted into the intestine. Renal handling of phosphate, especially the proximal tubules, therefore, plays an important role in maintaining the homeostatic balance of phosphate. Renal phosphate transport is active, saturable, and dependent on pH and sodium ions. However, fluctuation in serum phosphorus mostly results from changes in either the GFR or the rate of tubular reabsorption.

Serum phosphorus and calcium concentrations as well as PTH and vitamin D levels are intimately related to each other. Serum phosphorus indirectly controls PTH secretion via a negative feedback mechanism. With a decrease in serum phosphorus concentration, the conversion of calcidiol to calcitriol increases (which increases serum concentrations of both phosphorus and calcium). Both the intestinal absorption and renal reabsorption of phosphate are increased. The concomitant increase in serum calcium then directly decreases PTH secretion. This decrease in serum PTH concentration permits a further increase in renal phosphate reabsorption.[53]

A true phosphate imbalance may result from an abnormality in any of the previously discussed mechanisms and hormones for maintaining calcium and phosphate homeostasis. They may include altered intestinal absorption, altered number or activity of osteoclast and osteoblast cells in bone, changes in renal calcium and phosphate reabsorption, and IV infusions of calcium or phosphate salts.

## Hypophosphatemia

*Hypophosphatemia* indicates a serum phosphate concentration of <2.3 mg/dL (<0.74 mmol/L). The following three mechanisms commonly contribute to decreased serum phosphorus concentrations:

- Increased renal excretion
- Intracellular shifting
- Decreased phosphate or vitamin D intake

To identify the etiology of hypophosphatemia, the serum and urine phosphate concentrations should be evaluated simultaneously. Low urine and serum phosphates indicate either a diminished phosphate intake or excessive use of phosphate-binders. An increased urine phosphate suggests either hyperparathyroidism or renal tubular dysfunction. If the increased urine phosphate is accompanied by elevated total serum calcium, the presence of primary hyperparathyroidism or decreased vitamin D metabolism must be considered.

***Common causes.*** Hypophosphatemia commonly results from decreased renal reabsorption or increased GFR, a shift of phosphate from extracellular to intracellular fluid, alcoholism, or malnutrition. Phosphate is added to parenteral nutrition solutions for muscle growth and replenishment of hepatic glycogen storage in malnourished patients. The infusion of concentrated dextrose (eg, ≥5%) solution increases insulin secretion from the pancreas, which facilitates glucose and phosphate cell entry. Phosphate is used to form phosphorylated hexose intermediates during cellular utilization of glucose. An inadequate phosphate content in these nutritional fluids can decrease anabolism, glycolysis, and ATP and 2,3-DPG production.

Infusion of concentrated dextrose solutions or feeding can produce hypophosphatemia through intracellular phosphate shifting. Refeeding syndrome is a classic example of this presentation. This risk of hypophosphatemia is higher in patients who have chronic malnutrition or insufficient nutrient intake. Patients with cancer, chronic alcoholism, and anorexia nervosa and older adults are at risk for developing refeeding syndrome. Hypophosphatemia also can occur during treatment of hyperkalemia with IV regular insulin and dextrose. In addition, aluminum- and calcium-containing antacids, as well as magnesium hydroxide, are potent binders of intestinal phosphate and reduce its absorption. Their chronic use can lead to hypophosphatemia. Moreover, calcitonin, glucagon, and β-adrenergic agonists can decrease serum phosphorus concentrations. Thiazide and loop diuretics can increase renal phosphate excretion; however, this effect is often mild at typical doses for treating hypertension.

Other conditions known to cause hypophosphatemia include treatment of diabetic ketoacidosis, decreased absorption or increased intestinal loss, alcohol withdrawal, the diuretic phase of acute tubular necrosis, and prolonged respiratory alkalosis. To compensate for respiratory alkalosis, carbon dioxide shifts from intracellular to extracellular fluid. This shift increases the intracellular fluid pH, which activates glycolysis and intracellular phosphate trapping. Metabolic acidosis, in contrast, produces a minimal change in serum phosphorus.

***Uncommon causes.*** Burn patients often retain a great amount of sodium and water. During wound healing, diuresis often ensues, which results in a substantial loss of phosphate. Because anabolism also occurs during recovery, hypophosphatemia may be inevitable without proper replacement. A moderate reduction in serum phosphorus can occur from prolonged nasogastric suctioning, gastrectomy, small bowel or pancreatic disease resulting in malabsorption, and impaired renal phosphate reabsorption in patients with multiple myeloma, Fanconi syndrome, heavy-metal poisoning, amyloidosis, and nephrotic syndrome.[53,54]

***Intracellular hypophosphatemia.*** Severe phosphate depletion (<1 mg/dL or <0.32 mmol/L) can occur during insulin infusion in the management of diabetic ketoacidosis. Acidemia causes bone mineral mobilization, promotes intracellular organic substrate metabolism, and releases phosphate into the extracellular fluid. The glycosuria and ketonuria caused by diabetic ketoacidosis result in an osmotic diuresis that increases urinary phosphate excretion. The combined effects of these events may produce a normal serum phosphorus concentration but a severe intracellular deficiency. When diabetic ketoacidosis is corrected with insulin, phosphate accompanies glucose to move intracellularly. Serum phosphorus is usually reduced within 24 hours of treatment. As the acidosis is corrected, there is further intracellular shifting of phosphate to result in profound hypophosphatemia. The accompanying volume repletion may exacerbate the hypophosphatemia further.

*Clinical diagnosis.* Patients with a moderate reduction in serum phosphorus (2 to 2.3 mg/dL or 0.64 to 0.74 mmol/L) are often asymptomatic. Neurologic irritability may occur as the serum phosphorus concentration drops below 2 mg/dL (<0.64 mmol/L). Severe hypophosphatemia is often associated with muscle weakness, rhabdomyolysis, paresthesia, hemolysis, platelet dysfunction, and cardiac and respiratory failure.

Central nervous system effects may include encephalopathy, confusion, obtundation, seizures, and, ultimately, coma. The mechanism for these effects may involve decreased glucose use by the brain, decreased brain cell ATP, or cerebral hypoxia from increased oxygen-Hgb affinity, secondary to diminished erythrocyte 2,3-DPG content. This decreased content results in decreased glycolysis, which leads to decreased 2,3-DPG and ATP production. The decreased contents of 2,3-DPG and ATP result in an increased affinity of Hgb for oxygen, eventually leading to decreased tissue oxygenation. The ensuing cerebral hypoxia may explain the persistent coma often seen in patients with diabetic ketoacidosis. Hemolysis may occur, but it is rarely seen at serum phosphorus concentrations >0.5 mg/dL (>0.16 mmol/L).

### Hyperphosphatemia

*Hyperphosphatemia* occurs when a serum phosphorus concentration is >4.7 mg/dL (>1.52 mmol/L). There are three basic causes for elevated serum phosphorus concentrations:

- Decreased renal phosphate excretion
- Shift of phosphate from intracellular to extracellular fluid
- Increased intake of vitamin D or phosphate-containing products

Elevated phosphate concentrations also may result from reduced PTH secretion, increased body catabolism, and certain malignant conditions (eg, leukemias and lymphomas).

*Causes.* The most common cause of hyperphosphatemia is renal dysfunction, which commonly occurs as the GFR falls below 25 mL/min. CKD results in secondary hyperparathyroidism, which can further reduce renal phosphate elimination. Elevated serum phosphorus concentration increases the risk for deposition of insoluble calcium–phosphate complex in soft tissues (ie, metastatic calcification). This complexation may further reduce the serum concentration of ionized calcium and stimulate a further increase in PTH production and release. A sustained period of high PTH levels leads to excessive bone resorption, which increases the risk of bone fracture.[53-57]

Hyperphosphatemia can be caused by a shift of phosphate from intracellular to extracellular fluid. This shift of phosphate can result from massive cell break down after administering chemotherapy for leukemia or lymphoma and during rhabdomyolysis and septic shock. In addition, hyperthyroidism can elevate serum phosphorus by directly increasing renal tubular phosphate reabsorption.

*Clinical diagnosis.* Signs and symptoms of hyperphosphatemia commonly result from accompanying hypocalcemia and hyperparathyroidism (see Hypocalcemia section). Renal function may diminish if hyperphosphatemia is left untreated. In the presence of renal dysfunction, phosphate excretion is further reduced, which causes an even greater increase of serum phosphorus concentration and a further decline in serum calcium concentration[56,57] (**Minicase 4**).

---

## MINICASE 4

### A Case of Calcium and Phosphate Disorders in a Patient With Chronic Renal Failure

Michael S., a 72-year-old man, had a 1-week history of nausea, vomiting, and general malaise. His appetite has severely decreased over the past 2 months. He has a longstanding history of uncontrolled hypertension and type 2 diabetes mellitus as well as diabetic nephropathy, retinopathy, and neuropathy.

His physical examination reveals a BP of 160/99 mm Hg, diabetic retinopathic changes with laser scars bilaterally, and diminished sensation bilaterally below the knees. His laboratory values include the following results:

- Serum sodium, 146 mEq/L
- Potassium, 4.7 mEq/L
- Chloride, 104 mEq/L
- Total $CO_2$ content, 15 mEq/L
- SCr, 3.2 mg/dL (3.1 mg/dL from 1 month ago)
- BUN, 92 mg/dL
- Random blood glucose, 181 mg/dL

Because of his renal failure, additional laboratory tests were obtained:

- Calcium, 7.5 mg/dL
- Phosphorus, 9.1 mg/dL
- Albumin, 3.3 g/dL

Over the next several days, he reports finger numbness, tingling, and burning of extremities. He also has experienced increasing confusion and fatigue. A neurologic examination is positive for both Chvostek and Trousseau signs. Repeated laboratory tests show substantial changes in serum calcium (6.1 mg/dL) and phosphorus (10.4 mg/dL). His intact serum PTH is 280 pg/mL (10 to 65 pg/mL).

QUESTION: How would you characterize this patient's calcium and phosphorus disorders?

DISCUSSION: He has three laboratory abnormalities that are related specifically to calcium–phosphate metabolism: (1) hypocalcemia,

*Continued*

## MINICASE 4 (cont'd)

(2) hyperphosphatemia, and (3) secondary hyperparathyroidism. He is exhibiting classic signs and symptoms of hypocalcemia, such as finger numbness, tingling, burning of extremities, confusion, fatigue, and positive Chvostek and Trousseau signs.

Chronic kidney disease, as seen in this patient, is commonly associated with hypocalcemia, hyperphosphatemia, secondary hyperparathyroidism, and vitamin D deficiency. These calcium–phosphate abnormalities are responsible for the development of renal osteodystrophy. During the early stages of renal failure, renal phosphate excretion begins to decrease. His serum phosphorus concentration was increased, and the total serum calcium concentration became reduced, which stimulated the release of PTH and resulted in secondary hyperparathyroidism. The higher concentration of PTH reduced his renal tubular phosphate reabsorption, thereby increasing its excretion. The hyperparathyroidism helped to maintain his serum phosphorus and calcium concentrations within normal ranges during the early stage of renal failure (Figure 11-3).

As renal function continues to deteriorate (eGFR <30 mL/min), renal tubules cease to respond adequately to the high serum PTH concentration, resulting in hyperphosphatemia. In response to the hypocalcemia that followed, calcium was mobilized from the bone through the action of PTH. However, such a compensatory response was not sufficient because hypocalcemia and hyperphosphatemia continued. The persistent hyperphosphatemia could inhibit the conversion of calcidiol to calcitriol and further reduce the intestinal calcium absorption capacity. Therefore, hypocalcemia was worsened by the presence of hypovitaminosis D, which subsequently stimulated PTH secretion increasing mobilization of calcium from bone. The metabolic acidosis that is common in renal failure also may have contributed to the negative calcium balance in the bone.

This patient was relatively asymptomatic up to this point, primarily because these laboratory abnormalities developed over a long period of time and allowed the body to compensate. In the presence of nausea and vomiting and the lack of appetite, his oral calcium intake was probably reduced substantially, which may have enhanced his malaise. Because calcium is commonly reported as total calcium and not as the free or ionized fraction, his total serum calcium concentration must be corrected for his low serum albumin value. For every 1 g/dL reduction in serum albumin <4 g/dL, 0.8 mg/dL should be added to his serum calcium concentration. Therefore, with his serum albumin concentration of 3.3 g/dL, his initial serum calcium value of 7.5 mg/dL is equivalent to a total calcium concentration of 8.1 mg/dL. He does have true hypocalcemia, although the deficit is mild. It is important to note that his calcium and phosphorus derangements are severe. This patient has demonstrated neurologic signs of hypocalcemia. His EKG should be checked to determine if his cardiac rhythm is affected by hypocalcemia.

---

***Causes of spurious laboratory results.*** Hemolysis can occur during phlebotomy, which may lead to a falsely elevated serum phosphorus concentration. If the serum is not separated soon after phlebotomy, phosphate may be falsely decreased as it is taken up by the cellular components of blood.

Similar to what may occur to specimens for potassium concentration determination, when blood is allowed to clot with the use of nonheparinized tubes, phosphate may leach out of platelets and result in a falsely elevated concentration. In patients with thrombocytosis, phosphate concentrations should, therefore, be obtained from plasma (ie, heparinized tube) rather than serum (ie, nonheparinized tube) samples.

Serum phosphorus may vary by 1 to 2 mg/dL (0.32 to 0.64 mmol/L) after meals. Meals rich in carbohydrates can reduce serum phosphorus; meals with high phosphate contents, such as dairy products, can increase serum phosphorus. If accurate assessment of the phosphate concentration is necessary, the blood specimen should be obtained from the patient after fasting.

## TRACE ELEMENTS

### Copper

*Normal range: 70 to 140 mcg/dL (11 to 22 mmol/L) (men); 80 to 155 mcg/dL (13 to 24 mmol/L) (women) for serum or plasma copper; 20-50 mg/dL for serum ceruloplasmin depending on age and assay used*

#### Physiology

The relationship between copper homeostasis and human diseases was uncovered in 1912 shortly after Wilson disease was described. In the early 1930s, a link between copper deficiency and anemia was suspected, although the hypothesis was not proven at that time. In the 1970s, the physiologic functions of copper were better understood and its link to various disease states was better appreciated. An official dietary copper recommendation and adequate daily dietary intake was introduced for the first time in 1979. Copper deficiency is now a recognized concern in patients with bariatric surgery and small bowel resection.

Copper plays an integral part in the synthesis and functions of many circulating proteins and enzymes. In addition, copper is an essential factor for the formation of connective tissues, such as the cross-linking of collagen and elastin. Copper also regulates the cellular uptake and physiologic functions with iron.[58] In the CNS, copper is necessary for the formation or maintenance of myelin and other phospholipids. Cuproenzymes (copper-dependent enzymes) are crucial in the metabolism of catecholamines. For example, the functions of dopamine hydroxylase and monoamine oxidase are impaired by copper deficiency. Copper also affects the function of tyrosinase in melanin synthesis, which is responsible for the pigmentation of skin, hair, and eyes. Deficiency of tyrosinase results in albinism. Other physiologic functions of copper include thermal regulation, glucose metabolism, blood clotting (eg, factor V function), and protection of cells against oxidative damage.[58]

The normal adult daily intake of copper, based on a typical American diet, is about 2 to 3 mg. Plant copper is in the inorganic (free ionic) form, whereas meat (animal) copper is in the form of cuproproteins (copper–protein complex). Inorganic copper is absorbed in the upper GI tract (stomach and proximal duodenum) under acidic conditions. Cuproprotein copper is absorbed in the jejunum and ileum. Absorption of copper from the GI tract is a saturable process. The oral bioavailability of copper ranges from 15% to 97% and shows a negative correlation with the amount of copper present in the diet and total body copper status.

Once absorbed, copper is bound to a mucosal copper-binding protein called *metallothionein* (a sulfur-rich, metal-binding protein present in intestinal mucosa). From this protein, copper is slowly released into the circulation, where it is taken up by the liver and other tissues.[58-60] Animal data suggest that the liver serves as the ultimate depot for copper storage. Copper absorption may be reduced by a high intake of zinc (>50 mg elemental zinc/day), ascorbic acid, and dietary fiber. Oral zinc supplementation may induce the synthesis of intestinal metallothionein and form a barrier to copper ion absorption by trapping copper ions in the enterocytes and decreases their oral bioavailability. IV zinc supplementation is not expected to decrease oral copper absorption.

The normal adult body contains approximately 110 mg of copper. The highest tissue copper concentration is found in the muscle and skeletal tissues, followed by liver and brain. Copper in the muscle and skeletal tissues account for about 50% of the total body copper. The rest is distributed in the heart, spleen, kidneys, and blood (erythrocytes and neutrophils).[59,60]

In the plasma, copper is highly bound (95%) to ceruloplasmin (also known as ferroxidase I), a blue copper protein. This protein contains six to seven copper atoms per molecule. The fraction of plasma copper associated with ceruloplasmin seems to be relatively constant for the same individual. However, a significant interindividual variation exists. The remainder of the plasma copper is bound to albumin and amino acids or is free.[58] Copper is eliminated mainly by biliary excretion (average 25 mcg/kg/day), with only 0.5% to 3% of the daily intake in the urine.[59]

Ceruloplasmin is considered the most reliable indicator of copper status because of its large and relatively stable binding capacity with serum copper. Therefore, when evaluating copper status in the body, it is highly recommended that serum ceruloplasmin concentration should be assessed together with serum copper concentration.[60]

## Hypocupremia

Although it was thought that copper deficiency is relatively uncommon in humans, more cases have been reported recently in patients after bariatric surgery. Copper deficiency is also an increasingly recognized concern in patients with Crohn disease or short bowel syndrome.[61;62] *Hypocupremia* usually occurs with chronic diarrhea or malabsorption syndrome, such as after Roux-en-Y gastric bypass surgery, duodenal switch, and major resection of the small intestine or in low-birth-weight infants fed with cow's milk (rather than formulas).[61-63] Premature infants, who typically have low copper stores, are at a higher risk for developing copper deficiency under these circumstances.

Copper deficiency may occur in patients receiving long-term parenteral nutrition with insufficient trace element supplementation (eg, product shortages). Chronic malabsorption syndromes (eg, celiac disease and ulcerative colitis), protein-wasting enteropathies, short bowel syndrome, and the presence of significant bowel resection or bypass (eg, malabsorptive bariatric surgical procedures such as long-limb Roux-en-Y or jejunoileal bypass) are all potential risk factors resulting in copper deficiency. Individuals on a vegan diet may also be at risk because (1) meat is a major food source of copper and (2) plant sources often have high-fiber content that may interfere with copper absorption.[59]

Prolonged hypocupremia leads to a syndrome of neutropenia and iron-deficiency anemia, which is correctable with copper.[62] The anemia can be normocytic or microcytic and hypochromic. It results mainly from poor iron absorption and ineffective heme incorporation of iron. Neurologic symptoms are another common presentation of copper deficiency and may include gait ataxia, numbness, peripheral neuropathy, and psychosis.[62] Copper deficiency can affect any system or organs whose enzymes require copper for proper functioning. As such, copper deficiency may lead to abnormal glucose tolerance, arrhythmias, hypercholesterolemia, atherosclerosis, depressed immune function, defective connective tissue formation, demineralization of bones, and pathologic fractures.

Two well-known genetic defects are associated with impaired copper metabolism in humans. Menkes syndrome (also called *kinky-hair syndrome/steely-hair syndrome*) is an X-linked disorder that occurs in 1 out of every 50,000 to 100,000 live births. These patients have defective copper absorption and are commonly deceased by the age of 4 years. They have reduced copper concentrations in the blood, liver, and brain.[64,65] Most of them are children suffering from slow growth and retardation, defective keratinization and pigmentation of hair, hypothermia, and degenerative changes in the aortic elastin and neurons. Progressive nerve degeneration in the brain results in intellectual deterioration, hypotonia, and seizures. However, anemia and neutropenia, hallmark symptoms of nutritional copper deficiency, are not found in persons with Menkes syndrome. Administration of parenteral copper increases serum copper and ceruloplasmin concentrations but does not have any apparent effect on slowing disease progression.

Wilson disease is an autosomal recessive disease of copper storage. Its frequency is uncertain, but it is believed to be not as common as Menkes syndrome. Wilson disease appears to be associated with altered copper catabolism and excretion of ceruloplasmin copper into the bile. It is associated with elevated urinary copper loss and low plasma ceruloplasmin and low plasma copper concentrations. However, copper deposition occurs in the liver, brain, and cornea. If untreated, significant copper accumulation in these organs eventually leads to irreversible damage such as cirrhosis and neurologic impairment.[66]

## Hypercupremia

Copper excess, or *hypercupremia*, is not common in humans and usually occurs with a deliberate attempt to ingest large quantities of copper. The exact amount of copper that results in toxicity is unknown. Acute or long-term ingestion of >15 mg of elemental copper may lead to symptomatic copper poisoning.[67] Also, it has been reported that drinking water with 2 to 3 mg/L of copper is associated with hepatotoxicity in infants. Similar to other metallic poisonings, acute copper poisoning leads to nausea, vomiting, intestinal cramps, and diarrhea.[67] A larger ingestion can result in shock, hepatic necrosis, intravascular hemolysis, renal impairment, coma, and death. Elevated intrahepatic copper concentrations may be present in patients with primary biliary cirrhosis and biliary atresia.[68] Long-term parenteral nutrition (PN) use is also a risk factor for hepatic copper overload due to chronic, unregulated exposure of IV copper through the multitrace element mixture. For patients receiving chronic home parenteral nutrition, it is recommended that serum copper concentration is monitored to prevent copper toxicity.[69,70] Chronic cholestasis secondary to parenteral nutrition–associated liver disease has been suggested as the primary cause. Because copper plays an important role in the neurologic system, it has been suggested that copper-induced free radical–induced neurodegeneration may be a contributing factor for Alzheimer disease. At present, there is no known treatment for hypercupremia.

## Zinc

*Normal range: 50 to 150 mcg/dL (7.7 to 23 micromol/L) serum or plasma*

### Physiology

Next to iron, zinc is the most abundant trace element in the body. It is an essential nutrient that is a constituent of, or a cofactor to, many enzymes. These metalloenzymes participate in the metabolism of carbohydrates, proteins, lipids, and nucleic acids. As such, zinc influences the following processes[71]:

- Tissue growth and repair
- Cell membrane stabilization
- Bone collagenase activity and collagen turnover
- Immune response, especially T-cell–mediated response
- Sensory control of food intake
- Spermatogenesis and gonadal maturation
- Normal testicular function

The normal adult body contains 1.5 to 2.5 g of zinc. Aside from supplementation with zinc capsules, dietary intake is the only source of zinc for humans. Food sources of zinc include meat products, oysters, and legumes. Food-based zinc is largely bound to proteins and released by gastric acid and pancreatic enzymes. Ionic zinc found in zinc supplements is absorbed in the duodenum directly. Foods rich in calcium, dietary fiber, or phytate may interfere with zinc absorption, as can folic acid supplements.

After absorption, zinc is transported from the small intestine to the portal circulation where it binds to proteins such as albumin, transferrin, and other globulins. Circulating zinc is bound mostly to serum proteins; two-thirds are loosely bound to albumin and transthyretin, while one-third is bound tightly to α-2 macroglobulin.[53] Only 2% to 3% (3 mg) of zinc is either in free ionic form or bound to amino acids.[72,73]

Zinc can be found in many organs. Tissues high in zinc include liver, pancreas, spleen, lungs, eyes (retina, iris, cornea, and lens), prostate, skeletal muscle, and bone. Because of their mass, skeletal muscle (60% to 62%) and bone (20% to 28%) have the highest zinc contents among the body tissues.[71] Only 2% to 4% of total body zinc is found in the liver. In blood, 85% is in erythrocytes, although each leukocyte contains 25 times the zinc content of an erythrocyte.[71]

Plasma or serum zinc concentration is a poor indicator of total body zinc store. Because 98% of the total body zinc is present in tissues and end organs, the plasma zinc concentration tends to reflect the continuous shifting from intracellular sources (ie, zinc trafficking). Additionally, metabolic stress, such as infection, acute myocardial infarction, and critical illnesses increase intracellular shifting of zinc to the liver and lower serum zinc concentrations, even when total body zinc is normal. Conversely, plasma zinc concentrations may be normal during starvation or wasting syndromes due to release of zinc from tissues and cells.[71] Therefore, serum/plasma zinc concentration alone has little meaning clinically in patients with acute illnesses. It has been suggested that the rate of zinc turnover in the plasma provides better assessment of the body zinc status. This may be achieved by measuring 24-hour zinc loss in body fluids (eg, urine and stool). However, this approach is rarely practical for critically ill patients as renal failure is often present. Alternatively, zinc turnover and mobilization may be determined by adjusting plasma zinc concentrations with serum α-2 macroglobulin and albumin concentrations.[72,73] To more accurately assess the body zinc status, others have suggested monitoring the functional indices of zinc, such as erythrocyte alkaline phosphatase, serum superoxide dismutase, and lymphocyte 5′ nucleotidase. However, the clinical validity of these tests remains to be substantiated, especially in patients who are acutely ill.

Zinc undergoes substantial enteropancreatic recirculation and is excreted primarily in pancreatic and intestinal secretions. Diarrhea significantly increases zinc loss. Zinc is also lost dermally through sweat, hair and nail growth, and skin shedding. Except in certain disease states, only 2% of zinc is lost in the urine.

### Hypozincemia

In Western countries, zinc deficiency is rare from dietary insufficiency. Individuals with no acute illnesses whose serum zinc concentrations are <50 mcg/dL (<7.6 μmol/L) are at an increased risk for developing symptomatic zinc deficiency. It also must be emphasized that serum zinc exhibits a negative acute phase response. The presence of proinflammatory cytokines causes an intracellular and intrahepatic influx of zinc from the serum, which would lead to transient *hypozincemia*. Therefore, serum or plasma zinc concentration alone should not be used to assess zinc status in patients with acute illnesses or any acute inflammatory response. Given the caveats of measuring serum zinc concentrations in certain disease states, response to empirical zinc supplementation may be the only way of diagnosing this deficiency. In the presence of chronic diseases, it is difficult to determine if zinc deficiency is clinical or subclinical because of the reduced protein binding. Conditions leading to deficiency may be divided into five classes (**Table 11-12**):

- Low intake
- Decreased absorption
- Increased use
- Increased loss
- Unknown causes

Zinc deficiency is commonly caused by diarrhea and insufficient intake. Patients with increased ostomy output due to GI tract surgery are especially at risk for zinc deficiency. Acrodermatitis enteropathica is an autosomal, recessive disorder involving zinc malabsorption that occurs in infants of Italian, Armenian, and Iranian heritage. It is characterized by severe dermatitis, chronic diarrhea, emotional disturbances, and growth retardation.[71] Examples of malabsorption syndromes that may lead to zinc deficiency include Crohn disease, celiac disease, and short bowel syndrome.

Excessive zinc may be lost in the urine (hyperzincuria), as occurs in alcoholism, beta thalassemia, diabetes mellitus, diuretic therapy, nephrotic syndrome, sickle cell anemia, and treatment with parenteral nutrition. Severe or prolonged diarrhea (eg, inflammatory bowel diseases and GI graft versus host disease) may lead to significant zinc loss in the stool. Patients with end-stage liver disease frequently have depleted zinc storage due to decreased functional hepatic cell mass.

Because zinc is involved in a diverse group of enzymes, its deficiency manifests in numerous organs and physiologic systems (**Table 11-13**). Dysgeusia (lack of taste) and hyposmia (diminished smell acuity) are common. Pica is a pathologic craving for specific food or nonfood substances (eg, geophagia). Chronic zinc deficiency, as occurs in acrodermatitis enteropathica, leads to growth retardation, anemia, hypogonadism, hepatosplenomegaly, and impaired wound healing. Additional signs and symptoms of acrodermatitis enteropathica include diarrhea; vomiting; alopecia; skin lesions in oral, anal, and genital areas; paronychia; nail deformity; emotional lability; photophobia; blepharitis; conjunctivitis; and corneal opacities.

### Hyperzincemia

Zinc is one of the least toxic trace elements. Clinical manifestations of excess zinc, *hyperzincemia*, occur with chronic, high doses of a zinc supplement. However, patients with Wilson disease who commonly take high doses of zinc rarely show signs of toxicity. This may be explained by the stabilization of serum zinc concentrations during high-dose administration. As much as 12 g of zinc sulfate (>2,700 mg of elemental zinc) taken over 2 days has caused drowsiness, lethargy, and increased serum lipase and amylase concentrations. Nausea, vomiting, and diarrhea also may occur.[71]

## TABLE 11-12. Etiologies of Zinc Deficiency

Low intake
  Anorexia
  Nutritional deficiencies
  Alcoholism
  CKD
  Premature infants
  Certain vegetarian diets
  Exclusion of trace elements in parenteral nutrition
Decreased absorption
  Acrodermatitis enteropathica
  Malabsorption syndromes
  Bariatric surgery
  Short bowel syndrome
Increased use
  Adolescence
  Lactation
  Pregnancy
Increased loss
  Alcoholism
  β-thalassemia
  Cirrhosis
  Diabetes mellitus
  Diarrhea
  Diuretic therapy
  Enterocutaneous fistula drainage
  Exercise (long-term, strenuous)
  Glucagon
  Impaired enteropancreatic recycling
  Nephrotic syndrome
  Protein-losing enteropathies
  Sickle cell disease
Unknown causes
  Arthritis and other inflammatory diseases
  Down syndrome

## Manganese

*Normal range: Varies depending on assay method, sample (whole blood versus serum), and age. Whole blood method is preferred to detect toxicity. Normal whole blood manganese concentrations range from 4 to 15 mcg/L (72 to 270 nmol/L)*

### Physiology

Manganese is an essential trace element that serves as a cofactor for numerous diverse enzymes involved in carbohydrate, protein, and lipid metabolism; protection of cells from free radicals; steroid biosynthesis; and metabolism of biogenic amines.[74] Interestingly, manganese deficiency does not affect the functions of

**TABLE 11-13.** Signs and Symptoms of Zinc Deficiency

Signs
  Acrodermatitis enteropathica
  Anemia
  Anergy to skin test antigens
  Complicated pregnancy
    Excessive bleeding
    Maternal infection
    Premature or stillborn birth
  Decreased basal metabolic rate
  Decreased circulating $T_4$ concentration
  Decreased lymphocyte count and function
  Effect on fetus, infant, or child
    Congenital defects of skeleton, lungs, and CNS
    Fetal disturbances
    Growth retardation
  Hypogonadism
  Impaired neutrophil function
  Impairment and delaying of platelet aggregation
  Increased susceptibility to dental caries
  Increased susceptibility to infections
  Mental disturbances
  Pica
  Poor wound healing
  Short stature in children
  Skeletal deformities
Symptoms
  Acne and recurrent furunculosis
  Ataxia
  Decreased appetite
  Defective night vision
  Hypogeusia
  Hyposmia
  Erectile dysfunction
  Oral ulcers

$T_4$ = thyroxine.

most of these enzymes, presumably because magnesium may substitute for manganese in most instances.[74] In animals, manganese is required for normal bone growth, lipid metabolism, reproduction, and CNS regulation.[75,76]

Manganese plays an important role in the normal function of the brain, primarily through its effect on biogenic amine metabolism. This effect may be responsible for the relationship between brain concentrations of manganese and catecholamines.[74,75]

The manganese content of the adult body is 10 to 20 mg. Manganese homeostasis is regulated through control of its absorption and excretion. Plants are the primary source of food manganese because animal tissues have low contents. Manganese is absorbed from the small intestine by a mechanism similar to that of iron. However, only 3% to 4% of the ingested manganese is absorbed. Dietary iron and phytate may affect manganese absorption.[77]

Human and animal tissues have low manganese content. Tissues relatively high in manganese are the bone, liver, pancreas, and pituitary gland. Most circulating manganese is loosely bound to the β-1 globulin transmanganin, a transport protein similar to transferrin. With overexposure, excess manganese accumulates in the liver and brain, causing severe neuromuscular signs and symptoms.

Manganese is excreted primarily in biliary and pancreatic secretions. In manganese overload, other GI routes of elimination also may be used. Little manganese is lost in urine.

### Manganese Deficiency

Because of its relative abundance in plant sources, manganese deficiency is rare among the general population. Deficiency normally occurs after several months of deliberate manganese omission from the diet. Little is known regarding serum manganese concentrations and the accompanying disease states in humans.[78] Limited evidence suggests that manganese deficiency may be associated with bone demineralization and poor growth in children, skin rashes, hair depigmentation, decreased serum lipids, depression, and increased premenstrual pain in women.[79,80]

### Manganese Excess

Manganese is one of the least toxic trace elements. Overexposure primarily occurs from inhalation of manganese compounds (eg, manganese mines).[77] Long-term use of parenteral nutrition is a risk factor for hypermanganesemia caused by continued and unregulated exposure. The excess amount accumulates in the liver and brain, resulting in severe neuromuscular manifestations. Patients receiving home parenteral nutrition with trace elements daily for >6 months should have serum manganese concentration monitored.[69,70,81-83] Symptoms include encephalopathy and profound neurologic disturbances that mimic Parkinson disease.[84-86] These manifestations are not surprising because metabolism of biogenic amines is altered in both manganese excess and Parkinson disease. Other signs and symptoms include anorexia, apathy, headache, erectile dysfunction, and speech disturbances. Inhalation of manganese products may cause manganese pneumonitis.[77]

## Selenium

*Average range: Varies depending on assay method, sample (whole blood versus serum), and age. Concentrations in blood and urine reflect recent selenium intake. Normal whole blood selenium concentrations are typically between 150 and 240 ng/mL, typical normal serum selenium concentration is usually between 70 and 150 ng/mL for patients >1 year*

### Physiology

Selenium is a trace element that is naturally present in many foods and available as a dietary supplement. The primary physiologic role of selenium is to serve as an antioxidant, especially via the selenoprotein, glutathione peroxidase, to help protect cells from oxidative damage. In most cases, selenoprotein and glutathione work along with other cellular antioxidant defense mechanisms, such as ascorbate, tocopherol, and superoxide dismutase. Glutathione peroxidase activity is decreased in patients with selenium deficiency. Upon repletion of selenium, glutathione activity is restored.[87]

Selenium exists in the inorganic form (selenite) and organic form (selenomethionine and selenocysteine). The most common form of selenium in the active site of glutathione peroxidase is selenocysteine, which has independent activity that does not allow it to use hydrogen peroxide as a substrate. Selenomethionine is another common form of selenium in human cells.

The estimated dietary intake of selenium varies geographically due to dietary variance and characteristics of the soil. Food sources of selenium include Brazil nuts, seafoods, organ meats, breads, grains, poultry, and eggs. About 90% of selenium is absorbed as the organic form of selenomethionine in the human body and is available in that form in most dietary supplements. The injectable forms of selenium are selenious acid and sodium selenite.[79,88]

### Selenium Deficiency

Dietary selenium deficiency is rare in the United States and Canada and in isolation rarely causes illness. Patients with acute inflammation or uncontrolled chronic illnesses have lower selenium concentrations, likely due to increased oxidative stress associated with their diseases. Critically ill patients have low serum selenium concentration, and the magnitude of deficiency correlates with the severity of illness. Supplementation with large doses of antioxidant cocktail containing selenium has not been shown to improve survival or decreased ICU or hospital length of stay.[89,90] Patients undergoing long-term hemodialysis and patients living with human immunodeficiency virus (HIV) are also likely to develop selenium deficiency. For patients undergoing hemodialysis, selenium is removed from the blood. Due to uremia and dietary restrictions, patients may have low dietary intakes that may be supplemented. However, little evidence suggests that supplementation is beneficial in this patient population.[91] Patients living with HIV have low levels of selenium due to insufficient intake and malabsorption due to GI symptoms (ie, diarrhea). More evidence is needed to determine whether selenium supplementation can reduce the risk of mortality, hospitalization, and HIV transmission.[92]

Selenoproteins may help prevent oxidative modification of lipids, thus reducing inflammation and preventing platelet aggregation. However, it is yet to be determined if patients should supplement with selenium as a primary prevention or if it should be used as a tertiary prevention for patients who already have cardiovascular disease. There are some conflicting reports on whether selenium supplementation may increase the risk of advanced prostate cancer and skin cancer in men.[93]

### Selenium Excess

Inorganic and organic forms of selenium can have similar toxic effects. Tolerable upper intake levels for selenium vary based on age and geographic location. Common symptoms of acute selenium excess include garlic breath odor and a metallic taste in the mouth. For adults, serum selenium concentration >400 mcg could produce symptoms such as hair and nail loss, GI and neurologic symptoms, acute respiratory distress syndrome, tremors, kidney failure, and cardiac failure. Death from selenium toxicity is rare but can occur with excessive intake.[88,92] A case report of fatality was associated with a single oral ingestion of 10 g of sodium selenite (96% purity) in a 75-year-old man. The patient presented with cardiovascular collapse, hypoxemic respiratory failure, mild hypokalemia (3.4 mEq/L), and a serum selenium concentration of 5,370 ng/mL.[93]

## Chromium

*Average range: serum chromium 0.3 to 0.9 ng/mL; sample contamination (eg, use of regular blood collection tubes not designed for trace elements) may result in ranges from 2 to 5 ng/mL*

### Physiology

The main physiologic role of chromium is as a cofactor for insulin.[94] In its organic form, chromium potentiates the action of endogenous and exogenous insulin, presumably by augmenting its adherence to cell membranes.[49] The organic form is in the dinicotinic acid–glutathione complex or glucose tolerance factor (GTF).[79] Chromium is the metal portion of GTF; with insulin, GTF affects the metabolism of glucose, cholesterol, and triglycerides.[94] Therefore, chromium is important for glucose tolerance, glycogen synthesis, amino acid transport, and protein synthesis. Chromium also is involved in the activation of several enzymes

The adult body contains an average of 5 mg of chromium.[95] Food sources of chromium include brewer's yeast, spices, vegetable oils, unrefined sugar, liver, kidneys, beer, meat, dairy products, and wheat germ.[95] GTF is present in the diet and can be synthesized from inorganic trivalent chromium ($Cr^{+3}$) available in food and dietary supplements.[50] Chromium is absorbed via a common pathway with zinc; its degree of absorption is inversely related to dietary intake, varying from 0.5% to 2%.[79,94]

Chromium circulates as free $Cr^{3+}$, bound to transferrin and other proteins, and as the GTF complex. GTF is the biologically active moiety and is more important than total serum chromium concentration. Trivalent chromium accumulates in the hair, kidneys, skeleton, liver, spleen, lungs, testes, and large intestine. GTF concentrates in insulin-responsive tissues such as the liver.[79,94]

The metabolism of chromium is not well-understood for several reasons:

- Low concentrations in tissues
- Difficulty in analyzing chromium in biological fluids and tissue samples
- Presence of different chromium forms in food

Homeostasis is controlled by release of chromium from GTF and by dietary absorption. The kidneys are the main site of elimination, where urinary excretion is constant despite variability in the fraction absorbed.[94]

## Chromium Deficiency

It is important to stress that the body store of chromium cannot be reliably assessed. Serum or plasma chromium may not be in equilibrium with other pools. As with other trace elements, the risk for developing chromium deficiency increases over time with lack of oral intake and insufficient supply from other sources, such as a trace element-free parenteral nutrition solution.[69,70] Marginal deficiencies or defects in use of chromium may be present in elderly patients, patients with diabetes, or patients with atherosclerotic coronary artery disease.[95]

Hyperglycemia increases urinary losses of chromium. Coupled with marginal intake, a patient with type II diabetes is predisposed to chromium deficiency, which can further impair glucose tolerance.[94,96] Finally, multiparous women are at a higher risk than nulliparous women for becoming chromium deficient because, over time, chromium intake may not be adequate to meet fetal needs and maintain the mother's body store.

The manifestations of chromium deficiency may involve insulin resistance and impaired glucose metabolism. Such manifestations may present clinically in three stages as the deficiency progresses:

- Glucose intolerance is present but is masked by a compensatory increase in insulin release.
- Impaired glucose tolerance and lipid metabolism are clinically evident.
- Marked insulin resistance and symptoms associated with hyperglycemia are evident.

Chromium supplementation has been shown in patients with diabetes to increase insulin sensitivity, improve glucose control, and shorten the QTc interval, suggesting a potential favorable effect on cardiovascular risk. However, currently, no conclusive support demonstrates the benefit of chromium supplementation in patients with diabetes or persons with impaired glucose metabolism.

Chromium deficiency may lead to hypercholesterolemia and become a risk factor for developing atherosclerotic disease. Low chromium tissue concentrations have been associated with increased risk for myocardial infarction and coronary artery disease in both healthy subjects and patients with diabetes, although a cause-and-effect relationship has not been established.[96]

## Chromium Excess

Chromium has low toxicity with no established specific clinical symptoms or presentations. The clinical significance of a high body store of chromium is unknown. Patients receiving long-term home parenteral nutrition with a standard daily amount of chromium from the multitrace element admixture may have an increase serum chromium concentration; however, the clinical risk is unknown at this point.[69] Serum chromium concentrations may be increased in asymptomatic patients with metal-on-metal prosthetics.

# SUMMARY

Hyponatremia and hypernatremia may be associated with high, normal, or low total body sodium. Hyponatremia may result from abnormal water accumulation in the intravascular space (dilutional hyponatremia), a decline in both extracellular water and sodium, or a reduction in total body sodium with normal water balance. Hypernatremia is most common in patients with either an impaired thirst mechanism (eg, neurohypophyseal or pituitary lesion) or an inability to replace water depleted through normal insensible loss or from renal or GI loss. Neurologic manifestations are signs and symptoms often associated with sodium and water imbalance. The most common symptom of hyponatremia is confusion. However, if sodium continues to fall, seizures, coma, and death may result. Thirst is a common symptom of hypernatremia; decreased urine specific gravity, suggesting less concentrated urine, is often observed.

Hypokalemia and hyperkalemia may indicate either a true or an apparent (due to transcellular shifting) potassium imbalance. Hypokalemia can occur because of excessive loss from the kidneys (diuretics) or GI tract (vomiting or diarrhea). The most serious manifestation involves the cardiovascular system (ie, cardiac arrhythmias). Renal impairment, usually in the presence of high intake, commonly causes hyperkalemia. Like hypokalemia, the most serious clinical manifestations of hyperkalemia involve the cardiovascular system.

Serum chloride concentration may be used as a confirmatory test to identify abnormalities in fluid and acid–base balance. Hypochloremia may be diuretic induced and results from the concurrent loss of sodium and also contraction alkalosis. Signs and symptoms associated with these conditions are related to the abnormalities in fluid or acid–base balance and underlying causes rather than to chloride itself.

Hypomagnesemia usually results from excessive loss from the GI tract (eg, nasogastric suction, biliary loss, ileostomy or chronic diarrhea) or the kidneys (eg, diuresis). Magnesium depletion is usually associated with neuromuscular symptoms such as weakness, muscle fasciculation with tremor, tetany, and increased reflexes. Increased magnesium intake in the presence of renal dysfunction commonly causes hypermagnesemia. Neuromuscular signs and symptoms that are opposite to those caused by hypomagnesemia may be observed.

The most common causes of true hypocalcemia are disorders of vitamin D metabolism and PTH production. Severe hypocalcemia can be a medical emergency and lead to cardiac arrhythmias and tetany, with symptoms primarily involving the neuromuscular system.

The most common causes of hypercalcemia are malignancy and primary hyperparathyroidism. Symptoms often consist of vague GI reports such as nausea, vomiting, abdominal pain, anorexia, constipation, and diarrhea. Severe hypercalcemia can cause acute neurologic changes and possibly cardiac arrhythmias, which can be a medical emergency.

The most common causes of hypophosphatemia are decreased intake and increased renal loss. Although mild hypophosphatemia is usually asymptomatic, severe depletion (<1 mg/dL or <0.32 mmol/L) is typically associated with muscle weakness, rhabdomyolysis, paresthesia, hemolysis, platelet dysfunction, and cardiac and respiratory failure. The most common cause of hyperphosphatemia is renal dysfunction, often with a GFR <25 mL/min. Signs and symptoms, if present, primarily result from the ensuing hypocalcemia and hyperparathyroidism.

Hypocupremia is uncommon in adults but can occur in infants, especially those born prematurely. Also susceptible are infants who have chronic diarrhea or malabsorption syndrome or whose diet consists mostly of milk. Prolonged hypocupremia results in neutropenia and iron-deficiency anemia that is correctable with copper.

Copper excess is not common and may result from a deliberate attempt to ingest large quantities. Similar to other metallic poisonings, acute copper poisoning leads to nausea and vomiting, intestinal cramps, and diarrhea.

Likely candidates for zinc deficiency are infants; rapidly growing adolescents; menstruating, lactating, or pregnant women; persons with low meat intake; institutionalized patients; and patients receiving parenteral nutrition solutions without trace elements for prolonged periods. Because zinc is involved with a diverse group of enzymes, its deficiency manifests in different organs and physiologic systems. Zinc excess develops from chronic, high-dose zinc supplementation. Signs and symptoms include nausea, vomiting, diarrhea, drowsiness, lethargy, and increases in serum lipase and amylase concentrations.

Manganese deficiency can occur after several months of deliberate omission from the diet. Signs and symptoms include weight loss, slow hair and nail growth, color change in hair and beard, transient dermatitis, hypocholesterolemia, and hypotriglyceridemia. Manganese excess primarily occurs through inhalation of manganese compounds (eg, manganese mines). As a result of manganese accumulation, severe neuromuscular manifestations occur, including encephalopathy and profound neurologic disturbances, which mimic Parkinson disease. Inhalation of manganese products may cause manganese pneumonitis.

Chromium deficiency may be found in patients receiving prescribed chronic nutrition regimens that are low in chromium content. Insulin resistance and impaired glucose metabolism are the main manifestations.

## LEARNING POINTS

**1.** *What does an abnormal serum electrolyte concentration mean?*

**ANSWER:** An isolated abnormal serum electrolyte concentration may not always necessitate immediate treatment because it can be the result of a poor sample (hemolyzed blood sample), wrong timing (during an IV infusion or immediately after hemodialysis), or other confounding factors. Careful assessment of the patient's existing risk factors, history of illness, and clinical symptoms should be made to correctly interpret a specific laboratory result. Patients with abnormal serum electrolyte concentrations who are also symptomatic, especially with potentially life-threatening clinical presentations such as EKG changes, should be treated promptly. The cause or precipitating factor of the electrolyte abnormality should be identified and corrected, if possible.

**2.** *How should we approach a patient who has an abnormal serum sodium concentration?*

**ANSWER:** Alteration of serum sodium concentration can be precipitated by sodium alone (either excess or deficiency) or abnormal water regulation. It is important to fully assess the patient's sodium and fluid status, symptoms, physical exam findings, and medical, surgical, and medication history for factors that may precipitate sodium disorders. Because the homeostasis of sodium and water is closely regulated by the kidney, it may be useful to check urine electrolytes and osmolality to help establish the diagnosis and guide clinical management.

**3.** *What are the most common risk factors that can lead to hyperkalemia?*

**ANSWER:** The leading cause of hyperkalemia is renal function impairment, especially acute renal insufficiency and associated metabolic acidosis common in severe acute kidney injury. Two other important causes are drug-induced hyperkalemia (eg, ACE inhibitors, potassium-sparing diuretic) and high dietary intake (especially with CKD).

**4.** *What is the clinical significance of abnormal serum calcium and phosphorus concentrations?*

**ANSWER:** Severe hypocalcemia and hypercalcemia can result in neuromuscular problems. In addition, significant hypercalcemia may cause EKG changes and arrhythmias. Although hyperphosphatemia is not expected to cause any acute problems, severe hypophosphatemia can result in neurologic and CNS manifestations. In the presence of chronic hyperphosphatemia, especially in patients with CKD, the risk is increased for phosphorus to bind with calcium to form insoluble complexes that will result in soft tissue and vascular calcification. There is an increasing amount of evidence to show that such vascular calcification can increase the mortality and morbidity of CKD patients. Concurrent hypercalcemia further increases the serum calcium–phosphate product and exacerbates the calcification process.

**5.** *What is the most common clinical presentation of hypocupremia and what are the causes of copper deficiency?*

**ANSWER:** The most common clinical symptoms associated with hypocupremia are neurologic symptoms, which may present as ataxia, spasticity, muscle weakness, peripheral neuropathy, loss of vision, anemia, and leukopenia. The most common causes include intestinal malabsorption, post-bariatric surgery status, and decreased nutrient consumption.

## REFERENCES

1. Sterns RH, Spital A, Clark EC. Disorders of water balance. In: Kokko JP, Tannen RL, eds. *Fluids and Electrolytes*. 3rd ed. Philadelphia, PA: WB Saunders; 1996:63-109.

2. Kanbay M, Yilmaz S, Dincer N, et al. Antidiuretic hormone and serum osmolarity physiology and related outcomes: what is old, what is new, and what is unknown? *J Clin Endocrinol Metab*. 2019;104(11):5406-5420. PubMed

3. Wiig H, Luft FC, Titze JM. The interstitium conducts extrarenal storage of sodium and represents a third compartment essential for extracellular volume and blood pressure homeostasis. *Acta Physiol (Oxf)*. 2018;222(3). PubMed

4. Sterns RH, Nigwekar SU, Hix JK. The treatment of hyponatremia. *Semin Nephrol.* 2009;29(3):282-299.PubMed

5. Liamis G, Megapanou E, Elisaf M, Milionis H. Hyponatremia-inducing drugs. *Front Horm Res.* 2019;52:167-177.PubMed

6. Shepshelovich D, Schechter A, Calvarysky B, et al. Medication-induced SIADH: distribution and characterization according to medication class. *Br J Clin Pharmacol.* 2017;83(8):1801-1807.PubMed

7. de Bragança AC, Moyses ZP, Magaldi AJ. Carbamazepine can induce kidney water absorption by increasing aquaporin 2 expression. *Nephrol Dial Transplant.* 2010;25(12):3840-3845.PubMed

8. Sterns RH. Treatment of severe hyponatremia. *Clin J Am Soc Nephrol.* 2018;13(4):641-649.PubMed

9. Verbalis JG, Goldsmith SR, Greenberg A, et al. Diagnosis, evaluation, and treatment of hyponatremia: expert panel recommendations. *Am J Med.* 2013;126(10)(suppl 1):S1-S42.PubMed

10. Espinel CH. The FENa test. Use in the differential diagnosis of acute renal failure. *JAMA.* 1976;236(6):579-581.PubMed

11. McGee S, Abernethy WB 3rd, Simel DL. The rational clinical examination: is this patient hypovolemic? *JAMA.* 1999;281(11):1022-1029.PubMed

12. Seay NW, Lehrich RW, Greenberg A. Diagnosis and management of disorders of body tonicity-hyponatremia and hypernatremia: core curriculum 2020. *Am J Kidney Dis.* 2020;75(2):272-286.PubMed

13. Muhsin SA, Mount DB. Diagnosis and treatment of hypernatremia. *Best Pract Res Clin Endocrinol Metab.* 2016;30(2):189-203.PubMed

14. Palmer BF, Carrero JJ, Clegg DJ, et al. Clinical management of hyperkalemia. *Mayo Clin Proc.* 2020;S0025-6196(20)30618-2.

15. Nomura N, Shoda W, Uchida S. Clinical importance of potassium intake and molecular mechanism of potassium regulation. *Clin Exp Nephrol.* 2019;23(10):1175-1180.PubMed

16. Palmer BF, Clegg DJ. Physiology and pathophysiology of potassium homeostasis: core curriculum 2019. *Am J Kidney Dis.* 2019;74(5):682-695. PubMed

17. Halperin ML, Goldstein MB, eds. *Fluid, Electrolyte, and Acid-Base Physiology: A Problem-Based Approach.* 2nd ed. Philadelphia, PA: WB Saunders; 1994.

18. Long B, Warix JR, Koyfman A. Controversies in management of hyperkalemia. *J Emerg Med.* 2018;55(2):192-205.PubMed

19. Adrogué HJ, Madias NE. Changes in plasma potassium concentration during acute acid-base disturbances. *Am J Med.* 1981;71(3):456-467. PubMed

20. Unwin RJ, Luft FC, Shirley DG. Pathophysiology and management of hypokalemia: a clinical perspective. *Nat Rev Nephrol.* 2011;7(2):75-84. PubMed

21. Zieg J, Gonsorcikova L, Landau D. Current views on the diagnosis and management of hypokalaemia in children. *Acta Paediatr.* 2016;105(7):762-772.PubMed

22. Sawaya BP, Briggs JP, Schnermann J. Amphotericin B nephrotoxicity: the adverse consequences of altered membrane properties. *J Am Soc Nephrol.* 1995;6(2):154-164.PubMed

23. Zietse R, Zoutendijk R, Hoorn EJ. Fluid, electrolyte and acid-base disorders associated with antibiotic therapy. *Nat Rev Nephrol.* 2009;5(4):193-202.PubMed

24. Wile D. Diuretics: a review. *Ann Clin Biochem.* 2012;49(Pt 5):419-431. PubMed

25. Dick TB, Raines AA, Stinson JB, et al. Fludrocortisone is effective in the management of tacrolimus-induced hyperkalemia in liver transplant recipients. *Transplant Proc.* 2011;43(7):2664-2668.PubMed

26. Dobbin SJH, Petrie JR, Lean MEJ, McKay GA. Fludrocortisone therapy for persistent hyperkalaemia. *Diabet Med.* 2017;34(7):1005-1008.PubMed

27. Rein JL, Coca SG. "I don't get no respect": the role of chloride in acute kidney injury. *Am J Physiol Renal Physiol.* 2019;316(3):F587-F605.PubMed

28. Bandak G, Kashani KB. Chloride in intensive care units: a key electrolyte. F1000Res. 2017;6:1930. 29123653; PMCID: PMC5668919.

29. Barker ME. 0.9% saline induced hyperchloremic acidosis. *J Trauma Nurs.* 2015;22(2):111-116.PubMed

30. Berend K, van Hulsteijn LH, Gans RO. Chloride: the queen of electrolytes? *Eur J Intern Med.* 2012;23(3):203-211.PubMed

31. Handy JM, Soni N. Physiological effects of hyperchloraemia and acidosis. *Br J Anaesth.* 2008;101(2):141-150.PubMed

32. Alfrey AC. Normal and abnormal magnesium metabolism. In: Schrier RW, ed. *Renal and Electrolyte Disorders.* 6th ed. Philadelphia, PA: Lippincott Williams & Wilkins; 2003:278-302.

33. Katopodis P, Karteris E, Katopodis KP. Pathophysiology of drug-induced hypomagnesaemia. *Drug Saf.* 2020;43(9):867-880.PubMed

34. Topf JM, Murray PT. Hypomagnesemia and hypermagnesemia. *Rev Endocr Metab Disord.* 2003;4(2):195-206.PubMed

35. Chang WT, Radin B, McCurdy MT. Calcium, magnesium, and phosphate abnormalities in the emergency department. *Emerg Med Clin North Am.* 2014;32(2):349-366.PubMed

36. Thomas SH, Behr ER. Pharmacological treatment of acquired QT prolongation and torsades de pointes. *Br J Clin Pharmacol.* 2016;81(3):420-427.PubMed

37. Hoshino K, Ogawa K, Hishitani T, et al. Successful uses of magnesium sulfate for torsades de pointes in children with long QT syndrome. *Pediatr Int.* 2006;48(2):112-117.PubMed

38. Kraft MD, Btaiche IF, Sacks GS, Kudsk KA. Treatment of electrolyte disorders in adult patients in the intensive care unit. *Am J Health Syst Pharm.* 2005;62(16):1663-1682.PubMed

39. Kumar R. Calcium disorders. In: Kokko JP, Tannen RL, eds. *Fluids and Electrolytes.* 3rd ed. Philadelphia, PA: WB Saunders; 1996:391-419.

40. Hruska KA, Slatopolsky E. Disorders of phosphorus, calcium, and magnesium metabolism. In: Schrier RW, Gottschalk CW, eds. *Diseases of the Kidney.* 7th ed. Philadelphia, PA: Lippincott Williams & Wilkins; 2001:2607-2660.

41. Goltzman D, Mannstadt M, Marcocci C. Physiology of the calcium-parathyroid hormone-vitamin D Axis. *Front Horm Res.* 2018;50:1-13. PubMed

42. Popovtzer MM. Disorders of calcium, phosphorus, vitamin D, and parathyroid hormone activity. In: Schrier RW, ed. *Renal and Electrolyte Disorders.* 6th ed. Philadelphia, PA: Lippincott Williams & Wilkins; 2003:216-277.

43. Fleet JC. The role of vitamin D in the endocrinology controlling calcium homeostasis. *Mol Cell Endocrinol.* 2017;453:36-45.PubMed

44. Christakos S, Li S, De La Cruz J, et al. Vitamin D and the intestine: review and update. *J Steroid Biochem Mol Biol.* 2020;196:105501.PubMed

45. Dusso AS, Brown AJ, Slatopolsky E. Vitamin D. *Am J Physiol Renal Physiol.* 2005;289(1):F8-F28.PubMed

46. Gil Á, Plaza-Diaz J, Mesa MD, Vitamin D. Vitamin D: classic and novel actions. *Ann Nutr Metab.* 2018;72(2):87-95.PubMed

47. Dirks NF, Ackermans MT, Lips P, et al. The when, what & how of measuring vitamin d metabolism in clinical medicine. *Nutrients.* 2018;10(4):482.PubMed

48. Bove-Fenderson E, Mannstadt M. Hypocalcemic disorders. *Best Pract Res Clin Endocrinol Metab.* 2018;32(5):639-656.PubMed

49. Pepe J, Colangelo L, Biamonte F, et al. Diagnosis and management of hypocalcemia. *Endocrine.* 2020;69(3):485-495.

50. Asonitis N, Angelousi A, Zafeiris C, et al. Diagnosis, pathophysiology and management of hypercalcemia in malignancy: a review of the literature. *Horm Metab Res.* 2019;51(12):770-778.PubMed

51. Carrick AI, Costner HB. Rapid fire: hypercalcemia. *Emerg Med Clin North Am.* 2018;36(3):549-555.PubMed

52. Randall RE Jr, Strauss MB, McNeely WF. The milk-alkali syndrome. *Arch Intern Med.* 1961;107:163-181.PubMed

53. Dennis VW. Phosphate disorders. In: Kokko JP, Tannen RL, eds. *Fluids and Electrolytes.* 3rd ed. Philadelphia, PA: WB Saunders; 1996:359-390.

54. Halevy J, Bulvik S. Severe hypophosphatemia in hospitalized patients. *Arch Intern Med.* 1988;148(1):153-155.PubMed

55. Delmez JA, Slatopolsky E. Hyperphosphatemia: its consequences and treatment in patients with chronic renal disease. *Am J Kidney Dis*. 1992;19(4):303-317.PubMed

56. Leung J, Crook M. Disorders of phosphate metabolism. *J Clin Pathol*. 2019;72(11):741-747.PubMed

57. Vervloet MG, van Ballegooijen AJ. Prevention and treatment of hyperphosphatemia in chronic kidney disease. *Kidney Int*. 2018;93(5):1060-1072.PubMed

58. Chan S, Gerson B, Subramaniam S. The role of copper, molybdenum, selenium, and zinc in nutrition and health. *Clin Lab Med*. 1998;18(4):673-685.PubMed

59. Bost M, Houdart S, Oberli M, et al. Dietary copper and human health: current evidence and unresolved issues. *J Trace Elem Med Biol*. 2016;35:107-115.PubMed

60. Harvey LJ, Ashton K, Hooper L, et al. Methods of assessment of copper status in humans: a systematic review. *Am J Clin Nutr*. 2009;89(6):2009S-2024S.PubMed

61. Gabreyes AA, Abbasi HN, Forbes KP, et al. Hypocupremia associated cytopenia and myelopathy: a national retrospective review. *Eur J Haematol*. 2013;90(1):1-9.PubMed

62. Altarelli M, Ben-Hamouda N, Schneider A, Berger MM. Copper deficiency: causes, manifestations, and treatment. *Nutr Clin Pract*. 2019;34(4):504-513.PubMed

63. Kumar P, Hamza N, Madhok B, et al. Copper deficiency after gastric bypass for morbid obesity: a systematic review. *Obes Surg*. 2016;26(6):1335-1342.PubMed

64. Kodama H, Fujisawa C, Bhadhprasit W. *Pathology,* clinical features and treatments of congenital copper metabolic disorders: focus on neurologic aspects. *Brain Dev*. 2011;33(3):243-251.PubMed

65. Kaler SG. Inborn errors of copper metabolism. *Handb Clin Neurol*. 2013;113:1745-1754.PubMed

66. Bandmann O, Weiss KH, Kaler SG. Wilson's disease and other neurological copper disorders. *Lancet Neurol*. 2015;14(1):103-113.PubMed

67. Lindeman RD. Minerals in medical practice. In: Halpern SL, ed. *Quick Reference to Clinical Nutrition*. 2nd ed. Philadelphia, PA: JB Lippincott; 1987:295-323.

68. Sato C, Koyama H, Satoh H, et al. Concentrations of copper and zinc in liver and serum samples in biliary atresia patients at different stages of traditional surgeries. *Tohoku J Exp Med*. 2005;207(4):271-277.PubMed

69. Olson LM, Wieruszewski PM, Jannetto PJ, et al. Quantitative assessment of trace-element contamination in parenteral nutrition components. *JPEN J Parenter Enteral Nutr*. 2019;43(8):970-976.PubMed

70. Howard L, Ashley C, Lyon D, Shenkin A. Autopsy tissue trace elements in 8 long-term parenteral nutrition patients who received the current U.S. Food and Drug Administration formulation. *JPEN J Parenter Enteral Nutr*. 2007;31(5):388-396.PubMed

71. Robinson CH, Lawler MR, Chenoweth WL, et al, eds. *Normal and Therapeutic Nutrition*. 7th ed. New York, NY: Macmillan; 1990.

72. Foote JW, Delves HT. Albumin bound and alpha 2-macroglobulin bound zinc concentrations in the sera of healthy adults. *J Clin Pathol*. 1984;37(9):1050-1054.PubMed

73. de Haan KE, de Goeij JJ, van den Hamer CJ, et al. Changes in zinc metabolism after burns: observations, explanations, clinical implications. *J Trace Elem Electrolytes Health Dis*. 1992;6(3):195-201.PubMed

74. Hurley LS. Clinical and experimental aspect of manganese in nutrition. In: Prasad AR, ed. *Clinical, Biochemical, and Nutritional Aspects of Trace Elements*. New York, NY: Alan R Liss; 1982:369-378.

75. Freeland-Graves JH, Mousa TY, Kim S. International variability in diet and requirements of manganese: causes and consequences. *J Trace Elem Med Biol*. 2016;38:24-32.PubMed

76. Livingstone C. Manganese provision in parenteral nutrition: an update. *Nutr Clin Pract*. 2018;33(3):404-418.PubMed

77. National Health Institute Office of Dietary Supplement. Manganese Fact Sheet for Health Professionals. https://ods.od.nih.gov/factsheets /Manganese-HealthProfessional (accessed 2021 February 22).

78. Chen P, Bornhorst J, Aschner M. Manganese metabolism in humans. *Front Biosci*. 2018;23:1655-1679.PubMed

79. Nielsen FH. Manganese, molybdenum, boron, chromium, and other trace elements. In: Erdman JW Jr, Zeisel SH, eds. Present Knowledge in Nutrition. 10th ed. Hoboken, NJ: Wiley-Blackwell; 2012:586-607.

80. Nakamura M, Miura A, Nagahata T, et al. Low zinc, copper, and manganese intake is associated with depression and anxiety symptoms in the Japanese working population: findings from the Eating Habit and Well-Being Study. *Nutrients*. 2019;11(4):847.PubMed

81. Kirk C, Gemmell L, Lamb CA, et al. Elevated whole-blood manganese levels in adult patients prescribed "manganese-free" home parenteral nutrition. *Nutr Clin Pract*. 2020;35(6):1138-1142.PubMed

82. Dastych M, Dastych M Jr, Senkyrík M. Manganese in whole blood and hair in patients with long-term home parenteral nutrition. *Clin Lab*. 2016;62(1-2):173-177.PubMed

83. Abdalian R, Saqui O, Fernandes G, Allard JP. Effects of manganese from a commercial multi-trace element supplement in a population sample of Canadian patients on long-term parenteral nutrition. *JPEN J Parenter Enteral Nutr*. 2013;37(4):538-543.PubMed

84. Kamata N, Oshitani N, Oiso R, et al. Crohn's disease with Parkinsonism due to long-term total parenteral nutrition. *Dig Dis Sci*. 2003;48(5):992-994.PubMed

85. Peres TV, Schettinger MR, Chen P, et al. Manganese-induced neurotoxicity: a review of its behavioral consequences and neuroprotective strategies. *BMC Pharmacol Toxicol*. 2016;17(1):57.PubMed

86. Khan A, Hingre J, Dhamoon AS. Manganese neurotoxicity as a complication of chronic total parenteral nutrition. *Case Rep Neurol Med*. 2020;2020:9484028.PubMed

87. Combs GF Jr. Biomarkers of selenium status. *Nutrients*. 2015;7(4):2209-2236.PubMed

88. Manzanares W, Lemieux M, Elke G, et al. High-dose intravenous selenium does not improve clinical outcomes in the critically ill: a systematic review and meta-analysis. *Crit Care*. 2016;20(1):356. PubMed

89. Gudivada KK, Kumar A, Shariff M, et al. Antioxidant micronutrient supplementation in critically ill adults: a systematic review with meta-analysis and trial sequential analysis. Clin Nutr. 2020:S0261-5614(20)30348-4.

90. Tonelli M, Wiebe N, Hemmelgarn B, et al. Trace elements in hemodialysis patients: a systematic review and meta-analysis. *BMC Med*. 2009;7:25. PubMed

91. Sunde RA. Selenium. In: Bowman B, Russell R, eds. *Present Knowledge in Nutrition*. 9th ed. Washington, DC: International Life Sciences Institute; 2006:480-497.

92. Klein EA, Thompson IM Jr, Tangen CM, et al. Vitamin E and the risk of prostate cancer: the Selenium and Vitamin E Cancer Prevention Trial (SELECT). *JAMA*. 2011;306(14):1549-1556.PubMed

93. See KA, Lavercombe PS, Dillon J, Ginsberg R. Accidental death from acute selenium poisoning. *Med J Aust*. 2006;185(7):388-389.PubMed

94. Cefalu WT, Hu FB. Role of chromium in human health and in diabetes. *Diabetes Care*. 2004;27(11):2741-2751.PubMed

95. National Health Institute Office of Dietary Supplement. Chromium Fact Sheet for Health Professionals. https://ods.od.nih.gov/factsheets /chromium-HealthProfessional (accessed 2021 February 22).

96. Guallar E, Jiménez FJ, van 't Veer P, et al. Low toenail chromium concentration and increased risk of nonfatal myocardial infarction. *Am J Epidemiol*. 2005;162(2):157-164.PubMed

## QUICKVIEW | Sodium

| PARAMETER | DESCRIPTION | COMMENTS |
|---|---|---|
| **Common reference ranges** | | |
| Adults | 135-145 mEq/L (135–145 mmol/L) | Useful for assessment of fluid status |
| Pediatrics: premature neonates | 128–148 mEq/L (128–148 mmol/L) | |
| Pediatrics: older children | 138–145 mEq/L (138–145 mmol/L) | |
| **Critical value** | >160 or <120 mEq/L (>160 or <120 mmol/L) | Acute changes more dangerous than chronic abnormalities |
| **Natural substance?** | Yes | Most abundant cation in extracellular fluid |
| **Inherent activity?** | Yes | Maintenance of transmembrane electric potential |
| **Location** | | |
| Storage | Mostly in extracellular fluid | |
| Secretion/excretion | Filtered by kidneys, mostly reabsorbed; some secretion in distal nephron | Closely related to water homeostasis |
| **Major causes of...** | | |
| **High results** | Multiple (discussed in text) | Can occur with low, normal, or high total body sodium |
| Associated signs and symptoms | Mostly neurologic | |
| **Low results** | Multiple (discussed in text) | Can occur with low, normal, or high total body sodium |
| Associated signs and symptoms | Mostly neurologic | |
| **After insult, time to...** | | |
| Initial elevation or positive result | Hours to years, depending on chronicity | The faster the change, the more dangerous the consequences |
| Peak values | Hours to years, depending on chronicity | |
| Normalization | Days, if renal function is normal | Faster with appropriate treatment |
| **Drugs often monitored with test** | Diuretics, ACE inhibitors, aldosterone antagonists, angiotensin II antagonists, ADH analogs | Any drug that affects water homeostasis |
| **Causes of spurious results** | None | |

## QUICKVIEW | Potassium

| PARAMETER | DESCRIPTION | COMMENTS |
|---|---|---|
| **Common reference ranges** | | |
| Adults and children | 3.8–5 mEq/L (3.8–5 mmol/L) | Age: >10 days old |
| **Critical value** | >7 or <2.5 mEq/L (>7 or <2.5 mmol/L) | Acute changes more dangerous than chronic abnormalities; Depends on serum pH |
| **Natural substance?** | Yes | Most abundant cation; 98% in intracellular fluid |
| **Inherent activity?** | Yes | Control of muscle and nervous tissue excitability, acid–base balance, intracellular fluid balance |
| **Location** | | |
| Storage | 98% in intracellular fluid | |
| Secretion/excretion | Mostly secreted by distal nephron | Some via GI tract secretion |
| **Major causes of…** | | |
| **High results** | Renal failure (GFR <10 mL/min) | Especially with increased intake and concurrent acidemia |
| Associated signs and symptoms | Mostly cardiac | EKG changes, bradycardia, hypotension, cardiac arrest |
| **Low results** | Decreased intake or increased loss | Usually a combination of the two or concurrent alkalemia |
| Associated signs and symptoms | Affects primarily cardiac system | Table 11-7 |
| **After insult, time to…** | | |
| Initial elevation or positive result | Hours to years, depending on chronicity | Acute changes can be life-threatening |
| Peak values | Hours to years, depending on chronicity | |
| Normalization | Days, if renal function is normal | Faster with appropriate treatment |
| **Drugs often monitored with test** | Diuretics, ACE inhibitors, amphotericin B, angiotensin receptor antagonists, cisplatin, trimethoprim | Some drugs are administered as potassium salts; be aware of potassium-sparing medications |
| **Causes of spurious results** | Hemolyzed samples (falsely elevated) | High potassium content in erythrocytes |

## QUICKVIEW | Chloride

| PARAMETER | DESCRIPTION | COMMENTS |
|---|---|---|
| **Common reference ranges** | | |
| Adults and children | 95–103 mEq/L (95–103 mmol/L) | |
| **Critical value** | | Depends on underlying disorder |
| **Natural substance?** | Yes | |
| **Inherent activity?** | Yes | Primary anion in extracellular fluid and gastric juice, cardiac function, acid–base balance |
| **Location** | | |
| Storage | Extracellular fluid | Most abundant extracellular anion |
| Secretion/excretion | Passively follows sodium and water | Also influenced by acid–base balance |
| **Major causes of...** | | |
| **High results** | Dehydration | |
| | Acidemia | |
| Associated signs and symptoms | Associated with underlying disorder | |
| **Low results** | Nasogastric suction | |
| | Vomiting | |
| | Serum dilution | |
| | Alkalemia | |
| Associated signs and symptoms | Associated with underlying disorder | |
| **After insult, time to...** | | |
| Initial elevation or positive result | Hours to years, depending on chronicity | The faster the change, the more dangerous the consequences |
| Peak values | Hours to years, depending on chronicity | |
| Normalization | Days, if renal function is normal | Faster with appropriate treatment of underlying disorder |
| **Drugs often monitored with test** | Loop diuretics, chloride-containing IV fluids (eg, saline solution), parenteral nutrition, drugs that cause diarrhea | |
| **Causes of spurious results** | Bromides; iodides (falsely elevated) | |

## QUICKVIEW | Magnesium

| PARAMETER | DESCRIPTION | COMMENTS |
|---|---|---|
| **Common reference ranges** | | |
| Adults and children | 1.7–2.4 mg/dL (0.7–1 mmol/L)<br>1.4–2 mEq/L | |
| **Critical value** | >5 or <1 mEq/L (>2.5 or <0.5 mmol/L) | Acute changes more dangerous than chronic abnormalities |
| **Natural substance?** | Yes | |
| **Inherent activity?** | Yes | Enzyme cofactor, thermoregulation, muscle contraction, nerve conduction, calcium and potassium homeostasis |
| **Location** | | |
| Storage | 50% bone, 45% intracellular fluid, 5% extracellular fluid | |
| Secretion/excretion | Filtration by kidneys | 3%–5% reabsorbed |
| **Major causes of...** | | |
| **High results** | Renal failure | Usually in presence of increased intake |
| Associated signs and symptoms | Neuromuscular manifestations | Table 11-9 |
| **Low results** | Excessive loss from GI tract or kidneys | Alcoholism and diuretics |
| | Decreased intake | |
| Associated signs and symptoms | Neuromuscular and cardiovascular manifestations, including weakness, muscle fasciculation, tremor, tetany, increased reflexes, and EKG abnormalities | More severe with acute changes |
| **After insult, time to...** | | |
| Initial elevation or positive result | Hours to years, depending on chronicity | The faster the change, the more dangerous the consequences |
| Peak values | Hours to years, depending on chronicity | |
| Normalization | Days, if renal function is normal | Faster with appropriate treatment |
| **Drugs often monitored with test** | Diuretics, proton pump inhibitors | |
| **Causes of spurious results** | Hemolyzed samples (falsely elevated) | |

## QUICKVIEW | Calcium

| PARAMETER | DESCRIPTION | COMMENTS |
|---|---|---|
| **Common reference ranges** | | |
| Adults | Total calcium: 9.2–11 mg/dL (2.3–2.8 mmol/L) Ionized calcium: 4–4.8 mg/dL (1–1.2 mmol/L) | Approximately half of calcium in the blood is bound to serum proteins; only ionized (free) calcium is physiologically active |
| Children | Total calcium: 8–10.5 mg/dL (2–2.6 mmol/L) Ionized calcium: 1.16–1.45 mmol/L | Please refer to Chapter 23 for age-specific ranges for children |
| **Critical value** | >14 or <7 mg/dL (>3.5 or <1.8 mmol/L) | Also depends on serum albumin and pH values |
| **Natural substance?** | Yes | |
| **Inherent activity?** | Yes | Preservation of cellular membranes, propagation of neuromuscular activity, regulation of endocrine functions, blood coagulation, bone metabolism, phosphate homeostasis |
| **Location** | | |
| Storage | 99.5% in bone and teeth | Very closely regulated |
| Secretion/excretion | Filtration by kidneys | Small amounts excreted into GI tract from saliva, bile, and pancreatic and intestinal secretions |
| **Major causes of...** | | |
| **High results** | Malignancy | Also thiazide diuretics, lithium, vitamin D, teriparatide, and calcium supplements |
| | Hyperparathyroidism | More severe with acute onset |
| Associated signs and symptoms | Vague GI complaints neurologic and cardiovascular symptoms, and renal dysfunction | |
| **Low results** | Vitamin D deficiency CKD Hypoparathyroidism Hyperphosphatemia Acute pancreatitis Loop diuretics Calcitonin Zoledronic acid Denosumab | Hypocalcemia due to hypoalbuminemia is asymptomatic (ionized calcium concentration unaffected) |
| Associated signs and symptoms | Primarily neuromuscular (eg, fatigue, depression, memory loss, hallucinations, seizures, tetany) | More severe with acute onset |
| **After insult, time to...** | | |
| Initial elevation or positive result | Hours to years, depending on chronicity | The faster the change, the more dangerous the consequences |
| Peak values | Hours to years, depending on chronicity | |
| Normalization | Days, if renal function is normal | Faster with appropriate treatment |
| **Drugs often monitored with test** | Loop diuretics, calcitonin, vitamin D, calcium supplements, phosphate binders | |
| **Causes of spurious results** | Hypoalbuminemia | Ionized calcium concentration usually unaffected |

## QUICKVIEW | Phosphorus

| PARAMETER | DESCRIPTION | COMMENTS |
|---|---|---|
| **Common reference ranges** | | |
| Adults | 2.3–4.7 mg/dL (0.74–1.52 mmol/L) | |
| Children | 4–7.1 mg/dL (1.3–2.3 mmol/L) | See Chapter 23 for detailed listing of normal ranges based on patient's age |
| **Critical value** | >8 or <1 mg/dL (>2.6 or <0.3 mmol/L) | Acute changes more dangerous than chronic abnormalities |
| **Natural substance?** | Yes | Most abundant intracellular anion |
| **Inherent activity?** | Yes | Bone and tooth integrity, cellular membrane integrity, phospholipid synthesis, acid–base balance, calcium homeostasis, enzyme activation, formation of high-energy bonds |
| **Location** | | |
| Storage | Extracellular fluid, cell membrane structure, intracellular fluid, collagen, bone | 85% in bone |
| Secretion/excretion | Filtration by kidneys | Mostly reabsorbed |
| **Major causes of...** | | |
| **High results** | Decreased renal excretion | Renal failure is the most common cause |
| | Extracellular shifting | Rhabdomyolysis; tumor lysis syndrome |
| | Increased intake of phosphate or vitamin D | |
| Associated signs and symptoms | Due primarily to hypocalcemia and hyperparathyroidism | See Quickview for calcium (hypocalcemia) |
| **Low results** | Increased renal excretion | Also can occur in renal failure |
| | Intracellular shifting | Insulin use |
| | Decreased intake of phosphate or vitamin D | |
| Associated signs and symptoms | Bone pain, weakness, malaise, hypocalcemia, cardiac failure, respiratory failure | Usually due to diminished intracellular ATP and erythrocyte 2,3-DPG concentrations |
| **After insult, time to...** | | |
| Initial elevation or positive result | Usually over months to years | |
| Peak values | Usually over months to years | |
| Normalization | Over days with renal transplantation | |
| **Drugs often monitored with test** | Vitamin D, phosphate binders | |
| **Causes of spurious results** | Hemolyzed samples (falsely elevated) and methotrexate (falsely elevated) | |

2,3-DPG = 2,3-diphosphoglycerate.

## QUICKVIEW | Copper

| PARAMETER | DESCRIPTION | COMMENTS |
|---|---|---|
| **Common reference ranges** | | |
| Adults | 70–140 mcg/dL (11–22 µmol/L) (men); 80–155 mcg/dL (13–24 µmol/L) (women) | |
| Children | 20–70 mcg/dL (3.1–11 µmol/L) | 0–6 mo |
| | 90–190 mcg/dL (14.1–29.8 µmol/L) | 6 yr |
| | 80–160 mcg/dL (12.6–25.1 µmol/L) | 12 yr |
| **Critical value** | Not applicable | |
| **Natural substance?** | Yes | |
| **Inherent activity?** | Yes | Companion to iron enzyme cofactor, Hgb synthesis, collagen and elastin synthesis, metabolism of many neurotransmitters, energy generation, regulation of plasma lipid levels, cell protection against oxidative damage |
| **Location** | | |
| Storage | One-third in liver and brain; one-third in muscles; one-third in heart, spleen, kidneys, and blood (erythrocytes and neutrophils) | 95% of circulating copper is protein bound as ceruloplasmin |
| Secretion/excretion | Mainly by biliary excretion; only 0.5%–3% of daily intake found in urine | |
| **Major causes of...** | | |
| **High results** | Deliberate ingestion of large amounts (>15 mg of elemental copper); Wilson disease | Uncommon in humans |
| Associated signs and symptoms | Nausea, vomiting, intestinal cramps, diarrhea | Larger ingestions lead to shock, hepatic necrosis, intravascular hemolysis, renal impairment, coma, and death |
| **Low results** | Infants with chronic diarrhea | |
| | Malabsorption syndromes | Following bariatric surgery |
| | Decreased intake over months | |
| | Menkes syndrome | |
| Associated signs and symptoms | Neutropenia, iron-deficiency anemia, abnormal glucose tolerance, arrhythmias, hypercholesterolemia, atherosclerosis, depressed immune function, defective connective tissue formation, demineralization of bones | Can affect any system or organ whose enzymes require copper for proper functioning |
| **Drugs often monitored with test** | Copper supplements, possibly during chronic parenteral nutrition | Serum copper concentrations not routinely monitored |

## QUICKVIEW | Zinc

| PARAMETER | DESCRIPTION | COMMENTS |
|---|---|---|
| **Common reference ranges** | | |
| Adults and children | 50–150 mcg/dL (7.7–23 µmol/L) | Increased risk for developing symptomatic zinc deficiency |
| **Critical value** | <50 mcg/dL (<7.7 µmol/L) | |
| **Natural substance?** | Yes | |
| **Inherent activity?** | Yes | Enzyme constituent and cofactor; carbohydrate, protein, lipid, and nucleic acid metabolism; tissue growth; tissue repair; cell membrane stabilization; bone collagenase activity and collagen turnover; immune response; food intake control; spermatogenesis and gonadal maturation; normal testicular function |
| **Location** | | |
| Storage | Liver, pancreas, spleen, lungs, eyes (retina, iris, cornea, lens), prostate, skeletal muscle, bone, erythrocytes, neutrophils | 60%–62% in skeletal muscle, 20%–28% in bone, 2%–4% in liver |
| Secretion/excretion | Primarily in pancreatic and intestinal secretions; also lost dermally through sweat, hair and nail growth, and skin shedding | Except in certain disease states, only 2% lost in urine |
| **Major causes of...** | | |
| **High results** | Large intake | Uncommon in humans |
| Associated signs and symptoms | Drowsiness, lethargy, nausea, vomiting, diarrhea, increases in serum lipase and amylase concentrations | |
| **Low results** | Low intake (infants) | Rare from inadequate dietary intake in adults |
| | Decreased absorption (acrodermatitis enteropathica) | |
| | Increased used (rapidly growing adolescents and menstruating, lactating, or pregnant women) | |
| | Increased loss (hyperzincuria) | |
| Associated signs and symptoms | Manifests in numerous organs and physiologic systems | Table 11-13 |
| **Drugs often monitored with test** | Zinc supplements, possibly during chronic parenteral nutrition | Serum zinc concentrations not routinely monitored |
| **Causes of spurious results** | Hemolyzed samples; 24-hr intrapatient variability | High zinc content in erythrocytes and neutrophils |

## QUICKVIEW | Manganese

| PARAMETER | DESCRIPTION | COMMENTS |
|---|---|---|
| **Common reference ranges** | | |
| Adults | Varies depending on array method, whether sample is blood or serum, and patient age; typical whole blood manganese concentrations range from 4–15 mcg/L, or 72–270 nmol/L. | |
| Children | 2–3 mcg/L (36–55 nmol/L) | |
| | 2.4–9.6 mcg/L (44–175 nmol/L) | Newborn |
| | 0.8–2.1 mcg/L (15–38 nmol/L) | 2–18 yr |
| **Critical value** | Not applicable | |
| **Natural substance?** | Yes | |
| **Inherent activity?** | Yes | Enzyme cofactor; carbohydrate, protein, and lipid metabolism; protection of cells from free radicals; steroid biosynthesis; metabolism of biogenic amines; normal brain function |
| | | Magnesium may substitute for manganese in most instances |
| **Location** | | |
| Storage | Bone, liver, pancreas, pituitary gland | Circulating manganese loosely bound to transmanganin |
| Secretion/excretion | Primarily in biliary and pancreatic secretions; limited excretion in urine | Other GI routes also may be used in manganese overload |
| **Major causes of...** | | |
| **High results** | Long-term parenteral nutrition with daily multitrace elements; accidental exposure to manganese compounds, such as in manganese mines | One of least toxic trace elements |
| Associated signs and symptoms | Encephalopathy and profound neurologic disturbances mimicking Parkinson disease | Accumulates in liver and brain |
| **Low results** | After several weeks to months of omission from diet or parenteral nutrition | Rare from inadequate dietary intake |
| Associated signs and symptoms | Weight loss, slow hair and nail growth, hair color change, transient dermatitis, hypocholesterolemia, hypotriglyceridemia | Seen mostly in experimental subjects |
| **Drugs often monitored with test** | Manganese supplements, possibly during chronic parenteral nutrition | |

## QUICKVIEW | Chromium

| PARAMETER | DESCRIPTION | COMMENTS |
|---|---|---|
| **Common reference ranges** | | |
| Adults | 0.3–0.9 ng/mL, serum<br>0.7–28 ng/mL, whole blood | Analysis of chromium in biological fluids and tissues is difficult |
| Children | Unknown | Analysis of chromium in biological fluids and tissues is difficult |
| **Critical value** | Unknown | |
| **Natural substance?** | Yes | |
| **Inherent activity?** | Yes | Cofactor for insulin and metabolism of glucose, cholesterol, and triglycerides |
| **Location** | | |
| Storage | Hair, kidneys, skeleton, liver, spleen, lungs, testes, large intestines | Chromium circulates as free $Cr^{3+}$, bound to transferrin and other proteins, and as an organic complex |
| Secretion/excretion | Excretion in urine | Circulating insulin may affect excretion |
| **Major causes of...** | | |
| **Low results** | Decreased intake | |
| Associated signs and symptoms | Glucose intolerance; hyperinsulinemia; hypercholesterolemia; possibly, increased risk of cardiovascular disease | Mainly due to its role as insulin cofactor |
| **Drugs often monitored with test** | Chromium supplement, possibly during chronic parenteral nutrition | Serum chromium concentration not routinely monitored |

# 12

# Interpretation of Laboratory Tests Associated with the Assessment of Nutritional Status

*Lingtak-Neander Chan and Sharon Wu*

Identifying patients who are at risk for malnutrition and continually monitoring a patient's nutritional status are critical components of the comprehensive patient care plan. Research has confirmed that the presence of malnutrition consistently correlates with increased length of stay in the hospital and the intensive care unit (ICU), prolonged mechanical ventilation, increased risk for healthcare-associated infections and complications, delayed recovery from surgery, delayed wound healing, and increased mortality.[1-7] Malnutrition is also associated with increased use of healthcare resources and increases healthcare costs.[8] Implementation of optimal nutrition support therapy in a timely manner has been shown to improve patient outcomes and reduce costs to the healthcare system.[9] The Joint Commission has established standards related to nutritional screening and assessment that are applicable to patients in all acute care and long-term care facilities.[10]

Understanding a patient's nutritional status has a direct implication on the roles performed by pharmacists. A patient's malnutrition risk and clinical conditions determine the needs and urgency for specialized nutrition support, such as enteral and parenteral nutrition. Use of specialized nutrition support has implications on patient safety, such as optimization of fluid and electrolyte balance, determining route and method of drug administration, and addressing drug compatibility concerns. Additionally, patients with malnutrition are at increased risk for falls and frailty. Altered body composition such as sarcopenia, dehydration, edema, and end organ dysfunction may alter pharmacokinetic and pharmacodynamic response to pharmacotherapy. Therefore, identifying malnourished patients or those who are at risk for malnutrition may help pharmacists adjust and optimize pharmacotherapeutic approaches and decisions that can improve patient safety and outcomes.

The perception and understanding of malnutrition have evolved over time. Historically, the term *malnutrition* is mostly associated with starvation and famine leading to kwashiorkor and marasmus. Kwashiorkor, sometimes known as *edematous malnutrition*, is a form of protein-calorie malnutrition most commonly associated with hunger and starvation. Patients typically present with loss of muscle and generalized edema and a large, protuberant belly. Marasmus is also a form of protein-calorie malnutrition. It generally presents with overall weight loss with severe muscle mass depletion without edema. The two conditions are not mutually exclusive because marasmus may progress to kwashiorkor in some patients. With changes in the global economy and landscape and improvements in agriculture, healthcare, education, living standards, and high-risk medical/surgical interventions, the presentation of malnutrition has expanded. The presentation of malnutrition in modern days may not be limited to a lack of access to food in general. Instead, malnutrition more commonly presents as nutrient imbalance, undernutrition, micronutrient abnormalities, obesity, cachexia, frailty, and sarcopenia.[11] In particular, *sarcopenia*, or loss of muscle mass, is the current malnutrition-related research focus. Its prevalence is especially high among older adults, hospitalized patients, critically ill patients, and patients with cancer (**Table 12-1**).[12] The evolving changes also challenge the existing clinical definition of malnutrition. According to the tenth revision of International Classification of Diseases (ICD) codes, the clinical features that fit the diagnosis of malnutrition are still limited (**Table 12-2**) and do not fully address the current understanding of the etiology and presentation of malnutrition.

DOI 10.37573/9781585286423.012

**TABLE 12-1.** Prevalence of Sarcopenia Among Patient Populations Based on Recent Clinical Studies

| PATIENT POPULATION | PREVALENCE (%) |
|---|---|
| **Older adults** | |
| 60–70 years old | 5–13 |
| ≥ 80 years old | 11–50 |
| Adult patients admitted to medical and surgical floors | 5–25 |
| Adult patients admitted to the ICU | 60–70 |
| Patients with cancer | 15–60 |

**TABLE 12-2.** ICD-10 codes for Malnutrition

| CODES | DESCRIPTION |
|---|---|
| E40 | Kwashiorkor |
| E41 | Nutritional marasmus |
| E42 | Marasmic kwashoikor |
| E43 | Unspecified severe protein-calorie malnutrition |
| E44 | Protein-calorie malnutrition of moderate and mild degree |
| E45 | Retarded development following protein-calorie malnutrition |
| E46 | Unspecified protein-calorie malnutrition |

The current etiology-based disease definition accepted in the field of nutrition is that malnutrition is a syndrome that includes chronic starvation without inflammation (eg, anorexia nervosa or major depression with lack of interest in eating); chronic disease-associated malnutrition, when inflammation is chronic and of mild to moderate degree (eg, organ failure, pancreatic cancer, rheumatoid arthritis, or sarcopenic obesity); and acute disease or injury-associated malnutrition, when inflammation is acute and of severe degree (eg, major infection, burns, trauma, or closed head injury).[11] Since 2016, a group of international researchers have come together and started a workgroup called Global Leadership Initiative on Malnutrition (GLIM). This group aims to develop a consensus-based framework to define, describe, and record the occurrence of malnutrition that would be applicable worldwide.[13]

Inflammation is an important component in the current/modern definition of malnutrition. Inflammation alters food intake, nutrition absorption, and/or assimilation and leads to altered body composition and impairs certain biological functions.[14] Inflammation is a critical pathophysiological process that leads to or accelerates the loss of lean body mass and muscle size (ie, sarcopenia) and cellularity. Chronic inflammation may progress to severe functional loss, and increases morbidity and mortality. Therefore, identifying the presence and severity of inflammation is crucial to the screening, characterization, and assessment of malnutrition as well as developing a patient-specific therapeutic plan to reverse malnutrition and functional loss. It also affects what monitoring parameters, including laboratory surrogate markers, are more accurate and specific for monitoring progress and response toward nutritional interventions. Laboratory tests that are significantly impacted by inflammation may not accurately reflect a person's nutritional status and, therefore, are unreliable nutritional markers.

Serum visceral protein concentrations, such as albumin, prealbumin, transferrin, and retinol binding protein, have been extensively used as laboratory markers for malnutrition since the 1970s.[15,16] Each of these serum proteins has different physiologic characteristics (**Table 12-3**). However, the regulation, synthesis, and degradation of these serum proteins are all affected by other factors in addition to decreased nutrient intake. End organ dysfunction, specific nutrient deficiency, and inflammation all have a direct impact on the homeostasis of these compounds. With the current knowledge that malnutrition is associated with an inflammatory state, none of these visceral proteins is a sensitive or specific marker in the clinical assessment of a patient's nutritional status and response to nutrition therapy. They should not be used for nutritional assessment. The history of each of the visceral proteins as a nutrition marker and their respective limitations are discussed next.

## SERUM ALBUMIN

Albumin is a major serum protein that is exclusively synthesized in the liver. Its primary functions include maintaining colloidal osmotic pressure for plasma, serving as the carrier and binding protein for many physiologic compounds (eg, bilirubin; long-chain fatty acids; divalent cations such as calcium, magnesium and zinc; bile acids; vitamin D; sex hormones; cortisol; thyroxine; and catecholamines) and drugs, maintaining acid–base balance for plasma, and providing important extracellular antioxidant function of the plasma to scavenge free radicals generated under normal physiology.[17,18] The estimated total body albumin is ~280 g for an average adult, as determined by tracer method. Of the total albumin pool, ~40% is found in the intravascular space and the rest is distributed in the interstitial space of different vital organs, such as muscle, connective tissues, and skin. The average hepatic synthetic rate of albumin for a healthy adult is ~150 mg/kg/day (~10 to 15 g/day). The average total body turnover time is ~25 days.[18,19] Under normal physiology, renal and gastrointestinal (GI) loss of albumin should be less than 6% and 10% of the total body albumin pool, respectively. The rest of the turnover mechanism is not fully understood. Some studies have suggested that albumin undergoes degradation in the extravascular compartment.[20] When the synthetic and removal rate of albumin is at steady state, the serum albumin concentration is maintained between 3.5 and 4 g/dL.

With its hepatic origin and the early studies linking its serum changes with kwashiorkor, it has been assumed historically that serum albumin concentration reflects a person's nutritional status given the liver is the primary organ for plasma protein synthesis.[21,22] In 1977, it was first suggested by Blackburn et al that serum proteins, including albumin and transferrin, could

**TABLE 12-3.** Summary of General Physiologic Functions and Serum Half-Lives of Visceral Proteins Used Historically as Nutrition Markers

| VISCERAL PROTEIN AND NORMAL RANGE | SERUM HALF-LIFE (UNDER NORMAL PHYSIOLOGY) | PRIMARY FUNCTIONS | FACTORS THAT AFFECT PLASMA CONCENTRATION |
|---|---|---|---|
| Albumin (3.5–4.5 g/dL) | 14–20 days | Maintaining oncotic pressure of plasma<br>Transporting a number of divalent cations (eg, calcium)<br>Transporting a number of peptide hormones and biological compounds<br>Serving as an antioxidant molecule | Inflammation<br>Liver disease<br>Pregnancy |
| Transferrin (200–350 mg/dL) | 10 days | Transporting iron | Inflammation<br>Iron deficiency<br>Kidney disease<br>Pregnancy<br>Dehydration |
| Prealbumin (15–36 mg/dL) | 2–3 days | Transporting thyroxine in the plasma and across the blood–brain barrier<br>Serving as a carrier protein for retinol-binding protein | Inflammation<br>Liver disease<br>Kidney disease |
| Retinol-binding protein (40–60 mcg/mL) | 12 hr | Transporting vitamin A, specifically retinol | Inflammation<br>Vitamin A status<br>Prealbumin<br>Kidney disease |

be used as a marker of nutritional assessment for hospitalized patients.[23] With a number of studies published shortly after that also demonstrating a correlation between serum albumin concentration and prognosis of hospitalized patients, serum albumin was widely suggested as a clinical marker of malnutrition. In their retrospective study involving 500 consecutively admitted patients, Seltzer and colleagues showed that patients with a serum albumin concentration <3.5 g/dL on admission had statistically significant higher complication rates (33% versus 7.3%) and mortality rates (0.8% versus 0%) for that hospital stay. Compared with patients with serum albumin >3.5 g/dL, those with hypoalbuminemia were associated with a 4-fold increase in complications and a 6-fold increase in deaths. When the data were further compared between surgical versus nonsurgical patients, hypoalbuminemia was associated with a 9.7 times higher mortality rate for nonsurgical patients. Based on their findings, the authors called for using serum albumin as an "instant nutritional assessment information" that should be used for every hospital admission.[24] In the following year, a pivotal trial by Rheinhart et al showed a negative linear correlation between serum albumin concentration and 30-day mortality in 509 adult patients with hypoalbuminemia.[25] The hospital mortality rate for those with albumin <2.1 g/dL was more than 10 times higher

than for patients with albumin <3.4 g/dL. These findings paved the way in making serum albumin a routine laboratory test in assessing nutritional status of patients.

Contemporary research in clinical nutrition and metabolism has significantly increased our understanding of the pathophysiology of malnutrition and the physiological response to feeding. It is now clear that although serum albumin concentration may have a prognostic value in predicting survival, it is not a valid surrogate marker of total muscle mass or clinical response to feeding. Increased vascular permeability, changes in interstitial volume, and systemic inflammation can alter serum albumin concentration independent of liver function, nutrient intake, and nutrient utilization. Thus, it should not be used as a clinical marker for a patient's nutritional status.[15]

Hypoalbuminemia is a common presentation in hospitalized patients, especially among individuals who are critically ill. Multiple factors may contribute to decreased serum albumin concentration. The most important driving factor is inflammation associated with an acute phase response. Acute phase response may occur in acute illnesses (eg, trauma, sepsis, pancreatitis) and ongoing, uncontrolled chronic diseases (eg, gout, heart failure, inflammatory bowel disease, autoimmune diseases). In both situations, it is associated with increased plasma and cellular concentrations of proinflammatory cytokines (eg, tumor necrosis factor, interleukin-6). The inflammatory process can also be confirmed by the presence of nonspecific surrogate markers of inflammation, such as an elevated C-reactive protein concentration in the plasma.

It is proposed that inflammation affects serum albumin in at least three different mechanisms: (1) increased capillary permeability and leak resulting in serum albumin leaving the intravascular compartment to the interstitium; (2) hepatic reprioritization of protein synthesis—a process in which the liver increases the synthesis of other proteins and compounds essential for host defense and survival over visceral proteins such as albumin and transferrin; (3) increased degradation to immediately increase the free concentrations of hormones, cytokines, and other vital peptides available in the plasma to promote healing and recovery of the body as well as be recycled after serving specific physiologic functions, such as oxidation, glycation, or binding of other highly reactive substances that may be harmful to cells and tissues.[15,18,26-28] These mechanistic explanations are consistent with clinical observations. In fact, serum albumin concentration falls quickly shortly after injuries and acute illnesses. For example, in the pivotal study published by Rheinhart et al, the lowest serum albumin concentration was recorded in 48.9% of the patients within 1 week of hospital admission.[25] In an ICU study with nine mild-to-moderate critically ill adults (mean APACHE II score 7.5) with hypoalbuminemia, feeding patients with parenteral nutrition at 35 to 40 kcal/kg/day with 1.2 to 1.6 g/kg/day of protein did not change the mean serum albumin concentration (2.0 g/dL to 2.1 g/dL) or extend the shortened serum half-life of albumin (9.1 days).[29] Serum albumin concentration is inversely correlated with C-reactive protein concentration and remains low as long as plasma C-reactive protein concentration is elevated (**Figure 12-1**).[30] These results indicate that although albumin consistently shows a positive correlation

with survival, hypoalbuminemia is a more accurate reflection of the magnitude of systemic inflammation (and possibly severity of acute illnesses) experienced by a patient rather than a true, reliable surrogate marker of a patient's nutritional status.

A related topic is whether serial serum albumin concentrations can be used to reliably assess a patient's response to nutritional interventions and guide therapeutic changes to the nutrition support regimen. Despite the relatively small number of clinical studies, the results have failed to confirm a positive relationship. For example, Li et al showed that among older adults undergoing gastric cancer surgery, continuous feeding by either enteral or parenteral route at 30 kcal/kg/day for up to 7 days did not improve serum albumin concentration (3.4 versus 3.1 g/dL on days 1 and 7, respectively). The lack of improvement was likely due to the ongoing, uncontrolled systemic inflammation, as reflected by the continued increase in serum C-reactive protein concentration (2.9 to 11.6 mg/L on days 1 and 7, respectively).[31] Yeh et al also showed that changes in serum albumin concentration did not correlate with the adequacy of nutrient delivery and clinical response to feeding in patients in the surgical ICU.[32] Overall, serum albumin concentration has not been shown to be a sensitive marker of energy and protein intake adequacy, especially in hospitalized patients. Normalization of serum albumin concentration during the hospital stay or course of care may merely be a reflection of the resolution of inflammation (ie, optimal and positive response to the treatment of the current illness) and does not suggest an improvement of nutritional status or decreased need for nutrition intervention.

In summary, based on current knowledge and evidence, serum albumin concentration is significantly affected by inflammation. Hypoalbuminemia in patients is likely a reflection of ongoing and uncontrolled illness involving a heightened inflammatory state. Serum albumin concentration does not serve as a proxy measure of total body protein or total muscle mass and should not be used to assess nutritional status or guide nutritional intervention.

## SERUM PREALBUMIN

Prealbumin, also known as transthyretin, is another visceral serum protein that has been proposed as a useful laboratory marker for nutritional assessment. Prealbumin is also a hepatic plasma protein and is partly catabolized by the kidneys. Its primary functions include transport of thyroid hormones and retinol-binding protein both in the plasma and across the blood–brain barrier. It may also play a role in regulating epinephrine availability because it has binding affinity for this neuropeptide.[33] Recently, it has also been found to be a major binding protein for β-amyloid (Aβ) peptide in the brain, suggesting its neuroprotective effect or as a potential treatment target for Alzheimer disease.[34]

The interest of using prealbumin as a nutrition marker can be traced back to the early 1970s. In 40 hospitalized children with protein-calorie malnutrition, serum prealbumin concentration was found to be depleted but quickly reversible upon dietary protein replenishment and with a much faster response rate than albumin.[35] The higher degree of responsiveness in the

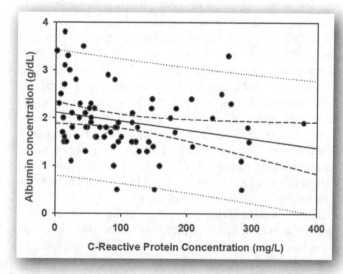

**FIGURE 12-1.** Serum albumin concentration is negatively correlated with C-reactive protein concentration, a marker of systemic inflammation. Data are based on adult patients admitted to the medical ICU.[30]

normalization of serum concentration can be attributed to its shorter biological half-life of 2 days, compared with 20 days for albumin.[36] In the following 30 years, numerous studies and conference proceedings have suggested and even emphasized the use of prealbumin as the preferred laboratory test to assess patient nutritional status and guide nutritional interventions.[37,38]

One of the major limitations of using prealbumin as a nutrition marker is that it is a negative acute phase reactant. It can be useful for estimating nutrition risk by identifying patients whose inflammatory state is heightened and can help determine whether these patients are at an increased risk of poor outcomes if nutritional intervention is not initiated. Because it is a visceral transport protein synthesized by the liver, however, it shares the same characteristics with albumin in response to stress and inflammatory response and thus is subject to the same limitations as a marker for nutritional status. Under acute stress conditions, the synthesis of prealbumin is abruptly depressed by a cytokine-directed hepatic reprioritization of metabolic and synthetic processes for plasma proteins as well as a redistribution of organ and tissue protein pools.[15,33] Additionally, prealbumin concentrations may be increased in renal dysfunction, corticosteroid therapy, or dehydration. Studies have also shown that prealbumin concentration does not correlated with anthropometric assessment findings in patients with cancer and eating disorders.[39,40]

Regarding its role for monitoring nutrition interventions and guiding nutrient provision, serum prealbumin is also found to be inconsistent and unreliable as a nutrition marker. Although some studies have suggested that prealbumin is more sensitive than transferrin and albumin as an indicator of adequate nutritional provision, additional studies have showed that prealbumin more accurately reflects systemic inflammation rather than adequacy of calorie and protein provision.[32,41-43] **Figure 12-2** summarizes the relationship between plasma concentration of prealbumin and

high-sensitivity C-reactive protein over time for 36 adult patients in the medical ICU. It shows that while a patient is under a heightened inflammatory state on ICU admission, prealbumin concentration is suppressed. As the patient's clinical status improved and C-reactive protein concentration dropped to <100 mg/L, prealbumin concentration increased significantly. However, as these patients experienced new clinical complications with C-reactive protein concentration rising once again, their prealbumin concentration also trended downward despite adequate caloric and protein provision through nutrition support (Figure 12-2).[44]

In summary, although prealbumin has been used and continues to be used as a laboratory marker for nutrition assessment and response to nutritional intervention, more recent knowledge and clinical data show that changes in its serum concentration are more likely related to system inflammation. Therefore, it should not be used to assess a patient's nutritional status. Its role as a surrogate marker for response to feeding is highly questionable and requires further investigation.

## SERUM TRANSFERRIN

Transferrin is another hepatic visceral protein with the primary function as a carrier protein for iron. Its expression is regulated by the iron status of the body, with increased expression in iron deficiency. Its use as a nutritional marker dates back in the 1970s. Its serum half-life is approximately 10 days, making it a more favorable serum marker than album.[45] However, it is also a negative acute phase reactant, and its serum concentration is increased with renal failure, pregnancy, anemia, and dehydration. Abrupt reduction in serum transferrin concentration in critically ill patients is common and is caused by inflammation and reprioritization of hepatic protein synthesis. Given the confounders that affect its homeostasis, transferrin is an unreliable marker for nutrition assessment. Studies have also shown conflicting results regarding its change in serum concentration in response to nutritional interventions.[46-49] Its use as a general malnutrition marker or as a marker for nutrition response is not recommended.

## OTHER HISTORICAL LABORATORY MARKERS

### Serum Retinol-Binding Protein

The use of retinol-binding protein as a laboratory marker to assess nutritional status was initially proposed by Ingenbleek and colleagues in 1975 in a study involving 37 children aged 18 to 30 months. All the patients in the study presented with protein-calorie malnutrition with clinical presentations including weight loss, growth failure, hair discoloration, skin lesions, diarrhea, and swollen limbs. Serial serum visceral protein concentrations were measured at baseline and weekly for 3 weeks after oral diet treatment was initiated. Serum viscera protein measured included albumin, transferrin, prealbumin, and retinol-binding protein. Retinol-binding protein was selected because it binds to prealbumin and has a short biologic half-life

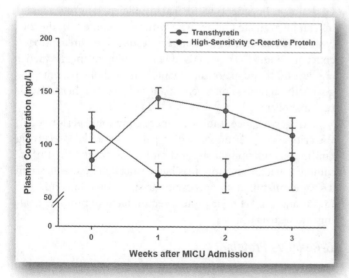

**FIGURE 12-2.** Comparison of longitudinal changes between transthyretin (prealbumin) and C-reactive protein (*n* = 36). A negative correlation is found between serum concentrations of prealbumin and C-reaction protein. Data based on Chan et al.[44]

of approximately 12 hours. It theoretically offers a benefit over prealbumin and transferring by having a faster turnover rate in detecting responses to feeding. Investigators found that prealbumin and retinol-binding protein had the most pronounced decline in their plasma concentration at baseline. The serum recovery rate after dietary intervention was initiated was comparable between the two proteins. By day 22, plasma retinol-binding protein concentration was increased by 3- to 4-fold from baseline. The authors suggested that retinol-binding protein is a more sensitive marker than albumin and transferrin in assessing nutritional status.[16]

Despite its potential benefits over other visceral proteins, there are an insufficient number of high-quality validation studies to confirm the role of retinol-binding protein in nutritional assessment across different patient populations. Additionally, retinol-binding protein is affected by a patient's vitamin A status and the presence of inflammation.[50,51] Currently, retinol-binding protein concentration should be considered a component of a comprehensive assessment for vitamin A status rather than a general laboratory marker for nutritional assessment.

## Total Lymphocyte Count

Total lymphocyte count has been used historically as a laboratory marker for nutritional assessment. Seltzer et al showed that an abnormal total lymphocyte count, defined as <1,500 cell/mm$^3$ of absolute lymphocyte, was associated with 1.8-fold increase in complications and a 4-fold increase in mortality among 500 hospitalized patients.[24] It is thought that malnutrition, especially protein-calorie malnutrition, may lead to decreased lymphocyte production by the body; however, this change is neither sensitive nor specific to malnutrition. Concomitant diseases and a severe stress reaction may also affect lymphocyte count and bone marrow response. Chronic deficiency in specific nutrients, such as hypocupremia from intestinal malabsorption, can also lead to lymphopenia. Although it continues to be used by some investigators as a marker of nutritional status, a consistent relationship between total lymphocyte count and malnutrition based on anthropometric assessment or validated nutrition screening tools is lacking.[52,53] Total lymphocyte count responds slowly to the correction of the nutritional status, even in the absence of other factors. Therefore, it is neither an accurate nor a clinically reliable laboratory marker as a diagnostic tool for malnutrition for assessment of response to nutritional support.

## Additional Laboratory Tests Used in Clinical Nutrition

### Nitrogen Balance Study

Nitrogen balance study is intended to assess the adequacy of protein intake and is the most established and accepted clinical procedure and laboratory assessment for this purpose in current practice and clinical research. Amino acids are important building blocks for tissues and other vital cellular components, such as transport proteins and peptide hormones. Protein synthesis involves the incorporation of an amine group into carbon molecules. By measuring the rate of dietary nitrogen entering and leaving the body and calculating the difference in a defined period, it can help optimize nutritional provision, especially for daily protein, which can, in turn, help prevent malnutrition by preserving or increasing body cell mass. Nitrogen balance study is the technique used to optimize dietary nitrogen (thus protein) intake.

Nitrogen is primarily eliminated from the body in the urine and feces. Other minor sources of nitrogen loss include dermal loss and daily tissue turnover such as from hair, nails, and secretions.[54] The nonurinary and fecal loss is generally considered negligible and clinically insignificant. Because most nitrogen loss is through the urine in the form of mostly urea but also as ammonium and creatinine, nitrogen balance study typically involves collecting 24-hour urine to quantify the urinary urea nitrogen (UUN). The following is the general equation to determine nitrogen balance:

$$\text{Nitrogen balance} = (\text{Total protein intake in grams}/6.25) - (\text{UUN in grams} + 4)$$

In this equation, *UUN* is the directly measured value from a 24-hour urine collection. The +4 is added to account for fecal and other minor sources of nitrogen loss based on historical data. Daily dietary protein intake in grams per day is divided by 6.25 because the metabolically active proteins in the human body, as well as in most dietary proteins, generally contain 16% nitrogen by weight.[55]

Based on the setup of this equation, ideal candidates for accurate nitrogen balance study include patients whose total protein intake can be fully and accurately quantified, who are preferably receiving full enteral or parenteral feeding, who have normal renal function, and who are not experiencing excessive nonurinary nitrogen loss, such as through diarrhea, open wounds, or GI drainage. In patients with renal insufficiency, nitrogen kinetics can be evaluated by analyzing nitrogen content in the dialyzed fluid and the rate of change in serum blood urea nitrogen concentration.[56-59] The details of determining nitrogen kinetics are beyond the scope of this chapter. In catabolic patients, the goal is the achieve a nitrogen balance of +2 or higher to facilitate anabolism.

Nitrogen balance studies are more commonly performed in the critical care setting, in which patients are likely receiving continuous nutritional support and an accurate timed urine sample collection is more feasible. Critically ill patients are in a severe inflammatory and catabolic state. Therefore, it is also important to meet their protein requirement to promote healing and recovery.

### C-Reactive Protein

C-reactive protein is a pentameric protein synthesized by the liver. It is released in response to inflammation; thus, it is a nonspecific positive acute phase reactant. Plasma C-reactive protein concentration is elevated in both acute and chronic inflammatory responses. It has a serum half-life of 19 hours.[60] Therefore, it can fluctuate throughout the course of a patient's treatment and offer some information on whether the patient's inflammatory state is worsening or improving. However, it must be interpreted according to patient-specific clinical context and presentation. No single value can be used to rule in or rule out a specific diagnosis or disease.

C-reactive protein is not a direct marker to reflect a patient's nutritional status. However, because the current consensus is that the etiology of malnutrition includes inflammation, determining plasma C-reactive protein concentration can help clinicians determine if a patient is at risk for malnutrition and prioritize the need for nutritional intervention.[11,13]

## WHAT ARE THE BEST APPROACHES TO ASSESS NUTRITION STATUS, DIAGNOSE MALNUTRITION, AND MONITOR NUTRITIONAL RESPONSE?

Based on the contemporary understanding and clinical definition of malnutrition, it appears that none of the laboratory tests historically or currently in use are sensitive markers for nutritional assessment and monitoring. Instead, changes in the serum concentrations of these visceral proteins reflect the magnitude of ongoing inflammation experienced by the patients. So, what are the optimal approaches in assessing nutritional status and response to nutritional interventions?

Malnutrition should be determined based on the presence of phenotypic or etiologic criteria. Phenotypic criteria include changes such as unintended weight loss of ≥5% within the past 6 months, lower body mass index (exact cutoff is being addressed by the GLIM workgroup and is likely to be region/demographic-specific), or reduced muscle mass as measured by validated body composition–measuring techniques, such as dual-energy absorptiometry, computed tomography, bioelectrical impedance analysis, magnetic resonance imaging, and ultrasound. Etiologic criteria include reduced food intake and the presence of systemic inflammation.[8,61] Importantly, the presence and the severity of inflammation should be routinely evaluated because they help determine a patient's malnutrition risk and prioritize the needs for nutritional intervention.

Ultimately, laboratory tests alone should not be used to replace a detailed nutritional assessment in determining a patient's malnutrition risk. The purpose of a nutritional assessment is to gather relevant information to provide evidence for the nutrition diagnosis and aid in the development of a patient-specific nutrition intervention plan. Assessing nutritional status and monitoring for clinical response to nutritional intervention require the application of basic clinical skills, which include collecting a detailed patient's history, performing physical examinations whenever possible, and using validated screening tools where applicable.[62,63] Detailed history-taking is a critical component of nutritional screening, assessment, and ongoing monitoring. It is important to identify risk factors that would increase a patient's malnutrition risk, such as inflammation, the use of certain medications (eg, corticosteroids, chemotherapeutics agents), and the presence of underlying

## TABLE 12-4. Factors Contributing to Increased Risk for Malnutrition in Patients

### Changes in Body Composition

Unintentional weight loss
  Moderate malnutrition: 5%–10% within 6 mo or 10%–20% beyond 6 mo
  Severe malnutrition: >10% within 6 mo or >20% beyond 6 mo
High or low body mass index
  Moderate malnutrition: <20 kg/m² if <70 yr; <22 kg/m² if ≥70 yr
  Severe malnutrition: <18.5 kg/m² if <70 yr; <20 kg/m² if ≥70 yr
Changes in intake
  Decreased or loss of appetite
  Swallowing difficulty
  Loss of smell or taste
  Dental problems
  Decreased food intake
  Severe dry mouth
Disease-related
  Inflammation (acute and/or chronic)
  Chronic diseases not being controlled
  Acute injuries and changes to the state of health
  Surgeries
  Significant decline or loss of visual acuity
  GI complications
Social and psychological factors
  Traumatic experience
  Depression
  Social isolation
  Neglect
  Grief
  Loss of companionship (eg, partners, pet)
Recent hospitalization
Economic hardship
Drug-induced changes in intake or GI tract functions

medical, health, or social conditions (eg, loss of dentition, depression, chronic nausea, dry mouth, lack of access to food) that could impair food intake or nutrient use (**Table 12-4**). Performing simple and basic physical examination, such as determining fluid status, adiposity, weight changes, and symptoms associated with specific nutrient deficiencies can help identify at-risk patients and expedite nutritional intervention. Finally, the use of validated nutritional assessment tools, such as Mini Nutritional Assessment or Subjective Global Assessment, can provide a comprehensive evaluation of a patient's malnutrition risk.

# SUMMARY

Inflammation is an important component of malnutrition that can lead to loss of muscle mass, impair physiologic and body function, and negatively impact clinical outcomes. Although a number of laboratory tests, such as albumin, prealbumin, and transferrin, are routinely used as surrogate markers of nutritional status, they mostly reflect the state of inflammation the body is experiencing and are neither accurate nor specific for nutritional assessment. Nutritional assessment should be performed by using a multicomponent comprehensive evaluation that includes history-taking, physical examination, and the use of a validated nutrition assessment tool rather than relying on a laboratory test or tests in isolation.

## MINICASE 1

Nancy M. is a 68-year-old woman admitted to the hospital for an aortic valve replacement and coronary artery bypass graft surgery. Her past medical history includes hypertension, type 2 diabetes mellitus, hypercholesterolemia, and chronic constipation. Her current medications include metformin, sitagliptin, simvastatin, fosinopril, and polyethylene glycol 3350.

Her height is 165 cm and weight is 89.4 kg. She has gained 2.5 kg in the last 2 weeks. Her vital signs on admission include blood pressure 110/85 mm Hg, heart rate 68 beats/min at regular rhythm, and a respiratory rate 12 breaths/min. Physical examination findings include +2 edema on both ankles and bilateral numbness in her thumb and first finger.

Her laboratory test results before surgery include a serum albumin concentration of 3.8 g/dL and a hemoglobin A1c concentration of 6.3%. All other laboratory values on the chemistry panel are within normal limits.

QUESTION: What is her malnutrition risk?

DISCUSSION: The fact that this patient is undergoing major cardiac surgery puts her at high risk for malnutrition. Cardiac surgery is a high-stress procedure. Underlying malnutrition is associated with increased postoperative mortality, especially in older adults. Fortunately, her chronic illnesses appear to be well controlled at this point. Additional history regarding her dietary habit, appetite, and approximate daily food intake should be obtained. Each of these independent factors affects her malnutrition risk.

Studies show that immediately after surgery, patients lose a substantial amount of muscle mass due to acute inflammation. The inflammation response will likely be reflected by an elevated C-reactive protein concentration and a decline in serum albumin concentration. Her nutritional status should be continually assessed by following daily intake, weight changes, and presence of any surgery-related complications. Serum albumin or prealbumin concentrations will not provide any patient-specific information regarding her ongoing nutritional status.

## MINICASE 2

Carrie M., a 32-year-old woman, presents to the emergency department with 1-day history of severe epigastric pain, nausea, dizziness, and fever. She rates the pain as 8 out of 10. She reports three episodes of vomiting within the past 12 hours. Before presenting to the hospital, she was in her usual state of health. Laboratory values obtained from her routine health maintenance visit from 6 months ago show normal findings for her liver function tests, including serum albumin, serum chemistry, and complete blood count.

Her past medical history includes Crohn disease since age 17 years, resulting in an extensive history of small bowel resection. Her current GI anatomy includes approximately 300 cm of functional small intestine and an intact colon. She tolerates an oral diet and takes four small meals daily with an oral protein supplementation. She has mild chronic diarrhea, which is usually well-controlled by diet at two to three soft bowel movements per day, and she takes loperamide three times a day and clonidine twice a day.

On admission, her weight is 65.7 kg, which has decreased by 1.1 kg from baseline measured 6 months ago. Her body mass index is 20.7 kg/m². Physical examination shows she has mild dehydration with no peripheral edema.

Pertinent laboratory findings are as follows:

- Albumin, 2.8 g/dL
- Prealbumin, 15 mg/dL
- Amylase, 880 units/L
- Lipase, 930 units/L
- C-reactive protein, 49 mg/dL

## MINICASE 2 (cont'd)

The patient is diagnosed with acute pancreatitis and admitted to the hospital for further management. Intravenous (IV) fluids and pain medication are started immediately.

QUESTION: Based on her underlying medical condition, clinical presentation, and laboratory findings, including serum albumin and prealbumin concentrations upon admission, does the patient have severe malnutrition necessitating immediate initiation of parenteral nutrition?

DISCUSSION: Acute pancreatitis is a disease associated with acute inflammation and catabolism. This is reflected by the elevated C-reactive protein concentration, which is common among patients with acute pancreatitis. The inflammation causes an acute decline in serum albumin and prealbumin concentrations because they are negative acute phase reactants. Therefore, the current albumin and prealbumin concentrations do not reflect this patient's nutritional status. Rather, these are additional markers besides C-reactive protein confirming the presence of acute inflammation.

The change of body weight from baseline is likely the result of dehydration. Along with acute pancreatitis, dehydration, vomiting, and fever are all independent factors associated with increased malnutrition risk. Therefore, this patient's nutritional status and intake should be carefully monitored in the next 24 to 48 hours. Nutritional interventions with protein provision should be initiated as tolerated. However, because she was in her usual state of health before admission and tolerated an oral diet at baseline, parenteral nutrition is not indicated at this point. Enteral nutrition should be first attempted after controlling vomiting and abdominal pain. Postpyloric feeding tube placement is more likely to increase enteral feeding tolerance without aggravating pain. This should be attempted along with IV fluid rehydration and electrolyte replacement, which are consistent approaches with the current practice standards for acute pancreatitis. Consistent with the current practice standards, if she is unable to tolerate enteral feeding in the next 3 to 5 days, parenteral nutrition would be considered.[64]

Serum albumin and prealbumin will remain suppressed as long as C-reactive protein concentration is elevated. Therefore, albumin and prealbumin should not be used during this time as a marker of nutritional response. Instead, her response to enteral feeding should be based on daily caloric and protein intake, GI symptoms, pain control, and general well-being. Additional protein supplementation is likely necessary upon hospital discharge as she continues to regain her appetite and reestablish an oral diet that is tolerated by her underlying medical condition.

## MINICASE 3

Frank K. is a 52-year-man who has systemic lupus erythematosus (SLE), hypertension, type 2 diabetes, chronic proteinuria, and chronic kidney disease (CKD) stage 5 and is currently receiving hemodialysis. The following laboratory results have been obtained as his dialysis care process:

- Hemoglobin, 10.5 g/dL
- Mean corpuscular volume, 77 fL
- Red cell distribution width, 19.9%
- Serum ferritin, 34 ng/mL
- Transferrin, 382 mg/dL
- Transferrin saturation, 28%

QUESTION: Based on this patient's medical history and laboratory results, what are his risk factors for malnutrition?

DISCUSSION: This patient has anemia based on his hemoglobin concentration, an unsurprising finding due to CKD. The results of the iron study suggest that he has iron deficiency, which can increase serum transferrin concentration. This finding makes serum transferrin an unreliable marker for nutritional status in this patient.

Nutritional status cannot be reliably assessed using retinol-binding protein because it is increased in CKD. Additionally, it is not uncommon that chronic inflammation is present in patient's CKD. Therefore, if his serum albumin concentration is below the normal range, it may be a reflection of uncontrolled systemic inflammation. This also makes hypoalbuminemia and hypo-prealbuminemia unreliable markers for malnutrition in CKD. Nutrition assessment for this patient should be based on a comprehensive clinical assessment using history, clinical findings, and a validated assessment tool.

This patient does have multiple risk factors for malnutrition, including SLE, hypertension, iron deficiency anemia, and CKD. SLE is associated with a chronic inflammatory state, which may have suppressive effect on appetite and oral intake. Along with proteinuria, this patient is at high risk for developing protein-calorie malnutrition. Therefore, his treatment plan must include suppressing chronic inflammation, reducing urinary protein loss, and optimizing calorie and protein intake. Ideally, in addition to body weight and oral intake monitoring, routine body composition assessment to prevent sarcopenia should be considered.

## MINICASE 4

Josha T. is a 39-year-old man has been admitted to the hospital after being hit by a bus while riding his bicycle to work. His injuries include multiple fractured ribs and blunt abdominal injury. He undergoes surgery upon admission to the hospital and is found to have a small intestinal perforation. Postoperatively, he is transferred to the trauma/surgical ICU for recovery and supportive care.

Because of abdominal trauma, parenteral nutrition is started on postoperation day 2. The parenteral nutrition prescription provides 2,350 kcal (35 kcal/kg) with 120 g (1.8 g/kg) of protein per day.

His serum albumin concentration on admission is 3.5 g/dL. On the day parenteral nutrition is initiated, his serum albumin level is 3.1 g/dL. Five days after parenteral nutrition therapy, his serum albumin concentration is still 3.1 g/L and prealbumin is 18 mg/dL. The surgical team consults with the clinical nutrition team to optimize nutrient provision and delivery. At this point, there is still substantial drainage from his small intestine; therefore, enteral feeding is not a feasible option.

QUESTION: How should the clinical nutrition team optimize nutrient provision and delivery for this patient?

DISCUSSION: Traumatic injury is associated with a profound systemic inflammation. Therefore, continued hypoalbuminemia in this patient, despite receiving 120 g of protein per day, is due to continued, unsuppressed inflammation. It does not reflect the patient's response to nutritional therapy. Neither serum albumin nor prealbumin should be used to determine the adequacy of nutritional intervention in this patient.

Because his renal function remains stable with an estimated glomerular filtration rate of 108 mL/min, the clinical nutrition team orders 24-hour urine collection for a nitrogen balance study. The next day, the clinical nutrition team assesses the result, which shows urine urea nitrogen output of 17.5 g in 24 hours. His blood urea nitrogen and serum creatinine concentrations remain stable at 19 mg/dL and 1.12 mg/dL, respectively. Under normal physiology with an assumed nonrenal nitrogen loss of 4 g/day, the total daily nitrogen output for this patient is approximately 21.5 g (17.5 g + 4 g). However, because he has continued fluid drainage from this small intestine, his actual nitrogen output is likely higher than 21.5 g/day. Based on his current parenteral nutrition prescription, his total nitrogen input is 120 g/6.25 g = 19.2 g. Therefore, he is currently in a negative nitrogen balance (at least −3 but probably higher).

In response to the nitrogen balance study, the clinical nutrition team suggests increasing the amino acid content from 120 to 150 g/day (equivalent to 24 g of nitrogen intake per day). In addition, indirect calorimetry is ordered to ensure that the patient is not overfed in total calories. The patient will continue to be monitored for vital signs, daily fluid and electrolyte balance, weight changes, ongoing inflammatory state, and clinical improvement. Repeat nitrogen balance study may be considered in a week if his clinical condition does not improve.

## REFERENCES

1. Gallagher-Allred CR, Voss AC, Finn SC, et al. Malnutrition and clinical outcomes: the case for medical nutrition therapy. *J Am Diet Assoc.* 1996;96(4):361-368.PubMed

2. Lew CCH, Yandell R, Fraser RJL, et al. Association between malnutrition and clinical outcomes in the intensive care unit: a systematic review. *JPEN J Parenter Enteral Nutr.* 2017;41(5):744-758.PubMed

3. Felder S, Braun N, Stanga Z, et al. Unraveling the link between malnutrition and adverse clinical outcomes: association of acute and chronic malnutrition measures with blood biomarkers from different pathophysiological states. *Ann Nutr Metab.* 2016;68(3):164-172.PubMed

4. Gomes F, Baumgartner A, Bounoure L, et al. Association of nutritional support with clinical outcomes among medical inpatients who are malnourished or at nutritional risk: an updated systematic review and meta-analysis. *JAMA Netw Open.* 2019;2(11):e1915138.PubMed

5. Correia MI, Hegazi RA, Higashiguchi T, et al. Evidence-based recommendations for addressing malnutrition in health care: an updated strategy from the feed. *J Am Med Dir Assoc.* 2014;15(8):544-550. PubMed

6. Sauer AC, Goates S, Malone A, et al. Prevalence of malnutrition risk and the impact of nutrition risk on hospital outcomes: results from nutrition day in the U.S. *JPEN J Parenter Enteral Nutr.* 2019;43(7): 918-926.PubMed

7. Lew CCH, Yandell R, Fraser RJL, et al. Association between malnutrition and clinical outcomes in the intensive care unit: a systematic review. *JPEN J Parenter Enteral Nutr.* 2017;41(5):744-758.PubMed

8. Jensen GL, Cederholm T, Correia MITD, et al. GLIM criteria for the diagnosis of malnutrition: a consensus report from the global clinical nutrition community. *JPEN J Parenter Enteral Nutr.* 2019;43(1):32-40. PubMed

9. Tyler R, Barrocas A, Guenter P, et al. Value of nutrition support therapy: impact on clinical and economic outcomes in the United States. *JPEN J Parenter Enteral Nutr.* 2020;44(3):395-406.PubMed

10. The Joint Commission. https://www.jointcommission.org/standards /standard-faqs/critical-access-hospital/provision-of-care-treatment-and -services-pc/000001652/. Accessed on June 5, 2021.

11. Jensen GL, Mirtallo J, Compher C; International Consensus Guideline Committee, et al. Adult starvation and disease-related malnutrition: a proposal for etiology-based diagnosis in the clinical practice setting from the International Consensus Guideline Committee. *JPEN J Parenter Enteral Nutr* 2010;34:156-159.

12. Peterson SJ, Braunschweig CA. Prevalence of sarcopenia and associated outcomes in the clinical setting. *Nutr Clin Pract.* 2016;31(1):40-48. PubMed

13. Cederholm T, Jensen GL, Correia MITD, et al. GLIM criteria for the diagnosis of malnutrition: a consensus report from the global clinical nutrition community. *Clin Nutr.* 2019;38(1):1-9.PubMed

14. Soeters PB, Reijven PL, van Bokhorst-de van der Schueren MA, et al. A rational approach to nutritional assessment. *Clin Nutr.* 2008;27(5):706-716.PubMed

15. Evans DC, Corkins MR, Malone A, et al. The use of visceral proteins as nutrition markers: an ASPEN position paper. *Nutr Clin Pract.* 2021;36(1):22-28.PubMed

16. Ingenbleek Y, Van Den Schrieck H-G, De Nayer P, et al. Albumin, transferrin and the thyroxine-binding prealbumin/retinol-binding protein (TBPA-RBP) complex in assessment of malnutrition. *Clin Chim Acta.* 1975;63(1):61-67.PubMed

17. Fasano M, Curry S, Terreno E, et al. The extraordinary ligand binding properties of human serum albumin. *IUBMB Life*. 2005;57(12):787-796. PubMed

18. Levitt DG, Levitt MD. Human serum albumin homeostasis: a new look at the roles of synthesis, catabolism, renal and gastrointestinal excretion, and the clinical value of serum albumin measurements. *Int J Gen Med*. 2016;9:229-255.PubMed

19. Levitt DG. The pharmacokinetics of the interstitial space in humans. *BMC Clin Pharmacol*. 2003;3:3.PubMed

20. Maxwell JL, Terracio L, Borg TK, et al. A fluorescent residualizing label for studies on protein uptake and catabolism in vivo and in vitro. *Biochem J*. 1990;267(1):155-162.PubMed

21. Cohen S, Hansen JD. Metabolism of albumin and gamma-globulin in kwashiorkor. *Clin Sci*. 1962;23:351-359.PubMed

22. Srikantia SG, Reddy V. Plasma volume and total circulating albumin in kwashiorkor. *J Pediatr*. 1963;63:133-137.PubMed

23. Blackburn GL, Bistrian BR, Maini BS, et al. Nutritional and metabolic assessment of the hospitalized patient. *JPEN J Parenter Enteral Nutr*. 1977;1(1):11-22.PubMed

24. Seltzer MH, Bastidas JA, Cooper DM, et al. Instant nutritional assessment. *JPEN J Parenter Enteral Nutr*. 1979;3(3):157-159.PubMed

25. Reinhardt GF, Myscofski JW, Wilkens DB, et al. Incidence and mortality of hypoalbuminemic patients in hospitalized veterans. *JPEN J Parenter Enteral Nutr*. 1980;4(4):357-359.PubMed

26. Roche M, Rondeau P, Singh NR, et al. The antioxidant properties of serum albumin. *FEBS Lett*. 2008;582(13):1783-1787.PubMed

27. Sheffield WP, Marques JA, Bhakta V, et al. Modulation of clearance of recombinant serum albumin by either glycosylation or truncation. *Thromb Res*. 2000;99(6):613-621.PubMed

28. Soeters PB, Wolfe RR, Shenkin A. Hypoalbuminemia: pathogenesis and clinical significance. *JPEN J Parenter Enteral Nutr*. 2019;43(2):181-193. PubMed

29. Spiess A, Mikalunas V, Carlson S, et al. Albumin kinetics in hypoalbuminemic patients receiving total parenteral nutrition. *JPEN J Parenter Enteral Nutr*. 1996;20(6):424-428.PubMed

30. Chan L-N, Sethi P, Mike LA, et al. Comparison of clinical characteristics and outcomes in medically ill icu (micu) patients according to serum zinc profile on admission [abstract]. *J Parentr Ent Nutr*. 2008;32(3):308.

31. Li B, Liu HY, Guo SH, et al. Impact of early enteral and parenteral nutrition on prealbumin and high-sensitivity C-reactive protein after gastric surgery. *Genet Mol Res*. 2015;14(2):7130-7135.PubMed

32. Yeh DD, Johnson E, Harrison T, et al. Serum levels of albumin and prealbumin do not correlate with nutrient delivery in surgical intensive care unit patients. *Nutr Clin Pract*. 2018;33(3):419-425.PubMed

33. Ingenbleek Y, Young V. Transthyretin (prealbumin) in health and disease: nutritional implications. *Annu Rev Nutr*. 1994;14:495-533.PubMed

34. Gião T, Saavedra J, Cotrina E, et al. Undiscovered roles for transthyretin: from a transporter protein to a new therapeutic target for Alzheimer's disease. *Int J Mol Sci*. 2020;21(6):2075.PubMed

35. Ingenbleek Y, De Visscher M, De Nayer P. Measurement of prealbumin as index of protein-calorie malnutrition. *Lancet*. 1972;2(7768):106-109. PubMed

36. Ingenbleek Y, Young VR. Significance of transthyretin in protein metabolism. *Clin Chem Lab Med*. 2002;40(12):1281-1291.PubMed

37. Mears E. Outcomes of continuous process improvement of a nutritional care program incorporating serum prealbumin measurements. *Nutrition*. 1996;12(7-8):479-484.PubMed

38. Bernstein L, Bachman TE, Meguid M, et al. Measurement of visceral protein status in assessing protein and energy malnutrition: standard of care. *Nutrition*. 1995;11(2):169-171.PubMed

39. Gürlek Gökçebay D, Emir S, Bayhan T, et al. Assessment of nutritional status in children with cancer and effectiveness of oral nutritional supplements. *Pediatr Hematol Oncol*. 2015;32(6):423-432.PubMed

40. Huysentruyt K, De Schepper J, Vanbesien J, et al. Albumin and pre-albumin levels do not reflect the nutritional status of female adolescents with restrictive eating disorders. *Acta Paediatr*. 2016;105(4):e167-e169. PubMed

41. Ota DM, Frasier P, Guevara J, et al. Plasma proteins as indices of response to nutritional therapy in cancer patients. *J Surg Oncol*. 1985;29(3):160-165.PubMed

42. Winkler MF, Gerrior SA, Pomp A, et al. Use of retinol-binding protein and prealbumin as indicators of the response to nutrition therapy. *J Am Diet Assoc*. 1989;89(5):684-687.PubMed

43. Davis CJ, Sowa D, Keim KS, et al. The use of prealbumin and C-reactive protein for monitoring nutrition support in adult patients receiving enteral nutrition in an urban medical center. *JPEN J Parenter Enteral Nutr*. 2012;36(2):197-204.PubMed

44. Chan L-N, Lee JK, Mike LA, et al. Assessing the prognostic value of serum transthyretin concentration (TTR) in medically ill ICU patients [abstract]. *J Parentr Ent Nutr*. 2008;32(3):319.

45. Keller U. Nutritional laboratory markers in malnutrition. *J Clin Med*. 2019;8(6):775.PubMed

46. Paillaud E, Bories PN, Le Parco JC, et al. Nutritional status and energy expenditure in elderly patients with recent hip fracture during a 2-month follow-up. *Br J Nutr*. 2000;83(2):97-103.PubMed

47. Church JM, Hill GL. Assessing the efficacy of intravenous nutrition in general surgical patients: dynamic nutritional assessment with plasma proteins. *JPEN J Parenter Enteral Nutr*. 1987;11(2):135-139.PubMed

48. Fletcher JP, Mudie JMA. A 2 year experience of a nutritional support service: prospective study of 229 non-intensive care patients receiving parenteral nutrition. *Aust N Z J Surg*. 1989;59(3):223-228.PubMed

49. Huang YC, Yen CE, Cheng CH, et al. Nutritional status of mechanically ventilated critically ill patients: comparison of different types of nutritional support. *Clin Nutr*. 2000;19(2):101-107.PubMed

50. Tanumihardjo SA, Russell RM, Stephensen CB, et al. Biomarkers of nutrition for development (BOND) vitamin: a review. *J Nutr*. 2016;146(9):1816S-1848S.PubMed

51. Larson LM, Namaste SM, Williams AM, et al. Adjusting retinol-binding protein concentrations for inflammation: biomarkers reflecting inflammation and nutritional determinants of anemia (BRINDA) project. *Am J Clin Nutr*. 2017;106(suppl 1):390S-401S.PubMed

52. Kuzuya M, Kanda S, Koike T, et al. Lack of correlation between total lymphocyte count and nutritional status in the elderly. *Clin Nutr*. 2005;24(3):427-432.PubMed

53. Mbagwu C, Sloan M, Neuwirth AL, et al. Preoperative albumin, transferrin, and total lymphocyte count as risk markers for postoperative complications after total joint arthroplasty: a systematic review. JAAOS: Global Res Rev 2020;4(9):pe19.00057.

54. Calloway DH, Odell AC, Margen S. Sweat and miscellaneous nitrogen losses in human balance studies. *J Nutr*. 1971;101(6):775-786. PubMed

55. Hoffer LJ. Human protein and amino acid requirements. *JPEN J Parenter Enteral Nutr*. 2016;40(4):460-474.PubMed

56. Misra M, Nolph K. A simplified approach to understanding urea kinetics in peritoneal dialysis. *J Ren Nutr*. 2007;17(4):282-285.PubMed

57. Kloppenburg WD, Stegeman CA, de Jong PE, et al. Anthropometry-based equations overestimate the urea distribution volume in hemodialysis patients. *Kidney Int*. 2001;59(3):1165-1174.PubMed

58. Kloppenburg WD, Stegeman CA, de Jong PE, et al. Relating protein intake to nutritional status in haemodialysis patients: how to normalize the protein equivalent of total nitrogen appearance (PNA)? *Nephrol Dial Transplant*. 1999;14(9):2165-2172.PubMed

59. Raimann JG, Ye X, Kotanko P, Daugirdas JT. Routine Kt/V and normalized protein nitrogen appearance rate determined from conductivity access clearance with infrequent postdialysis serum urea nitrogen measurements. *Am J Kidney Dis*. 2020;76(1):22-31.PubMed

60. Vigushin DM, Pepys MB, Hawkins PN. Metabolic and scintigraphic studies of radioiodinated human C-reactive protein in health and disease. *J Clin Invest.* 1993;91(4):1351-1357.PubMed

61. de van der Schueren MAE, Keller H, Cederholm T, et al. Global Leadership Initiative on Malnutrition (GLIM): guidance on validation of the operational criteria for the diagnosis of protein-energy malnutrition in adults. *Clin Nutr.* 2020;39(9):2872-2880.PubMed

62. Juby AG, Mager DR. A review of nutrition screening tools used to assess the malnutrition-sarcopenia syndrome (MSS) in the older adult. *Clin Nutr ESPEN.* 2019;32:8-15.PubMed

63. Mehta NM, Corkins MR, Lyman B, et al. Defining pediatric malnutrition: a paradigm shift toward etiology-related definitions. *JPEN J Parenter Enteral Nutr.* 2013;37(4):460-481.PubMed

64. Worthington P, Balint J, Bechtold M, et al. When is parenteral nutrition appropriate? *JPEN J Parenter Enteral Nutr.* 2017;41(3):324-377. PubMed

# 13

# Arterial Blood Gases and Acid–Base Balance

*Jeffrey F. Barletta*

Acid–base homeostasis is a fundamental component for the maintenance of normal metabolic function. Acid–base disorders, however, are extremely common in the intensive care unit, and rapid, careful assessment is required to prevent unwanted morbidity and mortality. This chapter provides a review of acid–base homeostasis, laboratory tests used to assess acid–base status, and a step-wise approach to classify acid–base disorders and their potential causes.

## ACID–BASE CHEMISTRY

An acid is a substance that can donate a proton (eg, $HCl \rightarrow H^+ + Cl^-$) whereas a base is a substance that can accept a proton (eg, $H^+ + NH_3 \rightarrow NH_4^+$). Every acid has a corresponding base. Every base has a corresponding acid. Some common acid–base pairs are carbonic acid/bicarbonate, ammonium/ammonia, monobasic/dibasic phosphate, and lactic acid/lactate.

The terms *acidemia* and *alkalemia* are used to describe an abnormal blood pH. Specifically, acidemia denotes a low blood pH whereas alkalemia denotes a high blood pH. The terms *acidosis* and *alkalosis*, on the other hand, refer to the process by which either acid or alkali accumulates. It is therefore possible to have an acidosis but not an acidemia. For this to occur (ie, acidosis without acidemia), a corresponding alkalosis must also be present.

The acidity of a body fluid is determined by the concentration of hydrogen ion ($H^+$). Normal $H^+$ concentration is approximately 40 nanoequivalents/liter. Because this is expressed in such small amounts (a nanoequivalent is one one-millionth of a milliequivalent), acid–base status is measured in pH units using a logarithmic scale. Normal blood pH is 7.4 with a range of 7.35 to 7.45. The range of pH values considered compatible with life is 6.8 to 7.8, which corresponds to a hydrogen ion concentration of only 16 to 160 nEq/L.[1] In general, the body tolerates acidemia much better than alkalemia. This is due to the fact that as pH decreases, a larger change in $H^+$ is required for a given change in pH.[2] In alkalemic states, small changes in $H^+$ can markedly affect pH. Furthermore, with alkalemia, the oxyhemoglobin dissociation curve shifts to the left and hemoglobin is less willing to release oxygen to the tissues (**Figure 13-1**).[3,4]

## ARTERIAL BLOOD GASES

Assessment of acid–base status is primarily determined using an arterial blood gas (ABG) measurement. ABG evaluation is typically performed in critically ill patients in whom complex disorders and treatment modalities can influence acid–base status (eg, mechanical ventilation). Outside the intensive care unit, many acid–base disorders are predicable (eg, respiratory acidosis in a patient with chronic obstructive pulmonary disease) and rarely require interpretation via an ABG. Arterial blood reflects how well the blood is being oxygenated by the lungs whereas venous blood reflects oxygen consumption by the tissues. It is important that arterial blood is used for these assessments because substantial differences may exist between the two, particularly

DOI 10.37573/9781585286423.013

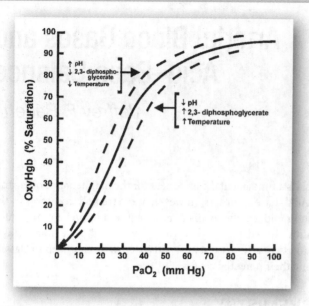

**FIGURE 13-1.** The oxyhemoglobin dissociation curve.

in the setting of critical illness.[5] Note that the "normal ranges" listed next are approximate and slight variability may be noted across different references or local laboratory standards.

## Arterial pH

*Normal range: 7.35 to 7.45*

The pH of arterial blood is the first value to consider when using an ABG to assess acid–base status. The pH is inversely related to hydrogen concentration. Generally speaking, pH values <7.35 represent acidemia and pH values >7.45 represent alkalemia, with 7.4 being the threshold for categorization during ABG assessment.

It is difficult to identify the pH value that will dictate the urgency whereby treatment must be initiated. Consequences of abnormal pH include arterial vasodilation, diminished myocardial contractility, impaired hepatic and renal perfusion, decreased oxygen-hemoglobin binding, and coma for acidemia; cerebral vasoconstriction, reduced contractility, increased oxygen-hemoglobin binding, decreased oxygen delivery, and coma are encountered with alkalemia. These deleterious effects become more prominent when pH is <7.2 or >7.55.[6]

## Arterial Partial Pressure of Carbon Dioxide

*Normal range: 35 to 45 mm Hg*

Evaluation of arterial partial pressure of carbon dioxide ($PaCO_2$) provides information about the adequacy of lung function in excreting carbon dioxide. The amount of carbon dioxide dissolved in the blood is directly proportional to the concentration of carbonic acid ($PaCO_2 \times 0.03 = H_2CO_3$). Elevations in $PaCO_2$ therefore contribute to acidosis. Changes to ventilatory status that alter carbon dioxide concentrations affect carbonic acid concentrations. Specifically, hypoventilation leads to a higher $PaCO_2$ whereas hyperventilation results in a lower $PaCO_2$. Regulation of ventilation is a major mechanism for respiratory compensation in the setting of primary metabolic disorders.

## Arterial Partial Pressure of Oxygen

*Normal range: 80 to 100 mm Hg*

Evaluation of the arterial partial pressure of oxygen ($PaO_2$) provides information about the level of oxygenation of arterial blood. The $PaO_2$ is important because it reflects not only the functional capabilities of the lungs but also the rate at which oxygen can enter the tissues. Although there is no set cutoff for defining hypoxemia because it is typically relative to metabolic requirements, most would define clinically significant hypoxia at <60 mm Hg. Factors that influence $PaO_2$ are the amount of ventilation, the fraction of inspired oxygen ($FiO_2$), the functional capacities of the lung, and the oxyhemoglobin dissociation curve.

The oxyhemoglobin dissociation curve describes the relationship between $PaO_2$ and oxygen saturation (Figure 13-1). Oxygen saturation is the percentage of hemoglobin binding sites in the bloodstream occupied by oxygen. During states of acidemia, this curve shifts to the right and hemoglobin has a decreased affinity for oxygen (resulting in increased unloading of oxygen). $PaO_2$ must therefore be higher to maintain a particular level of oxygen saturation. During alkalemia, on the other hand, this curve shifts to the left and hemoglobin's affinity for oxygen is increased, resulting in decreased oxygen delivery to tissues. Other factors that can influence the oxyhemoglobin dissociation curve are temperature and the amount of 2,3-diphosphoglycerate in red blood cells.

Although $PaO_2$ and oxygen saturation are both measurements of oxygenation, it is important to not confuse one with the other. For example, a $PaO_2$ of 80 mm Hg would typically not be considered abnormal because in most patients this is reflective of an oxygen saturation >93%. An oxygen saturation of 80%, on the other hand, would be considered critical and require immediate intervention. Oxygen saturation is expressed as a percentage and cannot exceed 100%. Conversely, $PaO_2$ is expressed in millimeters of mercury, and values that exceed 100 can exist (especially when supplemental oxygen is administered). The ratio of $PaO_2$ to $FiO_2$, which is referred to as PF ratio, is frequently used to evaluate respiratory status in patients receiving supplemental oxygen. A PF ratio in a healthy individual would be expected to be approximately 500 and values less than 300, 200, and 100 are encountered in mild, moderate, and severe acute respiratory distress syndrome, respectively.[7] Although $PaO_2$ assessment is crucial for determining pulmonary status, it does not directly impact acid–base balance.

## Arterial Bicarbonate

*Normal range: 22 to 26 mEq/L*

The concentration of $HCO_3^-$ reported from ABG is not a direct measurement but calculated using pH and $PaCO_2$ via the Henderson-Hasselbalch equation. It is important to compare this value (ie, bicarbonate reading from the ABG) with the total $CO_2$ content (commonly referred to as serum bicarbonate) on a basic metabolic panel from venous sampling. Under normal circumstances, bicarbonate from the ABG is approximately 1.5 to 3 mEq/L less than the total $CO_2$ content from a plasma electrolyte panel (higher end of this range for venous samples).[8]

Results should be interpreted with caution if this correlation does not exist.

# OTHER TESTS ASSOCIATED WITH ACID–BASE INTERPRETATION OR OXYGENATION

## Venous Total Carbon Dioxide Content (Serum Bicarbonate)

*Normal range: 22 to 30 mEq/L*

The total carbon dioxide content refers to the total of all carbon dioxide present in the blood. This consists of bicarbonate, dissolved $CO_2$, carbonic acid, and carbamino compounds.[8] Because roughly 95% of this is made up of bicarbonate, the term *serum bicarbonate* is often used interchangeably with *total carbon dioxide content*. Although the name total carbon dioxide content implies that it is a measure of acid (similar to $PaCO_2$), it is important to recognize that this test represents bicarbonate. Increases in total carbon dioxide content contribute to alkalosis. Clinicians should refer to this as serum bicarbonate and not carbon dioxide to avoid confusion with $pCO_2$ obtained on an ABG test.

## Anion Gap

*Normal range: 3 to 16 mEq/L*

The anion gap (AG) is a calculated value that is an estimate of the relative abundance of unmeasured anions. It is commonly used to determine the possible causes of metabolic acidosis. Anion gap is based on the principles of electrochemical balance; that is, the concentration of negatively charged anions must equal the concentration of positively charged cations. Anion gap is calculated using the following formula:

$$AG = Na^+ - (Cl^- + HCO_3^-) \qquad (1)$$

Whereas the normal value for AG can vary, values that exceed 16 mEq/L are generally indicative of anion accumulation (eg, lactate, pyruvate, acetoacetate). This is often due to lactic acidosis, ketoacidosis, toxic ingestions, or end-stage renal failure.

The AG is largely influenced by plasma albumin; therefore, an adjustment is required when hypoalbuminemia exists. For every decrement of 1 g/dL in serum albumin concentration, the calculated AG should be increased by 2.5.[9]

$$\text{Corrected AG} = \text{AG} + 2.5 \text{ (normal albumin}$$
$$\text{per local laboratory standard – measured albumin)} \qquad (2)$$

Anion gap interpretation may also be affected by serum phosphate, magnesium, calcium, and even some β-lactam antibiotics.[10] The influence of these confounding variables, coupled with the heterogeneity of critical illness, has led to questions regarding its diagnostic value.[11-13] Nevertheless, clinicians should consider the AG one method to assist with potential causes of metabolic acidosis and not the sole factor for decision-making at the bedside.

## Arterial Oxygen Saturation

*Normal range: 93% to 100%*

Arterial oxygen saturation is a measure of the fraction of hemoglobin molecules that are saturated with oxygen. Its relationship with $PaO_2$ is described using the oxyhemoglobin dissociation curve. Under normal circumstances (eg, pH, temperature, etc.), a $PaO_2$ of approximately 60 mm Hg corresponds to an arterial oxygen saturation ($SaO_2$) of 90%. Arterial oxygen saturation is the major determinant of arterial oxygen content ($CaO_2$) (normal range is roughly 17 to 20 mL/dL; Equation 3) and oxygen delivery ($DO_2$) (normal range is roughly 950 to 1,150 mL/min or 550 to 650 mL/min/m$^2$ when indexed to body surface area; Equation 4).

$$CaO_2 \text{ (mL/dL)} = 1.34 \times Hgb \text{ (g/dL)} \times SaO_2 \qquad (3)$$
$$+ [PaO_2 \text{ (mm Hg)} \times 0.003]$$

$$DO_2 \text{ (mL/min)} = CaO_2 \text{ (mL/dL)} \times CO \text{ (L/min)} \times 10 \qquad (4)$$

where *CO* is cardiac output.

## Serum Lactate

*Normal range: 0.6 to 2 mmol/L*

Lactate is a byproduct of anaerobic metabolism and often used as a surrogate for inadequate tissue perfusion. In fact, the Third International Consensus Definition for Sepsis and Septic Shock (Sepsis-3) lists lactate levels >2 mmol/L as part of the diagnostic criteria for septic shock (coupled with vasopressors to maintain MAP ≥65 mm Hg).[14] Levels >4 mmol/L are generally associated with increased mortality and used as a threshold to initiate aggressive fluid resuscitation.[15,16] Serial lactate levels are often used to assess adequacy of resuscitation and substantial decreases are associated with improved survival.[17,18] Lactate levels may first increase at the onset of resuscitation as it is flushed from the tissues to central circulation before being metabolized. Trends must therefore be assessed.

## Venous Oxygen Saturation

*Normal range: 65% to 75%*

The oxygen saturation in mixed venous blood describes the balance between systemic oxygen delivery and oxygen uptake. It can also be used as a target for resuscitation. Venous oxygen saturation ($SvO_2$) measurement is taken from a pulmonary artery catheter and sometimes referred to as *mixed venous oxygenation* because blood from the pulmonary artery is considered to be a mix of venous blood from all tissue beds. Decreases in $SvO_2$ indicate systemic oxygen delivery is impaired, which is often encountered in low-flow states (eg, heart failure, low cardiac index) or anemia.[19] In contrast, $SvO_2$ may be normal or high in patients with distributive shock.[19,20] This often represents an inability of the tissues to extract the oxygen that has been delivered.

A surrogate of $SvO_2$ is central venous oxygen saturation ($ScvO_2$). $ScvO_2$ is measured in the superior vena cava and reflects the oxygen saturation of venous blood from only the upper half of the body.[19] It must be obtained from a central venous catheter.

In general, $ScvO_2$ is typically 5% to 7% higher than $SvO_2$.[21] Target thresholds for $ScvO_2$ therefore are >70%.[22] High $ScvO_2$ values, however (ie, >90%), have been associated with poor outcomes.[23]

# ACID–BASE PHYSIOLOGY

## The Physiologic Approach (Henderson-Hasselbalch)

The physiologic approach is largely composed of the carbonic acid–bicarbonate buffering system and described by the Henderson-Hasselbalch equation.

$$pH = 6.1 + \log [HCO_3^- / (0.03 \times pCO_2)] \qquad (5)$$

In this equation, both $HCO_3^-$ and $pCO_2$ are independent variables, with $HCO_3^-$ representing the base and $pCO_2$ representing the acid. Disturbances that primarily affect $pCO_2$ concentrations are called *respiratory* whereas those that affect $HCO_3^-$ are called *metabolic*.

The pH is determined not by the absolute values of either but by the ratio of $HCO_3^-$ to $pCO_2$. That being said, both values may be largely abnormal (indicating an acid–base disorder is present) but pH may be in the normal range. In fact, a common pitfall is assuming an acid–base disorder can exist only when pH is abnormal.

## The Stewart Approach

A second theory originated from the principles proposed by Peter Stewart and is based on the concept of strong ion difference (SID) and the laws of electrical neutrality.[24]

$$SID + H^+ - HCO_3^- - CO_3^{2-} - A^- - OH^- = 0 \qquad (6)$$

where $A^-$ equals dissociated weak acids. This theory states that bicarbonate and hydrogen ions are the dependent variables and represent the effects rather than the causes of acid–base imbalances. The three independent variables that ultimately control blood pH are SID, $pCO_2$, and the total weak acid concentration.

Strong ions are the ones that are completely dissociated (eg, $Na^+$, $K^+$, $Ca^{2+}$, $Mg^{2+}$, $Cl^-$, lactate) as opposed to weak ions, which can exist in both charged and uncharged forms (eg, albumin, phosphate, $HCO_3^-$).[25] The SID is the difference between the sum of all the strong cations and strong anions.[12] Because not all strong ions can be measured, the apparent SID (aSID) can be calculated as follows:

$$aSID = (Na^+ + K^+ + Ca^{2+} + Mg^{2+}) - (Cl^- + lactate) \qquad (7)$$

In a healthy individual, the normal SID is approximately +40 to +42.[25,26] As such, this difference must be counterbalanced with an equal opposing charge obtained from $pCO_2$ and weak acids (eg, albumin and phosphate). This is referred to as the effective SID (eSID). The difference between the aSID and eSID is called the strong ion gap; in healthy individuals, it is equal to zero. When the aSID and eSID are not equal, as in a critically ill patient, the imbalance must be matched by a change in the concentration of another charged entity ($HCO_3^-$, $CO_3^{2-}$, $OH^-$, $H^+$).

This makes hydrogen and bicarbonate the dependent variables in this model.

In summary, the Stewart approach can be useful to explain pathophysiologic principles but is not associated with improved outcomes compared with the physiologic approach (ie, Henderson-Hasselbalch). As a result, the physiologic approach is more commonly used in bedside practice.

# REGULATION OF ACID–BASE HOMEOSTASIS

The metabolism of carbohydrates and fat results in the production of approximately 15,000 mmol of $CO_2$ per day. In addition, digestion of proteins and tissue metabolism results in the production of nonvolatile acids. For normal cellular function to occur, hydrogen ion concentration must be maintained within a narrow therapeutic range. In fact, the normal variance of hydrogen ion in extracellular fluid is <10 nEq/L.[2] The three mechanisms the body uses to maintain this tight therapeutic range are buffers, respiratory regulation, and renal regulation.

## Buffers

Buffers represent the first line of defense when an acid–base imbalance exists. A buffer is a substance that can absorb or donate hydrogen ions when in the presence of a strong acid or base and minimize resultant changes in pH. The principal extracellular buffer system in the body is the bicarbonate/carbonic acid system.

$$HCO_3^- + H^+ \leftrightarrow H_2CO_3 \leftrightarrow CO_2 + H_2O \qquad (8)$$

This system plays a central role because both $HCO_3^-$ and $CO_2$ can be regulated independently. Reactions in this system flow both ways depending on the concentration of each component. In this model, carbonic acid ($H_2CO_3$) and bicarbonate ($HCO_3^-$) exist in equilibrium with hydrogen ions. In the presence of carbonic anhydrase, carbonic acid is converted to $CO_2$. Carbon dioxide concentrations are regulated through ventilation (ie, the respiratory component) whereas bicarbonate concentrations are regulated through the kidney (ie, the metabolic component).

Other buffer systems that are present are the phosphate buffer system and intracellular and extracellular proteins. Both of these function more so as intracellular buffers.

## Respiratory Regulation

The second line of defense against acid–base disturbances is the respiratory system. Within minutes of detecting an imbalance, chemoreceptors located in the medulla of the brain can modify ventilation to either retain or eliminate $CO_2$. Specifically, an increase in ventilation decreases $CO_2$ while a decrease in ventilation increases $CO_2$. A new steady-state $PaCO_2$ is typically reached within hours.[1]

## Renal Regulation

The kidneys maintain acid–base homeostasis by regulating the concentration of bicarbonate in the blood. Approximately

4,300 mEq of bicarbonate is filtered to the kidney each day, all of which must be reabsorbed to maintain normal acid–base balance.[27] Approximately 90% of this reabsorption takes place in the proximal tubule and is catalyzed by carbonic anhydrase. The remaining 10% is reabsorbed in the more distal segments. Filtered bicarbonate combines with hydrogen ions secreted by the renal tubule cell to form carbonic acid. The enzyme carbonic anhydrase, located in the brush border of the renal tubule, catalyzes conversion of carbonic acid to carbon dioxide. The uncharged $CO_2$ readily crosses the cell membrane and passively diffuses into the renal tubule cell. Inside the cell, $CO_2$ is converted to carbonic acid in the presence of intracellular carbonic anhydrase. Carbonic acid dissociates into hydrogen ion (which is later secreted into the tubular lumen) and bicarbonate (which is reabsorbed into capillary blood). Drugs that inhibit carbonic anhydrase (eg, acetazolamide) interfere with this process by blocking the reabsorption of bicarbonate, hence creating a metabolic acidosis.

The second mechanism used by the kidney is excretion of the daily load of nonvolatile acids that are produced by the body (approximately 50 to 100 mEq/day).[27] This is accomplished by hydrogen ions combining with urinary buffers such as phosphates or with ammonia to form ammonium.

In general, renal compensation begins approximately 6 to 12 hours after an acid–base derangement, but full compensation takes roughly 3 to 5 days.[28]

# ARTERIAL BLOOD GAS INTERPRETATION

Acid–base disorders can be categorized based on the pH derangement (ie, acidosis and alkalosis) and the primary disorder leading to that derangement (ie, respiratory and metabolic). There are four classifications for acid–base disorders: metabolic acidosis, metabolic alkalosis, respiratory acidosis, and respiratory alkalosis. The term *respiratory* is used when the primary problem is related to abnormal $PaCO_2$ concentrations, whereas *metabolic* is used when the primary disorder is related to abnormalities in serum bicarbonate. For homeostasis to be maintained, there must be a compensatory response performed by the opposing system (respiratory for primary metabolic disorders and metabolic for primary respiratory disorders). This compensatory response, however, will neither completely correct nor overcorrect the primary disorder.

A simple disorder is considered to have a single disturbance with the expected degree of compensation. Mixed disorders, on the other hand, consist of a combination of disturbances that occurs simultaneously. While more than one metabolic disorder can coexist (eg, metabolic acidosis and metabolic alkalosis), there can only be one respiratory disorder at the same time.

Alternatively, clinicians should think of the following three groups when reviewing causes of acid–base disorders and resultant treatments: iatrogenic (eg, hyperchloremic metabolic acidosis from saline resuscitation), fixed feature of a preexisting disease process (eg, renal failure), or a liable feature of an evolving disease process (eg, lactic acidosis from shock).[29] While the conditions listed in each example may all be classified as metabolic acidosis, the treatment plans are inherently different.

# STEP-WISE APPROACH FOR ARTERIAL BLOOD GAS ASSESSMENT

## Step 1: pH Assessment

The first step in interpreting an ABG is to evaluate the pH and determine if an acidemia or alkalemia exists. A blood pH <7.4 is acidemia and >7.4 is alkalemia. As stated earlier, a normal pH does not mean that an acid base disorder does not exist.

## Step 2: Determine Primary Acid–Base Disorder

The second step is to determine if the primary acid–base disorder is respiratory or metabolic. To do this the clinician should (1) pose the question, "If the primary problem were respiratory, would the $PaCO_2$ be high or low?"; (2) use the principles of acid–base physiology to answer the question. Given $PaCO_2$ is considered to be an acid, primary respiratory acidosis occurs when $PaCO_2$ concentrations are high (>40 mm Hg), while primary respiratory alkalosis occurs when $PaCO_2$ concentrations are low; and (3) confirm the actual $PaCO_2$ value from the ABG.

The same approach can then be performed on the metabolic side by evaluating bicarbonate: (1) Pose the question, "If the primary problem were metabolic, would the $HCO_3^-$ be high or low?" (2) Use the principles of acid–base physiology to answer the question. Given $HCO_3^-$ is considered to be a base, primary metabolic acidosis occurs when $HCO_3^-$ concentrations are low (<24 mEq/L), while primary metabolic alkalosis occurs when $HCO_3^-$ concentrations are high. (3) Confirm the actual $HCO_3^-$ value from the ABG. If the primary problem appears to be both respiratory and metabolic, then a mixed disorder exists.

## Step 3: Compensatory Response

The third step is to evaluate the degree of compensation for the primary acid–based disturbance. Respiratory compensation can occur quickly after the detection of a primary metabolic problem (through adjustment in ventilatory rate), but metabolic compensation for a primary respiratory disorder occurs more slowly. Therefore, when primary respiratory disorders are detected, they are further classified as being either acute or chronic. From there, the expected change in either bicarbonate (for primary respiratory disorders) or $PaCO_2$ (for primary metabolic disorders) can be calculated using the appropriate compensation formula (**Table 13-1**). If the calculated expected value differs substantially from the actual value, then a secondary disorder is present.

## Step 4: Conditional Assessments for Metabolic Derangements

If a metabolic acidosis exists, the fourth step is to calculate the anion gap. The anion gap can be used to identify the cause of a metabolic acidosis. While the threshold for "high" will vary,

**TABLE 13-1.** Summary of Primary Acid–Base Disorders and Their Compensatory Response

| DISORDER | pH | PRIMARY ALTERATION | COMPENSATORY ALTERATION | NORMAL COMPENSATORY RESPONSE |
|---|---|---|---|---|
| Metabolic acidosis | ↓ | ↓ $HCO_3^-$ | ↓ $PaCO_2$ | Expected $PaCO_2 = (1.5 \times HCO_3^-) + (8 \pm 2)$ |
| Metabolic alkalosis | ↑ | ↑ $HCO_3^-$ | ↑ $PaCO_2$ | Expected $PaCO_2 = (0.7 \times HCO_3^-) + (21 \pm 2)$ |
| Respiratory acidosis | ↓ | ↑ $PaCO_2$ | ↑ $HCO_3^-$ | Acute: $\Delta pH = 0.008 \times \Delta PaCO_2$<br>$\Delta HCO_3^- = \Delta PaCO_2/10$<br>Chronic: $\Delta pH = 0.003 \times \Delta PaCO_2$<br>$\Delta HCO_3^- = 3.5 (\Delta PaCO_2)/10$ |
| Respiratory alkalosis | ↑ | ↓ $PaCO_2$ | ↓ $HCO_3^-$ | Acute: $\Delta pH = 0.008 \times \Delta PaCO_2$<br>$\Delta HCO_3^- = \Delta PaCO_2/5$<br>Chronic: $\Delta pH = 0.003 \times \Delta PaCO_2$<br>$\Delta HCO_3^- = \Delta PaCO_2/2$ |

values >16 are generally considered "positive." The following disorders have been associated with an anion gap acidosis: lactic acidosis, ketoacidosis, toxic ingestions, and end-stage renal failure. A classic mnemonic that is used to distinguish causes of anion gap acidosis is MUDPILES: methanol, uremia, diabetic ketoacidosis, paraldehyde or propylene glycol, isoniazid or iron, lactic acid, ethylene glycol, and salicylates. A more recent mnemonic is GOLD MARK: glycols (ethylene and propylene), oxoproline (associated with chromic acetaminophen ingestion), *l*-lactate (most common measured form of lactic acid), *d*-lactate (typically seen in patients with short gut syndromes), methanol, aspirin, renal failure, and ketoacidosis.[30]

If a metabolic alkalosis exists, then the clinician should determine if the disorder is chloride responsive or chloride resistant. This is performed by assessing the urinary Cl⁻. Urinary Cl⁻ concentrations <25 mEq/L are suggestive of chloride-responsive alkalosis while urinary Cl⁻ concentrations >40 mEq/L are chloride-resistant.[1] Chloride-responsive alkalosis typically responds to intravenous normal saline (0.9% sodium chloride) administration. Common causes of chloride-responsive alkalosis include vomiting, gastrointestinal losses, gastrointestinal drainage, and diuretics. Chloride-resistant alkalosis, on the other hand, does not respond to normal saline administration and is often reflective of mineralocorticoid excess or severe hypokalemia. Other causes include Bartter syndrome, Cushing syndrome, Gitelman syndrome, severe hypercalcemia, and severe magnesium deficiency.

## ACID–BASE DISORDERS

### Metabolic Acidosis

Metabolic acidosis is caused by the net retention of nonvolatile acids or loss of bicarbonate. On ABG, both the pH and the serum bicarbonate would be low and the $PaCO_2$ would decrease in an attempt to compensate. This would be manifested by an increase in respirations.

Traditionally, metabolic acidosis is classified by the anion gap, which can be used to identify the underlying cause. Metabolic acidosis with an increased anion gap commonly results from increased endogenous organic acid production whereas nonanion gap acidosis is often related to extensive loss of bicarbonate. Common causes of anion gap and nonanion gap acidosis are listed in **Table 13-2**. One cause of anion gap acidosis is lactic acidosis, which is further classified as being Type A (ie, hypoxic) or Type B (ie, nonhypoxic). Causes of Type A lactic acidosis include septic shock, mesenteric ischemia, hypoxemia, hypovolemic shock, carbon monoxide poisoning, and cyanide toxicity. Type B lactic acidosis can be caused by seizures, intoxication (eg, salicylate, ethylene glycol, propylene glycol), and medications (Table 13-2). A complete review of the patient's medication list should therefore be performed to rule out potential drug-induced causes.

Nonanion gap acidosis occurs when the decrease in bicarbonate ions corresponds with an increase in chloride ions to maintain electrical neutrality. A common cause of nonanion gap acidosis is hyperchloremic metabolic acidosis due to resuscitation with large volumes of normal saline. Nonanion gap acidosis is also encountered with renal tubular acidosis, excessive gastrointestinal loses (eg, diarrhea, fistula drainage, ureteral diversion), or iatrogenic causes (eg, parenteral nutrition, carbonic anhydrase inhibitors) (**Minicases 1 and 3**).

### Metabolic Alkalosis

Metabolic alkalosis is caused by a net gain of bicarbonate or loss of hydrogen ion from the extracellular fluid. It is characterized on ABG by an increase in both pH and bicarbonate values. Although some respiratory compensation occurs as a result of hypoventilation and $CO_2$ retention, the degree is relatively minor.

**TABLE 13-2.** Causes of Metabolic Acidosis

| ANION GAP | NONANION GAP |
|---|---|
| Lactic acidosis | Gastrointestinal losses |
|   Type A |   Diarrhea |
|     Septic shock |   Ureteral diversions |
|     Hypovolemic shock |   Fistulas |
|     Mesenteric ischemia | Medications and Iatrogenic |
|     Hypoxemia | Causes |
|     Severe anemia |   Intravenous sodium |
|     Carbon monoxide |   chloride (excessive doses) |
|     poisoning |   Parenteral nutrition |
|     Cyanide |   Carbonic anhydrous |
|   Type B |   inhibitors |
|     Medications |   Topiramate |
|       Nonnucleoside reverse- |   Cholestyramine |
|       transcriptase inhibitors | Renal tubular acidosis |
|       Metformin | |
|       Propofol | |
|       Linezolid | |
|       Niacin | |
|       Isoniazid | |
|       Iron | |
|       IV lorazepam (vehicle) | |
|       Sodium nitroprusside | |
|       (cyanide) | |
|     Seizures | |
|     Diabetes mellitus | |
|     Malignancy | |
|     Intoxication | |
| Poisonings | |
|   Salicylate | |
|   Ethylene glycol | |
|   Propylene glycol | |
|   Methanol | |
|   Toluene ingestion | |
|   Paraldehyde | |
| Ketoacidosis | |
|   Diabetic | |
|   Alcoholic | |
|   Starvation | |
|   Metabolic errors | |
| Renal failure | |

## MINICASE 1

## Patient Involved in a Motor Vehicle Collision

John W. is a 21-year-old man, previously healthy, who presents to the emergency department after a motor vehicle collision in which he sustained multiple rib fractures, a pelvic fracture, and a liver laceration. On physical exam, he is not following commands and is perseverating. His blood pressure on presentation is 81/42 mm Hg and his heart rate is 120 beats/min. He is aggressively resuscitated with normal saline and blood products (packed red blood cells, fresh frozen plasma, and platelets) and subsequently taken to the operating room for hemorrhagic shock. In the operating room, surgical hemostasis is achieved. The patient is extubated and admitted to the ICU on normal saline at a rate of 150 mL/hr. Laboratory values and ABG postop are as follows:

- pH, 7.32
- $PaCO_2$, 36 mm Hg
- $PaO_2$, 90 mm Hg
- $HCO_3^-$, 20 mEq/L
- Sodium, 149 mEq/L
- Potassium, 3.1 mEq/L
- Cl, 119 mEq/L
- Total carbon dioxide, 22 mEq/L
- Blood urea nitrogen (BUN) 22 mg/dL
- Serum creatinine (SCr), 0.9 mg/dL
- White blood cell count, 17,000 cells/mm³
- Albumin, 3 g/dL

QUESTION: What acid–base disorder does this patient present with? What is the most likely cause?

DISCUSSION: The pH of 7.32 indicates acidemia. Because both the $HCO_3^-$ and the $PaCO_2$ are low, the primary disorder is metabolic acidosis. This is consistent with the patient's admitting presentation of shock. The degree of respiratory compensation can be calculated using the formula $PaCO_2 = 1.5 \times HCO_3^- + 8 \pm 2$. In this example, the actual $PaCO_2$ (36 mm Hg) is within the range for expected $PaCO_2$ (36 to 40 mm Hg), indicating this is a simple disorder. The next step is to calculate the anion gap, which is 8 (corrected for hypoalbuminemia, 10.5), consistent with a nonanion gap metabolic acidosis. Common causes of nonanion gap metabolic acidosis are hyperchloremic acidosis due to resuscitation with normal saline, renal tubular acidosis, and excessive gastrointestinal losses. Because this patient received large amounts of normal saline secondary to hypotension and shock, this is the most likely cause. Treatment should consist of reevaluating the rate of IV fluid administration and changing to a balanced crystalloid solution such as lactated ringers.

## MINICASE 2

### Patient with Acute Respiratory Depression

Pat R. is an 80-year-old woman who is admitted to the hospital after falling and breaking her hip. On hospital day 2, she undergoes surgery to repair her hip. Postoperatively, her stay has been relatively unremarkable with the exception of pain control. Upon evaluation, her pain scores have been no lower than 8 out of 10 for which she has been receiving IV hydromorphone. On postoperative day 3, a "rapid assessment" code is called because her oxygen saturation falls to 81% and her respiratory rate is 4 breaths/min. The nurse states she has been receiving 2 mg of hydromorphone every 2 hours around the clock and her last dose was approximately 15 minutes ago. Her vital signs are heart rate 100 beats/min, blood pressure 110/70 mm Hg, temperature 37.6°C. Laboratory results, and ABG are as follows:

- Na, 136 mEq/L
- K, 5.1 mEq/L
- Chloride, 98 mEq/L
- Total carbon dioxide, 28 mEq/L
- BUN, 25 mg/dL
- SCr, 0.8 mg/dL

- ABG, pH 7.26
- $PaCO_2$, 58 mm Hg
- $PaO_2$, 55 mm Hg
- $HCO_3^-$, 26 mEq/L

QUESTION: What acid–base disorder does this patient present with? What is the most likely cause?

DISCUSSION: The pH of 7.26 indicates acidemia. Because the $PaCO_2$ and $HCO_3^-$ are both high, the primary cause is a respiratory acidosis. This is consistent with her clinical presentation of respiratory distress and inability to eliminate carbon dioxide. With respiratory acidosis, metabolic compensation is delayed and changes in $HCO_3^-$ are often minimal and rarely >31 mEq/L in the acute setting. In this example, the expected degree of compensation is appropriate for an acute disorder. The most likely cause of respiratory acidosis in this case is respiratory depression secondary to narcotic overuse. Treatment should consist of supplemental oxygen and reversal of hydromorphone with naloxone.

### TABLE 13-3. Causes of Metabolic Alkalosis

| CHLORIDE RESPONSIVE | CHLORIDE RESISTANT |
|---|---|
| Gastrointestinal losses | Mineralocorticoid excess |
| Vomiting | Exogenous steroids |
| Gastric drainage | Increased renin/aldosterone states |
| Nasogastric suctioning | |
| Chloride wasting diarrhea | Cushing syndrome |
| Diuretics | Liddle syndrome |
| Posthypercapnia | Bartter syndrome |

Metabolic alkalosis is delineated into two types: chloride responsive and chloride resistant (**Table 13-3**). A common drug-related cause of metabolic alkalosis is diuretic therapy. Diuretics cause a wasting of $Cl^-$ in association with sodium $(Na)^+$ and potassium $(K)^+$ without a proportional increase in bicarbonate excretion. In addition, volume depletion leads to hyperaldosteronism, $H^+$ secretion, and bicarbonate resorption (**Minicase 4**).

### Respiratory Acidosis

Respiratory acidosis is usually a direct result of hypoventilation; therefore, any situation associated with decreased respiratory rate can lead to its occurrence. It is, therefore, important to identify and treat the underlying cause (**Table 13-4**). Laboratory findings consistent with respiratory acidosis are decreased pH and increased $PaCO_2$. Because renal compensation is slower to respond, the increase in bicarbonate is only modest at first. With respiratory acidosis, the biggest threat to life is not from acidemia but from hypoxia. In patients breathing room air, $PaCO_2$ cannot exceed 80 mm Hg or else life-threatening hypoxia may result[10] (**Minicase 2**).

### Respiratory Alkalosis

Respiratory alkalosis is characterized by excessive elimination of $CO_2$ through hyperventilation. Laboratory derangements include increased pH and decreased $PaCO_2$. Renal compensation is characterized by inhibition of bicarbonate reabsorption, which is complete within several days. It is one of the most frequently encountered acid–base disorders and is associated with several pathologic conditions (**Table 13-5**).[10]

## SUMMARY

Acid–base disorders are highly prevalent in critically ill patients. Acid–base status is assessed measuring an arterial blood gas and evaluation of pH, $PaCO_2$, and $HCO_3^-$. Carbon dioxide is the most abundant acid that is controlled through respiratory regulation, whereas bicarbonate is the most abundant base and concentrations are maintained by the kidney. There are four primary acid–base disturbances that are categorized by the type (ie, acidosis versus alkalosis) and origin (metabolic versus respiratory). When evaluating for the presences of acid–base disorders, a systematic approach should be taken using data obtained from the ABG, serum electrolytes, and clinical presentation. Medications are frequently implicated in acid–base disorders; thus, careful assessment of the medication profile is necessary. These skills can be used to assist clinicians with the identification, prevention, and treatment of acid–base disorders.

## MINICASE 3

## Patient with Severe Abdominal Pain

Jill M. is a 67-year-old woman who presents to the hospital with reports of severe abdominal pain and distention that has been present for the last 2 days. She is tachycardic, tachypneic, and normotensive. Her temperature is 38.4°C. A computed tomography scan reveals a large amount of intraabdominal free air and she is taken to the operating room for an exploratory laparotomy. In the operating room, a colon perforation is noted with a significant amount of fecal contamination and pus. The colon is repaired and the wound is left open, with a wound-vac in place. She returns to the ICU, mechanically ventilated on maintenance IV fluids (normal saline at 100 mL/hr) and antibiotics. Postoperatively, her blood pressure remains low and is currently 88/56 mm Hg. A bolus of 0.9% sodium chloride is administered and a norepinephrine infusion is initiated. Pertinent laboratory values are as follows:

- Sodium, 146 mEq/L
- Potassium, 3.8 mEq/L
- Chloride, 112 mEq/L
- Total carbon dioxide, 16 mEq/L
- BUN, 38 mg/dL
- SCr, 1.3 mg/dL
- White blood cells, 21,000 cells/mm$^3$
- Albumin, 2.5 g/dL
- Lactate, 5.2 mmol/L

- ABG, pH 7.28
- $PaCO_2$, 38 mm Hg
- $PaO_2$, 72 mm Hg
- $HCO_3^-$, 14 mEq/L

QUESTION: What acid–base disorder does this patient present with? What is the most likely cause?

DISCUSSION: The pH is 7.28, which indicates acidemia. Because the $HCO_3^-$ is low and the $PaCO_2$ is low, the primary disturbance is metabolic acidosis. The expected degree of respiratory compensation, which is calculated using the formula expected $PaCO_2 = 1.5 \times HCO_3^- + 8 \pm 2$, is less than the actual $PaCO_2$; therefore, a secondary respiratory acidosis exists. Because the primary problem is a metabolic acidosis, the next step is to calculate the anion gap. The anion gap is 18 (corrected for albumin, 22); therefore, this is an anion gap, metabolic acidosis. Common causes of anion gap acidosis are lactic acidosis, ketosis, renal failure, and poisonings. Because this patient has an elevated lactate level and presents with an infection and hypotension requiring vasopressors, the most likely cause is lactic acidosis secondary to septic shock. The treatment plan should consist of fluid resuscitation and vasopressor support (as needed) to restore tissue perfusion along with broad-spectrum antibiotics. Low-dose corticosteroid therapy could be considered if hypotension persists despite fluids and vasopressor therapy.

## MINICASE 4

## Patient with Fever and Shortness of Breath

Beth D. is a 65-year-old woman who is admitted to the hospital with fever and shortness of breath. A pulse oximeter reveals an oxygen saturation of 89%, her chest radiograph demonstrates a right lower lobe infiltrate, and her blood pressure is 88/49 mm Hg. IV fluids are administered and she is subsequently intubated. She is admitted to the ICU with the diagnosis of sepsis secondary to pneumonia. Throughout her ICU stay, she has required a significant amount of IV fluids to maintain a mean arterial pressure (MAP) goal of 65 mm Hg with intermittent use of vasopressors. Currently, her blood pressure remains stable, but the cumulative fluid balance for her hospital stay is +10.6 L and the team would like to wean her off the ventilator; a furosemide infusion is administered. Over the next 48 hours, her daily fluid balance has been –5 L (day 1) and –3.8 L (day 2). Laboratory results and ABG reveal the following: pH 7.53, $PaCO_2$ 48 mm Hg, $PaO_2$ 65 mm Hg, and $HCO_3^-$ 35 mEq/L. The remainder of her laboratory results are as follows:

- Sodium, 141 mEq/L,
- Potassium, 4.2 mEq/L
- Chloride, 99 mEq/L
- Total carbon dioxide, 36 mEq/L
- BUN, 48 mg/dL
- SCr, 1.2 mg/dL
- Urine chloride, 7 mEq/L

QUESTION: What acid–base disorder does this patient present with? What is the most likely cause?

DISCUSSION: The pH is 7.53, which indicates alkalemia. Because the $HCO_3^-$ is high and the $PaCO_2$ is high, the primary problem is metabolic. The degree of compensation by the respiratory side is appropriate as per the formula expected $PaCO_2 = (0.7 \times HCO_3^-) + 21 \pm 2$. Because the primary problem is metabolic alkalosis, the next step is to determine if it is chloride responsive or resistant. This is done by assessing the urinary chloride. Because the urinary chloride is 7 mEq/L, this would be classified as chloride responsive. There are several potential causes of metabolic alkalosis in this patient. Diuretic administration can cause metabolic alkalosis through aldosterone secretion and increased chloride excretion. Loss of gastrointestinal fluid through nasogastric suction leads to a loss of hydrogen and chloride ions. In addition, parenteral nutrition can be an iatrogenic cause of alkalosis if excessive amounts of acetate are provided in the formula. The most likely cause in this patient is excessive diuresis secondary to the furosemide infusion. Treatment would first consist of discontinuing the diuresis. IV fluid administration can be considered but this may interfere with ventilator weaning. Instead, acetazolamide would be preferred to lower the serum bicarbonate.

## TABLE 13-4. Causes of Respiratory Acidosis

Central
  Opiates
  Sedatives
  Stroke
  Trauma
  Head injury
  Status epilepticus

Perfusion abnormalities
  Pulmonary embolism
  Cardiac arrest

Airway abnormalities
  Obstruction
  Asthma
  Chronic obstructive pulmonary disease
  Pneumonia
  Pulmonary edema
  Acute respiratory distress syndrome

Neuromuscular
  Brainstem or cervical cord injury
  Guillain-Barré syndrome
  Myastenia gravis

Parenteral nutrition

## TABLE 13-5. Causes of Respiratory Alkalosis

CNS-Respiratory Stimulation
  Anxiety
  Pain
  Fever
  Sepsis
  Pregnancy
  Progesterone derivatives
  Salicylates
  Cerebrovascular accidents

Hypoxemia
  Pneumonia
  Congestive heart failure
  High altitude
  Pulmonary edema
  Pulmonary embolism

is appropriate. If it is not, then a secondary disorder is present. Finally, if the primary problem is metabolic acidosis, or metabolic alkalosis, then the anion gap or urinary chloride, respectively, should be assessed to assist with identification of the possible cause.

3.  **How can the anion gap be used to assess acid–base disorders?**

    **ANSWER:** The anion gap is an estimate of the relative abundance of unmeasured anions. It can suggest the possible causes of metabolic acidosis, particularly if the disorder is secondary to an accumulation of nonvolatile acids or a net loss of bicarbonate. When the anion gap is normal, the acidosis is usually caused by a loss of bicarbonate ions; common causes include diarrhea, early renal insufficiency, and infusion of large amounts of isotonic saline. When the anion gap is elevated, causes may include lactic acidosis, ketoacidosis, end-stage renal failure, or certain toxic ingestions. Correction of the anion gap for hypoalbuminemia can improve the accuracy of this approach. The anion gap represents one factor that can help determine the etiologic cause of metabolic acidosis and should not be interpreted as absolute, especially in a complex intensive care unit (ICU) patient.

# LEARNING POINTS

1.  **Can an acid–base disorder exist if a patient presents with a normal pH?**

    **ANSWER:** Yes, an acid–base disorder can still exist even when the pH is within the normal range. pH is determined by the ratio of base to acid as opposed to the individual concentration of one (ie, acid or base) independently. Therefore, an acidosis can be present without an acidemia if a coexisting alkalosis is present. Conversely, an alkalosis can be present without an alkalemia if a coexisting acidosis is present. In these settings, evaluation of the $PaCO_2$ and $HCO_3$ reveals abnormal values (hence a pathophysiologic process), but each offsets the other and the net effect on pH is negligible. Careful evaluation of the patient's history, clinical presentation, physical exam, and laboratory values is necessary to identify the acid–base disorders that are present.

2.  **What are the steps to follow to assess an ABG?**

    **ANSWER:** The first step is to determine if an acidemia or alkalemia is present. This is done by evaluating the pH. Once the correct categorization is made, the second step is to determine if the primary cause is metabolic or respiratory. This is performed by assessing the $PaCO_2$ and the $HCO_3$ on the ABG. Once the primary cause is determined, the opposing side should compensate. The third step is to assess if the degree of compensation

# REFERENCES

1.  Berend K, de Vries AP, Gans RO. Physiological approach to assessment of acid-base disturbances. *N Engl J Med.* 2014;371(15):1434-1445.PubMed

2.  Marino PL. *Marino's The ICU Book.* 4th ed. Philadelphia, PA: Wolters Kluwer Health/Lippincott Williams & Wilkins; 2014.

3.  Adrogué HJ, Madias NE. Management of life-threatening acid-base disorders. Second of two parts. *N Engl J Med.* 1998;338(2):107-111. PubMed

4.  Narins RG, Emmett M. Simple and mixed acid-base disorders: a practical approach. *Medicine (Baltimore).* 1980;59(3):161-187.PubMed

5.  Weil MH, Rackow EC, Trevino R, et al. Difference in acid-base state between venous and arterial blood during cardiopulmonary resuscitation. *N Engl J Med.* 1986;315(3):153-156.PubMed

6.  Faridi AB, Weisberg LS. Acid-Base, Electrolyte and Metabolic Abnormalities. Parrillo JE, and Dellinger RP, eds. *Critical Care Medicine: Principles of Diagnosis and Management in the Adult*. 3rd ed. Philadelphia, PA: Mosby Elsevier; 2008:1203-1243.

7.  Ranieri VM, Rubenfeld GD, Thompson BT, et al. Acute respiratory distress syndrome: the Berlin Definition. *JAMA*. 2012;307(23):2526-2533. PubMed

8.  Wilson RF. *Critical Care Manual: Applied Physiology and Principles of Therapy*. 2nd ed. Philadelphia, PA: F.A. Davis Company; 1992.

9.  Figge J, Jabor A, Kazda A, et al. Anion gap and hypoalbuminemia. *Crit Care Med*. 1998;26(11):1807-1810.PubMed

10. Al-Jaghbeer M, Kellum JA. Acid-base disturbances in intensive care patients: etiology, pathophysiology and treatment. *Nephrol Dial Transplant*. 2015;30(7):1104-1111.PubMed

11. Gilfix BM, Bique M, Magder S. A physical chemical approach to the analysis of acid-base balance in the clinical setting. *J Crit Care*. 1993;8(4):187-197.PubMed

12. Kellum JA. Disorders of acid-base balance. *Crit Care Med*. 2007;35(11):2630-2636.PubMed

13. Salem MM, Mujais SK. Gaps in the anion gap. *Arch Intern Med*. 1992;152(8):1625-1629.PubMed

14. Singer M, Deutschman CS, Seymour CW, et al. The Third International Consensus definitions for sepsis and septic shock (sepsis-3). *JAMA*. 2016;315(8):801-810.PubMed

15. Aduen J, Bernstein WK, Khastgir T, et al. The use and clinical importance of a substrate-specific electrode for rapid determination of blood lactate concentrations. *JAMA*. 1994;272(21):1678-1685.PubMed

16. Levy MM, Evans LE, Rhodes A. The Surviving Sepsis Campaign Bundle: 2018 Update. *Crit Care Med*. 2018;46(6):997-1000.PubMed

17. Jansen TC, van Bommel J, Schoonderbeek FJ, et al. Early lactate-guided therapy in intensive care unit patients: a multicenter, open-label, randomized controlled trial. *Am J Respir Crit Care Med*. 2010;182(6):752-761.PubMed

18. Vincent JL, Dufaye P, Berré J, et al. Serial lactate determinations during circulatory shock. *Crit Care Med*. 1983;11(6):449-451.PubMed

19. Vincent JL, De Backer D. Circulatory shock. *N Engl J Med*. 2013;369(18):1726-1734.PubMed

20. Marik PE. Early management of severe sepsis: concepts and controversies. *Chest*. 2014;145(6):1407-1418.PubMed

21. Reinhart K, Kuhn HJ, Hartog C, et al. Continuous central venous and pulmonary artery oxygen saturation monitoring in the critically ill. *Intensive Care Med*. 2004;30(8):1572-1578.PubMed

22. Rhodes A, Evans LE, Alhazzani W, et al. Surviving Sepsis Campaign: International Guidelines for Management of Sepsis and Septic Shock: 2016. *Crit Care Med*. 2017;45(3):486-552.PubMed

23. Pope JV, Jones AE, Gaieski DF, et al. Multicenter study of central venous oxygen saturation (ScvO$_2$) as a predictor of mortality in patients with sepsis. *Ann Emerg Med*. 2010;55(1):40-46.e1.PubMed

24. Stewart PA. Modern quantitative acid-base chemistry. *Can J Physiol Pharmacol*. 1983;61(12):1444-1461.PubMed

25. Kellum JA. Determinants of blood pH in health and disease. *Crit Care*. 2000;4(1):6-14.PubMed

26. Morgan TJ. The meaning of acid-base abnormalities in the intensive care unit: part III. Effects of fluid administration. *Crit Care*. 2005;9(2):204-211. PubMed

27. Rose DB, Post TW. *Clinical Physiology of Acid-Base and Electrolyte Disorders*. 5th ed. New York, NY: McGraw-Hill; 2001.

28. Dzierba AL, Abraham P. A practical approach to understanding acid-base abnormalities in critical illness. *J Pharm Pract*. 2011;24(1):17-26.PubMed

29. Kaplan LJ, Frangos S. Clinical review: acid-base abnormalities in the intensive care unit. Part II. *Crit Care*. 2005;9(2):198-203.PubMed

30. Mehta AN, Emmett JB, Emmett M. GOLD MARK: an anion gap mnemonic for the 21st century. *Lancet*. 2008;372(9642):892.PubMed

## QUICKVIEW | Venous Total Carbon Dioxide Content (Venous Serum Bicarbonate)

| PARAMETER | DESCRIPTION | COMMENTS |
|---|---|---|
| **Common reference range** | | |
| Adults | 22–30 mEq/L | Venous bicarbonate can be 1.5–3 mEq/L higher than arterial measure of bicarbonate |
| **Critical value** | <10 mEq/L or >40 mEq/L | Reference range and critical values may vary based on local laboratory standards |
| **Inherent activity** | Yes | Primary substance responsible for buffering acids |
| **Location** | | |
| Production | Byproduct of typical cell metabolism | |
| Storage | Exchanged via circulation | |
| Secretion/excretion | Renal excretion (reabsorption occurs at proximal tubule) | |
| **Causes of abnormal values** | | |
| High | Metabolic alkalosis and respiratory acidosis | Change in $HCO_3^-$ is the primary cause of metabolic acid–base disorders. In contrast, change in $HCO_3^-$ is the primary method of compensation for respiratory disorders. |
| Low | Metabolic acidosis and respiratory alkalosis | |
| **Signs and symptoms** | | |
| High level | Related to primary process | |
| Low level | Related to primary process | |
| **After event, time to….** | | |
| Initial elevation | 6–12 hr to initiate compensation | Assumes acute insult |
| Peak values | None (will rise until pH balanced) | Assumes insult not yet removed |
| Normalization | 3–5 days to complete compensation | Assumes insult removed and nonpermanent damage |
| **Causes of spurious results** | Inadvertent venous sampling, delayed time to analysis | |

## QUICKVIEW | Arterial Partial Pressure of Carbon Dioxide

| PARAMETER | DESCRIPTION | COMMENTS |
|---|---|---|
| **Common reference range** | | |
| Adults | 35–45 mm Hg | |
| **Critical value** | >70 mm Hg (may require mechanical ventilation) | |
| **Inherent activity** | Yes | Primary volatile acid in the body |
| **Location** | | |
| Production | Generated intracellularly from carbon dioxide and water | |
| Storage | N/A | |
| Secretion/excretion | Excreted by the lungs during expiration | |
| **Causes of abnormal values** | | |
| High | Respiratory acidosis and metabolic alkalosis | Change is $PaCO_2$ is the primary cause of respiratory acid–base disorders. In contrast, change in $PaCO_2$ is the primary method of compensation for metabolic disorders. |
| Low | Respiratory alkalosis and metabolic acidosis | |
| **Signs and symptoms** | | |
| High level | Respiratory failure | |
| Low level | Related to primary process | |
| **After event, time to....** | | |
| Initial elevation | Minutes to hours | Assumes acute insult |
| Peak values | None | Assumes insult not yet removed |
| Normalization | Hours to days | Assumes insult removed and nonpermanent damage |
| **Causes of spurious results** | Inadvertent venous sampling, delayed time to analysis | Higher carbon dioxide content |

N/A = not applicable.

# 14

# Pulmonary Function and Related Tests

*Lori A. Wilken and Min J. Joo*

## OBJECTIVES

*After completing this chapter, the reader should be able to*

- Identify common pulmonary function tests and list their purpose and limitations

- Describe how pulmonary function tests are performed and discuss factors affecting the validity of the results

- Interpret commonly used pulmonary function tests, given clinical information

- Discuss how pulmonary function tests provide objective measurement to aid in the diagnosis of pulmonary diseases

- Discuss how pulmonary function tests assist with monitoring efficacy and toxicity of various drug therapies

Pulmonary function tests (PFTs) provide objective and quantifiable measures of lung function and are useful in diagnosing, evaluating, and monitoring respiratory disease. Diagnosing and monitoring many pulmonary diseases, including diseases of gas exchange, often require measuring the flow or volume of air inhaled and exhaled by the patient. Spirometry, a test that measures the movement of air into and out of the lungs during various breathing maneuvers, is the most frequently used PFT. Clinicians use spirometry to aid in the diagnosis of respiratory diseases such as asthma and chronic obstructive pulmonary disease (COPD). Other tests of lung function include lung volume assessment, carbon monoxide diffusion capacity (DLCO), exercise testing, and bronchial provocation tests. Arterial blood gases (ABGs) can be measured with PFTs and are useful for assessing lung function. (Interpretation of arterial blood gases is discussed in Chapter 13.) This chapter discusses the mechanics and interpretation of PFTs.

## ANATOMY AND PHYSIOLOGY OF LUNGS[1]

The purpose of the lungs is to take oxygen from the atmosphere and exchange it for carbon dioxide in the blood. The movement of air in and out of the lungs is called *ventilation*; the movement of blood through the lungs is termed *perfusion*.

Air enters the body through the mouth and nose and travels through the pharynx to the trachea. The trachea splits into the left and right main stem bronchi, which deliver inspired air to the respective lungs. The left and right lungs are in the pleural cavity of the thorax. These two spongy, conical structures are the primary organs of respiration. The right lung has three lobes, whereas the left lung has only two lobes, thus leaving space for the heart. Within the lungs, the main bronchi continue to split successively into smaller bronchi, bronchioles, terminal bronchioles, and finally alveoli. In the alveoli, carbon dioxide is exchanged for oxygen across a thin membrane separating capillary blood from inspired air.

The thoracic cavity is separated from the abdominal cavity by the diaphragm. The diaphragm, a thin sheet of dome-shaped muscle, contracts and relaxes during breathing. The lungs are contained within the rib cage but rest on the diaphragm. Between the ribs are two sets of intercostal muscles, which attach to each upper and lower rib. During inhalation, the intercostal muscles and the diaphragm contract, which enlarges the thoracic cavity. This action generates a negative intrathoracic pressure, allowing air to rush in through the nose and mouth down into the pharynx, trachea, and lungs. During exhalation, these muscles relax, and a positive intrathoracic pressure causes air to be pushed out of the lungs. Normal expiration is a passive process that results from the natural recoil of the expanded lungs. However, in people with rapid or labored breathing or airflow limitation, the accessory muscles and abdominal muscles often must contract to help force air out of the lungs more quickly or completely.

The ability of the lungs to expand and contract to inhale and exhale air is affected by the compliance of the lungs, which is a measure of the ease of expansion of the lungs and thorax. Processes that result in scarring of lung tissue (eg, pulmonary fibrosis) can decrease compliance, thus decreasing the flow and volume of air moved by the lungs, and increase the work to breathe. The degree of ease in which air travels through the airways is known as *resistance*. The length and radius of the airways

DOI 10.37573/9781585286423.014

as well as the viscosity of the gas inhaled determine resistance. A patient with a high degree of airway resistance may not be able to take a full breath in or exhale fully (some air may become trapped in the lungs).

To have an adequate exchange of the gases, there must be a matching of ventilation (V) and perfusion (Q) at the alveolar level. An average V:Q ratio, determined by dividing total alveolar ventilation (4 L/min) by cardiac output (5 L/min), is 0.8. A mismatch of ventilation and perfusion may result from a shunt or dead space. A shunt occurs when there is flow of blood adjacent to alveoli that are not ventilated. This could be physiologic (eg, at rest, some alveoli are collapsed or partially opened but perfused) or pathologic when alveoli are filled with fluid (eg, heart failure) or cellular debris (eg, pneumonia) or are collapsed (eg, atelectasis). A shunt can also occur when airways are obstructed by mucus or collapse on exhalation (eg, COPD). In a shunt, blood moves from the venous circulation to the arterial circulation without being oxygenated.

Dead space occurs when there is ventilation of functional lung tissue without adjacent blood flow for gas exchange. Dead space can be physiologic (eg, the trachea) or pathologic because of airflow limitation of blood flow (eg, pulmonary embolism). The body uses a few mechanisms to normalize the V:Q ratio, such as hypoxic vasoconstriction and bronchoconstriction. When the V:Q ratio is low, hypoxic vasoconstriction leads to decreased perfusion to the hypoxic regions of the lungs, thus redirecting perfusion to functional areas of the lungs, which leads to an increase in the V:Q ratio. When the V:Q ratio is high, the bronchi constrict in areas that are not well perfused, which leads to a decrease in the amount of ventilation to areas that are not well perfused, a decrease in the amount of alveolar dead space, and a decrease in the V:Q ratio.

For the respiration process to be complete, gas diffusion must occur between the alveoli and the pulmonary capillaries. By the diffusion mechanism, gases equilibrate from areas of high concentration to areas of low concentration. Hemoglobin (Hgb) releases carbon dioxide and adsorbs oxygen as it diffuses through the alveolar walls. If these walls thicken, diffusion is hampered, potentially causing carbon dioxide retention, hypoxia, or both. Membrane formation with secondary thickening of the alveolar wall may result from an acute or chronic inflammatory process such as interstitial pneumonia and pulmonary fibrosis. The pulmonary diffusing capacity is also reduced in the presence of a V:Q mismatch, loss of lung surface areas (eg, emphysema, lung resection), or decrease in oxygen-carrying capacity (eg, anemia). The various PFTs can measure airflow in or out of the lungs, indicate how much air is in the lungs, and provide information on gas diffusion or specific changes in airway tone or reactivity.

# CLINICAL USE OF PULMONARY FUNCTION TESTING

Pulmonary function tests are useful in many clinical situations.[2] They aid in the diagnostic differentiation of various pulmonary diseases. PFT results are divided into two types of pulmonary abnormalities: *obstructive* and *restrictive* lung diseases. Obstructive diseases (eg, asthma and COPD) decrease the flow rate of air (liters/minute) out of the lungs but have less impact on the total volume of air per breath. In restrictive diseases (eg, kyphosis or sarcoidosis), the lungs are limited in the amount of air they can contain. Restrictive diseases usually decrease the total volume of air per breath in a similar ratio to the flow rate of air. **Table 14-1** summarizes common pulmonary disease states with PFT results.

In addition, serial PFTs allow tracking of the progression of pulmonary diseases and the need for or response to various treatments. They also help to establish a baseline of respiratory function before surgical, medical, or radiation therapy. Subsequent serial measurements then aid in the detection and tracking of changes in lung function caused by these therapies. Similarly, serial PFTs can be used to evaluate the risk of lung damage from exposure to environmental or occupational hazards. **Table 14-2** summarizes the selected uses of PFTs.

# PULMONARY FUNCTION TESTS AND MEASUREMENTS

Pulmonary function tests use equations based on an individual's age, height, sex, and race (when available) to calculate reference values from the population. The reference values most commonly used for spirometry is the National Health and Nutrition Examination Survey III and, more recently, the Global Lung Function Initiative (GLI)-2012.[3] The individual's measurement is then compared with the calculated reference values and the lower limit of normal (LLN). The LLN value is set at the fifth percentile, indicating that if the measured value is less than the lower fifth percentile of a normal population, then it is considered reduced and may be associated with disease. Using both the reference measurement and the LLN helps decrease overdiagnosing by removing bias from age seen in fixed value cutoffs.[3]

## Spirometry

*Spirometry* is a PFT that helps detect airflow limitation that can be manifested in asthma or COPD. Spirometry measures the flow of air in volume per time. The physical forces of the airflow and the total amount of air inhaled and exhaled are converted by transducers to electrical signals, which are displayed on a computer screen.

During this maneuver, a *volume-time curve*—a plot of the volume exhaled against time—and a *flow-volume curve* or *flow-volume loop*—a diagram with flow (liters/second) on the vertical axis and volume on the horizontal axis (liters)—are generated as the report (**Figure 14-1**). After the data are generated, the patient's spirometry results are compared with the reference values. The flow-volume curve is visually useful for diagnosing airflow limitation. The Global Initiative for Chronic Obstructive Lung Disease (GOLD) strategy suggests suspecting COPD in patients >40 years old with symptoms and/or risk factors and recommends spirometry to definitively diagnose COPD.[5] Once diagnosed with COPD, spirometry, in conjunction with

**TABLE 14-1.** Pulmonary Disease States and Common PFT Results

| PULMONARY ABNORMALITY | PATHOPHYSIOLOGY | DISEASE STATE EXAMPLES | COMMON PFT RESULTS | | | | |
|---|---|---|---|---|---|---|---|
| | | | FEV$_1$/FVC | FEV$_1$ | FVC | RV | TLC |
| Obstructive lung disease, chronic | Fixed airflow limitation | Asthma with fixed airflow limitation, COPD, cystic fibrosis, bronchiectasis | Decreased | Decreased | Normal or decreased | Normal or increased | Normal or increased |
| Obstructive lung disease, reversible and stable | Reversible (eg, bronchoconstriction) | Asthma | Normal | Normal | Normal | Normal | Normal |
| Restrictive lung disease | Parenchymal infiltration or fibrosis | Idiopathic pulmonary fibrosis and other idiopathic interstitial pneumonias, drug induced, secondary to autoimmune diseases, sarcoidosis | Normal or increased | Decreased | Decreased | Decreased | Decreased |
| | Extrathoracic compression | Kyphosis, morbid obesity, ascites, chest wall deformities, pregnancy | Normal or increased | Decreased | Decreased | Decreased | Decreased |
| | Neuromuscular causes | Guillain-Barré syndrome, myasthenia gravis, muscular dystrophy, amyotrophic lateral sclerosis | Normal or increased | Decreased | Decreased | Decreased | Decreased |
| Mixed obstructive and restrictive | Combinations of restrictive and obstructive processes | Both restrictive and obstructive diseases | Decreased | Decreased | Decreased | Increased, normal, or decreased | Decreased |

FEV$_1$ = forced expiratory volume in 1 second; FVC = forced vital capacity; RV= residual volume; TLC = total lung capacity

symptoms and history of exacerbations, can be used to monitor disease state severity.[5] When asthma is suspected, spirometry can be used to assess for airflow variation and is recommended at the time of diagnosis, 3 to 6 months after starting treatment, at least every 1 to 2 years, and as needed to assess ongoing risk of exacerbations.[6]

## Spirometry Measurements

Spirometry routinely assesses forced vital capacity (FVC), forced expiratory volume in 1 second (FEV$_1$), and FEV$_1$/FVC.

### Forced Vital Capacity

The FVC is the total volume of air, measured in liters, forcefully and rapidly exhaled in one breath (from maximum inhalation to end of forced expiration). End of forced expiration is achieved when there is less than a 0.025 L change in volume for at least 1 second, or the forced expiratory time has reached 15 seconds, or the FVC is within 0.150 L of another FVC measurement if the patient is older than 6 years of age. When the full inhalation-exhalation procedure is repeated slowly—instead of forcefully and rapidly—it is called the *slow vital capacity* (SVC). This value is the maximum amount of air exhaled after a full and complete inhalation. In patients with normal airway function, FVC and SVC are usually similar and constitute the *vital capacity*. In patients with diseases such as COPD, the FVC may be lower than the SVC due to collapse of narrowed or floppy airways during forced expiration. Because of this, some interpretive strategies recommend using the FEV$_1$/SVC ratio to determine the presence of airflow limitation, especially for pronounced airflow limitation.[5]

### Forced Expiratory Volume in One Second

The full, forced inhalation-exhalation procedure was already described as the FVC. During this maneuver, the computer can discern the amount of air exhaled at specific time intervals of the FVC. By convention, $FEV_{0.5}$, $FEV_{0.75}$, $FEV_1$, $FEV_3$, and $FEV_6$ are the amounts of air exhaled after one-half, three-fourths, 1, 3, and 6 seconds, respectively. Usually, a patient's value is described in liters and as a percentage of a predicted value based on reference values adjusted for age, height, sex, and race. Of these

### TABLE 14-2. Selected Uses of PFTs

Diagnosis

    Evaluate signs and symptoms of respiratory disease

    Screen at-risk individuals for pulmonary disease

Evaluation

    Assess the health status before initiating physical activity or rehabilitation

    Determine preoperative risk of having pulmonary-related issues during surgery

Monitoring

    Describe the course of lung function from a respiratory disease

    Monitor respiratory changes for occupational or environmental exposure to toxins

    Assess therapeutic drug effectiveness (eg, inhaled corticosteroids or bronchodilators for asthma)

    Monitor adverse drug effects on pulmonary function (eg, amiodarone)

measurements, $FEV_1$ has the most clinical relevance, primarily as an indicator of airway function. A value ≥80% of the predicted normal value or greater than the LLN is considered normal. Normal values can be seen in patients with asthma when the disease is mild or well controlled. $FEV_1$ is an important value for predicting clinical outcomes, such as mortality, hospitalizations, and lung transplantation.[5] For children aged 6 years and younger, $FEV_{0.75}$ is used instead of $FEV_1$ if the maximal volume expired by time is less than 1 second.[4]

### Forced Expiratory Volume in One Second/Forced Vital Capacity

The ratio of $FEV_1$ to the FVC is used to estimate the presence and amount of airflow limitation in the airways. This ratio indicates the amount of air mobilized in 1 second as a percentage of the total amount of movable air. Normal, healthy individuals can exhale approximately 50% of their FVC in the first one-half second, about 80% in 1 second, and about 98% in 3 seconds. Patients with obstructive disease usually show a decreased ratio, and the actual percentage reduction varies with the severity of airflow limitation. In COPD, the GOLD strategy defines persistent airflow limitation as a postbronchodilator $FEV_1$/FVC ratio <0.70.[5] **Table 14-3** summarizes the definition of airflow limitation severity for COPD. **Minicase 1** discusses how spirometry is used to diagnose COPD.

Spirometry can also show airflow variability necessary for the diagnosis of asthma. However, frequency of asthma symptoms, quick-relief medication use, and level of medications required to control symptoms are also necessary to assess asthma severity.

Generally, the $FEV_1$/FVC is normal (or high) in patients with restrictive diseases. In mild restriction, the FVC alone may be decreased, resulting in a high ratio. Often in restrictive

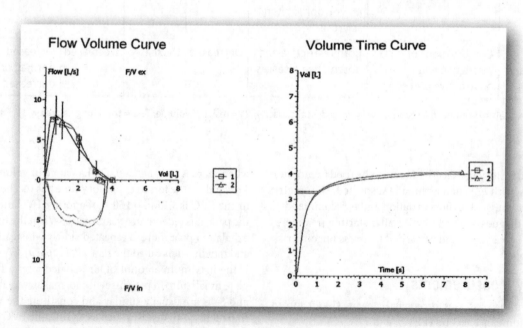

**FIGURE 14-1.** The flow-volume curve and volume-time curve from an effort meeting American Thoracic Society (ATS) acceptability criteria. The flow-volume curve has a deep inspiratory effort with a sharp complete expiratory flow. The volume-time curve demonstrates a plateau without complete flattening signifying the end of expiration or very-low flow.

lung disease, both the FVC and $FEV_1$ are similarly reduced compared with predicted values resulting in a normal ratio. It is important to note that this pattern is consistent with a restrictive pattern on spirometry, but lung volumes are needed to confirm restriction.

### Flow-Volume Curves

**Figure 14-2** shows several *flow-volume curves* in which the expiratory flow is plotted against the exhaled volume.

**TABLE 14-3.** Severity of Airflow Limitation for COPD with the Postbronchodilator $FEV_1$/FVC <0.7

| GOLD GRADE | SEVERITY | POSTBRONCHODILATOR $FEV_1$ (% PREDICTED) |
|---|---|---|
| 1 | Mild | ≥80 |
| 2 | Moderate | 50–79 |
| 3 | Severe | 30–49 |
| 4 | Very severe | <30 |

Refer to the Global Initiative for Chronic Obstructive Lung Disease (GOLDCOPD) 2022 Report[4] for more information.

As explained earlier, these curves are graphic representations of inspiration and expiration. The shape of the curve can indicate both the type of disease and the severity of airflow limitation. Obstructive changes result in decreased airflow, revealing a characteristic concave appearance. Restrictive changes result in a shape similar to that of a healthy individual, but the size is considerably smaller. The flow-volume loop also reveals mixed obstructive and restrictive disease by a combination of the two patterns.

### Standardization of Spirometry Measurements

Spirometry is performed by having a person breathe into a tube (mouthpiece) connected to a machine (spirometer) that measures the amount and flow of inhaled and exhaled air. Prior to performing spirometry, relative contraindications such as recent brain, eye, or sinus surgery are assessed.[4] Spirometry results depend greatly on the completeness and speed of the patient's inhalation and exhalation, so the importance of completely filling and emptying the lungs of air during the test is emphasized. During spirometry, nose clips are worn to minimize air loss through the nose. The patient is seated comfortably without leaning or slumping, and any restrictive clothing (such as ties or tight belts) is loosened or removed. The patient is coached to take a full deep breath in and then blast the air out as quickly and forcefully as possible and to keep blowing the air out, while

## MINICASE 1

## Using Spirometry to Diagnose Asthma and COPD

Debra T. is a 56-year-old woman who reports chronic cough and shortness of breath when walking up a few stairs. She has been admitted several times each year for COPD exacerbations and pneumonia. She has a 40 pack-year-history of tobacco use. She is allergic to dust mites and dogs and has had a history of asthma since childhood. Today, on exam, she is wheezing and has nasal congestion.

QUESTION: How do the results from this patient's spirometry test support the diagnosis of asthma and COPD?

DISCUSSION: A postbronchodilator measurement for $FEV_1$/FVC <0.70 is consistent with COPD using the GOLD criteria[4] in the right clinical setting. She has a postbronchodilator $FEV_1$/FVC of <0.70 at

0.643 consistent with a diagnosis of COPD. A postbronchodilator $FEV_1$ of 65.69% of her predicted is considered moderate airflow limitation or GOLD Grade 2 COPD.

Her $FEV_1$ increased by more than 12% and 200 mL, which are the criteria for a positive bronchodilator test. Patients with asthma and COPD can have a positive bronchodilator test, but patients with asthma usually have a more extreme response. In addition, her clinical picture substantiates a diagnosis of both asthma and COPD: significant smoking history and shortness of breath on exertion are common with COPD, whereas allergies are associated more with asthma. Many patients, like Debra T., have both asthma and COPD that can be detected with PFTs and need to be treated appropriately.

| | PREBRONCHODILATOR | | | POSTBRONCHODILATOR | | |
|---|---|---|---|---|---|---|
| PFT | LLN | MEASURED | % PREDICTED | MEASURED | % PREDICTED | % CHANGE |
| FVC (L) | 2.07 | 1.70 | 66 | 2.13 | 82.48 | +24.97 |
| $FEV_1$ (L) | 1.59 | 1.15 | 55.18 | 1.37 | 65.69 | 19.04 |
| $FEV_1$/FVC | 0.696 | 0.676 | | 0.643 | | |

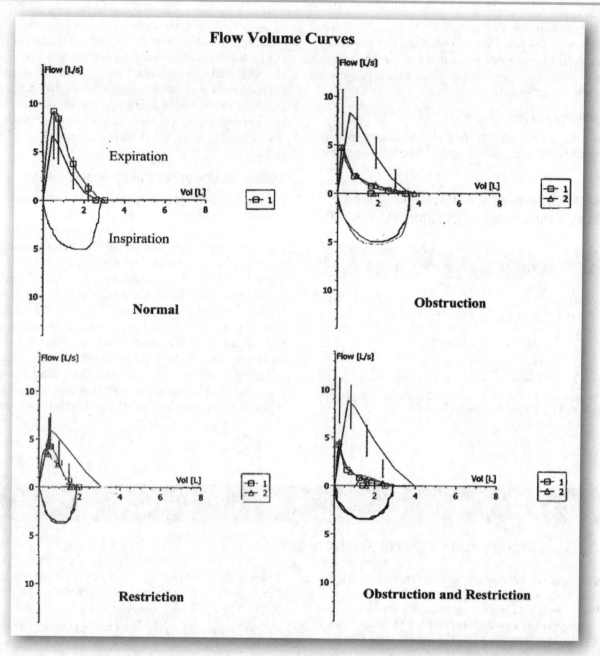

**FIGURE 14-2.** Flow-volume curves seen with obstructive and restrictive pulmonary diseases. This figure illustrates the flow-volume curves observed for normal adults: obstructive, restrictive, and mixed disease. Flow-volume curve number 1 represents baseline spirometry. Flow-volume curve number 2, if present, is a repeat of the spirometry after a bronchodilator is administered. (Refer to bronchodilator studies under Bronchodilator Responsiveness Test.) The curve with the vertical lines represents the predicted normal values. In these examples, there is no improvement in the flow-volume curves after bronchodilator administration. The normal flow-volume curve shows that the curve is larger than expected based on predicted values and is, therefore, normal. Concavity of the expiratory portion of the curve, consistent with limitation in flow compared with the predicted, is illustrated in the airflow limitation flow-volume curve. The restriction flow-volume curve shows a FVC that is smaller than expected. The predicted volume is approximately 3 L; however, the patient's FVC is 2 L. In restriction, although the forced expiratory flows are often decreased, there is no concavity such as seen in the airflow limitation curve. It is important to note that spirometry does not diagnose restriction. The flow-volume loop demonstrates findings such as this consistent with restriction; however, lung volumes are needed to define restriction. Concavity in the expiratory phase and a decreased FVC volume is consistent with a combination of an airflow limitation and restriction flow-volume curve.

maintaining an upright posture, until all the air is exhaled. The patient is then instructed to inspire with maximal effort until completely full. This maneuver can be repeated up to eight times in adults if needed to meet testing standards.

Like most medical tests, spirometry has seen changes over the years in equipment, computer support, and recommendations for standardization. In an effort to maximize the usefulness of spirometry results, the American Thoracic Society (ATS), in conjunction with the European Respiratory Society (ERS), developed standardizations of spirometry testing.[3,4] These recommendations are intended to decrease the variability of spirometry testing by improving the performance of the test. The recommendations cover equipment, quality control, the training and education of people conducting the test, and the training of patients performing the test. The recommendations also provide criteria for acceptability and usability of the patient's spirometry efforts and guidelines on interpreting the spirometry test results. For acceptability and usability of both the $FEV_1$ and FVC results, three criteria must be met. The first criterion is the back-extrapolated volume (BEV), which must be ≤5% of the FVC or 0.100 L, whichever is greater. BEV is the volume of gas exhaled before the start of forced expiration. The BEV would be too high if a patient leaked out air before maximal exhalation. Spirometers show the BEV calculation. The second criterion is the measurement must have no evidence of a faulty zero-flow setting, or airflow through the mouthpiece sensor before the start of the test. Newer spirometers use technology to detect this error and alert the user. The last criterion is there must be no glottic closure in the first second of expiration. Glottic closure appears like a flat line on the volume-time graph and shows a stop in airflow. Because the results of spirometry depend on the patient's effort, at least three acceptable efforts are obtained with a goal of having the two highest measurements of FVC and $FEV_1$ vary ≤0.150 L if the patient's age is >6 years and FVC and $FEV_1$ vary ≤0.100 L or 10% of the highest value, whichever is greater for patients 6 years of age and younger.[4]

### Bronchodilator Responsiveness Test

One of many tests that may be useful in the diagnostic workup of asthma is spirometry with *bronchodilator responsiveness to assess airflow variability*. Before the testing day, the patient is asked to hold short-acting β₂-agonists (SABA) for at least 4 hours; twice daily long-acting β₂-agonists (LABA) for at least 12 hours and once-daily LABA for at least 24 hours; and ultra-LABA for 36 hours and long-acting muscarinic antagonists for 48 hours.[4] Spirometry is performed at baseline and then again 15 to 30 minutes after the administration of an inhaled SABA. A positive bronchodilator response is defined as an improvement of the postbronchodilator $FEV_1$ and FVC by at least 12% and 200 mL from the prebronchodilator measurement.[7] The Global Initiative for Asthma defines airway reversibility in adults as an increase in $FEV_1$ of at least 12% and 200 mL from the prebronchodilator measurement, with more confidence of a positive test with an increase in $FEV_1$ of at least 15% and 400 mL from baseline. For children, an increase of at least 12% of predicted for the $FEV_1$

is considered positive.[6] Minicase 1 illustrates how spirometry is used to confirm COPD and how the bronchodilator reversibility study is useful for diagnosing asthma.

### Peak Expiratory Flow

The peak expiratory flow (PEF) is measured with a simple, inexpensive hand-held peak flow meter that can be used at a patient's home, in the clinician's office, or in the emergency department. Because PEF measures airflow through the upper airway over a shorter time and readings can vary depending on the patient's efforts and meter type, it is not the preferred test to detect airflow limitation.

When spirometry is not available, PEF can be used to help diagnose asthma by assessing diurnal variability.[6,8] Diurnal variability is indicative of asthma when the diurnal variability is >10% after 1 to 2 weeks in adults and >13% for children.[6] One can calculate diurnal variability by dividing [day's highest PEF minus day's lowest PEF] by the mean of these two values and then averaging these daily variability results over 1 week.[9] Twice-daily PEF is measured in the morning before using inhalers and in the afternoon or evening. Variability decreases after about 3 months of use an inhaled corticosteroid.

Peak flow meters are designed for both pediatric and adult patients with PEFR between 60 and 400 L/min for children and between 60 and 850 L/min for adults. PEFR is measured by having a patient perform the following steps:

1. Stand up.
2. Move the indicator on the peak flow meter to the end nearest the mouthpiece.
3. Hold the meter and avoid blocking the movement of the indicator and the holes on the end of the meter.
4. Take a deep breath in and then seal the mouth around the mouthpiece.
5. Blow out into the meter as hard and as fast as possible without coughing into the meter (like blowing out candles on a cake).
6. Examine the indicator on the meter to identify the number corresponding to the peak flow measurement.
7. Repeat the test two more times (remembering to move the indicator to the base of the meter each time).
8. Record the highest value of the three measurements in a diary (readings in the morning and afternoon are ideal).

To establish a patient's personal best peak flow rate, measure the peak flow rate over a 2-week period when asthma symptoms and treatment are stable. The highest value over the 2-week period is the personal best. Using the individual patient's personal best peak flow instead of predicted peak flow values is considered best practice. Asthma patients typically have lower peak flow readings than the healthy population, and using predicted values may result in overtreatment.

Using PEF for long-term monitoring is helpful for patients who have sudden asthma exacerbations or severe asthma. Improved asthma outcomes have been seen in asthma action plans, including personal best PEF. PEF is also helpful for

## MINICASE 2

## Six-Minute Walk Test

Charles O. is a 65-year-old man diagnosed with World Health Organization group 1 pulmonary arterial hypertension after completing a right-heart catheterization. He reports a persistent and progressive dyspnea on exertion with walking from room to room in his home with use of oxygen via nasal cannula at 6 L/min with exertion only. His medications were changed 6 months ago because he was experiencing side effects.

### Test 1. Baseline

|  | SpO$_2$ (%) | HEART RATE (beats/min) | BLOOD PRESSURE (mm Hg) | SUPPLEMENTAL OXYGEN (L/min) |
|---|---|---|---|---|
| Baseline on room air | 89 | 69 | 100/69 | Room air |
| Baseline on supplemental oxygen |  |  |  |  |
| Minute 1 | 90 | 96 |  | Room air |
| Minute 2 | 86 | 104 |  | Room air |
| Minute 3 | 83<br>85 | 109<br>112 |  | 2 L/min O$_2$ NC<br>4 L/min O$_2$ NC |
| Minute 4 | 89 | 114 |  | 6 L/min O$_2$ NC |
| Minute 5 | 89 | 115 |  | 6 L/min O$_2$ NC |
| Minute 6 | 90 | 115 | 104/69 | 6 L/min O$_2$ NC |
| Recovery 2nd minute | 89 | 65 | 106/75 | Room air |
|  |  |  |  |  |
| Distance walked | 274.3 m |  |  |  |
| Number of rests | 0 |  |  |  |
|  |  |  |  |  |
| Borg scale self-rate | Pretest | Posttest |  |  |
| Dyspnea | 2 | 5 |  |  |
| Fatigue | 2 | 5 |  |  |

NC = nasal cannula.

### Test 2. 6 Months Later

|  | SATURATION (%) | HEART RATE (beats/min) | BLOOD PRESSURE (mm Hg) | SUPPLEMENTAL OXYGEN (L/min) |
|---|---|---|---|---|
| Baseline on room air | 90 | 81 | 109/78 | Room air |
| Baseline on supplemental oxygen |  |  |  |  |
| Minute 1 | 91 | 88 |  | Room air |
| Minute 2 | 88 | 103 |  | Room air |
| Minute 3 | 86 | 113 |  | 3 L/min O$_2$ NC |
| Minute 4 | 88 | 115 |  | 4 L/min O$_2$ NC |
| Minute 5 | 90 | 116 |  | 6 L/min O$_2$ NC |

## MINICASE 2 (cont'd)

**Test 2.** 6 Months Later

| | SATURATION (%) | HEART RATE (beats/min) | BLOOD PRESSURE (mm Hg) | SUPPLEMENTAL OXYGEN (L/min) |
|---|---|---|---|---|
| Minute 6 | 90 | 118 | 108/81 | 6 L/min $O_2$ NC |
| Recovery 2nd minute | 90 | 70 | 112/79 | Room air |
| | | | | |
| Distance walked | 320 m | | | |
| Number of rests | 0 | | | |
| | | | | |
| Borg scale self-rate | Pretest | Posttest | | |
| Dyspnea | 2 | 3 | | |
| Fatigue | 2 | 4 | | |

NC = nasal cannula.

QUESTION: Do the results from this patient's 6-month 6MWT show an improvement in distance walked after his medications were changed?

DISCUSSION: According to the first 6MWT, the patient walked 274.3 meters. He required 6 L/min of oxygen with exercise. The patient's distance walked was 48% of the LLN. The patient became tachycardic with exertion, which improved after a 2-minute recovery period. The results of the second 6MWT show the patient walked for 320 m with no rests. The patient required 6 L/min supplemental oxygen with exertion. Comparing his 6MWT after starting the new medication regimen, the patient's 6-minute walk distance improved by 45.7 m and his oxygen requirement remained unchanged. A distance greater than a 30-m walk is considered clinically important.[20] The patient has improved with the medication change.

identifying environmental and occupational asthma triggers along with differentiating between asthma and anxiety symptoms.[6]

## Body Plethysmography

*Body plethysmography* is a method used to obtain lung volume measures. Lung volume tests indicate the amount of gas contained in the lungs at the various stages of inflation. The lung volumes and capacities may be obtained by several methods, including body plethysmography, gas dilution, and imaging techniques.[10] Different methods can have small but significant effects on the values reported. Gas dilution methods only measure ventilated areas, whereas body plethysmography measures both ventilated and nonventilated areas. Therefore, body plethysmography values may be larger in patients with nonventilated or poorly ventilated lung areas. Computed tomography (CT) and magnetic resonance imaging can estimate lung volumes with additional detail of the lung tissue. Because body plethysmography is the most used method, this technique is discussed in more detail.

In body plethysmography, a patient sits in an airtight box and is told to inhale and exhale to functional residual capacity (FRC), or the volume of gas remaining at the end of a normal breath. Inside, a mouthpiece contains a pressure transducer. This is done to measure the change in pressure within the box during respiration. It senses the intrathoracic pressure generated when the patient rapidly and forcefully puffs against the closed mouthpiece. These data are then placed into the equation for Boyle's law:

$$P_1 \times V_1 = P_2 \times V_2$$

where $P_1$ is pressure inside the box in which the patient is seated (atmospheric pressure), $V_1$ is volume of the box, $P_2$ is intrathoracic pressure generated by the patient, and $V_2$ is the calculated volume of the box at the end of chest expansion. The difference between this $V_2$ and the initial volume of the box is the change in the volume of the box which is the same as the change in the volume in the chest. Because temperature ($T_1$ and $T_2$) is constant throughout testing, it is not included in the calculations.

Using this change in volume in Boyle's law again, this test provides a measure of the FRC. Once the FRC is determined, the other lung volumes and capacities can be calculated based on this FRC and volumes obtained in static spirometry. After these data are generated, the patient's plethysmography results are usually compared with references from a presumed normal population. This comparison necessitates the generation of predicted values for that patient if he or she were completely normal and healthy. Through complex mathematical formulas, sitting and standing height, age, sex, race, barometric pressure, and altitude are factored in to give predicted values for the pulmonary functions being assessed. The patient's results are compared with the percentage of predicted values based on the results of these calculations.

## Lung Volumes and Lung Capacities

*Lung volumes* include tidal volume (TV), inspiratory reserve volume (IRV), expiratory reserve volume (ERV), and residual volume (RV). These four volumes in various combinations make up *lung capacities*, which include inspiratory capacity, FRC, SVC, and total lung capacity (TLC).

### Tidal Volume, Functional Residual Capacity, Expiratory Reserve Volume, and Residual Volume

The *tidal volume* is the amount of air inhaled and exhaled at rest in a normal breath. It is usually a small proportion of the lung volume and is infrequently used as a measure of respiratory disease. The IRV is the volume measured from the "top" of the TV (ie, initial point of normal exhalation) to the maximal inspiration. During exhalation, the ERV is the volume from the "bottom" of the TV (ie, initial point of normal inhalation) to maximal expiration. The RV is the volume of air left in the lungs at the end of forced expiration to the bottom of ERV. Without the RV, the lungs would collapse like deflated balloons. In diseases characterized by airflow limitation that trap air in the lungs (eg, COPD), the RV increases and the patient is less able to mobilize trapped air out of the lung. These four lung volumes are depicted in **Figure 14-3**.

### Inspiratory Capacity, Functional Residual Capacity, Slow Vital Capacity, and Total Lung Capacity

The *inspiratory capacity* is the volume measured from the point of the TV at which inhalation normally begins to maximal inspiration, and it is a summation of TV and IRV. The *functional residual capacity* is the sum of the ERV and RV, and it is the volume of gas remaining in the lungs at the end of the TV. It also may be defined as a balance point between chest wall forces that increase volume and lung parenchymal forces that decrease volume. An increased FRC represents hyperinflation of the lungs and usually indicates airflow limitation. The FRC may be decreased in diseases that affect many alveoli (eg, pneumonia) or by restrictive changes, especially those due to fibrotic pulmonary tissue changes. The *SVC* is the volume of air that is exhaled as much as possible after inhaling as much as possible. It is a summation of the IRV, TV, and ERV and is described in more detail in the Spirometry Measurements section. The *total lung capacity* is the summation of all four lung volumes (IRV + TV + ERV + RV). It is the total amount of gas contained in the lungs at maximal inhalation. Restrictive lung disease is defined as a TLC below the 5th percentile of normal predicted value with a normal FEV1/VC ratio.[7]

## Diffusion Capacity Tests

Tests of gas exchange measure the ability of gases to cross (diffuse) the alveolar-capillary membrane and are useful in assessing interstitial lung disease.[11] Typically, these tests measure the per-minute transfer of a gas, usually carbon monoxide (CO), from the alveoli to the blood. CO is used because it is a gas that is not normally present in the lung, has a high affinity for Hgb in red blood cells, and is easily delivered and measured. The diffusion capacity may be lessened after losses in the surface area of the alveoli or thickening of the alveolar-capillary membrane. Membrane thickening may be due to infiltration of inflammatory cells or fibrotic changes. These test results can be confounded by a loss of diffusion capacity due to poor ventilation, which may be related to closed or partially closed airways (as with airflow limitation) or to a ventilation-perfusion mismatch (as with pulmonary emboli or pulmonary hypertension). The diffusion capacity of the lungs to CO can be measured by either a single-breath test or steady-state test.

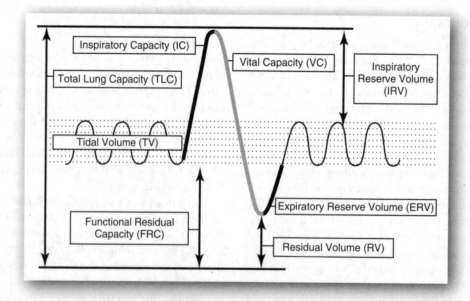

**FIGURE 14-3.** Lung volumes and capacities. Representation of various lung compartments based on a typical spirogram. Refer to Pellegrino et al[6] for more information.

In the single-breath test, the patient deeply inhales—to vital capacity—a mixture of 0.3% CO, a tracer gas such as 10% helium or 0.3% methane, and balanced air. After holding his or her breath for 10 seconds, the patient exhales fully, and the concentrations of CO and helium are measured during the end of expiration (ie, alveolar flow). These concentrations are compared with the inspired concentrations to determine the amount diffusing across the alveolar membrane. The mean value for CO is about 25 to 30 mL/min/mm Hg.

A normal DLCO using a cutoff of the percent predicted has not been standardized but 70% to 75% if often utilized. A normal DLCO is also considered when greater than the LLN for the patient. Diffusion capacity is decreased in diseases that cause alveolar fibrotic changes. Changes may be idiopathic, such as those seen with sarcoidosis or environmental or occupational disease (asbestosis and silicosis), or be induced by drugs (eg, nitrofurantoin, amiodarone, and bleomycin).[12,13] Anything that alters Hgb, decreases the red blood cell Hgb concentration, or changes diffusion across the red blood cell membrane may alter the DLCO. The DLCO also reflects the pulmonary capillary blood volume. An increase in this volume (pulmonary edema or asthma) may increase the DLCO. **Minicase 3** describes how PFTs are used to diagnose restrictive airway disease.

## Specialized Tests
### Bronchial Challenge Tests

*Bronchial challenge tests* (BCTs) are used to (1) aid in the diagnosis of asthma when the more common tests (symptom history, spirometry with reversibility) cannot confirm or reject the

---

# MINICASE 3

## Using Pulmonary Function Tests to Evaluate a Patient with Interstitial Lung Disease

Jacob K. is a 59-year-old man who presents to the medicine clinic with reports of progressive dyspnea on exertion and minimal dry cough for the past 3 months. He has a history of rheumatoid arthritis and was started on methotrexate 4 months ago. CT of the chest shows diffuse ground glass opacities consistent with active inflammation and some minimal fibrosis at the bases. He had a PFT performed over a year ago that was completely normal. A repeat PFT is ordered and includes spirometry, lung volumes, and diffusion capacity. His PFT reveals the following results and the flow-volume curve in Figure 14-2 labeled "Restriction."

QUESTION: How are these PFTs useful in the diagnosis, evaluation, and management of this patient?

DISCUSSION: Looking at his PFT in the following table, the FVC is 56% of predicted (reduced), the FEV$_1$ is 60% of predicted (reduced), and the FEV$_1$/FVC ratio is 0.85 (normal). This is consistent with a restrictive pattern. A TLC is 54% of predicted (reduced), verifying a restrictive pulmonary defect, and the DLCO is 50% of predicted (normal range is ≥70–75% of predicted). These findings are helpful in the diagnosis of interstitial lung disease in the setting of abnormal results on CT scan and change from previous normal spirometry. The severity of restriction can also be determined by the amount of decrease in TLC.[6]

| | PREBRONCHODILATOR | | | POSTBRONCHODILATOR | |
|---|---|---|---|---|---|
| PFT | LLN | MEASURED | % PREDICTED | MEASURED | % CHANGE |
| FVC (L) | 4.09 | 3.03 | 56 | 3.11 | +2 |
| FEV$_1$ (L) | 3.10 | 2.48 | 60 | 2.65 | +6 |
| FEV$_1$/FVC | | 0.82 | | 0.85 | +3 |
| SVC (L) | 4.09 | 3.06 | 57 | | |
| TLC (L) | 6.54 | 4.36 | 54 | | |
| RV (L) | 1.71 | 1.30 | 51 | | |
| DLCO (mL/min/mm Hg) | 22.06 | 15.99 | 50 | | |

He is diagnosed with methotrexate-induced lung disease. The methotrexate is discontinued, and he is treated with prednisone. After 3 months of therapy, a repeat PFT is performed. The FVC is 75% of predicted, the FEV$_1$ is 72% of predicted, and the FEV$_1$/FVC ratio is 0.80. The TLC has increased to 65%, and the DLCO has increased to 60% of predicted. The repeat PFT shows that he is improved. He reports improvement in his symptoms. The follow-up PFT is used to help evaluate the response to discontinuing the offending medication and establish a new pulmonary function status.

diagnosis, (2) evaluate the effects of drug therapy on airway hyperreactivity, and (3) evaluate potential drug effectiveness. A BCT measures the reactivity of the airways to known concentrations of agents that induce airway narrowing. Negative BCTs are useful in excluding the diagnosis of asthma more than confirming the diagnosis when a test is positive. Using this technique in research, the magnitude and duration of the effect of different drugs on the airways may be compared. BCTs are often referred to as *challenges* because the airways are challenged with increasing doses of methacholine, a synthetic derivative of acetylcholine, in a protocolized manner to determine whether there is a drop in the $FEV_1$. A decrease in the $FEV_1$ of 20% at specified doses is considered a positive test result.[14] The ERS has published guidelines for methacholine challenge testing to enhance the safety, accuracy, and validity of the test.[14]

Bronchial challenge testing begins by measuring baseline spirometry parameters to ensure it is safe to conduct the test. A BCT should not be performed if the $FEV_1$ is <60% of predicted.[14] Most BCTs then begin with nebulization of a solution of phosphate buffered saline. This both serves as a placebo to assess the airway effect of nebulization and establishes baseline airway function from which the amount of pulmonary function to be reduced is calculated. After each dose, spirometry efforts are performed based on ATS/ERS criteria. The challenge data are then summarized into a single number, the provocative dose causing a 20% fall in forced expiratory volume in 1 second ($PD_{20}$/mcg).

For methacholine, a $PD_{20}FEV_1$ of <6 mcg indicates severe airway hyperresponsiveness (AHR), 6–25 mcg indicates moderate AHR, 25–100 mcg indicates mild AHR, 100–400 mcg suggests borderline AHR, and >400 mcg is a normal AHR test and excludes asthma. During a BCT, patients may experience transient respiratory symptoms such as cough, shortness of breath, wheezing, and chest tightness. An inhaled, SABA or short-acting muscarinic antagonist may be administered to alleviate symptoms and quicken the return of the $FEV_1$ to the baseline value. Because BCTs can elicit severe, life-threatening bronchospasm, trained personnel and medications to treat severe bronchospasm should be on hand in the testing area.

### Exercise Challenge Test

The *exercise challenge test* is used to confirm or rule out exercise-induced bronchospasm (EIB) and to evaluate the effectiveness of medications used to treat or prevent EIB, which occurs usually in patients with normal PFTs who become symptomatic with exercise. The etiology of EIB is thought to be related to the cooling and drying of the airways caused by rapid breathing during exercise.

Exercise tests are usually done with a motor-driven treadmill (with adjustable speed and grade) or an electromagnetically braked cycle ergometer. Heart rate should be monitored throughout the test, nose clips should be worn, and the room air should be dry and cool to promote water loss from the airways during the exercise test. In most patients, symptoms are effectively blocked by use of an inhaled bronchodilator immediately before beginning exercise or other exertion causing the problem. After obtaining baseline spirometry, the exercise test is started

at a low speed that is gradually increased over 2 to 4 minutes until the heart rate is 80% to 90% of the predicted maximum or the work rate is at 100%. The duration of the exercise is age and tolerance dependent. Children <12 years generally take 6 minutes, while older children and adults take 8 minutes to complete the test. After the exercise is completed, the patient does serial spirometry at 5-minute intervals for 20 to 30 minutes. $FEV_1$ is the primary outcome variable. A 10% or more decrease in $FEV_1$ from baseline is generally accepted as an abnormal response, although some clinicians feel a 15% decrease is more diagnostic of EIB.[15]

### Six-Minute Walk Test

The *six-minute walk test* (6MWT) is a test used to measure the distance a patient can walk on a flat, hard surface in 6 minutes.[16] The results of the test are used to determine if a patient requires continuous oxygen at home. The results have also been correlated to a patient's quality of life and abilities to complete daily activities. The results of the 6MWT also help predict morbidity and mortality for patients with congestive heart failure, COPD, and primary pulmonary hypertension.[17-19] Pulmonary hypertension studies use this test to monitor the efficacy of interventions with medications.[20] Minicase 2 is an example of how a 6MWT is used to monitor a patient with pulmonary hypertension.

While performing the 6MWT, the patient is educated that the goal of the test is to walk as far as possible in 6 minutes, allowing the patient to select the intensity of exercise. Stopping and resting is allowed during the test. Reference equations for healthy adults have been published; however, large variations in the predicted values exist.[21] The minimal important difference for the 6MWT is 30 meters for adults with chronic respiratory disease.[21] Continuous pulse oximetry is recommended to capture the lowest arterial oxygen saturation ($SpO_2$). The lowest $SpO_2$ is a marker for prognosis and disease severity. The test is discontinued if the $SpO_2$ decreases to <80%. Heart rate measurements and heart rate recovery are recorded during the test. Poorer outcomes have been associated with reduced heart rate recovery in the first minute after the test. Use of the Borg scale to document dyspnea and fatigue before and after the 6MWT has good reliability when determining exercise limitations in patients with chronic respiratory disease. Practice tests, younger age, taller height, less weight, male sex, longer corridor length, and encouragement all improve test results. Unstable angina and myocardial infarction in the past 3 to 5 days and syncope and arterial oxygen saturation by pulse oximetry ≤85% are all contraindications for performing the 6MWT.[22] In practice, the 6MWT is also used to assess the amount of oxygen needed with exertion. Patients with mild-to-moderate pulmonary disease may have normal oxygen saturation at rest but poor saturation with exertion. An oxygen saturation of ≤88% indicates the need for supplemental oxygen.

### Carbon Monoxide Breath Test

Carbon monoxide is a poisonous gas emitted from anything burning, including cigarette smoke. As discussed in the Diffusion Capacity Tests section, CO binds more readily to Hgb than oxygen, causing increased fatigue and shortness of breath.

With a simple breath test by a handheld CO meter, the patient can see how much CO is in the body (parts per million [ppm]) and in the blood (% COHgb). In clinical studies, a result of ≤10 ppm often defines a nonsmoker; however, in clinical practice, depending on the meter used, the level is usually lower. A Cochrane Review found no significant increase in smoking abstinence rates with CO measurements.[23]

Testing exhaled CO is a simple breath test in which the patient holds his or her breath for 15 seconds and then exhales into a meter. The meter is able to indicate how much CO is in the patient's lungs and estimate how much is attached to Hgb in the patient's blood. The test is an objective value in which patients can visually see the effects of inhaling smoke when higher values of CO are detected. After 8 to 12 hours without smoking, CO levels become undetectable.

### Fractional Exhaled Nitric Oxide

Measurement of exhaled concentrations of nitric oxide is a noninvasive biomarker test of airway inflammation for both diagnosing and monitoring eosinophilic airway inflammation.[24] Various handheld devices using the patient's breath are available that include an electrochemical sensor to determine the exhaled nitric oxide concentration. *Fractional exhaled nitric oxide* (FENO) results of >50 parts per billion (ppb) in adults and >35 ppb in children younger than 12 years indicate eosinophilic inflammation with a high likelihood to respond to corticosteroids and certain add-on biologic asthma treatments.[25,26] As a monitoring test, FENO results are best interpreted as changes from baseline for each patient rather than using population normal readings. FENO measurements have many confounding factors, including smoking history, age, and sex. The test should be used in context with the patient history and as a tool with other diagnostic and monitoring tests.

## SUMMARY

This chapter discusses the importance of pulmonary function testing as it relates to the diagnosis, treatment, and monitoring of respiratory disease states. After a review of the anatomy and physiology of the lungs, the mechanics of obtaining PFTs were emphasized. By understanding these mechanics, a clinician can better understand the interpretation of PFTs, use findings from different PFTs to help differentiate among diagnoses, and assist in making optimal therapeutic recommendations. PFT results are not interpreted in isolation but need to be assessed within the context of the other findings from the medical history and from other laboratory or clinical test results. Clearly, PFTs are an important tool to aid the clinician in decision-making.

## LEARNING POINTS

### 1. What is a PFT?

**ANSWER:** A PFT is any test used to assess the function of the lungs (eg, spirometry, body plethysmography, 6MWT). The component of the PFT to be ordered is determined by the information needed. For example, spirometry is performed to reveal the presence of obstructive lung disease. Lung volumes determine the presence of restrictive lung disease, and the diffusion capacity test ascertains the adequacy of gas exchange.

### 2. Why is spirometry an important test in the diagnosis of COPD?

**ANSWER:** In COPD, postbronchodilator spirometry is necessary to determine the presence of persistent airflow limitation and the degree of disease severity. In the absence of COPD, other causes of symptoms should be considered. Physical exam and history alone are often not adequate to detect airflow limitation. Therefore, an objective test with spirometry is needed to confirm a clinical suspicion.

### 3. Does a significant bronchodilator response on spirometry testing differentiate asthma from COPD?

**ANSWER:** Traditionally, reversibility after bronchodilator use was considered a criterion to differentiate asthma and COPD. However, evidence has shown that a significant bronchodilator response is common in COPD as well, and this assessment is no longer used to differentiate between asthma and COPD. It is still a useful test when used in conjunction with a clinical history (eg, risk factors for COPD, presentation of shortness of breath, evidence of atopy), physical exam, and other PFTs to support a clinical suspicion of asthma and/or COPD.

### 4. How is restrictive lung disease diagnosed?

**ANSWER:** It is important to note that spirometry only can provide evidence consistent with restrictive disease, such as a decrease in $FEV_1$ and FVC with a normal or elevated $FEV_1/FVC$ ratio. However, restriction is a decrease in lung volume as defined by a decrease in the TLC, which is obtained by lung volume tests, such as body plethysmography. Test results are needed to diagnose restrictive lung disease.

## REFERENCES

1. Milavetz G, Teresi M. Pulmonary function and related tests. In Lee M, ed., *Basic Skills in Interpreting Laboratory Data*, 3rd ed. Bethesda, MD: American Society of Health-System Pharmacists; 2004.

2. Crapo RO. Pulmonary-function testing. *N Engl J Med.* 1994;331(1):25-30. PubMed

3. Culver BH, Graham BL, Coates AL, et al. American Thoracic Society Committee on Proficiency Standards for Pulmonary Function Report. An official American Thoracic Society technical statement. *Am J Respir Crit Care Med.* 2017;196(11):1463-1472.PubMed

4. Graham BL, Steenbruggen I, Miller MR, et al. Standardization of spirometry 2019 update: an official American Thoracic Society and European Respiratory Society technical statement. *Am J Respir Crit Care Med.* 2019;200(8):e70-e88.PubMed

5. Global Strategy for the Diagnosis, Management, and Prevention of Chronic Obstructive Pulmonary Disease. Global Initiative for Chronic Obstructive Lung Disease (GOLDCOPD) 2022 Report. http://www.goldcopd.org. Accessed February 1, 2022.

6. Global Initiative for Asthma. Global strategy for asthma management and prevention, 2020. http://www.ginasthma.org. Accessed Aug 3, 2020.

7. Pellegrino R, Viegi G, Brusasco V, et al. Interpretative strategies for lung function tests. *Eur Respir J.* 2005;26(5):948-968.PubMed

8. Dekker FW, Schrier AC, Sterk PJ, et al. Validity of peak expiratory flow measurement in assessing reversibility of airflow obstruction. *Thorax.* 1992;47(3):162-166.PubMed

9. Reddel HK, Taylor DR, Bateman ED, et al. An official American Thoracic Society/European Respiratory Society statement: asthma control and exacerbations: standardizing endpoints for clinical asthma trials and clinical practice. *Am J Respir Crit Care Med.* 2009;180(1):59-99.PubMed

10. Wanger J, Clausen JL, Coates A, et al. Standardisation of the measurement of lung volumes. *Eur Respir J.* 2005;26(3):511-522.PubMed

11. Graham BL, Brusasco V, Burgos F, et al. 2017 ERS/ATS standards for single-breath carbon monoxide uptake in the lung. *Eur Respir J.* 2017;49(1):1600016.PubMed

12. Cooper JA Jr, White DA, Matthay RA. Drug-induced pulmonary disease. Part 1: cytotoxic drugs. *Am Rev Respir Dis.* 1986;133(2):321-340.PubMed

13. Cooper JA Jr, White DA, Matthay RA. Drug-induced pulmonary disease. Part 2: noncytotoxic drugs. *Am Rev Respir Dis.* 1986;133(3):488-505. PubMed

14. Coates AL, Wanger J, Cockcroft DW, et al. ERS technical standard on bronchial challenge testing: general considerations and performance of methacholine challenge tests. *Eur Respir J.* 2017;49(5):1601526.PubMed

15. Parsons JP, Hallstrand TS, Mastronarde JG, et al. An official American Thoracic Society clinical practice guideline: exercise-induced bronchoconstriction. *Am J Respir Crit Care Med.* 2013;187(9):1016-1027. PubMed

16. Holland AE, Spruit MA, Troosters T, et al. An official European Respiratory Society/American Thoracic Society technical standard: field walking tests in chronic respiratory disease. *Eur Respir J.* 2014;44(6):1428-1446.PubMed

17. Cahalin LP, Mathier MA, Semigran MJ, et al. The six-minute walk test predicts peak oxygen uptake and survival in patients with advanced heart failure. *Chest.* 1996;110(2):325-332.PubMed

18. Kessler R, Faller M, Fourgaut G, et al. Predictive factors of hospitalization for acute exacerbation in a series of 64 patients with chronic obstructive pulmonary disease. *Am J Respir Crit Care Med.* 1999;159(1):158-164. PubMed

19. Kadikar A, Maurer J, Kesten S. The six-minute walk test: a guide to assessment for lung transplantation. *J Heart Lung Transplant.* 1997;16(3):313-319.PubMed

20. Klinger JR, Elliott CG, Levine DJ, et al. Therapy for pulmonary arterial hypertension in adults: update of the CHEST guideline and expert panel report. *Chest.* 2019;155(3):565-586.PubMed

21. Singh SJ, Puhan MA, Andrianopoulos V, et al. An official systematic review of the European Respiratory Society/American Thoracic Society: measurement properties of field walking tests in chronic respiratory disease. *Eur Respir J.* 2014;44(6):1447-1478.PubMed

22. American Thoracic Society. American College of Chest Physicians, ATS/ACCP statement on cardiopulmonary exercise testing. *Am J Respir Crit Care Med.* 2003;167:211-277.

23. Bize R, Burnand B, Mueller Y, et al. Biomedical risk assessment as an aid for smoking cessation. *Cochrane Database Syst Rev.* 2012;12:CD004705. PubMed

24. American Thoracic Society. Recommendations for standardized procedures for the online and offline measurement of exhaled lower respiratory nitric oxide and nasal nitric oxide in adults and children: 1999. *Am J Respir Crit Care Med.* 1999;160:2104-2117.

25. Dweik RA, Boggs PB, Erzurum SC, et al. An official ATS clinical practice guideline: interpretation of exhaled nitric oxide levels (FENO) for clinical applications. *Am J Respir Crit Care Med.* 2011;184(5):602-615. PubMed

26. Global Initiative for Asthma. GINA Difficult-to-treat and severe asthma in adolescent and adult patients diagnosis and management. A GINA pocket guide for health professionals. V 2.April 0, 2019. https://ginasthma.org/wp-content/uploads/2019/04/GINA-Severe-asthma-Pocket-Guide-v2.0-wms-1.pdf. Accessed October 25, 2020.

# 15

# Liver and Gastroenterology Tests

*Paul Farkas, Joanna Sampson, Matthew Slitzky, and Jason Altman*

## OBJECTIVES

*After completing this chapter, the reader should be able to*

- Discuss how the anatomy and physiology of the liver and pancreas affect interpretation of pertinent laboratory test results

- Classify liver test abnormalities into cholestatic and hepatocellular patterns and understand the approach to evaluating patients with these abnormalities

- Explain how hepatic and other diseases, as well as drugs and analytical interferences, cause abnormal laboratory test results for bilirubin

- Understand hepatic encephalopathy and the role of serum ammonia in its diagnosis

- Discuss the laboratory test abnormalities typically associated with hemochromatosis

- Design and interpret a panel of laboratory studies to determine if a patient has active, latent, or previous viral hepatitis infection

- Understand the significance and use of amylase and lipase in evaluating abdominal pain and pancreatic disorders

- Discuss the role of *Helicobacter pylori* in peptic ulcer disease and the tests used to diagnose it

- Discuss the tests and procedures used to diagnose *Clostridioides difficile* colitis

Hepatic and other gastrointestinal (GI) abnormalities can cause a variety of clinically significant diseases, in part because of their central role in the body's biochemistry. This chapter provides an introduction to common laboratory studies used to investigate these diseases. Studies of the liver are roughly divided into those associated with (1) synthetic liver function, (2) excretory liver function and cholestasis, (3) hepatocellular injury, and (4) detoxifying liver function and serum ammonia. Specific tests may also be used to investigate specific disease processes, including viral hepatitis, primary biliary cholangitis (PBC), and hemochromatosis. This chapter also covers several tests for specific nonhepatic disease processes, including pancreatitis, *Helicobacter pylori* infection, and *Clostridioides difficile* colitis.

## ANATOMY AND PHYSIOLOGY OF THE LIVER AND PANCREAS

### Liver

The liver, located in the right upper quadrant of the abdomen, is the largest solid organ in the human body. It has two sources of blood.

1. The hepatic artery, originating from the aorta, supplies arterial blood rich in oxygen.
2. Portal veins carry the venous blood from the intestines to the liver. They transport absorbed toxins, drugs, and nutrients directly to the liver for metabolism.

The liver is divided into thousands of lobules (**Figure 15-1**). Each lobule is comprised of plates of hepatocytes (liver cells) that radiate from the central vein much like spokes in a wheel. Between adjacent liver cells formed by matching grooves in the cell membranes are small bile canaliculi. The hepatocytes continually form and secrete bile into these canaliculi, which empty into terminal bile ducts. Subsequently, like tiny streams forming a river, these bile ducts empty into larger and larger ducts until they ultimately merge into the common bile duct. Bile then drains into the gallbladder for temporary storage or directly into the duodenum.

The liver is a complex organ with a prominent role in all aspects of the body's biochemistry. It takes up amino acids absorbed by the intestines, processes them, and synthesizes them into circulating proteins, including albumin and clotting factors. The liver is also involved in breaking down excess amino acids and processing byproducts, including ammonia and urea. The liver plays a similar role in absorbing carbohydrates from the gut, storing them in the form of glycogen, and releasing them as needed to prevent hypoglycemia. Most lipid and lipoprotein metabolism, including cholesterol synthesis, occurs in the liver. The liver is the primary location for detoxification and excretion of a wide variety of endogenous substances produced by the body (including sex hormones) as well as exogenous substances absorbed by the intestines (including a panoply of drugs and toxins). Thus, in patients with liver failure, standard dosing of some medications can lead to dangerously high serum concentrations and toxicity. The role of the liver in bilirubin metabolism is explored further later in the chapter.

DOI 10.37573/9781585286423.015

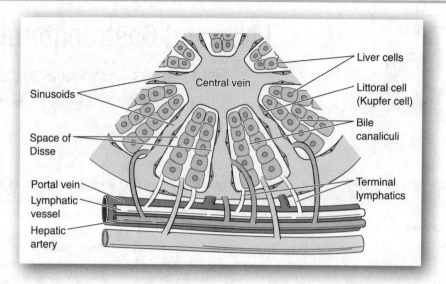

**FIGURE 15-1.** Basic structure of a liver lobule, including the lymph flow system comprised of the spaces of Disse and interlobular lymphatics. *Source:* Reproduced with permission from Guyton AC. *Medical Physiology*. 5th ed. Philadelphia, PA: WB Saunders; 1976.

With its double blood supply, large size, and critical role in regulating body metabolic pathways, the liver is affected by many systemic diseases. Although numerous illnesses affect the liver, it has tremendous reserve capacity and can often maintain its function despite significant disease. Furthermore, the liver is one of the few human organs capable of regeneration.

## Pancreas

The pancreas is an elongated gland located in the retroperitoneum. Its head lies in close proximity to the duodenum, and the pancreatic ducts empty into the duodenum. The pancreas has both exocrine glands (which secrete digestive enzymes into the duodenum) and endocrine glands (which secrete hormones directly into the circulation).

The pancreatic exocrine glands produce enzymes that aid in digestion of proteins, fats, and carbohydrates (including trypsin, chymotrypsin, lipase, and amylase). Insufficient enzyme production (ie, pancreatic exocrine insufficiency) is associated with malabsorption of nutrients, leading to progressive weight loss and severe diarrhea. The glands also produce many hormones, including insulin and glucagon. Insufficient insulin production leads to diabetes mellitus. Thus, the pancreas plays an important role in digestion and absorption of food as well as metabolism of sugar. Like the liver, the pancreas has a tremendous reserve capacity; >90% glandular destruction is required before diabetes or pancreatic insufficiency develops.

## INTRODUCTION TO LIVER TESTS AND THE LIVER FUNCTION TEST PANEL

Investigation of liver disease often begins with obtaining a panel of liver tests, generally referred to as the *LFT panel* or *liver function tests* (LFTs).[1] This panel may vary slightly between hospitals and laboratories but generally includes the aminotransferases

**TABLE 15-1.** Categories of Liver Tests

| PROCESS | MOST CLOSELY RELATED TESTS |
|---|---|
| Protein synthesis | Albumin<br>Prealbumin<br>PT/INR (clotting factors) |
| Excretion into the bile ducts and drainage into the duodenum (impairment of this process is defined as cholestasis) | Bilirubin<br>ALP<br>5′-nucleotidase<br>GGT |
| Hepatocellular injury | Aminotransferases:<br>AST<br>ALT |
| Detoxification | Ammonia ($NH_3+$) |

(previously referred to as *transaminases*), including aspartate aminotransferase (AST), alanine aminotransferase (ALT), bilirubin, alkaline phosphatase (ALP), and albumin. LFT is a misnomer because not all tests actually measure liver function (specifically, aminotransferases reflect liver injury).

Additionally, the liver has multiple functions, and different tests reflect these different functions. **Table 15-1** divides liver tests into rough categories. Although there is considerable overlap between these categories, these divisions may provide an initial framework for understanding the LFT panel.

This grouping of tests mirrors a division of liver diseases into two broad categories: cholestatic and hepatocellular. In cholestatic disease, there is an abnormality in the excretory function of the liver (ie, namely secretion of bile by hepatocytes and passage of bile through the liver and bile ducts into the duodenum). In hepatocellular disease, there is primary inflammation and damage to the hepatocytes themselves (eg, due to viral infection of the hepatocytes). These two categories may overlap because disease of the hepatocytes (hepatocellular processes), if severe enough, will also lead to derangement of bile secretion. However, the distinction between primarily cholestatic and primarily hepatocellular diseases and, in turn, LFT patterns, remains useful and fundamental. Further confusing is the fact that liver test results may be abnormal in patients with diseases that do not affect the liver.

The range of normal laboratory values used here is taken from *Harrison's Principles of Internal Medicine*, 19th edition.[2] Reference ranges may vary slightly between different laboratories, and most laboratories list their reference ranges along with laboratory results. Listed normal ranges are for adult patients; normal ranges for pediatric patients often have different values.

# TESTS OF SYNTHETIC LIVER FUNCTION

As discussed previously, one of the functions of the liver is to synthesize proteins that circulate in the blood, including albumin and clotting proteins. Measurement of the levels of these proteins in the blood provides a reflection of the ability of the liver to synthesize them. The liver has an enormous reserve function so that it may synthesize normal amounts of proteins despite significant liver damage. Therefore, tests of synthetic function are not sensitive to low levels of liver damage or dysfunction. Inadequate protein synthetic function is mainly limited to *hepatic cirrhosis*, which is scarring of the liver that can result from years of alcohol abuse, inflammation, or massive liver damage (eg, due to alcoholic liver disease, severe acute viral hepatitis, autoimmune hepatitis, unrecognized and untreated chronic hepatitis, or potentially lethal toxin ingestion). In these situations, measuring synthetic function may be useful in determining prognosis by reflecting the degree of hepatic failure. The most commonly used tests of protein synthetic function are albumin, prothrombin time (PT), and International Normalized Ratio (INR). An example of this is the Model for End-stage Liver Disease score, which uses the prothrombin time/INR (PT/INR) to help assess the severity of a patient's liver disease and has been used to prioritize patients awaiting liver transplants.

## Albumin

*Normal range: 4 to 5 g/dL (40 to 50 g/L)*
*Albumin* is a major plasma protein that is involved in maintaining plasma oncotic pressure and the binding and transport of numerous hormones, anions, drugs, and fatty acids. The normal serum half-life of albumin is about 20 days, with about 4% degraded daily.[3] Because of albumin's long half-life, serum albumin measurements are slow to fall after the onset of hepatic dysfunction (eg, complete cessation of albumin production results in only a 25% decrease in serum concentrations after 8 days). For this reason,

levels are often normal in acute viral hepatitis or drug-related hepatotoxicity. Alternatively, albumin is commonly reduced in patients with chronic synthetic dysfunction caused by cirrhosis.

Albumin levels may be low due to a variety of other abnormalities in protein synthesis, distribution, and excretion, in addition to liver dysfunction. These abnormalities include malnutrition/malabsorption; protein loss from the gut, kidney, or skin (as in nephrotic syndrome, protein-losing enteropathy, or severe burns, respectively); or increased blood volume (eg, following administration of large volumes of intravenous [IV] fluids). Albumin is a negative acute phase reactant, meaning that in the setting of systemic inflammation (eg, due to infection or malignancy), the liver produces less albumin, and there is a shifting of albumin out of the intravascular compartment. Severely ill, hospitalized patients commonly have low albumin levels due to a combination of poor nutrition, systemic inflammation, and IV fluid administration. In these patients, extremely low albumin concentrations carry a poor prognosis regardless of any particular liver disease. Although hypoalbuminemia is common in these patients, there is little evidence to support replacement simply for a low albumin concentration. Given the numerous causes of a low albumin level, it is important to interpret it within the context of each patient. For example, in a patient with metastatic cancer and no known liver disease, a low albumin level suggests decreased nutritional intake and advanced malignancy with systemic inflammation. Alternatively, in a patient with known cirrhosis, a low albumin level suggests severe chronic liver failure. While a low albumin level is commonly found in elderly patients with suboptimal nutrition, it may also suggest the presence of significant disease and requires further consideration and often investigation.

Hypoalbuminemia itself is usually not associated with specific symptoms or findings until concentrations become quite low. At very low concentrations (<2 to 2.5 g/dL), patients can develop peripheral edema, ascites, or pulmonary edema. Albumin normally generates oncotic pressure, which holds fluid in the vasculature. Under conditions of low albumin, fluid leaks from the vasculature into the interstitial spaces of subcutaneous tissues or into the body cavities. Calcium is bound to albumin, so a decrease in serum albumin may be associated with a decrease in total calcium concentrations, but the ionized (ie, free) calcium concentration usually does not change. In the presence of hypoalbuminemia, measuring an ionized calcium level helps sort this out. Finally, in the presence of low albumin concentration, the percentage of nonprotein bound medication in the bloodstream is increased for highly protein-bound agents (eg, phenytoin, warfarin, and salicylates). This could result in increased pharmacologic effects or adverse effects from usual doses of these medications.

Hyperalbuminemia is seen in patients with marked dehydration (which concentrates their plasma), in which it is associated with concurrent elevations in blood urea nitrogen (BUN) and hematocrit. Patients taking anabolic steroids may demonstrate truly increased albumin concentrations, but those on heparin or ampicillin may have falsely elevated results with some assays. Perhaps the most common cause of hyperalbuminemia is iatrogenic, overzealous use of parenteral albumin, which may be associated with fluid overload. Otherwise, hyperalbuminemia is not associated with any symptoms.

## Prealbumin (Transthyretin)

*Normal range: 17 to 34 mg/dL (170 to 340 mg/L)*
*Prealbumin* is similar to albumin in several respects: it is synthesized primarily by the liver, involved in the binding and transport of various solutes (thyroxin and retinol), and affected by similar factors that affect albumin levels. The primary difference between the two proteins is that prealbumin has a short half-life (2 days, compared with 20 days for albumin) and a smaller body pool than albumin, making the former more rapidly responsive than albumin.[4] Additionally, due to its high percentage of tryptophan and essential amino acids, prealbumin is more sensitive to protein nutrition than albumin and is less affected by liver disease or hydration status than albumin.[5] In practice, prealbumin is generally used to assess protein calorie nutrition, which is discussed in more detail in Chapter 12.[6]

## International Normalized Ratio and Prothrombin Time

*Normal range: INR 0.9 to 1.1; PT 12.7 to 15.4 seconds*
For an introduction to INR and PT, please see Chapter 17. These two tests measure the speed of a set of reactions in the extrinsic pathway of the coagulation cascade. Decreased synthesis or impaired activation of clotting factors correlates with prolonged reaction times and increased values of INR and PT. Both PT and INR are two different measures of the same set of reactions, with the INR being a derived index that takes into account variations between test reagents used in different laboratories. As such, INR is more precise and easily interpretable and replaces the use of the PT.

The liver is required for the synthesis of clotting factors (with the exception of factor VIII), many of which require a vitamin K cofactor for their activation. Therefore, either hepatic impairment or vitamin K deficiency may lead to a deficiency in activated clotting factors with subsequent prolongation of PT/INR. Both synthetic failure and vitamin K deficiency may also cause prolongation of activated partial thromboplastin time, which measures a different set of coagulation reactions in the intrinsic coagulation cascade, but to a much lesser degree than PT/INR.

The prolongation of PT/INR alone is not specific for liver disease. It can be seen in many situations, most of which interfere with the use of vitamin K, a cofactor required for the proper posttranslational activation of clotting factors II, VII, IX, and X. Because vitamin K is a fat-soluble vitamin, inadequate vitamin K in the diet or fat malabsorption as caused by cholestasis may cause hypovitaminosis. Many broad-spectrum antibiotics, including tetracyclines, may reduce vitamin K–producing flora in the gut. The anticoagulant agent warfarin interferes directly with vitamin K–dependent activation of clotting factors.

If the etiology of elevated PT/INR remains unclear despite obtaining additional coagulation tests, then the clinical approach is to provide parenteral vitamin K.[7] Although commonly given as a subcutaneous injection, vitamin K (10 mg) can be given by slow IV infusion in patients with prolonged PT/INR with

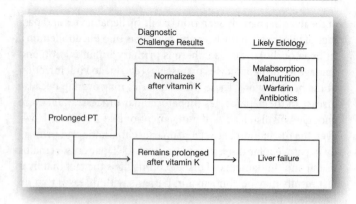

**FIGURE 15-2.** Evaluation of a prolonged PT/INR.

serious bleeding. If the PT/INR is prolonged due to malabsorption, warfarin, perturbed gut flora, or the absence of vitamin K in the diet, the PT/INR usually corrects by at least 30% within 24 hours. Alternatively, failure of PT/INR to normalize despite parenteral vitamin K suggests impaired synthetic liver function (**Figure 15-2**). Other factors that may cause a prolonged PT/INR that does not respond to parenteral vitamin K include inherited clotting factor deficiencies.

Because clotting factors are produced in excess of need and because the liver has tremendous synthetic reserves, only substantial hepatic impairment (>80% loss of synthetic capability) leads to decreased synthesis of these factors and subsequent clotting abnormalities. Thus, PT/INR, albumin, and prealbumin levels lack sensitivity and may remain normal in the face of substantial liver damage. However, they have considerable prognostic value if liver damage is sufficient to affect them. Unlike albumin (which responds slowly to hepatic insult), PT/INR responds within 24 hours to changes in hepatic status because of the short half-life of certain clotting proteins (ie, factor VII has a half-life of <6 hours). Thus, the PT/INR may become elevated days before other manifestations of liver failure and, likewise, may normalize before other evidence of clinical improvement. One use for determining PT/INR in liver disease is to provide prognostic data, generally in situations in which the cause of the elevated PT/INR is known; for example, with an acute acetaminophen overdose leading to hepatic failure.

In addition to serving as an LFT, PT/INR has direct clinical relevance in accessing a patient's tendency to bleed spontaneously or as a result of surgical or diagnostic procedures. Bleeding is a dramatic complication of hepatic failure. When the PT/INR is significantly elevated, bleeding may be controlled or at least diminished by coagulation factors or fresh frozen plasma, which contains the needed activated clotting factors and often corrects the PT/INR temporarily.

## CHOLESTATIC LIVER DISEASE

*Cholestasis* is a deficiency of the excretory function of the liver. As described previously, bile is normally secreted by hepatocytes into bile canaliculi, where it flows into larger bile ducts and eventually empties into the duodenum. Excretion of bile from the liver serves multiple purposes. Certain large lipophilic toxins, drugs, and endogenous substances are eliminated by secretion into the bile with eventual elimination in the feces. Bile salts also play an important role in dissolving and absorbing dietary fat-soluble vitamins and nutrients within the small intestine.

Failure of the excretory functions of the liver leads to a predictable set of consequences. Substances normally secreted in the bile accumulate, resulting in jaundice (from bilirubin), pruritus (from bile salts), or xanthomas (from lipid deposits in skin). Absence of bile salts to dissolve fat-soluble nutrients can lead to deficiencies of fat-soluble vitamins A, D, E, and K, which may result in osteoporosis (lack of vitamin D) and PT/INR elevation (lack of vitamin K).

Cholestatic syndromes may be subclassified as either disorders of hepatocytes and microscopic bile ducts (*intrahepatic cholestasis*) or anatomic obstruction of the macroscopic bile ducts (*extrahepatic cholestasis*).[8] The approach to a patient with cholestasis generally begins with a radiographic study, often a right upper-quadrant ultrasound, to look for dilation of bile ducts within or outside of the liver. Dilation of the bile ducts indicates extrahepatic cholestasis; otherwise, extrahepatic cholestasis is largely excluded, and the next step is to investigate for various causes of intrahepatic cholestasis.

## Intrahepatic Cholestasis

*Intrahepatic cholestasis* includes a variety of processes that interfere with hepatocyte secretion of bile as well as diseases of the microscopic and macroscopic bile ducts within the liver. Etiologies involving impaired hepatocyte secretion of bile overlap to some extent with hepatocellular diseases as noted previously; such processes include viral hepatitis (especially type A), alcoholic hepatitis, and even cirrhosis. Processes that cause a cholestatic pattern include a variety of drugs (**Table 15-2**), pregnancy, severe infection (cholestasis of sepsis), and certain nonhepatic neoplasms, especially renal cell carcinoma. Infiltrative processes of the liver produce a primarily cholestatic pattern, and these include granulomatous diseases and amyloidosis. PBC causes inflammatory scarring of the microscopic bile ducts, whereas sclerosing cholangitis is a similar process that may affect

**TABLE 15-2.** Classification of Liver Disease[a]

| HEPATOCELLULAR | CHOLESTATIC |
|---|---|
| Viral hepatitis | Intrahepatic |
| Autoimmune hepatitis | Systemic illness (ie, sepsis, CHF) |
| Impaired blood flow | Extrahepatic neoplasms (ie, renal cell) |
| Hypotension (shock liver) | |
| Congestive heart failure | Cholestasis of pregnancy |
| Metabolic diseases | Infiltrative liver diseases |
| Hemochromatosis | Granulomatous (sarcoid, TB) |
| Wilson disease | Lymphoma |
| Alcoholic hepatitis | Metastatic carcinoma |
| NAFLD | |

**TABLE 15-2.** Classification of Liver Disease[a], cont'd

| HEPATOCELLULAR | CHOLESTATIC |
|---|---|
| **Drugs include** | Inflammatory diseases of bile ducts |
| Acetaminophen | PBC |
| ACE inhibitors | PSC |
| Allopurinol | AIDS Cholangiopathy |
| Amiodarone | IgG4 associated disease |
| Antiepileptic agents | Benign postoperative jaundice. |
| Carbamazepine | **Drugs include** |
| Phenytoin | Allopurinol |
| Valproic acid | Antibiotics |
| Antimicrobial agents | Erythromycin |
| Amoxicillin– clavulanate | β-lactams |
| Azole antifungals | Rifampin |
| Dapsone | Cardiovascular |
| Fluoroquinolones | Amiodarone |
| INH | Captopril |
| Nitrofurantoin | Diltiazem |
| Protease inhibitors | Quinidine |
| Sulfonamides | Carbamazepine |
| Azathioprine | Hormonal agents |
| Cisplatin | Estrogens |
| Glyburide | Methyltestosterone |
| Heparin | Anabolic steroids |
| Labetalol | Niacin |
| Methotrexate | NSAIDs |
| Methyldopa | Penicillamine |
| Niacin | Phenothiazines |
| NSAIDs | Sulfa drugs |
| Phenothiazines | TPN (hyperalimentation) |
| Trazodone | Extrahepatic |
| Statin medications | Biliary stricture |
| Herbal medications | Gallstone-obstructing bile duct |
| Nutritional supplements | Tumors |
| Illicit drugs | Pancreatic cancer |
| Toxins | Cholangiocarcinoma of bile duct |
| | PSC |
| | AIDS cholangiopathy |

ACE = angiotensin-converting enzyme; INH = isoniazid; NAFLD = nonalcoholic fatty liver disease; TPN = total parenteral nutrition.
[a]Note that listings of drugs contain more commonly used agents and are not exhaustive. For any particular patient, potentially causative drugs should be specifically researched in the appropriate databases to determine any hepatotoxic effects, such as the National Library of Medicine database, LiverTox: Livertox.nih.gov/.

microscopic or macroscopic bile ducts. Masses within the liver, including tumors or abscesses, may block the flow of bile as well.

## Extrahepatic Cholestasis

*Extrahepatic cholestasis* involves obstruction of the larger bile ducts both inside and outside the liver. The most common cause is stones in the common bile duct; other causes include obstruction by strictures (after surgery), tumors (of the pancreas, ampulla of Vater, duodenum, or bile ducts), chronic pancreatitis with scarring of the ducts as they pass through the pancreas, and parasitic infections of the ducts. Another cause is primary sclerosing cholangitis (PSC), a disease-causing diffuse inflammation of the bile ducts, often both intrahepatic and extrahepatic. Of note is that PSC is associated with inflammatory bowel disease, especially involving the colon. Some patients with human immunodeficiency virus (HIV) can develop a picture similar to sclerosing cholangitis, referred to as *AIDS cholangiopathy*. Although previously referred to as *surgical cholestasis*, extrahepatic cholestasis can often be treated or at least palliated using endoscopic means (eg, dilation of strictures with or without stent placement). Another entity is immunoglobulin G (IgG) 4–related sclerosing cholangitis. This is an autoimmune disease, a variant of autoimmune hepatitis, often with elevated autoimmune markers (antinuclear antibody, abnormal serum protein electrophoresis). It can present with a picture of sclerosing cholangitis or even one mimicking cholangiocarcinoma, but the elevated autoimmune markers, especially elevated levels of IgG4, help make this distinction. Tissue biopsy reveals IgG4, plasma cell infiltrates, and interstitial fibrosis. Patients characteristically respond to glucocorticoids.

## Tests Associated with Excretory Liver Function and Cholestasis

Laboratory tests do not distinguish between intrahepatic and extrahepatic cholestasis. This distinction is usually made radiographically. In most instances of extrahepatic cholestasis, a damming effect causes dilation of bile ducts above the obstruction, which can be visualized via computed tomography (CT), magnetic resonance imaging (MRI), or ultrasound. Laboratory abnormalities primarily associated with cholestasis include elevation of ALP, 5′-nucleotidase, γ-glutamyl transpeptidase (GGT), and bilirubin.

## Alkaline Phosphatase

*Normal range: 33 to 96 units/L (0.56 to 1.63 μkat/L)*
*Alkaline phosphatase* (ALP) refers to a group of isoenzymes whose exact function remains unknown. These enzymes are found in many body tissues, including the liver, bone, small intestine, kidneys, placenta, and leukocytes. In the liver, they are found primarily in the bile canalicular membranes of the liver cells. In adults, most serum ALP comes from the liver and bone (~80%), with the remainder mostly contributed by the small intestine.

Normal ALP concentrations vary primarily with age. In children and adolescents, elevated ALP concentrations result from bone growth, which may be associated with elevations as high as three times the adult normal range. Similarly, increase during late pregnancy is due to placental ALP.[9] In the third trimester, concentrations often double and may remain elevated for 3 weeks postpartum.

The mechanism of hepatic ALP release into the circulation in patients with cholestatic disease remains unclear. Bile accumulation appears to increase hepatocyte synthesis of ALP, which eventually leaks into the bloodstream. ALP concentrations persist until the obstruction is removed and then normalize within 2 to 4 weeks.

Clinically, ALP elevation is associated with cholestatic disorders and, as mentioned previously, does not help to distinguish between intrahepatic and extrahepatic disorders. ALP concentrations more than four times normal suggest a cholestatic disorder, and 75% of patients with primarily cholestatic disorders have ALP concentrations in this range (**Table 15-3**). Concentrations of three times normal or less are nonspecific and can occur in all types of liver disease. Mild elevations, usually <1.5 times normal, can be seen in healthy patients and are less significant.

When faced with an elevated ALP concentration, a clinician must determine whether it is derived from the liver. One approach is to fractionate the ALP isoenzymes using electrophoresis, but this method is expensive and often unavailable. Thus, the approach usually taken is to measure other indicators of cholestatic disease, 5′-nucleotidase, or GGT. If ALP is elevated, an elevated 5′-nucleotidase or GGT indicates that at least part of the elevated ALP is of hepatic origin. Alternatively, a normal 5′-nucleotidase or GGT suggests a nonhepatic cause (Table 15-3).

**TABLE 15-3.** Initial Evaluation of Elevated ALP Concentrations in Context of Other Test Results

| ALP | GGT, 5′ NUCLEOTIDASE | AMINOTRANSFERASES (ALT AND AST) | DIFFERENTIAL DIAGNOSIS |
|---|---|---|---|
| Mildly elevated | Within normal limits | Within normal limits | Pregnancy; nonhepatic causes (Table 15-4) |
| Moderately elevated[a] | Markedly elevated | Within normal limits or minimally elevated | Cholestatic syndromes |
| Mildly elevated[b] | Mildly elevated | Markedly elevated | Hepatocellular disease |

[a]Usually more than four times normal limit.
[b]Usually less than four times normal limit.

**TABLE 15-4.** Some Nonhepatic Illnesses Associated with Elevated ALP

| BONE DISORDERS | OTHER DISORDERS AND DRUGS |
|---|---|
| Healing fractures | Acromegaly |
| Osteomalacia | Anticonvulsant drugs (eg, phenytoin and phenobarbital) |
| Paget disease | |
| Rickets | Hyperthyroidism/ hyperparathyroidism |
| Tumors | |
| | Lithium (bone isoenzymes) |
| | Neoplasia |
| | Oral contraceptives |
| | Renal failure |
| | Small bowel obstruction |
| | Pregnancy (third trimester) |
| | Sepsis |

Nonhepatic causes of elevated ALP include bone disorders (eg, healing fractures, osteomalacia, Paget's disease, rickets, tumors, osteoporosis, hypervitaminosis D, or vitamin D deficiency as caused by celiac sprue), hyperthyroidism, hyperparathyroidism, sepsis, diabetes mellitus, renal failure, and neoplasms (which may synthesize ALP ectopically, outside tissues that normally contain ALP) (**Table 15-4**). Some families have inherited elevated concentrations (two to four times normal), usually as an autosomal dominant trait.[10] Markedly elevated concentrations (more than four times normal) are generally seen only in cholestasis, Paget's disease, or infiltrative diseases of the liver. Because of an increase in intestinal ALP, serum ALP concentrations can be falsely elevated in patients with blood type O or B whose blood is drawn 2 to 4 hours after a fatty meal.[11] Alkaline phosphatase concentrations can be lowered by several conditions, including hypothyroidism, hypophosphatemia, pernicious anemia, and zinc or magnesium deficiency. Also, ALP may be confounded by a variety of drugs.

### 5′-Nucleotidase

*Normal range: 0 to 11 units/L (0 to 0.19 μkat/L)*

Although *5′-nucleotidase* is found in many tissues (including liver, brain, heart, and blood vessels), serum 5′-nucleotidase is elevated most often in patients with hepatic diseases. It has a response profile parallel to ALP and similar utility in differentiating between hepatocellular and cholestatic liver disease. Because it is only elevated in the face of liver disease, the presence of an elevated ALP together with a normal 5′-nucleotidase (or GGTP, see below) suggests that the ALP is elevated secondary to nonhepatic causes.

### γ-Glutamyl Transpeptidase

*Normal range: 9 to 58 units/L (0.15 to 0.99 μkat/L)*

*γ-glutamyl transpeptidase* (GGT, also GGTP), a biliary excretory enzyme, can also help determine whether an elevated ALP is of hepatic etiology. Similar to 5′-nucleotidase, it is not elevated in

bone disorders, adolescence, or pregnancy. It is rarely elevated in conditions other than liver disease.

Generally, GGT parallels ALP and 5′-nucleotidase levels in liver disease. Additionally, GGT concentrations are usually elevated in patients who abuse alcohol or have alcoholic liver disease. Therefore, this test is potentially useful in differential diagnosis, with a GGT/ALP ratio >2.5 being highly indicative of alcohol abuse.[12] With abstinence, GGT concentrations often decrease by 50% within 2 weeks.

Although it is often regarded as the most sensitive test for cholestatic disorders, GGT is unlike 5′-nucleotidase in that GGT lacks specificity. Not all GGT elevations are of hepatic origin. GGT is found in the liver, kidneys, pancreas, spleen, heart, brain, and seminal vesicles. Elevations may occur in pancreatic diseases, myocardial infarction, severe chronic obstructive pulmonary diseases, some renal diseases, systemic lupus erythematosus, hyperthyroidism, certain cancers, rheumatoid arthritis, and diabetes mellitus. GGT may be confounded in patients on a variety of medications, some of which overlap with the medications that confound ALP test results. Thus, elevated GGT (even with concomitant elevated ALP) does not necessarily imply liver injury when 5′-nucleotidase is normal, but rather both elevations in GGT and ALP may be caused by a common confounding medication (eg, phenytoin, barbiturates) or medical condition (eg, myocardial infarction).

### Bilirubin

*Total bilirubin: 0.3 to 1.3 mg/dL (5.1 to 22 μmol/L)*

*Indirect (unconjugated, insoluble) bilirubin: 0.2 to 0.9 mg/dL (3.4 to 15.2 μmol/L)*

*Direct (conjugated, water soluble) bilirubin: 0.1 to 0.4 mg/dL (1.7 to 6.8 μmol/L)*

Understanding the various laboratory studies of *bilirubin* requires knowledge of the biochemical pathways for bilirubin production and excretion (**Figure 15-3**). Bilirubin is a breakdown product of heme pigments, which are large, insoluble organic compounds. Most of the body's heme pigments are located in erythrocytes (red blood cells), in which they are a component of hemoglobin. Breakdown of erythrocytes releases hemoglobin into the circulation (which is converted to bilirubin, predominantly in the spleen), where it is initially a large lipophilic molecule bound to albumin.

The liver plays a central role in excretion of bilirubin, similar to its role in the metabolism and excretion of a wide variety of lipophilic substances. Prior to excretion, bilirubin must be converted into a form that is water soluble. The liver achieves this by covalently linking it to a water-soluble sugar molecule (glucuronic acid) using an enzyme glucuronyl transferase. The conjugate of bilirubin linked to glucuronic acid is water soluble, so it may then be excreted into the bile and eventually eliminated in the feces. Incidentally, bilirubin and some of its breakdown products are responsible for coloring feces brown (such that with complete obstruction of the bile ducts or cessation of bile synthesis by the liver, the stool takes on a pale color). With progressive cholestasis, there is increased renal excretion of the water-soluble bilirubin, coloring the urine dark brown.

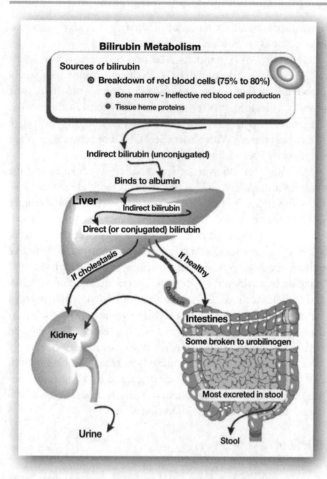

**Bilirubin Metabolism**

**Sources of bilirubin**
- Breakdown of red blood cells (75% to 80%)
  - Bone marrow - Ineffective red blood cell production
  - Tissue heme proteins

Indirect bilirubin (unconjugated)

Binds to albumin

**Liver**    Indirect bilirubin

Direct (or conjugated) bilirubin

If cholestasis          If healthy

**Kidney**

**Intestines**
Some broken to urobilinogen

Most excreted in stool

Urine                    Stool

**FIGURE 15-3.** Overview of bilirubin production and metabolism. Most bilirubin is produced by the breakdown of heme pigments in erythrocytes (red blood cells) and, to a lesser extent, other tissues. The indirect bilirubin is carried in the circulation to the liver, where it is conjugated and becomes direct or conjugated bilirubin. In healthy individuals, conjugated bilirubin is largely excreted via the biliary system into the gut. In individuals with disease, it will "back up" into the circulation, causing elevated levels of direct/conjugated bilirubin and, ultimately, jaundice. (Courtesy of Esta Farkas.)

## Indirect Versus Direct Bilirubin

The total amount of bilirubin in the serum can be divided into *direct* and *indirect* fractions. Bilirubin conjugated to glucuronic acid (water-soluble bilirubin) reacts quickly in the van der Bergh reaction and is thus called *direct-reacting* or *direct bilirubin*. Alternatively, unconjugated bilirubin, because it is water insoluble, requires the presence of dissolving agents to be detected by this assay and is thus called *indirect-reacting* or *indirect bilirubin*. Although this nomenclature system is slightly awkward, it is the standard terminology used in clinical practice today. Labs generally measure the total bilirubin and the direct bilirubin. Indirect bilirubin may be determined by subtracting the direct from the total bilirubin. Only the water-soluble direct bilirubin

can be excreted in the urine; therefore, urine dipsticks only will measure this fraction. In fact, urine dipsticks may be more sensitive than most serum tests for detecting a slight elevation of direct bilirubin.

Elevated bilirubin causes abnormal yellow coloration of the skin and sclera of the eyes (collectively, these symptoms are referred to as jaundice or icterus). Excess carotenes (eg, due to large amounts of carrot consumption) may cause a similar effect on the skin but spare the eyes. Icterus usually becomes visible when total bilirubin concentrations exceed 2 to 4 mg/dL. In infants, extremely elevated concentrations of bilirubin (for example, >20 mg/dL) may have neurotoxic effects on the developing brain, but in adults a direct toxic effect of bilirubin is quite rare.

The first step in evaluating an elevated serum bilirubin is to determine if only the indirect fraction is elevated or if there is involvement of the direct fraction. Given the sequential location of these two molecules within the pathway of bilirubin metabolism, elevated levels of the molecules may have markedly different significance (**Table 15-5**).

### Indirect Hyperbilirubinemia (Unconjugated, Insoluble)

*Indirect bilirubin* is mostly produced by the breakdown of erythrocytes and is removed from the circulation by conversion to direct bilirubin by glucuronyl transferase in the liver. Therefore, elevated levels may result from increased breakdown of red blood cells (hemolysis) or reduced hepatic conversion to direct bilirubin. Patients with primarily *unconjugated hyperbilirubinemia* (>70% indirect) generally do not have serious liver disease. The most common causes of elevated indirect bilirubin are hemolysis, Gilbert syndrome, Crigler-Najjar syndrome, and various drugs, including probenecid and rifampin. In infants, this can be physiologic (neonatal jaundice), although very high levels may require medical intervention.

Hemolysis refers to increased destruction of erythrocytes, which increases the production of indirect bilirubin and may overwhelm the liver's ability for conjugation and excretion. However, the liver's processing mechanisms are intact so that serum bilirubin generally does not rise dramatically (rarely >5 mg/dL). Hemolysis may result from a wide variety of hematologic processes, including sickle cell anemia, spherocytosis, hematomas, mismatched blood transfusions, and intravascular fragmentation of blood cells. Evaluation includes various hematologic tests, as described in further detail in Chapter 16.

Gilbert syndrome is an inherited, benign trait present in 3% to 5% of the population. It is due to reduced production of hepatic glucuronyl transferase enzymes, resulting in intermittent elevation of indirect bilirubin and mild jaundice (increased with fasting, stress, or illness). The primary significance is that it may cause elevation of bilirubin when there is in fact no significant hepatic or hematologic disease. Bilirubin elevation is generally mild, with values <5 mg/dL.

### Direct Hyperbilirubinemia (Conjugated, Soluble)

*Conjugated hyperbilirubinemia* is defined as bilirubinemia with >50% in the direct fraction (although absolute levels of unconjugated bilirubin may also be elevated). In the normal course of

**TABLE 15-5.** Evaluation of Elevated Bilirubin Concentrations in Context of Other Test Results

| TOTAL BILIRUBIN | DIRECT BILIRUBIN | INDIRECT BILIRUBIN | ALT, AST, GGT | DIFFERENTIAL DIAGNOSIS |
|---|---|---|---|---|
| Moderately elevated | Within normal limits or low | Moderately elevated | Within normal limits | Hemolysis,[a] Gilbert syndrome,[a] Crigler-Najjar syndrome,[b] neonatal jaundice |
| Moderately elevated | Moderately elevated | Within normal limits | Within normal limits | Congenital syndromes[c]: Dubin-Johnson[d] and Rotor |
| Mildly elevated | Mildly elevated | Moderately elevated | Moderately elevated | Hepatobiliary disease |

[a]Usually indirect bilirubin is <4 mg/dL but may increase to 18 mg/dL.
[b]Usually indirect bilirubin is >12 mg/dL but may go as high as 45 mg/dL.
[c]These syndromes are distinguished in the laboratory by liver biopsy.
[d]Usually direct bilirubin is 3 to 10 mg/dL.

bilirubin metabolism, direct bilirubin is synthesized in hepatocytes by conjugating indirect bilirubin and secreted into bile. Therefore, elevated direct bilirubin implies hepatic or biliary tract disease that interferes with secretion of bilirubin from the hepatocytes or clearance of bile from the liver.

*Direct hyperbilirubinemia* is generally classified as a positive cholestatic liver test, although as discussed earlier, it may be elevated to some extent in hepatocellular processes as well. In cholestatic disease, elevated bilirubin is primarily conjugated, whereas in hepatocellular processes significant increases in both conjugated and unconjugated bilirubin may result. The most reliable method of determining the cause of hyperbilirubinemia considers the magnitude and pattern of abnormalities in the entire liver function panel. It should be noted that direct bilirubin is generally readily cleared by the kidney, such that its levels rarely rise very high, even in severe cholestatic disease if a patient has normal renal function. Very rarely, congenital disorders (eg, Dubin-Johnson and Rotor syndromes) may cause elevations of primarily conjugated bilirubin.

It should be noted that a gray area exists between indirect and direct hyperbilirubinemia. Most authors agree that >50% direct bilirubin indicates direct hyperbilirubinemia whereas <30% direct fraction indicates indirect hyperbilirubinemia. For cases in which the fraction falls between 30% and 50%, other liver tests and hematologic tests may be required to determine the etiology.

Patients with elevated direct bilirubin levels may have some binding of bilirubin to albumin, referred to as *δ bilirubin*. This explains delayed resolution of jaundice during recovery from acute hepatobiliary diseases; while the "free" bilirubin is rapidly metabolized, the bilirubin linked to albumin is metabolized at a much slower rate. Δ bilirubin has a half-life of 14 to 21 days, which is similar to albumin.[13]

## HEPATOCELLULAR INJURY

As discussed earlier, the liver is a large organ with diverse biochemical roles, which require its cells to be in close communication with the bloodstream. These properties place the hepatocytes at risk for injury due to a variety of processes. Toxin and drug metabolism produce cascades of metabolic byproducts, some of which may damage hepatocytes. Likewise, the liver plays a central role in the body's biochemical homeostasis, so metabolic disorders tend to involve the liver. Finally, the close relationship of hepatocytes to the blood supply places them at risk for a variety of infectious agents.

*Hepatitis* is a term that technically refers to a histologic pattern of inflammation of hepatocytes. It may also be used to refer to a clinical syndrome caused by diffuse liver inflammation. The laboratory reflection of hepatitis is a hepatocellular injury pattern, which is marked primarily by elevated aminotransferases.

There are multiple causes of hepatitis. One common type is viral hepatitis, which is classified A, B, C, D (δ hepatitis), or E based on the causative virus. These viruses, and the tests for them, are discussed in detail in the Viral Hepatitis section. Less common viral hepatitis may be caused by the Epstein-Barr virus, herpes virus, or cytomegalovirus.

Hepatitis may also be caused by various medications, and drug-induced hepatitis can be either acute or chronic. Some drugs commonly implicated in cellular hepatotoxicity are listed in Table 15-2. In addition, elevation of aminotransferases has been reported in patients receiving heparin.[14] ALT is elevated in up to 60% of these patients, with a mean maximal value of 3.6 times the baseline. A vast number of drugs can cause hepatic injury, especially drugs that are extensively metabolized by the liver. Although numerous drugs may result in aminotransferase elevations, such elevations are usually minor, transient, not associated with symptoms, and of no clinical consequence.

Perhaps the most common cause of abnormal aminotransferases in ambulatory patients is fatty liver.[15] Estimates are 30% to 46% of adults in the United States have fatty liver, which can vary from hepatic steatosis (fat in the liver) to nonalcoholic steatohepatitis (NASH), in which the extra fat in the liver is associated with inflammation. It is potentially serious because up to one-fourth of these patients can progress to having cirrhosis. Fatty liver and NASH are mostly related to increased body mass index, but they can also be associated with rapid weight loss or drugs such as tamoxifen, amiodarone, diltiazem, nifedipine, corticosteroids, and petrochemicals. Fatty liver/NASH can be seen in patients with hepatitis C and patients on total parenteral nutrition, and it is associated with hypothyroidism and short bowel syndrome.

It is important to note that although mild hepatic inflammation is often of minimal significance, it may signal the presence of a chronic and serious disease process. Some other causes of hepatic inflammation and injury are listed in Table 15-2.

It is often difficult to determine the exact etiology of hepatic inflammation or hepatitis. A careful history—especially for exposure to drugs, alcohol, or toxins—and detailed physical examination are crucial. Additional laboratory studies are usually necessary to distinguish one form of hepatitis from another (**Figure 15-4**). Radiologic testing or liver biopsy may be indicated, not only to determine the etiology of the liver disease but also to help determine the indications for (and results of) therapy and prognosis.

## Aminotransferases: Aspartate Aminotransferase and Alanine Aminotransferase

*AST: 12 to 38 units/L (0.2 to 0.65 μkat/L); ALT: 7 to 41 units/L (0.12 to 0.70 μkat/L) (normal values for either test vary from laboratory to laboratory but tend to be in the range of <30 units/L for men and <20 units/L for women)*

The *aminotransferases* (also known as *transaminases*) are used to assess hepatocellular injury and include AST (formerly serum glutamic-oxaloacetic transaminase) and ALT (formerly

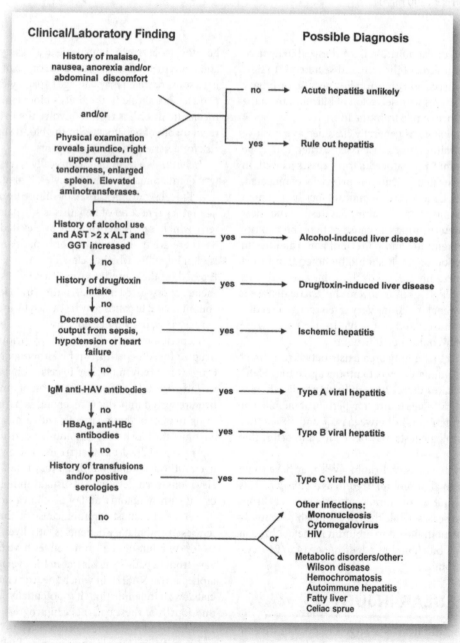

**FIGURE 15-4.** Algorithm for differential diagnosis of suspected hepatitis.

serum glutamic-pyruvic transaminase). These enzymes are primarily located inside hepatocytes, where they assist with various metabolic pathways. They are released into the serum in greater quantities when there is hepatocyte damage, are very sensitive, and may be elevated even with minor levels of hepatocyte damage. However, this renders them relatively nonspecific, and slightly elevated levels may not be clinically significant (particularly in an ill, hospitalized patient who is on many medications and has a variety of active medical problems).

Aminotransferases are often slightly increased in cholestatic liver diseases, but in this situation, they are generally overshadowed by a greater elevation of cholestatic liver tests (ie, ALP and total bilirubin to produce a predominantly cholestatic pattern of liver tests). If both aminotransferases and cholestatic tests are elevated in a similar pattern, it suggests a severe hepatocellular process, which interferes with bile secretion at the level of the hepatocytes. Finally, it should be noted that aminotransferases may rise into the thousands within 24 to 48 hours after common bile duct obstruction, after which they decline rapidly. This is one instance in which a cholestatic process may transiently cause a hepatocellular injury LFT profile.

Both AST and ALT have half-lives of 17 and 47 hours, respectively, so they reflect *active* hepatocyte damage and not, for example, damage to hepatocytes that occurred weeks, months, or years previously. This may lead to some counterintuitive relationships between aminotransferase levels and the overall state of the liver. For example, a drop in aminotransferase levels in the setting of acute massive (*fulminant*) hepatitis may reflect a depletion of viable hepatocytes with poor prognosis. Extremely high concentrations (>1,000 units/L) are usually associated with acute viral hepatitis, severe drug or toxic reactions, or ischemic hepatitis (inadequate blood flow to the liver). Lesser elevations are caused by a vast number of hepatic insults and are less specific.

The ratio of AST to ALT may be of value in diagnosing alcoholic hepatitis, in which the AST is generally at least twice the ALT, and the AST is rarely >300 units/L. In alcoholic liver disease, this is due, in part to a deficiency of pyridoxal 5′-phosphate, which favors production of ALT over AST.[16] Alcoholic liver disease is also suggested by an elevation in GGT, as previously reviewed.

AST is not solely located in hepatocytes but rather is also found in cardiac muscle, skeletal muscle, kidneys, brain, lungs, intestines, and erythrocytes. Consequently, AST may be elevated due to a variety of situations, including musculoskeletal diseases (eg, muscular dystrophy, dermatomyositis, heavy exercise, trichinosis, gangrene, and muscle damage secondary to hypothyroidism), myocardial infarction, renal infarction or failure, brain trauma or cerebral infarction, hemolysis, pulmonary embolism, necrotic tumors, burns, and celiac sprue. ALT is more localized to the liver than AST, so it is more specific to liver injury. Elevation of AST without elevation of the ALT or other liver test abnormality suggests cardiac or muscle disease. A muscular origin of aminotransferases may also be indicated by increases in aminotransferases >300 International Units/L with concomitant increases in serum creatine kinase activity.

Measurement of AST may be affected by a bewildering variety of medications. Almost any prescription drug (as well as various herbal compounds and illegal drugs) can cause an elevation of aminotransferases, and the significance of these elevations is often unclear. Furthermore, the in vitro assay may be confounded by a variety of factors, including uremia, hyperlipidemia, and hemolysis.[17] False elevations in the in vitro test may also be seen in patients on acetaminophen, levodopa, methyldopa, tolbutamide, para-aminosalicylic acid, or erythromycin.

Other factors may interfere with the test's accuracy. Levels may be elevated to two to three times normal by vigorous exercise in male patients and decreased to about half following dialysis. Complexing of AST with immunoglobulin (known as *macro-AST*) may occasionally produce a clinically irrelevant elevation of AST.[18] Testing for macro-AST is not a clinical laboratory test used in practice. Given the array of factors that can cause an abnormal result, unexplained false-positive results often occur. In healthy individuals, an isolated elevated ALT returns to normal in repeat studies one-half to one-third of the time. For this reason, prior to an evaluation of mildly elevated aminotransferases in low-risk healthy patients, a practitioner should check for an elevation of more than one test (ie, both AST and ALT) or repeated elevations of a single test.

# TESTS ASSOCIATED WITH DETOXIFICATION

## Hepatic Encephalopathy

*Hepatic encephalopathy* refers to a potentially reversible diffuse metabolic dysfunction of the brain that may occur in acute or chronic liver failure.[19] Clinically, it ranges from subtle changes in personality to coma and death. The etiology of hepatic encephalopathy remains controversial. Many theories ascribe a major role to ammonia. Most ammonia enters the portal circulation from the intestines, where it is formed by bacterial catabolism of protein within the gut lumen as well as conversion of serum glutamine into ammonia by enterocytes of the small intestine. Normally, the liver removes >90% of this ammonia via first-pass metabolism before it can enter the systemic circulation.[20] In liver failure, ammonia, along with possibly other toxic substances, may avoid this first-pass metabolism and gain immediate access to the brain, where it has a variety of toxic effects. While the exact role of ammonia in terms of hepatic encephalopathy is not clear, it is of interest that current treatment seems focused on lowering serum ammonia levels.

### Ammonia

*Normal range: 19 to 60 mcg/dL (11 to 35 μmol/L)*
*Ammonia* levels do not correlate well with hepatic encephalopathy in the setting of chronic liver failure (ie, patients with cirrhosis). This is likely because hepatic encephalopathy also involves an increase in the permeability of the blood–brain barrier to ammonia. There is a large overlap between ammonia levels in patients with and without hepatic encephalopathy among patients with chronic liver disease, making it a poor test in this situation.[21] Although a very high ammonia level (ie, >250 mcg/dL) is suggestive of hepatic encephalopathy, most patients with

cirrhosis suspected of having encephalopathy have normal or slightly elevated ammonia levels, which adds little diagnostic information. Generally, hepatic encephalopathy is a clinical diagnosis based on history, physical exam, and exclusion of other possibilities. Psychometric testing is becoming increasingly available to assist in confirming this diagnosis. Recent articles have questioned the value of checking ammonia levels in terms of their utility in guiding therapy.[22]

Some recent studies have suggested that ammonia levels may have more significance in the setting of acute liver failure (eg, due to overwhelming infection of the liver by viral hepatitis). In these patients, the degree of ammonia elevation correlates with the severity of hepatic encephalopathy and the likelihood of death, and it may be a useful marker for predicting which patients may require emergent liver transplant.[23]

Ammonia concentration may also be elevated in patients with Reye syndrome, inborn disorders of the urea cycle, various medications (most notably valproic acid), impaired renal function, ureterosigmoidostomy, or urinary tract infections with bacteria that convert urea to ammonia. In patients with cirrhosis or mild liver disease, elevated ammonia and hepatic encephalopathy may be precipitated by such factors as increased dietary protein, GI bleeding, constipation, and *H pylori* infection. Patients with vascular shunts or bypass procedures in which blood flow is directed from the portal circulation directly into the systemic circulation (as in transjugular intrahepatic portosystemic shunt) are more likely to develop hepatic encephalopathy.

## VIRAL HEPATITIS

The onset of acute *viral hepatitis* may be dramatic and present as an overwhelming infection, or it may pass unnoticed by the patient. In the usual prodromal period, the patient often has a nonspecific flu-like illness that may include nausea, vomiting, fatigue, or malaise. This period may be followed by clinical hepatitis with jaundice. During this time, the most abnormal laboratory results are usually the aminotransferases, which can be in the thousands. Bilirubin may be quite elevated, while ALP only mildly so.

The major types of viral hepatitis are reviewed here, but they are often clinically indistinguishable. Thus, serologic studies of antibodies, molecular assays to detect viral genetic material, and knowledge of the epidemiology and risk factors for these different viruses (**Table 15-6**) are central to diagnosis.

### Type A Hepatitis

*Hepatitis A virus* (HAV) is spread primarily by the fecal–oral route by contaminated food or water or by person-to-person contact. It has an incubation period of 3 to 5 weeks with a several-day prodrome (preicteric phase) before the onset of jaundice and malaise, or the icteric phase. The icteric phase generally lasts 1 to 3 weeks, although prolonged courses do occur. Hepatitis A is responsible for about 50% of acute hepatitis in the United States (more than all other hepatotropic viruses combined), generally due to person-to-person contact within community-wide outbreaks. Between 2016 and 2018, reports of hepatitis A infections in the United States increased by 294%

**TABLE 15-6.** Groups at Higher Risk of Infection by Various Hepatitis Viruses

| |
|---|
| **Hepatitis A virus** |
| Persons in contact with infected persons |
| Daycare workers and attendees |
| Institutionalized persons |
| Travelers to countries with high rate of hepatitis A infections |
| Military personnel |
| Men who have sex with men |
| IV drug users |
| **Hepatitis B virus** |
| Persons in contact with infected persons |
| Unvaccinated healthcare professionals and morticians |
| Hemodialysis patients |
| Men who have sex with men |
| IV drug users |
| Multipartner heterosexuals |
| Tattooed/body-pierced persons |
| Newborns of HBsAg-carrier mothers |
| **Hepatitis C virus** |
| Dialysis patients |
| Healthcare professionals |
| IV drug use (primary cause)* (even once) |
| Intranasal drug use |
| Recipients of clotting factors before 1987 |
| Recipients of transfusion or organ transplant before July 1992 |
| Tattooed/body-pierced persons |
| Children born to HCV-positive mothers |
| **Hepatitis D virus** |
| Only individuals with chronic HBV infection |
| **Hepatitis E virus** |
| Travelers to Latin America, Egypt, India, and Pakistan |
| Persons in contact with infected persons |

*Even one isolated incident of injection drug use can lead to Hepatitis C.

compared with 2013 to 2015; this increase reflects outbreaks involving individuals who report drug use or homelessness, men who have sex with men, and contaminated food items.[24]

Unlike types B, C, and D hepatitis virus, HAV does not cause chronic disease, and recovery usually occurs within 1 month. Many patients who get type A hepatitis never become clinically ill. Perhaps 10% of all patients become symptomatic, and only 10% of those patients become jaundiced. Fulminant hepatic failure occurs in <1% of cases. Most patients have a full recovery, but there is a substantial mortality risk in elderly patients and very young patients, in patients with chronic hepatitis B or C, and in patients with chronic liver disease of other etiologies.

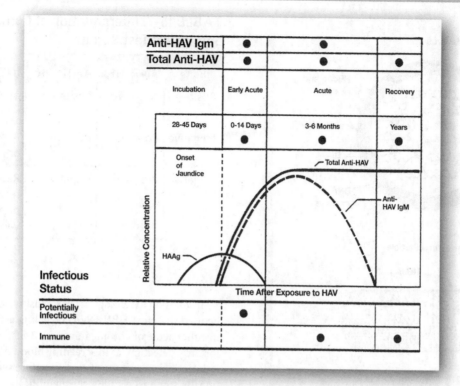

**FIGURE 15-5.** Temporal relationships of serologies for type A hepatitis with onset of jaundice and infectious status. Anti-HAV IgM is the IgM antibody against HAV. HAAg is the hepatitis A antigen (virus). Total anti-HAV is primarily IgG antibodies (and some IgM in acute phase) against HAV. *Source:* Adapted with permission from Abbott Laboratories, North Chicago, IL.

A vaccine for HAV is available. It is recommended for those from or traveling to endemic regions (ie, Central and South America), men who have sex with men, users of street drugs, those with occupational exposure, patients requiring clotting factor concentrates, and patients with chronic liver diseases. This vaccine is increasingly being recommended as a universal vaccine for pediatric patients. Although this vaccine is generally preferred for postexposure prophylaxis, use of immunoglobulin should be considered in the very young (<12 months) or patients who cannot receive the vaccine.

Presently, the only two tests available to measure antibodies to HAV are immunoglobulin M (IgM) or total (all isotypes of) antibody. Detection of IgM is the more clinically relevant test as it reveals acute or recent infection. These antibodies are present at the onset of jaundice and decline within 12 (but usually 6) months. Total antibody, which is comprised of antibody of all isotypes against HAV, indicates present or previous infection or immunization (**Figure 15-5**).

## Type B Hepatitis

*Hepatitis B virus* (HBV) is a DNA virus spread by bodily fluids, most commonly as a sexually transmitted disease, but also via contaminated needles (as with parenteral drug abuse or needle stick accidents), shared razor blades or toothbrushes, nonsterile tattooing or body piercing, blood products, or vertical transmission (transmission from mother to child, generally at birth). This disease is 50 to 100 times more contagious than HIV. The incubation period of HBV varies from 2 to 4 months, much longer than that of HAV. Geographically, there is a markedly increased prevalence of hepatitis B in Southeast Asia, China, and sub-Saharan Africa, with 10% to 20% of the populations being hepatitis B carriers. In contrast, the incidence of hepatitis B carriers in the United States is approximately 0.4%.

The clinical illness is generally mild and self-limited but can be quite severe. Unfortunately, up to 5% of infected adults and 90% of infected neonates develop a chronic illness. Chronic HBV infection is often mild but may progress to cirrhosis, liver failure, or hepatocellular carcinoma, thereby contributing to premature death in 15% to 25% of cases.

### Viral Antigens and Their Antibodies

Three HBV antigens and antibody systems are relevant to diagnosis and management: surface antigen (HBsAg), core antigen (HBcAg), and e antigen (HBeAg). HBsAg is present on the outer surface of the virus, and neutralizing hepatitis B surface antibodies (anti-HBs) directed against this protein are central to natural and vaccine-induced immunity (**Figure 15-6**). Neither HBcAg nor HBeAg are on the surface of the virion, and thus antibodies against these antigens are not protective. Nevertheless, antibodies are directed against these proteins and may serve as markers of infection. Of these antigens, only HBsAg and HBeAg can be detected in the serum by conventional techniques. HBsAg is detected for a greater window of time during

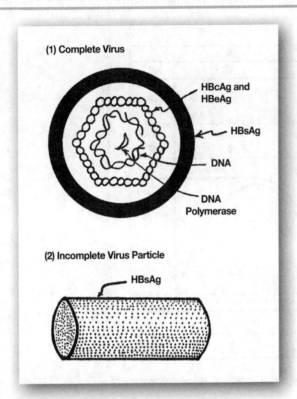

(1) Complete Virus

HBcAg and
HBeAg

HBsAg

DNA

DNA
Polymerase

(2) Incomplete Virus Particle

HBsAg

**FIGURE 15-6.** Hepatitis B virus and its antigenic components. The complete and infectious virus (1), originally known as the Dane particle, is composed of the outer layer (HBsAg) and inner nucleocapsid core. The inner core is comprised of HBcAg intermeshed with HBeAg and encapsulates the viral DNA. HBeAg may be an internal component or degradation product of the nucleocapsid core. An incomplete and noninfectious form (2) is composed exclusively of HBsAg and is cylindrical in shape.

infection and reveals active infection. Detection of HBeAg indicates large amounts of circulating HBV; these patients are 5 to 10 times more likely to transmit the virus than are HBeAg-negative persons.

In response to infection with HBV, the body may produce anti-HBs, hepatitis B core antibody (anti-HBc), and hepatitis B e-antibody (anti-HBe). All of these antibodies can be detected in clinical laboratories, and in the case of anti-HBcAg, separate tests are available to detect IgM or total antibody (all isotypes). Anti-HBs are associated with resolved type B hepatitis or patients who have responded to vaccination for HBV. Anti-HBc is a bit more challenging to interpret, as it can be seen in acute type B hepatitis, after recovery from type B hepatitis (often in concert with anti-HBs), and in chronic infection (often with HBsAg and HBeAg), and there can be false-positive results as well. As shown in **Table 15-7** and **Figure 15-7**, levels of antigens and antibodies show complex patterns in the course of HBV infection and thus can yield considerable information about the infection's course and chronology.

**TABLE 15-7.** Interpretation of Common Hepatitis B Serological Test Results

| HBsAg | ANTI-HBs | ANTI-HBc | INTERPRETATION |
|---|---|---|---|
| Positive | Negative | Positive | Acute infection or chronic hepatitis B |
| Negative | Positive | Positive | Resolving hepatitis B or previous infection |
| Negative | Positive | Negative | Resolving or recovered hepatitis B or patient after vaccination |

In addition to serological tests, sensitive molecular assays may be used to detect HBV DNA, revealing active viral replication in either acute or chronic infection. These assays may be useful for early detection, as in screening blood donors, because DNA is detectible an average of 25 days before seroconversion. Additionally, some assays allow the quantification of serum viral load, which may be used in the decision to treat and, subsequently, monitor therapy. Presently, eight genotypes of HBV have been identified, which can be of real value in terms of determining appropriate therapy for chronic infection. For example, genotype A—most prevalent in the United States—seems to respond better to interferon than the others, and patients with this genotype might benefit from starting with interferon as opposed to the oral agents available. Genotype C is more prevalent in Asia. For the details of these assays (PCR, RNA:DNA hybrid capture assay, nucleic acid cross-linking assay, and branched DNA assay), refer to a review by Pawlotsky et al.[25]

### Acute Type B Hepatitis

HBsAg titers usually develop within 4 to 12 weeks of infection and may be seen even before elevation of aminotransferases or clinical symptoms (Figure 15-7). Subsequently, HBsAg levels decline as anti-HBs titers develop, which indicates resolution of the acute symptomatic infection and development of immunity. In between the decline of HBsAg and the rise of anti-HBs, there is often a window when neither is present during which time anti-HBc may be used to diagnose infection. IgM anti-HBc may be used to reveal acute infection as opposed to a flare of chronic HBV.

### Chronic Type B Hepatitis

The development of chronic hepatitis B is suggested by the persistence of elevated LFTs (aminotransferases) and is supported by persistence of HBsAg for >6 months. Persistence of HBeAg also suggests chronic infection, but some chronically infected patients produce anti-HBe and, subsequently, clear HBeAg well after the acute phase is over (late seroconversion; **Figure 15-8**). Clearance of HBeAg is associated with a decrease in viral DNA and some degree of remission in chronic hepatitis B. However, this can be confusing because HBeAg is a precore

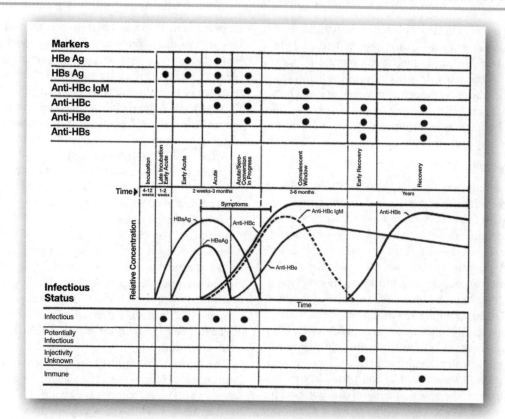

**FIGURE 15-7.** Serological profile, including temporal relationships integrated with infectious status and symptoms, in 75% to 85% of patients with acute type B hepatitis. *Source:* Adapted with permission from Abbott Laboratories, North Chicago, IL.

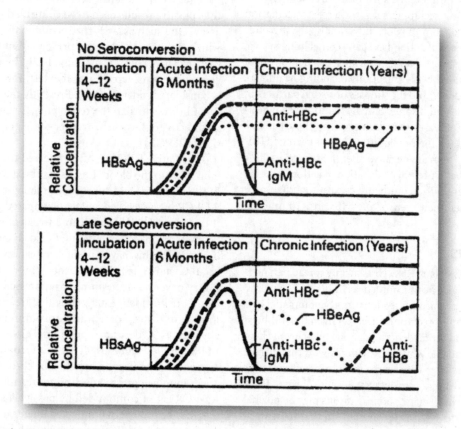

**FIGURE 15-8.** Serological profiles of patients who chronically carry HBV. *Source:* Reproduced with permission from Abbott Laboratories, North Chicago, IL.

protein, and in patients infected with certain mutations developed during the course of the disease (precore and core promoter), HBeAg may not be produced. Yet even in the face of anti-HBe, there may be active disease with ongoing fibrosis and development of cirrhosis. Although chronically infected individuals usually lack anti-HBs, in some cases low levels of nonneutralizing antibodies may be present. Additionally, low levels of IgM anti-HBc may persist.

### Hepatitis B Vaccine

The *HBV vaccine* consists of recombinant HBsAg, which, although not infectious, stimulates the production of protective anti-HBs. Generally, this is a safe vaccine, with efficacy of >90%. Presently, it is recommended as a standard vaccine for neonates. The hepatitis B vaccine is administered in a total of three doses, given at 0, 1, and 6 months. In those who were not vaccinated at birth, it is indicated for people at high risk of acquiring type B hepatitis or its complications including neonates of mothers with hepatitis B, men who have sex with men, injection drug abusers, dialysis patients, healthcare workers, patients with HIV, family and household contacts of patients with type B hepatitis, sexually active people with multiple partners, and patients with chronic liver disease. It should also be considered in patients about to undergo chemotherapy or other forms of immunosuppression. More recent efforts, especially in endemic countries, are leading to this being accepted as a universal vaccine. This vaccine, for example, is often required for students in the United States before entering the public school system.

A vaccine product directed against both HAV and HBV is available. In analyzing serologic data, successful vaccination may be distinguished from previous infection by the presence of anti-HBs and absence of antibodies against other antigens (eg, HBcAg, HBeAg). Testing for antibodies after vaccination is not generally recommended, with exceptions including healthcare workers, dialysis patients, and the spouses or sexual partners of infected patients. Although some patients fail to develop antibodies for a number of reasons, including anergy, these patients should be evaluated for the possibility of occult chronic HBV infection if antibody tests are negative after the second vaccine series. The vaccine has a prolonged duration of action. Routine booster injections are not recommended except, perhaps, for dialysis patients when their titers of anti-HBs are <10 International Units/L.

## Type C Hepatitis

*Hepatitis C virus* (HCV) is an RNA virus mainly spread parenterally, although it may also be transmitted vertically and sexually.[26] Although 70% to 80% of acute infections are asymptomatic, 70% to 80% of patients develop chronic disease. Given the mildness of the acute attack and the tendency to develop into chronic hepatitis, it is understandable why many patients with this disease first present decades later with cirrhosis or, more commonly, chronic elevations of aminotransferases. Because chronic HCV infection is often asymptomatic and LFT results may be normal or intermittently elevated, it is recommended that patients at high risk for HCV be screened appropriately. Patients for whom screening would be appropriate include those born in the United States between 1945 and 1965, patients with a history of illegal drug use. Additionally, patients who received clotting factors before 1987 or blood products or organ transplants before July 1992, are HIV positive, have a history of hemodialysis, or have evidence of liver disease (elevated ALT) should be screened. These guidelines are rapidly changing. Presently, the U.S. Preventive Services Task Force recommends universal screening for everyone between the ages of 18 and 79 years.

Acute hepatitis C is often asymptomatic, and when symptoms are present, they are mild. Diagnosis of acute hepatitis C, however, is important as evidence suggests that prompt treatment with antiviral medications can prevent progression to chronic hepatitis C in most cases.

In chronic hepatitis C infection, the LFT results are usually minimally elevated, with ALT and AST values commonly in the 60 to 100 International Units/L range. These values can fluctuate and occasionally return to normal for a year or more, only to rebound when next checked. The primary clinical concern in chronic HCV is that if untreated, within 20 years 20% to 30% of patients develop cirrhosis and 1% to 5% develop hepatocellular carcinoma.

The first screening test used is often an enzyme-linked immunosorbent assay (ELISA) assay for anti-HCV, which detects antibodies against a cocktail of HCV antigens. Positive test results can be seen in patients who have passively acquired these antibodies (but not the infection), as a result of blood transfusions, or as children of mothers with hepatitis C. Because of possible cross-reactivity with one of the antigens in the assay, this test has a considerable false-positive rate, and thus positive results need to be confirmed with a more specific assay. One such assay is the recombinant immunoblot assay, which is similar to ELISA in principle, but tests antibody reactivity to a panel of antigens individually. Binding to two or more antigens is considered a positive test. Binding to one antigen is considered indeterminate. Presently the approach to a positive ELISA is to skip the recombinant immunoblot assay and go directly to the reverse transcriptase polymerase chain reaction (RT-PCR) assay.

Qualitative RT-PCR, often referred to as just *PCR*, detects viral RNA in the blood. It is a sensitive assay that may be used in the diagnosis and subsequent management of hepatitis C. RT-PCR has several advantages compared with serologic tests. It can detect HCV within 1 to 2 weeks of exposure and weeks before seroconversion, presentation of symptoms, or the elevation of LFTs. This may be useful because seroconversion only has occurred in 70% to 80% of patients at the onset of symptoms, and it may never occur in immunosuppressed patients. Additionally, there is evidence suggesting that treating acute hepatitis C may be of value. Some immunocompromised patients with hepatitis C (as described previously) may have false-negative ELISA studies, and thus RT-PCR is recommended for consideration in patients with hepatitis or chronic liver disease who are immunosuppressed. Furthermore, unlike serologic assays, RT-PCR is not confounded by passively acquired antibodies that may be present in uninfected infants or recipients of blood products, and RT-PCR can distinguish between resolved and chronic infection.

Once a diagnosis of HCV infection is established, various quantitative molecular assays that monitor viral load may be useful in following viral titers during treatment or assessing the likelihood of response to therapy. A major consideration with these tests is that the methodology is not yet standardized, and there is laboratory-to-laboratory variability. These tests are not preferred for initial diagnosis because they are less sensitive than qualitative RT-PCR. They include a quantitative PCR assay and a branched-chain DNA assay (for more information, see Pawlotsky et al.[25]). Presently, most laboratories report HCV PCR measurements in International Units/milliliter, with pretreatment levels often in the millions.

There are at least six major genotypes of the type C virus and multiple subtypes. Viral genotype determination is useful because genotype may help direct the antiviral regimen needed, length of therapy, as well as predict the likelihood of response to treatment. Recent release of several new oral antiviral agents has improved treatment in terms of being well tolerated by the patients and yielding eradication rates >90%. Length of treatment may vary depending not only on genotype but also on presence of cirrhosis and previous exposure to other medications. Genotype determination may be done via direct sequencing or hybridization of PCR amplification products.

## Type D Hepatitis

*Hepatitis D virus* (HDV) is caused by a defective virus that requires the presence of HBsAg to cause infection. Therefore, people only can contract type D hepatitis concomitantly with HBV infection (coinfection) or if chronically infected with HBV (superinfection). Coinfection presents as an acute infection that may be more severe than HBV infection alone. Alternatively, the picture of superinfection is that of a patient with known or unknown chronic HBV who develops an acute flare with worsening liver function and increases in HBsAg. Acute coinfection is usually self-limited with rare development of chronic hepatitis, while superinfection becomes chronic in >75% of cases and increases the risk of negative sequelae, such as cirrhosis. Transmission of HDV is generally by parenteral routes, although no obvious cause can be determined in some cases.

Testing for HDV is usually only indicated in known cases of HBV infection. The single, widely available assay detects anti-HDV antibodies of all isotypes (**Figure 15-9**). This test is unable to distinguish between acute, chronic, or resolved infection and lacks sensitivity because only about 38% of infected patients have detectible anti-HDV within the first 2 weeks of illness. Because seroconversion may occur as late as 3 months after infection, testing may be repeated if the clinical picture suggests HDV. Tests are also available for HDV RNA, and stains are available to assess the D antigen in hepatocytes.

## Type E Hepatitis

*Hepatitis E virus* (HEV) is generally similar to hepatitis A. It is a hardy, protein-coated RNA virus that is spread by the fecal–oral route, often by contaminated food or water. Like HAV, HEV causes an acute illness that is generally self-limited. HEV is endemic in parts of Asia and has become increasingly detected in the United States. Unlike HAV, HEV is notable for a predilection for causing life-threatening illness in women who are in their third trimester of pregnancy. Recently, testing for antibodies to hepatitis E has become available, including HEVAg or hepatitis E antigen. Work is underway to develop a vaccine for hepatitis E.

## PRIMARY BILIARY CHOLANGITIS

*Primary biliary cholangitis* (PBC), previously called primary biliary cirrhosis, is a chronic disease involving progressive destruction of small intrahepatic bile ducts leading to cholestasis and progressive fibrosis over a period of decades. Ultimately, it can progress to cirrhosis and liver failure, necessitating transplantation.[27] Ninety percent of affected individuals are women, with onset occurring in adulthood. The etiology of the disease is unknown, although it seems to involve an autoimmune component and is associated with a variety of autoimmune disorders, including Sjögren's syndrome, rheumatoid arthritis, and scleroderma, and thyroid diseases. The initial symptoms of the disease are often those of progressive cholestasis with fatigue, pruritus, jaundice, and deficiencies in fat-soluble vitamins.

The most useful laboratory test in diagnosing PBC is the detection of antimitochondrial antibodies (AMA), with a sensitivity of 95%. This assay is also highly specific, although patients with autoimmune and drug-induced hepatitis occasionally have low antibody titers. PBC usually presents with a predominantly cholestatic laboratory picture, initially with an elevated ALP and GGT, and later, with an elevated total bilirubin. Aminotransferases tend to be minimally elevated or normal (**Minicase 1**).

## HEMOCHROMATOSIS

*Hemochromatosis* is an iron overload state involving the liver and other organs. If left untreated, hemochromatosis can lead to cirrhosis, cardiac failure, diabetes, and hepatocellular carcinoma.[28] Its presentation is often subtle, and most cases are discovered either in patients undergoing evaluation of abnormal aminotransferases or presenting with a positive family history of hemochromatosis. Iron overload can be either by a primary or secondary disorder. Hereditary hemochromatosis (also referred to as *classic* or *primary hemochromatosis*) is inherited in an autosomal recessive fashion and involves dysregulated handling of iron absorption from the GI tract. Up to 90% of affected individuals have inherited two alleles carrying the mutant C282Y genotype on chromosome 6. Persons of northern European descent have the highest risk, with a greater likelihood in men. Secondary hemochromatosis is generally the result of iatrogenic iron overload from repeated blood transfusions used as therapy for disorders such as thalassemias, sideroblastic anemias, myelodysplastic syndromes, and congenital dyserythropoietic anemias.[29]

Hemochromatosis remains an underdiagnosed disease entity. Many patients report nonspecific symptoms leading to a delay in diagnosis and treatment for up to several years. The classically reported clinical manifestations of hemochromatosis included the

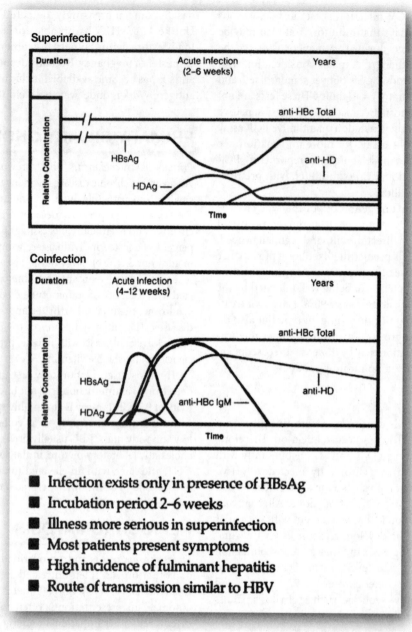

**FIGURE 15-9.** Two serological profiles of patients infected with HDV. HDAg = hepatitis D antigen (the virus); anti-HD = antibodies against HDV. *Source:* Reproduced with permission from Abbott Laboratories, North Chicago, IL.

triad of bronze skin, diabetes, and cirrhosis but were infrequent at the time of disease diagnosis. Now more commonly, patients experience malaise, fatigue, arthralgias, hepatomegaly, and elevated aminotransferase levels when diagnosis is confirmed.

Diagnosis typically begins with laboratory assessment of serum ferritin and transferrin iron saturation levels in patients found to have chronically elevated liver enzymes and clinical suspicion of hemochromatosis.[30] A transferrin iron saturation level of >60% in men or 50% in women may suggest this, although the American Association for the Study of Liver Diseases guidelines suggests 45% as a cutoff.[31] Ferritin levels tend to be elevated as well, >200 ng/mL in men and 150 ng/mL in women. Hemochromatosis gene testing can then be performed

on these patients or individuals at risk for hereditary hemochromatosis based on family history. This diagnosis can be suggested in patients who are homozygous for the C282Y gene or compound heterozygote with a copy of the C282Y gene and a copy of the H63D gene. Early diagnosis of hereditary hemochromatosis is important so that therapy can be started before end organ involvement is evident and is associated with improved outcomes.[32] Therapeutic phlebotomies to decrease serum ferritin levels may result in a normal life expectancy. Management of secondary hemochromatosis is usually through chelation therapy, but life expectancy may be shorter and related to the need for continued transfusion therapy to treat the primary disorder (**Minicases 2 through 11**).

## MINICASE 1

## Cholestasis in a Middle-Aged Woman

Gwen V., a 52-year-old woman, presents for her routine annual medical examination. She has no new medical complaints. In the past, she was diagnosed with osteoporosis and started on alendronate as well as supplemental vitamin D. She denies alcohol use, illicit drug use, or use of other vitamins or herbal supplements. Her physical examination is entirely normal. Routine laboratory evaluation includes a normal CBC, lipid profile, and renal function. Her liver profile is abnormal, with an elevated ALP of 330 International Units/L. Her AST, ALT, and bilirubin are normal.

An ultrasound of her liver and biliary system is normal. Additional bloodwork shows that her GGT is abnormally elevated at 562 International Units/L. Additional workup demonstrates negative serologies for viral hepatitis, negative ANA, and ASM. Her AMA titer is positive at 1:280. She is told she has primary biliary cirrhosis, needs a liver biopsy, and seeks another opinion.

QUESTION: What disease does she have, and how do we diagnose her? Does she need a liver biopsy?

DISCUSSION: Gwen V. has a cholestatic picture with elevations in ALP and GGTP. Her negative ultrasound helps exclude biliary obstruction. Her positive AMA is a further clue to her diagnosis. Prior to 2014, the diagnostic term was indeed primary biliary cirrhosis. This was an unfortunate term because many of these patients do not have cirrhosis at all. Currently, the correct diagnostic term is *primary biliary cholangitis* (PBC), which is classified as an autoimmune disease of the liver. Over the course of decades there can be continued inflammation of the small bile ducts in the liver, leading to scarring and ultimately cirrhosis. The disease is much more common in women and is often associated with other autoimmune diseases, especially thyroid disease.

Diagnosis requires two out of the three criteria:

1. Cholestatic liver tests
2. Abnormal serum AMA over 1:40
3. Characteristic findings on liver biopsy

Thus, our patient does not need a liver biopsy because she meets the criteria for PBC. Management would include treatment with ursodiol and following up with her lab results. If her ALP remains elevated, a newer treatment with obeticholic acid might be considered. Patients with PBC may have a higher incidence of osteoporosis, as our patient does. Additionally, lipids may be abnormal.

## MINICASE 2

## Case of a Prolonged International Normalized Ratio and Low Serum Albumin

Jane M., a 50-year-old woman, presents to her physician with reports of increasing fatigue and a 20-lb weight loss over the past 4 months. Initial evaluation shows an albumin of 2 g/dL and an INR of 2.3. Jane M. is referred for evaluation of possible cirrhosis. On further questioning, she denies any history of hepatitis, exposure to hepatotoxins, alcohol use, family history of liver disease, or liver disease.

Jane M.'s physical examination does not suggest liver disease; there is no evidence of ascites, palmar erythema, asterixis, hepatomegaly, splenomegaly, or spider angiomata. It is noted that she has pedal edema. Liver function studies are otherwise normal: ALT 12 International Units/L, AST 20 International Units/L, total bilirubin 1 mg/dL, and ALP 56 International Units/L.

An IM dose of vitamin K 10 mg corrects the INR within 24 hours. Workup shows that Jane M. has malabsorption due to sprue, a disease of the small bowel. With proper dietary management, her symptoms resolve and she gains weight. At a follow-up visit 3 weeks later, her albumin concentration is 3.7 g/dL and her edema has resolved.

QUESTION: Why did Jane M. develop a low albumin and a prolonged PT? What caused her pedal edema?

DISCUSSION: This case demonstrates that although low albumin and a prolonged PT suggest advanced liver disease, other causes need to be considered. Administration of vitamin K promptly corrected Jane M.'s INR, suggesting malabsorption of vitamin K. If she had cirrhosis, her PT would not have corrected with the vitamin K. Similarly, her hypoalbuminemia was not due to her liver's inability to synthesize albumin but to the malabsorptive disorder that was interfering with protein absorption. Therefore, Jane M. had a low albumin and elevated INR in the absence of liver disease. Her pedal edema was due to hypoalbuminemia secondary to malabsorption.

## PANCREATIC INFLAMMATION/ PANCREATITIS

*Pancreatitis* refers to inflammation of the pancreas (either acute or chronic) and is the most common disease associated with this gland.[33] Although there are multiple causes of pancreatitis, the clinical presentation is often the same. Acute pancreatitis generally presents with severe midepigastric abdominal pain developing over an hour, often radiating to the back. The pain tends to be continuous and can last for several days.

This condition is often associated with nausea and vomiting; in severe cases, fever, ileus, and hypotension can occur. Ultimately, there can be progressive anemia, hypocalcemia, hypoglycemia, hypoxia, renal failure, systemic inflammatory response

## MINICASE 3

### Jaundice Caused by Oral Contraceptives

Amber S., a 16-year-old girl, is found by her pediatrician to be slightly jaundiced during a routine school physical. She denies any history of liver disease, abdominal pain, illicit drug abuse, alcohol use, or abdominal trauma. Laboratory evaluation shows a moderately elevated bilirubin of 2.3 mg/dL along with ALP and GGT concentrations about four times normal. Her AST is 23 International Units/L.

Amber S. denies being on any medications (except for vitamins) or being exposed to toxins. Nothing suggests the possibility of a neoplastic or infectious process (temperature of 98.9°F and WBC count of $7.5 \times 10^3$ cells/mm$^3$). Ultrasound of the liver and biliary system is normal with no evidence of biliary dilation.

Her parents take her to a pediatric hepatologist. After much discussion (and threat of a liver biopsy), Amber S. tearfully reveals that she went to a local family planning clinic and is using birth control pills.

QUESTION: How might oral contraceptives cause a cholestatic picture? What is the importance of the ultrasound? What is the usual outcome of patients who develop jaundice while taking oral contraceptives?

DISCUSSION: This case demonstrates that oral contraceptives, primarily because of their estrogen content, can cause alterations in cholestatic test results (manifested by an elevated bilirubin, GGT, and ALP) with relatively normal aminotransferases. The ultrasound helps to distinguish between intrahepatic and extrahepatic cholestasis. The absence of biliary dilation suggests intrahepatic cholestasis. The normal AST suggests that jaundice is not due to hepatitis.

Cholestasis from oral contraceptives is generally benign and reverses promptly when the medication is withdrawn. Patients often omit mentioning use of birth control pills.

## MINICASE 4

### Abnormal Liver Function Tests

Dana D., a 36-year-old executive, is referred to a prominent medical center for a second opinion. Her physician finds an elevated AST of 180 International Units/L on a routine screening exam. Dana D. has no symptoms; her physical examination has been normal, without any signs of liver disease or hepatomegaly.

Additional studies show an ALT of 60 International Units/L, a markedly elevated GGT of 380 International Units/L, and a minimally elevated ALP of 91 International Units/L. Her WBC count is elevated at $20 \times 10^3$ cells/mm$^3$. After much discussion, she reveals that she has been drinking 1 pint of vodka a day.

Dana D. enrolls in Alcoholics Anonymous and stops drinking. Three months later, her test results are normal: ALT 28 International Units/L, GGT 54 International Units/L, and ALP 54 International Units/L.

QUESTION: What findings suggest alcoholic liver disease? Why did all of Dana D.'s laboratory test results return to normal? What else might have happened in this situation?

DISCUSSION: This case demonstrates several aspects of alcoholic liver disease. The diagnosis is suggested by an elevated AST out of proportion to the ALT (generally an AST/ALT ratio of ≥2), as well as by

a markedly elevated GGT with a normal (or virtually so) ALP. AST and ALT levels generally are <300. An elevated mean corpuscular volume (MCV), if present, also would support this diagnosis. Patients with alcoholic liver disease may have markedly elevated WBC counts.

Alcoholic liver disease tends to have several different stages. The earliest manifestation may be just a "fatty liver," which is generally reversible with cessation of alcohol intake. Alcoholic hepatitis and cirrhosis can follow with continued excessive alcohol intake. Unfortunately, alcoholic cirrhosis can develop without any warning signs. If Dana D. had alcoholic cirrhosis, stopping alcohol consumption probably would not have significantly altered her abnormal test results.

Clinicians should remember that a patient does not need to be an "obvious" alcoholic to develop alcoholic cirrhosis. Women are more susceptible to the hepatotoxic effects of alcohol than men, and as few as two or three drinks a day can cause significant liver disease in susceptible persons, this being due to differences in alcohol metabolism. Of note, 12 oz of beer, 5 oz of wine, and 1.5 oz of "spirits" all have about 14 g of alcohol and thus are equivalent in terms of risk of alcoholic liver disease.

## MINICASE 5

## A Jaundiced College Student

Jacob N., a 19-year-old college student, anxiously reports to the infirmary when his girlfriend notices that he has become yellow. He feels well and has a normal physical examination. On discussion, he indicates that he has recently embarked on a rigorous crash diet in anticipation of winter break in Florida.

The evaluation shows an elevated total bilirubin of 4.8 mg/dL, with a direct bilirubin of 0.48 mg/dL. The absence of hemolysis is established by microscopic examination of a blood smear, normal reticulocyte count, and lactate dehydrogenase (LDH), which is 112 International Units/L. Jacob N.'s other LFT results are normal: ALT 21 International Units/L and ALP 76 International Units/L.

QUESTION: What was the most likely cause of Jacob N.'s signs and symptoms? How should his condition be managed? What is his prognosis?

DISCUSSION: Elevated bilirubin concentrations do not necessarily indicate severe liver disease. In this case, the unconjugated bilirubin was substantially elevated. The normal ALT and ALP rule out hepatocellular and cholestatic liver diseases. If done, AST would have been normal. The normal LDH, red blood cell microscopic exam, and reticulocyte count rule out hemolysis as a cause of the elevated unconjugated bilirubin. The normal LDH is also consistent with a lack of intrinsic liver disease.

Jacob N. should be reassured that he has Gilbert syndrome and might become somewhat jaundiced with fasting or acute or chronic illness. Gilbert syndrome is not associated with any symptoms, is totally benign, and requires no treatment. When a patient has an elevated bilirubin, a practitioner should always obtain LFTs before providing a diagnosis or performing unnecessary tests.

## MINICASE 6

## Hepatic Encephalopathy

Stephen F., a 47-year-old man with alcoholism, is admitted to a hospital after being found on a park bench surrounded by empty beer bottles. Known to have cirrhosis, Stephen F. is thought to be showing signs of hepatic encephalopathy as he slowly lapses into a deep coma over the first 4 days of hospitalization. His physical examination is significant in that he has hepatomegaly and splenomegaly.

Laboratory evaluation shows a negative urine drug screen for central nervous system (CNS) depressants with serum glucose mildly elevated at 120 mg/dL. All serum electrolytes are normal: sodium, 140 mEq/L; potassium, 4 mEq/L; chloride, 98 mEq/L; carbon dioxide, 25 mEq/L; and magnesium, 1.5 mEq/L. Stephen F.'s blood alcohol concentration on admission is 150 mg/dL (normal: 0 mg/dL). His serum GGT is 321 International Units/L, and his AST is 87 International Units/L.

Unfortunately, efforts at treating hepatic encephalopathy do not reverse his coma. Further examination and testing are undertaken when it is noted that his ammonia concentration is normal at 48 mcg/dL. Then, a large bruise is noticed on the side of Stephen F.'s head, and a CT scan reveals a large subdural hematoma. With surgical treatment of the hematoma, he promptly awakes and asks for more beer.

QUESTION: How does one establish the diagnosis of hepatic encephalopathy for this patient? What is the role of the serum ammonia concentration in the diagnosis?

DISCUSSION: This case demonstrates that the diagnosis of hepatic encephalopathy is not always straightforward. Hepatic encephalopathy is only one cause of altered mental function in patients with advanced liver disease. Other causes may include accumulation of drugs with CNS depressant properties, head trauma, hypoglycemia, delirium tremens, and electrolyte imbalances. The diagnosis of hepatic encephalopathy is suggested by the following:

- Elevated ammonia concentrations
- Presence (in early stages) of asterixis or a flapping tremor of the hands
- Absence of other causative factors
- Characteristic electroencephalographic findings (rarely used)

The response to therapy (usually correction of electrolyte imbalances, rehydration, and lactulose and/or rifaximin) further supports this diagnosis. Serum ammonia concentrations, therefore, are just one piece of this puzzle. An elevated concentration suggests, but does not establish, this diagnosis. Furthermore, although normal ammonia concentrations may cause one to question the diagnosis of hepatic encephalopathy, they can occur in this condition.

## MINICASE 7

### Laboratory Diagnosis of Acute Hepatitis

Michael C., a 45-year-old executive, presents to his physician after noticing that he has been turning yellow. Other than increased fatigue, he says he feels well. His physical examination is normal except for his jaundice and tenderness over a slightly swollen liver. Initial laboratory studies show elevations of the aminotransferases, with an ALT of 1,235 International Units/L and an AST of 2,345 International Units/L. His total bilirubin is 18.6 mg/dL.

The tentative diagnosis is acute hepatitis. However, Michael C. has not had any transfusions, used parenteral drugs, or had recent dental work. No exposure to medications or occupational exposure accounts for the disease, and there is no family history of liver disease. Careful review of his history offers no explanation for his development of hepatitis.

Ultimately, serologies show a positive HBsAg and anti-HBc antibody. A diagnosis of acute type B hepatitis is established. After much questioning, Michael C. reveals that he had a "brief encounter" with a prostitute on a recent business trip. His wife is treated with the vaccine and hepatitis B immunoglobulin, a γ-globulin with high concentrations of antibodies to HBsAg, and she does not develop hepatitis.

QUESTION: How is this diagnosis established? How should Michael C. be followed, and what is the likely outcome?

DISCUSSION: This case demonstrates why a determination of the etiology of hepatitis is often difficult. The practitioner must obtain a detailed history of exposures to medicines, drugs, alcohol, infected people, family members with similar illness, and ongoing medical illness. In this case, the exposure to the prostitute put Michael C. at risk for hepatitis B, C, and D and for HIV. The diagnosis is established by the serologies. If just the anti-HBc antibody had been present, he could have

- been in the "window" of the acute phase of the disease where this antibody is positive and HBsAg is negative
- previously recovered from hepatitis B
- been a chronic carrier

Although the additional presence of HBsAg helps to secure the diagnosis, the clinical picture must be considered. Both HBsAg and anti-HBc also can be positive in patients with chronic hepatitis B. Determination of the type of hepatitis has prognostic value and, in this case, allows administration of prophylactic medications to people who might have been exposed.

| HBSAG | ANTI-HBS | ANTI-HBC | INTERPRETATION |
|-------|----------|----------|----------------|
| Positive | Negative | Positive | Acute infection or chronic hepatitis B |
| Negative | Positive | Positive | Resolving hepatitis B or previous infection |
| Negative | Positive | Negative | Resolving or recovered hepatitis B or patient after vaccination |

There is no generally accepted drug therapy for type B acute viral hepatitis. Michael C. should have repeated physical examinations and repeat laboratory testing for albumin, INR, AST, ALT, and bilirubin. There is a >1% chance that he will develop fulminant hepatitis and die. Most likely, he will recover completely, with his LFTs normalizing over 1 to 2 months. However, there is a 10% to 20% chance that he will develop chronic hepatitis, which could lead to cirrhosis.

## MINICASE 8

### Laboratory Diagnosis of Hepatitis Type C

Katherine M., a 48-year-old woman, receives a notice 2 weeks after donating blood that it could not be used because her aminotransferases are elevated and a test for hepatitis C is positive. She is referred to a specialist; her ALT is 87 International Units/L, her AST is 103 International Units/L, and her bilirubin is 0.8 mg/dL.

A liver biopsy demonstrates chronic active hepatitis. After considerable discussion, Katherine M. is placed on oral drug therapy for hepatitis C. After 3 months of therapy, however, her

aminotransferases are not responding, and she is referred for a second opinion.

Viral hepatitis C infection is excluded when her laboratory results are repeated, and she is found to have negative titers to detect HCV RNA (PCR). Additional history is then obtained. Katherine M. reluctantly tells her local family physician that about 6 months previously, she had a positive skin test for tuberculosis (TB) after discovering that her partner is HIV positive. She also says she sought treatment

## MINICASE 8 (cont'd)

in a nearby city, had been placed on isoniazid, and finished the prescription but never returned to the clinic.

QUESTION: What are the roles of the second-generation and third-generation tests in the diagnosis of hepatitis C? What other nonviral forms of hepatitis can present as chronic hepatitis?

DISCUSSION: This case demonstrates several points. Many patients with chronic active hepatitis remain totally asymptomatic—their disease first being detected during routine blood work or when symptoms of cirrhosis or liver failure develop. Now that all blood donors are checked for hepatitis C and abnormal aminotransferases, many patients with chronic liver disease are detected before symptoms are present. Unfortunately, however, blood banks tend to use the less expensive and less accurate ELISA testing for hepatitis C, which (as in this case) gives many false-positive results. Before starting therapy or establishing a diagnosis of type C hepatitis, a practitioner should confirm the diagnosis with RT-PCR.

A similar picture also may be seen in autoimmune hepatitis, Wilson disease, $\alpha$1-antitrypsin deficiency, and hemochromatosis. Isoniazid, a common medication for TB, can cause serious liver damage that may be clinically and histologically indistinguishable from viral chronic active hepatitis. Therefore, aminotransferases need to be carefully monitored in patients on this drug. This problem tends to occur in patients over the age of 50, particularly women.

The aminotransferases may only be minimally elevated, as in this patient. Generally, hepatitis develops after about 2 to 3 months of drug therapy. With withdrawal of the medication, the numbers usually return to normal over an additional 1 to 2 months. When the diagnosis of chronic active hepatitis is considered, a patient's medications must be carefully reviewed.

## MINICASE 9

## A Case of Acute Liver Failure

Matthew Z., an 18-year-old high school senior, notices he is becoming increasingly tired and somewhat weak. He initially is taken to a local clinic where he is reassured that most likely he is getting the "flu" and is sent home. Over the next day, he becomes progressively weaker, and his family notices that he is becoming yellow. He is taken to his physician.

He denies being on any medications or supplements. There is no family history of liver disease. Matthew Z. denies alcohol use. There has been no recent history of unusual travel.

Initial physical examination is unremarkable except for his being markedly icteric (jaundiced) and his liver being somewhat enlarged.

Laboratory findings include ALT 1,354 International Units/L, AST 1,457 International Units/L, and total bilirubin 12.5 mg/dL. Serum ALP is 245 International Units/L.

The tentative diagnosis is acute viral hepatitis. However, as more laboratory results come back, this diagnosis is increasingly under question because they show negative serologies for hepatitis A, B, C, and E. Evaluation for autoimmune hepatitis is negative as well with a negative antinuclear antibody (ANA) and antismooth muscle antibody. Serologies for mononucleosis and cytomegalovirus are negative as well.

Matthew Z. is admitted to the hospital; over the next 2 days, his total bilirubin progressively climbs to 23.4 mg/dL and his INR increases to 4. He becomes increasingly confused and lethargic, and a serum ammonia level is found to be elevated at 348 mcg/dL.

A diagnosis of acute liver failure is made, and he is transferred to a liver transplant center where he admits that in the days before the onset of his illness, he had visited his girlfriend in college and they both took some ecstasy (MDMA, 3,4-methylenedioxy-N-methylamphetamine).

QUESTION: What is acute liver failure and what generally causes it?

DISCUSSION: Acute liver failure refers to the rapid development (typically within 8 weeks) of severe liver injury with associated failure of the liver to perform its usual synthetic/detoxifying functions. In this case, it is evident by the elevated bilirubin, prolonged INR, and the development of hepatic encephalopathy. There are many potential causes, such as drug or toxin related, with acetaminophen being among the most common culprits. Viral hepatitis can cause this picture, as can ischemia of the liver, sepsis, autoimmune hepatitis, malignancy, and certain conditions associated with pregnancy.

MDMA hepatotoxicity is increasingly common in young people, as this drug is increasingly used. It can cause subclinical liver damage, including fibrosis, and is rarely associated with a picture of fulminant liver failure as in Matthew Z. Treatment is largely supportive and may involve liver transplantation.

## MINICASE 10

## A Case of Drug-Induced Hepatotoxicity

Darcie D. is a 43-year-old executive who presents to her doctor because she is not feeling well. She has become increasingly fatigued, lost her appetite, and just feels "sick."

Her past medical history is generally unremarkable; she does not smoke, drinks only socially, and does not take any medications or supplements. Physical examination is entirely normal.

Screening laboratory tests include a normal complete blood count (CBC), BUN, serum creatinine, and serum electrolytes. LFT results, however, are remarkable: ALT 257 International Units/L and AST 397 International Units/L. Her bilirubin is elevated at 2.3 mg/dL, and alkaline phosphatase is elevated at 367 units/L.

Additional laboratory findings include negative serologies for hepatitis A, B, and C. Tests to rule out autoimmune hepatitis (ANA, AMA) are negative, and tests to exclude hemochromatosis (iron, TIBC, and ferritin) are also normal.

Darcie D. presents again to her doctor's office, and on further questioning, she says that 3 weeks before, while on a business trip to California, she developed a bad cold and had been given azithromycin "Z-pak" at a local clinic. Over the next 2 weeks, Darcie's D.'s laboratory results gradually return to normal, and she reports feeling better.

QUESTION: Is it common for patients to develop symptomatic hepatitis weeks to months after exposure to hepatotoxins?

DISCUSSION: When we think of hepatotoxic agents (drugs, supplements, toxins), we tend to limit our thinking to a patient's current exposures. Usually, this alone solves our diagnostic dilemma. It is useful, however, to realize that often hepatoxicity can present weeks (occasionally months) after exposure. One classic agent that can present this way is amoxicillin–clavulanate. Azithromycin can present with jaundice, abdominal pain, pruritus, and evidence of hepatocellular injury weeks after a brief exposure. Treatment is generally supportive.

## MINICASE 11

## A Case of Nonalcoholic Steatohepatitis

Allen K., a 48-year-old corporate executive, presents for his required company physical examination. He had no medical complaints, has a negative past medical history, and is not taking any medications. He denies alcohol use.

Physical exam reveals weight 240 lb and height 5'10". His blood pressure is elevated at 154/98. The rest of his physical examination is normal.

Laboratory data include a normal CBC and kidney function, fasting glucose 129 mg/dL, and elevated cholesterol. His LFT results are elevated with ALT 134 International Units/L and AST 105 International Units/L. His serum bilirubin, albumin, ALP, and INR are all normal.

He is referred for evaluation of his abnormal liver panel, and further testing shows no evidence of viral hepatitis, hemochromatosis, or autoimmune liver disease. The possibility of fatty liver is raised, and a liver biopsy is performed, which shows NASH with early cirrhosis.

QUESTION: What is NASH, and how is it treated?

DISCUSSION: Our society is experiencing a marked increase in the incidence of obesity. Many of these patients develop what is defined as metabolic syndrome, which must have three of the following factors: abdominal obesity, elevated blood pressure, impaired glucose tolerance, or hyperlipidemia. Obese patients, particularly those with the metabolic syndrome, are at a higher risk of developing nonalcoholic fatty liver disease or fatty liver. Some patients with fatty liver can progress to NASH and ultimately to cirrhosis and liver failure. Progression to NASH is usually associated with abnormal LFTs. As in this case most patients who progress to cirrhosis have no symptoms to suggest progressive liver disease at the time the diagnosis is ultimately made. Although many drugs have been tried in these cases, ultimately the only accepted treatment is weight loss through diet and occasionally surgery, including laparoscopic gastric bypass, gastric sleeves, or banding. Fatty liver also can be caused by rapid weight loss, parenteral nutrition, medications (such as steroids, estrogens, amiodarone), and short bowel syndrome.

syndrome (SIRS), and death. Clinicians face the challenge of rapidly establishing this diagnosis, because many conditions (eg, ulcers, biliary disease, myocardial infarction, and intestinal ischemia or perforation) can present in a similar manner.

Chronic pancreatitis, generally due to chronic inflammation of the pancreas leading to progressive fibrosis and calcification, can lead to the development of diabetes mellitus or malabsorption caused by deficiencies in the production of pancreatic hormones (insulin) or enzymes.

Gallstones and alcohol abuse are causative factors in 60% to 80% of acute pancreatitis cases. Medications can also cause acute pancreatitis (**Table 15-8**). Other possible causes include trauma (a typical example being an injury due to a bicycle handlebar), penetrating ulcers, hypercalcemia, hypertriglyceridemia, pancreatic neoplasm, and hereditary or autoimmune pancreatitis. Often, however, it is impossible to determine the definite cause of a patient's attack. The tests discussed in this section, amylase and lipase, are primarily used to diagnose pancreatitis, although they may be clinically useful in the diagnosis of other pathologies. Of note is that lipase is increasingly the test of choice in the diagnosis of pancreatitis.

## Amylase

*Normal range: 20 to 96 units/L (method dependent) (0.34 to 1.6 μkat/L)*

*Amylase* is an enzyme that helps break starch into its individual sugar molecules. The most frequent clinical use of measuring serum amylase levels is in the diagnosis of acute and chronic pancreatitis. Although amylase levels have long been used for this diagnosis, increasingly lipase (see later discussion) is preferred in part due to its longer half-life and greater specificity.

### TABLE 15-8. Selected Drugs That May Cause Pancreatitis[a]

| | |
|---|---|
| 5-ASA drugs | Nitrofurantoin |
| ACE inhibitors | Pentamidine |
| Antiviral medications | Ranitidine |
| Asparaginase | Sitagliptin |
| Atypical antipsychotics | Statins |
| Azathioprine | Sulfonamides |
| Cimetidine | Sulindac |
| Corticosteroids | Tetracycline |
| Didanosine | Thiazides |
| Estrogens | Valproic acid |
| Exenatide | |
| Furosemide | |
| Isoniazid | |
| Mercaptopurine | |
| Methyldopa | |
| Metronidazole | |

ASA = acetylsalicylic acid.
[a]A good review on drug induced pancreatitis, with a much more inclusive list is seen in Jones MR, Hall OM, Kaye AM, et al. Drug induced pancreatitis: A review. *Ochsner J*; 2015 (Spring); 15:45–51.

As with any serum protein, concentrations result from the balance between entry into circulation and rate of clearance. Most circulating amylase originates from the pancreas and salivary glands. These sources are responsible for approximately 40% and 60% of serum amylase, respectively. However, the enzyme is also found in the lungs, liver, fallopian tubes, ovary, testis, small intestine, skeletal muscle, adipose tissue, thyroid, tonsils, and certain cancers, and various pathologies may increase secretion from these sources. The kidneys are responsible for about 25% of the metabolic clearance, with the remaining extrarenal mechanisms being poorly understood. The serum half-life is between 1 and 2 hours. Patients with azotemia can have decreased amylase clearance and elevated amylase levels. More than half of the patients who have a low creatinine clearance between 13 and 39 mL/min have elevated amylase levels. Although there is no amylase activity in neonates and only small amounts at 2 to 3 months of age, concentrations increase to the normal adult range by 1 year of age.

Amylase concentrations rise within 2 to 6 hours after the onset of acute pancreatitis and peak after 12 to 30 hours if the underlying inflammation has not recurred. In uncomplicated disease, these concentrations frequently return to normal within 3 to 5 days. More prolonged, mild elevations occur in up to 10% of patients with pancreatitis and may indicate ongoing pancreatic inflammation or associated complications (eg, pancreatic pseudocyst).

Although serum amylase concentrations do not correlate with disease severity or prognosis, a higher amylase may indicate a greater likelihood that the patient has pancreatitis. For example, serum amylase concentrations may increase up to 25 times the upper limit of normal in acute pancreatitis, while elevations from opiate-induced spasms of the sphincter of Oddi generally are <2 to 10 times the upper limit of normal. Unfortunately, the magnitude of enzyme elevation can overlap in these situations, and ranges are not very specific. Most guidelines require a 3-fold elevation in amylase (or lipase) as one of the criteria for establishing this diagnosis. The other two criteria are characteristic symptoms and an abnormal imaging study. Two criteria are generally required.

Amylase has a relatively low sensitivity, with about 20% of patients with acute pancreatitis having normal levels. This is especially common in patients with alcoholic pancreatitis or pancreatitis due to hypertriglyceridemia. Additionally, amylase has relatively low specificity and may be elevated in a wide range of conditions. These include a variety of diseases of the pancreas, salivary glands, GI tract (including hepatobiliary injury, perforated peptic ulcer, and intestinal obstruction or infarction), and gynecologic system (eg, ovarian or fallopian cysts) as well as pregnancy, trauma, renal failure, various neoplasms, and diabetic ketoacidosis. Additionally, alcohol and a variety of medications including, but not limited to, aspirin, cholinergics, thiazide diuretics, and oral contraceptives may also cause increased values.[34] In diagnosing acute pancreatitis, other useful laboratory tests include lipase because it is confounded by fewer factors and fractionation of serum amylase into pancreatic and salivary isoenzymes (although its use has been questioned).

Another condition that may cause elevated amylase concentrations is *macroamylasemia*, a benign condition present in 2% to 5% of patients with hyperamylasemia. In this condition, amylase molecules are bound by immunoglobulins or complex polysaccharides, forming aggregates that are too large to enter the glomerular filtrate and be cleared by the kidneys. This results in serum concentrations up to 10 times the normal limit. Macroamylasemia can be detected by fractionating serum amylase or by measuring urine amylase.

Urine amylase concentrations (normal range: <32 International Units for a 2-hour collection or <384 International Units for a 24-hour collection) usually peak later than serum concentrations, and elevations may persist for 7 to 10 days. This is useful if a patient is hospitalized after acute symptoms have subsided at which point serum amylase may already have returned to normal, leaving only urinary amylase to indicate pancreatitis. As discussed next, lipase may also persist after serum amylase levels decline. Urine amylase levels may also be useful in revealing macroamylasemia, in which case serum amylase is elevated, while urinary amylase is normal or decreased. However, this pattern of elevated serum amylase without elevated urinary amylase is also consistent with renal failure.

One cause of amylase's relatively low sensitivity is that marked hypertriglyceridemia may cause amylase measurements to be artificially low, masking an elevation in serum amylase. This finding is clinically relevant because hypertriglyceridemia (>800 mg/dL) is a potential cause of acute pancreatitis. In this situation, serial dilution of the serum specimen can eliminate the assay interference of hypertriglyceridemia, and elevated amylase values can be identified and measured. Fortunately, urinary amylase and serum lipase would typically be abnormal in this situation, which is another way to assess patients suspected of having elevated serum amylase levels.

## Lipase

*Normal range: 3 to 43 units/L (0.51 to 0.73 μkat/L)*

*Lipase* is an enzyme secreted by the pancreas that is transported from the pancreatic duct into the duodenum where it aids in fat digestion. Lipase catalyzes the hydrolysis of triglycerides into fatty acids and a monoglyceride that are more readily absorbed by the small intestine. Although mostly secreted by the pancreas, lipase can also be found in the tongue, esophagus, stomach, small intestine, leukocytes, adipose tissue, lung, breast milk, and liver. In healthy individuals, serum lipase tends to be mostly of pancreatic origin.

Lipase initially parallels amylase levels in acute pancreatitis, increasing rapidly and peaking at 12 to 30 hours. However, lipase has a half-life of 7 to 14 hours so that it declines much more slowly, typically returning to normal after 8 to 14 days. Thus, one utility of lipase (similar to urinary amylase) is the detection of acute pancreatitis roughly ≥3 days after onset, at which point amylase levels may no longer be elevated. As with amylase, peak lipase concentrations typically range from three to five times the upper limit of the reference range.

A comparison of the sensitivity and specificity of amylase versus lipase, and the use of these tests alone or in combination, is debated. This issue is complicated by the fact that the sensitivity and specificity of any laboratory test varies depending on where the cutoff is chosen (eg, choosing a higher cutoff increases specificity at the cost of lower sensitivity). In general, serum lipase appears to be superior, particularly with respect to specificity. However, simultaneous determination of both lipase and amylase may increase overall specificity because different factors confound the different assays. For example, an elevated amylase with a normal lipase suggests amylase of salivary origin or may represent macroamylasemia. Similarly, an elevated lipase with normal amylase has often been shown not to be due to pancreatitis, although in the case of pancreatitis it could be caused by delayed laboratory evaluation or artificial lowering of amylase levels by hypertriglyceridemia.[35]

Lipase concentrations may be elevated in patients with nonpancreatic abdominal pain, such as a ruptured abdominal aortic aneurysm, and a variety of disorders of the alimentary tract and liver, such as intestinal infarction. This is because lipase is located in these organs. Renal failure, nephrolithiasis, diabetic ketoacidosis, and alcoholism are conditions in which lipase elevations tend to be present but usually in concentrations less than three times the upper limit of the reference range. Drug-induced elevations in lipase can be attributed to opioids (codeine, morphine), nonsteroidal antiinflammatory drugs (NSAIDs; indomethacin), and cholinergics (methacholine and bethanechol). In the condition of macrolipasemia, similar to macroamylasemia but far less frequent, macromolecular complexes of lipase to immunoglobulin prevent excretion and elevate serum lipase concentrations.[36]

## Other Test Results in Pancreatitis

In severe cases of acute pancreatitis, occasionally several days after the insult, fat necrosis may result in the formation of organic soaps that bind calcium. Serum calcium concentrations then decrease (low albumin may also contribute), sometimes enough to cause tetany. When pancreatitis is of biliary tract origin, typical elevations in ALP, bilirubin, AST, and ALT are seen. Some researchers believe that in acute pancreatitis an increase of ALT to three times baseline or higher is relatively specific for gallstone-induced pancreatitis.

Pancreatitis also may be associated with hemoconcentration and subsequent elevations of the BUN or hematocrit. Depending on the severity of the attack, lactic acidosis, azotemia, anemia, hyperglycemia, hypoalbuminemia, or hypoxemia may also occur.

Despite the performance of amylase and lipase assays for acute pancreatitis, the sensitivity and specificity of these tests are often regarded as unsatisfactory, and in some patients, pancreatitis is only diagnosed on autopsy. For this reason, several new tests have been investigated (eg, serum trypsin and trypsinogen), although they are not yet widely available. Ultimately, it is recognized that the lack of sensitivity for both amylase and lipase implies that these tests can be used to support a diagnosis of acute pancreatitis but may not definitively provide a secure diagnosis, particularly if the levels are not dramatically elevated. Recent practice guidelines suggest that two of the following are needed to diagnose acute pancreatitis: (1) characteristic symptoms; (2) elevation of amylase or lipase to at least three times normal; (3) characteristic findings on imaging (usually CT or MRI) (**Minicase 12, Minicase 13**).

# MINICASE 12

## Diagnosing Pancreatitis

James T., a 55-year-old man, develops a vague but persistent epigastric pain that radiates to his back. He notes that his appetite is "off," and his clothes are getting much looser on him. His pain is not related to eating, activity, or position.

He presents to his primary care physician, who documents that he lost about 25 lb in the past year. His physical examination is unremarkable. Laboratory data show a normal CBC, renal function, and LFTs. His amylase and lipase are both elevated, with a serum amylase of 189 units/L and a lipase of 390 units/L. Serum calcium and triglycerides are normal.

There are no identifiable precipitating causes noted. The first consideration is that he might have acute or even chronic pancreatitis.

A CT scan shows a pancreatic mass. He is referred to a surgeon for consideration of surgery, with a presumptive diagnosis of pancreatic carcinoma. James T. and his family, however, get a second opinion. Further workup shows an elevated ANA and a serum IgG4 markedly elevated at 464 mg/dL (normal being up to 140 mg/mL).

The diagnosis of autoimmune pancreatitis is suggested, and James T. is offered a pancreatic biopsy. He elects for a 2-week trial of steroids.

Prednisone is started at 40 mg/day. Two weeks later, he reports feeling better, and his CT demonstrates a marked reduction in the size of his mass.

QUESTION: How do we diagnose autoimmune pancreatitis?

DISCUSSION: Autoimmune pancreatitis is a new recognized disease in which patients can present with findings often indistinguishable from pancreatic cancer or chronic pancreatitis. The diagnosis is suggested if other autoimmune diseases are present, including Sjögren syndrome, autoimmune thyroid diseases, and autoimmune renal diseases. In this patient, the presence of a markedly elevated IgG4 level is highly suggestive of this autoimmune disease. The biopsy would likely have been diagnostic. However, a rapid response to steroids is virtually diagnostic of this condition. In some cases, the steroids can be tapered down, and some patients require ongoing immunosuppressive therapy, usually with azathioprine.

The importance of making this diagnosis is in providing appropriate therapy and avoiding what would have been extensive, life-changing surgery. The patient's steroids were tapered over a period of time, and his CT results did revert to normal.

# MINICASE 13

## Abdominal Pain in a Young Woman

Betsy L., a 32-year-old woman, presents with a sudden onset of severe epigastric pain radiating to her back. She has tried antacids without any relief. This began after a night of heavy partying and drinking. Her past history is otherwise unremarkable. She and her family deny a history of chronic alcohol abuse. Physical examination shows some tenderness in her epigastric area, which is otherwise benign. Lab studies showed a normal CBC, and her lipase is markedly elevated at 1,382 units/L, with an elevated ALT of 592 units/L and an AST of 649 units/L. Her total bilirubin is elevated at 2.8 mg/dL. Serum lipid profile and calcium are normal. She is admitted to the hospital with a diagnosis of alcohol-induced pancreatitis.

QUESTION: Does she really have alcoholic pancreatitis? What else might be going on here?

DISCUSSION: Typically, alcoholic pancreatitis does not occur just after an occasional episode of binge drinking; it is generally seen in people with a long history of chronic alcohol abuse. Her LFT results are markedly abnormal, suggesting a hepatobiliary etiology. Additionally, serum lipase levels >1,000 do not suggest alcoholic-induced pancreatitis but suggest a surgical cause of her pancreatitis. In this case there were no medications that could have caused her

attack and no history of abdominal trauma. Her lipids and calcium were normal.

An ultrasound of her abdomen showed gallstones in a somewhat inflamed gall bladder, dilated biliary ducts, and a 1-cm stone in her distal bile duct. An endoscopic retrograde cholangiopancreatography was undertaken with removal of the stone, and subsequently she underwent a laparoscopic cholecystectomy.

Gallstone disease is one of the two most common causes of acute pancreatitis in the United States, the other being alcohol. The mechanism, while not completely understood, seems to be the passing of a stone from the gallbladder, down the common bile duct, and through the ampulla. In the ampulla, it may serve to block the pancreatic duct, and indeed sometimes a stone will lodge at that site. Additionally, it may cause reflux of bile into the pancreatic duct. In most cases, by the time of diagnosis, the offending stone has passed, and the approach would be to remove the gallbladder (preferably during the same hospitalization) to prevent recurrent attacks. In this case, the stone had not passed, and it was removed endoscopically prior to the surgery.

# ULCER DISEASE

Up to 10% of the U.S. population develops duodenal or gastric *ulcers* at some point in life. Previously, ulcers were believed to be primarily due to acid. Traditional therapy with antacids, histamine-2-antagonists, and proton pump inhibitors (PPIs) have been effective in treating ulcers, but they are not as effective in preventing recurrences, in part because they do not eradicate the underlying bacterial cause.

## Helicobacter pylori

*H pylori* has been identified as a cause of ulcer disease, and studies into its detection and treatment are still in a state of rapid development.[37] *H pylori* is a gram-negative bacillus, usually acquired during childhood, that establishes lifelong colonization of the gastric epithelium in affected individuals. Transmission seems to be by the fecal–oral or oral–oral route. Prevalence increases with age and correlates with poor sanitation. By the age of 50, 40% to 50% of people in developed countries and >90% of people in developing countries harbor these bacteria.[38]

*H pylori* infection may be found in >90% of patients with duodenal ulcers and >80% of patients with gastric ulcers. Furthermore, the bacterium has been associated with the development of gastritis, gastric cancer, and certain types of gastric lymphoma. The most common lymphoma associated with *H pylori* is mucosa-associated lymphoid tissue, which is often curable just by treating the underlying *H pylori* infection. However, most infected individuals (>70%) are asymptomatic, and eradication therapy remains a controversial subject for asymptomatic colonization. From the other perspective, *H pylori*-infected individuals have a 10% to 20% chance of developing peptic ulcers and a 1% to 2% chance of developing gastric cancer during their lifetime. Candidates for screening for *H pylori* include those with active ulcer disease, history of ulcer disease, and certain gastric lymphomas. Screening should be considered prior to long-term therapy with aspirin or NSAIDs or in patients under the age of 60 with chronic dyspepsia. One problem in managing patients with *H pylori* infection is that treatment is not always successful in eradicating this bacterium, in part due to increasing resistance to antibiotics. In the United States, rates of resistance to metronidazole (20% to 40%) and clarithromycin (10% to 15%) have been documented.

## Helicobacter pylori-*Associated Gastric Cancer*

*H pylori*-associated gastric cancers account for about 5.5% of all cancers worldwide and about one-fourth of all infection-associated cancers. Its colonization is a key component for the development of gastric cancer; however, other factors, such as atrophic changes in the stomach, are needed for this to occur. Atrophic gastritis, characterized by chronic inflammation of the gastric mucosa, decreases and ultimately inhibits the ability of the stomach to secrete acid. Eradication of *H pylori* infection before atrophic changes occur can provide protection from gastric cancer. Individuals who have already suffered irreversible atrophic changes may still receive some benefit but should be considered at risk even after eradication. Currently, there is no effective *H pylori* vaccine available, so bacterial eradication must be executed with antibiotic therapy.

### Diagnosis

The diagnostic tests for *H pylori* are classified as *noninvasive* (serology, urea breath test, and fecal antigen test) or *invasive* (histology, culture, and rapid urea test)—the latter depending on upper endoscopy and biopsy. The serological test for *H pylori* detects circulating IgG antibodies against bacterial proteins. It has a relatively low sensitivity and specificity (80% to 95%) but has advantages of being widely available and inexpensive. Although useful to establish an initial diagnosis of *H pylori*, it should not be used to monitor the success of eradication therapy because antibody titers decrease slowly in the absence of bacteria.

The urea breath test is based on the ability of the bacteria to produce urease, an enzyme that breaks down urea and releases ammonia and carbon dioxide as its products. In the breath test, $^{13}C$- or $^{14}C$-labeled urea is given by mouth. If the bacteria are present, the radiolabeled urea is metabolized to radiolabeled $CO_2$, which may be measured in exhaled air. The tests have high sensitivity and specificity (both 90% to 95% for $^{13}C$ and 86% to 95% for $^{14}C$). However, the $^{14}C$ isotope has the drawback of being radioactive, and the $^{13}C$ isotope requires the use of sophisticated detection methods such as isotope ratio mass spectrometry (although samples are stable and may be sent off for analysis).

The fecal antigen test detects *H pylori* proteins in stool via ELISA. It has high sensitivity and specificity, both 90% to 95%. Like the urea breath test, the fecal antigen test is a very accurate noninvasive measure that is used primarily to monitor the success of eradication therapy. The fecal antigen test may not be appropriate for patients with active GI bleeding because of a cross-reactivity with blood constituents in the immunoassay, which can produce a high incidence of false-positive results. Patients undergoing urea breath tests or fecal antigen tests need to discontinue PPIs for 2 weeks before these tests are conducted because PPIs may decrease the numbers of *H pylori* in the stomach and decrease test accuracy.

Upper endoscopy with biopsy of gastric tissue and subsequent histologic examination has high sensitivity and specificity (88% to 95% and 90% to 95%, respectively) with the added advantage of allowing detection of gastritis, intestinal metaplasia, or other histologic features. Although not commonly performed, biopsy specimens may also be used to culture *H pylori*. By performing various tests on the cultured bacteria, this test may be rendered highly specific (95% to 98%), but the bacterium is difficult to culture, making this the least sensitive test (80% to 90%). The main advantage of culture is that it allows for antibiotic sensitivity testing, which can help optimize therapy and possibly prevent treatment failure. A rapid urease test (also known as the *Campylobacter-like organism test*) involves incubating a biopsy specimen in the presence of urea and a pH indicator. As mentioned previously, *H pylori* metabolizes urea, releasing ammonia, which in this case may be detected by its effect of increasing the pH. This test allows for rapid results (eg, 1-hour incubation time following endoscopy), high sensitivity and specificity (both 90% to 95%, respectively), and low cost. One proposed strategy is to take several biopsies at the time of endoscopy and first check the rapid urease test, sending specimens for detailed pathologic analysis only if the urease test is negative (or tissue diagnosis is needed to sort out other diagnoses).

All of these tests, with the exception of serology, tend to be confounded by factors that lower bacterial burden. In patients with achlorhydria or patients being treated with antisecretory drugs (eg, PPIs), increased stomach pH decreases bacterial levels and may lead to false-negative results. Similarly, use of bismuth or antibiotics (including recent, unsuccessful eradication therapy) may decrease test sensitivity. Recommendations advise waiting 2 to 3 months after finishing therapy before performing these tests to determine whether H pylori has been successfully eradicated and additionally holding PPIs for 2 weeks.

Although GI bleeding may confound the rapid urease test and the fecal antigen test, urea breath tests remain a viable diagnostic option in patients with active bleeding, detecting 86% of H pylori-positive patients.

# COLITIS

Colitis—acute or chronic inflammation of the colon—often presents quite dramatically with profound and bloody diarrhea, urgency, and abdominal cramping. It is generally distinguished from noninflammatory causes of diarrhea on the basis of physical signs, including fever, abdominal tenderness, and an elevated white blood cell (WBC) count in the blood.

There are many causes of colitis. Infectious colitis may be caused by invasive organisms, including Campylobacter jejuni, Shigella, Salmonella, and invasive Escherichia coli. Amoeba can present in this manner, as can certain infections associated with HIV/AIDS; for example, cytomegalovirus and herpes virus have also been found to cause a colitis picture. Recently COVID-19 has been found to be associated with diarrheal symptoms, including a colitis picture.[39] Noninfectious colitis includes ischemic colitis, drug-induced colitis (as with gold salts or NSAIDs), inflammatory bowel disease (Crohn's disease or ulcerative colitis), and radiation injury. C difficile colitis, which is discussed in the next section, is a relatively new disease that has emerged as a major cause of hospital-acquired infection over the past 40 years, largely caused by the widespread use of broad-spectrum antibiotics.

## Clostridioides Difficile (Pseudomembranous Colitis)

C difficile colitis is a toxin-induced bacterial disease, which has become increasingly common and progressively more difficult to treat. Most infections follow antibiotic use, which reduces the normal bacterial flora of the colon and produces a niche for supra-infection by C difficile.[40] As such, C difficile infection only became common following widespread use of broad-spectrum antibiotics in the 1960s. C difficile infection is most commonly associated with, but not limited to, exposure to fluoroquinolones, clindamycin, cephalosporins, and β-lactamase inhibitors. Clinical symptoms of infection range from an asymptomatic carrier state to chronic diarrhea, acute colitis, and life-threatening colitis with sepsis. Attacks can occur weeks after antibiotic therapy. Severe C difficile colitis is marked by a characteristic appearance of pseudomembranes, which consist of inflammatory exudates or yellowish plaques on the colonic mucosa and is thus referred to as pseudomembranous colitis. Milder cases present with inflammation limited to the superficial colonic epithelium; however, in severe cases there can be necrosis of the full thickness of the colonic wall.[41]

Clostridia species have the ability to form spores that can survive extreme environmental conditions and remain viable for years. Spores tend to persist within the hospital environment where they may infect patients receiving antibiotics, causing C difficile to be the most common cause of infectious diarrhea in hospitalized patients.

C difficile produces clinical disease by secreting various toxins within the colon. Toxins A and B are the most common toxins produced, with >90% of pathogenic strains producing toxin A. These toxins affect the permeability of enterocytes, trigger apoptosis, and stimulate inflammation. Some emerging strains also produce a binary toxin, which is associated with a more severe illness. The bacterium itself is not pathogenic, and some strains of C difficile do not produce toxins and are therefore harmless.

About 3% of healthy adults and 20% of hospitalized patients are asymptomatically colonized with C difficile bacteria. Unlike other similar hospital-infections (eg, Staphylococcus aureus), asymptomatic carriage of C difficile bacteria actually reduces the likelihood of developing clinical disease, even after antibiotic exposure. This is probably because people who are asymptomatically colonized have developed antibodies that neutralize the C difficile toxins or have harmless strains of C difficile, which produce no toxin (yet occupy a niche in the colon preventing infection by toxigenic strains).

Recently, several outbreaks have resulted from a new strain of C difficile bacteria that is resistant to fluoroquinolones (eg, ciprofloxacin, moxifloxacin).[42] This strain expresses a binary toxin (until now generally not seen in clinical isolates) and upregulates its expression of toxins A and B by about 20-fold. Clinically, this correlates with ominous increases in morbidity and mortality. The continued emergence of C difficile strains with resistance to commonly used antibiotics and increased expression of virulence factors suggests that this bacterium will continue to be a serious complication of antibiotic use until a toxin vaccine can be developed. Current treatment consists of metronidazole (oral or IV) or vancomycin (oral or rectal), depending on severity; however, 20% to 30% of patients who receive therapy will face recurrent C difficile infection. Fidaxomicin, a more recently U.S. Food and Drug Administration–approved narrow spectrum macrolide for C difficile infection, may serve as a beneficial alternative therapy.[43] A newer approach to treatment of C difficile involves fecal transplantation, in which stool is "donated" by a healthy donor and instilled into the GI tract of the infected patient.

Prevention of C difficile infection is largely based on avoidance of antibiotic therapy, unless absolutely necessary, and careful handwashing in hospitals and other institutional settings (including in-home patient care). C difficile spores are somewhat resistant to alcohol-based hand disinfectants, so washing with soap and water is preferred.

## Diagnosis

The diagnosis of *C difficile* can be challenging. There are a variety of tests available that vary in sensitivity, specificity, cost, availability, and timeliness. One important consideration is that patients with pseudomembranous colitis may deteriorate rapidly, so making a prompt and accurate diagnosis is important. In situations that clearly point to a diagnosis of *C difficile* in an acutely ill patient, it may be reasonable to initiate treatment on an empirical basis before the test results are even available. Hospitals and labs seem to have their own specific algorithms in terms of testing for *C difficile*. Diagnosis may also be made during lower endoscopy on encountering the characteristic white or yellow pseudomembranes on the colonic wall.

Generally, the most commonly used initial tests for *C difficile* infection are the ELISA assays for toxin or *C difficile* antigen within the stool. These tests are available in various commercial kits and have the advantage of being rapid, producing results within hours, and relatively inexpensive. Tests detect toxin A or both toxins A and B and have high specificity (typically >95%) but variable sensitivity (60% to 95%). For this reason, a negative test may be followed by one to two repeat tests to increase the composite sensitivity to the 90% range and exclude infection with more certainty. Testing for both toxins has a diagnostic advantage over testing for toxin A because a minority of strains are toxin A-negative and toxin B-positive. Alternatively, a negative test result is often confirmed with a PCR study (see later discussion).

Enzyme-linked immunosorbent assays for *C difficile* common antigen (glutamate dehydrogenase) have improved sensitivity but are less specific because they detect nontoxigenic species as well as some species of closely related anaerobes. Therefore, a positive assay for *C difficile* antigen does not prove pseudomembranous colitis and must be followed up with a toxin assay to prove the presence of a pathogenic *C difficile* strain. The advantage of this assay for *C difficile* antigen is that the sensitivity is better, such that a single negative assay may be used to exclude the presence of pseudomembranous colitis. The availability, performance, and appropriate use of these assays may vary among hospital laboratories, and inquiries should be made with the laboratory regarding which tests are available and the appropriate strategy for their use.

The "gold standard" test for pseudomembranous colitis has been the detection of toxin A or B in stool samples by demonstrating their cytopathic effect in cell cultures and inhibition of cytopathic effect by specific antiserum. Referred to as *cell cytotoxicity assay*, this test has excellent sensitivity (94% to 100%) and specificity (99%). However, these performance characteristics may be laboratory dependent. Moreover, this test is limited by high cost, a requirement for meticulously maintained tissue culture facilities, and a time delay of 1 to 3 days.

*C difficile* can also be cultured from stools with selective medium and identified with more traditional microbiologic techniques, including colony morphology, fluorescence, odor, gram stain, and signature gas liquid chromatography.

Interestingly, this is not the most sensitive test for the organism. In addition, the bacterium is named *difficile* because of *difficulty* in culturing it. Another drawback is that isolated bacteria must then be tested for toxin production to avoid confusing it with nontoxic *C difficile* strains. Altogether, these factors make bacterial culture and toxin profiling a costly, time-consuming process; thus, they are rarely used. The primary advantage of this approach is that it isolates the organism, allowing genetic tests, which may aid in tracking mutant strains and determining the source of epidemics.

Nucleic acid amplification tests, including RT-PCR assays for the gene toxin A or B, not only provide fast and accurate diagnosis of *C difficile* but also provide the ability to identify if the pathogen is in the epidemic 027/NAP1/BI strain.[44] This test is rapidly becoming a standard test for initial evaluation of *C difficile* infections. More typically it is being used if the initial test results (toxin, antigen studies) are negative. One issue with these tests is that they can detect asymptomatic carriers and should only be used in patients with frequent loose stools (**Minicase 14**).

## SUMMARY

Analysis of liver tests is complex and may be frustrating. Most tests in the LFT panel check for the presence of two broad categories of liver diseases—cholestasis versus hepatocellular injury. Therefore, an abnormal value may raise more questions than it answers. None of the tests is 100% sensitive or specific, and most may be confounded by a variety of factors. How, then, can these tests be used to answer clinical questions with any certainty?

Probably the most important point to bear in mind when interpreting LFTs is that they are but one piece of the puzzle. Correct interpretation relies on interpreting the test within the greater context of the patient, other laboratory data, historical information, and the physical exam.[2,19] For example, mildly elevated bilirubin and ALP in the setting of a critically ill, septic patient is likely cholestasis of sepsis and does not necessarily require extensive evaluation. The same set of laboratory tests (mildly elevated bilirubin and ALP) in an ambulatory patient could be a sign of serious chronic illness such as PBC. However, if this same ambulatory patient had a history of normal LFTs and had recently started taking a medication known to cause cholestasis, then the abnormality would most likely be a side effect of the medication. Thus, the same set of liver tests in three different settings may have widely differing significance.

It is also important to interpret an abnormal value within the context of other laboratory tests, which is why LFTs are often obtained as a group (ie, the LFT panel). For example, a mildly elevated AST in the setting of an otherwise normal LFT panel might be of nonhepatic origin (eg, muscle disease). Alternatively, a mildly elevated AST combined with mildly elevated ALT might raise a concern about a mild hepatocellular process, perhaps chronic viral hepatitis or NASH. Finally, mildly elevated ALT and AST in combination with dramatically elevated ALP and bilirubin would point instead to a cholestatic process.

## MINICASE 14

### Antibiotic-Induced Pseudomembranous Colitis

Julia T., a 36-year-old woman, presents to her physician after several days of crampy abdominal pain, diarrhea, persistent fever up to 102.5°F, and chills. On physical examination, she is well hydrated. Her abdomen is soft and nontender. Stools are sent for pathogenic bacterial cultures, including *Shigella*, *Salmonella*, *Campylobacter*, entero-invasive *E coli*, and *Yersinia*; meanwhile, Julia T. is given a prescription for diphenoxylate.

Twenty-four hours later, Julia T. presents to the emergency department (ED) doubled over with severe abdominal pain. Her abdomen is distended and tender with diffuse rigidity and guarding. Clinically, she is dehydrated. Her WBC count is elevated at 23,000 cells/mm³ (3.54 to 9.06 × 10³ cells/mm³), and her BUN is 34 mg/dL. Abdominal radiographs show a dilated colon (toxic megacolon) and an ileus. She then tells the ED physician that about 6 weeks earlier, she had taken two or three of her sister's amoxicillin pills because she had thought she was developing a urinary tract infection. Although pseudomembranous colitis is tentatively diagnosed, Julia T. cannot take oral medication because of her ileus. Therefore, IV metronidazole and rectal vancomycin are started. She continues to get sicker, however, and early the next day, most of her colon is removed (the rectum was left intact), and an ileostomy is created.

QUESTION: What is the time course of pseudomembranous colitis? Did the use of diphenoxylate influence the outcome?

DISCUSSION: Pseudomembranous colitis can occur even after only one or two doses of a systemic antibiotic or after topical antibiotic use. Moreover, it can occur weeks after the last dose of antibiotic. A complete history of antibiotic use is critical when dealing with patients with diarrhea.

Diphenoxylate or loperamide use in the face of colitis is associated with an increased risk, although small, of toxic megacolon. In this medical emergency, the colon has no peristalsis. Together with the inflammation in the colon wall (colitis), toxic megacolon often leads to progressive distention. If untreated, perforation and death ensue. The development of a megacolon or ileus in this patient is especially worrisome because the best treatment—oral antibiotics—would be of little benefit. However, IV metronidazole is excreted into the bile in adequate bactericidal levels to eradicate the bacteria. Unfortunately, in the absence of peristalsis, its benefit would be questionable.

Therefore, liver tests should always be interpreted with a clear understanding of the clinical context and other laboratory abnormalities. Although the LFT panel rarely yields an exact diagnosis, it may indicate the type of process (eg, cholestatic versus hepatocellular) and the severity of the process (eg, fulminant liver failure versus mild hepatic inflammation), which leads the practitioner to a group of possibilities that may be further evaluated based on the information at hand, along with other laboratory tests or studies (eg, radiographs, endoscopic procedures, or tissue biopsies) as needed. The diagnostic yield of these tests also depends on their appropriateness and the thoughtfulness of their selection. Liver studies obtained to answer a specific clinical question (eg, "Does this patient have liver inflammation due to initiation of statin medications?") are more likely to yield interpretable information than a less guided question ("Is this patient sick?").

Some other aspects of gastroenterology and related laboratory tests are also reviewed in this chapter. Amylase and lipase may reflect pancreatic inflammation; *H pylori* may be related to ulcer disease; and *C difficile* is a major cause of hospital-acquired colitis. Although these tests are less convoluted than the LFT panel, it is still paramount to obtain them in a thoughtful manner and interpret the results in the appropriate clinical setting. For example, colonization with *H pylori* may be of little acute significance in an asymptomatic patient, whereas it may mandate an immediate course of multiple antibiotics in a patient with recurrent gastric ulcer bleeding.

## LEARNING POINTS

1. **Why is the term *liver function test* a misnomer?**

   **ANSWER:** Often, the term is used to describe a panel of tests, including AST, ALT, bilirubin, ALP, and albumin. However, the term is a misnomer because most of these tests do not measure liver function. The liver has several functions and different tests reflect these different functions. The following table divides liver tests into rough categories by function and type.

   | FUNCTION/TYPE | LABORATORY TESTS |
   |---|---|
   | Synthetic liver function | Albumin, prealbumin, PT/INR |
   | Excretory function | ALP, 5′ nucleotidase, GGT, bilirubin |
   | Hepatocellular injury | AST, ALT |
   | Detoxification | Ammonia |

2. **What common disorders cause isolated increased indirect bilirubinemia versus direct bilirubinemia? Explain the pathophysiologic cause of the laboratory abnormality in each case.**

   **ANSWER:** Indirect bilirubin is produced by the breakdown of erythrocytes. Indirect bilirubin is delivered to the liver, where it is converted to direct bilirubin by glucuronyl transferase. Thus, an elevated level of indirect bilirubin may result from increased breakdown of red blood cells (hemolysis) or reduced hepatic conversion of indirect bilirubin to direct bilirubin. Common causes include hemolysis, Gilbert syndrome, and drugs, such as probenecid or rifampin.

Increased direct bilirubin usually implies hepatic disease, which interferes with secretion of bilirubin from the hepatocytes or clearance of bile from the liver. There are exceptions to this, Dubin-Johnson syndrome and Rotor syndrome being two benign abnormalities of bilirubin metabolism and excretion. Direct hyper-bilirubinemia, especially in the presence of other abnormalities in the LFT profile, is generally classified as reflecting hepatic cholestasis, although it may also be due to a hepatocellular process. In cholestatic disease, the bilirubin is primarily conjugated, whereas in hepatocellular processes, significant increases in both conjugated and unconjugated bilirubin may result. Cholestasis may be intrahepatic or extrahepatic. Intrahepatic cholestasis may be due to viral hepatitis, reactions to different medications, alcoholic hepatitis or cirrhosis, pregnancy, severe infection, or PBC. Extrahepatic cholestasis involves obstruction of the larger bile ducts either inside or outside of the liver, which can be due to strictures, stones, or tumors.

### 3. What is the relative importance of AST and ALT tests in terms of diagnosing hepatocellular disease?

**ANSWER:** Elevations of AST and ALT generally reflect inflammation in the liver. However, they are not associated with prognosis (higher levels do not suggest a worse prognosis) or with etiology. Although there is value in assessing the ratios of these two (for example an AST/ALT ratio of over two may suggest alcoholic liver disease), these tests do not "tell the whole story." Evaluating a patient with suspected liver disease is a complex undertaking. The history must be obtained in detail, including present and past medications, supplements, vitamins, occupational exposure, underlying diseases, history of surgical procedures, history of transfusions, and drug use.

### 4. How is acute pancreatitis diagnosed?

**ANSWER:** The clinical presentation of acute pancreatitis generally consists of epigastric pain, often radiating to the back. There can be associated nausea, vomiting, diaphoresis, and fever. The challenge here is that these symptoms are not specific at all. Similar complaints can be seen with biliary disease, ulcers, gastritis, small bowel problems, or compromised blood supply to the gut. At times there can be overlap. Gallstones can migrate down the common bile duct, causing pancreatitis. Ulcers can penetrate the duodenum and invade the pancreas also causing pancreatitis. To establish a diagnosis of pancreatitis one looks for three things. First, the clinical picture should be consistent with this diagnosis. Second, a serum lipase or amylase should be over three times normal (realizing that these tests are not specific). Third, it is often of value (especially if the first two criteria are not both present) to have an advanced imaging study, either MRI or CT, showing pancreatitis. Generally, two of the three criteria should be present before diagnosing acute pancreatitis.

# REFERENCES

1. Kwo PK, Cohen SM, Lim JK. ACG clinical guideline: evaluation of abnormal liver chemistries. *Am J Gastroenterol.* 2017;112:18-25.

2. Kasper DL, Fauci AS, Hauser SL, et al. *Harrison's Principles of Internal Medicine.* 19th ed. New York, NY: McGraw Hill; 2015.

3. Chopra S, Griffin PH. Laboratory tests and diagnostic procedures in evaluation of liver disease. *Am J Med.* 1985;79:221-230.

4. Neyra NR, Hakim RM, Shyr Y, et al. Serum transferrin and serum prealbumin are early predictors of serum albumin in chronic hemodialysis patients. *J Ren Nutr.* 2000;10:184-190.

5. Spiekerman AM. Nutritional assessment (protein nutriture). *Anal Chem.* 1995;67:429R-436R.

6. Mittman N, Avram MM, Oo KK, et al. Serum prealbumin predicts survival in hemodialysis and peritoneal dialysis: 10 years of prospective observation. *Am J Kidney Dis.* 2001;38:1358-1364.

7. Giannini EG, Testa R, Savarino V. Liver enzyme alteration: a guide for clinicians. *CMAJ.* 2005;172:367-379.

8. Green RM, Flamm S. AGA technical review on the evaluation of liver chemistry tests. *Gastroenterology.* 2002;123:1367-1384.

9. Birkett DJ, Done J, Neale FC, et al. Serum alkaline phosphatase in pregnancy: an immunologic study. *Br Med J.* 1966;1:1210-212.

10. Wilson JW. Inherited elevation of alkaline phosphatase activity in the absence of disease. *N Engl J Med.* 1979;301:983-984.

11. Pratt DS, Kaplan MM. Evaluation of abnormal liver-enzyme results in asymptomatic patients. *N Engl J Med.* 2000;342:1266-1271.

12. Kaplan MM, Matloff DS, Selinger MJ, et al. Biochemical basis for serum enzyme abnormalities in alcoholic liver disease. In: Chang NC, Chan NM, eds. Early Identification of Alcohol Abuse. NIAAA Research Monograph 17. Rockville, MD, US Department of Health and Human Services; 1985:186-198.

13. Friedman LS, Keefee EB. *Handbook of Liver Disease.* 3rd ed. Philadelphia, PA: Elsevier Saunders; 2012.

14. Dukes GE, Sanders SW, Russo J, et al. Transaminase elevations in patients receiving bovine or porcine heparin. *Ann Intern Med.* 1984;100:646-650.

15. Chalasani N, Younossi Z, Lavine JE, et al. The diagnosis and management of nonalcoholic fatty liver disease: practice guideline from the American Association for the Study of Liver Diseases. *Hepatology.* 2018;67(1):328-357.

16. Diehl A, Boitnott J, Van Duyn M, et al. Relationship between pyridoxal 5′-phosphate deficiency and aminotransferase levels in alcoholic hepatitis. *Gastroenterology.* 1984;86:632-636.

17. Cohen GA, Goffinet JA, Donabedian RK, et al. Observations on decreased serum glutamic oxaloacetic transaminase (SGOT) activity in azotemic patients. *Ann Intern Med.* 1976;84:275-280.

18. Chtioui H, Mauerhofer O, Gunther B, et al. Macro-AST in an asymptomatic young patient. *Ann Hepatol.* 2010;9:93-95.

19. Vilstrup H, Amodio P, Bajaj J, et al. Hepatic encephalopathy in chronic liver disease: 2014 practice guideline by the American Association for the Study of Liver Diseases and the European Association for the Study of the Liver. *Hepatology.* 2014 60:715-733.

20. Chtioui H, Mauerhofer O, Gunther B, et al. Macro-AST in an asymptomatic young patient. *Ann Hepatol.* 2010;9:93-95.

21. Ong JP, Aggarwal A, Krieger D, et al. Correlation between ammonia levels and the severity of hepatic encephalopathy. *Am J Med.* 2003;114:188-193.

22. Haj M, Rockey DC. Ammonia levels do not guide clinical management of patients with hepatic encephalopathy caused by cirrhosis. *Am J Gastroenterol.* 2020;115:723-728.

23. Bhatia V, Singh R, Acharya SK. Predictive value of arterial ammonia for complications and outcome of acute liver failure. *Gut.* 2006;55:98-104.

24. Foster MA, Hofmeister MG, Kupronis BA, et al. Increase in hepatitis A virus infections, United States, 2013-2018. *MMWR Morb Mortal Wkly Rep.* 2019;68:413.

25. Pawlotsky JM. Molecular diagnosis of viral hepatitis. *Gastroenterology.* 2002;122:554-568.

26. AASLD-ISDA Hepatitis C Guidance Panel. Hepatitis C Guidance 2019 Update: American Association for the Study of Liver Disease-Infectious Disease Society of America recommendations for testing, managing, and treating hepatitis C virus infection. *Hepatology.* 2019;71:686-709.

27. Lindor K, Bowlus CL, Boyer J, et al. Primary biliary cholangitis: 2018 practice guidance from the American Association for the Study of Liver Diseases. *Hepatology.* 2019;69(1):394-419.

28. Kowdley KV, Brown KE, Ahn J, et al. ACG clinical guideline: hereditary hemochromatosis. *Am J Gastroenterol.* 2019;114:1202-1208.

29. Siddique A, Kowdley K. Review article: the iron overload syndromes. *Aliment Pharmacol Ther.* 2012; 35:876-893.

30. Cherfane C, Hollenbeck R, Go J, et al. Hereditary hemochromatosis: missed diagnosis or misdiagnosis? *Am J Med.* 2013;126:1010-1015.

31. Bacon B, Adams P, Kowdley K, et al. Diagnosis and management of hemochromatosis: 2011 practice guideline by the American Association for the Study of Liver Disease. *Hepatology.* 2011;54(1):328-343.

32. Salgia R, Brown K. Diagnosis and management of hereditary hemochromatosis. *Clin Liver Dis.* 2015;19:187-198.

33. Tenner S, Baillie J, DeWitt J, et al. American College of Gastroenterology guideline: management of acute pancreatitis. *Am J Gastroenterol.* 2013; 108(9):1400-1415.

34. Frossardl JL, Steer ML, Pastor CM. Acute pancreatitis. *Lancet.* 2008;371: 143-152.

35. Frank B, Gottlieb K. Amylase normal, lipase elevated: Is it pancreatitis? *Am J Gastroenterol.* 1999;94:463-469.

36. Bode C, Riederer J, Brauner B, et al. Macrolipasemia: a rare cause of persistently elevated serum lipase. *Am J Gastroenterol.* 1990;85:412-416.

37. Chey WD, Leontiadis GI, Howden CW, et al. ACG clinical guideline: treatment of *Helicobacter pylori* infection. *Am J Gastroenterol.* 2017;112: 212-238.

38. Logan RP, Walker MM. Epidemiology and diagnosis of *Helicobacter pylori* infection. *Br Med J.* 2001;323:920-922.

39. Pan L, Mu M, Yang P, et al. Clinical characteristics of COVID-19 patients with digestive symptoms in Hubei, China: a descriptive cross-sectional, multicenter study. *Am J Gastroenterol.* 2020;115(5):766-733.

40. Surawicz CM, Brandt L, Binion DG, Ananthakrishnan AN. Guidelines for diagnosis, treatment, and prevention of Clostridium difficile infections. *Am J Gastroenterol.* 2013; 108(4):478-489.

41. Lee VR. *Clostridium difficile* infection in older adults: a review and update on its management. *Am J Geriatr Pharmacother.* 2012;10:14-24.

42. Kelly CP, LaMont JT. *Clostridium difficile*: more difficult than ever. *N Engl J Med.* 2008;359:1932-1940.

43. Louie TJ, Miller MA, Mullane KM, et al. Fidaxomicin vs vancomycin for *Clostridium difficile* infection. *N Engl J Med.* 2011;364:422-432.

44. Bababy NE, Stiles J, Ruggiero,P et al. Evaluation of the Cephoid Xpert *Clostridium difficile* Epi assay for diagnosis of *Clostridium difficile* infection and typing of the NAP1 strain at a cancer hospital. *J Clin Microbiol.* 2010;48:4519-4524.

## QUICKVIEW | Albumin

| PARAMETER | DESCRIPTION | COMMENTS |
|---|---|---|
| **Common reference ranges** | | |
| Adults | 4–5 g/dL (40–50 g/L) | |
| Pediatrics | 1.9–4.9 g/dL (19–49 g/L) | <1 yr old |
| | 3.4–4.2 g/dL (34–42 g/L) | 1–3 yr old |
| **Critical value** | <2.5 g/dL (<25 g/L) | In adults |
| **Natural substance?** | Yes | Blood protein |
| **Inherent activity?** | Increases oncotic pressure of plasma; carrier protein | |
| **Location** | | |
| Production | Liver | |
| Storage | Serum | |
| Secretion/excretion | Catabolized in liver | Half-life, approximately 20 days |
| **Major causes of...** | | |
| **High or positive results** | Dehydration | |
| | Anabolic steroids (rare) Iatrogenic (administration of albumin) | |
| Associated signs and symptoms | Limited to underlying disorder | No toxicological activity |
| **Low results** | Decreased hepatic synthesis | Seen in liver disease |
| | Malnutrition or malabsorption | Substrate deficiency |
| | Protein losses Pregnancy or chronic illness | Via kidney in nephrotic syndrome or via gut in protein-losing enteropathy |
| Associated signs and symptoms | Edema, pulmonary edema, ascites | At levels <2–2.5 g/dL or <20–25 g/L |
| **After insult, time to...** | | |
| Initial depression or positive result | Days | |
| Lowest values | Weeks | Half-life, approximately 20 days |
| Normalization | Weeks | Assumes insult removed and no permanent damage |
| **Drugs often monitored with test** | Parenteral nutrition | Goal is increased levels |
| **Causes of spurious results** | | |
| Falsely elevated | Ampicillin and heparin | |
| Falsely lowered | Supine patients, icterus, penicillin | |

## QUICKVIEW | Prothrombin Time/International Normalized Ratio

| PARAMETER | DESCRIPTION | COMMENTS |
|---|---|---|
| **Common reference ranges** | | |
| Adults and pediatrics | INR: 0.9–1.1 | |
| | PT: 12.7–15.4 sec | |
| **Critical value** | INR: >5 | Unless on warfarin |
| **Natural substance?** | Yes | |
| **Inherent activity?** | Indirect measurement of coagulation factors | |
| **Location** | | |
| Production | Coagulation factors produced in liver | |
| Storage | Carried in bloodstream | |
| Secretion/excretion | None | |
| **Major causes of...** | | |
| **Prolonged elevation** | Liver failure | Liver unable to produce coagulation factors; prolonged PT or increased INR does not correct with vitamin K |
| | Malabsorption or malnutrition | Vitamin K aids in activation of coagulation factors and is not absorbed; defect corrects with parenteral vitamin K supplementation |
| | Warfarin | Corrects with vitamin K supplementation |
| | Antibiotics | Interfere with vitamin K production by bacteria in the GI tract or metabolism or activation of clotting factors |
| Associated signs and symptoms | Increased risk of bleeding and ecchymosis | Easy bruising |
| **Low results** | None | |
| **After insult, time to...** | | |
| Initial elevation or positive result | 6–12 hr | |
| Peak values | Days to weeks | Depends on etiology |
| Normalization | 4 hr if vitamin K responsive (due to malabsorption, maldigestion, warfarin) but 2–4 days if due to liver disease and liver disease reverses | |
| **Drugs often monitored with test** | Warfarin | |
| **Causes of spurious results** | Improper specimen collection | |

## QUICKVIEW | Alkaline Phosphatase

| PARAMETER | DESCRIPTION | COMMENTS |
|---|---|---|
| **Common reference ranges** | | |
| Adults | 33–96 units/L<br>0.56–1.63 ukat/L | Varies with assay<br>Elevated in pregnancy |
| Pediatrics | Varies; can be 2-fold to 3-fold higher than in adults | Elevated with developing bone |
| **Natural substance?** | Yes | Metabolic enzyme (intracellular) |
| **Inherent activity?** | Elevation alone causes no symptoms | Intracellular activity only |
| **Location** | | |
| Production | Intracellular enzyme | |
| Storage | Liver, placenta, bone, small intestine, leukocytes | These tissues are rich in ALP |
| Secretion/excretion | None | |
| **Major causes of...** | | |
| **High or positive results** | Cholestasis | Hepatic; associated with elevation of GGT |
| | Bone disease | Paget disease, bone tumors, rickets, osteomalacia, healing fracture |
| | Pregnancy | Placental ALP |
| | Childhood | Related to bone formation |
| Associated signs and symptoms | Limited to underlying disorder | Reflects tissue or organ damage |
| **Low results** | Vitamin D intoxication | |
| | Scurvy | |
| | Hypothyroidism | |
| Associated signs and symptoms | Limited to underlying disorder | |
| **After insult, time to...** | | |
| Initial elevation or positive result | Hours | |
| Peak values | Days | |
| Normalization | Days | Assumes insult removed and no ongoing damage |
| **Drugs often monitored with test** | None | |
| **Causes of spurious results** | Blood drawn after fatty meal and prolonged serum storage | |

## QUICKVIEW | Aspartate Aminotransferase

| PARAMETER | DESCRIPTION | COMMENTS |
|---|---|---|
| **Common reference ranges** | | |
| Adults | 12–38 International Units/L (0.2–0.64 µkat/L) | Varies with assay |
| Newborns/infants | 30–100 International Units/L (0.5–1.67 µkat/L) | Varies with assay |
| **Critical value** | >80 International Units/L (1.34 µkat/L) | Two times upper limit of normal |
| **Natural substance?** | Yes | Metabolic enzyme |
| **Inherent activity?** | None in serum | Intracellular activity only |
| **Location** | | |
| Production | Intracellular enzyme | |
| Storage | Liver, cardiac muscle, kidneys, brain, pancreas, lungs | These tissues are rich in AST |
| Secretion/excretion | None | |
| **Major causes of...** | | |
| **High or positive results** | Hepatitis | Elevated in any disease with hepatocyte inflammation (liver cells) |
| | Hemolysis | Elevated in any disease with damage to tissues rich in enzyme |
| | Muscular diseases | |
| | Myocardial infarction | |
| | Renal infarction | |
| | Pulmonary infarction | |
| | Necrotic tumors | |
| Associated signs and symptoms | Varies with underlying disease | Reflects tissue or organ damage |
| **Low results** | None | |
| **After insult, time to...** | | |
| Initial elevation or positive result | 2–6 hr | |
| Peak values | 24–48 hr (without further cell damage) | With extensive liver or cellular damage, levels can go up to thousands |
| Normalization | 24–48 hr | Assumes insult removed and no ongoing damage |
| **Drugs often monitored with test** | Isoniazid, statins, allopurinol, methotrexate, ketoconazole, and valproic acid | Monitoring frequency varies with drug |
| **Causes of spurious results** | | |
| Falsely elevated | Heparin, levodopa, methyldopa, tolbutamide, para-aminosalicylic acid, erythromycin, diabetic ketoacidosis | |
| Falsely lowered | Metronidazole, trifluoperazine, vitamin $B_6$ deficiency | |

HMG-CoA = 3-hydroxy-3-methylglutaryl-CoA lyase.

## QUICKVIEW | Alanine Aminotransferase

| PARAMETER | DESCRIPTION | COMMENTS |
|---|---|---|
| **Common reference ranges** | | |
| Adults | 7–41 International Units/L (0.12–0.68 µkat/L) | Varies with assay |
| Newborns/infants | 6–40 International Units/L (0.1–0.67 µkat/L) | Decreases to adult values within a few months |
| **Critical value** | >60 International Units/L (>1 µkat/L) | >2 times normal limit |
| **Natural substance?** | Yes | Metabolic enzyme |
| **Inherent activity?** | None in serum | Intracellular activity only |
| **Location** | | |
| Production | Intracellular enzyme | |
| Storage | Liver, muscle, heart, kidneys | These tissues are rich in ALT |
| Secretion/excretion | | Normally contained intracellularly, but with cell damage, serum concentrations increase |
| **Major causes of…** | | |
| **High or positive results** | Hepatitis | Elevated in any disease with hepatocyte inflammation (liver cells) |
| | Hemolysis | Elevated in any disease with damage to tissues rich in enzymes |
| | Muscular diseases | |
| | Myocardial infarction | |
| | Renal infarction | |
| Associated signs and symptoms | Varies with underlying disease | Reflects tissue or organ damage |
| **Low results** | Patients deficient in vitamin $B_6$ | |
| Associated signs and symptoms | None | |
| **After insult, time to…** | | |
| Initial elevation or positive result | 2–6 hr | |
| Peak values | 24–48 hr (without further cell damage) | With extensive liver or cellular damage, levels can go up to thousands |
| Normalization | 24–48 hr | Assumes insult removed and no ongoing damage |
| **Drugs often monitored with test** | Isoniazid and cholesterol-lowering agents (eg, statins, allopurinol, ketoconazole, valproic acid, and methotrexate) | Monitoring frequency varies with drug |
| **Causes of spurious results** | Heparin (false elevation) | |

## QUICKVIEW | Bilirubin

| PARAMETER | DESCRIPTION | COMMENTS |
|---|---|---|
| **Common reference ranges** | | |
| Adults | Total: 0.3–1.3 mg/dL (5.1–22.2 µmol/L)<br>Indirect: 0.2–0.9 mg/dL<br>Direct: 0.1–0.4 mg/dL | Varies slightly with assay |
| Children | 2–4 mg/dL (34.2–68.4 µmol/L) | 24-hr infant |
| | 5–6 mg/dL (85.5–102.6 µmol/L) | 48-hr infant |
| | 0.3–1.3 mg/dL (5.1–22.2 µmol/L) | >1 mo old |
| **Critical value** | >4 mg/dL (>68.4 µmol/L) | In adults |
| **Natural substance?** | Yes | Byproduct of Hgb metabolism |
| **Inherent activity?** | Yes | CNS irritant or toxin in high levels in newborn (not adult) |
| **Location** | | |
| Production | Liver | |
| Storage | Gallbladder | Excreted into bile |
| Secretion/excretion | Stool and urine | Bilirubin and urobilinogen |
| **Major causes of…** | | |
| **High or positive results** | Liver disease, both hepatocellular and cholestatic | |
| | Hemolysis | |
| | Metabolic abnormalities (eg, Gilbert syndrome) | |
| Associated signs and symptoms | Jaundice | |
| **Low results** | No important causes | |
| **After insult, time to…** | | |
| Initial elevation or positive result | Hours | |
| Peak values | 3–5 days | Assumes insult not removed |
| Normalization | Days | Assumes insult removed and no evolving damage |
| **Drugs often monitored with test** | None | |
| **Causes of spurious results** | Fasting, levodopa, phenelzine, methyldopa, ascorbic acid (false elevation) | |

## QUICKVIEW | Ammonia

| PARAMETER | DESCRIPTION | COMMENTS |
|---|---|---|
| **Common reference ranges** | | |
| Adults and pediatrics | 19–60 mcg/dL (11–35 µmol/L) | Varies with assay |
| Newborns | <100 mcg/dL (71.4 µmol/L) | Varies with assay |
| **Critical value** | Varies, generally 1.5 upper limit of normal | |
| **Natural substance?** | Yes | Product of bacterial metabolism of protein (in the gut) |
| **Inherent activity?** | Probably | Progressive deterioration in neurologic function |
| **Location** | | |
| Production | In gut (by bacteria) | |
| Storage | None | |
| Secretion/excretion | Liver metabolizes to urea | Urea cycle; diminished in cirrhosis |
| **Major causes of...** | | |
| **High or positive results** | Liver failure | |
| | Reye syndrome | |
| | Metabolic abnormalities (urea cycle) | |
| Associated signs and symptoms | Hepatic encephalopathy | |
| **Low results** | No important causes | |
| **After insult, time to...** | | |
| Initial elevation or positive result | Hours | |
| Peak values | No peak value; rises progressively | |
| Normalization | Days | After appropriate therapy or resolution of underlying liver disease |
| **Drugs often monitored with test** | Valproic acid | |
| **Causes of spurious results** | Sensitive test (discussed in text) | |

# 16

# Hematology: Red and White Blood Cell Tests

*Michael D. Katz and Timothy C. Jacisin*

## OBJECTIVES

*After completing this chapter, the reader should be able to*

- Describe the physiology of blood cell development and bone marrow function

- Discuss the interpretation and alterations of hemoglobin, hematocrit, and various red blood cell indices in the evaluation of macrocytic, microcytic, and normocytic anemias

- Describe the significance of abnormal erythrocyte morphology, including sickling, anisocytosis, and nucleated erythrocytes

- Name the different types of leukocytes and describe their primary functions

- Calculate the absolute number of various types of leukocytes from the white blood cell count and differential

- Interpret alterations in the white blood cell count, differential, and CD$_4$ lymphocyte count in acute bacterial infections, parasitic infections, and human immunodeficiency virus infection

- Identify potential causes of neutropenia and neutrophilia

This chapter reviews the basic functions and expected laboratory values of erythrocytes (red blood cells [RBCs]) and leukocytes (white blood cells [WBCs]). It also discusses, in an introductory manner, selected disorders of these two cellular components of blood. It must be remembered that the ability of laboratory medicine to discriminate between leukocytes is increasing, and many methods considered investigational in this edition may become routine components of blood examination in the future.

## PHYSIOLOGY OF BLOOD CELLS AND BONE MARROW

The cellular components of blood are derived from pluripotential stem cells located in the bone marrow that can differentiate into RBCs, WBCs, and platelets (**Figure 16-1**). *Bone marrow* is a highly structured and metabolically active organ that normally produces 2.5 billion RBCs, 1 billion granulocytes, and 2.5 billion platelets/kilogram of body weight daily.[1] Production can vary greatly from nearly 0 to 5 to 10 times normal. Usually, however, levels of circulating cells remain in a relatively narrow range (**Table 16-1**).[2]

In a fetus and child, blood cell formation or hematopoiesis occurs in the marrow of virtually all bones as well as in liver, spleen, and other visceral organs. With maturation, the task of hematopoiesis ceases in the liver and shifts to flat bones of the axial skeleton, such as the skull, ribs, pelvis, and vertebrae. The long bones, such as the femur and humerus, do not produce a large amount of blood cells in adulthood

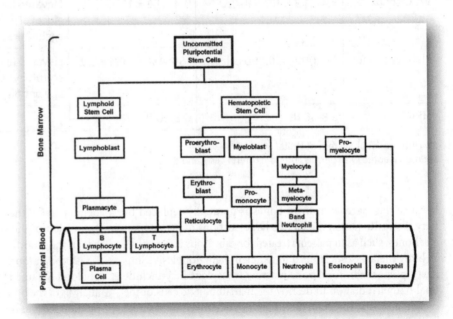

**FIGURE 16-1.** Schematic diagram of hematopoiesis.

DOI 10.37573/9781585286423.016

**TABLE 16-1.** Reference Ranges and Interpretative Comments for Common Hematologic Tests (Typical CBC)

| TEST NAME | RANGE[a] REFERENCE | SI UNITS | COMMENTS |
|---|---|---|---|
| RBC | Men: $4.5–5.9 \times 10^6$ cells/µL<br>Women: $4.1–5.1 \times 10^6$ cells/µL | $4.5–5.9 \times 10^{12}$ cells/L<br>$4.1–5.1 \times 10^{12}$ cells/L | |
| Hgb | Men: 14–17.5 g/dL<br>Women: 12.3–15.3 g/dL | 140–175 g/L or<br>8.68–10.85 mmol/L<br>123–153 g/L or<br>7.63–9.49 mmol/L | Amount of Hgb in given volume of whole blood; indication of oxygen-transport capacity of blood; may be falsely elevated in hyperlipidemia |
| Hct | Men: 42% to 50%<br>Women: 36% to 45% | 0.42–0.5<br>0.36–0.45 | Percentage volume of blood comprised of RBCs; usually approximately three times Hgb |
| RBC indices MCV | 80–96 fL/cell | 80–96 fL/cell | Hct/RBC: average size of RBCs in a specimen; decreased in iron deficiency; increased in vitamin $B_{12}$ and folate deficiency, cold agglutinins, reticulocytosis, hyperglycemia, and leukemias |
| MCH | 27–33 pg/cell | 27–33 pg/cell | Hgb/RBC: average amount of Hgb in RBCs in a specimen; decreased in iron deficiency; increased in vitamin $B_{12}$ and folate deficiency |
| MCHC | 33.4–35.5 g/dL | 334–355 g/L | Hgb/Hct: average concentration of Hgb in RBCs in a specimen; decreased in iron deficiency, increased in hyperlipidemia and cold agglutinins |
| Reticulocyte count | 0.5% to 2.5% of RBCs | 0.005–0.025 | Immature RBCs; increased in acute blood loss and hemolysis; decreased in untreated iron, vitamin $B_{12}$, and folate deficiency |
| RDW | 11.5% to 14.5% | 0.115–0.145 | Measure of variation in RBC volumes (anisocytosis): the larger the width percent, the greater the variation in size of RBCs; increased in early iron deficiency anemia and mixed anemias |
| WBC count | $4.4–11.3 \times 10^3$ cells/µL | $4.4–11.3 \times 10^9$ cells/L | Elevated by neutrophil demargination with exercise, glucocorticoids, epinephrine; decreased with cold agglutinins |
| Platelet count | 150,000–450,000 cells/µL | $150–450 \times 10^9$ cells/L | Elevated in presence of RBC fragments and microcytic erythrocytes; decreased in presence of large numbers of giant platelets and platelet clumps |
| MPV | 6.8–10 fL | 6.8–10 fL | |

SI = International System of Units.
*Source*: Adapted with permission from references 7 and 8.

because the marrow in these bones is gradually replaced by fatty tissue. Radiation directed to large portions of hematopoietic bones, such as in patients treated for cancerous lesions such as bony metastases, can lead to deficient hematopoiesis. Similarly, preparation for a bone marrow transplant may include total body irradiation to destroy the hematopoietic cells of the recipient so that the grafted cells are not destroyed by residual host defenses.

Although most hematopoiesis occurs in the marrow, modern methods of identifying cellular characteristics have demonstrated that pluripotential cells—identified by a cellular expression of the surface marker CD34—also normally circulate in the blood.[3]

Although most of this chapter discusses laboratory analysis of blood obtained from the vein (peripheral venipuncture), an analysis of the bone marrow itself may be needed to diagnose or monitor various disease states, most commonly leukemias. Bone marrow specimens are usually obtained from the posterior iliac crest of the pelvis or, less commonly, from the sternum. Bone marrow sampling can involve an aspirate, a core biopsy, or both.

The biopsy provides the advantage of examining the structure of the marrow stroma as well as the spatial relationship of the various hematopoietic cells.[4]

Blood pluripotential (stem) cells become increasingly differentiated in the bone marrow until they are committed to develop further into erythrocytes, platelets, or various leukocytes (Figure 16-1). Many regulatory proteins, including colony-stimulating factors, are involved in the differentiation and proliferation phases of hematopoiesis, but their functions and interrelationships are not yet fully understood. In addition to the colony-stimulating factors mentioned previously, proteins that stimulate hematopoiesis include erythropoietin, thrombopoietin, and various interleukins. Inhibitors of hematopoiesis are not as well defined but include interferons and lymphotoxins. When considering the response of neutrophils or erythrocytes to exogenously administered hematopoietic stimulants (eg, filgrastim, epoetin alfa), it is important to recall that normal physiologic hematopoietic regulation is more complex than the effect of one therapeutic protein would suggest. WBC formation involves local production of a combination of signaling proteins by cells of the hematopoietic microenvironment (eg, macrophages, T lymphocytes, osteoblasts, fibroblasts, and endothelial cells). Leukocyte-stimulating proteins, such as granulocyte-colony stimulating factor and granulocyte-macrophage colony-stimulating factor, are normally directed toward adjacent or closely approximated differentiating hematopoietic cells.[3] In contrast, renal synthesis of the hormone erythropoietin is increased when oxygen tension in one or both kidneys decreases. Once it is released into the systemic circulation, erythropoietin stimulates erythrocyte precursors in the blood-forming areas of bone marrow.

Committed blood precursor cells undergo further differentiation in the bone marrow until they develop into mature cells. These developmental stages can be identified by differing morphologic or immunochemical staining characteristics. These same imaging techniques are used to identify the developmental phenotype of the cancerous WBCs of leukemia and lymphoma. Generally, only mature cellular forms are found in the circulating blood, and it is from this blood that clinical specimens are usually taken. As discussed later, the presence of immature forms of WBCs or RBCs in the blood typically indicates the presence of a pathologic process.

# COMPLETE BLOOD COUNT

The *complete blood count* (CBC) is a frequently ordered laboratory test. It supplies useful information regarding the concentration of the different cellular and noncellular elements of blood and applies to multiple disorders. CBC is a misnomer because concentrations of cells/microliter, not counts, are measured and reported, and many hematologic tests are not included. Functionally, the CBC can be thought of as a routine or screening blood analysis given several tests are performed.

Most clinical laboratories use an automated method to determine the CBC. Results are usually accurate, reproducible, and rapidly obtained. Numerous measured and calculated values are included in a CBC (Table 16-1). These results traditionally include the following values:

- Erythrocyte count or RBC
- Leukocyte count or WBC
- Hemoglobin (Hgb)
- Hematocrit (Hct)
- RBC (Wintrobe) indices: mean cell (corpuscular) volume (MCV), mean Hgb content, mean cell Hgb concentration (MCHC), and RBC distribution width (RDW)
- Platelet estimate or count and mean platelet volume
- Reticulocyte count
- Erythrocyte sedimentation rate (ESR)

When a "CBC with differential" is ordered, the various types of WBCs are also analyzed (see White Blood Cell Count and Differential section). The reliability of the results can be doubtful if (1) the integrity of the specimen is questionable (inappropriate handling or storage) or (2) the specimen contains substances that interfere with the automated analysis. Grossly erroneous results are usually flagged for verification by another method. Manual microscopic review of the blood smear may be used to resolve unusual automated results (and if the counts are lower in specific pathologic or spurious myeloid conditions).[1]

Note that laboratory value reference ranges vary slightly among laboratories.

## Red Blood Cell Count

*Normal adult range: men, 4.5 to 5.9 × 10⁶ cells/μL (4.5 to 5.9 × $10^{12}$ cells/L); women, 4.1 to 5.1 × 10⁶ cells/μL (4.1 to 5.1 × $10^{12}$ cells/L)*

The *red blood cell (RBC) count* is the number of red cells in a given volume of blood. The international unit for reporting blood cells is for a 1-L volume, but it is still common to see values reported in cells/microliter (μL), or less commonly in cells/cubic millimeter ($mm^3$). After puberty, women have slightly lower counts (and Hgb/Hct) than men, partly because of their menstrual blood loss and because of higher concentrations of androgens (an erythropoietic stimulant) in men. The RBC count in all anemias is by definition below the normal range, and this decrease causes a proportionate decrease in Hct and Hgb. In clinical practice, the Hgb and Hct are more commonly used to define the presence or absence of anemia. The reticulocyte is the cell form that precedes the mature RBC or erythrocyte. During the entire maturation process, Hgb is produced, gradually filling the cytoplasm. The reticulocyte does not contain a nucleus but possesses remnants of the nucleus or endoplasmic reticulum. The mature erythrocyte contains neither an organized nucleus nor nucleic acids. Reticulocytes persist in the circulation for 1 to 2 days before maturing into erythrocytes.[2,5,6]

Mature erythrocytes have a median lifespan of 120 days under normal conditions. They are removed from the circulation by macrophages in the liver, spleen, bone marrow, and other reticuloendothelial organs. The erythrocytes are tested for flexibility, size, and integrity in these organs as the cells pass through areas of osmotic, pH, or hypoxic stress.[5]

Variability in the size of RBCs is termed *anisocytosis*, and variation in the normal biconcave disc shape is termed *poikilocytosis*. Such abnormalities are seen with iron deficiency or periods of increased erythrocyte production and RBC damage.[6]

## White Blood Cell Count

*Normal range: 4.4 to 11.3 × 10³ cells/μL (4.4 to 11.3 × 10⁹ cells/L)*

The *white blood cell count* is an actual count of the number of leukocytes in a given volume of blood. Unlike RBCs, leukocytes have a nucleus and normally represent five different mature cell types. The various percentages of the five mature and WBC types comprise the WBC differential, which is discussed later in this chapter.

## Hemoglobin

*Normal range: men 14 to 17.5 g/dL (140 to 175 g/L); women 12.3 to 15.3 g/dL (123 to 153 g/L)*

The *hemoglobin* (Hgb) value is the amount of this metalloporphyrin-protein contained in a given volume (100 mL or 1 L) of whole blood. The Hgb concentration provides a direct indication of the oxygen-transport capacity of the blood. As the major content of the RBCs, Hgb is proportionately low in patients with anemia. Fluid volume must be taken into consideration because Hgb and Hct are sensitive to the volume status of a patient, making the setting of the evaluation paramount in its interpretation (ambulatory versus acute care versus critical care).

## Hematocrit

*Normal range: men 42% to 50% (0.42 to 0.5); women 36% to 45% (0.36 to 0.45)*

The *hematocrit* (Hct), also known as the packed cell volume, is the percentage volume of blood that is composed of erythrocytes. To manually perform the Hct test, a blood-filled capillary tube is centrifuged to settle the erythrocytes. Then, the percentage volume of the tube that is composed of erythrocytes is calculated.[7] The Hct is usually about three times the value of the Hgb, but disproportion can occur when cells are substantially abnormal in size or shape. Like Hgb, Hct is usually low in patients with anemia and is useful in evaluation for surgical procedures and reversal of coagulopathies.

## Red Blood Cell Indices

Because the following laboratory tests specifically assess RBC characteristics, they are called *RBC indices*. These indices, which assess the size and Hgb content of the RBC, may be useful in the evaluation of anemias, polycythemia, and nutritional disorders. The MCV is measured directly, whereas the MCHC and MCH are calculated from the Hgb, MCV, and RBC count using predetermined formulas. Because of its dependence on cell size, MCH is rarely used in clinical practice, whereas the MCHC is sometimes used to assess RBCs for their Hgb concentration and color.

### Mean Corpuscular Volume

*Normal range: 80 to 96 fL/cell (80 to 96 fL/L SI)*

The *mean cell (corpuscular) volume* (MCV) is an estimate of the average volume of RBCs and is the most clinically useful of the RBC indices. It can be calculated by dividing the Hct by the RBC count, but it is now determined by averaging the directly measured size of thousands of RBCs with modern hemocytometry instruments.

Abnormally large cells have an increased MCV and are called *macrocytic*. Vitamin $B_{12}$ and folate deficiency cause the formation of macrocytic erythrocytes, which corresponds to a true increase in MCV. In contrast, a false increase in MCV may be observed when a patient has reticulocytosis, an increase in the number of reticulocytes in the peripheral blood, because reticulocytes are larger than mature erythrocytes.[7,8] The MCV may also be falsely increased in hyperglycemia due to osmotic expansion of the erythrocyte. When erythrocytes are mixed with diluting fluid to perform the test, the cells swell because the diluent is relatively hypotonic compared with the patient's hyperglycemic blood. Abnormally small cells with a decreased MCV are called *microcytic*. A decrease in the MCV implies some abnormality in Hgb synthesis. The most common cause of microcytosis is iron deficiency.[9] Some patients have simultaneous microcytic and macrocytic anemias (eg, iron and folic acid deficiencies), and in those patients, the MCV may not be predictive of the patient's overall status.

### Mean Corpuscular Hemoglobin

*Normal range: 27 to 33 pg/cell*

The *mean cell (corpuscular) hemoglobin* (MCH) is a measure of the oxygen-carrying capacity (ie, Hgb) of each cell. It is calculated as the quotient of Hgb/RBC. The presence of Hgb adds color to the erythrocyte and picks up the dyes of RBC stains for microscopic viewing. Cells that have decreased amounts of Hgb are referred to as being *hypochromic*, such as in iron deficiency.

### Mean Corpuscular Hemoglobin Concentration

*Normal range: 33.4 to 35.5 g/dL (334 to 355 g/L)*

The *mean cell (corpuscular) hemoglobin concentration* (MCHC) is the Hgb divided by the Hct, and this calculation is usually around 33 g/dL (330 g/L) because the Hct is usually three times the Hgb. Some laboratories do not report the MCH, as the MCHC reports the Hgb per volume of blood rather than per erythrocyte and, therefore, provides a more direct index of the oxygen carrying capacity of the blood. Iron deficiency is the only anemia in which the MCHC is routinely low although it can also be decreased in other disorders of Hgb synthesis.[7,8] In this case, RBCs are described as hypochromic (pale). MCHC can be falsely elevated in hyperlipidemia. The Wintrobe indices are averages for the patient's blood, and normal values may be reported by automated methods, even in the presence of a mixed (normal + abnormal) erythrocyte population.

### Red Blood Cell Distribution Width

*Normal range: 11.5% to 14.5% (0.115 to 0.145)*

The *RBC distribution width* (RDW) is an indication of the variation in RBC size, termed *anisocytosis*.[8] The RDW is reported as the coefficient of variation of the MCV (standard deviation/mean value). This value is used primarily with other tests to differentiate iron deficiency anemia from thalassemias and to identify the presence of a mixed anemia. The RDW increases in macrocytic anemias and in early iron deficiency, often before other tests show signs of this kind of anemia. However, it is not specific for iron deficiency anemia. Mild forms of thalassemia often are microcytic but have a normal or only slightly elevated RDW.

## Platelet Count and Mean Platelet Volume

*Normal range: 150,000 to 450,000 cells/μL (150 to 450 × 10⁹ cells/L)*

The *platelet estimate* or *count*, often included routinely in the CBC with differential, and *mean platelet volume* are discussed with other coagulation tests in Chapter 17.

## Reticulocyte Count

*Normal range: 0.5% to 2.5% of RBCs (0.005 to 0.025)*

Reticulocytes are almost-mature RBC that contain nuclear fragments. Normally, only a small number of reticulocytes are in the peripheral circulation. When the bone marrow increases the production of RBC, more reticulocytes are released into the peripheral circulation. In anemia, the *reticulocyte count* or *reticulocyte index* (RI) reflects not only the level of bone marrow production but also a decline in the total number of mature erythrocytes that normally dilute the reticulocytes. Therefore, the reticulocyte count would double in a person whose bone marrow production is unchanged but whose Hct has fallen from 46% to 23%. The RI corrects for the transient increase in reticulocyte release that may be seen even in hypoproliferative anemias. It is calculated as follows:

RI = measured % reticulocytes × (patient's Hct/normal Hct)

where a normal RI is <3%.[7]

In persons with anemia secondary to acute blood loss or hemolysis, even the corrected reticulocyte count is increased.[5,7] This increase reflects an attempt by the bone marrow to compensate for the lack of circulating erythrocytes by speeding bone marrow production and release of RBCs. In contrast, persons with untreated anemia secondary to iron, folate, or vitamin $B_{12}$ deficiency are unable to increase their reticulocyte count appropriate to the degree of their anemia. Appropriate treatment of an anemia should be accompanied by an increase in the reticulocyte count, typically in 5 to 7 days.

The reticulocyte count can be useful in identifying drug-induced bone marrow suppression in which the percentage of circulating reticulocytes may be close to zero.

## ERYTHROCYTE SEDIMENTATION RATE

*Normal range: men 1 to 15 mm/hr; women 1 to 20 mm/hr (increases with age)*

Numerous physiologic and disease states are associated with the rate at which erythrocytes settle from blood, termed the *erythrocyte sedimentation rate* (ESR). Erythrocytes normally settle slowly in plasma but settle rapidly when they aggregate because of electrostatic forces. Each cell normally has a net negative charge and repels other erythrocytes because like charges repel each other. Many plasma proteins are positively charged and are attracted to the surface charge of one or more erythrocytes, thereby promoting erythrocyte aggregation.[10] Nonmicrocytic anemia, pregnancy, multiple myeloma, and various inflammatory diseases (including infections) can increase the ESR. Sickle cell disease, high doses of corticosteroids, liver disease, microcytosis, carcinomas, and congestive heart failure can decrease the ESR.[7]

Although the ESR may be used to confirm a diagnosis supported by other tests, it is rarely used alone for a specific diagnosis. Rather, the ESR is sometimes useful as a nonspecific biomarker for monitoring the activity of inflammatory conditions (eg, temporal [giant cell] arteritis, polymyalgia rheumatica, rheumatoid arthritis, and osteomyelitis).[10] The ESR is often higher when the disease is active due to increased amounts of circulating proteins, termed *acute phase reactants* (eg, fibrinogen), and falls when the intensity of the disease decreases.

The ESR is usually measured using either the Wintrobe or the Westergren method. Anticoagulated blood is diluted and placed in a vertical glass tube of standard size. After 1 hour, the distance from the plasma meniscus down to the top of the erythrocyte column is recorded as the ESR in millimeters per hour.[10,11]

## LABORATORY ASSESSMENT OF ANEMIA

The functions of the erythrocyte are to transport and protect Hgb, the molecule used for oxygen and carbon dioxide transport. *Anemia* is practically defined by a decrease in either the Hct or the Hgb concentration below the normal range for age and gender. Anemia is not a disease in itself but a manifestation of an underlying disease process. Appropriate treatment of the patient with anemia must include identification and treatment of the underlying cause of the condition. Signs and symptoms of anemia depend on its severity (how low is the Hgb/Hct or H/H) and the rapidity with which it has developed. Severe, acute blood loss results in more dramatic symptoms than an anemia that took months to develop because with chronic loss some compensatory adaptation may occur. Patients with mild anemia are often asymptomatic (ie, absence of pallor, weakness, and fatigue), but severely symptomatic patients may manifest shortness of breath, tachycardia, and palpitations even at rest. The presence of patient signs and symptoms must always be considered when interpreting test results.

Anemia can be caused by decreased production, increased destruction, or loss of RBC.[12,13] The first two situations can often be differentiated by the reticulocyte count, which is decreased in the former and increased in the latter. The MCV is commonly used to characterize the possible etiology of anemia. This method is useful because different causes of anemia lead to different erythrocyte morphology. **Figure 16-2** outlines this approach. Only the more common causes of anemia are included, but others can be fit into this outline. Other laboratory tests that are useful in differentiating the anemias are described later. Usual laboratory findings are also included in each section (**Table 16-2**).

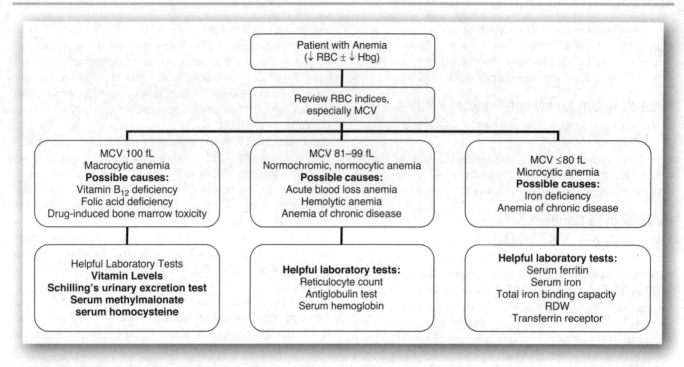

**FIGURE 16-2.** Use of erythrocyte morphology in differential diagnosis of anemia.

**TABLE 16-2.** Qualitative Laboratory Findings for Various Types of Anemia[a]

| | VITAMIN $B_{12}$ DEFICIENCY | FOLATE DEFICIENCY | IRON DEFICIENCY | ACUTE BLOOD LOSS | HEMOLYTIC ANEMIA | ANEMIA OF CHRONIC DISEASE |
|---|---|---|---|---|---|---|
| RBC | ↓ | ↓ | ↓ | ↓ | ↓ | ↓ |
| Hgb | ↓ | ↓ | ↓ | ↓ | ↓ | ↓ |
| Hct | ↓ | ↓ | ↓ | ↓ | ↓ | ↓ |
| MCV | ↑ | ↑ | ↓ | ↔ | ↔ | ↔↓ |
| MCH | ↑ | ↑ | ↓ | ↔ | ↔ | ↔↓ |
| MCHC | ↔ | ↔ | ↔ | ↔ | ↔ | ↔↓ |
| RDW | ↑ | ↑ | ↑ | ↔ | ↔ | ↔ |
| Reticulocyte count | ↓ | ↓ | ↓ | ↑ | ↑ | ↔↓ |
| Serum vitamin $B_{12}$ | ↓ | ↔ | | | | |
| Serum folate | ↔ | ↓ | | | | |
| Serum methylmalonate | ↑ | ↔ | | | | |
| Serum homocysteine | ↑ | ↑ | | | | |
| Ferritin | | | ↓ | | | ↔ |
| Serum iron | | | ↓ | | | ↓ |
| TIBC | | | ↑ | | | ↓ |
| Transferrin saturation | | | ↓ | | | |
| Serum haptoglobin | | | | | ↓ | |
| Plasma-free Hgb | | | | | ↑ | |
| Autoantibodies | | | | | + | |

[a]Some tests with no change (↔) are left empty for clarity. Autoantibodies positive for antibody-mediated immune hemolysis. Patients with multiple causes of anemia, such as iron deficiency and inflammation, may have a confusing laboratory picture.

# Macrocytic Anemia

*Macrocytic anemia* is a lowered Hgb value characterized by abnormally enlarged erythrocytes. The two most common causes are vitamin $B_{12}$ and folic acid deficiencies. Drugs that cause macrocytic anemia mainly interfere with proper use, absorption, and metabolism of these vitamins (**Table 16-3**) (**Minicase 1**).

## Vitamin $B_{12}$ Deficiency

*Vitamin $B_{12}$* is also known as *cobalamin*. The normal daily requirement of vitamin $B_{12}$ is 2 to 5 mcg.[14-16] It is stored primarily in the liver, which contains approximately 1 mcg of vitamin/g of liver tissue. Overall, the body has $B_{12}$ stores of approximately 2,000 to 5,000 mcg. Therefore, if vitamin $B_{12}$ absorption suddenly ceased in a patient with normal liver stores, several years would pass before any abnormalities occurred because of vitamin deficiency.

## TABLE 16-3. Examples of Causes of Drug-Induced Macrocytic Anemia

### ALTERED FOLATE ABSORPTION

| | |
|---|---|
| Alcohol | Aminosalicylic acid |
| Antimalarials | Erythromycin |
| Estrogen | Oral contraceptives |
| Ampicillin and other penicillins | Phenytoin |
| Nitrofurantoin | Tetracyclines |

### VITAMIN $B_{12}$ MALABSORPTION

| | |
|---|---|
| Colchicine | Isoniazid |
| Metformin | Neomycin |
| Para-aminosalicylic acid | Proton pump inhibitors |

### ALTERED PURINE METABOLISM

| | |
|---|---|
| Allopurinol | Azathioprine |
| Fludarabine | Cladribine |
| Mercaptopurine | Methotrexate |
| Mycophenolate mofetil | Pentostatin |
| Thioguanine | |

### ALTERED PYRIMIDINE SYNTHESIS

| | |
|---|---|
| Capecitabine | Cytosine arabinoside |
| Fluorouracil | Gadolinium |
| Gemcitabine | Hydroxyurea |
| Leflunomide | Methotrexate |
| Mercaptopurine | Nitrous oxide |
| Teriflunomide | Trimethoprim |

### VITAMIN $B_{12}$ INACTIVATION

Nitrous oxide

### UNCLEAR MECHANISM

| | |
|---|---|
| Imatinib | Sunitinib |

*Source*: Adapted with permission from references 14–16,18.

---

# MINICASE 1

## Anemia with Increased Mean Cell Volume

Anna B., a 45-year-old woman with alcoholism, is admitted to the hospital because of pneumonia. Her physical exam reveals an emaciated patient with ascites, dyspnea, fever, cough, and weakness. No cyanosis, jaundice, or peripheral edema is evident. Her peripheral neurologic exam is within normal limits, as are her serum electrolytes, urea nitrogen, creatinine, and glucose. The following CBC results are obtained:

| TEST NAME | RESULT | REFERENCE RANGE |
|---|---|---|
| RBC | $3 \times 10^6$ cells/µL | $4.1$–$5.1 \times 10^6$ cells/µL for women |
| WBC | $4.6 \times 10^3$ cells/µL | $4.4$–$11.3 \times 10^3$ cells/µL |
| Hgb | 10.3 g/dL | 12.3–15.3 g/dL for women |
| Hct | 30.9% | 36% to 45% for women |
| MCV | 110.8 fL/cell | 80–96 fL/cell |
| RDW | 15.4% | 11.5% to 14.5% |
| Platelets | 174,000 cells/µL | 150,000–450,000 cells/µL |
| Neutrophils | 68% | 45% to 73% |
| Bands | 6% | 3% to 5% |
| Monocytes | 11% | 2% to 8% |
| Eosinophils | 2% | 0% to 4% |
| Basophils | 2% | 0% to 1% |
| Lymphocytes | 11% | 20% to 40% |

QUESTION: What abnormalities are present? What is the likely cause?

DISCUSSION: The patient has anemia, evidenced by the low RBC, Hgb, and Hct. The increased MCV identifies this as a macrocytic anemia. The RDW is elevated, indicating variability in the size of the erythrocytes. These findings are typical of folic acid deficiency, a common finding in persons with alcoholism due to poor nutrition. Folic acid deficiency is more common than vitamin $B_{12}$ deficiency because body stores of folic acid are not as large. However, vitamin $B_{12}$ deficiency must also be ruled out as it may arise with or without a concurrent folate deficiency. Vitamin $B_{12}$ deficiency

*Continued*

## MINICASE 1 (cont'd)

may arise from poor nutrition but is more commonly caused by disorders such as pernicious anemia. It is critical that both serum folate and vitamin $B_{12}$ concentrations be measured in this patient to guide appropriate supplementation. Replenishment of folate in a patient with vitamin $B_{12}$ deficiency may temporarily improve the values of the CBC, but failure to appropriately replenish vitamin $B_{12}$ can lead to irreversible brain and nerve damage.

The absorption of vitamin $B_{12}$ is complex, and the mechanisms responsible are still being defined. Vitamin $B_{12}$ is ingested mostly in meats, eggs, and dairy products. Therefore, strict vegans may develop vitamin $B_{12}$ deficiency over time if supplements are not ingested. Some supplements have forms of $B_{12}$, such as those made by the blue-green algae *Spirulina*, which are active vitamins in bacterial assays but are not active vitamins for humans. Other cobamides structurally related to cobalamin are found in plasma after ingesting other animal and plant-based foods. Only the cobamide with an attached 5,6-dimethylbenzimidazole group is correctly termed *cobalamin* and is active in humans.[14]

Dietary $B_{12}$ is usually bound nonspecifically to food proteins, and gastric acid and pepsin are required to hydrolyze the vitamin from the protein. Aging patients with decreasing stomach acid production may be less able to free vitamin $B_{12}$ from meat protein. Freed $B_{12}$ is bound with high affinity to protein R, which is a large protein secreted in saliva. The cobalamin–protein R complex moves to the duodenum, where proteases denature protein R and allow the freed vitamin to bind to intrinsic factor, which is secreted by the parietal cells of the stomach and is resistant to the intestinal proteases. Patients may develop autoantibodies to intrinsic factor and thereby develop vitamin $B_{12}$ deficiency. The $B_{12}$–intrinsic factor complex binds to cubulin at the ileal epithelium. The $B_{12}$ translocates, dissociates, and then enters the circulation bound to transcobalamin, which is largely homologous with intrinsic factor.[14] When vitamin $B_{12}$ deficiency occurs, there are several steps in the absorption of vitamin $B_{12}$ that may be responsible for the deficiency.

Vitamin $B_{12}$ deficiency may arise from inadequate intake of the vitamin or from a deficiency of the intrinsic factor required for the effective ileal absorption of the vitamin. Inadequate dietary intake is a rare cause of vitamin $B_{12}$ deficiency, usually occurring only in vegans who abstain from all animal food, including milk and eggs.[15,16] Defective production of intrinsic factor is a common cause of the deficiency.[14-16] The gastric mucosa can fail to secrete intrinsic factor because of atrophy, especially in elderly persons, due to autoimmune diseases or due to surgical removal of the stomach. Disorders that affect the ileum, such as Crohn disease, also may impair $B_{12}$ absorption.

***Clinical and laboratory diagnosis.*** Vitamin $B_{12}$ is necessary for deoxyribonucleic acid (DNA) synthesis in all cells, for the synthesis of neurotransmitters, and for metabolism of homocysteine. Therefore, $B_{12}$ deficiency leads to signs and symptoms involving many organ systems.[14] The most notable symptoms involve the following systems:

- Gastrointestinal (GI) tract (eg, loss of appetite, smooth and sore tongue, and diarrhea or constipation)
- Central nervous system (eg, paresthesias in fingers and toes, loss of coordination of legs and feet, tremors, irritability, somnolence, abnormalities of taste and smell and dementia)
- Hematopoietic system (anemia)

Nuclear maturation retardation occurs in the developing cells in the bone marrow due to slowed DNA synthesis. The morphologic result—cells with an immature and enlarged nuclei (megaloblasts) but a cytoplasm that matures normally—causes mature cells to be larger than normal. The resulting anemia is called a *macrocytic, megaloblastic anemia*, which has both morphologic characteristics of nuclear maturation retardation.[14] Visual inspection of smears of both peripheral blood and bone marrow reveals characteristic megaloblastic changes in the appearance of erythrocytes and WBCs. The development of neutrophils is also affected, which results in large cells with hypersegmentation (more than three nuclear lobes).[17] A mild pancytopenia (decreased numbers of all blood elements) also occurs. The usual laboratory test results associated with vitamin $B_{12}$ deficiency are listed in Table 16-2.

In the past, vitamin $B_{12}$ concentrations were measured using a microbiologic assay and a cobalamin-dependent organism. The assay has largely been replaced by a competitive displacement assay using radioactive cobalamin and intrinsic factor. Unfortunately, because of cross-reactivity with other cobamides, approximately 5% of patients have cobalamin concentrations that appear to be within the normal range yet can be shown to have hematologic/neurologic signs of deficiency. Metabolic intermediates homocysteine and methylmalonate may be more sensitive indicators of $B_{12}$ deficiency. In the presence of inadequate $B_{12}$, these two compounds accumulate because of the cobalamin dependence of their metabolizing enzymes, methionine synthase and methylmalonyl-CoA-mutase, respectively. An elevated methylmalonate and homocysteine concentration in the presence of normal RBC folate is strongly indicative of a pure deficiency of $B_{12}$.

Historically, the Schilling test, which involves oral administration of radiolabeled $B_{12}$, was used to determine if impaired absorption is the reason for the cobalamin deficiency. However, with the advent of assays to measure autoantibodies targeting intrinsic factor and/or gastric parietal cells, this test is now rarely used. The availability of intramuscular injections of vitamin $B_{12}$ obviates the need to specify the defect in $B_{12}$ absorption, and such injections are favored in patients with impaired $B_{12}$ absorption, regardless of the cause.

*Pernicious anemia* is a specific disease associated with $B_{12}$ deficiency characterized by atrophic gastritis associated with antibodies against intrinsic factor and gastric parietal cells. In addition to causing $B_{12}$ deficiency pernicious anemia is associated with gastric cancer. Gastrectomy (removal of all or part of the stomach) can also lead to vitamin $B_{12}$ deficiency because the procedure removes the production site of intrinsic factor.

Achlorhydria from gastrectomy or drugs such as proton pump inhibitors can decrease the release of $B_{12}$ from food. Defective or deficient absorption of the intrinsic factor–vitamin $B_{12}$ complex can be caused by inflammatory disease of the small bowel, ileal resection, and bacterial overgrowth in the small bowel.[14-16] Administration of colchicine, neomycin, and para-aminosalicylic acid can also lead to impaired absorption of vitamin $B_{12}$ (Table 16-3).[15,16,18]

### Folic Acid Deficiency

*Folic acid* is also called *pteroylglutamic acid*. Folates refer to folic acid or reduced forms of folic acid that may have variable numbers of glutamic acid residues attached to the folic acid molecule. The folates present in food are mainly in a polyglutamic acid form and must be hydrolyzed in the intestine to the monoglutamate form to be absorbed efficiently. The liver is the chief storage site. Adult daily requirements are approximately 50 mcg of folic acid, equivalent to about 400 mcg of food folates. Folate stores are limited, and anemia arising from a folate-deficient diet occurs in 4 to 5 months.[14-16]

Inadequate dietary intake is the major cause of folate deficiency. Folates are found in green, leafy vegetables such as spinach, lettuce, and broccoli. Inadequate intake can have numerous causes: alcoholics often have poor nutritional intake of folic acid; certain physiologic states such as pregnancy require an increase in folic acid; malabsorption syndromes (mentioned in the section on vitamin $B_{12}$) can lead to defective absorption of folic acid; and celiac sprue can lead to folate malabsorption. Patients with chronic hemolysis, such as in sickle cell disease, and patients undergoing hemodialysis also may develop folate deficiency[15,16]

Certain medications (eg, methotrexate, trimethoprim–sulfamethoxazole, and triamterene) can act as folic acid antagonists by interfering with the conversion of folic acid into its metabolically active form, tetrahydrofolic acid. Phenytoin and phenobarbital administration can interfere with the intestinal absorption or use of folic acid (Table 16-3).[15,16,18]

Folic acid is required as the intermediate for one-carbon transfers in several biochemical pathways, including the thymidine required for DNA synthesis. After absorption, folate is reduced to tetrahydrofolate, and a carbon in one of several oxidation states is attached for transfer. The formation of methyltetrahydrofolate requires vitamin $B_{12}$ as a cofactor for the methyl group transfer. Methyltetrahydrofolate is required for the conversion of homocysteine to methionine, which is subsequently used as a methyl donor in many synthetic pathways that include the production of critical neurotransmitters and amino acids.

***Clinical and laboratory diagnosis.*** Because folic acid is necessary for DNA synthesis, a deficiency causes a maturation retardation in the bone marrow similar to that caused by vitamin $B_{12}$ deficiency. Folic acid deficiency is also characterized by a macrocytic, megaloblastic anemia.[14-16] However, with folic acid deficiency, pancytopenia does not develop as consistently as it does with vitamin $B_{12}$ deficiency.

Folate supplementation in patients with a folate deficiency provides folate for the nonmethyl transfer steps that do not require vitamin $B_{12}$. High doses of folic acid can often, at least partially, reverse megaloblastic anemia in patients with $B_{12}$ deficiency but do not reverse the neurologic sequelae. Although folate deficiency is more common and easily treated, it is critical to correctly identify the cause of a megaloblastic anemia so that any vitamin $B_{12}$ deficiency is appropriately treated.

### Folate Concentration

*Normal range: serum folate 5 to 25 mcg/L (11.33 to 56.65 nmol/L); RBC folate 166 to 640 mcg/L (376.16 to 1450.24 nmol/L)*

The *folate concentration* in both serum and in RBCs is used to assess folate homeostasis. A low serum folate indicates negative folate balance and can be expected to lead to folate deficiency when hepatic folate stores are depleted. Although in most patients the serum folate alone is adequate for assessment, in patients who were recently administered folate supplementation, the RBC folate concentration may be more indicative of folate status.

## Microcytic Anemia

### Iron Deficiency

*Microcytic anemia*, or anemia with abnormally small erythrocytes, is most commonly caused by iron deficiency. Decreased MCV is a late indicator of the deficiency (Figure 16-2). Daily requirements are approximately 1 mg of elemental iron for each 1 mL of RBCs produced, so daily iron requirements are approximately 20 to 25 mg for erythropoeisis.[19-21] Most iron needed within the body is obtained by recycling metabolized Hgb. RBCs have an average lifespan of approximately 120 days. When old or damaged erythrocytes are taken up by macrophages in the liver, spleen, and bone marrow, the Hgb molecule is broken down and iron is extracted and stored with proteins. Only about 5% of the daily requirement (1 mg) is newly absorbed to compensate for losses caused by fecal and urinary excretion, sweat, and desquamated skin (**Minicase 2**).

Menstruating women require more iron because of increased blood losses. Iron requirements vary among women but average 2 mg/day. Orally ingested iron is absorbed in the GI tract, which should permit just enough iron absorption to prevent excess or deficiency. Typically, 5% to 10% of oral intake is absorbed (normal daily dietary intake: 10 to 20 mg).[21]

Dietary iron exists primarily in the ferric state. Because ferrous iron is more bioavailable, dietary ferric iron is reduced by gastric acid to ferrous iron. Patients with inadequate gastric acid secretion due to underlying diseases or medications such as proton pump inhibitor may develop iron deficiency due to decreased absorption.[21]

Recent research indicates that hepatic hepcidin[22] is the primary controller of GI iron absorption, with an inverse relationship between hepcidin level and iron absorption. Hepcidin blocks the transmembrane iron transporter ferroportin. Hepcidin levels are low in the presence of iron deficiency and increase with iron therapy. Hepcidin levels are increased in the presence of inflammatory states. Hepcidin is being studied as a biomarker for the diagnosis of iron deficiency to optimize oral iron replacement therapy and predict failure of oral iron therapy.

## MINICASE 2

## Anemia and Iron Stores

Denise T. is a 25-year-old woman seen in a community health clinic for a routine checkup. Her family history includes a sister with sickle cell disease. She has not been affected personally but has not been tested to determine her sickling genotype. She describes painful menstrual periods and takes aspirin for them. She also admits to a pica of ingesting cornstarch throughout the day. The following laboratory test results are obtained:

| TEST NAME | RESULT | REFERENCE RANGE |
|---|---|---|
| RBC | $3.3 \times 10^6$ cells/µL | $4.1–5.1 \times 10^6$ cells/µL for women |
| WBC | $5.1 \times 10^3$ cells/µL | $4.4–11.3 \times 10^3$ cells/µL |
| Hgb | 8.3 g/dL | 12.3–15.3 g/dL for women |
| Hct | 26% | 36% to 45% for women |
| MCV | 78 fL/cell | 80–96 fL/cell |
| RDW | 16.1% | 11.5% to 14.5% |
| Platelets | 195,000 cells/µL | 150,000–450,000 cells/µL |
| Neutrophils | 52% | 45% to 73% |
| Bands | 3% | 3% to 5% |
| Monocytes | 2% | 2% to 8% |
| Eosinophils | 1% | 0% to 4% |
| Basophils | 0% | 0% to 1% |

| TEST NAME | RESULT | REFERENCE RANGE |
|---|---|---|
| Lymphocytes | 42% | 20% to 40% |
| Serum iron | 44 mcg/dL | 50–150 mcg/dL |
| TIBC | 451 mcg/dL | 250–410 mcg/dL |
| Transferrin saturation | 14% | 20% to 50% |
| Serum ferritin | 5.2 mcg/L | 10–20 mcg/L |

QUESTION: What hematologic abnormalities are apparent from these results?

DISCUSSION: This patient demonstrates an anemia as manifested by the decreased RBC, Hgb, and Hct. Her WBC and platelet counts are normal. The RDW is elevated, indicating increased variability of erythrocyte size (anisocytosis). Because the MCV is low, this microcytic, hypochromic form of anemia is most likely due to iron deficiency. This is corroborated by the iron studies, which indicate a low serum iron and transferrin saturation. Serum ferritin is also decreased, indicating that her iron stores are markedly reduced. The TIBC is increased both because of increased transferrin production and decreased iron available to bind to the protein.

There may be multiple causes of her iron deficiency. Most commonly, the combination of low dietary iron and blood loss from menstruation increases the frequency of iron deficiency anemia in women. An additional possibility is occult blood loss from GI ulcerations caused by aspirin. An exacerbating factor for this woman is her starch pica (craving for unusual food). In addition to the high caloric intake associated with this particular pica, the starch decreases the bioavailability of ingested iron, decreasing the ability of the patient to absorb dietary or supplemental iron. Given the pica, parenteral iron may be considered.

Iron deficiency is usually due to inadequate dietary intake in children and increased iron requirements in adults. Poor dietary intake, especially in situations that require increased iron (eg, pregnancy), is a common cause. Other causes of iron deficiency include the following factors:

- Blood loss due to excessive menstrual discharge
- Peptic ulcer disease
- Hiatal hernia
- Gastrectomy
- Gastritis due to the ingestion of alcohol, aspirin, and nonsteroidal antiinflammatory drugs
- Bacterial overgrowth of the small bowel
- Inflammatory bowel disease
- Occult bleeding from GI cancers
- Starch or clay pica

Ionized, soluble iron is toxic because of its ability to mediate the formation of oxidative species. Iron is therefore bound to proteins both in and outside of cells. *Ferritin* is the iron-protein storage complex (**Figure 16-3**). In the normal adult, approximately 500 to 1,500 mg of total body iron is stored as ferritin and 2,500 mg is contained in Hgb.[19] When the total quantity of extracted iron exceeds the amount that can be stored as ferritin, the excess iron is stored in an insoluble form called *hemosiderin*.

The serum ferritin concentration reflects total body iron stores and is the most clinically useful method to evaluate patients for iron deficiency. Because ferritin is an acute phase reactant, serum ferritin concentrations can be increased by

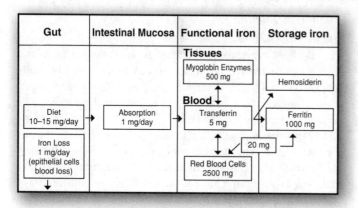

**FIGURE 16-3.** Intake, loss, and recycling of iron and iron storage forms.

critical illness, chronic infections, fever, and inflammatory disorders such as rheumatoid arthritis, hepatitis, and malignancies. The transport of iron in plasma and extracellular fluid occurs with two ferric ions bound to the protein transferrin, which when not binding iron or other metals, is termed *apotransferrin*. Transferrin binds to specific membrane transferrin receptors where the complex enters the cell and releases the iron. Apotransferrin is released when the apotransferrin-receptor complex returns to the surface of the cell.

The tendency of ferritin to be falsely elevated with inflammatory processes has led to recent interest in using soluble transferrin receptor concentrations as an alternative marker of iron deficiency. The circulating receptor fragment is considered to reflect total body receptor expression and is elevated in times of increased erythropoiesis such as sickle cell anemia, thalassemias, and chronic hemolysis. If such causes of increased erythropoiesis can be excluded, elevated concentrations of circulating transferrin receptor are thought to reflect iron deficiency. The use of transferrin receptor concentrations may help determine if decreased ferritin concentrations are due to iron deficiency or anemia of chronic (inflammatory) disease.[19]

*Clinical and laboratory diagnosis.* The first change observed in the development of iron deficiency anemia is a loss of storage iron (hemosiderin). If the deficiency continues, a loss of plasma iron occurs. The decrease in plasma iron stimulates an increase in transferrin synthesis. When enough iron has been depleted such that supplies for erythropoiesis are inadequate, anemia develops. The RDW rises, often before the MCV decreases, to a notable degree. If the iron deficiency persists, the RBCs become smaller than usual (microcytic—low MCV) and not as heavily pigmented as normal RBCs because they contain less Hgb than normal erythrocytes (hypochromic-low mean hemoglobin content and MCHC). Patients present with progressively worsening weakness, fatigue, pallor, shortness of breath, tachycardia, and palpitations. Numbness, tingling, and glossitis also may exist.[13,21] Laboratory results for iron deficiency anemia are listed in Table 16-2. With adequate iron therapy, the maximal daily rate of Hgb regeneration is 0.3 g/dL, or approximately 1%/day in Hct.

### Serum Ferritin

*Normal range: >10 to 200 ng/mL (>10 to 200 mcg/L)*

Loss of storage iron (hemosiderin) was traditionally evaluated by iron-stained bone marrow aspirate. *Serum ferritin* has largely replaced these invasive tests as an indirect measure of iron stores. Serum ferritin concentrations are markedly reduced in iron deficiency anemia (3 to 6 mcg/L) and elevated in the setting of inflammation.

### Serum Iron and Total Iron-Binding Capacity

*Serum iron normal range: 50 to 150 mcg/dL (9 to 26.9 µmol/L);*
*TIBC normal range: 250 to 410 mcg/dL (44.8 to 73.4 µmol/L);*
*transferrin saturation 20% to 50%*

The *serum iron* concentration measures iron bound to transferrin. This value represents about one-third of the *total iron-binding capacity* (TIBC) of transferrin.[20] The TIBC measures the iron-binding capacity of transferrin protein and is an indirect indicator of iron stores. In iron deficiency anemia, TIBC is increased due to a compensatory increase in transferrin synthesis. This increase leads to a corresponding decrease in the percent transferrin saturation that can be calculated by dividing the serum iron by the TIBC and then multiplying by 100. For example, a person with a serum iron concentration of 100 mcg/dL and a TIBC of 300 mcg/dL has a transferrin saturation of 33%. Iron deficient erythropoiesis exists whenever the percent transferrin saturation is 15% or less.

Other disease states besides iron deficiency that can alter serum iron and TIBC are critical illness, infections, cancers, and inflammatory diseases[7,23]. Anemia from these diseases is sometimes called *anemia of chronic disease* or *anemia of inflammation*. Serum iron and TIBC both decrease in these disorders, unlike in iron deficiency anemia in which serum iron decreases but TIBC increases (**Minicase 2**).

Patients with renal failure often have anemia because of inadequate renal production of erythropoietin.[24] These patients, particularly those receiving hemodialysis, may have iron deficiency in addition to the anemia caused by their renal disease. In these patients, the transferrin saturation (TSat) is used to determine if the patient has iron deficiency.

## Normochromic, Normocytic Anemia

This classification encompasses numerous etiologies. Three causes are discussed: acute blood loss anemia, hemolytic anemia, and anemia of chronic disease.

### Acute Blood Loss Anemia

Patients who suffer from acute hemorrhage may experience a dramatic drop in their whole blood volume. In this situation, the Hct is not a reliable indicator of the extent of anemia. It is a measure of the amount of packed RBCs per unit volume of the blood, not the total body amount of RBCs. The total whole blood volume may be markedly reduced, but in the acute phase of the hemorrhage, the Hct may be normal or even slightly increased. Usually, the Hgb and Hct are decreased by the time a CBC is obtained. Also, patients with hemorrhage often receive

IV crystalloid fluids such as normal saline or lactated Ringer's solution to maintain intravascular volume. The drop in these patients' Hgb and Hct is partly iatrogenic, caused by dilution of the patient's RBCs with the IV fluid.

In patients with normal bone marrow, the production of RBCs increases in response to hemorrhage, resulting in reticulocytosis. If the patient is transfused, each unit of packed RBCs administered should increase the Hgb by 1 g/dL if the bleeding has stopped. Table 16-2 shows the usual laboratory findings in acute blood loss anemia (**Minicase 3**).

## MINICASE 3

### Anemia and Low Platelet Count

Michael T., a 50-year-old man with a long history of alcohol abuse, cirrhosis, and esophageal varices, is brought to the emergency department (ED) by concerned family members. The family says that he suddenly began coughing up bright red blood. As he is moved to a bed in the ED, he begins coughing and vomiting large amounts of bright red blood. A stat CBC reveals the following values:

| TEST NAME | RESULT | REFERENCE RANGE |
|---|---|---|
| RBC | $2.91 \times 10^6$ cells/µL | $4.5–5.9 \times 10^6$ cells/µL for men |
| WBC | $6.6 \times 10^3$ cells/µL | $4.4–11.3 \times 10^3$ cells/µL |
| Hgb | 8 g/dL | 14–17.5 g/dL for men |
| Hct | 28.2% | 42% to 50% for men |
| MCV | 92.4 fL/cell | 80–96 fL/cell |
| RDW | 14.1% | 11.5% to 14.5% |
| Platelets | 75,000 cells/µL | 150,000–450,000 cells/µL |

QUESTION: What does this CBC indicate?

DISCUSSION: The presence of bright blood (as opposed to dark, "coffee ground" material) in the emesis indicates an acute and active bleed—either from a gastric ulcer or from esophageal varices. The CBC is consistent with acute blood loss. At the onset of bleeding, the RBC, Hgb, and Hct may show minimal changes. Here, the RBC, Hgb, and Hct are all moderately decreased, and the red cell indices are within normal limits, supporting a recent history of significant blood loss. The platelet count is also decreased, which may have led to the increasing risk of bleeding. Esophagogastroduoedenoscopy revealed that the bleeding was caused by ruptured esophageal varices.

## Hemolytic Anemia

Hemolysis, the lysis of RBCs, often leads to irregularly shaped or fragmented erythrocytes, termed *poikilocytosis*. If hemolysis is rapid and extensive, severe anemia can develop, yet RBC indices (MCV and MCHC) remain unchanged in the short term. Patients with normal bone marrow respond with an increase in erythrocyte production to replace the lysed cells, and reticulocytosis is present. Specialized tests, called *antiglobulin tests*, can be useful in determining immune causes of hemolytic anemia.

Plasma (free) Hgb measures the concentration of Hgb circulating in the plasma unattached to RBCs. It is almost always elevated in the presence of intravascular hemolysis. Haptoglobin, an acute-phase reactant, binds free Hgb and carries it to the reticuloendothelial system. In the presence of intravascular hemolysis, the serum haptoglobin concentration is decreased. Concomitant corticosteroid therapy may confound interpretation because many diseases associated with in vivo hemolysis are treated with corticosteroids. Serum haptoglobin may be normal or elevated in hemolysis if the patient is receiving steroids. If the increase in serum haptoglobin is from steroids, other acute-phase reactants, such as hepcidin or ferritin, will also be elevated. Serum haptoglobin is also elevated in patients with biliary obstruction and nephrotic syndrome. It is variably decreased in folate deficiency, sickle cell anemia, thalassemia, hypersplenism, liver disease, estrogen therapy, and pregnancy.[8]

Immune hemolytic anemias are caused by the binding of antibodies and complement components to the erythrocyte cell membrane with subsequent lysis.[25,26] The method used to detect autoantibodies already bound to erythrocytes is a direct antiglobulin test (DAT), sometimes referred to as the *direct Coombs test*. The DAT is performed by combining a patient's RBCs with rabbit or goat antihuman globulin serum, which contains antibodies against human immunoglobulins and complement.[23] If the patient's RBCs are coated with antibody or complement, the antibodies in the antiglobulin serum bind to the immunoglobulins coating the RBCs, leading to the agglutination of the RBCs. The DAT is the only test that provides definitive evidence of immune hemolysis.[25] The DAT can also be used to investigate possible blood transfusion reactions.

The method used to detect antibodies present in serum is an indirect antiglobulin test (IAT, indirect Coombs). Patient serum is combined with several types of normal erythrocytes of known antigenic expression. Any antibodies able to bind to the antigens expressed on these sample RBCs adhere after the serum is washed away. Antihuman immune globulin is then added and binds to any of the patient's immune globulin that is present on the erythrocytes, followed by agglutination.[25]

The antiglobulin tests are sensitive, but a negative result does not eliminate the possibility of antibodies bound to erythrocytes. A low concentration of antibodies may give a false-negative reaction. Numerous conditions and medications can be associated with immune hemolytic anemia (**Table 16-4**).[26,27] Medications can induce antibody formation by three mechanisms[25-27] that result in a hemolytic anemia.

***Autoimmune type.*** Methyldopa and procainamide are infrequently used cardiovascular drugs that may induce the

**TABLE 16-4.** Causes of Immune Hemolytic Anemia

**Neoplasm**
    Chronic lymphocytic leukemia
    Lymphoma
    Multiple myeloma

**Rheumatologic disorders**
    Systemic lupus erythematosus
    Rheumatoid arthritis

**Medication**
    **Autoimmune type**
        Levodopa, mefenamic acid, methyldopa, procainamide
    **Innocent bystander type**
        Cefotaxime, ceftazidime, ceftriaxone, chlorpromazine, doxepin, fluorouracil, isoniazid, quinidine, quinine, rifampin, sulfonamides, thiazides, chlorpropamide
    **Hapten type 1**
        Cephalosporins, penicillins

**Infections**
    *Mycoplasma*
    Viruses

*Source:* Adapted with permission from References 25–29.

formation of antibodies directed specifically against normal RBC proteins. This autoimmune state can persist for up to 1 month after drug administration has been discontinued. This mechanism is known as a true autoimmune type of antibody formation and is detected using the DAT.

***Innocent bystander type.*** Antibodies to the drugs quinine and quinidine are examples of the immune complex (innocent bystander) mechanism. Each drug forms a drug–protein complex with plasma proteins to which antibodies are formed. This drug–plasma protein–antibody complex attaches to RBCs and fixes complement, which leads to lysis of the cells.[25,26] In this situation, the RBC is an innocent bystander. Examples of other drugs implicated in causing this type of hemolytic anemia are listed in Table 16-4.

***Hapten type 1.*** The hapten (penicillin) type 1 mechanism is involved when a patient has produced antibodies to penicillin. If the patient receives penicillin at a future date, some penicillin can bind to the RBC membrane. The antipenicillin antibodies, in turn, bind to the penicillin bound to the RBC, and hemolysis can result.

### Glucose-6-Phosphate Dehydrogenase Deficiency Anemia

*Glucose-6-phosphate dehydrogenase* (G6PD) is an intracellular enzyme that forms the nicotinamide adenine dinucleotide phosphate needed by the erythrocyte to synthesize the antioxidant glutathione. Variants of this enzyme are more commonly found in African Black (Gd$^{A-}$), Mediterranean, and Asian populations (Gd$^{Med}$) than in white populations. These variants have

an impaired ability to resist the oxidizing effect of drugs and collateral oxidative exposure to the granulocytic response to infections. Thus, exposure of patients with G6PD deficiency to oxidizing drugs or an infection can lead to a dramatic, non-immunologic hemolysis.[28] Examples of drugs that can lead to hemolysis in G6PD-deficient patients include dapsone, primaquine, rasburicase, phenazopyridine, methylene blue, and nitrofurantoin. A more complete list of offending medications and their relative risk can be found at https://www.g6pd.org/G6PD Deficiency/SafeUnsafe.aspx.

Assessment of at-risk patients for signs of hemolysis (anemia, hemoglobinemia, dark urine, and back pain) is appropriate. Routine genotyping of patients aids in drug selection and monitoring; for example, it aids before prescribing dapsone for *Pneumocystis juroveci* prophylaxis in a patient with human immunodeficiency virus (HIV) infection.

### Anemia of Inflammation (Anemia of Chronic Disease)

Mild-to-moderate anemia often accompanies various infections, inflammatory illnesses, or neoplastic diseases that last more than 1 to 2 months.[23,30] Chronic infections include pulmonary abscesses, tuberculosis, endocarditis, pelvic inflammatory disease, and osteomyelitis. Chronic inflammatory illnesses (eg, rheumatoid arthritis and systemic lupus erythematosus), solid tumors, and hematologic malignancies (eg, Hodgkin disease, leukemia, and multiple myeloma) are also associated with anemia. Because these disorders as a group are common, anemia due to chronic disease (also called anemia of chronic inflammation) is also common. Although anemia of chronic disease is more commonly associated with normocytic, normochromic anemia, it can also cause microcytic anemia. Table 16-2 shows the usual laboratory results found in anemia of inflammation.

The pathogenesis of this anemia is not totally understood. Various investigations have found that the erythrocyte lifespan is shortened and that the bone marrow does not increase erythrocyte production to compensate for the decreased longevity. While iron stores are normal or even elevated, iron use is impaired. Although erythrocytes are frequently normal size, microcytosis can develop. One distinguishing feature between early iron deficiency anemia and microcytic anemia of chronic disease is the normal serum ferritin that is present in the latter.[23,30]

In patients with chronic kidney disease (CKD), anemia is associated with decreased renal production of erythropoietin, decreased RBC lifespan, impaired RBC production, and, in patients receiving hemodialysis, blood loss with subsequent iron deficiency and folate deficiency.[24,30] In the presence of sufficient iron stores, erythrocyte-stimulating agents (ESA), such as epoetin alfa and darbepoetin, may be used to decrease a patient's need for blood cell transfusions. In patients with CKD and anemia, a trial of IV or oral iron is recommended regardless of whether they are receiving an ESA, particularly if the TSat is ≤30% and the ferritin is ≤500 ng/mL. In pediatric patients, thresholds of TSat ≤20% and ferritin ≤ 100 ng/mL are used to determine the need for a trial of iron replacement.[24] More conservative use and dosing of ESAs is recommended by recent guidelines based on evidence that ESAs increase the risk for serious adverse cardiovascular events. ESA use should be individualized to use the lowest dose of ESA sufficient to reduce the need for transfusion. Patients with CKD who are not on dialysis should consider starting ESA treatment only when the Hgb level is <10 g/dL and reduce or stop the ESA dose if the Hgb level exceeds 10 g/dL. For patients on dialysis, ESA treatment should be initiated when the Hgb level is <10 g/dL, and the ESA dose should be reduced or interrupted if the Hgb level approaches or exceeds 11 g/dL. Monitoring of Hgb levels should be done at least weekly until stable and then monitored monthly.[24]

Use of ESA therapy in patients with cancer has become controversial because of the increased risk of thromboembolism and mortality. Recent guidelines recommend use of ESA therapy only with great caution in patients with malignancy, such as in patients with incurable malignancies and Hgb <10 g/dL.[24,31] As with patients with CKD, dosing should be individualized to use the lowest dose of ESA sufficient to reduce the need for transfusion.

Anemia of critical illness[32] is common in critically ill patients and is similar to anemia of inflammation, but in a compressed time frame. Critically ill patients have decreased RBC life span and production, with the additional problem of blood loss due to frequent phelobotomies and potential hemorrhagic losses in surgical and trauma patients. Anemia of critical illness is associated with adverse patient outcomes, and it is not clear if transfusion and/or ESA therapy improves outcomes.

## Hemoglobinopathies

Several diseases arise from abnormal synthesis of the α or β subunits of Hgb. The most common types of anemias related to these *hemoglobinopathies* include sickle cell trait/disease and thalassemias. Sickle cell disease is caused by the substitution of a valine amino acid for glutamate on the β chain of Hgb. The heterozygous (trait) carrier state involving valine substitution on one β chain is thought to provide a resistance to clinical manifestations and sequelae of malaria. Homozygous persons with both β chains carrying the valine substitution are at increased risk of developing a sickling of RBCs. This occurs most commonly under circumstances of hypoxia, infection, dehydration, or acidosis. Deoxygenated Hgb molecules polymerize into rod-like structures within the RBC, deforming the cell into an arched, rigid sickle-shaped cell. These erythrocytes are not able to deform and pass through the capillaries or reticuloendothelial system. Hypoxia, ischemia, and even infarction occur in tissues downstream of these sites of impaired blood flow. Severe pain is usually present during these "sickle crises," and pain management is often needed in addition to hydration, transfusion, and other treatments. Diagnosis is made by inspection of the peripheral blood smear and by electrophoresis of the patient's Hgb.[33]

Thalassemias are a more diverse group of hemoglobinopathies most commonly associated with persons of ancestry arising in the Mediterranean, Middle East, South Asia, and Asia regions. Unlike the chemical change caused by the valine substitution in sickle cell patients, thalassemias are characterized by a deficiency or absence of one of the subunits of the Hgb. Because there are two α and two β Hgb subunits in the normal Hgb tetramer, an inability to produce adequate amounts of one of the subunits would clearly lead to difficulty in synthesizing intact, complete Hgb molecules.[34]

Thalassemias are often diagnosed by a peripheral blood smear, which shows small, pale erythrocytes, sometimes in very high numbers. Some of the RBCs are nucleated, reflecting the intense pressure on erythropoiesis in the bone marrow to provide oxygen-carrying capacity to the body even if it requires releasing immature, nucleated erythrocyte precursors. The type of thalassemia present is determined using electrophoresis.

# WHITE BLOOD CELL COUNT AND DIFFERENTIAL

White blood cells are divided into two general classifications:

1. Granulocytes or phagocytes (leukocytes that engulf and digest other cells)
2. Lymphocytes (leukocytes involved in the recognition of non-self cells or substances)

The functions of these general leukocyte classes are interrelated. For example, immunoglobulins produced by B lymphocytes are needed to coat or opsonize encapsulated bacteria so that T cells and neutrophils can more effectively identify, adhere, and destroy them.

When a WBC count and differential is ordered for a patient, the resulting laboratory report provides the total WBCs in a given volume of blood plus the relative percentages each cell type that contribute to the total. Therefore, the percentages of the WBC subtypes must add up to 100%. If one cell type increases or decreases, percentages of all other types change in the opposite direction. **Table 16-5** is a general breakdown of the different types of WBCs and their usual percentages in peripheral blood.

The WBC count and differential is one of the most widely performed clinical laboratory tests. Large, clinical laboratories commonly use automated methods for determining the WBC differential, but manual differential counts may still be used. Automated instruments count thousands of cells and can report not only the relative percentages of the various WBC types but also the absolute numbers, Hgb, RBC, platelets, and RBC indices. When reviewing a WBC differential, one must be aware of not only the relative percentages of cell types but also the absolute numbers. The percentages viewed in isolation can lead to incorrect conclusions.

Numerous cluster of differentiation (CD) surface markers have been characterized on leukocytes and their precursors. CD molecules are surface proteins or glycoproteins that are typically immunologically characterized by their unique epitopes. The function of only a minority of the hundreds of CD molecules identified on human cells have been determined; however, their expression on specific cell types can permit identification of abnormal cell types and allow targeted treatment at cells expressing the CD molecule.

## Granulocytes

*Granulocytes* are phagocytic cells and derive their name from the presence of granules within the cytoplasm. The granules store lysozymes and other chemicals needed to oxidize and

## TABLE 16-5. Normal WBC Count and Differential

| CELL TYPE | NORMAL RANGE |
|---|---|
| Total WBC count | 4.4–11.3 × 10³ cells/μL |
| Polymorphonuclear neutrophils ("polys," "segs," PMN) | 45% to 73% |
| Band neutrophils ("bands," "stabs") | 3% to 5% |
| Lymphocytes | 20% to 40% |
| Monocytes | 2% to 8% |
| Eosinophils | 0% to 4% |
| Basophils | 0% to 1% |

PMN = polymorphonuclear cells.

enzymatically destroy foreign cells. Granulocytic leukocytes include neutrophils, eosinophils, and basophils. Monocytes are phagocytic cells that mature into macrophages, which are predominantly found in tissue rather than in the circulation. When a peripheral smear of blood is prepared, three types of granulocytes are named by the staining characteristics of their cytoplasmic granules[8,35]:

1. Neutrophils, which retain neutral stains and appear light tan
2. Eosinophils, which retain acidic dyes and appear red-orange
3. Basophils, which retain basic dyes and appear dark blue to purple

Granulocytes are formed in large numbers from the pluripotential stem cells in the bone marrow. They undergo numerous differentiation and proliferation steps in the marrow and are usually released into the peripheral blood in their mature form. A common exception is the appearance of banded neutrophil during an infection, as discussed later. Neutrophils, eosinophils, and basophils die in the course of destroying ingested organisms or particles, forming purulent material or pus. On the other hand, monocytes and macrophages do not usually need to sacrifice themselves when destroying target cells.

### Neutrophils

*Normal range: PMN leukocytes 45% to 73% or 0.45 to 0.73; bands 3% to 5% or 0.03 to 0.05*

*Neutrophils* are also termed *segmented neutrophils* ("segs") or *polymorphonuclear cells* (PMNs, "polys"). The less mature form of the neutrophil with a crescent-shaped nucleus is a band cell. Bands derive their name from the morphology of their nucleus, which has not yet segmented into multiple lobes. Less mature forms of the neutrophil, such as the metamyelocyte and myelocyte, are normally found in the bone marrow but not in the peripheral blood. The neutrophil is a phagocytic cell that exists to ingest and digest foreign cells and proteins (eg, bacteria and fungi).

The absolute segmented neutrophil count is the percentage of neutrophils and bands multiplied by the WBC count. The reference range for absolute counts can be estimated by multiplying the normal range of percentages for the particular type of WBC by the upper and lower limits of the total WBC count. Absolute neutrophil counts of <1,000/μL represent neutropenia, with counts of <500/μL and 100/μL considered severe and absolute neutropenia, respectively. Because of the risk of rapidly progressing, life-threatening infection, antimicrobials may be started after cytotoxic chemotherapy if the absolute neutrophil count is <500/μL and the patient develops a fever.[36]

Under normal conditions, about 90% of the neutrophils are stored in the bone marrow. When released, neutrophils normally circulate for several hours before eventually marginating by the adhering to vascular endothelium in the spleen and other organs. This dynamic process of margination, with the potential for demargination, causes large shifts in the measured neutrophil count because only the granulocytes that are circulating at the time are measured by a venipuncture. Neutrophils spend only about 6 to 8 hours in the circulation, after which they move through the endothelium into the tissue. Unless used to engage a foreign body or sustained by the cytokine milieu, neutrophils then undergo programmed cell death, a noninflammatory process termed *apoptosis*.

During an acute infection, there is an increase in the percentage of neutrophils because they initially demarginate from the endothelium and are released from the bone marrow.[37,38] Demarginated neutrophils are mature, so initially the percent of band neutrophils will remain normal. However, as less mature neutrophils are released from the marrow, usually in response to bacterial infection, the percent of band neutrophils increases. The increase percent of band cells in infections is termed a *left shift*. This term may be due to the traditional order in which the manual differential count was reported. It may also arise from the use of a left-to-right sequence in figures describing the process of neutrophil differentiation from the stem cell (Figure 16-1).

When the neutrophils and bands are elevated, the percentage of lymphocytes decreases. Ratios of only 10% to 15% lymphocytes may appear in these patients, but this relative lymphopenia arises from the concomitant increase in total WBCs and likely does not reflect an absolute lymphopenia. An exception is a neutrophilia caused by glucocorticoid treatment, which will cause a drop in the absolute lymphocyte count because of its lymphotoxic effect while increasing the absolute neutrophil count due to demargination.

### Eosinophils and Basophils

*Normal range: eosinophils 0% to 4% or 0 to 0.04; basophils 0% to 1% or 0 to 0.01*

The functions of *eosinophils* and *basophils* are not completely known. Eosinophils are present in large numbers in the intestinal mucosa and lungs, two locations in which foreign proteins enter the body. Eosinophils can phagocytize, kill, and digest bacteria and yeast. Elevations of eosinophils counts are highly suggestive of parasitic infections and allergic diseases, including some forms of asthma.

Basophils are present in small numbers in the peripheral blood and are the most long-lasting granulocyte in blood, with a circulating lifespan of approximately 2 weeks.[2] They contain heparin, histamine, and leukotriene B$_4$.[39] Many signs and symptoms of allergic responses can be attributed to specific mast cell and basophil products. Basophils are probably involved in immediate hypersensitivity reactions (eg, extrinsic, or allergic, and asthma) in addition to delayed hypersensitivity reactions. Basophils may be increased in chronic inflammation and in some types of leukemia.

### Monocytes/Macrophages

*Normal range: monocytes 2% to 8% or 0.02 to 0.08*
*Monocytes* leave the circulation in 16 to 36 hours and enter the tissues, where they mature into macrophages. *Macrophages* are present in lymph nodes, alveoli of the lungs, spleen, liver, and bone marrow, comprising the reticuloendothelial system.[40] Macrophages, both those circulating and those that have migrated out of the blood, participate in the removal of foreign substances from the body. In addition to attacking foreign cells, they are involved in the destruction of old erythrocytes, denatured plasma proteins, and plasma lipids. Tissue macrophages also salvage iron from the Hgb of old erythrocytes and return the iron to transferrin for delivery to the bone marrow. Under appropriate stimuli, monocytes/macrophages are transformed into antigen-presenting cells (also termed *dendritic cells*). These transformed macrophages are an important component of both cell-mediated (T lymphocytes) and soluble (B lymphocyte) immune activity against antigens.[40] Macrophages express a variety of chemokine receptors and secrete a variety of substances, including enzymes, a variety of interleukins, tumor necrosis factor-$\alpha$, interferons, and a variety of tissue and vascular growth factors.

## Lymphocytes and Plasma Cells

*Normal range: lymphocytes 20% to 40% or 0.2 to 0.4*
*Lymphocytes* make up the second major group of leukocytes. They are characterized by a far less granular cytoplasm and relatively large, smooth nuclei. These cells give specificity and memory to the body's defense against foreign invaders.[41] There are three subgroups of lymphocytes:

1. T lymphocytes (T cells)
2. B lymphocytes (B cells)
3. Natural killer cells (NK cells)

Lymphocytes are not phagocytic, but the NK and T-cell subtypes are cytotoxic by virtue of complement activation and antibody-dependent cell-mediated cytotoxicity. Morphologic differentiation of lymphocytes is difficult; visual inspection of a blood smear cannot uniformly distinguish between T, B, and NK cells. Fortunately, lymphocytes can be distinguished by the presence of CD lineage-specific membrane markers. Thus, mature T cells have CD3 and CD5, B cells have CD20, and NK cells have CD56 membrane markers.[41] Individual CD moieties may be surface proteins, enzymes, or adhesion molecules, to name a few. Labeled antibodies to specific CD molecules identify the lineage of the lymphocyte, either in blood or in tissue.

Identification of the subtype of lymphocytes is not a routine clinical hematology test at present; they are reported simply as lymphocytes by automated counting instruments. However,

in research applications and for the diagnosis and guidance of targeted treatment of leukemias and lymphomas, subtypes can be both counted and sorted by an automated process termed *fluorescence-activated cell sorting*. The WBC layer is separated by centrifugation and exposed to one or more CD antibodies tagged with fluorescent dyes. The labeled cells are given an electrostatic charge and then flow individually past one or more lasers that induce the labeled cells to glow at wavelengths specific to the dye staining each cell. This method is general and can be used to count and sort virtually any cell that can be labeled with a fluorescent tag.[42]

With the help of T cells, B cells recognize foreign substances and are transformed into plasma cells, capable of producing antibodies (discussed later). **Table 16-6** lists the types of disorders in which lymphocytes are increased or decreased.

### T Lymphocytes

*T lymphocytes* are responsible for cell-mediated immunity and are the predominant lymphocytes in circulation and in tissue. They require partial maturation in the embryonic thymus, hence, the name *T cell*. In addition to identifying infections, they oversee delayed hypersensitivity (seen with the skin test for tuberculosis) and rejection of transplanted organs.[41,43] For a foreign antigen to be recognized by T cells, it must be "presented" by macrophages or dendritic cells on one of two complex, individualized molecules termed *major histocompatibility complexes* (MHC1 and MHC2).

T cells can be further divided into helper and cytotoxic (or suppressor) cells, which, respectively, express the CD4 and CD8 markers. CD4 helper cells are not cytotoxic but on recognizing an antigen will activate and produce cytokines such as IL-2, which stimulate nearby immune cells, including macrophages and CD8 T cells, B cells, and NK cells.

CD4 T-helper cells can again be divided into T$^1_H$ and T$_{H2}$ subtypes. The T$^1_H$ subtype mediates the activation of macrophages and the delayed hypersensitivity response, while the T$_{H2}$ subtype appears primarily responsible for B-cell activation. The cellular specificity of these subtypes appears to arise primarily from their distinct pattern of cytokine production.

Human immunodeficiency virus binds specifically to the CD4 receptor but does not elicit the desired antiviral response in most patients. This infection leads to destruction of this subset of T cells and a reversal of the CD4/CD8 ratio (normally >1). The CD4 lymphocyte count and viral load measured by viral RNA are inversely related and correlate with overall prognosis. Although the CD4 count remains a useful surrogate marker in monitoring the course and treatment of patients infected with HIV, viral loads are routinely measured. The lack of adequate numbers of active T-helper cells that activates other immune cells leads to an increased susceptibility to numerous opportunistic infections, cancer, and progression to acquired immune deficiency syndrome.[44,45] T cells are the primary mediator for host rejection of transplanted solid organs,[47] such as heart, lung, kidney, liver, and pancreas grafts. The perioperative and postoperative treatment of solid organ graft recipients is directed toward minimizing the antigraft T-cell response, while not ablating the T-cell population to the point of causing life-threatening infections. In practice, this is a narrow path plagued by viral and

**TABLE 16-6.** Quantitative Disorders of White Blood Cells[35,41,43,47,50,51,34]

| WBC ABNORMALITY | TYPICAL THRESHOLD (CELLS/μL) | POSSIBLE CAUSES | |
|---|---|---|---|
| Neutrophilia | >12,000 | Acute bacterial infection | |
| | | Trauma | |
| | | Myocardial infarction | |
| | | Chronic bacterial infection | |
| | | Epinephrine, lithium, G-CSF, GM-CSF, glucocorticosteroids | |
| Neutropenia | <1,500 | Radiation exposure | |
| | | Medications: | |
| | | Antineoplastic cytotoxic agents | |
| | | Captopril | Carbamazepine |
| | | Cephalosporins | Chloramphenicol |
| | | Clozapine | Diclofenac |
| | | Ganciclovir | Levamisole |
| | | Methimazole | Penicillins |
| | | Phenothiazines | Procainamide |
| | | Propylthiouracil | Ticlopidine |
| | | Vancomycin | Zidovudine |
| | | Tricyclic antidepressants | |
| | | Sulfamethoxazole–trimethoprim | |
| | | Overwhelming acute bacterial infection | |
| | | Vitamin $B_{12}$ or folate deficiency | |
| | | Salmonellosis | |
| | | Pertussis | |
| Eosinophilia | >350 | Allergic disorders/asthma | |
| | | Parasitic infections | |
| | | Leukemia | |
| | | Medications | |
| | | Angiotensin-converting enzyme inhibitors | |
| | | Antibiotics (or any allergic reaction to a drug) | |
| Eosinopenia | <50 | Acute infection | |
| Basophilia | >300 | Chronic inflammation | |
| | | Leukemia | |
| Monocytosis | >800 | Recovery state of acute bacterial infection | |
| | | Tuberculosis (disseminated) | |
| | | Endocarditis | |
| | | Protozoal or rickettsial infection | |
| | | Leukemia | |
| Lymphocytosis | >4,000 | Infectious mononucleosis | |
| | | Viral infections (eg, rubella, varicella, mumps, cytomegalovirus) | |
| | | Pertussis | |
| | | Tuberculosis | |
| | | Syphilis | |
| | | Lymphoma | |
| Lymphopenia | <1,000 | HIV type 1 | |
| | | Radiation exposure | |
| | | Corticosteroids | |
| | | Lymphoma (Hodgkin disease) | |
| | | Aplastic anemia | |

G-CSF = granulocyte-colony stimulating factor; GM-CSF = granulocyte-macrophage colony-stimulating factor.
*Source*: Adapted with permission from references 34,35,41,43,47,50,51.

fungal infections that cause substantial morbidity and mortality in graft recipients.

Typically, T-cell populations in graft recipients[46] are not measured, and drug titration is based on biopsies of the transplanted organ, drug concentrations of the immunosuppressants, and blood counts. Anti–T-cell treatments employed in transplant recipients include corticosteroids; Muromonab-CD3 (OKT3), an anti-CD3 antibody directed against the CD3 marker found on T cells; antihuman lymphocyte immunoglobulin; and inhibitors of T-cell activation such as cyclosporine, tacrolimus, or mycophenolate. Because these immunoglobulin products are typically obtained from nonhuman species, they can cause severe allergic reactions and are usually effective for only a short period.

### B Lymphocytes

B cells are named after similar avian lymphocytes that required maturation in an organ termed the *Bursa of Fabricius*. There is no equivalent organ in humans, and maturation of B lymphocytes occurs in the bone marrow. Quiescent, circulating B cells express one form of antibody, immunoglobulin M (IgM). When stimulated by activated T cells or antigen-presenting cells, B cells are transformed into plasma cells that will produce one of five immunoglobulin types: IgA, IgD, IgE, IgG, or IgM.[47]

The two antibodies most commonly associated with the development of immunity to foreign proteins, viruses, and bacteria are IgM and IgG. IgE is associated with the development of immediate hypersensitivity reactions, such as anaphylaxis and allergic diseases, including asthma. IgA is secreted into the lumen of the GI tract and helps avoid sensitization to foods, and IgD is bound to the lymphocyte cell membrane.[47] Abnormal immunoglobulins can typically be detected using serum and/or urine protein electrophoretic gels and urine immunofixation. Monoclonal hyperimmunoglobulinemias are identified by single electrophoretic peaks and are typically associated with plasma (B) cell premalignant or malignant disorders. Polyclonal hyperimmunoglobulinemias can be associated with infections and inflammatory reactions.

Lymphopenia and hypogammaglobulinemia (a decrease in the total quantity of immunoglobulin) are seen as a consequence of corticosteroid treatment, transplant rejection prophylaxis, and anticancer treatment, but they can also paradoxically arise from leukemias. In general, lymphopenia is more common in chemotherapy regimens that include high doses of corticosteroids, which bind to a receptor on lymphocytes and are lymphotoxic, even to the point of initiating cellular apoptosis.[47] Interestingly, although HIV-1 infections lead to lymphopenia, other viral infections (eg, infectious mononucleosis, hepatitis, mumps, varicella, rubella, herpes simplex, herpes zoster, and influenza) often increase the number of circulating lymphocytes (lymphocytosis)[48,49] (**Minicase 4**). Severe malnutrition also may result in lymphopenia.

### Natural Killer Cells

*Natural killer cells* (NK) are derived from T-cell lineage but are not as restricted in requiring MHC identification of the target cell. NK cells are thought to be particularly important for cytotoxic effects on virally infected cells and cancer cells.

## Leukocyte Disorders

Patients can suffer from three major classes of *leukocyte disorders*: functional, quantitative, and myeloproliferative. *Functional* disorders involve defects in recognition, metabolism, cytotoxic effects, signaling, and other related activities. Routine laboratory values are not intended to evaluate these abnormalities and are not discussed further here.

*Quantitative* disorders involve too few or too many leukocytes. Possible causes are listed in Table 16-6. Neutropenia is usually considered to exist when the neutrophil count is <1,500 or 1,000 cells/μL.[36,50] When the neutrophil count is <500 cells/μL, normal defense mechanisms are significantly impaired, and the patient is at increased risk of bacterial and fungal infections. A neutrophil count <100/μL is termed *absolute neutropenia* or *agranulocytosis*. This is often encountered after cytotoxic chemotherapy is administered and after regimens intended to ablate the bone marrow in preparation for a stem cell transplant. An infection is probable if agranulocytosis is prolonged or severe, so patients at risk are monitored closely for infection and administered broad spectrum antimicrobials when fever or other signs of infection are seen. When infections do occur in such patients, they can be difficult to successfully treat—even with normally effective antibiotics—because the number and phagocytic activity of the neutrophils are impaired.

Agranulocytosis[51] may be seen as a specific toxic drug effect (such as seen with propylthiouracil) or as part of a broader myelopoietic disorder (such as aplastic anemia). Aplastic anemias (inadequate production of blood cells by the bone marrow) have multiple causes including drug, toxin, or radiation exposure; congenital defect; or age-related fatty or fibrotic bone marrow replacement. The word *anemia* in this term is misleading because production of other blood cell types can also be decreased resulting in pancytopenia. Because some cases of aplastic anemia are autoimmune in nature, some patients are treated with immunosuppressive therapy.

Myelodysplastic anemias are characterized by abnormal maturation of RBCs and WBCs. These are typically classified by the World Health Organization system[52] based on the marrow morphology identified from a bone marrow aspirate. The usual treatment course is supportive care (ie, transfusions or stem cell transplant in patients for whom this is feasible).

Neutrophilia (increased circulating neutrophils) is caused by both an increased release from the bone marrow and a shift of marginated cells into the circulation. This rapid rise in the number of circulating cells can be caused by acute infections, trauma, or administration of epinephrine or corticosteroids. Neutrophilia exceeding 50,000 cells/μL is termed "leukemoid reaction" and can be seen with a variety of underlying inflammatory conditions. While sometimes mistaken for leukemia, the neutrophils in leukemoid reactions typically are mature cells rather than the highly immature cells seen in leukemias.

## Myeloproliferative Disorders
### Leukemias

Neoplasms of the bone marrow cells most commonly involve a leukocyte line and are termed *leukemias*. Leukemias are

## MINICASE 4

### Anemia and Lymphopenia

Donna L. is a 55-year-old woman with a history of rheumatoid arthritis and type 2 diabetes mellitus who presents to her physician for a routine physical examination. She is feeling well and has no complaints, other than the soreness routinely associated with the arthritis in her hands. She has normal vital signs, and other than the stigmata of her moderate rheumatoid arthritis, she has a normal physical examination. She takes the following oral medications routinely:

- Prednisone 5 mg once daily with dinner
- Metformin 750 mg once daily with dinner
- Methotrexate 10 mg weekly
- Acetaminophen 650 mg q 6 hr PRN for hand pain

The physician draws a comprehensive metabolic panel and a CBC with differential and platelet count. The results of the CBC with differential and platelet count are as follows:

| TEST NAME | RESULT | REFERENCE RANGE |
|---|---|---|
| RBC | $4 \times 10^6$ cells/µL | $4.1–5.1 \times 10^6$ cells/µL for women |
| WBC | $9.6 \times 10^3$ cells/µL | $4.4–11.3 \times 10^3$ cells/µL |
| Hgb | 13.3 g/dL | 12.3–15.3 g/dL for women |
| Hct | 37.9% | 36% to 45% for women |
| MCV | 105.5 fL/cell | 80–96 fL/cell |
| MCH | 39.2 pg/cell | 27–33 pg/cell |
| RDW | 15% | 11.5% to 14.5% |
| Platelets | 304,000 cells/µL | 150,000–450,000 cells/µL |

| TEST NAME | RESULT | REFERENCE RANGE |
|---|---|---|
| Neutrophils | 76% | 45% to 73% |
| Bands | 5% | 3% to 5% |
| Monocytes | 7% | 2% to 8% |
| Eosinophils | 2% | 0% to 4% |
| Basophils | 1% | 0% to 1% |
| Lymphocytes | 9% | 20% to 40% |

QUESTION: What abnormalities are present, and what is their cause and resolution?

DISCUSSION: This patient has somewhat low RBC count and Hgb as well as elevated MCV and MCH, indicating a macrocytic anemia. She also has a high WBC count with increased neutrophil and decreased lymphocyte counts. She is not showing signs of infection. The macrocytic anemia could be caused by vitamin $B_{12}$ or folate deficiency. Treatment with methotrexate, an antifolate drug, is the likely cause. The differential diagnosis can be made by obtaining blood assays for vitamin $B_{12}$ and folate. Many clinicians prescribe 5 mg oral folate daily except for methotrexate dosing days, and this would be an appropriate recommendation for this patient as well.

The lymphopenia and neutrophilia are likely caused by the prednisone therapy. Glucocorticoids are known to cause demargination of neutrophils from the vascular endothelium, leading to a relative neutrophilia. Glucocorticoids are also lymphotoxic, typified in their use for treatment of lymphocytic malignancies. No treatment is indicated in this patient, but monitoring for opportunistic infections, such as candidiasis, needs to be ongoing. The corticosteroid-induced changes in lymphocyte and neutrophil counts are expected to return to normal after the cessation of the steroid dosing.

---

broadly classified as being acute or chronic, and leukemias are either of myeloblastic (granulocytic lineage) or lymphoblastic (lymphocytic) lineage.[52;53] The clinical course and biology of various leukemias varies. Almost all leukemias fall within one of four categories:

1. Acute myelogenous
2. Acute lymphoblastic
3. Chronic myelogenous
4. Chronic lymphocytic

Although the clinical course varies among these neoplasms, a common denominator is the proliferation of the neoplastic cell line and displacement of normal hematopoiesis. The neoplastic cells may arise from cells of varying levels of differentiation of either a granulocytic or lymphocytic lineage. Morphology and CD membrane markers vary among individuals but are

fairly uniform throughout the disease course in a given patient. The morphology and CD membrane markers of cells obtained from the diagnostic bone marrow aspirate and flow cytometry, respectively, are used to assign a French-American-British (FAB) classification of M0 through M7 to subtype acute myelogenous leukemia or to diagnose acute lymphoblastic leukemia. Other morphologic features and surface marker combinations are used to characterize the other leukemias.

Multiple (plasma cell) myeloma is notable in that it is a plasma cell neoplasm of the bone marrow. The monoclonal neoplastic plasma cells produce a single immunoglobulin isotype (IgG, IgA, light chain only, IgD, IgE, or rarely IgM). This single, monoclonal protein is referred to as the *M-protein*. The M-protein is usually identified using serum protein electrophoresis. The specific immunoglobulin type can be defined with a subsequent step of serum immunofixation with protein-specific antibody (eg, anti-IgG). Other laboratory findings associated with multiple myeloma include Bence Jones protein (light chain) in urine, hypercalcemia, increased ESR, normochromic, normocytic anemia, and coagulopathy.[54]

Chronic *myeloproliferative* disorders[55] involve an abnormal proliferation of more mature bone marrow cells. Excessive or uncontrolled proliferation of all cell lines leads to polycythemia vera, a malignancy when erythrocyte overproduction is the most prominent abnormality. Chronic myelogenous leukemia is characterized by a chromosomal translocation [t(9:22), "Philadelphia chromosome"] that creates a fusion product (BCR/ABL) resulting in autonomous tyrosine kinase activity, a growth-signaling enzyme. Patients with chronic lymphocytic leukemia present with increased numbers of circulating mature B lymphocytes, which are monoclonal.

Patients with chronic leukemias may live for several years with minimal treatment because of the indolent nature of the disease. At some point, a patient typically develops a transformation of the disease into a life-threatening accelerated phase or blast crisis. Fortunately, with the development of tyrosine kinase inhibitors and other targeted medications, this fatal complication can now often be substantially delayed. Although the chronic leukemias are less aggressive than the acute leukemias, they are less curable with chemotherapy, and stem cell transplantation is appropriate in selected patients.

### Lymphomas

A lymphoma is a neoplasm of lymphocytic lineage, which typically predominates in lymph nodes forming tissue masses rather than being primarily located in the bone marrow. The lymphomas are classified into two main groups: (1) non-Hodgkin lymphoma (NHL), and (2) Hodgkin lymphoma. The pattern of tissue involvement—termed either *diffuse* or *follicular* (nodular)—and the cytology of the neoplastic lymphoid cells (primarily the size and appearance of the cell nucleus) are used to morphologically subclassify non-Hodgkin lymphoma.[56] The World Health Organization classification[57] of NHL also uses CD surface markers, cytogenetics, and molecular and genetic studies to further define subcategories of NHL. Non-Hodgkin lymphomas can also be practically divided into aggressive and indolent forms. The aggressive lymphomas grow and spread quickly but are generally more likely to be eradicated with current, intensive chemotherapy. In contrast, the slower-growing, indolent lymphomas are not as responsive and are more difficult to cure, but these often have a long disease course. Hodgkin lymphoma is generally a more treatable lymphoma. The neoplastic cellular element is termed the *Reed-Sternberg cell*. This is a large cell with a lobulated nucleus and prominent nucleoli. It is typically surrounded by a nonneoplastic population of lymphocytes, eosinophils, neutrophils, plasma cells, and macrophages.

Lymphomas predictably involve T-lymphocyte or B-lymphocyte precursors, and many express CD marker characteristics of mature lymphocytes. Identification of the CD20 marker on B-cell lymphomas provides an opportunity to treat these patients with recombinant antibodies specific to this surface marker. Differentiation between a T-cell leukemia and a peripheral T-cell lymphoma likely requires the identification of CD phenotypes.

## SUMMARY

This chapter presents a brief characterization of the lineage and function of RBCs and WBCs. Normal laboratory values have been presented, but it is important to realize that normal ranges vary slightly depending on the laboratory conducting the analysis and the population being studied. Hematologic conditions are common, resulting in widespread use of hematologic tests such as the CBC in all patient care settings. Proper interpretation of these commonly used tests is important for the clinician to provide a correct assessment of the patient's condition, choose the most appropriate therapy, and monitor the outcomes of that therapy.

## ACKNOWLEDGMENTS

The authors and editors would like to acknowledge the contributions of Dr. Paul R. Hutson, who authored this chapter in previous editions of this textbook.

## LEARNING POINTS

1. ***How do iron deficiency and nutrient deficiency (folate and vitamin B$_{12}$) differ in their presentation in a CBC?***

   **ANSWER:** As expressed by the term *anemia*, in each of these circumstances, the Hgb and Hct are low. Iron deficiency is characterized by small (microcytic, low MCV) and pale (hypochromic) RBCs. In contrast, both folate and vitamin B$_{12}$ deficiency classically present with larger (macrocytic, elevated MCV) erythrocytes. Patients with vitamin B$_{12}$ deficiency may also have abnormalities in WBC and platelets.

2. ***What are the roles of transferrin, ferritin, TIBC, and TSat, and how are these laboratory values interpreted?***

   **ANSWER:** Transferrin's primary role is to transport iron to the bone marrow for erythrocyte synthesis, while in the process protecting intervening tissue from the reactivity of the metal ion. Ferritin serves as the storage form of iron. Ferritin protein not bound to iron is termed *apoferritin*. Most of the iron-binding protein in the plasma is transferrin, and the serum TIBC is an indirect measure of the transferrin concentration. With iron deficiency, the liver synthesizes more transferrin. Thus, the residual, unbound capacity of the transferrin (and thus TIBC) is increased, while the percentage saturation of receptors on the transferrin molecules (transferrin saturation, TSat) is decreased. With less tissue stores of iron, the ferritin level is decreased in iron deficiency. In anemia of chronic disease, the plasma iron and transferrin concentrations are both low, and the TSat may be decreased or normal. Liver disease or malnutrition can also slow the production of transferrin, which may complicate the interpretation of the TIBC.

3. ***What are typical reasons why WBC counts are elevated, and how can the differential cell count help clarify the cause?***

   **ANSWER:** A sustained elevation of the WBC count is typically due to metabolic stress, infections, certain medications, or leukemias. Infections, corticosteroids, epinephrine, and exercise cause a demargination of neutrophils from the endothelium, causing a transient, increased percentage of neutrophils, but in most cases a normal absolute lymphocyte count. Corticosteroids cause neutrophil demargination but are also lymphotoxic, so the absolute lymphocyte count decreases. Bacterial infections are associated with an increase in the percentage and absolute number of neutrophils and to the release of less mature neutrophils (band cells) from the bone marrow.

**4. What are common, unintended drug-induced alterations in RBC and WBC counts and function?**

ANSWER: RBC counts can be reduced by nonsteroidal antiinflammatory drug–induced GI bleeding or by hemolytic anemia in patients with G6PD deficiency treated with various oxidizing drugs. RBC and WBC (and platelet) counts are commonly decreased following cytotoxic chemotherapy, but the impact on WBCs is greater, especially for neutrophils, because of their faster turnover and shorter lifespan. Macrocytic, hypochromic anemia can be caused by treatment with antifolates such as methotrexate, or chronic treatment with antibiotics inhibiting DNA synthesis such as trimethoprim. Corticosteroids are lymphotoxic and decrease the lymphocyte count but also lead to a higher apparent neutrophil count due to their drug-induced demargination from the endothelium. Some medications, such as propylthiouracil and clozapine, can cause a sudden, dramatic reduction in neutrophils, resulting in agranulocytosis.

# REFERENCES

1. Gulati GL, Ashton JK, Hyun BH. Structure and function of the bone marrow and hematopoiesis. *Hematol Oncol Clin North Am.* 1988;2(4):495-511.PubMed
2. Finch CA, Harker LA, Cook JD. Kinetics of the formed elements of human blood. *Blood.* 1977;50(4):699-707.PubMed
3. Kushansky N. Hematopoietic stem cells, progenitors and cytokines. In: Kaushansky K, Lichtman MA, Prchal JT, et al, eds. *Williams Manual of Hematology.* 9th ed. New York: McGraw-Hill; 2016. https://accessmedicine-mhmedical-com.ezproxy3.library.arizona.edu/content.aspx?bookid=1581&sectionid=94302625. Accessed June 28, 2020.
4. Ryan DH. Examination of the Marrow. In: Kaushansky K, Lichtman MA, Prchal JT, et al, eds. *Williams Manual of Hematology.* 9th ed. New York, NY: McGraw-Hill; https://accessmedicine-mhmedical-com.ezproxy3.library.arizona.edu/content.aspx?bookid=1581&sectionid=94301405. Accessed June 28, 2020.
5. Prchal JT, Thiagarajan P. Erythropoiesis. In: Kaushansky K, Lichtman MA, Prchal JT, et al, eds. *Williams Manual of Hematology.* 9th ed. New York, NY: McGraw-Hill; 2016. https://accessmedicine-mhmedical-com.ezproxy3.library.arizona.edu/content.aspx?bookid=1581&sectionid=94303394. Accessed June 28, 2020.
6. Narla M. Structure and Composition of the Erythrocyte. In: Kaushansky K, Lichtman MA, Prchal JT, et al, eds. *Williams Manual of Hematology.* 9th ed. New York, NY: McGraw-Hill; 2016. https://accessmedicine-mhmedical-com.ezproxy3.library.arizona.edu/content.aspx?bookid=1581&sectionid=94303279. Accessed June 28, 2020.
7. Mais DD. Diseases of Red Blood Cells. In: Laposata M, ed. *Laposata's Laboratory Medicine: Diagnosis of Disease in the Clinical Laboratory.* 3rd ed. New York, NY: McGraw-Hill; 2019. https://accessmedicine-mhmedical-com.ezproxy3.library.arizona.edu/content.aspx?bookid=2503&sectionid=201362558. Accessed June 28, 2020.
8. Vajpayee N, Graham SS, Bem S. Basic examination of the blood and bone marrow. In: McPherson RA, Pincus MR, eds. *Henry's Clinical Diagnosis and Management by Laboratory Methods.* 23rd ed. Philadelphia, PA: WB Saunders; 2016:510-539.
9. Tefferi A, Hanson CA, Inwards DJ. How to interpret and pursue an abnormal complete blood cell count in adults. *Mayo Clin Proc.* 2005;80(7):923-936.PubMed
10. Sox HC Jr, Liang MH. The erythrocyte sedimentation rate. Guidelines for rational use. *Ann Intern Med.* 1986;104(4):515-523.PubMed
11. Laposata M, Nichols JH, Steele P, et al. Methods. In: Laposata M, ed. *Laposata's Laboratory Medicine: Diagnosis of Disease in the Clinical Laboratory.* 3rd ed. New York, NY: McGraw-Hill; 2019. https://accessmedicine-mhmedical-com.ezproxy3.library.arizona.edu/content.aspx?bookid=2503&sectionid=201361411. Accessed June 28, 2020.
12. Quigley JC, Means RT, Glader B. The birth, life and death of red blood cells: Erythropoiesis, the mature red blood cell and cell destruction. In: Greer JP, Rodgers MD, Glader B, et al, eds. *Wintrobe's Clinical Hematology.* 14th ed. Philadelphia, PA: Lippincott Williams & Wilkins; 2018:90-130.
13. Cascio MJ, DeLoughery TG. Anemia. Evaluation and diagnostic tests. *Med Clin North Am.* 2017;101(2):263-284.PubMed
14. Green R. Folate, cobalamin, and megaloblastic anemias. In: Kaushansky K, Lichtman MA, Prchal JT, et al, eds. *Williams Manual of Hematology.* 9th ed. New York, NY: McGraw-Hill; 2016. https://accessmedicine-mhmedical-com.ezproxy3.library.arizona.edu/book.aspx?bookid=1581#94301184. Accessed June 28, 2020.
15. Green R, Datta Mitra A. Megaloblastic anemias. Nutritional and other causes. *Med Clin North Am.* 2017;101(2):297-317.PubMed
16. Socha DS, DeSouza SI, Flagg A, et al. Severe megaloblastic anemia: vitamin deficiency and other causes. *Cleve Clin J Med.* 2020;87(3):153-164.PubMed
17. Neutrophils N-CA. In: Lichtman MA, Shafer MS, Felgar RE, et al, eds. *Lichtman's Atlas of Hematology.* New York, NY: McGraw-Hill; 2016. https://accessmedicine-mhmedical-com.ezproxy3.library.arizona.edu/content.aspx?bookid=1630&sectionid=116917108, Accessed June 28, 2020.
18. Hesdorffer CS, Longo DL. Drug-induced megaloblastic anemia. *N Engl J Med.* 2015;373(17):1649-1658.PubMed
19. Ganz T. Iron metabolism. In: Kaushansky K, Lichtman MA, Prchal JT, et al, eds. *Williams Manual of Hematology.* 9th ed. New York, NY: McGraw-Hill. https://accessmedicine-mhmedical-com.ezproxy3.library.arizona.edu/content.aspx?bookid=1581&sectionid=101238028, Accessed June 28, 2020.
20. Ganz T. Iron deficiency and overload. In: Kaushansky K, Lichtman MA, Prchal JT, et al, eds. *Williams Manual of Hematology.* 9th ed. New York, NY: McGraw-Hill. https://accessmedicine-mhmedical-com.ezproxy3.library.arizona.edu/content.aspx?bookid=1581&sectionid=94304160, Accessed June 28, 2020.
21. DeLoughery TG. Iron deficiency anemia. *Med Clin North Am.* 2017;101(2):319-332.PubMed
22. Camaschella C. Iron deficiency. *Blood.* 2019;133(1):30-39.PubMed
23. Fraenkel PG. Anemia of inflammation: a review. *Med Clin North Am.* 2017;101(2):285-296.PubMed
24. Kidney Disease: Improving Global Outcomes (KDIGO) Anemia Work Group. KDIGO clinical practice guideline for anemia in chronic kidney disease. *Kidney Int.* 2012;2(suppl):279-335.
25. Packman CH. Hemolytic anemia resulting from immune injury. In: Kaushansky K, Lichtman MA, Prchal JT, et al, eds. *Williams Manual of Hematology.* 9th ed. New York, NY: McGraw-Hill; https://accessmedicine-mhmedical-com.ezproxy3.library.arizona.edu/content.aspx?bookid=1581&sectionid=94305662, Accessed June 28, 2020.
26. Liebman HA, Weitz IC. Autoimmune hemolytic anemia. *Med Clin North Am.* 2017;101(2):351-359.PubMed
27. Garratty G, Arndt PA. Drugs that have been shown to cause drug-induced immune hemolytic anemia or positive direct antiglobulin tests: some interesting findings since 2007. *Immunohematology.* 2014;30(2):66-79.PubMed

28. Haley K. Congenital hemolytic anemias. *Med Clin North Am.* 2017;101(2): 361-374.PubMed

29. Youngster I, Arcavi L, Schechmaster R, et al. Medications and glucose-6-phosphate dehydrogenase deficiency: an evidence-based review. *Drug Saf.* 2010;33(9):713-726.PubMed

30. Ganz T. Anemia of Chronic Disease. In: Kaushansky K, Lichtman MA, Prchal JT, Levi MM, Press OW, Burns LJ, Caligiuri M. eds. *Williams Manual of Hematology.* 9th ed. New York, NY: McGraw-Hill. https://accessmedicine-mhmedical-com.ezproxy3.library.arizona.edu/content .aspx?bookid=1581&sectionid=94303965, Accessed June 28, 2020.

31. Hayden SJ, Albert TJ, Watkins TR, et al. Anemia in critical illness: insights into etiology, consequences, and management. *Am J Respir Crit Care Med.* 2012;185(10):1049-1057.PubMed

32. Bohlius J, Bohlke K, Castelli R, et al. Management of cancer-associated anemia with erythropoiesis-stimulating agents: ASCO/ASH clinical practice guideline update. *J Clin Oncol.* 2019;37(15):1336-1351.PubMed

33. Piel FB, Steinberg MH, Rees DC. Sickle cell disease. *N Engl J Med.* 2017;376(16):1561-1573.PubMed

34. Viprakasit V, Ekwattanakit S. Clinical classification, screening and diagnosis for thalassemia. *Hematol Oncol Clin North Am.* 2018;32(2):193-211.PubMed

35. Aster JC, Berliner N. Leukocyte function and nonmalignant leukocyte disorders. In: Aster JC, Bunn H, eds. *Pathophysiology of Blood Disorders,* 2nd ed. New York, NY: McGraw-Hill; 2017. https://accessmedicine -mhmedical-com.ezproxy3.library.arizona.edu/content.aspx?bookid =1900&sectionid=137395503. Accessed June 28, 2020.

36. National Comprehensive Cancer Network NCCN Guidelines. Prevention and treatment of cancer-related infections, Version 2.2020, https://www .nccn.org/professionals/physician_gls/pdf/infections.pdf. Accessed June 28, 2020.

37. Strausbaugh LJ. Hematologic manifestations of bacterial and fungal infections. *Hematol Oncol Clin North Am.* 1987;1(2):185-206.PubMed

38. McKenzie SB, Laudicina RJ. Hematologic changes associated with infection. *Clin Lab Sci.* 1998;11(4):239-251.PubMed

39. Serafin WE, Austen KF. Mediators of immediate hypersensitivity reactions. *N Engl J Med.* 1987;317(1):30-34.PubMed

40. Smith CW. Production, distribution, and fate of monocytes and macrophages. In: Kaushansky K, Lichtman MA, Prchal JT, et al, eds. *Williams Manual of Hematology.* 9th ed. New York, NY: McGraw-Hill; 2016. https://accessmedicine-mhmedical-com.ezproxy3.library.arizona .edu/content.aspx?bookid=1581&sectionid=101238988. Accessed June 28, 2020.

41. Muthusamy N, Caligiuri MA. The structure of lymphocytes and plasma cells. In: Kaushansky K, Lichtman MA, Prchal JT, et al, eds. *Williams Manual of Hematology.* 9th ed. New York, NY: McGraw-Hill; 2016. https:// accessmedicine-mhmedical-com.ezproxy3.library.arizona.edu/content .aspx?bookid=1581&sectionid=108067702. Accessed June 28, 2020.

42. Porwit A. Clinical flow cytometry. In: Greer JP, Rodgers MD, Glader B, et al, eds. *Wintrobe's Clinical Hematology.* 14th ed. Philadelphia, PA: Lippincott Williams & Wilkins; 2018:17-46.

43. McClanahan F, Gribben J. Functions of T lymphocytes: t-cell receptors for antigen. In: Kaushansky K, Lichtman MA, Prchal JT, et al, eds. *Williams Manual of Hematology.* 9th ed. New York, NY: McGraw-Hill; https:// accessmedicine-mhmedical-com.ezproxy3.library.arizona.edu/content .aspx?bookid=1581&sectionid=108068314. Accessed June 28, 2020.

44. Moir S, Chun TW, Fauci AS. Pathogenic mechanisms of HIV disease. *Annu Rev Pathol.* 2011;6:223-248.PubMed

45. Panel on Antiretroviral Guidelines for Adults and Adolescents. Guidelines for the use of antiretroviral agents in adults and adolescents with HIV. Department of Health and Human Services. http://www .aidsinfo.nih.gov/ContentFiles/AdultandAdolescentGL.pdf. Accessed June 28, 2020.

46. Callus R, Buttigieg J, Anastasi AA, Halawa A. Basic concepts in kidney transplant immunology. *Br J Hosp Med (Lond).* 2017;78(1):32-37.PubMed

47. Kipps TJ. Functions of B lymphocytes and plasma cells in immunoglobulin production. In: Kaushansky K, Lichtman MA, Prchal JT, et al, eds. *Williams Manual of Hematology.* 9th ed. New York, NY: McGraw-Hill; 2016. https://accessmedicine-mhmedical-com.ezproxy3 .library.arizona.edu/content.aspx?bookid=1581&sectionid=108068055. Accessed June 28, 2020.

48. Baranski B, Young N. Hematologic consequences of viral infections. *Hematol Oncol Clin North Am.* 1987;1(2):167-183.PubMed

49. Friedman AD. Hematologic manifestations of viral infections. *Pediatr Ann.* 1996;25(10):555-560.PubMed

50. Dale DC, Welte K. Neutropenia and neutrophilia. In: Kaushansky K, Lichtman MA, Prchal JT, et al, eds. *Williams Manual of Hematology.* 9th ed. New York, NY: McGraw-Hill; 2016. https://accessmedicine -mhmedical-com.ezproxy3.library.arizona.edu/content.aspx?bookid =1581&sectionid=101238861. Accessed June 28, 2020.

51. Curtis BR. Drug-induced immune neutropenia/agranulocytosis. *Immunohematology.* 2014;30(2):95-101.PubMed

52. Arber DA, Orazi A, Hasserjian R, et al. The 2016 revision to the World Health Organization classification of myeloid neoplasms and acute leukemia. *Blood.* 2016;127(20):2391-2405.PubMed

53. Blum W, Bloomfield CD. Acute myeloid leukemia. In: Jameson J, Fauci AS, Kasper DL, et al, eds. *Harrison's Principles of Internal Medicine.* 20th ed. New York, NY: McGraw-Hill; 2018:677-686.

54. O'Donnell E, Cottini F, Raje N, et al. Myeloma. In: Kaushansky K, Lichtman MA, Prchal JT, et al, eds. *Williams Manual of Hematology.* 9th ed. New York, NY: McGraw-Hill; 2016:1645-1681.

55. Liesveld JL, Lichtman MA. Chronic myelogenous leukemia and related disorders. In: Kaushansky K, Lichtman MA, Prchal JT, et al, eds. *Williams Manual of Hematology.* 9th ed. New York, NY: McGraw-Hill; 2016:1331-1380.

56. Gascoyne R, Skinnider B. *Pathology* of lymphomas. In: Kaushansky K, Lichtman MA, Prchal JT, et al, eds. *Williams Manual of Hematology.* 9th ed. New York, NY: McGraw-Hill; 2016:1511-1526.

57. de Leval L, Jaffe ES. Lymphoma Classification. *Cancer J.* 2020;26(3): 176-185.PubMed

# 17

# Hematology: Blood Coagulation Tests

*Lea E. Dela Peña*

## OBJECTIVES

*After completing this chapter, the reader should be able to*

- Describe the role of platelets, the coagulation cascade, and fibrinolytic system in normal hemostasis

- List the laboratory tests used to assess platelets and discuss factors that may influence their results

- List the laboratory tests used to assess coagulation and explain their use in evaluating anticoagulant therapy

- List the laboratory tests used to assess clot degradation and disseminated intravascular coagulation and discuss their limitations

- Interpret results and suggest follow-up action given results of laboratory tests used for evaluating coagulation and anticoagulant therapy in a case description

- Discuss the availability and use of point-of-care testing devices specifically for platelet and coagulation tests

Normal hemostasis involves a complex interaction among the vascular subendothelium, platelets, coagulation factors, and proteins that promote clot formation, clot degradation, and inhibitors of these substances. Disruption in normal hemostasis can result in bleeding or excessive clotting. Bleeding can be caused by trauma or damage to vessels, acquired or inherited deficiencies of coagulation factors, or physiologic disorders of platelets, whereas excessive clotting can result from abnormalities of the vascular endothelium, alterations in blood flow, or deficiencies in clotting inhibitors.

Clinicians must monitor the hemostasis process in individual patients to ensure their safety from an imbalance in this complex system. For example, practitioners routinely order platelet tests in patients on certain antineoplastic medications to assess for thrombocytopenia. Likewise, clinicians may closely monitor coagulation tests for patients receiving certain anticoagulants to prevent thromboembolic or hemorrhagic complications; however, it should be noted that not all anticoagulants are routinely monitored, nor are all laboratory tests available for routine clinical use. Overall, the hemostatic process is intricate and requires a clinician knowledgeable in its dynamics for quality assessment.

This chapter reviews normal coagulation physiology, common tests used to assess coagulation and hypercoagulable states, and factors that alter coagulation tests.

## PHYSIOLOGIC PROCESS OF HEMOSTASIS

Normal *hemostasis* involves the complex relationship among participants that promotes clot formation (platelets and the coagulation cascade), inhibits coagulation, and dissolves the formed clot. Each phase of the process is briefly reviewed.

### Clot Formation

Numerous mechanisms promote and limit coagulation. Factors that promote coagulation include malignancy, pregnancy, obesity, immobilization, damage to the blood vessel wall, and causes of low blood flow or venous stasis. Certain medications may also increase risk of thrombosis, including estrogen, tamoxifen, thalidomide, and erythropoietin.[1] Normal blood flow dilutes activated clotting factors and results in their degradation in various tissues (eg, liver) and by proteases. However, when low flow or venous stasis is present, activated clotting factors may not be readily cleared.

#### Platelets

*Platelets* are nonnucleated, disk-shaped structures, 1 to 5 μm in diameter, that are formed in the extravascular spaces of bone marrow from megakaryocytes. Megakaryocyte production and maturation are promoted by the hormone thrombopoietin, which is synthesized in the bone marrow and liver. Two-thirds of the platelets are found in the circulation and one-third is found in the spleen; however, in splenectomized patients, nearly 100% is in the circulation.

The average human adult makes approximately 100 billion platelets per day, with the average platelet circulating for 7 to 10 days. On aging, platelets are destroyed by the spleen, liver, and bone marrow. Throughout their lifespan, platelet function is affected by numerous factors, such as medications, vitamins, foods, spices, and systemic conditions, including chronic renal disease and hematologic disorders

DOI 10.37573/9781585286423.017

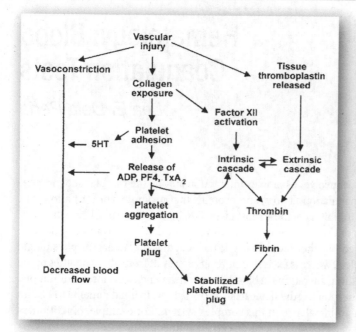

**FIGURE 17-1.** Relationship between platelets and the clotting cascade in the generation of a stabilized fibrin clot. 5HT = serotonin; ADP = adenosine diphosphate; $TxA_2$ = thromboxane $A_2$.

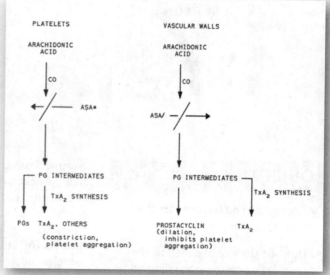

**FIGURE 17-2.** Formation of thromboxane $A_2$, prostaglandins, and prostacyclin in platelets and vascular endothelial cells. CO = cyclooxygenase; ASA* = low-dose, irreversible, inactivation of platelet cyclooxygenase; ASA/= high-dose inactivation of platelet cyclooxygenase.

(eg, myeloproliferative and lymphoproliferative diseases, dysproteinemias, and the presence of antiplatelet antibodies).

The primary function of platelets is to regulate hemostasis, but platelets also play a prominent role in the pathologic formation of arterial thrombi. Three processes (platelet adhesion, activation, and aggregation) are essential for arterial thrombus formation. The surface of normal blood vessels inhibits platelet function, thereby preventing thrombosis; however, endothelial injury to the vasculature, caused by flow abnormalities, trauma, or the rupture of atherosclerotic plaque in the vessel wall, starts the process of platelet plug formation. Subendothelial structures, such as collagen, then become exposed (**Figure 17-1**), which can result in platelet adhesion mediated by von Willebrand factor (vWF); platelet adhesion is enhanced by substances such as epinephrine, thrombin, adenosine diphosphate (ADP), and serotonin.[2] Circulating vWF acts as a binding ligand between the subendothelium and glycoprotein Ib receptors on the platelet surface.

Once adhesion occurs, platelets change shape and activation occurs. Activated platelets release their contents—including nucleotides, adhesive proteins, growth factors, and procoagulants—which promotes platelet aggregation and completes the formation of the hemostatic plug.[3] This process is mediated by glycoprotein IIb/IIIa receptors on the platelet surface, with fibrinogen acting as the primary binding ligand bridging between platelets. Platelets have numerous glycoprotein IIb/IIIa binding sites, which are an attractive option for antiplatelet drug therapy.[2] However, the platelet plug is not stable and can be dislodged. To form a more permanent hemostatic plug, the clotting system must be stimulated. By releasing

platelet factor (PF) 3, platelets initiate the clotting cascade and concentrate activated clotting factors at the site of vascular (endothelial) injury.

Prostaglandins (PGs) play an important role in platelet function. **Figure 17-2** displays a simplified version of the complex arachidonic acid pathways that occur in platelets and on the vascular endothelium. Thromboxane $A_2$, a potent stimulator of platelet aggregation and vasoconstriction, is formed in platelets. In contrast, prostacyclin ($PGI_2$), produced by endothelial cells lining the vessel luminal surface, is a potent inhibitor of platelet aggregation and a potent vasodilator that limits excessive platelet aggregation.

Cyclooxygenase and $PGI_2$ are clinically important. An aspirin dose of 50 to 81 mg/day acetylates and irreversibly inhibits cyclooxygenase in the platelet. Platelets are rendered incapable of converting arachidonic acid to PGs. This effect of low-dose aspirin lasts for the lifespan of the exposed platelets (8 to 12 days). Vascular endothelial cells also contain cyclooxygenase, which converts arachidonic acid to $PGI_2$. Aspirin in high doses (3,000 to 5,000 mg) inhibits the production of PG2.[4] However, because the vascular endothelium can regenerate $PGI_2$, aspirin's effect is much shorter here than on platelets. Thus, aspirin's effect at high doses may both inhibit platelet aggregation and block the aggregation inhibitor $PGI_2$. This phenomenon is the rationale for using low doses of aspirin (75 to 162 mg/day) to help prevent MI.

In summary, a complex interaction between the platelet and blood vessel wall maintains hemostasis. Once platelet adhesion occurs, the clotting cascade may become activated. After thrombin and fibrin are generated, the platelet plug becomes stabilized with insoluble fibrin at the site of vascular injury.

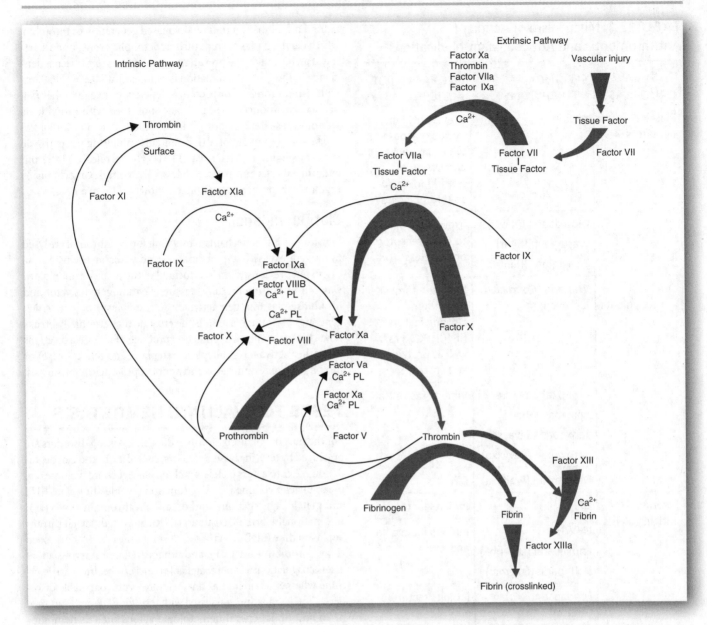

**FIGURE 17-3.** Coagulation cascade. a = activated factor; Ca = calcium; PL = phospholipid. *Source*: Adapted with permission from Davie EW, Fujikawa K, Kisiel W. The coagulation cascade; initiation, maintenance, and regulation. *Biochemistry*. 1991;30:10363–10370. Copyright © 1991. The American Chemical Society.

## Coagulation Cascade

The ultimate goal of the *coagulation cascade* (**Figure 17-3**) is to generate fibrin from thrombin. Fibrin forms an insoluble mesh surrounding the platelet plug. Platelets concentrate activated clotting factors at the site of vascular injury.

In addition to the direct effects and feedback mechanisms of thrombin shown in Figure 17-3, thrombin also stimulates platelet aggregation and activates the fibrinolytic system.

***Additional factors within the pathway.*** Factors such as calcium and vitamin K play an intricate role within the various pathways in the coagulation cascade. Calcium is essential for the platelet surface binding of several factors within the pathway. Vitamin K facilitates the calcium binding function of

factors II, VII, IX, and X via carboxylation. These processes are critical in activating proteins within the pathway.

## Inhibition of Coagulation

Mechanisms that limit *coagulation* include the natural inhibitors such as antithrombin (AT) and the vitamin K-dependent proteins C and S, tissue factor pathway inhibitor (TFPI), and the fibrinolytic system. Endothelial cells produce several substances that have antithrombotic and anticoagulant effects, which may also activate the fibrinolytic system.[2] Several medications also can inhibit coagulation by acting on (1) platelets, such as aspirin and P2Y$_{12}$ inhibitors or (2) one or more clotting factors, such as warfarin; low molecular weight heparins

**TABLE 17-1.** Mechanism of Action of Antithrombotic and Anticoagulant Medications

| DRUG CLASS | SPECIFIC MEDICATIONS | MECHANISM OF ACTION |
|---|---|---|
| Platelet inhibitors | Aspirin | Irreversibly inhibits cyclooxygenase-1, which prevents conversion of arachidonic acid to thromboxane $A_2$ |
| | Clopidogrel (Plavix) Prasugrel (Effient) Ticagrelor (Brilinta) | Irreversibly binds to $P2Y_{12}$ receptors on platelets |
| Oral anticoagulants | Warfarin (Coumadin, Jantoven) | Inhibits vitamin K-dependent clotting factors (II, VII, IX, X) as well as protein C and protein S |
| | Rivaroxaban (Xarelto) Apixaban (Eliquis) Edoxaban (Savaysa) Betrixaban (Bevyxxa) | Inhibits factor Xa |
| | Dabigatran (Pradaxa) | DTI |
| Parenteral anticoagulants | UFH | Inhibits factor IIa |
| | LMWH: Enoxaparin (Lovenox) Dalteparin (Fragmin) | Inhibits factors IIa and Xa |
| | Fondaparinux (Arixtra) | Inhibits factor Xa |
| | Bivalirudin (Angiomax) Argatroban | DTI |

(LMWHs); unfractionated heparin (UFH); direct oral anticoagulants (DOACs); fondaparinux; and direct thrombin inhibitors (DTIs). **Table 17-1** lists the mechanism of action of these classes of drugs and provides specific examples.

High concentrations of thrombin, in conjunction with thrombomodulin, activate protein C, which can then inactivate cofactors Va and VIIIa. Thus, there is a negative feedback mechanism that blocks further thrombin generation and subsequent steps in the coagulation cascade. Protein S is another of the body's natural anticoagulants and serves as a cofactor for protein C. AT inactivates thrombin as well as factors IX, X, and XI, and this process can be hastened by heparin. Heparin and AT combine one-to-one, and the complex neutralizes the activated clotting factors and inhibits the coagulation cascade. Deficiencies in these

natural inhibitors can result in increased generation of thrombin, which can lead to recurrent thromboembolic events often starting at a young age; the prevalence of protein C or protein S deficiency in the general population is estimated at <0.5%.[5,6] Patients with either protein C or protein S deficiency are at a higher risk of warfarin-induced skin necrosis compared with individuals without these deficiencies.[7-10] TFPI impedes the binding of tissue factor (TF) to factor VII, essentially inhibiting the extrinsic pathway (Figure 17-3). UFH and LMWHs can release TFPI from endothelial cells and from platelets.[2] The complex mechanisms that limit thrombus formation are shown in **Figure 17-4**.

## Clot Degradation

Fibrinolysis is the mechanism by which formed thrombi are lysed to prevent excessive clot formation and vascular occlusion. As discussed previously, fibrin is formed in the final common pathway of the clotting cascade. Tissue plasminogen activator and urokinase plasminogen activator activate plasminogen, which generates plasmin. Plasmin is the enzyme that eventually breaks down fibrin into fibrin degradation products (FDPs). Medications can either activate (eg, alteplase, reteplase, and tenecteplase) or inhibit (eg, tranexamic acid and aminocaproic acid) fibrinolysis.

## TESTS TO EVALUATE HEMOSTASIS

For the purpose of discussion, bleeding and clotting disorders are organized by tests that assess platelets, coagulation, and clot degradation. Tests to assess platelets include platelet count, volume (eg, mean platelet volume [MPV]), function (eg, bleeding time [BT] and platelet aggregation), and others. Prothrombin time (PT)/International Normalized Ratio (INR), activated partial thromboplastin time (aPTT), activated clotting time (ACT), fibrinogen assay, thrombin time (TT), and others are laboratory tests that assess coagulation; a hypercoagulable panel can be drawn to determine whether a patient has one or more hypercoagulable disorders. Clot degradation is assessed with tests for FDPs and D-dimer.

In addition, general hematologic values such as hemoglobin (Hgb), hematocrit (Hct), red blood cell (RBC) count, and white blood cell count, as well as urinalysis and stool guaiac tests may be important to obtain when evaluating blood and coagulation disorders; some of these tests are further discussed in Chapter 16. **Table 17-2** is a summary of common tests used to evaluate bleeding disorders and monitor anticoagulant therapy.

## Platelet Tests
### Platelet Count

*Normal range: 150,000 to 450,000/μL (150 to 450 × 10⁹/L)*
The only test to determine the number or concentration of platelets in a blood sample is the *platelet count*, through either manual (rarely done) or automated methods. Interferences with platelet counts include RBC fragments, platelet clumping, and platelet satellitism (platelet adherence to white blood cells). Automated platelet counts are performed on anticoagulated whole blood. Most instrumentation that performs hematologic profiles provides platelet counts. Platelets and RBCs are passed through an aperture, generating an electric pulse with a magnitude related to the size of the cell/particle. The pulses are counted, and the

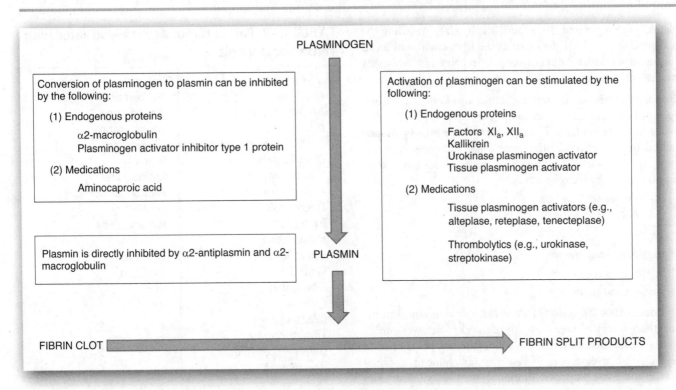

**FIGURE 17-4.** Endogenous and exogenous factors that inhibit or activate plasminogen's conversion to plasmin.

**TABLE 17-2.** Summary of Coagulation Tests for Hemorrhagic Disorders and Anticoagulant Drug Monitoring

| DISORDER OR DRUG | PLATELET COUNT | PT/INR | APTT | TT | COMMENTS |
|---|---|---|---|---|---|
| Thrombocytopenic purpura | Low | WNL | WNL | | |
| Glanzmann thrombasthenia | WNL | WNL | WNL | | Platelets appear normal |
| von Willebrand disease | Low or WNL | WNL | WNL or prolonged | | Factor VIII levels low or WNL, vWF (antigen level and activity) low or WNL |
| Fibrinogen deficiency | WNL | Prolonged | Prolonged | Prolonged | Fibrinogen levels decreased |
| Warfarin therapy | WNL | Prolonged | WNL or prolonged | | |
| Heparin therapy | WNL | WNL or prolonged | Prolonged (UFH) WNL or prolonged (LMWH) | Prolonged | Platelet count may decrease |
| DTI | WNL | WNL to prolonged | Prolonged | Prolonged | |
| Direct Xa inhibitors | WNL | WNL to prolonged | | WNL | |
| Vascular purpura | WNL | WNL | WNL | | Normal platelet count distinguishes this from other forms of purpura, such as TTP or ITP |

ITP= idiopathic thrombocytopenic purpura; TTP= thrombotic thrombocytopenic purpura; WNL= within normal limits.

platelets are separated from the RBCs by size, providing the platelet count and MPV as well as the RBC count and mean corpuscular volume. An abnormal platelet count can have many causes, which are listed in the next sections.

***Thrombocythemia.*** Thrombocythemia, also known as *thrombocytosis* or *elevated platelet count*, may be considered either primary or secondary. Primary thrombocytosis is usually caused by myeloproliferative neoplasms and other hematologic malignancies.[11] Secondary or reactive thrombocytosis may be caused by factors such as:[3,11]

- Malignancy
- Infection
- Trauma
- Iron-deficiency anemia
- Inflammation
- Postsurgical state

Values of 500,000 to 800,000/μL are not uncommon. Thrombocythemia may be seen with any of the chronic myeloproliferative neoplasms, essential thrombocythemia, polycythemia vera, chronic myelogenous leukemia, or idiopathic myelofibrosis. Clinical consequences of thrombocythemia include arterial or venous thromboses, skin and mucous membrane hemorrhages, and microcirculatory disturbances such as headaches, paresthesias, and erythromelalgia.[11] Additionally, patients with thrombocythemia may have abnormalities in platelet function studies, which can manifest as bleeding problems.

***Thrombocytopenia.*** The main causes of thrombocytopenia, or decreased platelet count, are (1) increased destruction or consumption of platelets, (2) decreased production, and (3) sequestration.[3] Mucosal and cutaneous bleeding is the most common clinical consequence of thrombocytopenia; however, patients with only modest decreases in platelet counts may be asymptomatic. When the platelet count falls below 20,000/μL, the patient is at risk for spontaneous bleeding. Platelet transfusions are often initiated when counts fall below 10,000/μL, but this number can vary based on individual patient risk factors and clinical situation.[12] Bleeding may occur at higher platelet counts (eg, 50,000/μL) if trauma occurs. The most common cause of death in a patient with severe thrombocytopenia is central nervous system bleeding, such as intracranial hemorrhage.

Numerous drugs have been associated with thrombocytopenia (**Table 17-3**).[13,14] However, heparin and antineoplastics are the most common ones implicated. Thrombocytopenia is also common with radiation therapy. Many drugs associated with thrombocytopenia alter platelet antigens, resulting in the formation of antibodies to platelets (eg, heparin, penicillin, and gold). Several diseases, such as thrombotic thrombocytopenic purpura, idiopathic thrombocytopenic purpura, disseminated intravascular coagulation (DIC), and hemolytic-uremic syndrome, result in rapid destruction of platelets. Other causes of thrombocytopenia include viral infections; pernicious, aplastic, and folate or B$_{12}$-deficiency anemias; complications of pregnancy; massive blood transfusions; exposure to dichlorodiphenyltrichloroethane; and human immunodeficiency virus infections.

Heparin-induced thrombocytopenia (HIT) is an antibody-mediated adverse reaction to heparin, occurring in 1 in 5,000

**TABLE 17-3.** Partial List of Agents Associated with Thrombocytopenia

| Anti-infective | Cardiac |
|---|---|
| Acyclovir | Abciximab |
| Amphotericin B | Amiodarone |
| Ampicillin | Atorvastatin |
| Ceftriaxone | Clopidogrel |
| Ciprofloxacin | Digoxin |
| Clarithromycin | Eptifibatide |
| Ethambutol | Hydrochlorothiazide |
| Fluconazole | LMWH |
| Isoniazid | Procainamide |
| Itraconazole | Quinidine |
| Linezolid | Simvastatin |
| Oxacillin | Tirofiban |
| Piperacillin | UFH |
| Quinine | |
| Rifampin | |
| Trimethoprim/ sulfamethoxazole | |
| Vancomycin | |
| **Antiseizure** | **Pain** |
| Carbamazepine | Acetaminophen |
| Phenobarbital | Diclofenac |
| Phenytoin | Ibuprofen |
| Valproic acid | Naproxen |
| **Psychiatric** | **Other** |
| Diazepam | Antineoplastics |
| Haloperidol | Interferon-α |
| Lithium | |
| Mirtazapine | |

*Source*: Adapted with permission from references 13 and 14.

hospitalized patients, that may cause venous and arterial thrombosis.[15] Specifically, this is due to the development of immunoglobulin G antibodies that bind to the heparin PF4 complex. Patients receiving UFH generally have 10-fold greater risk of developing HIT than patients receiving LMWH because it does not bind to PF4 as well as UFH, which is thought to be due to the smaller size of LMWH compared with UFH.[16] Therefore, the heparin-PF4 complex is less likely to form with LMWH, and there are fewer immunoglobulin G antibodies generated. The frequency or risk of HIT is influenced by certain factors, such as heparin preparation, route, dose, and duration of heparin therapy, patient population, gender, previous history of heparin exposure, and the animal source of heparin (bovine versus porcine).[17]

The 4Ts score is a clinical prediction tool to determine the probability of HIT. This tool requires the clinician to evaluate the degree of thrombocytopenia, timing of platelet count fall, presence of thrombosis or other clinical sequelae, and other causes for thrombocytopenia; a score of 0 to 2 is assigned for each of the four items based on specific patient characteristics to determine the probability of HIT occurring in that particular patient. Thus, the score range is 0 to 8. A score of 0 to 3, 4 to 5, or 6 to 8 suggests

**TABLE 17-4.** Incidence of HIT According to Patient Characteristics and Recommendations for Monitoring Platelets

| RISK OF DEVELOPING HIT | | >1% | 0.1% TO 1% | <0.1% |
|---|---|---|---|---|
| Patient characteristics/ examples | CHEST | Postoperative patients on prophylactic dose or therapeutic dose UFH ≥4 days<br><br>Cardiac surgery patients | Medical patients on prophylactic or therapeutic-dose UFH or LMWH ≥4 days<br><br>Postoperative patients on prophylactic or therapeutic dose LMWH ≥4 days<br><br>Patients receiving UFH flushes<br><br>Obstetrics patients<br><br>Intensive care patients | N/A |
| | ASH | Surgical and trauma patients receiving UFH | Medical and obstetrical patients receiving UFH<br><br>Patients receiving LMWH after major surgery or major trauma | Medical and obstetrical patients receiving LMWH<br><br>Patients receiving LMWH after minor surgery or trauma<br><br>Patients receiving fondaparinux |
| Frequency of platelet counts | CHEST | Every 2–3 days from days 4–14, or until heparin is discontinued, whichever occurs first | Routine monitoring is not recommended | Routine monitoring is not recommended |
| | ASH | If patient has received heparin in the last 30 days prior to current regimen, begin monitoring on day 0, when heparin is initiated<br><br>If patient has not received heparin in the last 30 days prior to current regimen, monitor at least every other day from days 4–14, or until heparin is discontinued, whichever occurs first | If patient has received heparin in the last 30 days prior to current regimen, begin monitoring on day 0, when heparin is initiated<br><br>If patient has not received heparin in the last 30 days prior to current regimen, monitor every 2–3 days from days 4–14, or until heparin is discontinued, whichever occurs first | |

ASH = American Society of Hematology
*Source*: Adapted with permission references 20 and 21.

a low, moderate, or high probability of HIT, respectively.[18] HIT is manifested both by clinical and serological features, and diagnosis of HIT is usually made when antibody formation is detected by an in vitro assay plus one or more of the following: unexplained decrease in platelet count, venous or arterial thrombosis, limb gangrene, necrotizing skin lesions at the heparin injection site, acute anaphylactoid reactions occurring after intravenous (IV) heparin bolus administration, and/or bleeding.[17,19]

There are two types of tests to help diagnose HIT: (1) the enzyme-linked immunosorbent assay (ELISA), which identifies anti-PF4/heparin antibodies, and (2) functional assays, such as the C-serotonin release assay or the heparin-induced platelet activation assay—both of which detect antibodies that induce heparin-dependent platelet activation.[15,20] The ELISA test has

high sensitivity, low specificity, and wide availability, with a relatively rapid turnaround time compared with the functional assays, which makes it a good screening test.[18] By contrast, the functional assays have high specificity, which are useful for confirming a positive ELISA test but are technically difficult, have a higher cost, and have longer turnaround time.[18]

The typical onset for HIT is 5 to 10 days after the start of heparin; however, onsets occurring either earlier or later than this have been reported. Rapid-onset HIT occurs when platelet counts fall within 24 hours of heparin initiation, which is typically the result of repeated heparin exposure within the past 100 days, and thus patients still have circulating HIT antibodies. Delayed-onset HIT, in which thrombocytopenia occurs several days after discontinuation of heparin, can also occur. **Table 17-4** outlines the patient

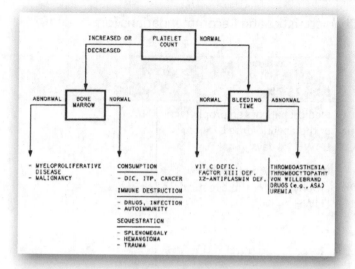

**FIGURE 17-5.** Assessment of abnormalities of homeostasis based on platelet count, bone marrow exam, and BT.

characteristics associated with the risk of developing HIT as well as recommendations for monitoring platelet counts.[20,21]

### Mean Platelet Volume

*Normal range: 7 to 11 fL (varies with laboratory)*
*Mean platelet volume* (MPV)—the relationship between platelet size and count—is most likely used by clinicians in assessing disturbances of platelet production. MPV is useful in distinguishing between hypoproductive and hyperdestructive causes of thrombocytopenia (**Figure 17-5**). Despite the widespread availability of this platelet index, many clinicians do not use it in clinical decision-making. In the past, this disuse was attributed to difficulties with the laboratory measurement of indices.

Many laboratories routinely report the MPV as part of the complete blood count, especially if a differential is requested. In general, lower platelet counts are common with higher platelet volumes because an inverse relationship exists between the platelet count and the MPV. This inverse relationship correlates with platelet production within the bone marrow. Although MPV is most valuable in distinguishing hypoproductive from hyperdestructive causes of thrombocytopenia, a definitive diagnosis cannot be made based on MPV alone. In thrombocytopenia, an elevated MPV suggests no problem with platelet production, when in fact, production is reflexively increased. Conversely, a normal or low MPV suggests impaired thrombopoiesis. Determination of MPV requires a blood collection tube containing an anticoagulant. Usually, such tubes contain the anticoagulant ethylenediamine tetraacetic acid (EDTA), which causes an inflation of the MPV.[22] **Table 17-5** lists conditions that affect the MPV.[23,24]

### Platelet Function

Simply stated, the *platelet function* tests look at the ability of platelets to aggregate and form a clot. Abnormalities of platelet function may be either inherited or acquired and can be caused by medications, the platelet milieu, and inherent platelet defects; platelet counts are usually normal.[25] Bleeding as a result of an inherited versus acquired

**TABLE 17-5.** Conditions Associated with Alterations in MPV

| INCREASE IN MPV | DECREASE IN MPV |
|---|---|
| Diabetes mellitus | Ulcerative colitis |
| Hypertension | HIV infection |
| Familial hyperlipidemia | Hypersplenism |
| Nonalcoholic fatty liver disease | Aplastic anemia |
| MI | Rheumatoid arthritis |
| Unstable angina | Systemic lupus erythematosus |
| Decompensated heart failure | Ankylosing spondylitis |
| Ischemic stroke | |
| VTE | |
| Preeclampsia | |
| Rheumatoid arthritis | |
| Ankylosing spondylitis | |
| Psoriasis | |
| Pulmonary arterial hypertension | |
| Thyroid disorders | |
| Chronic obstructive pulmonary disease | |
| Obstructive sleep apnea | |
| Renal failure | |
| Sepsis | |
| Erythropoietin | |

HIV = human immunodeficiency virus.
*Source*: Adapted with permission from references 23 and 24.

abnormality may be difficult to prove. Common bleeding sites in patients with disorders of platelet function include ecchymosis of the skin, epistaxis, gingival bleeding, and menorrhagia; gastrointestinal (GI) hemorrhage and hematuria are less common and usually have an associated underlying pathology.

Although the sites of bleeding may be predictable, the severity is not predictable in patients with inherited disorders of platelet function. Unfortunately, the risk of bleeding and bleeding patterns in patients with acquired platelet dysfunction are less predictable and more difficult to distinguish. Because both inherited and acquired etiologies increase the risk of bleeding, patients overtly bleeding without a clear cause or without an invasive procedure should be evaluated for one of these platelet function disorders.

## Bleeding Time

*Normal range: 2 to 9 minutes*

Bleeding time (BT) is a measure of platelet function and has been used to assess bleeding risk, but this test is neither specific nor sensitive; thus, it does not help differentiate among the types of problems seen in disorders of primary hemostasis, such as von Willebrand disease and platelet function defects. Because BT is neither specific nor sensitive, its use has been declining, and some institutional clinical laboratories no longer perform this test. Additionally, the test is invasive and must be performed by a trained healthcare worker. To perform the test, small cuts are made on the forearm of the patient, and the time it takes to stop bleeding is measured. Several factors can prolong the BT, including thrombocytopenia, certain medications, and conditions such as uremia and macroglobulinemia. Most acquired disorders affecting BT are related to medications that decrease platelet numbers or reduce platelet function, including aspirin, P2Y$_{12}$ inhibitors (clopidogrel, prasugrel, ticagrelor), GPIIb/IIIa inhibitors (abciximab, eptifibatide, tirofiban), and phosphodiesterase inhibitors (dipyridamole). Although BT is influenced by some drugs, it is not used to monitor drug therapy. The increase in BT caused by aspirin may have beneficial effects in the treatment and prevention of cardiovascular disease.

**Platelet aggregation.** With the many drawbacks of the BT, there was a need for a test that could aid in the diagnosis of defects in platelet function. The ability of platelets to aggregate is most commonly measured by preparing a specimen of platelet-rich plasma and warming it to 98.6°F (37°C) with constant stirring. This test is performed with an aggregometer that measures light transmission through a sample of platelets in suspension. After a baseline reading is obtained, a platelet-aggregating agonist (eg, epinephrine, collagen, ADP, or arachidonic acid) is added. As platelets aggregate, more light passes through the sample. The change in optical density can be measured photometrically and recorded as an aggregation curve, which is then printed on a plotter. Although light transmittance aggregometry (LTA) testing is the gold standard in platelet function analysis, it has requirements for specially trained personnel, large sample volume, and sample preparation, and it is costly.[22]

Interpretation of platelet aggregation tests involves a comparison of the patient's curves with the corresponding curves of a normal control. To eliminate the optical problems of turbidity with lipemic plasma, the patient and the normal control should be fasting. Patients should not take medications that affect platelet aggregation (eg, aspirin, nonsteroidal anti-inflammatory drugs, P2Y$_{12}$ inhibitors) for approximately 7 to 14 days before the test because they may interfere with test results. Other drugs that may affect platelet function are listed in **Table 17-6**.[26]

Novel point-of-care (POC) technologies are available and allow for rapid and meaningful evaluation of platelet function, although major differences between devices do exist. These devices can assess the effects of medications such as aspirin, P2Y$_{12}$ inhibitors, and GP IIb/IIIa antagonists on platelet function and help predict the incidence of major adverse cardiac events in patients treated with medications affecting platelet function.[27] Further studies of each individual device are needed to elucidate

**TABLE 17-6.** Medications and Drug Classes That May Cause Abnormalities of Platelet Function

| | |
|---|---|
| Angiotensin-Converting Enzyme Inhibitors | Nitroglycerin |
| Aspirin | NSAIDs |
| β-blocking agents | Omega fatty acids |
| Calcium channel blockers | Penicillins |
| Cephalosporins | Phenothiazines |
| Chemotherapeutic agents | P2Y$_{12}$ inhibitors |
| Ethanol | SSRIs |
| Heparin | Statins |
| Nitrofurantoin | Tricyclic antidepressants |

NSAIDs = nonsteroidal anti-inflammatory drugs; SSRIs = selective serotonin reuptake inhibitors.
*Source:* Adapted with permission from reference 26.

the exact place in therapy of these in monitoring antiplatelet medications.

### Other Platelet Tests

The measurement of platelet-specific substances, such as PF4 (normal values 1.7 to 20.9 ng/mL) and β-thromboglobulin (normal levels 6.6 to 47.9 ng/mL), can now be performed by radioimmunoassay or enzyme immunoassay.[28] High concentrations of these substances may be observed with coronary artery disease, acute MI, and thrombosis, in which platelet lifespan is reduced. Because numerous drugs can potentially cause thrombocytopenia, detection of antibodies directed by specific drugs against platelets may help to determine the culprit. Platelet survival can be measured by injecting radioisotopes that label the platelets. Serial samples can then determine platelet survival, which is normally 8 to 12 days.

**Pharmacogenomics and clopidogrel metabolism.** Genetic variability in the genes coding for CYP2C19 may have an effect on clopidogrel efficacy and safety; this concept is covered in more detail in Chapter 6. There are commercially available assays to test for these variants in CYP2C19.[29,30] Guidelines do not recommend routine platelet function testing or genetic testing in all patients taking clopidogrel; instead, they recognize a possible role for testing patients who undergo high-risk percutaneous coronary intervention (PCI) procedures, such as those involving bifurcating left main artery.[31-33]

## COAGULATION TESTS

*Coagulation tests* are useful in the identification of deficiencies of coagulation factors responsible for bleeding as well as thrombotic disorders. The most commonly performed tests, including PT, INR, aPTT, and ACT, are used to monitor anticoagulant therapy. Numerous high-precision automated laboratory methods are available to perform these tests. However, an overall lack of standardization across coagulation testing can lead to considerable variation in test results and their interpretation. Normal and therapeutic ranges established for one test method are not necessarily interchangeable with other methods, especially when differences in endpoint detection or reagents exist. Therefore, it is important to interpret test results based on the specific performance characteristics of the method used to analyze samples.

Coagulation studies may be used to assess certain bleeding disorders, such as hemophilia A (factor VIII deficiency) or hemophilia B (factor IX deficiency). These deficiencies, which are inherited, sex-linked recessive traits, primarily affect males and cause >90% of hemophilia cases. Other bleeding disorders include von Willebrand disease—the most common hereditary bleeding disorder—and deficiencies in fibrinogen or factors II, V, VII, X, XI, XIII, and a combination of these factors.

Patients with thrombotic disorders may have their hypercoagulability evaluated with specific assays for the following conditions[5,6]:

- Antiphospholipid antibody syndrome (APS)—lupus anticoagulant, anticardiolipin antibody
- AT
- Protein C
- Protein S
- Prothrombin G20210A mutation
- Activated protein C (APC) resistance mutation (factor V Leiden)
- Homocysteine polymorphisms

These tests are often performed in panels because the presence of more than one predisposition to thrombosis further increases the risk for thrombosis. Normal reference ranges for AT and proteins C and S are often reported as a percent of normal activity, with 100% being the mean normal value. For AT, the normal activity level is 80% to 130%; for both proteins C and S, normal activity levels are 70% to 140%. Deficiencies can result in frequent, recurrent thromboembolic events in patients with these disorders. Because these deficiencies are rare, their respective assays are not discussed here in detail. The use for thrombophilia testing is controversial with no clear guidelines on which patients should be tested.[5,6,34] Negative results may falsely reassure patients and/or clinicians that the risk of recurrent venous thromboembolism (VTE) is low, leading to discontinuation of anticoagulants, which may put the patient at risk for thrombosis; positive results may lead to continued anticoagulation due to overestimation of the risk of recurrent VTE with the specific thrombophilia, which can put the patient at risk for bleeding.[34] Acquired, transient deficiencies of any of these inhibitors may be observed during thrombotic states. Therefore, these parameters should not be assessed during the acute phase of thrombosis or while the patient is currently on anticoagulant therapy because a false-positive result may occur. It is recommended to test for AT, protein C, protein S, and APC resistance after the thrombosis has been resolved when the patient is off heparin or

warfarin for a few weeks or off DOACs for at least five half-lives[6]; the test for prothrombin G20210A mutation and factor V Leiden is not affected by current anticoagulant therapy[6] (**Minicase 1**). The results of thrombophilia testing should be used along with other risk factors for recurrent VTE to help determine whether a patient should continue anticoagulants.

## MINICASE 1

### Risk of Recurrent Venous Thromboembolism

Juan R., a 55-year-old man, presents to the anticoagulation clinic to discuss the possible continued need for anticoagulation. He recently completed 3 months of warfarin therapy for a first event deep vein thrombosis. He reports that he has started a new job that does not allow him to readily come in for INR appointments, so he is asking about converting to a DOAC if he needs to stay on anticoagulant medication. He weighs 85 kg and is 72″ tall with reduced renal function. Laboratory results 4 weeks after stopping warfarin are as follows:

| LABORATORY RESULTS | NORMAL RESULTS | PATIENT RESULTS |
|---|---|---|
| PT | 10–13 sec | 11.6 sec |
| INR | 0.9–1.1 | 0.9 |
| Estimated glomerular filtration rate | >60 mL/min | 42 mL/min |
| D-dimer | <0.5 mcg/mL | 1.3 mcg/mL |

QUESTION: How should his lab results be interpreted for his risk of recurrent VTE? Should any additional lab work be performed? What are his options for future anticoagulation if needed?

DISCUSSION: The D-dimer is elevated, which means the patient is at higher risk of recurrent VTE and an extended duration of anticoagulation can be considered. The patient and clinician may elect to do a hypercoagulable panel to see if he has any of the conditions for thrombophilia. Because he has been off warfarin for 4 weeks, there is less likelihood of a false-positive result for tests such as protein C deficiency, protein S deficiency, AT, or APC resistance. This patient can be started on a DOAC or warfarin if extended duration of anticoagulation is selected. The patient would need to be counseled on the benefits and drawbacks of DOACs, including fewer dietary issues, fewer drug interactions, higher cost, and need for adherence to therapy due to short half-lives of these agents. If he decides to stay with warfarin, he may be able to do patient self-monitoring or PST after the anticoagulation clinic assesses his ability to perform such care.

**TABLE 17-7.** Summary of Interpreting Laboratory Tests with DOACs

| | TESTS THAT MAY BE USED FOR QUALITATIVE ASSESSMENT OF DOACs | TESTS THAT MAY BE USED FOR QUANTITATIVE ASSESSMENT OF DOACs | TESTS NOT RECOMMENDED |
|---|---|---|---|
| DTIs (dabigatran) | aPTT: normal to prolonged<br>TT: prolonged | ECT<br>dTT | PT: normal to prolonged<br>Anti-Xa: no effect |
| Factor Xa inhibitors (apixaban, edoxaban, rivaroxaban, betrixaban) | PT: normal to prolonged (recommended for rivaroxaban only)<br>Anti-Xa (if not calibrated to a specific DOAC or if calibrated to UFH or LMWH) | Anti-Xa (only if calibrated to a specific DOAC) | aPTT: normal to prolonged<br>TT: no effect<br>ECT: no effect<br>dTT: no effect |

*Source*: Adapted with permission from references 35 and 39.

Activated protein C resistance due to the factor V Leiden mutation is the most prevalent hereditary predisposition to venous thrombosis. It is present in approximately 5% of the general white population and is less common or rare in other ethnic groups.[6] Prothrombin G20210A mutation is the second most common hereditary predisposition to venous thrombosis. DNA-based methods, such as polymerase chain reaction–based assay, are used to determine the presence or absence of a specific mutation at nucleoside position 20210 in the prothrombin gene. A normal test result would show absence of the G20210A mutation.

Although routine laboratory monitoring is not indicated with DOACs, there are some clinical instances when laboratory assessment could be considered, including a thrombotic or hemorrhagic event, perioperative management, suspicion of overdosage/toxicity, renal/hepatic dysfunction, extremes of body weight, trauma, questionable adherence to therapy, concomitant administration with significant drug interactions, advanced age, and after attempted reversal of anticoagulation.[35] Although therapeutic concentrations of the actual drug associated with optimal outcomes have not been established for the DOACs, certain coagulation tests are better suited to assess qualitative (presence or absence of drug) versus quantitative (estimates of drug levels) information for specific DOACs, which are discussed in detail later and summarized in **Table 17-7**.

Careful attention to blood collection technique, sample processing, and laboratory quality control is critical for reliable coagulation test results. Blood is collected in syringes or vacuum tubes that contain heparin, EDTA, or sodium citrate. Because heparin and EDTA interfere with several clotting factors, only sodium citrate is used for coagulation and platelet tests. Errors in coagulation can be significant unless quality assurance is strict concerning specimen collection, reagents, controls, and equipment. Factors that promote clotting and interfere with coagulation studies are as follows:

- Tissue trauma (searching for a vein)
- Prolonged use of tourniquet
- Small-bore needles
- Vacuum tubes
- Heparin contamination from indwelling catheters
- Slow blood filling into collection tube

***Bleeding risk and test results.*** The major determinants of bleeding are the intensity of the anticoagulant effect, the underlying patient characteristics, the use of drugs that interfere with hemostasis (Tables 17-3, 17-6, and 17-8), and the length of anticoagulant therapy. When evaluating anticoagulation treatment, one must weigh the potential for decreased thrombosis risk versus increased bleeding risk. Serious bleeding can occur in patients prone to bleeding, even when the anticoagulant response is in the therapeutic range. The risk of bleeding is usually higher earlier in therapy (eg, when both heparin and warfarin are given together, which may be related to excessive anticoagulation). Also, patients who have a coexisting disease that elevates PT, aPTT, or both (eg, liver disease) are often at much higher risk of bleeding. In these patients, the use and intensity of anticoagulation that should be employed are controversial. Patient on oral anticoagulants who experience GI bleeding are more likely to receive a diagnosis of GI cancer.[36,37] Thus, patients on anticoagulation medication who have GI bleeding should undergo further evaluation to assess possibility of a GI malignancy. More information about these types of tests can be found in Chapter 15.

### Prothrombin Time/International Normalized Ratio

*Normal range for PT: 10 to 13 seconds but varies based on reagent-instrument combinations; normal range for INR: 0.8 to 1.1; therapeutic range for INR depends on indication for anticoagulation; most indications: 2 to 3*

The *prothrombin time* (PT), also called *ProTime*, test is used to assess the integrity of the extrinsic and common pathways (factors II, V, VII, X). Deficiencies or inhibitors of extrinsic and common pathway clotting factors results in a prolonged PT; however, it should be noted that the PT is more sensitive to deficiencies in the extrinsic pathway (factor VII) compared with the common pathway (factors V, X, II, and fibrinogen).[38]

***Assay performance characteristics, standardization, and reporting.*** The PT is dependent on the thromboplastin source and test method used to detect clotting. Thromboplastin reagents are derived from animal or human sources and include recombinant products. Factor sensitivity is highly dependent on the source of the thromboplastin and can exhibit variability between different lots of the same reagent. Some thromboplastin reagents are less sensitive to changes in factor activity. This means that it takes a more significant decrease in factor activity to produce a prolongation of the PT. Differences in reagent sensitivity, combined with the influence of endpoint detection, affect clotting time results both in the normal and therapeutic ranges. Large differences in factor sensitivity between comparative methods can result in conflicting interpretation of results, both in the assessment of factor deficiencies and adequacy of anticoagulation therapy. Heparin also may prolong PT because it affects factor II in the common pathway; the addition of a heparin neutralizing agent to the blood sample can blunt this effect at heparin concentrations up to 2 units/mL.[38] However, at higher concentrations of heparin—whether due to higher doses of heparin or sample collection issues—the neutralizing agent may not be enough, and the PT may be prolonged. These "crossover" effects may have to be considered when oral and parenteral anticoagulants are given concomitantly for several days to avoid premature discontinuation of the parenteral agent. The PT is not as sensitive as the aPTT for dabigatran; PT levels may be normal or prolonged while a patient is on dabigatran, so this is not a useful test for monitoring or measuring dabigatran levels. In terms of the oral factor Xa inhibitors, the PT is more sensitive to rivaroxaban compared with apixaban or edoxaban; therapeutic doses of rivaroxaban can result in a normal or prolonged PT level.[35] The PT is not sensitive enough for assessing apixaban or edoxaban therapy.[35]

Because PT results can vary widely depending on the thromboplastin source, the INR is the standardized reporting method for monitoring warfarin therapy. The INR is calculated according to the following equation:

$$INR = (\text{patient PT/mean normal PT})^{ISI}$$

where the *International Sensitivity Index* (ISI) expresses the sensitivity of the thromboplastin reagent compared with the World Health Organization reference standard. The more sensitive or responsive the reagent, the lower the ISI. Theoretically, an INR result from one laboratory should be comparable to an INR result from a different laboratory although the PTs may be different. The INR should not be used as a test for DOAC monitoring because the ISI is specific for vitamin K antagonists.[35,39]

Although the INR system has greatly improved the standardization of the PT, one can still expect differences in INRs reported with two different methods, particularly in the upper therapeutic and supratherapeutic ranges. The greater the differences in the ISI values for two comparative methods, the more likely differences will be noted in the INR. Laboratories and anticoagulation clinics should review the performance characteristics of the PT method used to evaluate their specific patient populations and report changes in methods to healthcare professionals, particularly those monitoring anticoagulant therapy.

***Monitoring warfarin therapy.*** Both the PT and INR may be reported when monitoring warfarin therapy, although clinically only the INR is used to adjust therapy. Warfarin exerts its anticoagulant effects by interfering with the synthesis of vitamin K-dependent clotting factors (II, VII, IX, and X) and the natural anticoagulant proteins C, S, and Z. Specifically, warfarin inhibits vitamin K-reductase and vitamin K epoxide reductase (VKOR), which blocks the activation of vitamin K to its reduced form. Reduced vitamin K is needed for the carboxylation of clotting precursors of factors II, VII, IX, and X. Noncarboxylated clotting factor precursors are nonfunctional, and thus an anticoagulated state is achieved.[40] Warfarin is manufactured as a racemic mixture of (*S*)- and (*R*)-enantiomers; the *S*-enantiomer is more potent than the *R*-enantiomer at inhibiting VKOR, which is why the *S*-enantiomer is responsible for most of the anticoagulant effects of warfarin. The *S*-enantiomer is metabolized largely by CYP2C9, whereas the *R*-enantiomer is metabolized mostly by CYP1A2, and CYP3A4; other CYP enzymes also are involved in the metabolism of warfarin although to a lesser extent.

Current guidelines from various organizations recommend an INR of 2 to 3 for most indications.[41-43] A higher INR of 2.5 to 3.5 is recommended for, but not limited to, patients with mechanical prosthetic heart valves in the mitral position and patients with recurrent thromboembolic events.[44-46] Results below the therapeutic range indicate that the patient is at increased risk for clotting, and warfarin doses may need to be increased. Results above the therapeutic range indicate the patient is at risk for bleeding and warfarin doses may need to be decreased. Numerous drugs, disease states, and other factors prolong or shorten the INR in patients receiving warfarin by various mechanisms of action (**Table 17-8**).

***Pharmacogenomics and oral anticoagulant therapy.*** Genetic variability in the genes coding for CYP2C9, VKOR complex subunit 1 (VKORC1), and CYP4F2 can influence warfarin dosing by altering its pharmacokinetics and pharmacodynamics.[47,48] CYP2C9 and VKORC1 have a larger influence compared with CYP4F2. More information regarding CYP2C9 and VKORC1 can be found in Chapter 6. The CYP4F2 enzyme normally plays a role in the conversion of vitamin K to vitamin $KH_2$, which is needed to carboxylate the clotting factor precursors; patients with the CYP4F2*3 variant may need higher warfarin dose requirements compared with noncarriers.[48]

U.S. Food and Drug Administration–approved warfarin pharmacogenomics testing devices are available, including one that is marketed as direct-to-consumer; each one tests for the CYP2C9*2 and CYP2C9*3 variants, and some may test for the VKORC1 variants.[29,30] Genetic testing, if used, should be used along with patient characteristics, clinical considerations, and continued INR monitoring for optimal outcomes associated with warfarin use.

Although genetic variants have not been well studied regarding the DOACs, some potential genes may influence a patient's response to these medications. Single nucleotide polymorphisms

**TABLE 17-8.** Select Factors Altering Pharmacokinetics and Pharmacodynamics of Warfarin

| ANTICOAGULANT EFFECT POTENTIATED | ANTICOAGULANT EFFECT COUNTERACTED |
|---|---|
| Low vitamin K intake | Increased vitamin K intake |
| Reduced vitamin K absorption in fat malabsorption | |
| Drug interactions | Drug interactions |
| Aminoglycosides | Barbiturates |
| Amiodarone | Carbamazepine |
| Azole antifungals | Cholestyramine |
| Cephalosporins | Colestipol |
| Fluoroquinolone antibiotics | Methimazole |
| Macrolide antibiotics | Nafcillin |
| Metronidazole | Propylthiouracil |
| Sulfa antibiotics | Rifampin |
| Tetracyclines | |
| Thyroid hormones | |
| Heart failure exacerbation | |
| Hepatic disease | |
| Pyrexia | |
| Alcohol (acute consumption or binge drinking) | Alcohol (chronic consumption) |

*Source:* Adapted with permission from reference 39.

on the CESI and ABCB1 genes can affect peak and trough levels for dabigatran, which may be associated with rates of bleeding.[49] Genetic variations in ABCB1 and CYP3A4 may alter drug levels of rivaroxaban, whereas ABCB1 and SULTA1A may alter drug levels of apixaban.[49] Edoxaban was shown to have little interpatient variability due to genetic variations in the factor X, ABCB1, CYP2C9, and VKORC1 genes.[49] Further studies are needed to elucidate potential genetic influences in the dosing of DOACs and associated clinical outcomes.

### Activated Partial Thromboplastin Time

*Normal range: varies by manufacturer, generally between 25 and 35 sec; therapeutic range for heparin-treated patients is 1.5 to 2.5 times control aPTT*

The *activated partial thromboplastin time* (aPTT) is used to screen for deficiencies and inhibitors of the intrinsic pathway

(factors VIII, IX, XI, and XII) as well as factors in the final common pathway (factors II, V, and X). The aPTT also is commonly used as a surrogate assay to monitor UFH and DTIs. The aPTT, reported as a clotting time in seconds, is determined by adding an aPTT reagent, containing phospholipids and activators, and calcium to the patient's blood sample.

Factor and heparin sensitivity as well as the precision of the aPTT test depend both on the reagents and instrumentation. In addition, some aPTT reagents are formulated for increased sensitivity to lupus anticoagulants. Despite numerous attempts to standardize the aPTT, little progress has been made. The difficulty in part may reflect differences in opinion as to the appropriate heparin sensitivity, the need to have lupus anticoagulant sensitivity for targeted patient populations, and suitable factor sensitivity to identify deficiencies associated with increased bleeding risk. Normal and therapeutic ranges must be established for each reagent instrument combination, and ranges should be verified with changes in a lot of the same reagent. Laboratory errors may cause either prolongation or shortening of the aPTT; these may include an inappropriate amount and concentration of anticoagulant in the collection tube, time between collection of the blood specimen and performance of the assay, inappropriate collection site (ie, through a venous catheter, which contains heparin), and inappropriate timing of blood collection.[50]

***Causes of aPTT prolongation.*** In addition to reagent specific issues impacting aPTT responsiveness, hereditary diseases or other acquired causes may prolong aPTT test results. Causes of aPTT prolongation include the following[2,51]:

Hereditary causes

1. Deficiency of factor VIII, IX, XI, XII, prekallikrein, or high-molecular weight kininogen (PT is normal)
2. Deficiency of fibrinogen or factor II, V, or X (PT also is prolonged)

Acquired causes

1. Lupus anticoagulant (PT usually normal)
2. Heparin (PT less affected than aPTT; PT may be normal)
3. Bivalirudin, or argatroban (PT usually also prolonged)
4. Dabigatran (less accurate at higher dabigatran concentrations)
5. Liver dysfunction (PT affected earlier and more than aPTT)
6. Vitamin K deficiency (PT affected earlier and more than aPTT)
7. Warfarin (PT affected earlier and more than aPTT)
8. DIC (PT affected earlier and more than aPTT)
9. Specific factor inhibitors (PT normal except in the rare case of an inhibitor against fibrinogen, factor II, V, or X)

***Use of aPTT to monitor heparin.*** Although used to detect clotting factor deficiencies, the aPTT is used primarily for monitoring therapeutic heparin therapy and may be used to qualitatively monitor dabigatran therapy. The generally accepted therapeutic range of heparin is an aPTT ratio of 1.5 to 2.5 times the control value.[40] Given the interpatient and intrapatient variability that can result from aPTT reagents, alternative means of monitoring heparin therapy are being scrutinized. This 1.5 to 2.5 aPTT ratio corresponds to the following concentrations[39]:

- A plasma heparin concentration of 0.2 to 0.4 units/mL by assay using the protamine titration method
- A plasma heparin concentration of 0.3 to 0.7 units/mL by assay using the inhibition of factor Xa

Unfractionated heparin should be given by continuous IV infusion or subcutaneous injection, with exact dosing dependent on the indication. The aPTT should be drawn at baseline, 6 hours after continuous IV heparin is begun, and 6 hours after each subsequent dosage adjustment because this interval approximates the time to achieve steady-state levels of heparin. Institutions may have their own specific heparin dosing nomogram or base their nomogram on one used in clinical studies; using a nomogram also allows quick fine-tuning of anticoagulation by nurses without continuous physician input.

Activated partial thromboplastin time determinations obtained earlier than 6 hours, when a steady-state concentration of heparin has not been achieved, may be combined with heparin concentrations for dosage individualization using non–steady-state concentrations. This approach has been demonstrated to reduce the incidence of subtherapeutic aPTT ratios significantly during the first 24 hours of therapy.[52,53] This finding is important because the recurrence rate of thromboembolic disease increased when aPTT values were not maintained >1.5 times patient baseline aPTT during the first 24 hours of treatment.[54,55]

Heparin concentration measurements may provide a target plasma therapeutic range, especially in unusual coagulation situations such as pregnancy, in which the reliability of clotting studies is questionable. In this setting, shorter-than-expected aPTT results in relation to heparin concentration measurements may be indicative of increased circulating levels of factor VIII and increased fibrinogen levels.[56] Patients may have therapeutic heparin concentrations measured by whole blood protamine sulfate titration or by the plasma anti-Xa heparin assay. However, they may have aPTTs not significantly prolonged above baseline. This difference has been referred to as a dissociation between the aPTT and the heparin concentration.[57] Many of these patients have short pretreatment aPTT values.

Current recommendations for patients with decreased aPTT results on heparin are that such patients be managed by monitoring heparin concentrations using a heparin assay to avoid unnecessary dosage escalation without compromising efficacy. These patients, referred to as *pseudoheparin resistant*, may be identified as having a poor aPTT response (to an adequate heparin concentration >0.3 units/mL via plasma anti-Xa assay) despite high doses of heparin (>50,000 units/24 hours; usual dose is 20,000 to 30,000 units/24 hours). When higher doses of heparin (>1,500 units/hour) are required to maintain therapeutic aPTT values, high concentrations of heparin-binding protein or phase reactant proteins bind and neutralize heparin. Additionally, thrombocytosis, or AT deficiency, may exist.

Another use for the aPTT is to demonstrate both efficacy and safety with LMWH, which have several indications. However, clinically, the anti-Xa levels are more routinely used for this class of medications. LMWH has a pharmacokinetic and pharmaco-dynamic profile, which makes routine monitoring unnecessary

in most circumstances. Exceptions include special populations, such as those patients with renal failure or severe obesity who are at risk for being overdosed when weight-adjusted regimens are used. Both PT and aPTT times are not significantly prolonged at recommended doses of LMWHs. However, both efficacy and safety can be demonstrated by assaying anti-Xa levels.

*Decreased aPTT levels.* Although most attention has been focused on causes of prolonged aPTT levels, there is growing evidence of adverse events associated with decreased aPTT levels, including VTE, myocardial infarction (MI), hyperthyroidism, diabetes, spontaneous abortion, and death.[58] Clotting factors of the intrinsic pathway, as well as vWF levels and activity, have been elevated in some patients presenting with decreased aPTT levels, which provides some evidence that patients with decreased aPTT levels are hypercoagulable.[59] There is no definitive answer whether a shortened aPTT is a cause, a consequence, or just an association with these other conditions. To rule out whether a shortened aPTT is due to a laboratory error, such as inappropriate specimen collection, repeat testing should be performed.

Heparin alone has minimal anticoagulant effects; when it is combined with AT (normal range: 80% to 120%), the inhibitory action of AT on coagulation enzymes is magnified 1,000-fold, resulting in the inhibition of thrombus propagation. Patients who are AT deficient (<50%) may be difficult to anticoagulate, as seen with DIC (**Minicase 2**). The DIC syndrome is associated not only with obvious hemorrhage but also occult diffuse thrombosis.

*Oral anticoagulant effect on aPTT.* Although warfarin mildly elevates aPTT, aPTT is not used to monitor warfarin therapy. Therefore, if warfarin is started in a patient receiving heparin, the clinician should expect some elevation in aPTT. The aPTT provides qualitative information on dabigatran but not quantitative information; clinicians should note that a normal aPTT does not mean there is no clinically important dabigatran activity occurring in a patient.[40] The aPTT is even less sensitive than PT for the oral factor Xa inhibitors and thus cannot be recommended for either qualitative or quantitative assessment for these agents.[35,60]

## Activated Clotting Time

*Normal range: 70 to 180 seconds but varies*
Activated clotting time (ACT), also known as *activated coagulation time*, is frequently used to monitor heparin or DTIs when high doses are required, such as during invasive procedures like cardiopulmonary bypass graft surgery, percutaneous transluminal coronary angioplasty, PCI extracorporeal membrane oxygenation, valve replacements, and carotid endarterectomy. In most cases, an ACT is obtained from a POC machine using whole blood; thus, it may be run directly in the operating room as well as at the bedside when rapid heparinization is required (eg, hemodialysis unit, operating room, and cardiac catheterization laboratories).

Activated clotting time responsiveness remains linear in proportion to an increasing dose of heparin, whereas the aPTT has a log-linear relationship to heparin concentration. Corresponding ACT values up to 400 seconds demonstrate this dose-response relationship, but ACT lacks reproducibility for values in excess

## MINICASE 2

### A Case of Disseminated Intravascular Coagulation

Teresa G., a 36-year-old woman in her third trimester of pregnancy, is hospitalized with clinical suspicion of DIC because of acute onset of respiratory failure, circulatory collapse, and shock. The following laboratory values for her are obtained:

| LABORATORY RESULTS | NORMAL RANGE | PATIENT RESULTS |
|---|---|---|
| PT | 10–13 sec | 16 sec |
| aPTT | 25–35 sec | 59 sec |
| TT | 25–35 sec | 36 sec |
| Hgb | 12.3–15.3 g/dL | 9.8 g/dL |
| Hct | 36% to 45% | 27.7% |
| Platelet count | 150,000–450,000/µL | 64,000/µL |
| MPV | 7–11 fL | 17 fL |
| FDP (latex) | <10 mcg/mL | 120 mcg/mL |
| AT | 80% to 120% | 57% |
| D-dimer | <0.5 mcg/mL | 2.04 mcg/mL |

QUESTION: What laboratory tests are used to determine if a patient is experiencing DIC? What are the expected laboratory results for these tests?

DISCUSSION: Laboratory findings of DIC may be highly variable, complex, and difficult to interpret. Scoring systems have been developed to aid in diagnosing DIC.[70-73] Both PT and aPTT should be prolonged (and they are prolonged in this patient), but this may not always occur. Therefore, the usefulness of both PT and aPTT determinations may be helpful in making the diagnosis. TT is prolonged as expected. The platelet count is typically and dramatically decreased. Her MPV is inversely related to her decreased platelet count as expected, suggesting a hyperdestructive phenomenon versus a hypoproliferative state. Although FDPs are elevated, this rise is not solely pathognomonic for DIC. Increased D-dimer levels are strongly suggestive of DIC. AT determination reveals a considerable decrease consistent with DIC. Decreased AT is useful and reliable for diagnosis of DIC in the absence of D-dimer testing ability.

of 600 seconds as well as low concentrations of heparin. ACT test results can be influenced by the following factors[61]:

- Testing device
- Testing technique
- Sample temperature
- Heparin potency
- Platelet count and function
- Factor deficiencies
- Hypothermia

The main indication for using ACT over aPTT involves patients receiving high-dose heparin or DTIs. The DOACs prolong the ACT, but reproducibility is poor for the factor Xa inhibitors, and sensitivity is low for dabigatran; thus, this test is not recommended for qualitative or quantitative measurements of these agents.

### Anti-Xa

*Normal range: varies based on specific anticoagulant used for treatment of existing VTE; heparin: 0.3 to 0.7 International Units/mL; LMWH: 0.5 to 1 International Units/mL (twice daily therapeutic dosing); 1 to 2 International Units/mL (once daily therapeutic dosing); 0.2–0.5 International Units/mL (prophylactic dosing); fondaparinux, rivaroxaban, apixaban, edoxaban, betrixaban: not established*

The anti-Xa level may be used to monitor LMWH when given in therapeutic doses; however, routine monitoring is not usually done because LMWH has a more predictable dose-response relationship than UFH. This assay is recommended to be drawn 4 hours after administration of a therapeutic weight-adjusted dose of LMWH, when anti-Xa activity has peaked. An effective plasma concentration range is approximately 0.5 to 1.1 plasma anti-Xa units/mL for twice-daily therapeutic subcutaneous dosing of LMWH, or 1 to 2 International Units/mL for once-daily therapeutic dosing of LMWH. The target range for prophylactic dosing is not as well defined as for therapeutic dosing, but 0.2 to 0.5 International Units/mL has been suggested.[62] When ordering an anti-Xa test, it is imperative that the correct calibrator is used to ensure correct results; for example, the LMWH calibrator cannot be used to measure anti-Xa activity of fondaparinux. The anti-Xa level may be used as a quantitative assessment for the oral factor Xa inhibitors as long as the specific drug calibrator is used; if the specific calibrator is not used, the anti Xa level can only serve as a qualitative assessment test. Dabigatran has no effect on anti-Xa levels. Currently, some laboratories may not have specific calibrators for the oral factor Xa inhibitors, which limits the usefulness of this test (**Minicase 3**).

### Fibrinogen Assay

*Normal range: 200 to 400 mg/dL (5.8 to 11.8 µmol/L)*

Although the PT and aPTT are used to screen for deficiencies in the intrinsic, extrinsic, and common pathways, the *fibrinogen assay* is most commonly used to assess fibrinogen concentration. Fibrinogen assays are performed by adding a known amount of thrombin to a dilution of patient plasma. The fibrinogen concentration is determined by extrapolating the patient's clotting time to a standard curve. Elevated fibrinogen levels may be related to pregnancy or acute phase reactions and may be associated with an increased risk of cardiovascular disease.[63] Decreased fibrinogen is associated with DIC and hepatic cirrhosis; PT and aPTT levels also may be

## MINICASE 3

### Direct Oral Anticoagulant Monitoring

Genevieve H., a 67-year-old woman, is hospitalized with reports of chest pain and must undergo emergency surgery. Her home medications include rivaroxaban, metoprolol, atorvastatin, and lisinopril.

The following laboratory parameters are obtained prior to surgery:

| LABORATORY STUDY | NORMAL RANGE | PATIENT RESULTS |
| --- | --- | --- |
| PT | 10–13 sec | 35.6 sec |
| INR | 0.9–1.1 | 1.28 |
| aPTT | 21–45 sec | 69 sec |
| TT | 17–25 sec | 23 sec |

QUESTION: What specific test result(s) can be used to assess this patient's DOAC therapy? What are the expected results for these tests if a patient is taking a DOAC such as rivaroxaban?

DISCUSSION: She shows elevations in her PT, INR, and aPTT, while her TT is within normal limits. The PT can be used as a qualitative measurement for rivaroxaban; results may be normal to elevated if rivaroxaban is present in this patient's system. An anti-Xa level calibrated for rivaroxaban is the only test that can quantitatively assess how much drug is in the patient's system. The INR, although slightly elevated, is noncontributory to this patient's findings given she is not on a vitamin K antagonist. The aPTT is also elevated, but this test has not been shown to be a reliable indicator of either qualitative or quantitative assessments of oral factor Xa inhibitors such as rivaroxaban. The TT is normal given this test is not affected by oral factor Xa inhibitors; the TT assesses the ability to convert fibrinogen to fibrin and is not affected by issues in the extrinsic or intrinsic pathways of the coagulation system.

increased due to decreased fibrinogen levels, and patients may have symptomatic bleeding. Additionally, supratherapeutic heparin concentrations >1 unit/mL may result in falsely low fibrinogen concentration measurements. TT (discussed later) is the most sensitive test for fibrinogen deficiency, and it is prolonged when fibrinogen concentrations <100 mg/dL. However, the actual fibrinogen concentration occasionally must be determined. Fibrinogen levels are usually drawn as part of a DIC panel, to further explore reasons for an elevated PT or aPTT level, or to further evaluate unexplained bleeding in a patient.

### Thrombin Time

*Normal range: 17 to 25 seconds but varies according to thrombin concentration and reaction conditions*

The *thrombin time* (TT), also known as *thrombin clotting time*, measures the time required for a plasma sample to clot after the addition of bovine or human thrombin and is compared with that of a normal plasma control. Deficiencies in both the intrinsic and extrinsic systems do not affect TT, which assesses only the final phase of the common pathway or essentially the ability to convert fibrinogen to fibrin.

Prolongation of TT may be caused by hypofibrinogenemia, dysfibrinogenemia, heparin, DTIs, or the presence of FDPs. The TT is ultrasensitive to heparin and dabigatran; therefore, it only is useful to show whether these drugs are present in the blood sample—not as a monitoring test or to quantify drug levels; a normal TT can exclude the presence of dabigatran. With thrombolytic therapy, laboratory monitoring may not prevent bleeding or ensure thrombolysis. However, some clinicians recommend measuring TT, fibrinogen, plasminogen activation, or FDPs to document that a lytic state has been achieved. Typically, TT is >120 seconds 4 to 6 hours after "adequate" thrombolytic therapy.

The dilute thrombin time (dTT) is a test that compensates for the extreme sensitivity of the TT to heparin and dabigatran by diluting the patient's blood sample with normal plasma. Neither TT nor dTT is a useful monitoring test for the oral factor Xa inhibitors.

### Ecarin Clotting Time

The *ecarin clotting time* (ECT) test is a specific assay for thrombin generation. It is used to monitor parenteral DTIs and can be used as a quantitative assessment for dabigatran (Table 17-7). Ecarin is a type of snake venom that can activate prothrombin; it is added to plasma, which cleaves prothrombin to meizothrombin, a serine protease similar to thrombin. Ecarin is a type of snake venom that can activate prothrombin.[35] DTIs inhibit meizothrombin so the ECT can quantify the amount of DTI in the body by measuring the time for meizothrombin to convert fibrinogen into fibrin. Thus, a longer ECT corresponds to higher drug concentrations. ECT is not affected by other anticoagulants such as warfarin, heparin, or factor Xa inhibitors.

### Clot Degradation Tests

*Clot degradation tests* are useful in assessing the process of fibrinolysis. These tests include FDPs and D-dimer, which can be used to diagnose DIC or thrombosis and monitor the safety and efficacy of thrombolytic therapy. Thrombolytics (eg, alteplase, reteplase, and tenecteplase) are exogenous agents that lyse clots already formed. They are used in the treatment of acute cerebrovascular accidents, MI, VTE, and peripheral arterial occlusion. The mechanism by which they activate fibrinolysis can variably impact circulating proteins (hence, the necessity for close monitoring to minimize bleeding complications and ensure efficacy). Numerous laboratory parameters have been evaluated for this purpose, including PT, aPTT, BT, fibrinogen, FDPs, and D-dimer. These laboratory parameters are discussed throughout this chapter and in **Minicase 4**.

## MINICASE 4

## A Patient on Thrombolytic Therapy

Alfred F., a 44-year-old man, has clinical signs and symptoms and electrocardiogram findings consistent with acute anterior-wall MI requiring PCI. However, he presents to a hospital without PCI capabilities. He receives reteplase between the transit time to the nearest hospital with PCI capability. Subsequently, he is started on a heparin infusion. The following pretherapy and posttherapy coagulation laboratory results are obtained:

| LABORATORY STUDY | NORMAL RESULTS | PRETHERAPY | POSTTHERAPY |
|---|---|---|---|
| PT | 10–13 sec | 12.2 sec | 17 sec |
| aPTT | 25–35 sec | 35 sec | 69 sec |
| Fibrinogen | 200–400 mg/dL | 300 ng/mL | 22 ng/mL |
| FDP (latex) | <10 mcg/mL | <10 mcg/mL | >160 mcg/mL |
| D-dimer | <0.5 mcg/mL | <0.5 mcg/mL | <0.6 mcg/mL |
| Plasminogen | 80% to 120% | 70% | 22% |

QUESTION: What might explain the elevated FDP? What accounts for the fall in the plasminogen level on completion of the lytic therapy? Finally, why is the D-dimer concentration not elevated in proportion to the greatly elevated FDP concentration?

DISCUSSION: The elevated posttherapy PT and aPTT are consistent with heparin therapy after receiving reteplase. The FDP concentration is elevated because reteplase resulted in fibrinogenolysis. Many FDPs are generated in this setting. By the nature of thrombolytic therapy, plasminogen is converted to plasmin, accounting for the decline in the plasminogen percentage. Because thrombolytic therapy was unsuccessful in full clot lysis (with predominate fibrinogenolysis), the D-dimer concentration is not greatly elevated. For this assay to have been more elevated, degradation products arising from cross-linked fibrin (fibrinolysis) would have had to be present. Fibrinogen concentrations should be followed periodically in patients receiving thrombolytic agents.

DIAGNOSTIC FOLLOW-UP: If TT, PT, or aPTT is prolonged and if circulating inhibitors or bleeding disorders are suspected, further tests are usually performed. These tests may include assays for specific clotting factors to determine if a specific deficiency exists. For example, hemophilia or autoimmune diseases may be associated with inhibitors such as antifactor VIII and the lupus anticoagulant.

### Fibrin Degradation Products

*Normal range: <10 mcg/mL or <10 mg/L but varies with assay* Excessive activation of thrombin leads to overactivation of the fibrinolytic system and increased production of *fibrin degradation products* (FDPs). Excessive degradation of fibrin and fibrinogen also increases FDPs. This increase can be observed with DIC or thrombolytic drugs. FDPs can be monitored during thrombolytic therapy, but they may not be predictive of clot lysis. False-positive reactions may occur in healthy women immediately before and during menstruation and in patients with advanced cirrhosis or metastatic cancer.

### D-Dimer

*Normal range: <0.5 mcg/mL (<3 nmol/L) but varies with specific assay*
D-*dimer* is a marker of thrombotic activity and is formed when thrombin initiates the transition of fibrinogen to fibrin and activates factor XIII to cross-link the fibrin formed; when plasmin digests the cross-linked fibrin, D-dimer is formed. The D-dimer test is specific for fibrin, whereas the formation of FDPs (discussed previously) may be either fibrinogen or fibrin derived following plasmin digestion (**Figure 17-6**).

The D-dimer is often used to help diagnose or rule out thrombosis in the initial assessment of a patient suspected of having acute thromboembolism; results are typically elevated if a patient is positive for VTE. However, D-dimer is a sensitive but nonspecific marker for VTE because other causes such as malignancy, DIC, infection, inflammation, and pregnancy also can elevate the D-dimer levels.[64,65] Thus, a positive result does not necessarily confirm a diagnosis of VTE, but a negative result can help rule out VTE. Clinical correlation is essential, and further diagnostic workup is warranted with a positive test result to rule out other disorders as causes for abnormal levels. Various guidelines recommend using D-dimer as one possible diagnostic aid in patients with a low or moderate probability for first event VTE as determined by calculating the pretest probability through a validated scoring system such as the Wells or Geneva score; if the D-dimer result is positive, further testing, including imaging studies, is recommended.[66,67] D-dimer levels can increase by age and some studies have suggested using a different cut-off point for patients ≥50 years old. Using this approach, the cut-off for patients <50 years old remains <0.5mcg/mL, but for patients ≥50 years old the cut-off would be 10 times the patient's age.[65,68,69] Using the age-adjusted cut-offs may increase the diagnostic efficacy and specificity of the D-dimer without losing its sensitivity.[65] In patients who have a high pretest probability for VTE, the D-dimer test is not recommended, and patients should have an imaging test done instead.[64,66,67]

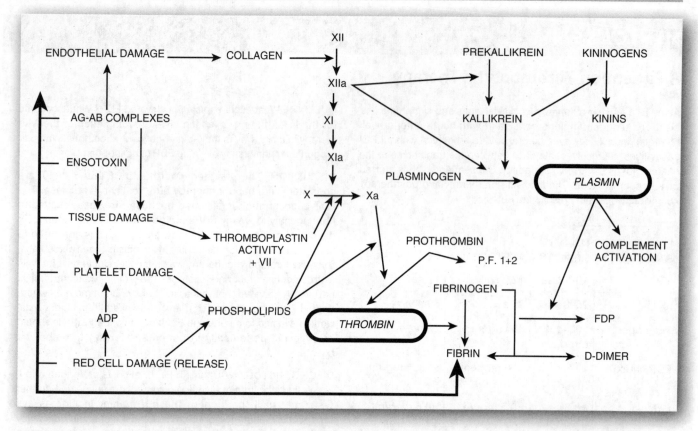

**FIGURE 17-6.** Formation of D-dimers in DIC triggered by amniotic fluid embolism. *Source:* Reprinted from Bick RL. Disseminated intravascular coagulation: objective criteria for clinical and laboratory diagnosis and assessment of therapeutic response. *Semin Thromb Hemost.* 1996;22:69–88. Copyright © 1996. SAGE Publications, Inc.

In addition, to diagnose or rule out VTE, D-dimer has been used for its predictive value for recurrent thromboembolism in patients treated for first event idiopathic VTE. Recurrent VTE risk prediction models, such as DASH, Vienna, and HERDOO 2, include the D-dimer test into their calculations.[65] Patients with normal levels of D-dimer 1 month after stopping anticoagulation therapy for a first-event idiopathic VTE have a lower risk for VTE recurrence, whereas elevated levels of D-dimer put patients at higher risk of VTE recurrence.[65] Thus, in patients with elevated levels of D-dimer, an extended duration of anticoagulation therapy could be considered (**Minicase 1**).

D-dimer is also a common test used as an aid to diagnose and evaluate patients with DIC. Several scoring systems for DIC based on clinical and laboratory data have been developed, which include specific laboratory measurements such as platelet counts, PT, fibrinogen, and FDPs.[70-73] The clinical and laboratory results are given specific scores, and when added up, indicate whether a patient is likely to have DIC. Although a D-dimer test is not specifically mentioned in some scoring systems, it is often used as a fibrin degradation marker, and it is a simple and quick test to perform. **Table 17-9** provides a list of the laboratory parameters, including the D-dimer, used to diagnose DIC (**Minicase 4**).

## Near-Patient or Point-of-Care Testing Devices

Several *point-of-care testing* (POCT) devices are available for different coagulation tests, such as PT/INR, ACT, D-dimer, and platelet function tests. More information about POCT can be found in Chapter 4. POCT uses whole blood, a sample that may be more physiologically relevant and result in a more accurate assessment of true coagulation potential.

Point-of-care coagulation testing offers specific clinical advantages, especially when used to monitor antithrombotic therapy because test results can be combined with clinical presentation to make more timely decisions regarding therapeutic intervention. This is especially significant in emergency departments, cardiac catheterization laboratories, surgical settings, and critical care units, in which immediate turnaround time is essential to patient care decisions. With newer antithrombotic options, these technologies will become increasingly relevant and may aid in making decisions for major bleeding events and prior to emergency surgery. Although many of the newer drugs do not require routine monitoring, the availability of rapid interventional testing may be critical to the selection of certain therapies for target patient populations, particularly when these drugs have a long half-life or cannot be completely reversed. Concomitant therapy is being used increasingly in cardiac patients, especially during cardiac intervention; thus, the potential for

**TABLE 17-9.** Laboratory Differential Diagnosis of DIC

| MONITORING PARAMETER | DIC | PRIMARY FIBRINOLYSIS | TTP | CHRONIC LIVER DISEASE |
|---|---|---|---|---|
| FDP | ↑ | ↑ | WNL to ↑ | WNL to ↑ |
| D-dimer | ↑ | ↑ | WNL | WNL |
| PT | ↑ | ↑ | WNL | ↑ |
| aPTT | ↑ | ↑ | WNL | WNL to ↑ |
| Fibrinogen | ↓ | ↓ | WNL | Variable |
| Platelet count | ↓ | WNL | WNL to ↓ | ↓ |
| LFTs | WNL | WNL | WNL | ↑ |
| BUN | ↑ | WNL | ↑ | WNL |

↓ = decreased; ↑ = increased; BUN = blood urea nitrogen; LFTs = liver function tests; WNL = within normal limits.

thrombotic or hemorrhagic problems may be increased without the ability to rapidly confirm coagulation status, both at the initiation of therapy and at the conclusion of a procedure.

In outpatient settings, POCT may be not only clinically beneficial but also more cost-effective and convenient than central laboratory testing, particularly in oral anticoagulation clinics and home healthcare settings. Patients can be informed of their INR results and subsequent dosing instructions within minutes, which is an obvious time-saving element. Certain patient variables may limit the accuracy of results obtained from the currently available POC devices for INR monitoring. These include concurrent use of LMWH or UFH, presence of antiphospholipid antibodies, and Hct levels above or below device-specific boundaries.

Patient self-testing (PST) and patient self-management (PSM) for INR are options for properly selected and trained patients on long-term warfarin therapy. PST is when a patient tests their own INR but rely on a clinician for interpretation of results and any modifications to the current regimen. PSM is when patients test their own INR and adjust their own therapy, usually based on an algorithm, which offers more patient autonomy and control over their own dosages. Benefits seen in both PST and PSM include lower VTE recurrence, increased time in therapeutic range, and increased patient satisfaction; additionally, there was a mortality benefit seen in PSM but not PST.[74] Although there are benefits to a PST/PSM model of care, including increased convenience to the patient, there also are issues that limit the widespread use of PST and PSM in the United States. These include reimbursement from insurance companies, lack of large-scale randomized trials using a U.S. population, low levels of awareness or understanding among healthcare practitioners and patients about these options, and areas with limited resources.[67] Additionally, the cost-effectiveness of PST/PSM is not well defined. Higher costs are associated with the cost of the test strip as well as increased testing frequency, but this may be offset by the convenience of PST/PSM,

especially for patients who live far away from testing facilities, who have difficulty with scheduled appointments, or who frequently travel.[67] Appropriate patient selection is essential for PST/PSM to be effective; ideal patient candidates or their caregivers should have manual dexterity, have visual acuity, demonstrate competency to perform the test, have the confidence and ability to responsibly participate in self-care, and have the ability to complete a structured training course.[74,75] The American Society of Hematology and the Anticoagulation Forum both endorse PST and/or PSM for appropriate patients.[74;75]

## SUMMARY

Many factors contribute to normal hemostasis, including interactions among vascular subendothelium, platelets, coagulation factors, natural anticoagulant proteins C and S, and substances that promote clot degradation, such as tissue plasminogen activator. In the clinical setting, the impact of these and other considerations must be evaluated. Disorders of platelets or clotting factors can result in bleeding, which may necessitate the monitoring of specific clotting tests.

Coagulation tests such as aPTT, ACT, and PT/INR are used to monitor heparin and warfarin therapies. Laboratory monitoring for DOACs is an emerging area with certain tests used for qualitative versus quantitative assessments of these agents. In general, coagulation tests are used for patients receiving anticoagulants, thrombolytics, and antiplatelet agents. The availability of rapid diagnostic tests to manage LMWH, DTIs, and platelet inhibitor drugs may influence the selection of these newer therapies. Other indications for routine use of these tests include primary coagulopathies and monitoring of drugs that may cause bleeding abnormalities. Finally, other available tests (eg, D-dimer and AT level determinations) may improve diagnostic assessment of patients with DIC and ensure appropriate treatment selection.

## ACKNOWLEDGMENTS

The contribution of material written by James B. Groce III, Julie B. Lemus, and Sheila M. Allen in previous editions of this book is gratefully acknowledged.

## LEARNING POINTS

### 1. What is the INR in relation to PT?

**ANSWER:** PT results are not standardized as various reagent sources and test methods are used when performing this test among differing laboratories. The INR is a calibration method developed to standardize the reported PT results. The method considers the sensitivity of individual reagents as well as the clot detection instrument used, designated as ISI. Although INR reporting has improved the standardization of the PT, potential problems (eg, ISI calibration, sample citrate concentration) still remain. Thus, laboratories should review the performance of their individual methods used in reporting PT/INRs and inform clinicians who are interpreting these results of any changes.

### 2. How can the D-dimer be used for diagnosis of VTE?

**ANSWER:** In patients who have a low to moderate probability for a VTE, as calculated through a validated scoring system, the D-dimer can be drawn; if the result is positive, then further imaging is needed to confirm the diagnosis. The D-dimer is a sensitive but nonspecific marker for VTE, so a positive result does not confirm a diagnosis of VTE, but a negative result helps rule out VTE. In patients with high probability for VTE, the D-dimer test should not be performed; instead, imaging tests should be done. The D-dimer can be also be used as a way to help predict the risk of recurrent VTE and determine whether anticoagulation should be continued long term. In instances like this, the D-dimer should be drawn after the patient stops anticoagulation; if the D-dimer level is elevated, the patient is at increased risk of VTE recurrence and can be considered for extended duration of anticoagulation.

### 3. Which laboratory tests may be used to monitor DOACs?

**ANSWER:** No one single test can universally monitor DOAC medications. Certain tests are better suited for qualitative measurements, which show whether the medication is present in the body, whereas other tests are better suited for quantitative measurements, which show actual levels of medication in the body. Qualitative measurements of dabigatran can be done through aPTT, whereas quantitative measurements of dabigatran can be done with either the dTT or the ECT. Qualitative information for the oral factor Xa inhibitors can be measured using the PT (only for rivaroxaban), while anti-Xa levels can be used for quantitative information if calibrated to a specific oral factor Xa inhibitor; if the anti-Xa test is not specifically calibrated, then this test can only be used as a qualitative assessment for these medications.

## REFERENCES

1. Ramot Y, Nyska A, Spectre G. Drug-induced thrombosis: an update. *Drug Saf.* 2013;36(8):585–603.PubMed

2. Konkle BA. Bleeding and Thrombosis. In: Jameson J, Fauci AS, Kasper DL, et al, eds. *Harrison's Principles of Internal Medicine.* 20th ed. New York, NY: McGraw-Hill; 2018. https://accesspharmacy.mhmedical.com/content.aspx?bookid=2129&sectionid=192014303. Accessed July 9, 2020.

3. Konkle BA. Disorders of Platelets and Vessel Wall. In: Jameson J, Fauci AS, Kasper DL, et al, eds. *Harrison's Principles of Internal Medicine.* 20th ed. New York, NY: McGraw-Hill; 2018. https://accesspharmacy.mhmedical.com/content.aspx?bookid=2129&sectionid=192018598. Accessed July 9, 2020.

4. Fuster V, Sweeny JM. Aspirin: a historical and contemporary therapeutic overview. *Circulation.* 2011;123(7):768–778.PubMed

5. Colucci G, Tsakiris DA. Thrombophilia screening: universal, selected, or neither? *Clin Appl Thromb Hemost.* 2017;23(8):893–899.PubMed

6. Connors JM. Thrombophilia testing and venous thrombosis. *N Engl J Med.* 2017;377(12):1177–1187.PubMed

7. Eby CS. Warfarin-induced skin necrosis. *Hematol Oncol Clin North Am.* 1993;7(6):1291–1300.PubMed

8. Broekmans AW, Bertina RM, Loeliger EA, et al. Protein C and the development of skin necrosis during anticoagulant therapy. *Thromb Haemost.* 1983;49(3):251.PubMed

9. Wattiaux MJ, Hervé R, Robert A, et al. Coumarin-induced skin necrosis associated with acquired protein S deficiency and antiphospholipid antibody syndrome. *Arthritis Rheum.* 1994;37(7):1096–1100.PubMed

10. Moreb J, Kitchens CS. Acquired functional protein S deficiency, cerebral venous thrombosis, and coumarin skin necrosis in association with antiphospholipid syndrome: report of two cases. *Am J Med.* 1989;87(2):207–210.PubMed

11. Tefferi A, Pardanani A. Essential thrombocythemia. *N Engl J Med.* 2019;381(22):2135–2144.PubMed

12. Squires JE. Indications for platelet transfusion in patients with thrombocytopenia. *Blood Transfus.* 2015;13(2):221–226.PubMed

13. Greene EM, Hagemann TM. Drug-Induced Hematologic Disorders. In: DiPiro JT, Yee GC, Posey L, et al., eds. *Pharmacotherapy: A Pathophysiologic Approach.* New York, NY: McGraw-Hill; https://accesspharmacy.mhmedical.com/content.aspx?bookid=2577&sectionid=235639814. Accessed July 17, 2020.

14. Bakchoul T, Marini I. Drug-associated thrombocytopenia. *Hematology (Am Soc Hematol Educ Program).* 2018;2018(1):576–583.PubMed

15. Barlow A, Barlow B, Reinaker T, et al. Potential role of direct oral anticoagulants in the management of heparin-induced thrombocytopenia. *Pharmacotherapy.* 2019;39(8):837–853.PubMed

16. Salter BS, Weiner MM, Trinh MA, et al. Hearpin-induced thrombocytopenia: a comprehensive clinical review. *J Am Coll Cardiol.* 2016;67(21):2519–2532.PubMed

17. Arepally GM. Heparin-induced thrombocytopenia. *Blood.* 2017;129(21):2864–2872.PubMed

18. East JM, Cserti-Gazdewich CM, Granton JT. Heparin-induced thrombocytopenia in the critically ill patient. *Chest.* 2018;154(3):678–690. PubMed

19. Warkentin TE, Greinacher A. Management of heparin-induced thrombocytopenia. *Curr Opin Hematol.* 2016;23(5):462–470.PubMed

20. Cuker A, Arepally GM, Chong BH, et al. American Society of Hematology 2018 guidelines for management of venous thromboembolism: heparin-induced thrombocytopenia. *Blood Adv.* 2018;2(22):3360–3392.PubMed

21. Linkins LA, Dans AL, Moores LK, et al. Treatment and prevention of heparin-induced thrombocytopenia: antithrombotic therapy and prevention of thrombosis. 9th ed. American College of Chest Physicians

Evidence-Based Clinical Practice Guidelines. *Chest*. 2012;141:(2 suppl): e495S-530S.

22. Vinholt PJ, Hvas AM, Nybo M. An overview of platelet indices and methods for evaluating platelet function in thrombocytopenic patients. *Eur J Haematol*. 2014;92(5):367–376.PubMed

23. Leader A, Pereg D, Lishner M. Are platelet volume indices of clinical use? A multidisciplinary review. *Ann Med*. 2012;44(8):805–816.PubMed

24. Noris P, Melazzini F, Balduini CL. New roles for mean platelet volume measurement in the clinical practice? *Platelets*. 2016;27(7):607–612. PubMed

25. Rice TW, Wheeler AP. Coagulopathy in critically ill patients: part 1. Platelet disorders. *Chest*. 2009;136(6):1622–1630.PubMed

26. Scharf RE. Drugs that affect platelet function. *Semin Thromb Hemost*. 2012;38(8):865–883.PubMed

27. Michelson AD, Frelinger AL 3rd, Furman MI. Current options in platelet function testing. *Am J Cardiol*. 2006;98(10A):4N-10N.PubMed

28. Kaplan KL, Owen J. Plasma levels of β-thromboglobulin and platelet factor 4 as indices of platelet activation in vivo. *Blood*. 1981;57(2): 199–202.PubMed

29. U.S. Food and Drug Administration. Medical devices direct to consumer tests. https://www.fda.gov/medical-devices/vitro-diagnostics/direct-consumer-tests. Updated December 20, 2019. Accessed July 10, 2020.

30. U.S. Food and Drug Administration. Medical devices nucleic acid based tests. https://www.fda.gov/medical-devices/vitro-diagnostics/nucleic-acid-based-tests. Updated July 7, 2020. Accessed July 10, 2020.

31. Amsterdam EA, Wenger NK, Brindis RG, et al. 2014 AHA/ACC guideline for the management of patients with non-ST-elevation acute coronary syndromes: a report of the American College of Cardiology/American Heart Association Task Force on Practice Guidelines. *J Am Coll Cardiol*. 2014;64(24):e139-e228.PubMed

32. Levine GN, Bates ER, Blankenship JC, et al. 2011 ACCF/AHA/SCAI Guideline for Percutaneous Coronary Intervention. A report of the American College of Cardiology Foundation/American Heart Association Task Force on Practice Guidelines and the Society for Cardiovascular Angiography and Interventions. *J Am Coll Cardiol*. 2011;58(24):e44-e122.PubMed

33. Levine GN, Bates ER, Bittl JA, et al. 2016 ACC/AHA guidelines focused update on duration of dual antiplatelet therapying patients with coronary artery disease: a report of the American College of Cardiology/American Heart Association task force on clinical practice guidelines. *J Am Coll Cardiol*. 2016;68(10):1082–1115.PubMed

34. Stevens SM, Woller SC, Bauer KA, et al. Guidance for the evaluation and treatment of hereditary and acquired thrombophilia. *J Thromb Thrombolysis*. 2016;41(1):154–164.PubMed

35. Conway SE, Hwang AY, Ponte CD, Gums et al. Laboratory and clinical monitoring of direct acting oral anticoagulants: what clinicians need to know. *Pharmacotherapy*. 2017;37(2):236–248.PubMed

36. Clemens A, Strack A, Noack H, et al. Anticoagulant-related gastrointestinal bleeding: could this facilitate early detection of benign or malignant gastrointestinal lesions? *Ann Med*. 2014;46(8):672–678. PubMed

37. Asiimwe A, Li JJ, Weerakkody G, et al. Diagnoses of gastrointestinal cancers after gastrointestinal bleeding in patients receiving clopidogrel or warfarin. *Curr Drug Saf*. 2013;8(4):261–269.PubMed

38. Kamal AH, Tefferi A, Pruthi RK. How to interpret and pursue an abnormal prothrombin time, activated partial thromboplastin time, and bleeding time in adults. *Mayo Clin Proc*. 2007;82(7):864–873.PubMed

39. Gosselin RC, Adcock DM, Bates SM, et al. International Council for Standardization in Haematology (ICSH) recommendations for laboratory measurement of direct oral anticoagulants. *Thromb Haemost*. 2018;118(3):437–450.PubMed

40. Nutescu EA, Burnett A, Fanikos J, et al. Pharmacology of anticoagulants used in the treatment of venous thromboembolism. *J Thromb Thrombolysis*. 2016;41(1):15–31.PubMed

41. Lip GYH, Banerjee A, Boriani G, et al. Antithrombotic therapy for atrial fibrillation. CHEST guideline and expert panel report. *Chest*. 2018;154(5):1121–1201.PubMed

42. Kearon C, Akl EA, Ornelas J, et al. Antithrombotic therapy for VTE disease. CHEST guideline and expert panel report. *Chest*. 2016;149(2):315–352.PubMed

43. January CT, Wann LS, Calkins H, et al. 2019 AHA/ACC/HRS focused update of the 2014 AHA/ACC/HRS guideline for the management of patients with atrial fibrillation. *J Am Coll Cardiol*. 2019;74(1):104–132. PubMed

44. Nishimura RA, Otto CM, Bonow RO, et al. 2017 Focused update of the 2014 AHA/ACC guideline for the management of patients with valvular heart disease. *J Am Coll Cardiol*. 2017;70:252–289.PubMed

45. Whitlock RP, Sun JC, Fremes SE, et al. Antithrombotic and thrombolytic therapy for valvular disease: antithrombotic therapy and prevention of thrombosis. 9th ed. American College of Chest Physicians Evidence-Based Clinical Practice Guidelines. *Chest*. 2012;141(suppl):e576S-600S

46. Streiff MB, Agnelli G, Connors JM, et al. Guidance for the treatment of deep vein thrombosis and pulmonary embolism. *J Thromb Thrombolysis*. 2016;41(1):32–67.PubMed

47. Johnson JA, Cavallari LH. Warfarin pharmacogenetics. *Trends Cardiovasc Med*. 2015;25(1):33–41.PubMed

48. Johnson JA, Caudle KE, Gong L, et al. Clinical pharmacogenetics implementation consortium (CPIC) guideline for pharmacogenetics-guided warfarin dosing: 2017 update. *Clin Pharmacol Ther*. 2017;102(3):397–404.PubMed

49. Kanuri SH, Kreutz RP. Pharmacogenomics of novel direct oral anticoagulants: newly identified genes and genetic variants. *J Pers Med*. 2019;9(1):7.PubMed

50. Marlar RA, Clement B, Gausman J. Activated partial thromboplastin time monitoring of unfractionated heparin therapy: issues and recommendations. *Semin Thromb Hemost*. 2017;43(3):253–260.PubMed

51. Favaloro EJ, Kershaw G, Mohammed S, Lippi G. How to optimize activated partial thromboplastin time (APTT) testing: solutions to establishing and verifying normal reference intervals and assessing APTT reagents for sensitivity to heparin, lupus anticoagulant, and clotting factors. *Semin Thromb Hemost*. 2019;45(1):22–35.PubMed

52. Groce JB 3rd, Gal P, Douglas JB, Steuterman MC. Heparin dosage adjustment in patients with deep-vein thrombosis using heparin concentrations rather than activated partial thromboplastin time. *Clin Pharm*. 1987;6(3):216–222.PubMed

53. Kandrotas RJ, Gal P, Douglas JB, Groce JB 3rd. Rapid determination of maintenance heparin infusion rates with the use of non-steady-state heparin concentrations. *Ann Pharmacother*. 1993;27(12):1429–1433.PubMed

54. Basu D, Gallus A, Hirsh J, Cade J. A prospective study of the value of monitoring heparin treatment with the activated partial thromboplastin time. *N Engl J Med*. 1972;287(7):324–327.PubMed

55. Hull RD, Raskob GE, Hirsh J, et al. Continuous intravenous heparin compared with intermittent subcutaneous heparin in the initial treatment of proximal-vein thrombosis. *N Engl J Med*. 1986;315(18):1109–1114. PubMed

56. Groce JB. Heparin and low molecular weight heparin. In: Murphy JE, ed. *Clinical Pharmacokinetics*. 2nd ed. Bethesda, MD: American Society of Health-System Pharmacists; 2001:165–198.

57. Levine MN, Hirsh J, Gent M, et al. A randomized trial comparing activated thromboplastin time with heparin assay in patients with acute venous thromboembolism requiring large daily doses of heparin. *Arch Intern Med*. 1994;154(1):49–56.PubMed

58. Lippi G, Salvagno GL, Ippolito L, et al. Shortened activated partial thromboplastin time: causes and management. *Blood Coagul Fibrinolysis*. 2010;21(5):459–463.PubMed

59. Mina A, Favaloro EJ, Mohammed S, et al. A laboratory evaluation into the short activated partial thromboplastin time. *Blood Coagul Fibrinolysis*. 2010;21(2):152–157.PubMed

60. Samuelson BT, Cuker A, Siegal DM, et al. Laboratory assessment of the anticoagulant activity of direct oral anticoagulants. *Chest.* 2017;151(1):127–138.PubMed

61. Bolliger D, Tanaka KA. Point-of-care coagulation testing in cardiac surgery. *Semin Thromb Hemost.* 2017;43(4):386–396.PubMed

62. Wei MY, Ward SM. The anti-factor Xa range for low molecular weight heparin thromboprophylaxis. *Hematol Rep.* 2015;7(4):5844.PubMed

63. Kakafika AI, Liberopoulos EN, Mikhailidis DP. Fibrinogen: a predictor of vascular disease. *Curr Pharm Des.* 2007;13(16):1647–1659.PubMed

64. Johnson ED, Schell JC, Rodgers GM. The D-dimer assay. *Am J Hematol.* 2019;94(7):833–839.PubMed

65. Weitz JI, Fredenburgh JC, Eikelboom JW. A test in context: D-dimer. *J Am Coll Cardiol.* 2017;70(19):2411–2420.PubMed

66. Bates SM, Jaeschke R, Stevens SM, et al. Diagnosis of DVT: antithrombotic therapy and prevention of thrombosis, 9th ed: American College of Chest Physicians Evidence-Based Clinical Practice Guidelines. *Chest.* 2012; 141:e351s-418s.

67. Lim W, Le Gal G, Bates SM, et al. American Society of Hematology 2018 guidelines for management of venous thromboembolism: diagnosis of venous thromboembolism. *Blood Adv.* 2018;2(22):3226–3256.PubMed

68. Righini M, Van Es J, Den Exter PL, et al. Age-adjusted D-dimer cutoff levels to rule out pulmonary embolism: the ADJUST-PE study. *JAMA.* 2014;311(11):1117–1124.PubMed

69. Douma RA, le Gal G, Söhne M, et al. Potential of an age adjusted D-dimer cut-off value to improve the exclusion of pulmonary embolism in older patients: a retrospective analysis of three large cohorts. *BMJ.* 2010;340:c1475.PubMed

70. Levi M, Toh CH, Thachil J, et al. Guidelines for the diagnosis and management of disseminated intravascular coagulation. *Br J Haematol.* 2009;145(1):24–33.PubMed

71. Wada H, Asakura H, Okamoto K, et al. Expert consensus for the treatment of disseminated intravascular coagulation in Japan. *Thromb Res.* 2010;125(1):6–11.PubMed

72. Di Nisio M, Baudo F, Cosmi B, et al. Diagnosis and treatment of disseminated intravascular coagulation: guidelines of the Italian Society for Haemostasis and Thrombosis (SISET). *Thromb Res.* 2012;129(5):e177-e184.PubMed

73. Wada H, Thachil J, Di Nisio M, et al. The Scientific Standardization Committee on DIC of the International Society on Thrombosis Haemostasis. Guidance for diagnosis and treatment of DIC from harmonization of the recommendations from three guidelines. *J Thromb Haemost.* 2013;11:761–767.

74. Witt DM, Nieuwlaat R, Clark NP, et al. American Society of Hematology 2018 guidelines for management of venous thromboembolism: optimal management of anticoagulation therapy. *Blood Adv.* 2018;2(22):3257–3291.PubMed

75. Witt DM, Clark NP, Kaatz S, et al. Guidance for the practical management of warfarin therapy in the treatment of venous thromboembolism. *J Thromb Thrombolysis.* 2016;41(1):187–205.PubMed

## QUICKVIEW | Platelet Count

| PARAMETER | DESCRIPTION | COMMENTS |
|---|---|---|
| **Common reference ranges** | | |
| Adults | 150,000–450,000/μL (150–450 × 10$^9$/L) | |
| **Critical value** | >800,000 or <20,000 μL (>800 × 10$^9$/L or <20 × 10$^9$/L) | |
| **Inherent activity** | Determines the number or concentration of platelets in a blood sample | |
| **Location** | | |
| Production | Bone marrow | Also can be produced by lungs and other tissues |
| Storage | Not stored | Two-thirds found in circulation, one-third found in spleen |
| Secretion/excretion | Destroyed by spleen, liver, bone marrow | |
| **Causes of abnormal values** | | |
| High | Primary causes<br>  Myeloproliferative neoplasms<br>Secondary (reactive) causes<br>  Acute hemorrhage<br>  Infection<br>  Inflammation<br>  Iron deficiency anemia<br>  Diseases: splenectomy, rheumatoid arthritis, occult malignancy | |
| Low | Hypersplenism<br>Severe B$_{12}$, folate deficiency<br>Diseases: TTP, ITP, DIC, aplastic anemia, myelodysplasia, leukemia<br>Drugs | Table 17-2<br>Table 17-3 |
| **Signs and symptoms** | | |
| High | Thrombosis: CVA, DVT, PE, portal vein thrombosis | |
| Low | Bleeding: mucosal, cutaneous | CNS bleeding (ie, intracranial hemorrhage) is the most common cause of death in patients with severe thrombocytopenia |
| **After event, time to...** | | |
| Initial elevation | Days to weeks | |
| Peak values | Days to weeks | |
| Normalization | Weeks to months | |
| **Causes of spurious results** | Values outside 50,000–500,000/μL (50 × 10$^9$/L to 500 × 10$^9$/L) | Need to review the peripheral blood smear to confirm automated platelet counts in these instances |
| | Hct <20 or >50% | |

CNS = central nervous system; CVA = cerebrovascular accident; DVT = deep vein thrombosis; PE = pulmonary embolism.

## QUICKVIEW | PT and INR

| PARAMETER | DESCRIPTION | COMMENTS |
|---|---|---|
| **Common reference ranges** | | |
| Adults | PT 10–13 sec<br>INR 0.8–1.1 | INR therapeutic ranges vary if patient is on warfarin and depending on indication for warfarin; usual therapeutic ranges are either 2–3 or 2.5–3.5 |
| Children | PT <16 sec | PT levels in the newborn are generally prolonged compared with adults; however, by 6 mo of age, levels are comparable to adults |
| **Critical value** | PT >15 sec | Unless on warfarin |
| | INR—depends on indication, but >5 is commonly used as a critical value | |
| **Inherent activity** | Indirect measure of coagulation factors, particularly factor VII, which has the shortest half-life and thus is affected the most rapidly by warfarin | |
| **Location** | | |
| Production | Coagulation factors produced in liver | |
| Storage | Not stored | |
| Secretion/excretion | None | |
| **Causes of abnormal values** | | |
| High | Diseases: liver disease<br>Malabsorption/malnutrition<br>Drug: warfarin | Table 17-8 |
| Low | None | Table 17-8 |
| **Signs and symptoms** | | |
| High | Increased risk of bleeding and ecchymosis | Risk increases as PT or INR value increases |
| Low | Potential thrombosis if on vitamin K antagonist | |
| **After event, time to...** | | |
| Initial elevation | 6–12 hr | |
| Peak values | Days to weeks | |
| Normalization | Hours to days | Depends, if reversed with vitamin K |
| **Causes of spurious results** | Improper laboratory collection | |
| **Additional info** | Used to monitor warfarin | Target levels depend on indication for warfarin |
| | May be used as a qualitative assessment of rivaroxaban | Only use the PT, not the INR |

## QUICKVIEW | aPTT

| PARAMETER | DESCRIPTION | COMMENTS |
|---|---|---|
| **Common reference ranges** | | |
| Adults | 25–35 sec | May vary by reagent/instrument used |
| **Critical value** | >100 sec, but depends on specific reagent | |
| **Inherent activity** | Used to monitor UFH activity | If patient is on UFH for treatment of deep venous thrombosis or pulmonary embolism, aim for 1.5–2.5 times control aPTT |
| **Location** | | |
| Production | Coagulation factors produced in liver | |
| Storage | Not stored | Two-thirds found in circulation, one-third found in spleen |
| Secretion/excretion | None | |
| **Causes of abnormal values** | | |
| High | Hereditary: deficiency of factors II, V, VIII, IX, X, XI, XII, HMWK, prekallikrein, fibrinogen | |
| | Acquired: lupus anticoagulant, heparin, DTIs, liver dysfunction, vitamin K deficiency, warfarin, DIC | aPTT not used to monitor warfarin therapy |
| Low | Laboratory testing drawn before 6 hr if on heparin, ATIII deficiency | |
| **Signs and symptoms** | | |
| High | Increased risk of hemorrhage | Risk increases as aPTT increases |
| Low | Thrombosis | |
| **After event, time to...** | | |
| Initial elevation | 6–12 hr | |
| Peak values | Hours to days | |
| Normalization | Hours to days | |
| **Causes of spurious results** | Improper laboratory collection | Need to do manual counts in these instances |
| **Additional info** | Used to monitor heparin | Dosing nomograms vary by institution |
| | May be used as a qualitative assessment of dabigatran | |

HMWK = high-molecular weight kininogen.

## QUICKVIEW | anti-Xa

| PARAMETER | DESCRIPTION | COMMENTS |
|---|---|---|
| **Common reference ranges** | | |
| Adults | 0.3–0.7 International Units/mL, for UFH<br>0.5–1 International Units/mL for twice-daily LMWH<br><br>1–2 International Units/mL for once-daily LMWH<br>0.2–0.5 International Units/mL for prophylactic dosing LMWH | For establishment of therapeutic heparin range using blood samples from heparinized patients<br><br><br>Values may vary depending on LMWH preparation used |
| **Inherent activity** | Used to establish therapeutic heparin range and monitor LMWH activity | |
| **Location** | | |
| Production | Coagulation factors produced in liver | |
| Storage | Not stored | |
| Secretion/excretion | None | |
| **Causes of abnormal values** | | |
| High | Overdosage of LMWH<br><br>Poor renal function | |
| Low | Laboratory testing drawn prior to 4 hr after dose is administered<br><br>Underdosage of LMWH | |
| **Signs and symptoms** | | |
| High | Increased risk of bleeding and bruising | |
| Low | Potential thrombosis | |
| **After event, time to...** | | |
| Initial elevation | 0–4 hr | |
| Peak values | 4 hr | |
| Normalization | Hours to days | |
| **Causes of spurious results** | Improper timing of collection | Should be drawn 4 hr after dose is administered |
| **Additional info** | Used to monitor LMWH<br><br>May be used as quantitative assessment of oral factor Xa inhibitors | Must be calibrated to the specific DOAC |

# 18

# Infectious Diseases: Bacteria

*Sharon M. Erdman, Rodrigo M. Burgos,*
*and Keith A. Rodvold*

*(continued on page 404)*

DOI 10.37573/9781585286423.018

The assessment, diagnosis, and treatment of a patient with an infection may appear to be an overwhelming task to some clinicians. This may be partly due to the nonspecific presentation of many infectious processes; the continuously changing taxonomy, diagnostic procedures, and antimicrobial susceptibility patterns of infecting organisms; and the continuous introduction of new antimicrobials to the existing large collection of anti-infective agents. This chapter focuses on the laboratory tests used for the diagnosis of the most common infections caused by bacteria.

Information regarding white blood cells (WBCs) and their role in infection is discussed in Chapter 16; laboratory tests used in the diagnosis of viral hepatitis, *Helicobacter pylori* gastrointestinal (GI) infection, and *Clostridioides difficile* pseudomembranous colitis are addressed in Chapter 15; and lab tests used for the diagnosis of viral, fungal, and mycobacterial infections are discussed in Chapter 19. Lastly, information regarding the clinical utility of the erythrocyte sedimentation rate (ESR) and C-reactive protein (CRP) as they relate to inflammatory diseases and infections are also addressed in Chapter 20.

## BACTERIA

*Bacteria* are small, unicellular, prokaryotic organisms that contain a cell wall but lack a well-defined nucleus. They are a diverse group of microorganisms that exist in different shapes and morphologies with varying rates of pathogenicity. Bacteria are a common cause of infection in both the community and hospital setting, and can cause infection in patients with normal or suppressed immune systems. Bacteria must be considered potential causative pathogens in any patient presenting with signs and symptoms of infection.

### Specimen Collection and Identification of Bacteria

Several factors should be considered when choosing an appropriate antimicrobial regimen for the treatment of infection, including patient characteristics (eg, immune status, age, end-organ function, comorbidities, drug allergies, and severity of illness), drug characteristics (eg, spectrum of activity, pharmacokinetics, penetration to the site of infection, and proven clinical efficacy), and infection characteristics (eg, site/type of infection [suspected or known] and potential causative organism(s)). Therefore, appropriate diagnosis is a key factor in selecting appropriate empiric and directed antibiotic therapy for the treatment of an infection. In the case of a suspected infection, appropriate culture specimens should be obtained for laboratory testing from the suspected site of infection *before* antibiotics are initiated, if possible, in an attempt to isolate and identify the causative pathogen. Special attention should be placed on specimen collection and timely transport to the laboratory because the accuracy of the results is limited by the quality and integrity of the submitted specimen.[1-4] **Table 18-1** lists common biologic specimens that may be submitted to the microbiology laboratory for bacteriologic analysis.[1-4]

When a specimen from the suspected site of infection is submitted to the microbiology laboratory, several microbiologic tests are performed to aid in the identification of the infecting bacteria. The most common laboratory tests used for the identification of bacteria include direct microscopic examination using specialized stains

## OBJECTIVES

- Define minimum inhibitory concentration, $MIC_{50}$, $MIC_{90}$, minimum inhibitory concentration susceptibility breakpoint, and minimum bactericidal concentration

- Describe the information that is used to construct a cumulative antibiogram; discuss the clinical utility of the cumulative antibiogram when choosing empiric antibiotic therapy for the treatment of a patient's infection

- List the laboratory tests that may be performed for the diagnosis of infections due to miscellaneous or uncommon organisms such as *Borrelia burgdorferi*, *Treponema pallidum*, and *Legionella pneumophila*

- Describe the clinical utility of laboratory tests routinely performed for the diagnosis of infection in the following situations: (1) cerebrospinal fluid when meningitis is suspected, (2) respiratory secretions when lower respiratory tract infections are suspected, (3) urine, prostatic secretions, or genital secretions when a genitourinary tract infection is suspected, and (4) otherwise sterile fluid when infection is suspected (eg, synovial fluid, peritoneal fluid)

(eg, Gram stain, fluorescent stains such as acridine orange or auramine-rhodamine stains) and bacterial culture techniques to foster growth of the microorganism. Once bacteria grow in culture, additional tests are then performed to identify the infecting organism and determine susceptibility of the bacteria to various antimicrobial agents.

### Gram Stain

*Gram stain* is the most common staining method used for the microscopic examination of bacteria and is most appropriate for the evaluation of body fluids (eg, cerebrospinal fluid [CSF], pleural, synovial, etc.), respiratory tract secretions, and wound/abscess swabs or aspirates.[4] The Gram stain classifies bacteria into one of two groups, gram-positive or gram-negative, based on their reaction to an established series of dyes and decolorizers. The difference in stain uptake between gram-positive and gram-negative bacteria is primarily due to differences in their bacterial cell wall composition and permeability.[5-8] Although the Gram stain does not provide an exact identification of the infecting organism (eg, *Klebsiella pneumoniae* versus *Serratia marcescens*), it does provide rapid (within minutes) preliminary information about the potential infecting organism that can be used to guide empiric antibiotic therapy while waiting for culture results, which may take 24 to 48 hours or more. The Gram stain is useful for characterizing most clinically relevant bacteria but is unable to detect intracellular bacteria (eg, *Chlamydia*), bacteria without cell walls (eg, *Mycoplasma*), and organisms that are too small to be visualized with light microscopy (eg, spirochetes).[6-8]

The current Gram stain methodology is a slight modification of the original process developed by Hans Christian Gram in the late 19th century.[5-8] The Gram stain procedure involves several staining and rinsing steps that can be performed within a few

**TABLE 18-1.** Common Biologic Specimens Submitted for Culture

**Abscess, lesion, wound, pustule:** swab or aspirate

**Blood**

**Bone marrow**

**Body fluids:** amniotic, abdominal, bile, pericardial, peritoneal, pleural, or synovial by needle aspiration

**Bone:** biopsy of infected area

**CSF:** by lumbar puncture or directly from shunt (eg, ventriculoperitoneal shunt)

**Cutaneous:** hair or nail clippings, skin scrapings, aspiration of leading edge of skin infection; biopsy

**Ear:** middle ear fluid specimen by myringotomy; outer ear specimen by swab or biopsy

**Eye:** conjunctival swab, corneal scrapings, aqueous or vitreous fluid

**Foreign bodies:** intravenous catheter tip by roll plate method; prosthetic heart valve, prosthetic joint material, intrauterine device, etc.

**GI tract:** gastric aspirate for acid fast bacilli (AFB), gastric biopsy for *H pylori*, rectal swab, stool cultures, stool specimen for *C difficile*

**Genital tract:** cervical, endometrial, urethral, vaginal, or prostatic secretions; ulcer biopsy

**Respiratory tract:** sputum, tracheal aspirate, BAL, pharyngeal or nasopharyngeal swab, sinus aspirate

**Tissue:** biopsy

**Urine:** clean-catch midstream, straight-catheterized, suprapubic aspirate

BAL = bronchoalveolar lavage.
*Source:* References 1–4.

minutes. The first step involves applying, drying, and heat-fixing a thin smear of a biological specimen to a clean glass slide. Once the slide has cooled, it is then rinsed with crystal or gentian violet (a purple dye) followed by Gram's iodine, decolorized with an ethanol or acetone rinse, and then counterstained with safranin (a pink or red dye), with a gentle tap water rinse performed between each of these steps. The slide is then blotted dry and examined under a microscope using the oil immersion lens. If bacteria are present, they are examined for stain uptake, morphology (round = coccus, rod = bacillus), and organization (eg, pairs, clusters). Gram-positive bacteria stain purple due to retention of the crystal violet-iodine complex in their cell walls, whereas gram-negative bacteria stain red because they do not retain crystal violet and are counterstained by safranin.[5,6,9] The results of the Gram stain (eg, gram-positive cocci in pairs or gram-negative rods) may provide information about the possible infecting organism before the culture results become available and, in some situations, may also be used to guide empiric antibiotic therapy. **Table 18-2** lists the most likely bacteria based on Gram stain results.[10,11] Once culture and susceptibility results are available, the initial empiric antibiotic regimen can be de-escalated, if necessary, to target the infecting bacteria (directed therapy).

**TABLE 18-2.** Preliminary Identification of Medically Important Bacteria Using Gram Stain Results

| GRAM STAIN RESULT | LIKELY BACTERIAL PATHOGEN |
|---|---|
| **Gram-positive (stain purple)** | |
| Gram-positive cocci in clusters | *Staphylococcus* spp.<br>**Coagulase-positive:** *S aureus*<br>**Coagulase-negative:** *S epidermidis, S hominis, S saprophyticus, S haemolyticus, S lugdunensis,* etc. |
| Gram-positive cocci in pairs | *Streptococcus pneumoniae* |
| Gram-positive cocci in chains | Viridans (α-hemolytic) streptococci (*S milleri, S mutans, S salivarius, S mitis,* etc.)<br>Group (β-hemolytic) streptococci (*S pyogenes* [group A], *S agalactiae* [group B], groups C, F, and G streptococci)<br>*Finegoldia magna, Peptostreptococcus* spp., *Peptoniphilus* spp., *Parvimonas micra* |
| Gram-positive cocci in pairs and chains | *Enterococcus* spp. (*E faecalis, E faecium, E durans, E gallinarum, E avium, E casseliflavus, E raffinosus*) |
| **Gram-positive bacilli** | |
| Nonspore-forming | *Corynebacterium* spp. (*C diphtheriae, C jeikeium, C striatum,* etc.)<br>*Lactobacillus* spp.<br>*Listeria monocytogenes*<br>*Cutibacterium* spp. |
| Spore-forming | *Bacillus* spp. (*B anthracis, B cereus,* etc.)<br>*Clostridium* spp. (*C perfringens, C tetani*)<br>*Clostridioides* spp. (*C difficile*)<br>*Streptomyces* spp. |
| Branching, filamentous | *Actinomyces* spp. (*A israelii*)<br>*Erysipelothrix rhusiopathiae*<br>*Nocardia* spp. (*N asteroides*) |
| **Gram-negative (stain red)** | |
| Gram-negative cocci | *Neisseria* spp. (*N gonorrhoeae, N meningitidis,* etc.)<br>*Veillonella* spp. (*V parvula*) |
| Gram-negative coccobacilli | *Haemophilus* spp. (*H influenzae, H parainfluenzae, H ducreyi,* etc.)<br>*Moraxella catarrhalis* |
| **Gram-negative bacilli** | |
| Lactose-fermenting | *Aeromonas hydrophila*<br>*Citrobacter* spp. (*C freundii, C koseri*)<br>*Enterobacter* spp. (*E cloacae, E asburiae, E gergoviae, E taylorae*)<br>*Escherichia coli*<br>*Klebsiella* spp. (*K pneumoniae, K oxytoca, K aerogenes*)<br>*Pasteurella multocida*<br>*Vibrio cholerae* |
| Nonlactose-fermenting | *Acinetobacter* spp.<br>*Alcaligenes* spp.<br>*Burkholderia cepacia*<br>*Morganella morganii*<br>*Proteus* spp. (*P mirabilis, P vulgaris*)<br>*Pseudomonas* spp. (*P aeruginosa, P putida, P fluorescens*)<br>*Salmonella* spp. (*S typhi, S paratyphi, S enteritidis, S typhimurium*)<br>*Serratia marcescens*<br>*Shigella* spp. (*S dysenteriae, S sonnei*)<br>*Stenotrophomonas maltophilia* |

*(continued)*

**TABLE 18-2.** Preliminary Identification of Medically Important Bacteria Using Gram Stain Results, cont'd

| GRAM STAIN RESULT | LIKELY BACTERIAL PATHOGEN |
| --- | --- |
| Other gram-negative bacilli | *Bacteroides* spp. (*B fragilis, B thetaiotaomicron, B ovatus, B distasonis*)<br>*Brucella* spp.<br>*Bordetella* spp.<br>*Campylobacter jejuni*<br>*Francisella tularensis*<br>*Helicobacter pylori*<br>*Legionella* spp. |
| **Gram-variable (stain both gram-positive and gram-negative in the same smear)** | |
| Gram-variable bacilli | *Gardnerella vaginalis* |

*Source*: References 10,11.

In addition to providing a clue about the potential infecting organism, the Gram stain helps to determine the *presence* of bacteria in a biological specimen obtained from normally sterile body fluids (eg, CSF, pleural fluid, synovial fluid, and urine directly from the bladder) and from specimens in which infection is suspected (eg, abscess aspirate, wound swabs, sputum, and tissue); the number or relative quantity of infecting bacteria; the presence of WBCs; and the quality of the submitted specimen (eg, large numbers of epithelial cells in a sputum or urine sample may signify contamination).[1,4,6,7,9]

### Culture and Identification

The results from the Gram stain provide preliminary information regarding the potential infecting bacteria. For the bacteria to be definitively identified, the clinical specimen is also processed to facilitate bacterial growth in culture and then observed for growth characteristics (eg, type of media, aerobic versus anaerobic, shape and color of colonies) and reactions to biochemical testing. Under normal circumstances, the results of bacterial culture are typically available within 24 to 48 hours of specimen setup and processing.

For bacteria to be grown successfully in culture, the specific nutritional and environmental growth requirements of the bacteria must be taken into consideration.[3,4,8,12,13] Several clinical microbiology textbooks and reference manuals are available that can assist the microbiology laboratory with the selection of appropriate culture media and environmental conditions to facilitate the optimal growth of bacteria based on specimen type and suspected bacteria.[3,4,8,12]

Several types of primary culture media are available that enhance or optimize bacterial growth including nutritive media (blood or chocolate agar), differential media, selective media, and supplemental broth.[1,3,8,12,13] The most commonly used bacterial growth media are listed in **Table 18-3**.[1,3,8,12,13] Blood and chocolate agar plates are *nutritive* or *enrichment* media because they support the growth of many different types of aerobic and anaerobic bacteria. Blood agar is also considered to be *differential* media because it can distinguish between organisms based on certain growth characteristics, such as the differentiation

between streptococci based on hemolysis patterns. MacConkey, eosin methylene blue, colistin nalidixic acid, and phenylethyl alcohol agar plates are considered *selective* media because they preferentially support the growth of specific organisms (eg, gram-negative or gram-positive bacteria) through the use of antimicrobials, dyes, or alcohol incorporated into their media. Trypticase soy broth and thioglycollate broth are considered *supplemental* media because they are used for subculturing bacteria detected on agar plates or as back-up cultures to agar plates for the detection of small quantities of bacteria in biological specimens.

Once a clinical specimen is processed on growth media, the plates must be incubated in the appropriate environment to support bacterial growth. The environmental factors that should be controlled during incubation include oxygen or carbon dioxide content, temperature, pH, and moisture content of the medium and atmosphere.[1,12,13] The oxygen requirements for growth differ among organisms. Strict aerobic bacteria, such as *Pseudomonas aeruginosa*, grow best in ambient air containing 21% oxygen and a small amount of carbon dioxide.[1] Strict anaerobes, such as *Bacteroides* spp., are unable to grow in an oxygen-containing environment and require a controlled environment containing 5% to 10% carbon dioxide for optimal growth. Facultative anaerobes, such as *Escherichia coli* and some streptococci, can grow in the presence or absence of oxygen. Overall, most clinically relevant bacteria grow best at 35°C to 37°C (the temperature of the human body), with a pH of 6.5 to 7.5, and in an atmosphere rich in moisture, which is why agar plates are sealed (to trap moisture) and humidified incubators are used.[12] Bacteria grown successfully in culture appear as colonies on the agar plates.

Bacterial identification is based on the results of genotypic and phenotypic testing.[12] Genotypic bacterial identification tests use molecular techniques for the detection of a particular gene or RNA product that is characteristic of specific bacteria. Phenotypic bacterial identification tests involve the observation of the physical and metabolic properties of a bacteria, including the evaluation of colony characteristics (size, pigmentation, shape, and surface appearance); the assessment of culture

**TABLE 18-3.** Commonly Used Bacterial Growth Media

| GROWTH MEDIUM | COMPOSITION | USES |
|---|---|---|
| **Agars** | | |
| Blood agar, SBA | 5% sheep blood | The most commonly used all-purpose medium with ability to grow most bacteria, fungi, and some mycobacteria; also used for determination of hemolytic activity of streptococci |
| Chocolate agar, enriched | 2% hemoglobin or Iso-VitaleX in peptone base | All-purpose medium that supports growth of most bacteria; especially useful for growth of fastidious bacteria, such as *Haemophilus* spp., *Brucella* spp., and pathogenic *Neisseria* spp. |
| EMB or Mac agar | Peptone base with sugars and dyes that yield differentiating biochemical characteristics | Included in primary setup of nonsterile specimens; selective isolation of gram-negative bacteria; differentiates between lactose-fermenting and nonlactose-fermenting enteric bacteria |
| PEA or CNA agar | Nutrient agar bases with supplemental agents to inhibit growth of aerobic gram-negative bacteria | Included in primary setup of nonsterile specimens; selective isolation of gram-positive cocci and bacilli as well as anaerobic gram-positive cocci or gram-negative bacilli |
| **Broths** | | |
| TSB | All-purpose enrichment broth | Used for subculturing bacteria from primary agar plates; supports the growth of many fastidious and nonfastidious bacteria |
| Thioglycollate broth | Pancreatic digest of casein, soy broth, and glucose | Supports the growth of aerobic, anaerobic, microaerophilic, and fastidious bacteria |

CNA = colistin-nalidixic acid; EMB = eosin methylene blue; Mac = MacConkey; PEA = phenylethyl alcohol; SBA = sheep blood agar; TSB = trypticase soy broth.
*Source:* References 1,3,8,12,13.

media and environmental conditions that supported bacterial growth; the changes that occurred to the culture media as a result of bacterial growth; the aroma of the bacteria; the Gram stain result of individual colonies; and the results from biochemical testing.[3,12] Biochemical tests for bacterial identification are either enzyme based, in which the presence of a specific enzyme is measured (eg, catalase, oxidase, indole, or urease tests), or based on the presence and measurement of metabolic pathways or byproducts (eg, oxidative and fermentation tests or amino acid degradation).[3,12] Examples of biochemical tests include the presence of catalase in the organism or the ability of a bacteria to ferment glucose. Most biochemical tests are performed using manual or automated commercial (preferred) identification systems.[12,14] Some of the commercial identification systems consist of multicompartment biochemical tests in a single microtiter tray so that several biochemical tests can be performed simultaneously.[12,14] Information derived from the macroscopic examination of the bacteria and the results of biochemical tests are then combined to determine the specific identity of the bacteria. Using traditional methodology, bacterial identification is usually achieved within 24 to 48 hours of detection of bacterial growth.[12,13]

Numerous rapid diagnostic tests are available for identification of bacteria (with some tests also detecting several pertinent bacterial resistance genes) directly from clinical specimens such as blood, stool, respiratory secretions, or body fluids (ie, saliva, urine, CSF) using a variety of methodologies that have all been designed to substantially decrease the time to organism identification (with results in 15 minutes to 12 hours) when compared with traditional bacterial culture and identification methods.[3,11,14,15] Rapid diagnostic tests are highly sensitive and specific and have become important tools for antimicrobial stewardship programs because they allow for quicker antimicrobial de-escalation/discontinuation and implementation of infection control procedures, such as isolation, when necessary.[3,11,14,15] Rapid diagnostic tests are usually more costly than traditional bacterial identification methods; however, when they are used in conjunction with antimicrobial stewardship programs, the cost-effectiveness of many of the tests have been justified through faster optimization of antimicrobial therapy, improved patient outcomes, and overall lower hospital costs.[15,16]

The currently available rapid bacterial identification tests are immunologically based, nucleic acid (NA) based (nonamplified and amplified), or proteomic based.[3,12,14,16] Immunologic methods use immunofluorescent or enzyme-linked immunosorbent assay antigen or antibody detection. Immunologically based rapid bacterial identification tests are available for the detection of group A streptococcus (pharyngeal), *Streptococcus pneumoniae* (urine, respiratory), *Neisseria gonorrhoeae* (urethral, cervical), *Neisseria meningitidis* (CSF), *L. pneumophila* (urine), influenza/ respiratory syncytial virus (RSV) (nasopharyngeal), and other viruses (see respective sections within this chapter and Chapter 19 for additional information).

Some commonly used nonamplified bacterial identification methods using NA probes include peptide NA fluorescence in situ hybridization (PNA-FISH; PNA FISH and QuickFISH [Opgen, Gaithersburg, MD]), and Verigene (Luminex, Austin, TX).[3,14,16] PNA-FISH and QuickFISH detect species-specific RNA using fluorescent probes and can differentiate between commonly encountered bacteria from positive blood cultures after Gram stain. PNA-FISH and QuickFISH kits are available to differentiate between *Staphylococcus aureus* and coagulase-negative staphylococci from blood culture bottles with gram-positive cocci in clusters; *Enterococcus faecalis* versus *Enterococcus faecium* versus other enterococci from blood cultures positive for gram-positive cocci in pairs and chains; *E coli*, *K pneumoniae* versus *P aeruginosa* from blood cultures positive for gram-negative rods; and *Candida albicans/Candida parapsilosis* versus *Candida krusei/Candida glabrata* from blood cultures positive for yeast. PNA-FISH results are available within 90 minutes whereas QuickFISH results are available within 20 minutes of blood culture positivity.

Verigene (Luminex, Austin TX) is a novel microarray, multiplex test using NA extraction and array hybridization in a conserved genetic region of the bacteria or virus to differentiate among different species. Several Verigene tests are currently available for the rapid identification of bacteria (and viruses) causing infection in the bloodstream, respiratory tract, and GI tract. The Verigene Gram-Positive Bloodstream Infection Test (Luminex) can identify 13 different gram-positive bacterial species and the presence of three notable gram-positive resistance gene markers, namely *mecA* (methicillin-resistance), *vanA/ vanB* (vancomycin resistance) within 2.5 hours of blood culture positivity.[3,16] The Verigene Gram-Negative Bloodstream Infection Test (Luminex) can identify nine different gram-negative bacteria and the presence of six resistance gene markers (CTX-M β-lactamase and several carbapenemases) within 2 hours of blood culture positivity. Verigene tests are also available for rapid pathogen identification (within 2 hours) of respiratory tract infections (Verigene Respiratory Pathogens Flex Test with three bacterial and 13 viral targets); GI infections (Verigene Enteric Pathogens Test with five bacterial, two viral, and two toxin targets); and *C difficile* (with the ability to detect the presence of toxin A, toxin B, and polymerase chain reaction [PCR] ribotype 027 hypervirulent strain).

Multiple amplified NA-based tests, including PCR and other methods, are available for the rapid identification of bacteria (and occasionally the presence of resistance gene markers) and viruses.[16] Currently, the most comprehensive test is the FilmArray multiplex PCR system (BioFire Diagnostics, Salt Lake City,

UT), which integrates sample preparation, amplification, detection, and analysis into one process with results available within 1 hour.[3,16] FilmArray is available in several U.S. Food and Drug Administration (FDA)–approved panels for the quick identification of the causative pathogens of meningitis/encephalitis, bloodstream infections, respiratory tract infections, and GI tract infections (https://www.biofiredx.com/ products/filmarray/).

Lastly, matrix-assisted laser desorption-ionization time-of-flight (MALDI-TOF) mass spectrometry is a proteomic-based rapid pathogen identification test that has become widely used by many clinical microbiology labs because it is an inexpensive test that provides the quick identification of a large number of clinically relevant pathogens.[3,14] The bacteria are placed on a target plate with a matrix solution and then pulsed with a laser. The mass of the ionized particles produced by the laser differx based on the organism, and the pathogen and relative quantity within the sample can be identified within 10 to 30 minutes using a library of standard reference species.[14,16]

## Colonization, Contamination, or Infection

The growth of an organism from a submitted biologic specimen does not always indicate the presence of infection; it may represent the presence of *colonization or contamination*.[9,11] **Table 18-4** lists the anatomic sites, fluids, and tissues of the human body that are sterile, including the bloodstream, the CSF, internal organs and tissues, bone, synovial fluid, peritoneal fluid, pleural fluid, pericardial fluid, and urine taken directly from the bladder or kidney. Alternatively, other body sites, particularly those with a direct connection to the outside environment, are naturally colonized with microorganisms called *normal flora*. Normal bacterial flora can be found on the skin, in the oral cavity, and in the respiratory, GI, and genitourinary tracts and may be recovered from clinical specimens obtained from these areas. Examples of bacteria that typically colonize these body sites are listed in **Table 18-5**.[11,17] Typically, normal flora are harmless bacteria that rarely cause infection. They are often located in the same areas of the body as pathogenic bacteria and are thought to provide protection by inhibiting the growth of pathogenic organisms through competition for nutrients and by stimulating the production of cross-protective antibodies.[11,17] However, normal flora may potentially become pathogenic and cause infection in patients with suppressed immune systems or after translocation to normally sterile body sites during trauma, intravascular line

## TABLE 18-4. Normally Sterile Body Sites

| Bloodstream |
| --- |
| CSF |
| Pericardial fluid |
| Pleural fluid |
| Peritoneal fluid |
| Synovial fluid |
| Bone |
| Urine (directly from the bladder or kidney) |

**TABLE 18-5.** Body Sites with Normal Colonizing Bacterial Flora

| SKIN | ORAL CAVITY |
|---|---|
| *Corynebacterium* spp. | *Actinomyces* spp. |
| *Cutibacterium* spp. | *Prevotella* spp. |
| *Staphylococcus* spp. (especially coagulase-negative staphylococci) | Viridans streptococci |
|  | Anaerobic streptococci |
|  | *Veillonella* spp. |
| *Streptococcus* spp. |  |

| RESPIRATORY TRACT | GI TRACT (COLON) |
|---|---|
| Viridans streptococci | *Bacteroides* spp. |
| Anaerobic streptococci | *Clostridium* spp. |
| *Haemophilus* spp. | *Escherichia coli* |
| *Neisseria* spp. | *Klebsiella pneumoniae* |
| *Moraxella* spp. | *Enterococcus* spp. |
|  | Anaerobic streptococci |

| GENITOURINARY TRACT |
|---|
| *Lactobacillus* spp. |
| *Streptococcus* spp. |
| *Staphylococcus* spp. |
| *Corynebacterium* spp. |
| *Enterobacterales* |
| *Mycoplasma hominis* |
| *Bacteroides* spp. |
| *Prevotella* spp. |

*Source:* References 11,17.

insertion, or surgical procedures, especially when the skin is not adequately cleansed in the latter two situations. Alternatively, pathogenic bacteria may occasionally *colonize* body sites, where they are present but do not invade host tissue or elicit signs and symptoms of infection (**Table 18-6**).

*Contamination* occurs when an organism is accidentally introduced into a biologic specimen during specimen collection, transport, or processing.[1,3,4,9,11] Bacteria that cause contamination typically originate from the skin of the patient (especially if the skin is not adequately cleaned before specimen acquisition), the clinician, or the laboratory technician but may also come from the environment. The most common contaminant is coagulase-negative staphylococci (especially *Staphylococcus epidermidis*), which is an organism that normally colonizes the skin.[17] Other common contaminants of blood culture specimens include *Micrococcus* spp., *Cutibacterium acnes*, and most *Bacillus* and *Corynebacterium* spp.[17]

*Infection* occurs when an organism is present and invades or damages host tissues, eliciting a host response and producing signs and symptoms consistent with an infectious process. When determining the presence of infection in an individual patient, several factors should be considered, such as the clinical condition of the patient (eg, fever and purulent discharge), the presence of laboratory signs of infection (eg, high WBC

**TABLE 18-6.** Clinical, Laboratory, and Radiographic Signs and Symptoms of Infection

| CLINICAL |
|---|

**Localized**

Pain and inflammation at site of infection: erythema, swelling, warmth

Purulent discharge (wound, vaginal, urethral discharge)

Sputum production and cough (pneumonia)

Diarrhea

Dysuria, frequency, urgency, suprapubic tenderness, costovertebral angle tenderness (UTI)

Headache, nuchal rigidity, photophobia, Brudzinski's sign, Kernig's sign (meningitis)

**Systemic**

Fever

Chills, rigors

Malaise

Tachycardia

Tachypnea

Hypotension

Mental status changes

| LABORATORY |
|---|

Increased WBC count: peripherally and/or at the site of infection

Decreased WBC count: occasionally, patients present with leukopenia

Increased neutrophil percentage, including an increase in immature neutrophils (bands or stabs) in the WBC differential called a "shift to the left"

Hypoxemia (pneumonia)

Elevated lactate

Positive Gram stain and/or culture from site of infection

Elevated ESR and CRP

Elevated procalcitonin levels

Positive antigen or antibody test, positive PCR test, elevated antibody titers

| RADIOGRAPHIC |
|---|

Chest radiograph with consolidation, infiltrate, effusion, or cavitary nodules (lung infection)

Bone radiograph or MRI: periosteal elevation or bone destruction (osteomyelitis)

CT/MRI: rim-enhancing lesions (abscess)

CT = computed tomography; MRI = magnetic resonance imaging.

count), and the results of radiographic and microbiologic tests.[18] Table 18-6 describes some of the local and systemic clinical signs and symptoms, laboratory findings, and radiographic findings that may be present in a patient with infection. The exact clinical, laboratory, and radiographic signs of infection differ based on the site of infection, the age of the patient, and the severity of the infection. For example, a patient with pneumonia usually exhibits a fever, productive cough, shortness of breath, tachypnea, leukocytosis, and an infiltrate on chest radiograph, whereas a patient with an uncomplicated urinary tract infection (UTI) typically experiences urinary frequency, urgency, dysuria, and pyuria. It is important to note that the typical signs and symptoms of infection may not be present in elderly persons or in patients who are immunocompromised (eg, patients with neutropenia and patients with acquired immune deficiency syndrome).

False-positive culture results can lead to the use of additional laboratory tests, radiographic tests, unnecessary antibiotics, increased length of hospitalization, and patient costs; therefore, every positive culture should warrant an evaluation for clinical significance. The diagnosis of infection should be suspected in any patient with a positive culture accompanied by clinical, laboratory, and radiographic findings suggestive of infection. Luckily, certain bacteria have a propensity to cause infection in particular body sites and fluids, as demonstrated in **Table 18-7**.[4,18,19] This information

## TABLE 18-7. Common Pathogens by Site of Infection

| MOUTH | SKIN AND SOFT TISSUE | BONE AND JOINT |
|---|---|---|
| Anaerobic streptococci<br>*Peptococcus* spp.<br>*Peptostreptococcus* spp.<br>*Actinomyces israelii* | *Staphylococcus aureus*<br>*Streptococcus pyogenes*<br>*Staphylococcus epidermidis*<br>*Pasteurella multocida*<br>*Clostridium* spp. | *Staphylococcus aureus*<br>*Streptococcus pyogenes*<br>*Streptococcus* spp.<br>*Staphylococcus epidermidis*<br>*Neisseria gonorrhoeae*<br>Gram-negative bacilli |
| **INTRA-ABDOMINAL** | **URINARY TRACT** | **UPPER RESPIRATORY TRACT** |
| *Escherichia coli*<br>*Proteus mirabilis*<br>*Klebsiella* spp.<br>*Enterococcus* spp.<br>*Bacteroides* spp.<br>*Clostridium* spp. | *Escherichia coli*<br>*Proteus mirabilis*<br>*Klebsiella* spp.<br>*Enterococcus* spp.<br>*Staphylococcus saprophyticus* | *Streptococcus pneumoniae*<br>*Haemophilus influenzae*<br>*Moraxella catarrhalis*<br>*Streptococcus pyogenes* |
| **LOWER RESPIRATORY TRACT, COMMUNITY-ACQUIRED** | **LOWER RESPIRATORY TRACT, HOSPITAL-ACQUIRED** | **MENINGITIS** |
| *Streptococcus pneumoniae*<br>*Haemophilus influenzae*<br>*Moraxella catarrhalis*<br>*Klebsiella pneumoniae*<br>*Legionella pneumophila*<br>*Mycoplasma pneumoniae*<br>*Chlamydia pneumoniae* | **Early onset (within 4 days of hospitalization)**<br>  *Klebsiella pneumoniae*<br>  *Escherichia coli*<br>  *Enterobacter* spp.<br>  *Proteus* spp.<br>  *Serratia marcescens*<br>  *Haemophilus influenzae*<br>  *Streptococcus pneumoniae*<br>  MSSA<br>**Late onset (> 4 days after hospitalization)**<br>  Pathogens above plus MDR organisms:<br>  *Acinetobacter* spp.<br>  *Pseudomonas aeruginosa*<br>  MRSA<br>  *Legionella pneumophila* | *Streptococcus pneumoniae*<br>*Neisseria meningitidis*<br>*Haemophilus influenzae*<br>Group B Streptococcus<br>*Escherichia coli*<br>*Listeria monocytogenes* |

MDR = multidrug resistant; MRSA = methicillin-resistant *Staphylococcus aureus*; MSSA = methicillin-susceptible *Staphylococcus aureus*.
*Source:* References 4,18,19.

can be used to determine if the bacteria isolated from a culture is a commonly encountered pathogen at the particular site of infection.[8] For instance, the growth of *S pneumoniae* from the sputum of a patient with signs and symptoms consistent with community-acquired pneumonia (CAP) is a significant finding because *S pneumoniae* is the most common cause of CAP. However, the growth of *S epidermidis* from a blood or wound culture from an asymptomatic patient should be evaluated for clinical significance because it may represent contamination of the submitted specimen.[11,18] The information in Table 18-7 regarding the most common causative organisms by infection site can also be used to select empiric antibiotic therapy before culture results are available by guiding the selection of an antibiotic regimen with activity against the most common causative bacteria at the suspected site of infection, as illustrated in **Minicase 1**.[19]

Occasionally, culture results may be negative in patients with infection, particularly in the setting of previous antibiotic use, improper specimen collection, or the submission of inadequate specimens. In this setting, the clinical condition of the patient may establish the presence of infection despite negative cultures, and the suspected site of infection should help guide antibiotic therapy based on most likely causative organisms that typically cause infection at that site.[9]

## Antimicrobial Susceptibility Testing

Once an organism has been cultured from a biologic specimen, further testing is performed in the microbiology laboratory to determine antibiotic susceptibility of the infecting organism to help direct and streamline antimicrobial therapy. Because of the continued emergence of resistance in some bacteria, susceptibility testing is imperative for determining the antimicrobial agents that should be used for the treatment of the patient's infection. Several methods are available for determining antibiotic susceptibility of a particular organism by either directly measuring the activity of an antibiotic against the organism or detecting the presence of a specific resistance gene/mechanism in the organism, as described in **Table 18-8**.[9,11,20-25] Microbiology laboratories often use several different methods for susceptibility testing to accurately determine the activity of antibiotics against many different types of bacteria (eg, aerobic, anaerobic, and fastidious). The Clinical and Laboratory Standards Institute (CLSI) continuously updates and publishes standards and guidelines for the susceptibility testing of aerobic and anaerobic bacteria to assist microbiology laboratories in determining the specific antibiotics and test methods that should be used for particular organisms or specific clinical situations/infections.[26-28]

## Methods That Directly Measure Antibiotic Activity

Several tests directly measure the activity of an antibiotic against a particular organism. *Quantitative* tests measure the exact concentration of an antibiotic necessary for inhibiting the growth of

---

## MINICASE 1

### Choosing Empiric Antibiotic Therapy for Hospital-Acquired Pneumonia

Marie A., a 68-year-old woman with no known drug allergies, is admitted to the general medical floor of University Hospital for management of a right cerebral vascular accident after stabilization in the emergency department. Prior to admission, she was living at home with her husband and was previously healthy without recent hospitalizations or antibiotic therapy within the past few years. She continues to have left-sided hemiparesis and has been deemed to be an aspiration risk by physical therapy/occupational therapy. On hospital day 3, she develops a temperature of 102.3°F, chills, tachypnea, a productive cough, and shortness of breath requiring supplemental oxygen via nasal cannula. Her physical exam reveals an increased respiration rate (RR) of 24 breaths/min and decreased breath sounds in the right middle lobe. Her laboratory results reveal a total WBC count of 18,000 cells/mm³ with 70% neutrophils, 19% bands, 7% lymphocytes, and 4% monocytes. Her chest radiograph demonstrates right middle lobe consolidation consistent with pneumonia. An expectorated sputum sample is obtained for Gram stain and culture. The Gram stain reveals >25 WBC/hpf, <10 epi/hpf, and many gram-negative rods. Her physician asks you to recommend empiric antibiotic therapy to treat her pneumonia before the final culture results are available.

QUESTION: What is the most likely causative organism of this patient's pneumonia, and which empiric antibiotic therapy would you choose based on the Gram stain results?

DISCUSSION: This patient most likely has early-onset (within 4 days of hospitalization) HAP, in which the most common causative organisms (Table 18-7) include *S pneumoniae; H influenzae*; gram-negative bacteria such as *K pneumoniae, E coli, Enterobacter* spp., *S marcescens*, and *Proteus* spp.; *S aureus* (methicillin-susceptible *Staphylococcus aureus*); and atypical bacteria such as *L pneumophila* (especially in patients with diabetes mellitus, underlying lung disease, renal failure, or suppressed immune systems). Based on the Gram stain results (Table 18-2) demonstrating the presence of gram-negative rods (not unexpected because gram-negative bacteria are the most common cause of HAP overall), the most likely causative organisms include *K pneumoniae, E coli, Enterobacter* spp., *S marcescens*, or *Proteus* spp. Based on the most recent Infectious Diseases Society of America guidelines for the management of HAP, the patient should receive empiric therapy with piperacillin–tazobactam, cefepime, or a fluoroquinolone (levofloxacin) because she is not at high risk for mortality from HAP (not on ventilatory support or in septic shock) and does not have risk factors for a multidrug-resistant organism.[19] The antibiotic regimen can be modified to more directed therapy, if possible, once the results of the culture and susceptibility are available.

## TABLE 18-8. Antimicrobial Susceptibility Testing Methods

**Methods that directly measure antibiotic activity**

*Dilution susceptibility tests:* broth macrodilution (tube dilution), broth microdilution, agar dilution

*Disk diffusion:* Kirby-Bauer

*Antibiotic concentration gradient methods:* Etest

*Other specialized tests:*

Measure bactericidal activity: MBC testing, time-kill studies, SBT

Susceptibility testing of antibiotic combinations (synergy testing): checkerboard technique, time-kill curve technique, disk diffusion, Etest

**Methods that detect the presence of antibiotic resistance or resistance mechanisms**

β-lactamase detection

Detection of HLAR

Agar screens for detection of MRSA or VRE

Chloramphenicol acetyltransferase detection

Molecular methods involving NA hybridization and amplification

Penicillin-binding protein (PBP) 2a

Inducible clindamycin resistance

Etest = epsilometer test; HLAR = high-level aminoglycoside resistance; MBC = minimum bactericidal concentration; NA = nucleic acid; SBT = serum bactericidal tests; VRE = vancomycin-resistant enterococci.
*Source*: References 9,11,20–25.

the bacteria whereas *qualitative* tests measure the comparative inhibitory activity of several antibiotics against the organism. The format of the reported test results and interpretation of susceptibility from each of these methods is different depending on the methodology used. The advantages and disadvantages of the different antimicrobial susceptibility testing methods are listed in **Table 18-9**.[9,11,20,25,29,30]

### Dilution Methods (Macrodilution and Microdilution)

Several dilution methods measure the activity of an antibiotic against a particular organism. Both broth dilution and agar dilution methods quantitatively measure the in vitro activity of antibiotics against a particular organism, with results reported as the minimum inhibitory concentration (MIC). Broth dilution can be performed using *macrodilution* or *microdilution*, in which the main differences between the methods include the volume of broth used, the number of antibiotics that can be simultaneously tested, and the manner in which the test results are generated and reported. The agar dilution method differs in that it is performed using solid growth media.

**Broth macrodilution.** Broth macrodilution, or the tube-dilution method, is one of the oldest methods of antimicrobial susceptibility testing and is often considered the gold

standard. This method is performed in test tubes containing 2-fold serial dilutions of the antibiotic being tested for susceptibility (with concentrations typically representing clinically achievable serum or site concentrations of the antibiotic in mcg/mL) in a liquid growth media (1 mL of broth or greater) to which a standard inoculum ($5 \times 10^5$ CFU/mL) of the infecting bacteria is added.[9,20,25-27,29] The test tubes are incubated for 16 to 24 hours at 35°C and then examined macroscopically for the presence of turbidity or cloudiness, which is an indication of bacterial growth.[11,20,25,27,29] The test tube containing the lowest antibiotic concentration that completely inhibits visible growth (the broth in the tube appears clear to the unaided eye) represents the MIC in mcg/mL (**Figure 18-1**).[9,20,25,27,29]

The CLSI has established interpretive criteria for MIC results of each antibiotic against each bacteria as susceptible (S), susceptible-dose dependent (SDD), intermediate (I), and resistant (R). The MIC value that separates or defines these categories for an antibiotic are known as *MIC breakpoints*.[20,21,25,26] MICs have been categorized as S, SDD, I, and R to help predict the probable response of a patient's infection to a particular antibiotic.[9,21,25,26] Bacteria that are categorized as susceptible to a given antibiotic will, most likely, be eradicated during treatment of the infection because concentrations of the antibiotic represented by the MIC are easily achievable using standard doses of the antibiotic. Susceptible-dose dependent is a category applied to specific antibiotic-organism pairs (eg, cefepime and *Enterobacterales*) in which several approved or routinely used dosing options are available. Bacteria that are categorized as SDD require treatment with higher and/or more frequent doses (usually higher doses than were used when establishing the S breakpoint) to achieve higher drug exposures for treatment of the infection. Intermediately susceptible bacteria display higher MICs, and successful treatment may be achieved if higher than normal doses of an antibiotic are used or if the antibiotic concentrates at the site of infection.[25] In clinical practice, antibiotics that display intermediate susceptibility are rarely used for treatment of infection because clinical response is unpredictable; however, they may be considered for treatment when the organism displays resistance to all other agents tested. Lastly, organisms that are resistant to an antibiotic display extremely high MICs that exceed the normal achievable serum concentrations of the antibiotic, even if maximal doses are used, resulting in a poor clinical response. In general, it is the responsibility of the clinician to determine if a drug listed as susceptible from an individual isolate susceptibility report is useful for the treatment of a particular infection based on the pharmacokinetic parameters (site penetration) and clinical efficacy studies of the antibiotic for that infection type.

Minimum inhibitory concentration breakpoints for each antibiotic and bacteria are different because they are based on achievable serum concentrations of the antibiotic with normal dosing; the inherent susceptibility of the organism to the antibiotic; the site of infection and ability of the antibiotic to obtain adequate concentrations at that site; pharmacodynamic analysis with Monte Carlo simulations to predict efficacy; and the results of antibiotic clinical trials evaluating efficacy based on organism MIC.[20,21,26,27] The safe and effective dose of each antibiotic is

**TABLE 18-9.** Advantages and Disadvantages of Antimicrobial Susceptibility Testing Methods

| METHOD | ADVANTAGES | DISADVANTAGES |
|---|---|---|
| Agar dilution | An exact MIC is generated<br><br>Several isolates can be tested simultaneously on the same plate at a relatively low cost<br><br>Susceptibility of fastidious bacteria can be determined because agar supports their growth | Time-consuming<br><br>Antibiotic plates need to be prepared manually when needed and can be stored only for short periods of time<br><br>Plates are not commercially available; must be prepared by the laboratory |
| Broth macrodilution (tube dilution) | An exact MIC is generated<br><br>The MBC can also be determined, if desired | Each antibiotic is tested individually<br><br>Method is labor and resource intensive |
| Broth microdilution (automated) | Simultaneously tests several antibiotics<br><br>Less labor and fewer resources are used<br><br>Commercially prepared trays or cards can be used | MIC range (rather than exact MIC) is typically reported<br><br>The number of antibiotics and concentrations that are tested are predetermined and limited |
| Disk diffusion (Kirby-Bauer) | Simultaneously tests several antibiotics | Exact MICs cannot be determined<br><br>Cannot be used for fastidious or slow-growing bacteria |
| Etest | An exact MIC is generated<br><br>Easy to perform<br><br>Several antibiotics can be tested on the same plate | Relatively expensive<br><br>Not all antibiotics are available as Etest strips |

Etest = epsilometer test; MIC = minimum inhibitory concentration.
*Source:* References 9,11,20,25,29,30.

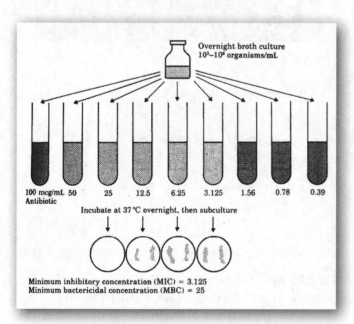

**FIGURE 18-1.** Broth macrodilution susceptibility testing for MIC and MBC. (*Source:* Reprinted with permission from Graman PS, Menegus MA. Microbiology laboratory tests. In: Betts RF, Chapman SW, Penn RL, eds. *A Practical Approach to Infectious Diseases.* 5th ed. Philadelphia, PA: Lippincott, Williams and Wilkins; 2003:929–956.)

typically determined using pharmacokinetic, safety, and efficacy data gathered during preclinical stages of drug development. Because each antibiotic has its own unique pharmacokinetic profile and recommended dosage range, it is not surprising that each antibiotic achieves different serum concentrations after standard dosing. For example, intravenously administered piperacillin–tazobactam achieves higher serum concentrations and area under the serum concentration time curve than intravenously administered levofloxacin. Therefore, the MIC susceptibility breakpoint for piperacillin–tazobactam against *Enterobacterales* is higher (≤16 mcg/mL) than levofloxacin (≤0.5 mcg/mL).[26]

As mentioned previously, there are other factors to consider when MIC breakpoints are established. Some antibiotics are inherently more active against an organism than others, which is reflected by a lower MIC required to inhibit bacterial growth. The site of infection may predict the potential usefulness of the antibiotic depending on its ability to achieve adequate concentrations at the site of infection. An antibiotic might display potent in vitro activity against a particular organism but may be ineffective in vivo due to poor penetration to the site of infection. In fact, there are a few clinical situations in which the site of infection is directly incorporated into the MIC susceptibility interpretation of an antibiotic, such as in the case of meningitis caused by *S pneumoniae* in which the interpretation of ceftriaxone and penicillin susceptibility are determined using meningitis MIC breakpoints (which are lower).[26] Monte Carlo simulations may also be performed to help establish MIC breakpoints. Analyses are performed using population pharmacokinetic data of the antibiotic and bacteria MIC distribution data from susceptibility studies to evaluate the percentage of time the antibiotic will achieve adequate pharmacodynamic indices for the treatment of that organism in a simulated population. Lastly, results from clinical trials evaluating antibiotic efficacy are also considered in MIC breakpoint determination where a correlation is made between clinical efficacy and the MIC value of the infecting organism. For example, what MICs were observed in patients with clinical success versus clinical failure?

Broth macrodilution is useful because an exact MIC of the infecting organism can be derived. The results of broth macrodilution are reported as the MIC of the antibiotic against the infecting organism with its corresponding interpretive category (S, I, and R). However, broth macrodilution is rarely used in microbiology laboratories because the methodology is resource and labor intensive, making it impractical for everyday use.

An additional step can be performed on the broth macrodilution test to determine the actual antibiotic concentration that kills 99.9% of the bacterial inoculum, which is also known as the minimum bactericidal concentration (MBC).[20,22,24] Samples from all of the test tubes that did not exhibit visible growth are subcultured on agar plates and incubated at 35°C for 18 to 24 hours (Figure 18-1).[9,22] The plate representing the lowest antibiotic concentration that does not support the growth of any bacterial colonies is defined as the MBC. Because a higher concentration of an antibiotic may be necessary to kill the organism rather than just inhibit its growth, the MIC will be equal to or lower than the MBC. The determination of the MBC is not routinely performed in clinical practice and may be considered in rare clinical circumstances, such as during the treatment of severe or life-threatening infections (eg, endocarditis, meningitis, osteomyelitis, or sepsis in immunocompromised patients) in patients who are not responding to therapy.[9,22,24]

***Broth microdilution.*** Broth microdilution susceptibility testing was developed to overcome some of the limitations of the broth macrodilution method and has become the most commonly used method for susceptibility testing of bacteria in microbiology laboratories.[11,20,25,27,29] Instead of using standard test tubes with 2-fold serial dilutions of antibiotics, this method uses manually prepared or commercially prepared disposable microtiter cassettes or trays containing up to 96 wells that can simultaneously test the susceptibility of up to 12 antibiotics depending on the product used.[11,20,25,27,29] Several examples of microtiter trays are shown in **Figure 18-2A** and **B**.[20] The wells in the broth microdilution trays contain a smaller volume of broth (0.05 to 0.1 mL) to support bacterial growth than broth macrodilution (1 mL or more). The microtiter tray is inoculated with a standardized inoculum of the infecting organism and incubated for 16 to 20 hours. The tray is then examined for bacterial growth by direct visualization using light boxes, direct visualization using reflecting mirrors, or automated, computer-assisted readers. The MIC represents the microdilution well containing the lowest antibiotic concentration that completely inhibits visible bacterial growth (eg,

did not produce turbidity). Several companies commercially supply broth microdilution panels that contain broth with appropriate antibiotic concentrations according to guidelines for conventional broth dilution methods. Some examples of manual/semiautomated systems include Sensititre OptiRead or Vizion System (Thermo Fisher Scientific, Waltham, MA) and MicroScan autoSCAN-4 (Beckman Coulter, Brea, CA). Examples of fully automated systems include Vitek 2 or Vitek-Legacy (bioMérieux Diagnostics, Marcy-l'Étoile, France), MicroScan WalkAway *plus* System (Beckman Coulter), Sensititre ARIS 2X (Thermo Fisher Scientific), and the Phoenix Automated Microbiology System (BD, Franklin Lakes, NJ).[20] Some of these systems also have been designed to identify bacteria and are able to provide more rapid susceptibility results (within 8 hours) due to shortened incubation times.

Because of the size constraints of the broth microdilution panels, only a limited number of antibiotics and concentrations can be incorporated into the trays. Typically, drugs that have

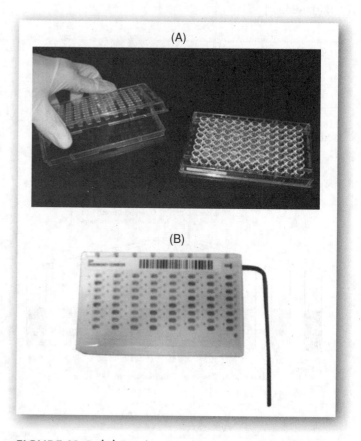

**FIGURE 18-2.** (A) Broth microdilution susceptibility panel containing 96 reagent wells and a disposable tray inoculator. (B) Example of the Vitek 2 antimicrobial susceptibility test card with 64 wells with multiple concentrations of up to 22 antibiotics. (*Source:* Reprinted with permission from Tile PM, ed. *Bailey and Scott's Diagnostic Microbiology*. 14th ed. St Louis, MO: Mosby Inc; 2017:177–204.)

inherent activity against the class of bacteria being tested (eg, gram-positive versus gram-negative) are included in the trays. For example, when determining the susceptibility of gram-negative bacteria, it is impractical to include antibiotics in the microdilution trays that do not have activity against these organisms, such as penicillin, nafcillin, or vancomycin. The same holds true for susceptibility testing of gram-positive organisms, where it would be impractical to test the susceptibility of piperacillin or ceftazidime against *S aureus* because these agents have limited antistaphylococcal activity. In addition, the trays are not large enough to incorporate the full range of antibiotic concentrations usually tested during broth macrodilution. Therefore, the concentrations incorporated into the wells for each antibiotic often reflect the CLSI interpretive category breakpoints of S, I, and R for the particular antibiotic-organism combination.

The results of broth microdilution tests are reported as either an exact MIC or MIC range with corresponding CLSI interpretation. In this case, an MIC range may be reported due to the limited antibiotic concentrations tested for each antibiotic. For example, if bacterial growth is not detected in the lowest concentration tested of a particular antibiotic using broth microdilution, the MIC would be reported as less than or equal to that concentration tested. The MIC could be much lower, but the exact MIC could not be determined because lower concentrations of the antibiotic were not tested because of the size constraints of the microdilution trays.

The advantages of broth microdilution include the ability to test the susceptibility of multiple antibiotics simultaneously, the ease of use when commercially prepared microdilution trays are used, rapid results with the automated methods, and decreased cost/labor.[20,25,27] The disadvantages of broth microdilution include the lack of flexibility of antibiotics available in commercially prepared microdilution trays, the limitation on the number of concentrations that can be tested for each antibiotic due to size constraints of the trays, and the reporting of an MIC range (on many occasions) rather than the true MIC against an infecting organism.[20,25]

***Agar dilution.*** Agar dilution is another quantitative susceptibility testing method that uses 2-fold serial dilutions of an antibiotic incorporated into agar growth medium, with each concentration placed into individual Petri dishes.[20,25,29] The surface of each plate is inoculated with a standardized bacterial inoculum ($1 \times 10^4$ CFU/mL) and incubated for 18 to 20 hours at 35°C. The susceptibility of several different bacteria can be evaluated simultaneously on the plates. The MIC is represented by the plate with the lowest concentration of antibiotic that does not support visible growth of the bacteria. The advantages of agar dilution include the ability to simultaneously test the susceptibility of several different bacteria, the ability to perform susceptibility testing of fastidious organisms given agar adequately supports their growth, and the generation of an exact MIC of the infecting bacteria. However, agar dilution is not commonly used in most microbiology laboratories because it is resource and labor intensive. In addition, the antibiotic plates are not commercially available and must be prepared before each susceptibility test because they can only be stored for short periods of time.[20,25,29]

### Disk Diffusion Method (Kirby-Bauer)

The *disk diffusion method* is a well-standardized and highly reproducible qualitative method of antimicrobial susceptibility testing. It was developed in 1966, before broth microdilution by Kirby and Bauer, in response to the need for a more practical susceptibility test capable of measuring the susceptibility of multiple antibiotics simultaneously.[20,25,28,29] Commercially prepared, filter paper disks containing a fixed concentration of an antibiotic are placed on solid media agar plates inoculated with a standardized inoculum of the infecting organism (1 to 2 × $10^8$ CFU/mL). The plates are large enough to accommodate up to 12 different antibiotic disks at the same time (**Figure 18-3**).[20] The plate is inverted to avoid moisture accumulation on the agar surface and incubated for 16 to 18 hours in ambient air at 35°C. During this incubation time, the antibiotic diffuses out of the disk into the surrounding media, with the highest concentration closest to the disk, as the bacteria multiply on the surface of the plates.[20,25,29] The bacteria grow only in areas on the plate where the concentrations of the antibiotic are too low to inhibit bacterial growth. At the end of incubation period, the plates are examined for the inhibition of bacterial growth by measuring the diameter (in millimeters) of the clear zone of inhibition surrounding each filter paper disk. In general, the larger the zone size, the more active the antibiotic is against the organism.

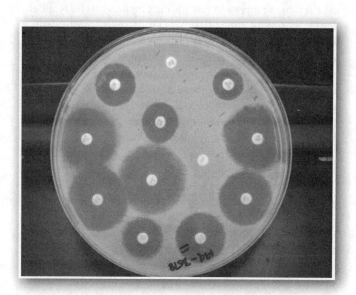

**FIGURE 18-3.** A disk diffusion test where the diameters of all zones of inhibition are measured and those values are translated to categories of susceptible, intermediate, or resistant using the tables published by the CLSI. (*Source*: Reprinted with permission from Tile PM, ed. *Bailey and Scott's Diagnostic Microbiology*. 14th ed. St Louis, MO: Mosby Inc; 2017:177–204.)

The diameter of the zone of inhibition has been correlated to the MIC of the antibiotic from broth or agar dilution against the infecting organism using regression analysis.[20,25,28,29] CLSI has established interpretive criteria based on this relationship to categorize zone diameters as S, I, and R for each antibiotic against each organism.[25,28,29] The results of disk diffusion test are considered qualitative because they only reveal the zone of inhibition and comparative activity of an antibiotic rather than an exact MIC.

The disk diffusion susceptibility test allows the simultaneous testing of several antibiotics in a relatively easy and inexpensive manner and provides flexibility in determining the antibiotics that will be tested for susceptibility, provided a filter paper disk for the desired antibiotic is available. However, the major disadvantages of disk diffusion include inability to generate an exact MIC and difficulty in determining the susceptibility of fastidious or slow-growing organisms.

### Antibiotic Concentration Gradient Methods

**Epsilometer test.** The Epsilometer test, or Etest (bioMérieux) combines the benefits of broth microdilution with the ease of disk diffusion.[11] The Etest method simultaneously evaluates the activity of numerous concentrations of an antibiotic using a single plastic strip impregnated on one side with a known, predefined concentration gradient of an antibiotic. One side of the Etest strip is marked with a numeric scale that depicts the concentration of antibiotic at that location on the reverse side of the test strip.[9,20,25] Like disk diffusion, the Etest strip is applied onto a solid media agar plate that has been inoculated with a standardized concentration of the infecting bacteria. Several Etest strips can be placed on the same agar plate to provide the simultaneous susceptibility testing of several antibiotics.[9,20,25] During overnight incubation, bacteria multiply on the agar plates as the antibiotic diffuses out of the Etest strip according to the concentration gradient. Bacterial growth occurs only in areas on the agar plate in which drug concentrations are below those required to inhibit growth. An elliptical zone of growth inhibition forms around the Etest strip where the MIC is read as the drug concentration where the ellipse intersects the plastic strip (**Figure 18-4A** and **B**).[20,25]

Etest results are reported as the exact MIC of the infecting bacteria with the corresponding CLSI susceptibility interpretation. The MIC results derived from the Etest correlate well with the results obtained using other susceptibility testing methods.[9,20,25] The advantages of the Etest method include its ease of use and the ability to evaluate the susceptibility of several antibiotics simultaneously as well as the fact that the results yield an exact MIC, and the laboratory can choose the antibiotics to be tested. However, the Etest method is considerably more expensive than disk diffusion or broth microdilution methods, the results may be reader-dependent, and testing is limited to only those antibiotics for which an Etest strip is commercially available.

The Etest is currently used by some microbiology laboratories for the susceptibility testing of fastidious bacteria, such as *S pneumoniae*, *H influenzae*, and anaerobes, as well as for testing antibiotics in which a routine susceptibility test is not available (eg, antibiotic is not on standard broth microdilution panels used by the hospital) and when an exact MIC result is preferred.[9,25]

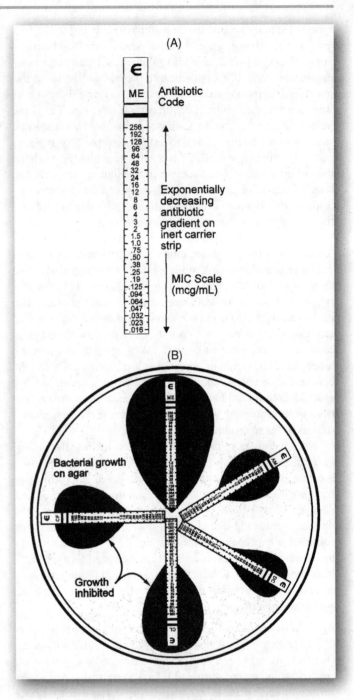

**FIGURE 18-4.** The Etest. (A) Individual Etest strips are placed on an inoculated agar surface. (B) After incubation, the MIC is read where the ellipse crosses the strip at the arrow. (*Source:* Reprinted with permission from Tile PM, ed. *Bailey and Scott's Diagnostic Microbiology.* 14th ed. St Louis, MO: Mosby Inc; 2017:177–204.)

### Specialized Susceptibility Tests

Additional tests may be performed in the microbiology laboratory to provide further information on the activity of an antibiotic against an organism. These specialty susceptibility tests may measure the bactericidal activity of the antibiotic (eg, MBC testing, time-kill curves, and serum bactericidal tests [SBTs]) or the activity of a combination of antibiotics against an infecting organism (eg, synergy testing using the checkerboard technique or time-kill studies). These tests are not routinely performed in most microbiology laboratories due to biological and technical difficulties, complexity in the interpretation of the results, and uncertain clinical applicability.[22-24,31]

***Testing methods for determining bactericidal activity.*** Several methods measure the direct killing activity of an antibiotic against an organism and, if used, should be performed only for antibiotics that are generally considered to be bactericidal. As noted earlier, there are only a limited number of clinical circumstances in which this information may be useful. The determination of bactericidal activity may have the best clinical utility in the treatment of infections at anatomic sites where host defenses are minimal or absent, such as endocarditis, meningitis, and osteomyelitis, as well as in the treatment of severe and life-threatening infections in immunocompromised patients.[9,20,22-24,31] Testing methods that determine the bactericidal activity of an antibiotic include the MBC test, time-kill assays, and SBTs.[20,22-24,31]

The MBC is the lowest concentration of an antibacterial agent that kills 99.9% of the bacterial inoculum, which represents a ≥3 log reduction in the original inoculum.[11,22] The methodology for determination of the MBC has been previously described in detail in the section on broth macrodilution because it is an extension of that test. CLSI has developed guidelines to standardize the methodology for MBC testing.[31] If the MBC is ≥32 times higher than the MIC or exceeds the achievable serum concentrations of the antibiotic, "tolerance" may be observed.[20] Tolerance occurs when a normally bactericidal antibiotic only can inhibit the growth of bacteria based on MBC testing. MBC testing is not routinely performed by most laboratories because it is labor intensive with limited clinical use.[20,22,31]

Time-kill studies, also known as *time-kill curves*, measure the rate of bacterial killing over a specified period of time, which is in contrast to the MBC that measures the bactericidal activity at a single point in time following an incubation period.[20,24,31] For time-kill studies, a standardized bacterial inoculum is placed into test tubes containing broth with several different concentrations of an antibiotic (usually the MIC and multiples of the MIC in separate tubes). Samples of the antibiotic-broth solutions are obtained at predetermined time intervals to evaluate the number of viable bacterial colonies present over the 24-hour incubation period.[11,20,24,31] The number of viable bacteria present at each time point are plotted over time to determine the rate and extent of bacterial killing of the antibiotic against the organism. A ≥3 log reduction in viable bacterial counts is representative of bactericidal activity.[11,20,24,31] Because it is labor and resource intensive, this test is not routinely performed in many clinical microbiology laboratories, but it is often used in the research setting.

The SBT, or Schlichter's test, is similar to MIC and MBC testing, except the SBT measures the bacterial killing activity of the patient's serum against their infecting organism after receiving a dose of an antibiotic.[9,20,23,24,31-33] The methodology is similar to determining the MIC using broth macrodilution, but dilutions of the patient's serum are used instead of 2-fold serial dilutions of an antibiotic.[9,24,31-33] The patient's serum is obtained at predefined intervals before and after a dose of an antibiotic, specifically at the time of expected peak concentration and at the time of expected trough concentration. The patient's serum is then serially diluted and inoculated with a standardized concentration of the infecting organism. The SBT is the highest dilution of the patient's serum that reduces the original standardized bacterial inoculum by ≥99.9%. The results of the SBT are reported as a titer, which represents the number of 2-fold serial dilutions of the patient's serum that led to bacterial killing (eg, SBT = 1:16), with a higher titer indicating better activity against the organism.[20,22,24,31-33] The CLSI has developed methodology standards for performance of the SBT.[31,33] However, this test is not routinely performed by most microbiology laboratories because of technical difficulties. In addition, limited inconclusive data has been published regarding the clinical usefulness of SBTs in guiding therapy (only a few studies in the treatment of endocarditis, osteomyelitis, and serious infections in febrile neutropenia).[22-24,31-33]

***Antimicrobial combination testing (synergy testing).*** In the treatment of bacterial infections, there are several clinical situations in which combination antimicrobial therapy may be used. The decision to use combination therapy is primarily based on the severity of infection, the causative organism, and the type of infection. The potential benefits of combination antibiotic therapy include (1) expanding the antimicrobial spectrum of activity, especially empiric therapy for a life-threatening infection or for the treatment of polymicrobial infections; (2) producing synergistic bactericidal activity with the combination that is not observed with each agent alone, such as the use of ampicillin and gentamicin for the treatment of Enterococcal endocarditis; and (3) decreasing the emergence of resistant organisms, which has been observed in the treatment of tuberculosis (TB).[24] Routine antimicrobial susceptibility tests measure the activity of an antibiotic against a particular organism. There are several tests, however, that evaluate the effects of combination antimicrobial therapy against an infecting organism (*synergy testing*), with the results being expressed as one of three types of activity[11,20]:

1. **Synergy:** The activity of the antimicrobial agents in combination is significantly greater than the additive effects of each agent alone.

2. **Indifference:** The activity of the antimicrobial agents in combination is similar to the additive effects of each agent alone.

3. **Antagonism:** The activity of the antimicrobial agents in combination is less than the additive effects of each agent alone.

Therefore, before two antibiotics are used together, it may be useful to determine the effects of the combined antibiotics against the infecting organism, especially because some antibacterial combinations may produce suboptimal effects.

Synergy testing of an antimicrobial combination can be performed using the checkerboard technique, the time-kill curve technique, the disk diffusion assay, or the Etest method, with the checkerboard and time-kill curve techniques being most often used.[20,24] The checkerboard technique is performed in macrodilution tubes or microdilution plates containing serial dilutions of the antibiotics alone and in combination. The tubes or plates are incubated with a standardized inoculum of the infecting bacteria for 24 hours. The effect of the antibiotic combination is determined by comparing the MICs of the agents when used in combination with the MICs of each agent alone. A synergistic combination displays lower MICs than when each agent is used alone. The time-kill curve method for combination therapy is similar to the time-kill curve method used to determine the rate of bacterial killing of a single agent, except that two antibiotics are added to the tubes in fixed concentrations. The effect of the antibiotic combination is determined by comparing the time-kill rates of combination therapy with the time-kill rates of each agent alone. A synergistic combination displays 100-fold or more killing activity than the most potent agent tested alone.[11,20] In the clinical setting, synergy testing methods are not routinely performed due to their tedious, time-consuming methodologies, their expense, and their limited clinical applicability in predicting clinical outcome.[11,20,24]

## Methods Detecting the Presence of Antibiotic Resistance Mechanisms

### Detection of β-Lactamase Activity

To date, more than 2,700 different β-lactamase enzymes have been characterized.[34] β-lactamase enzymes can be chromosomally-, plasmid-, or transposon-mediated and may be produced constitutively or inducibly. These enzymes cause hydrolysis of the cyclic amide bond in the β-lactam ring and, depending on the type of enzyme, may result in inactivation of one or numerous β-lactam antibiotics. It is important to understand the consequences of detecting a particular β-lactamase enzyme in an organism because certain enzymes produce resistance only to certain antimicrobials.[20,23,34,35]

Several methods detect the presence of β-lactamase enzyme depending on the organism and type of β-lactamase enzyme suspected. Some tests directly detect the presence of β-lactamase activity whereas others predict the presence of certain β-lactamase enzymes (such as the inducible AmpCs or the extended-spectrum β-lactamases [ESBLs]) based on resistance patterns and MICs derived from routine susceptibility tests.

The assays that directly detect β-lactamase activity include the acidimetric, iodometric, and chromogenic tests, which all measure the presence of β-lactamase enzyme by observing a color change based on reactions to different substrates.[20,36] The chromogenic test is the most common test used by microbiology laboratories because of its reliability in detecting β-lactamase enzymes produced by many different bacteria.[20,36] The chromogenic tests use chromogenic cephalosporins (nitrocefin, cefesone, or cefinase) incorporated into filter paper disks or strips that produce a color change when they are hydrolyzed by β-lactamase enzymes present in a clinical specimen once inoculated onto the disk or strip. Test tube assays using chromogenic cephalosporins can also be also used. A positive reaction using one of these direct β-lactamase tests for *H influenzae*, *Moraxella*

*catarrhalis*, and *N gonorrhoeae* predicts resistance to only penicillin, ampicillin, and amoxicillin but not to other β-lactam antibiotics that are more stable to β-lactamase enzymes. A positive β-lactamase test for *Staphylococcus* spp. predicts resistance to penicillin, ampicillin, amoxicillin, carbenicillin, ticarcillin, and piperacillin.

Extended-spectrum β-lactamases are plasmid-encoded β-lactamase enzymes (eg, TEM, SHV, CTX-M) that hydrolyze most penicillins, cephalosporins (except the cephamycins and cefepime), and aztreonam.[35] Historically, routine susceptibility tests using CLSI breakpoints did not reliably detect ESBL-producing organisms. Therefore, new CLSI interpretive criteria using lower MIC breakpoints for several cephalosporins and aztreonam for *Enterobacterales* were recently introduced to better detect resistance and obviate the need for ESBL screening and confirmatory tests (except for infection control or epidemiologic purposes). CLSI guidelines also outline criteria for performing screening and confirmatory tests for ESBLs that involve MIC and disk diffusion screening breakpoints for particular antibiotics using β-lactamase inhibitors.[21,23,26-28,36,37] However, false-negative results may occur with these phenotypic ESBL confirmatory tests in the presence of an AmpC enzyme, which is not inhibited by clavulanic acid.[23] Several automated susceptibility test systems, such as Vitek 2 and the Phoenix System, contain phenotypic ESBL detection tests that, when used with expert system software, are able to accurately detect ESBLs.[37]

AmpC β-lactamases are chromosomal- or plasmid-mediated β-lactamase enzymes that hydrolyze first-, second-, and third-generation cephalosporins and cephamycins, and also display resistance to some currently available β-lactamase-inhibitors, such as clavulanic acid, sulbactam, and tazobactam. Several gram-negative bacteria, such as *S marcescens*, *P aeruginosa*, indole-positive *Proteus* spp., *Acinetobacter* spp., *Citrobacter freundii*, and *Enterobacter* spp. (often referred to as the *SPICE* or *SPACE* bacteria) contain chromosomally-mediated, inducible AmpC enzymes that, when hyperproduced, can also hydrolyze penicillins and aztreonam in addition to the cephalosporins and cephamycins listed previously.[37] AmpC hyperproduction can occur during the treatment of infection due to one of these organisms, especially when a strong inducer such as ceftazidime or clavulanic acid is used.[35] Plasmid-mediated AmpC enzymes have also been reported in *Klebsiella* spp., *Proteus mirabilis*, *Citrobacter koseri*, and *Salmonella* spp., and often display an antibiotic susceptibility profile similar to chromosomally-mediated AmpC hyperproducers.[37] All SPICE and SPACE bacteria should be assumed to be AmpC producers, so specific detection of AmpC production is not recommended.[37] However, plasmid-mediated AmpC β-lactamases can be detected by demonstrating cephamycin hydrolysis using the AmpC disk test, the modified Hodge test (MHT), or the three-dimensional test.[37]

Carbapenemase enzymes have also emerged that may be chromosomal- (*Stenotrophomonas maltophilia*) or plasmid-mediated (eg, *Pseudomonas aeruginosa*, *Acinetobacter* spp., *Klebsiella pneumoniae*, etc.). Several plasmid-mediated carbapenemase enzymes have been characterized (KPC, VIM, OXA-4, NDM, and IMP) that hydrolyze carbapenems and most other β-lactam antibiotics, as well as display resistance to multiple other antibiotic classes.[34,37] The modified Hodge test can be used for carbapenemase detection on isolates with elevated carbapenem MICs; however, it cannot differentiate between carbapenemase types.[23,37]

Because of the wide diversity of β-lactamase enzymes and the potential limitations of phenotypic ESBL-, AmpC-, and carbapenemase detection methods, several commercial tests have been developed to aid in the detection these enzymes, some of which include the RAPIDEC CARBA NP (bioMérieux, Durham, NC; phenotypic, colorimetric test that detects KPC, NDM, VIM, IMP, and OXA-48), Check-MDR assay (Wageningen, The Netherlands; microarray that detects TEM, SHV, CTX-M, some AmpCs, and NDM, VIM, IMP, OXA-48, and KPC), Expert CarbaR (Cepheid, Sunnyvale, CA; PCR that detects NDM, VIM, IMP, and OXA-48), FilmArray (bioMérieux; PCR that detects only KPC), and the Verigene (Luminex; PCR that detects CTX-M, KPC, NDM, VIM, OXA-48, and IMP).[38]

As mentioned earlier, the CLSI recently lowered the cephalosporin and carbapenem breakpoints for *Enterobacterales* in an attempt to better identify antibiotics with predictable efficacy against bacteria with multiple resistance mechanisms and eliminated the recommendation to perform specialized testing to detect ESBL-, AmpC-, or carbapenemase-mediated resistance. However, this recommendation has gained considerable criticism from many clinicians and microbiologists because detection of the exact mechanism of resistance is thought to be important for both treatment and epidemiologic purposes.[37]

## High-Level Aminoglycoside Resistance

Aminoglycosides display relatively poor activity against *Enterococcus* spp. due to poor intracellular uptake (intrinsic, moderate-level resistance), so they should not be used alone in the treatment of infections due to enterococci. In addition, enterococci can acquire resistance to aminoglycosides through acquisition of genes that code for aminoglycoside-modifying enzymes (acquired resistance), which often leads to elevated aminoglycoside MICs (high-level aminoglycoside resistance or HLAR).[23] Aminoglycosides (primarily gentamicin or streptomycin) may be considered with ampicillin, penicillin, or vancomycin to provide synergistic bactericidal activity, especially in the treatment of Enterococcal endocarditis or Enterococcal osteomyelitis. However, supplemental testing should be performed to detect the presence of HLAR, which predicts the lack of synergism between gentamicin or streptomycin and cell wall active agents against *Enterococcus* spp.[20,23]

The presence of HLAR can be evaluated using agar dilution (agar plates) or broth microdilution (wells) using high concentrations of gentamicin (500 mcg/mL) and streptomycin (2000 mcg/mL).[23] The plates or wells are inoculated with a standardized suspension of the infecting *Enterococcus* spp. and incubated for 24 hours in ambient air.[23] The growth of one or more *Enterococcus* spp. colonies on the agar plate or in the broth

microdilution well demonstrates the presence of HLAR, signifying that the corresponding aminoglycoside cannot be used with a cell-wall active agent to achieve synergistic bactericidal activity. HLAR can also be detected using a disk diffusion method in which disks containing high concentrations of gentamicin (120 mcg) and streptomycin (300 mcg) are used.[23] HLAR to gentamicin also confers resistance to tobramycin, netilmicin, and amikacin but not necessarily streptomycin, which should be tested independently.[23] Testing for HLAR is usually performed only on Enterococcal isolates from infections that may require combination bactericidal activity, such as bacteremia, endocarditis, osteomyelitis, or meningitis.[23]

## Tests for the Detection of MRSA, VISA, VRSA, and VRE

Several tests are available that can quickly detect or confirm the presence of methicillin-resistant *S aureus* (MRSA) or vancomycin-resistant enterococci (VRE). For the detection or confirmation of MRSA, the cefoxitin disk diffusion test, oxacillin–salt agar screening tests, culture-based chromogenic media, rapid latex agglutination (LA) tests, or molecular methods using real-time PCR can be used.[23,30,39]

The cefoxitin disk diffusion test is performed using routine CLSI procedures, with modified interpretive criteria used to detect *mecA*-mediated resistance in MRSA in which MRSA is reported for *S aureus* strains with a zone size of ≤21 mm.[23,28] This test has also been useful in detecting methicillin-resistance in some coagulase-negative staphylococci.[23] The oxacillin–salt agar screening tests have been widely used for the detection of *mecA*-mediated resistance MRSA, but they appear to lack sensitivity for the detection of strains that exhibit heteroresistance.[23] A standard inoculum of *S aureus* is inoculated onto an agar plate containing Mueller-Hinton agar supplemented with 4% sodium chloride and 6 mcg/mL of oxacillin and incubated in ambient air at 33°C to 35°C for 24 hours.[23] The growth of more than one colony indicates MRSA, which also confers resistance to nafcillin, oxacillin, cloxacillin, dicloxacillin, and all cephalosporins excluding ceftaroline. However, this test is not recommended for the detection of methicillin-resistance in other *Staphylococcus* spp.[23]

Selective chromogenic media are available to detect MRSA from surveillance specimens, all of which produce a characteristic pigment in the presence of MRSA with results available within 24 hours.[23] There are also numerous rapid commercial LA tests to detect MRSA in clinical specimens by using highly specific monoclonal antibodies for the detection of penicillin-binding protein (PBP) 2a (also termed *PBP 2'*), the protein encoded by the *mecA* gene in MRSA.[23,39]

Several molecular tests for the detection of MRSA are commercially available that detect the *mecA* resistance determinant.[38] Depending on the test, they may be used for surveillance testing (detecting colonization) or for the diagnosis of infection. Some examples of common molecular MRSA surveillance tests include the GeneOhm MRSA Assay (BD), the Xpert MRSA (Cepheid, Sunnyvale, CA), and the LightCycler MRSA Advanced Test (Roche Diagnostics, Indianapolis, IN), which all are FDA-approved PCR assays for the rapid, direct detection of nasal colonization by MRSA for the prevention and control of MRSA infection in healthcare institutions.[23,30,38,39] These assays can detect the presence of MRSA directly from nasal swab specimens within 2 hours using real-time PCR that couples primers specific for *mecA* and the *S aureus*-specific gene *orfX* (sensitivity 93%, specificity 96%).[39] Several PCR-based tests also exist for the diagnosis of infection due to MRSA and include the GeneOhm StaphSR Assay (BD; blood cultures), the XPert MRSA/SA BC and SSTI tests (Cepheid; blood cultures and skin/soft tissue infections), the Verigene Gram-Positive Blood Culture Nucleic Acid Test (Luminex), and the mecA XpressFISH (OpGen, Gaithersburg, MD), with results typically available within 1 to 2 hours of culture positivity.[38]

The CLSI reference broth microdilution method can accurately detect vancomycin intermediate *S aureus* (VISA, MIC 4 to 8 mcg/mL) and vancomycin-resistant *S aureus* (VRSA, MIC ≥16 mcg/mL) but may not consistently detect the presence of heteroresistant VISA.[23] The use of brain heart infusion (BHI) agar plates with 6 mcg/mL of vancomycin (VRE screening plates described below) can be considered for the detection of *S aureus* strains with an MIC of ≥8 mcg/mL but is not useful for VISA strains with an MIC of 4 mcg/mL.[23] Lastly, the disk diffusion test is unable to accurately detect VISA strains but detects VRSA strains mediated by *vanA*.[23]

Current automated susceptibility testing methods, including the Vitek 2 system and the BD Phoenix, are able to accurately detect the presence of VRE.[23] VRE can also be detected using the vancomycin agar screen test, and is often performed on rectal swab specimens to detect carriers of VRE. A standard inoculum of the infecting *Enterococcus* spp. is inoculated onto an agar plate supplemented with BHI broth containing vancomycin 6 mcg/mL and incubated in ambient air for 24 hours.[20,23] The presence of any growth demonstrates the presence of VRE. This test is most useful for detecting acquired vancomycin resistance (eg, *vanA* or *vanB*) in *E faecalis* and *E. faecium*, but it is not as useful for strains that display intrinsic resistance to vancomycin (eg, *vanC*), such as *E. gallinarum* and *E. casseliflavus*, in which MICs range from 8 to 16 mcg/mL (intermediate) and growth is variable on agar screening plates.

## D-Zone Test for Detecting Inducible Clindamycin Resistance

Clindamycin resistance in staphylococci, *S pneumoniae*, and β-hemolytic streptococci is typically mediated by expression of the *erm* gene, which also confers resistance to macrolides, lincosamides, and streptogramin b (called MLS$_b$-type resistance). MLS$_b$ resistance can be either constitutive or inducible, especially in staphylococci.[20,23] Staphylococci (and β-hemolytic streptococci if susceptibility is performed) that are macrolide resistant but clindamycin susceptible should be evaluated for inducible clindamycin resistance using the D-zone test.[20,23] The D-zone test is a disk diffusion procedure in which a 15-mcg erythromycin disk is placed 12 mm (streptococci) or 15 to 26 mm (staphylococci) apart from a 2-mcg clindamycin disk on an agar plate inoculated with the infecting organism.[20,23] If inducible clindamycin resistance is present in the organism, the clindamycin zone of inhibition will be flattened

on the side nearest the erythromycin disk, demonstrating the letter D in appearance. Organisms that display a flattening of the clindamycin zone are D-zone test positive and should be reported resistant to clindamycin in the final organism susceptibility report.

## Special Considerations for Fastidious, Anaerobic, or Miscellaneous Bacteria

The susceptibility testing of fastidious bacteria (eg, *H influenzae*, *N gonorrhoeae*, and *S pneumoniae*) and anaerobes cannot be performed using standard broth microdilution, disk diffusion, or automated susceptibility testing methods because these organisms require more complex growth media and environmental conditions to support bacterial growth.[36,40,41] The cultivation of fastidious bacteria or anaerobes may require media with supplemental nutrients, prolonged incubation times, and incubation in atmospheres with higher $CO_2$ concentrations.[36,40,41] Microbiology reference texts and CLSI standards have been developed to outline specific methodologies (broth dilution, disk diffusion, and automated methods), quality control guidelines, and interpretive breakpoint criteria that should be used for the susceptibility testing of these bacteria.[21,25-29,36,40,41]

The clinical significance of anaerobes as a cause of infection is more widely appreciated, and the susceptibility of anaerobes to various anti-infective agents is no longer predictable.[9,40-43] The handling and processing of biologic specimens for anaerobic culture and susceptibility testing are extremely crucial to the validity of the results because most anaerobic bacteria of clinical importance are intolerant to oxygen.[9,40] Specimens should be collected in appropriate anaerobic transport systems (commercially available vials or tubes) that contain specialized media and atmospheric conditions to support the growth of the anaerobic bacteria until the specimen is processed in the laboratory.[40] Once collected, the specimens should be transported to the laboratory within minutes to hours of collection, processed for culture in anaerobic jars or chambers in the appropriate growth media, and incubated in anaerobic atmospheric conditions. The clinical specimens that provide the best yield for anaerobic culture include aspirated or tissue biopsy specimens.[40]

The identification of anaerobic bacteria by an individual hospital laboratory may be performed using one of three methods: (1) presumptive identification based on information from the primary growth plates, including the Gram stain results, patterns of growth on selective or differential media, plate and cell morphology, and results of various rapid spot and disk tests; (2) definitive identification based on the results of individual biochemical tests that detect the presence of preformed enzymes found in certain anaerobes; and (3) rapid identification of anaerobes using commercially available NA detection panels or MALDI-TOF.[40,41] Many hospital laboratories do not have the resources for commercially available, anaerobic bacteria identification systems and rely on the first two methods for presumptive identification of anaerobic bacteria. If necessary, clinical isolates can be sent to a reference laboratory for further testing.

Most clinical microbiology laboratories do not currently offer routine susceptibility testing of anaerobic bacteria because of the uncommon occurrence of pure anaerobic infections, the uncertain role of anaerobes in mixed infections, the previous predictable susceptibility of anaerobic bacteria to antibiotics, the previous lack of standardization of antimicrobial susceptibility testing of anaerobes, and the technical difficulties in performing the tests.[40-42] However, it is becoming apparent that routine antimicrobial susceptibility testing of anaerobic bacteria is necessary due to the increasing incidence of serious infections caused by anaerobic bacteria, the emerging resistance of anaerobic bacteria to multiple antibiotic agents, and the poor clinical outcomes observed when ineffective antibiotics are used for the treatment of infections caused by anaerobes.[40-43]

The susceptibility testing of anaerobic bacteria has undergone numerous methodological modifications and standardization over the past several years.[41-43] The CLSI has recently published a standard outlining the clinical situations where anaerobic susceptibility testing should be considered, the methods of susceptibility testing that should be used, when and how surveillance susceptibility reporting should be performed, and the antibiotic agents that should be tested for susceptibility.[42]

Susceptibility testing for anaerobes should be performed in patients with serious or life-threatening infections such as endocarditis, brain abscess, osteomyelitis, joint infection, refractory or recurrent bacteremia, and infection of prosthetic devices or vascular grafts.[40-42] Susceptibility testing should also be performed in patients with persistent or recurring anaerobic infections despite appropriate antibiotic therapy.[41,42] Lastly, susceptibility testing of anaerobic bacteria should be periodically performed within geographic areas or individual institutions to monitor regional susceptibility patterns of anaerobic bacteria over time.[40-42]

The recommended anaerobic susceptibility testing methods include agar dilution and broth microdilution using supplemented *Brucella* broth, both of which can be reliably performed by most clinical microbiology laboratories.[40-43] The agar dilution method is the gold standard reference method that can be used for susceptibility testing of any anaerobic bacteria, whereas the broth microdilution method has been validated only for antimicrobial susceptibility testing of *Bacteroides spp.* and *Parabacteroides spp.*[41,42] In contrast to agar dilution, the broth microdilution method can evaluate the susceptibility of multiple antibiotics simultaneously, and several microdilution panels are now commercially available for routine susceptibility testing, including Anaerobe Sensititre panel (ANO2, Thermo Fisher Scientific) and Oxoid ANA MIC Panel (Thermo Fisher Scientific). The general methodology for each of these tests is similar to those described previously for aerobic bacteria. Etest strips can also be used for anaerobe susceptibility testing, and results appear to correlate well with agar dilution. In addition, β-lactamase testing of anaerobes can be performed according to CLSI guidelines using chromogenic disks.[41-43]

Because routine antimicrobial susceptibility of anaerobes is not performed by all hospital microbiology laboratories or for all anaerobic isolates, antibiotic therapy for infections caused by anaerobes is usually selected empirically based on susceptibility

reports published by reference laboratories.[41,42] However, if susceptibility testing is performed on an individual anaerobic isolate, the results should be used to guide the anti-infective therapy for the patient.

Lastly, several miscellaneous (often uncommon) pathogenic bacteria are difficult to detect or cultivate using the standard microbiologic procedures outlined previously. These organisms often pose a diagnostic dilemma because they often require specialized testing for identification. It is beyond the scope of this chapter to describe all specialized testing methods that are available to detect these organisms; however, an abbreviated list can be found in **Table 18-10**.[4,13,44-61]

## Methods for Reporting Susceptibility Results
### Individual Isolate Susceptibility Reports

When a bacterial isolate is recovered from a clinical specimen, the identification and susceptibility results are compiled in a report that is available electronically or via a hard copy in the patient's chart. The bacterial identification and antibiotic susceptibility report often contains the following information: the patient's name, medical record number, the date and time of specimen collection, the source of specimen (eg, blood, wound, urine), the bacteria that were identified (if any), and the list of antibiotics tested for susceptibility with the MIC or disk diffusion result and CLSI interpretive category, as shown in **Figure 18-5**.[20,62] Additionally, the site of blood culture collection (eg, drawn peripherally versus central line) and the time to positivity are occasionally reported. In some hospitals, the individual isolate susceptibility report may also contain information regarding the usual daily dose and cost of antibiotics.

Once bacterial culture and susceptibility results are available, this information should be used to change the patient's empiric antibiotic regimen, which usually covers a broad spectrum of bacteria, to a more *directed* antibiotic regimen targeting the infecting bacteria and antibiotic susceptibility (de-escalation). The directed antibiotic regimen should be chosen based on clinical and economic factors, some of which include the severity of infection, the site of infection, the activity (MIC value) of the antibiotic against the infecting organism, the proven efficacy of the antibiotic in the treatment of the particular infection, the overall spectrum of activity of the antibiotic (a narrow spectrum agent is preferred), the end-organ function of the patient, the presence of drug allergies, the route of administration (oral versus parenteral), the daily cost of the antibiotic, and so on. The susceptibility report provides some of the information necessary for the de-escalation of antibiotic therapy, namely, the site of infection, the infecting organism(s), and the susceptibility of the infecting organism(s).

As seen in the sample susceptibility report in Figure 18-5, several antibiotics may display activity against the infecting bacteria, often with different MICs. It is not always advantageous to choose the antibiotic with the lowest MIC against a particular organism on a susceptibility report. As discussed earlier in this chapter, antibiotics have different MIC breakpoints corresponding to S, I, and R (and SDD for select antibiotics) for

**TABLE 18-10.** Laboratory Tests for the Detection of Miscellaneous Organisms

| ORGANISM | TYPE OF ORGANISM | CLINICAL FINDINGS AND INFECTIONS | DIAGNOSTIC METHOD | POSITIVE RESULT | REFERENCE |
|---|---|---|---|---|---|
| *Bordetella pertussis* (Whooping cough) | Bacteria | Upper respiratory tract symptoms, characteristic whooping cough, pneumonia | Culture | Growth within 3–7 days; more sensitive when performed early in course of infection | 44 |
| | | | DFA, ELISA | Rapid detection of *B. pertussis* antibodies; should be used in conjunction with culture due to variable specificity | |
| | | | PCR | Direct detection in 1–2 days; most sensitive when performed early in course of infection | |
| *Borrelia burgdorferi* (Lyme disease) | Spirochete | Erythema migrans, pericarditis, arthritis, neurologic disease | Culture | Not routinely performed due to difficulty and low sensitivity; long incubation (hold cultures for up to 12 wk) | 13,45,46 |
| | | | ELISA (or rarely IFA); first step screening test | Measures IgM (appears within 1–2 wk) and IgG (appears within 4–6 wk) antibodies against *B burgdorferi* | |
| | | | WB if ELISA borderline or positive, second step confirmatory test | Measures IgM and IgG antibodies against *B burgdorferi* | |
| | | | PCR (confirm) | Can detect low numbers of spirochetes; especially useful in synovial fluid | |
| *Brucella* spp. | Bacteria | Systemic infection (can involve any organ); spondylitis, arthritis, endocarditis | Culture | Growth within 7 days, but cultures should be held for 3 wk | 47 |
| | | | SAT, MAT | Detects antibodies to most *Brucella* spp.; titer of ≥1:160 is diagnostic in conjunction with appropriate clinical scenario | |
| | | | ELISA | Useful for detection of chronic or past brucellosis; most useful for diagnosis of neurobrucellosis | |
| | | | PCR | Detection of *Brucella*-specific DNA sequences; not routinely available in most laboratories | |

**TABLE 18-10.** Laboratory Tests for the Detection of Miscellaneous Organisms, cont'd

| ORGANISM | TYPE OF ORGANISM | CLINICAL FINDINGS AND INFECTIONS | DIAGNOSTIC METHOD | POSITIVE RESULT | REFERENCE |
|---|---|---|---|---|---|
| *Chlamydia pneumoniae* | Atypical bacteria | Upper respiratory tract infections, pharyngitis; pneumonia | Culture | Monoclonal antibodies detect organism in culture | 4,13,48 |
| | | | CF | 4-fold rise in antibody titer between paired sera (acute and convalescent samples) | |
| | | | MIF | 4-fold rise in antibody titer between paired sera (acute and convalescent samples) or a single serum sample with an IgM titer of 1:16 or an IgG titer 1:512 | |
| | | | PCR | Detection of *C pneumoniae* DNA | |
| *Clostridioides difficile* (Pseudomembranous colitis) | Anaerobic bacteria | Pseudomembranous colitis, diarrhea | Toxigenic culture using CCFA growth media | Growth within 48 hr; most sensitive test | 49 |
| | | | CCNA or EIA toxin test | Detection of toxin A or B activity; cell cytotoxicity test more sensitive than EIA | |
| | | | PCR | Rapid sensitive and specific detection of *Clostridioides difficile tcdB* gene | |
| | | | Glutamate dehydrogenase (GDH) assays | Detects GDH, an enzyme present in all *Clostridioides difficile* isolates; cannot differentiate between toxigenic and nontoxigenic strains | |
| *Coxiella burnetti* (Q fever) | Bacteria | Acute or chronic systemic illness, pneumonia, hepatitis, endocarditis | Culture with DFA | Growth in 6–14 days, organism detected by DFA | 13,48 |
| | | | IFA, EIA, CF | IgM titer of 1:50 or an IgG titer of 1:200 | |
| *Cryptosporidium parvum* | Protozoa | Acute diarrhea (self-limiting to severe), abdominal pain, dehydration | Modified acid fast, Ziehl-Neelsen or Kinyoun staining | Detection of oocysts in stool or intestinal scrapings | 50 |
| | | | DFA using a monoclonal antibody against oocyst | Detection of oocysts in stool or intestinal scrapings | |
| | | | EIA | Detection of *C. parvum* antigen in stool or intestinal scrapings | |
| | | | PCR | Detection and differentiation of *Cryptosporidium* spp. | |

*(continued)*

**TABLE 18-10.** Laboratory Tests for the Detection of Miscellaneous Organisms, cont'd

| ORGANISM | TYPE OF ORGANISM | CLINICAL FINDINGS AND INFECTIONS | DIAGNOSTIC METHOD | POSITIVE RESULT | REFERENCE |
|---|---|---|---|---|---|
| *Ehrlichia* spp. | Bacteria | HME - fever, myalgia, headache, malaise, rash (more common in children), nausea, vomiting, diarrhea, leukopenia, thrombocytopenia, elevated hepatic transaminases; may be life-threatening | IFA serology | 4-fold rise in antibody titer between paired sera (acute and convalescent samples) | 48,51,52 |
| | | | Peripheral blood smear Wright-Giemsa or Diff-Quik stain | Detect morulae (cytoplasmic vacuoles) | |
| | | | PCR | Detection of *E chaffeensis* or *E phagocytophilum* DNA sequences | |
| *Entamoeba histolytica* | Protozoa | Amebiasis: intestinal (colitis, diarrhea) and extraintestinal (liver abscess) | Stool exam for ova and parasites | Detection of trophozoites and cysts | 50 |
| | | | Serology (IFA) | Detection of *E histolytica* antibodies with titer ≥1:200 | |
| | | | Antigen detection on fresh stool samples | Detection of *E histolytica* or *E dispar* specific antigen | |
| | | | PCR | Detection and differentiation of *E histolytica* or *E dispar* | |
| *Giardia* spp. | Protozoa | Acute diarrhea (self-limiting to severe), malabsorption syndromes, low-grade fever, chills, abdominal pain | Stool exam for ova and parasites | Detection of trophozoites and/or cysts | 50 |
| | | | Wet preps or stains of duodenal material | Detection of trophozoites and/or cysts | |
| | | | EIA, DFA, or ICA antigen detection assays | Detection of trophozoite and/or cyst antigens | |
| *Helicobacter pylori* | Bacteria | Peptic ulcer disease | Urea breath test | Positive test indicative of the presence of organism | 53 |
| | | | LA serologic tests | Detect IgG antibodies against *H pylori* | |
| | | | Stool antigen tests using monoclonal antibodies (ELISA) | Detection of *H pylori* antigen | |
| | | | Urease test on antral biopsy specimen | Positive test indicative of active infection | |
| | | | PCR | Detection of *H pylori* DNA | |

**TABLE 18-10.** Laboratory Tests for the Detection of Miscellaneous Organisms, cont'd

| ORGANISM | TYPE OF ORGANISM | CLINICAL FINDINGS AND INFECTIONS | DIAGNOSTIC METHOD | POSITIVE RESULT | REFERENCE |
|---|---|---|---|---|---|
| *Legionella pneumophila* | Atypical bacteria | Pneumonia | Culture using specialized media | Growth in 3–5 days | 4,54 |
| | | | DFA staining | Binds to *L. pneumophila* antigen to produce fluorescence | |
| | | | IFA serology | 4-fold rise in antibody titer between paired sera (acute and convalescent samples) | |
| | | | Urinary antigen detection (EIA, RIA, ICA) | Detects *Legionella pneumophila* serogroup 1 antigen only | |
| | | | PCR | Detection of *Legionella* spp. DNA | |
| *Leishmania* spp. | Protozoa | Cutaneous, mucocutaneous, or visceral (VL, kala-azar) infection; can infect reticuloendothelial system | Giemsa staining and light microscopy | Amastigotes within the specimen | 55 |
| | | | Culture | Growth of promastigotes | |
| | | | IFA, DAT, ELISA (VL) | Detection of antileishmanial antibodies in blood or serum | |
| | | | LA (VL) | Detection of leishmanial antigen in urine | |
| | | | PCR (VL) | Detection of *Leishmania* DNA | |
| *Leptospira* spp. | Spirochetes | Leptospirosis (self-limiting with fevers, chills, myalgia, headache, aseptic meningitis); icteric leptospirosis (severe form associated with jaundice, bleeding, and renal failure) | Dark-field microscopy or immunofluorescence | Detection of motile leptospires | 13,46 |
| | | | Culture | Growth within 6 wk | |
| | | | Serology using MAT | 4-fold or greater rise in agglutinating antibody titer between paired sera (acute and convalescent samples) | |
| | | | ELISA | Detection of leptospiral antibodies | |
| | | | PCR | Detection of leptospiral DNA | |
| *Mycoplasma hominis* | Atypical bacteria | Urogenital tract infections, including prostatitis, PID, bacterial vaginosis, urethritis; systemic infection in neonates and immunocompromised patients | Culture using selective media | Growth within 5 days | 13,56 |

*(continued)*

**TABLE 18-10.** Laboratory Tests for the Detection of Miscellaneous Organisms, cont'd

| ORGANISM | TYPE OF ORGANISM | CLINICAL FINDINGS AND INFECTIONS | DIAGNOSTIC METHOD | POSITIVE RESULT | REFERENCE |
|---|---|---|---|---|---|
| *Mycoplasma pneumoniae* | Atypical bacteria | Pneumonia, tracheobronchitis, pharyngitis | EIA, IFA, CF serology | 4-fold or greater rise in antibody titer between paired sera (acute and convalescent samples) | 4,13,56 |
| | | | NAAT, PCR | Detection of *M pneumoniae* DNA | |
| *Plasmodium falciparum, P. vivax, P. ovale, P. malariae* (Malaria) | Protozoa | Symptoms include high fever (cyclic with *P. vivax, P. ovale, P. malariae*), chills, nausea, vomiting, severe headache, anemia, abdominal pain; life-threatening with *P. falciparum* | Thick and thin blood films stained with Giemsa or Wright's stain (gold standard) | Presence of malarial parasites | 55 |
| | | | Fluorescent-assisted microscopy with acridine orange | Detection of fluorescence when dyes are taken up by the nucleus of the parasite | |
| | | | ICA antigen assays | Detection of malaria-specific antigens | |
| | | | PCR | Detection of malaria-specific DNA sequences | |
| *Pneumocystis jirovecii* (*carinii*; PCP) | Fungus with protozoal characteristics | Pneumonia, extrapulmonary infection | Microscopic exam after Giemsa or methenamine silver stain of induced sputum, BAL specimen, or tissue biopsy | Detection of trophic or cystic forms | 57 |
| | | | DFA or IFA | Detection of cysts or trophozoites | |
| | | | PCR | Detection of *P jirovecii*-specific DNA | |
| | | | 1,3-β-D-glucan serum test | Positive values >100 pg/mL | |
| *Rickettsia rickettsii* (Rocky Mountain spotted fever) | *Rickettsia* | Fever, chills, headache and rash in patient with recent tick bite; myalgias, malaise, nausea, vomiting, abdominal pain, focal neurologic findings; small vessel vasculitis may result in life-threatening complications | IFA (gold standard) | 4-fold or greater rise in IgM or IgG antibody titers between paired sera (acute and convalescent samples) | 48,52 |
| | | | EIA or LA | Detection of IgM or IgG antibodies | |
| | | | PCR | Detection of *R rickettsii* DNA sequences | |

**TABLE 18-10.** Laboratory Tests for the Detection of Miscellaneous Organisms, cont'd

| ORGANISM | TYPE OF ORGANISM | CLINICAL FINDINGS AND INFECTIONS | DIAGNOSTIC METHOD | POSITIVE RESULT | REFERENCE |
|---|---|---|---|---|---|
| *Strongyloides stercoralis* | Parasite | Abdominal infection; disseminated infection (hyperinfection syndrome with pneumonitis, sepsis) | Stool exam for ova and parasites | Detection of adult worms, eggs, and/or larvae | 58 |
| *Taenia solium* | Tapeworm | Neurocysticercosis (infection within brain tissue) causing seizures, headache, focal neurologic deficits; muscular and subcutaneous abscesses | Serology by EITB | Detection of antibodies to *T solium* glycoprotein antigens | 59 |
| | | | ELISA on CSF | Detection of anticysticercal antibodies or cysticercal antigens | |
| *Toxoplasma gondii* (Toxoplasmosis) | Protozoa | Encephalitis, myocarditis, lymphadenitis, polymyositis, chorioretinitis, toxoplasmosis during pregnancy, congenital toxoplasmosis | Serology testing | Positive IgG antibody | 60,61 |
| | | | Giemsa or Diff-Quik stain of CSF or body fluid/tissue | Demonstration of tachyzoites | |
| | | | PCR | Detection of *T gondii*-specific DNA | |
| *Ureaplasma urealyticum* | Atypical bacteria | Urogenital tract infections, including prostatitis, PID, bacterial vaginosis, urethritis; systemic infection in neonates and immunocompromised | Culture using selective media | Growth within 5 days | 13,56 |
| | | | PCR | Detection of NA or gene targets | |

BAL = bronchoalveolar lavage; CCFA = cycloserine cefoxitin fructose agar; CCNA = cell cytotoxicity neutralization assay; CF = complement fixation; DAT = direct agglutination test; EITB = enzyme-linked immunoelectrotransfer blot; GDH = glutamate dehydrogenase; HME = human monocytic ehrlichiosis; ICA = immunochromatographic assay; IFA = immunofluorescent assay/indirect fluorescent antibody; MAT = microagglutination test; MIF = microimmunofluorescence; NAAT = nucleic acid amplification test; O&P = ova and parasites; PID = pelvic inflammatory disease; RIA = radioimmunoassay; SAT = serum agglutination test; VL = visceral leishmaniasis; WB = western blot.
*Source:* References 4,13,44–61.

each bacterium based on several factors. Some drugs, such as piperacillin–tazobactam, are assigned higher MIC breakpoint values for susceptibility because they achieve higher serum and site concentrations than other antibiotics. Because of this, a simple number comparison of the MIC between antibiotics should not be performed. The choice of antibiotic should be based on the knowledge of the MICs that are acceptable for a

particular antibiotic–bacteria combination, the site of infection, the penetration of the antibiotic to the site of infection, as well as the clinical and economic parameters listed previously. In the sample report in Figure 18-5, oxacillin (nafcillin) or cefazolin would be an acceptable choice for the treatment of *S aureus* bacteremia in a patient without drug allergies because these agents are active against the infecting organism, have

**Patient Name:** Jane Doe
**Medical Record Number:** 1111111
**Specimen Collection Date and Time:** Dec 12, 2014, 0730
**Specimen Type:** Blood
**Organism Identification:** *Staphylococcus aureus*

**ANTIMICROBIAL SUSCEPTIBILITY**

| Antibiotic | MIC (mcg/mL) | Interpretive Category |
|---|---|---|
| Penicillin | ≥16 | Resistant |
| Ampicillin/Sulbactam | ≤4 | Susceptible |
| Cefazolin | ≤8 | Susceptible |
| Oxacillin | 0.5 | Susceptible |
| Trimethoprim/Sulfa | ≤10 | Susceptible |
| Vancomycin | ≤0.5 | Susceptible |
| Clindamycin | ≤0.5 | Susceptible |
| Erythromycin | ≤0.5 | Susceptible |

**FIGURE 18-5.** Example of microbiology laboratory report with bacterial identification and antibiotic susceptibility.

been demonstrated to be effective in the treatment of systemic staphylococcal infections, have a relatively narrow spectrum, and are inexpensive. **Minicase 2** is an example illustrating the use of a bacterial culture and susceptibility report in the antibiotic decision-making process.

The decision regarding the specific antibiotics that will be routinely reported in an individual susceptibility report for a bacterial isolate is typically based on input from a hospital or institutional multidisciplinary committee (eg, Antimicrobial Subcommittee, Infectious Diseases Subcommittee, Antimicrobial Stewardship Team) comprised of infectious diseases physicians, infectious diseases pharmacists, and representatives from the Infection Control Committee and the microbiology laboratory. The choice of specific drugs to report is often based on the hospital formulary, the level of control of antibiotic use that is desired, and the tests that are used by the microbiology laboratory for susceptibility testing. Tables that outline the antibiotics that should be routinely tested and reported for each bacterium can be found in the CLSI Performance Standards and Guidelines for Antimicrobial Susceptibility Testing.[21,26-28]

Several methods can be used for reporting antibiotic susceptibility of individual bacterial isolates, including general reporting, selective reporting, and cascade reporting. *General reporting* involves reporting all antibiotics that were tested for susceptibility against the organism without any restrictions. *Selective reporting* involves reporting certain antibiotic susceptibility test results on an individual bacterial isolate based on defined criteria, such as the bacteria identified, the site of infection, antibiotics available on the hospital formulary, etc. An example of selective reporting would be the exclusion of cefazolin from the susceptibility report of a CSF sample growing *E coli* because cefazolin is not a suitable treatment option for meningitis. *Cascade reporting* involves the preferential release of susceptibility information for first-line choices for the treatment of a particular

organism or infection (usually narrow spectrum and inexpensive), with the reporting of second-line antibiotic susceptibility results (usually broad spectrum and costly) only if the first-line agents are inactive against the infecting organism or are inappropriate for the treatment of the particular infection. An example of cascade reporting is the reporting of amikacin susceptibility results against *P aeruginosa* only if the organism displays resistance to both gentamicin and tobramycin, which are less expensive aminoglycoside agents. Both selective reporting and cascade reporting are often used as antimicrobial stewardship activities to control the inappropriate use of broad-spectrum or expensive antibiotics.[62]

## Hospital Susceptibility Reports (Hospital Cumulative Antibiograms)

Most hospitals prepare and publish an annual cumulative report of antimicrobial susceptibility profiles of the bacteria that have been isolated from patients within their hospital, healthcare system, or institution, called a *cumulative antibiogram*. For the cumulative antibiogram to be clinically useful, the susceptibility data from patient isolates should be appropriately collected, analyzed, and reported according to the CLSI guidelines, which are outlined in **Table 18-11**.[62]

The cumulative antibiogram contains information on the percent of isolated bacteria that were susceptible to antibiotics tested over the time frame of the antibiogram, as illustrated in **Figure 18-6**.[62] This percent susceptibility information is derived by dividing the number of organisms susceptible to a particular antibiotic by the total number of single-patient isolates collected and reported (with duplicate patient isolates removed). The calculations can be performed either manually or through the use of automated systems that have been programmed using appropriate definitions to remove duplicate patient isolates. Cumulative antibiograms usually contains separate data tables for the susceptibility reporting of gram-positive, gram-negative, and anaerobic bacteria (if performed).

The specific data published in the cumulative antibiogram should be based on input from the hospital/healthcare system's multidisciplinary committee (eg, Infectious Diseases Subcommittee, Antimicrobial Stewardship Committee) that is often comprised of infectious diseases physicians, infectious disease pharmacists, infection preventionists, and the microbiology laboratory. The cumulative antibiogram report typically contains information on the antibiotic susceptibility patterns of isolates obtained from patients in the hospital (either admitted with infection or who developed infection in the hospital) but may also include the susceptibility of organisms causing infection in outpatients if the hospital/medical center also serves a substantial outpatient population. In addition, each hospital or healthcare system may further stratify their susceptibility data by various parameters, such as patient care unit (eg, Burn Unit, MICU, Pediatric Unit, Med-Surg Unit, outpatient clinic, nursing home), patient age, site of infection (eg, bloodstream isolates, UTI isolates), patient characteristics (eg, cystic fibrosis, transplant patients, hematology/oncology patients), or by organism (eg, susceptibility of *S aureus*). For

## MINICASE 2

## Using Laboratory Test Results to Guide the Choice of a Directed Antibiotic Regimen for the Treatment of Pyelonephritis

Diana J., a 27-year-old woman, presents to the urgent care clinic with reports of urinary frequency and urgency, pain on urination, and hematuria for the past 2 days. She also reports fever of 101.6°F and intractable nausea and vomiting during the past 24 hours. At presentation, she is febrile (102.3°F), hypotensive (90/60 mm Hg), and lethargic; physical exam reveals right costovertebral angle and suprapubic tenderness. A urine dipstick performed in the clinic is leukocyte esterase positive, and a urine pregnancy test is negative. Because she appears ill, the clinic physician sends the patient to the local emergency department (ED) for admission. Her past medical history is significant for recurrent UTIs, with three episodes over the past 6 months that have required antibiotic therapy, including oral trimethoprim–sulfamethoxazole and oral ciprofloxacin. She reports no known drug allergies. Upon admission to the ED, urinalysis, urine culture, and blood cultures are performed.

QUESTION: What is an appropriate recommendation for empiric antibiotic therapy for this patient?

DISCUSSION: Based on her presenting symptoms and the findings on her physical examination, this patient most likely has acute pyelonephritis, an upper tract UTI, making the acquisition of urinalysis, urine culture, and blood cultures important for guiding directed antimicrobial treatment. This is especially important in this patient because she has received multiple recent courses of antibiotics for her past UTIs, which put her at risk for infection with resistant bacteria. Because she is hypotensive and is experiencing significant nausea and vomiting, she should initially receive empiric parenteral antibiotic therapy that displays activity against the likely causative organisms of pyelonephritis and has proven efficacy in the treatment of complicated UTIs (eg, ceftriaxone because she does not have any antibiotic allergies). The patient should receive ceftriaxone as empiric therapy, which can be de-escalated to cefazolin based on the results of the blood and urine culture and susceptibility test results that follow.

URINALYSIS: Yellow, cloudy; pH 7; specific gravity 1.015; protein negative; RBC trace; WBC 50 to 100/hpf; leukocyte esterase positive; nitrite positive.

Midstream Urine Culture/Susceptibility: > 100,000 CFU/mL of *E coli*

| ANTIBIOTIC TESTED | MIC RESULT | CLSI INTERPRETATION |
|---|---|---|
| Ampicillin | >32 mcg/mL | R |
| Ampicillin–sulbactam | 8 mcg/mL | S |
| Cefazolin | 1 mcg/mL | S |
| Ceftriaxone | 1 mcg/mL | S |
| Imipenem | 1 mcg/mL | S |
| Gentamicin | 0.5 mcg/mL | S |
| Ciprofloxacin | 4 mcg/mL | R |
| Trimethoprim–sulfamethoxazole | >4/76 mcg/mL | R |

R = resistant; S = susceptible.

Blood Culture/Susceptibility: *E coli*

| ANTIBIOTIC TESTED | MIC RESULT | CLSI INTERPRETATION |
|---|---|---|
| Ampicillin | >32 mcg/mL | R |
| Ampicillin–sulbactam | 8 mcg/mL | S |
| Cefazolin | 1 mcg/mL | S |
| Ceftriaxone | 1 mcg/mL | S |
| Imipenem | 1 mcg/mL | S |
| Gentamicin | 0.5 mcg/mL | S |
| Ciprofloxacin | 4 mcg/mL | R |
| Trimethoprim–sulfamethoxazole | >4/76 mcg/mL | R |

R = resistant; S = susceptible.

some organisms, the cumulative antibiogram only will contain information regarding the presence of bacterial resistance mechanisms, particularly when routine susceptibility testing is difficult to perform, such as in the case of *H influenzae* in which the percentage of isolates that produce β-lactamase enzyme during the time period of the cumulative antibiogram will be reported. Other information that may be incorporated into a cumulative antibiogram includes graphs demonstrating resistance trends, antibiotic dosing guidelines, recommended empiric antibiotic choices based on infection type, and antibiotic cost data.[62]

The cumulative antibiogram is a useful tool for selecting *empiric* antibiotic therapy, where an antibiotic is selected based on the local susceptibility patterns of the most likely infecting organism causing the patient's infection (Table 18-7) while waiting for the results of culture and susceptibility tests, as described

**TABLE 18-11.** CLSI Recommendations for Cumulative Antibiogram Development

1. To serve as a continuously useful tool to guide appropriate empiric antibiotic therapy, the cumulative antibiogram should be compiled, analyzed, and reported at least annually.

2. Only the first clinical isolate of a given species of bacteria per patient per analysis period (annually if that is the time frame of the antibiogram) should be included in the cumulative susceptibility report regardless of site of isolation, susceptibility pattern of the bacteria, or other phenotypic characteristics. The inclusion of duplicate clinical isolates from the same patient will lead to overreporting of bacterial resistance.

3. To provide a reasonable statistical estimate of susceptibility, only species of bacteria in which at least 30 isolates have been collected, tested, and reported during the time period of the antibiogram should be included.

4. Data from isolates recovered during surveillance cultures (eg, MRSA and VRE), environmental cultures, or other nonpatient sources should not be included in the antibiogram.

5. The cumulative susceptibility report should include all antibiotics that were tested for susceptibility, regardless of whether they were reported in the final susceptibility report for the individual patient.

6. Only bacterial isolates for which all routine antibiotics have been tested for susceptibility should be included. Results of agents selectively or supplementally tested should not be included in the cumulative susceptibility report. For example, if only isolates resistant to primary agents were then analyzed for susceptibility to secondary agents, this will bias the resistance results toward higher levels of resistance to the secondary agents.

7. Data may be stratified and reported by age, unit in which the isolate was collected (eg, MICU, SICU, outpatient clinic), or anatomic site of collection (eg, blood isolates, CSF isolates, and urine isolates) as long as duplicate patient isolates are removed and there are a sufficient number of isolates collected (> 30) during the time frame of the antibiogram.

MICU = medical intensive care unit; SICU = surgical intensive care unit.
*Source*: Reference 62.

**ANTIBIOTIC SUSCEPTIBILITIES Jan.–Dec. 2015** — Numbers are percent susceptible (# isolates)

Antibiotic Formulary Status: Bold = FORMULARY; Upper/Lower = RESERVED

Pharmacy (x2549); Microbiology (x5529)

| Antibiotic | Acinetobacter calcoaceticus (11) | Enterobacter aerogenes (12) | Enterobacter cloacae (30) | Escherichia coli (271) | Haemophilus influenzae (63) | Klebsiella pneumoniae (67) | Proteus mirabilis (37) | Pseudomonas aeruginosa (101) | Staphylococcus aureus (153) | Enterococci (gp D strep) (97) | Enterococcus faecium (12) | Usual dose | Cost/day (includes administration costs) |
|---|---|---|---|---|---|---|---|---|---|---|---|---|---|
| **AMPICILLIN** | | | | 73 | 73 | | 100 | | | 97 | | 1–2 g IV q 6 hr | $4–5 |
| AMOXICILLIN-CLAVULANATE | | | | | 95 | | | | | | | 250–500 mg PO TID | $4–6 |
| **CEFAZOLIN** | | | | 97 | | 97 | 100 | | 87 | | | 500 mg IV q 8 hr | $6 |
| **CEFOTETAN** | | | 63 | 100 | | 100 | 100 | | | | | 1–2 g IV q 12 hr | $18–35 |
| Ceftazidime | 100 | 92 | | | | | | 98 | | | | 1–2 g IV q 8 hr | $31–61 |
| Ceftriaxone | | 92 | 86 | 100 | 100 | 100 | 100 | | | | | 1–2 g IV q 24 hr | $25–50 |
| Cefuroxime | | 92 | 72 | 99 | 97 | 98 | 100 | | | | | 750 mg IV q 8 hr | $14 |
| Ciprofloxacin | 100 | 100 | 100 | 100 | | 100 | 100 | 95 | 90 | 78 | | 250–750 mg PO BID | $4–9 (only oral form available) |
| **CLINDAMYCIN** | | | | | | | | | 91 | | | 600 mg q 8 hr | IV - $9   PO - $8 |
| **ERYTHROMYCIN** | | | | | | | | | 72 | | | 500 mg q 6 hr | IV - $7   PO - $0.20 |
| **GENTAMICIN** | 91 | 100 | 100 | 100 | | 100 | 100 | 92 | | | | 80 mg IV q 8 hr | $5 |
| Imipenem | 100 | 100 | 100 | | | | | 91 | | | | 500 mg IV q 8-6 hr | $60–79 |
| **METRONIDAZOLE** | | | | | | | | | | | | 500 mg q 6 hr | IV - $7   PO - $.50 |
| **OXACILLIN** | | | | | | | | | 87 | | | 2 g IV q 6 hr | $10 |
| **NITROFURANTOIN** | | | 100 | 99 | | | | | | 99 | 95 | 50–100 mg PO q 6 hr for urine isolates only | $2–3 |
| **PENICILLIN G** | | | | | | | | | | | | 1 million units IV q 4 hr | $9 |
| **TETRACYCLINE** | | | 85 | 85 | | 92 | | | 92 | | | 250–500 mg PO q 6 hr | $0.20 |
| **TICARCILLIN** | 100 | 83 | 63 | 74 | | | 100 | 89 | | | | 3 g IV q 4 | $48 |
| Ticarcillin-clavulanate | Activity superior to ticarcillin versus staph, most gram neg. rods and anaerobes (including B. fragilis). Activity same as ticarcillin versus Pseudomonas, Acinetobacter, Enterobacter. | | | | | | | | | | | 3.1 g IV q 6 hr | $43 |
| Tobramycin | 100 | 100 | | | | | 100 | | | | | 80 mg IV q 8 hr | $18 |
| **TRIMETHOPRIM-SULFAMETHOXAZOLE** | 91 | 100 | 97 | 92 | 92 | 90 | 97 | | 94 | | | 20 mL IV q 12 hr / 1 DS Tab PO BID | IV - $3   PO - $0.15 |
| Vancomycin | | | | | | | | | 99 | 100 | 92 | 1 g IV q 12 hr | $15 |

**FIGURE 18-6.** Example of a hospital antibiogram report.

in **Minicase 3**.[62] Antibiotic therapy must often be initiated at the suspicion of infection because many infectious diseases are often acute where a delay in treatment may result in significant morbidity or mortality (eg, meningitis and pneumonia). Once the culture and susceptibility results of the infecting bacteria are

known, antibiotic therapy should be deescalated or directed, if necessary, to an agent with more targeted activity against the organism

### Surveillance Susceptibility Testing of Large Numbers of Isolates

Surveillance susceptibility testing is a useful method to monitor the susceptibility of bacteria to antimicrobial agents over time and can be performed in an individual hospital or within a geographic location (eg, regionally, nationally, and internationally).[20] Surveillance studies typically report the overall susceptibility of the bacteria to particular antibiotics using CLSI breakpoints, along with other susceptibility parameters, such as the $MIC_{50}$ and the $MIC_{90}$. To determine the $MIC_{50}$ or $MIC_{90}$, the MIC values from the bacterial population studied are arranged in ascending order, where the $MIC_{50}$ is the MIC value representing 50% of the bacterial population (the MIC value of the isolate that represents 50% of the bacterial population studied) and the $MIC_{90}$ is the MIC that represents 90% of the bacterial population (the MIC value of the isolate that represents 90% of the bacterial population studied). The $MIC_{90}$ value is usually higher than the $MIC_{50}$ value. This information is useful for detecting the emergence of subclinical antibiotic resistance in which the $MIC_{50}$ and $MIC_{90}$ of a particular agent may be increasing over time but are still below the MIC susceptibility breakpoint.

### Additional Considerations When Interpreting Susceptibility Results

The successful treatment of a patient's infection involves an understanding of the interactions among the patient, the infecting organism, and the antibiotic. It is important to note that antimicrobial susceptibility testing only measures one of these factors, namely, the activity of the antibiotic against the infecting organism in a laboratory setting. The current methodologies for antibiotic susceptibility testing are unable to reproduce the interaction between the antibiotic and the bacteria at the site of infection in which a multitude of host factors (eg, immune system function, concomitant disease states) and drug factors (eg, pharmacokinetic parameters, including concentration of free drug at the site of infection and protein binding) play an integral role.

## LABORATORY TESTS USED FOR DIAGNOSIS OF SPECIFIC INFECTIONS

### Bacterial Meningitis

Meningitis is an infectious diseases medical emergency requiring prompt, accurate diagnosis and treatment. Meningitis may be caused by bacteria, viruses, fungi, or mycobacteria, and it produces a resulting clinical presentation of acute or chronic meningitis depending on the causative organism. In a patient with suspected meningitis, a lumbar puncture is performed to obtain CSF for laboratory analysis to aid in the diagnosis of the infection, including the potential causative organism.[2,63-67] In patients who

---

## MINICASE 3

### Using the Cumulative Antibiogram to Choose Empiric Antibiotic Therapy

David M. is a 45-year-old man who sustained multiple traumatic injuries after a motorcycle accident. He has required multiple surgeries over the past 10 days for fracture stabilization. In the last 12 hours, he has spiked a temperature to 39°C and has developed shaking chills. His other vital signs are stable, and his physical exam does not demonstrate any significant focal findings. Urinalysis, urine culture, and blood cultures are performed to determine the potential etiology for his new fever. In addition, a chest radiograph is obtained, which does not demonstrate any pulmonary infiltrates. The microbiology laboratory calls the surgical floor later that day to report that the blood culture results are positive for gram-negative rods. The patient is allergic to penicillin (nonurticarial rash); the local hospital antibiogram is pictured in Figure 18-6.

QUESTION: What empiric antibiotic therapy should be used to treat this patient's gram-negative rod bacteremia while waiting for the culture and susceptibility results?

DISCUSSION: Nosocomial gram-negative bacteremia is a potentially life-threatening infection that requires early, aggressive antibiotic therapy. The choice of whether to use monotherapy or combination therapy while waiting for culture and susceptibility results in this setting often depends on the clinical condition of the patient and local susceptibility patterns. Combination antibiotic therapy might be considered initially if the patient is critically ill (septic shock) from the bacteremia because it might provide some synergistic antibacterial activity as well as enhanced coverage against a wide range of potential infecting bacteria. Based on the hospital antibiogram in Figure 18-6, it is desirable to choose an antibiotic that displays good activity (>85% susceptible) against gram-negative bacteria isolated at the institution (eg, *P aeruginosa*, *E coli*, *K pneumoniae*, *S marcescens*, and *Enterobacter cloacae*) and choose an antibiotic with proven efficacy in the treatment of bacteremia. Because the patient is clinically stable and displays only a rash to penicillin, some useful therapeutic options based on review of the hospital antibiogram include meropenem, ceftazidime, or cefepime. If the patient were to clinically deteriorate on monotherapy, an aminoglycoside (tobramycin) or a fluoroquinolone (ciprofloxacin) could be added to the carbapenem or cephalosporin while waiting for the culture and susceptibility results. The antibiotic regimen could then be modified to more directed therapy, if possible, once the final culture and susceptibility results were available.

present with papilledema, altered consciousness, new-onset seizures, or focal neurologic findings, a head computed tomography may be performed prior to the lumbar puncture to exclude the presence of a space-occupying lesion, which may put the patient at risk for brain herniation after lumbar puncture.[63,66] A lumbar puncture involves the aseptic insertion of a spinal needle into the subarachnoid space at the lumbar spine level (between L3, L4, or L5) for the aspiration of 5 to 20 mL of CSF for analysis.[63,64] When inserting the spinal needle, the opening pressure may be measured (normal opening pressure is 50 to 195 mm $H_2O$ in adults) and is often elevated in patients with meningitis (especially *C neoformans* meningitis) and concomitant cerebral edema or intracranial focus of infection.[63,66] The CSF should be placed in three to four separate sterile screw-cap tubes and immediately transported to the laboratory for rapid processing. The first two tubes of CSF are used for microbiologic (eg, Gram stain, fungal stains, acid-fast bacilli stain, culture, and antigen detection) and chemical studies (eg, general appearance, glucose, and protein), whereas the last tubes are used for determination of the WBC count and differential. The typical CSF chemistry, hematology, and microbiologic findings in patients with meningitis caused by different pathogens are listed in **Table 18-12**.[63-67]

### Chemistry and Hematology

In patients with meningitis, the CSF often appears cloudy because of the presence of WBCs, protein, and bacteria.[66] The chemistry and hematology results from the CSF analysis directly correlate with the probability of infection so that negative findings exclude the likelihood of meningitis in almost all cases.[63,65,66] Patients with acute bacterial meningitis often demonstrate marked abnormalities in the chemistry analysis of the CSF, with protein concentrations of >100 mg/dL and glucose concentrations <45 mg/dL (or a CSF/blood glucose ratio of <0.5) due, in part, to disruption of the blood–brain barrier.[63,66]

Hematologic analysis of the CSF involves measurement of the WBC count with corresponding differential. Patients with acute bacterial meningitis often demonstrate an elevated CSF WBC count (>1,000 cells/mm³) with a neutrophilic predominance (>80% neutrophils). In contrast, patients with viral, fungal, or mycobacterial meningitis often display lower CSF WBC counts (5 to 1,000 cells/mm³) with a predominance of lymphocytes. In cases of a traumatic lumbar puncture (surrounding blood vessels are damaged during needle insertion), peripheral blood can enter the subarachnoid space and contaminate the CSF, making interpretation of the CSF WBC difficult. When interpreting the CSF WBC count after a traumatic tap, there should be one WBC for every 500 to 1,000 RBCs (based on blood composition); this ratio should be used to calculate a corrected CSF WBC during CSF analysis/interpretation.

### Cerebrospinal Fluid Stain and Culture

For patients with suspected bacterial meningitis, a Gram stain and culture should be performed on CSF. Gram stain will demonstrate an organism in 60% to 90% of patients with bacterial meningitis and is helpful in selecting appropriate empiric antibiotic therapy.[2,63,65-67] However, the sensitivity of the CSF Gram stain diminishes to 40% to 60% in patients who have received antibiotics prior to the lumber puncture (also known as *partially treated meningitis*).[2,65] In patients with meningitis caused by viruses, fungi, or mycobacteria, the Gram stain is usually negative, and specialized tests should be used, such as the India ink stain or cryptococcal antigen test for the detection of *Cryptococcus neoformans* or the acid-fast stain for the detection of *Mycobacterium tuberculosis*.

### TABLE 18-12. Typical CSF Findings in Patients with Meningitis

| | NORMAL | BACTERIAL MENINGITIS | VIRAL INFECTION | FUNGAL MENINGITIS | TUBERCULOUS MENINGITIS |
|---|---|---|---|---|---|
| Opening pressure (mm $H_2O$) | <180 | >195 | | | |
| WBCs (count/mm³) | 0–5 <30 (newborns) | 1,000–20,000 (mean 800) | 50–2,000 (mean 80) | 20–2,000 (mean 100) | 5–2,000 (mean 200) |
| WBC differential | No predominance | ≥80% PMNs | >50% lymphs, 20% PMNs | >50% lymphs | >80% lymphs |
| Protein (mg/dL) | <50 | >100 | 30–150 | 40–150 | >50 |
| Glucose (mg/dL) (CSF/blood glucose ratio) | 45–100 (two-thirds of serum) | <45 (< one-half of serum) | 45–70 | 30–70 | <40 |
| Gram stain (% positive) | | 60–90 | Negative | Negative | 37–87 (AFB smear) |

PMNs = polymorphonuclear leukocytes; lymphs = lymphocytes.
*Source*: References 63–67.

All CSF specimens should be processed for culture based on the type of meningitis (acute versus chronic) and the organism suspected of causing the infection. In patients with bacterial meningitis, the cultures are often positive within 24 to 48 hours. In patients with nonbacterial meningitis, culture specimens should be incubated for longer periods of time (up to 2 to 6 weeks), because some organisms take longer to grow.

### Other Specialized Tests

Several specialized tests may be performed on CSF specimens to aid in the detection of the causative organism, including bacterial antigen detection using LA, latex fixation, or enzyme immunoassay (EIA); fungal antigen detection; antibody detection; and bacterial, viral, or mycobacterial PCR assays.[63-67]

Bacterial antigen testing on CSF specimens is a rapid diagnostic test with results available within 10 to 15 minutes. Commercially available tests use antibody-coated particles that bind to specific capsular antigens of the most common pathogens that cause acute bacterial meningitis, including *S pneumoniae, N meningitidis, H influenzae* type B, and group B streptococci. The tests are performed by combining CSF (although they can also be performed using urine or serum) with antibody-coated particles and observing for agglutination, which signifies the presence of the bacterial antigen in the specimen. If visible agglutination does not occur, either the antigen is not present or it is present in insufficient amounts to cause detectable agglutination. Routine bacterial antigen detection of CSF specimens is not currently recommended because the results lack high specificity/sensitivity (not better than the traditional Gram stain), have an inadequate negative predictive value, and their use has rarely impacted patient treatment or been demonstrated to be cost-effective.[3,63,67] However, bacterial antigen testing may be useful in patients with negative Gram stains or in patients who have received previous antimicrobial therapy.[2,63-65,67]

Nucleic-acid amplification tests, including PCR, are rapid and accurate tests for the diagnosis of meningitis due to bacteria, viruses, and fungi.[66,67] CSF PCR results are often positive early in the course of infection and even remain positive during the first week of therapy.[66] Several commercial PCR assays are available that amplify small amounts of specific DNA of the target organism followed by subsequent identification and verification. The FilmArray meningitis/encephalitis panel (BioFire Diagnostics, Salt Lake City, UT) is a multiplex PCR with high sensitivity of 94.2% and specificity of 99.8% that rapidly (<1 hr) detects 14 common causes (six bacteria [*Escherichia coli* K1, *Haemophilus influenzae, Listeria monocytogenes, Neisseria meningitidis, Streptococcus agalactiae, Streptococcus pneumoniae*]; seven viruses [Cytomegalovirus, Enterovirus, Herpes simplex virus 1, Herpes simplex virus 2, Human herpesvirus 6, Human parechovirus, Varicella zoster virus], and *Cryptococcus neoformans*) of meningitis/encephalitis directly from CSF.[66,67]

### Streptococcal Pharyngitis

Acute pharyngitis is one of the most common infections encountered in medicine and can occur in both children and adults. Acute pharyngitis can be caused by several organisms (eg, bacteria and viruses), which produce similar signs and symptoms of infection. Antibiotic therapy is recommended only for patients with pharyngitis caused by bacteria, especially group A streptococci (*Streptococcus pyogenes*).[68] Because group A strep pharyngitis comprises only a small percentage (20% to 30%) of patients with acute pharyngitis, it is important that a rapid, reliable diagnostic test be available to avoid unnecessary antibiotic use in patients with acute viral pharyngitis.[68]

The gold standard diagnostic test for acute pharyngitis caused by group A streptococcus is the throat culture, which often takes 1 to 2 days for results. Therefore, rapid antigen detection tests (RADTs) have been developed to expedite and confirm the diagnosis of group A streptococcal pharyngitis, with most tests yielding results within 15 minutes.[68,69] Positive RADT test results expedite the initiation of antibiotic treatment in the appropriate patient. Several RADT tests are commercially available, with the newer tests employing EIA or chemiluminescent DNA probes (>95% specificity and ≥90% sensitivity).[68,69] There are limited studies comparing the performance of different RADT tests to throat culture (the gold standard), so current recommendations suggest that traditional throat culture be performed in children and adolescents with a negative RADT test result to definitively exclude group A streptococcal pharyngitis.[68,69]

## Pneumonia

Several obstacles make the diagnosis of bacterial pneumonia quite difficult. First, the respiratory tract is colonized with bacteria that may or may not be contributing to the infectious process. When obtaining a sample for culture, lower respiratory tract secretions can become contaminated with secretions or bacteria colonizing the upper respiratory tract; therefore, expectorated sputum samples should be evaluated to determine if contamination with saliva or upper respiratory tract flora has occurred (assessing of the adequacy of the sample).[1,2,4,6,7,70,71] If bacteria other than normal respiratory flora are isolated, the clinician must determine the relative importance and significance of the organism(s) as a potential cause of pneumonia, in addition to assessing the patient for signs and symptoms of pneumonia. It is estimated that 40% to 60% of hospitalized patients with CAP are unable to produce a sputum sample; and 40% to 60% of produced samples that are submitted are judged as being inadequate.[70] For this reason, in some patients, adequate sputum specimens are difficult to obtain without invasive procedures. Invasive procedures, such as BAL or protected specimen brush (PSB), are occasionally used to aid in the diagnosis of pneumonia in patients who are unable to expectorate an adequate sputum sample (especially in patients not responding to appropriate empiric therapy), in immunocompromised patients, and in patients with hospital-acquired pneumonia (HAP) or ventilator-associated pneumonia (VAP).[2,19,70,71] Despite the best efforts at obtaining a lower respiratory tract sputum specimen for culture, as many as 30% to 50% of patients with pneumonia have negative culture results.[70,71]

To obtain an adequate expectorated sputum sample, the patient should be instructed to provide sputum generated from a deep cough. All expectorated sputum samples should be screened to ensure that the specimen is adequate and has not been contaminated by saliva or upper respiratory tract flora prior to processing for culture.[2,70,71] Information used to assess the adequacy of an expectorated sputum sample is derived from visualization of the Gram stain of the specimen. Expectorated sputum specimens that contain >25 WBCs/hpf (unless the patient is neutropenic) and <10 squamous epithelial cells/hpf are considered adequate for further processing and culture.[4,70,71] Samples with >10 epithelial cells/hpf are representative of upper respiratory tract contamination (saliva) and should not be processed for culture. The sputum Gram stain from an adequate sputum specimen may be used to guide empiric antibiotic therapy when the specimen is purulent and contains a predominant organism. Antibiotic therapy should be modified based on the culture results, especially if they reveal an infecting organism.

Because of the difficulty with collection and low yield with sputum culture, several rapid direct detection tests have been developed, including urinary antigen detection (*Streptococcus pneumoniae* and *Legionella pneumophila* serogroup 1) or NA-based methods on respiratory specimens.[70,71] The *S pneumoniae* urinary antigen test may be useful in hospitalized patients who are unable to produce a sputum sample, in patients with severe pneumonia requiring intensive care unit admission, in patients at risk for pneumococcal pneumonia (eg, asplenic, alcohol abuse, liver disease), in patients with pneumonia and concomitant pleural effusion, and in patients who have received antibiotics before a specimen for culture has been obtained.[70,71] Several NA-based rapid (in 1 hour) detection methods are commercially available for the detection of respiratory viruses and bacteria capable of causing upper and lower respiratory tract infections, and include tests such as the Verigene Respiratory Pathogens Flex Test (Luminex; detects three *Bordetella* spp. and 13 viral targets, including adenovirus, influenza, parainfluenza, rhinovirus, and RSV), the FilmArray Respiratory EZ Panel (BioFire Diagnostics; detects coronavirus, adenovirus, five influenza, human rhinovirus/enterovirus, parainfluenza, RSV, human metapneumovirus, *B pertussis, M pneumoniae*, and *C pneumoniae*), the FilmArray Respiratory Panel (BioFire Diagnostics; detects four coronaviruses, adenovirus, five influenza, human rhinovirus/enterovirus, four parainfluenza viruses, RSV, human metapneumovirus, *B pertussis, B parapertussis M pneumoniae*, and *C pneumoniae*), and the FilmArray Pneumonia Panel (BioFire Diagnostics; detects eight viruses, 18 bacteria associated with HAP and seven genetic markers of resistance).[70] Additionally, serologic tests may also be used in the diagnosis of pneumonia caused by atypical bacteria such as *L pneumophila, Mycoplasma pneumoniae*, or *Chlamydia pneumoniae* because they are difficult to culture in the laboratory.[2,3,70,71]

In patients with HAP or VAP, semiquantitative analysis of tracheal aspirates or sputum cultures or quantitative analysis from BAL specimens may occasionally be performed to differentiate between infection and colonization based on the history of prior antibiotic use and the number of organisms recovered in the sputum specimen.[19] Diagnostic thresholds for pneumonia based on colony counts recovered from a quantitative BAL specimen may differ among institutions. Studies evaluating quantitative BAL or PSB specimens for the diagnosis of HAP or VAP use a diagnostic threshold between $10^3$ and $10^5$ CFU/mL of an organism for the diagnosis of pneumonia.[2,19,70]

# Genitourinary Tract Infections
## Urinary Tract Infections

*Urinary tract infections* (UTIs) are common infections, prompting >8 million office visits and more than 100,000 hospitalizations per year.[72-75] UTIs are especially common in female patients because of the close proximity of the urethra (which is shorter than in male patients) to the perirectal and vaginal regions, which are both colonized with bacteria. Because of this anatomic difference, bacteria are able to easily ascend the urethra in female patients and potentially cause infection in the bladder (cystitis) and upper urinary tract (pyelonephritis). In addition, hospitalized patients (male and female) with indwelling urinary catheters are at increased risk for developing UTIs, with approximately 20% of catheterized patients developing a UTI, even with only short-term catheterization.[73,76]

Under normal circumstances, urine within the bladder is sterile because all anatomic sites within the urinary tract above the urethra are not colonized with bacteria. However, the urethra is colonized with bacteria. If noninvasive urine collection methods are used for specimen collection, urine travels through the urethra and may inadvertently collect bacteria while passing through this nonsterile environment. Therefore, diagnostic criteria have been developed to discriminate between infection, bacterial colonization, or bacterial contamination based on quantitative bacterial colony counts from urine cultures and the presence of inflammatory cells and epithelial cells in the urinalysis.[72-74]

Urine samples for urinalysis and culture can be collected several ways. The most common method involves the collection of a clean-catch, midstream urine sample. Before obtaining the sample, the patient should be instructed to clean and rinse the periurethral area with a mild detergent and then retract the labial folds or penile foreskin when beginning to urinate. The patient should attempt to collect the urine in a sterile cup at the midpoint of the urine stream, collecting the urine sample a few seconds after the start of urination.

Other methods for specimen collection involve invasive procedures, such as obtaining urine via bladder catheterization (straight catheter) or via suprapubic bladder aspiration. Both of these methods avoid the potential contamination of the urine specimen by the urethra because the urine is collected directly from the bladder. In hospitalized patients with short-term indwelling urinary catheters, urine specimens should be collected directly from the urinary catheter by aspirating the catheter port or tubing (representing freshly voided urine) rather than obtaining the specimen from the collection bag (urine collected over a period of time).[4,72,73,76] In patients with long-term indwelling urinary catheters, the catheter should be exchanged with the urine sample collected upon insertion of the new catheter.[76] In all cases, urine samples should be immediately transported to the laboratory for processing.

Urine samples from women with acute uncomplicated cystitis are usually only evaluated using screening tests because the results are rapidly available and are useful at excluding the presence of a UTI.[72] The most common rapid screening tests include commercially available reagent test strips, or urine dipsticks, that contain the leukocyte esterase test and the nitrate reductase test, and provide a negative predictive value of 98%.[72,73] The leukocyte esterase test detects the presence of leukocyte esterase, which is an enzyme found in neutrophils. The nitrate reductase test detects the presence of urinary nitrite produced by the reduction of nitrate by nitrate-reducing enzymes of common urinary tract pathogens (primarily *Enterobacterales*).[72-74] Positive results from either the leukocyte esterase test or nitrate reducatase test lead to initiation of treatment for a UTI without the need for urine culture in women with symptoms suggesting acute uncomplicated cystitis.

The urine from patients with recurrent UTIs, complicated/upper tract UTIs, or catheter-associated UTIs is typically evaluated using a urinalysis (microscopic examination) and urine culture. The urinalysis is a rapid test that involves the macroscopic and microscopic examination of the urine sample for color, clarity, specific gravity, and the presence of protein, glucose, RBCs, WBCs, bacteria, and epithelial cells. The urinalysis is performed either manually or with automated instruments. Urinalysis findings suggestive of a UTI include specimen cloudiness and the presence of pyuria (>10 WBC/mm³).[72-74] The detection of pyuria, hematuria, proteinuria, or bacteriuria in the urinalysis may be an indication of infection, but none of these alone is specific for infection. The presence of squamous epithelial cells (>2 to 5 epithelial cells/mm³) in a urine sample suggests poor specimen collection and possible contamination.

The urine culture remains the hallmark laboratory test for the diagnosis of UTIs, with quantitative cultures providing the most useful data for determining the clinical significance of isolated bacteria. To establish the diagnosis of a UTI, urine cultures from midstream urine samples should display >10⁵ CFU/mL of a single potential uropathogen with concomitant pyuria on urinalysis; however, some women with symptomatic cystitis may have lower colony counts of bacteria (10³).[73] Colony counts of >10³ CFU/mL with pyuria are considered clinically relevant in urine specimens from patients with indwelling urethral catheters or intermittent catheterization, from men, or from children.[72,75] Urine specimens obtained by suprapubic aspiration that display >10² CFU/mL with pyuria are indicative of the presence of infection.[72,73,76]

### Prostatitis

Bacterial prostatitis can present as an acute or chronic infection that typically occurs in men >30 years of age.[74] The diagnosis of acute bacterial prostatitis is often based on clinical presentation and the presence of bacteria in a urine specimen. Digital palpation of the prostate and prostatic massage to express purulent secretions are not recommended for the diagnosis of acute bacterial prostatitis because it may induce bacteremia. Conversely, the diagnosis of chronic bacterial prostatitis often cannot be established based on clinical grounds alone because the symptoms are nonspecific and the prostate is often not acutely inflamed. Therefore, the diagnosis of chronic prostatitis is classically established through the analysis of sequential urine and prostatic fluid cultures.[74,77] Initially, two samples of urine are obtained for culture—one sample on initiation of urination (VB-1) and one sample obtained at midstream (VB-2). Next,

prostate fluid is obtained for culture by massaging the prostate to produce expressed prostatic secretions. Lastly, a urine sample (VB-3) is obtained after prostatic secretions have been obtained and sent for culture. The diagnosis of chronic bacterial prostatitis is made when the expressed prostatic secretion sample contains > 10 times the quantity of bacteria cultured from VB-1 or VB-2 or if the VB-3 contains 10 times the quantity of bacteria cultured from VB-1 or VB-2.[74,77]

## Sexually Transmitted Diseases

### Gonorrhea

Infection due to *N gonorrhoeae* is the second most common notifiable sexually transmitted disease (STD) reported in the United States, with most infections involving the mucosa of the cervix, the urethra, the rectum, and the pharynx.[78,79] Infections caused by *N gonorrhoeae* include localized, uncomplicated, or complicated genital infections (eg, urethritis, cervicitis, endometritis, pelvic inflammatory disease [PID] in women, and urethritis or epididymitis in men), pharyngitis, anorectal infections, and disseminated infection (eg, septic arthritis and meningitis) in both men and women.[78,79] Women with genital tract infection and patients with pharyngeal infection are often asymptomatic, while men with urethritis often display symptoms of dysuria and urethral discharge. In addition, patients with *N gonorrhoeae* are often coinfected with other STDs, such as *Chlamydia trachomatis*, syphilis, or *Trichomonas vaginalis;* therefore, the diagnosis and treatment of all possible STDs in the patient and their sexual partners are important public health considerations in the control of STDs.[78]

The diagnosis of infection due to *N gonorrhoeae* can be established using Gram-stained smears, culture, or nonculture techniques detecting cellular components (only NA amplification tests [NAATs] are currently recommended for routine use; EIA and DNA probe tests are no longer recommended) of urethral, endocervical, or urine specimens (NAAT only) that detect cellular components of *N gonorrhoeae*.[4,78-81]

A presumptive diagnosis of gonorrhea can be made using direct microscopic examination of a clinical specimen using a Gram stain and oxidase test, in which gram-negative, oxidase-positive diplococci are demonstrated.[78-81] In addition, the presence of neutrophils on a Gram stain of a urethral specimen is also helpful in establishing the presumptive diagnosis of urethritis.[79] The Gram stain is both sensitive and specific for the presumptive diagnosis of *N gonorrhoeae* as a point-of-care test for symptomatic men with urethral discharge but is not as useful as a single diagnostic test in asymptomatic men or when evaluating endocervical or pharyngeal specimens.[78,79] Additional tests, such as culture, should be performed to confirm the identification of the organism.

Culture on selective media remains the diagnostic standard for the identification of *N gonorrhoeae*.[79,80] Culture is recommended for the diagnosis of gonorrhea from urethral, endocervical, vaginal, pharyngeal, or rectal swab (plastic or wire shafts with rayon, Dacron, or calcium alginate tips) specimens and should be performed on specimens from all patients (and sexual partners) with suspected gonococcal infections.[79] Culture is also used as a confirmatory test in patients who have suspected gonorrhea based on positive Gram-stained smears or nonculture tests if the specimen has been adequately maintained. However, culture is not optimal in all circumstances due to the tenuous viability of the organism during storage and transport, which is what led to the development of nonculture tests for the detection of gonorrhea.[79] Occasionally, susceptibility testing is performed on *N gonorrhoeae* isolates, especially in patients with suspected or documented treatment failure, to guide the choice of antibiotic therapy, as well as for epidemiologic purposes.[78] In either case, patients are typically given empiric therapy with an antibiotic that demonstrates excellent activity against gonorrhea, keeping in mind that the incidence of β-lactamase-producing, penicillin-resistant gonococci is increasing.

In many clinical settings, nonculture tests for the detection of *N gonorrhoeae* have replaced traditional culture. Nonculture tests include NAATs, which are able to amplify organism-specific DNA sequences, and the NA hybridization (probe) test, which hybridizes any complementary rRNA that is present in the specimen (cannot differentiate organisms).[78,79] Several NAATs for the detection of *N gonorrhoeae* are commercially available and have been designed to detect RNA or DNA sequences using amplification techniques (even on nonviable organisms). These tests have been FDA-approved for the detection of *N gonorrhoeae* in endocervical and vaginal swabs from women, urethral swabs from men, and urine samples from men and women; because the tests are different, the product information for each individual test should be consulted to dictate the collection methods and clinical specimen type that is suitable for each test.[78,79] These tests are also useful for the detection of *N gonorrhoeae* from clinical specimens that have not been adequately maintained during transport or for collection for culture methods to be used. The major drawback of nonculture techniques for the detection of gonorrhea is that they cannot provide information on antibiotic susceptibility of the organism.[81]

## Chlamydia

*Chlamydia trachomatis* is the most frequently reported infectious disease in the United States, with >1.3 million cases reported to the Centers for Disease Control and Prevention in 2010.[78,79] Infection with *C trachomatis* is now a reportable communicable disease in the United States, with the highest prevalence in persons aged ≤24 years.[78] *C trachomatis* can cause a number of infections, including cervicitis, endometritis, and PID in women; and urethritis, epididymo-orchitis, prostatitis, and proctitis (via receptive anal intercourse) in men.[78] Infection with *C trachomatis* is also thought to contribute to female infertility and ectopic pregnancies. It is estimated that more than $500 million is spent annually on the direct costs associated with the management of *C trachomatis* infections.[79]

Most patients with chlamydial infections are asymptomatic, so screening is necessary to detect the presence of the organism.[78,79] Because of the asymptomatic nature of chlamydia, it is thought that the current rates of reporting underestimate the true incidence of infection due to this organism. Chlamydia screening is now recommended annually in all sexually active women aged <25 years and other women at increased risk for infection (eg, new sexual partner, multiple sexual partners,

sexual partner with an STD).[78] In addition, chlamydia screening is also recommended in patients with other STDs because chlamydia often coexists with other STD pathogens.

Culture and nonculture methods are available for the detection of chlamydia. Culture involves the inoculation of the biologic specimen onto a confluent monolayer of cells that support the growth of *C trachomatis*. The culture is evaluated at 24 to 72 hours for the presence of intracellular inclusions using a fluorescent monoclonal antibody stain, which occur as a result of *C trachomatis* infection.[79] Cell culture is not routinely used by most laboratories because of lack of standardization, technical difficulty, cost, and length of time to yield results (at least 48 hours). Therefore, other nonculture approaches for the laboratory diagnosis of chlamydia have been developed, including the direct fluorescent antibody (DFA) test and NAATs.[80]

Direct fluorescent antibody testing involves the staining of a biologic specimen with a fluorescein-labeled monoclonal antibody that binds to *C trachomatis*-specific antigens (elementary bodies).[80] If the patient is infected with *C trachomatis*, the antibodies will react with the elementary bodies of the chlamydia in the secretions to produce fluorescence. DFA tests require significant technologist time for performance, so they are typically only used as a confirmatory test to other antigen detection tests.[80]

The other nonculture test used for the detection of *C trachomatis* is the NAAT, which has largely replaced tissue culture and DFA testing because of greater sensitivity and specificity.[78,79,81] Several commercially available NAATs for the detection of *C trachomatis* have been designed to detect RNA or DNA sequences using PCR, ligase chain reaction, and various amplification techniques. These tests have been FDA approved for the detection of *C trachomatis* in endocervical or vaginal swabs from women, urethral swabs from men, and rectal swab or first catch urine samples from men and women.[78,79]

## Syphilis

The spirochete *T pallidum* is the causative pathogen of an STD known as *syphilis*. There are a number of clinical manifestations and stages of syphilis that are based primarily on presenting symptoms and the natural history of the infection[46,78,81]:

1. **Primary syphilis:** characterized by painless ulcers called *chancres* that are typically located at the site of inoculation or initial infection (usually in genital area) and spontaneously resolve over 1 to 8 weeks.

2. **Secondary syphilis:** characterized by systemic symptoms, including fever, weight loss, malaise, headache, lymphadenopathy, and a mucocutaneous skin rash (generalized or localized, often involving the palms or the soles of the feet) resulting from hematogenous or lymphatic spread of the organism. If untreated, the manifestations resolve within 4 to 10 weeks.

3. **Latent syphilis:** occurs after secondary syphilis, in which the organism is still present, but the patient is without symptoms. Latent syphilis acquired within the preceding year is categorized as early latent syphilis, whereas syphilis acquired more than 1 year ago or of unknown duration is categorized as late latent syphilis. This subclinical infection can be detected only by serologic tests.

4. **Late/tertiary syphilis and neurosyphilis:** occurs in approximately 35% of untreated patients up to 10 to 25 years after initial infection; clinical manifestations are caused by progressive inflammatory disease that can involve the CNS (categorized as neurosyphilis) or outside the CNS (referred to as tertiary syphilis) including cardiovascular lesions (ascending aorta) and granuloma-like lesions (gummas) in the skin, bone, or visceral organs.

*T pallidum* cannot be grown in culture; therefore, the diagnosis of syphilis involves the direct detection of the spirochete in biologic specimens by microscopy or the detection of treponemal-specific antibodies using serologic testing.

Direct detection methods can be performed on appropriate clinical specimens obtained from suspicious genital or skin lesions, including lesion exudate or tissue. The direct detection of *T pallidum* using dark-field microscopy involves the immediate examination (within 20 minutes of collection) of the biologic specimen under a microscope with a dark-field condenser, looking for the presence of motile spirochetes, where *T pallidum* appears as 8- to 10-μm spiral-shaped organisms.[4,46,81] Another test for the direct detection of *T pallidum* is the direct fluorescent antibody (DFA-TP) test in which the biologic specimen is combined with fluorescein-labeled monoclonal or polyclonal antibodies specific for *T pallidum* and examined by fluorescence microscopy.[46,78] The interaction between the antibodies and treponemal-specific antigens produces fluorescence that can be visualized using microscopy.

There are two types of serologic tests that are used for the diagnosis of syphilis – *nontreponemal* and *treponemal* antibody tests. The use of only one type of serologic test is not sufficient for the diagnosis of syphilis (may result in false-negative or false-positive diagnoses), so persons with a reactive nontreponemal test result should undergo treponemal antibody testing to confirm the diagnosis.[78]

The *nontreponemal* antibody tests include the Venereal Disease Research Laboratory (VDRL) test and the rapid plasma reagin (RPR) test.[46,81] Both the VDRL and RPR measure the presence of reagin, an antibody-like protein produced in patients with syphilis. However, reaginic antibodies are also produced in patients with other infections and conditions including autoimmune diseases, leprosy, TB, malaria, pregnancy, and injection drug use, so false-positive RPR results may occur.[46,81] Both the RPR and VDRL tests are flocculation tests in which visible clumps are produced in the presence of the reagin antibody (*T pallidum*) in the submitted specimen. For the VDRL test, the biologic specimen (serum, CSF) is combined with cardiolipin-lecithin coated cholesterol particles on a glass slide and examined microscopically.[46] If the reagin antibody is present in the biologic specimen, visual clumping occurs and is reported as reactive (medium and large clumps). The VDRL can be performed on serum and CSF as a quantitative test in which dilutions of the biologic specimen can be evaluated for reactivity; the dilution that produces a fully reactive result is reported as the VDRL titer (eg, 1:8 or 1:32). Therefore, the VDRL titer can be used to monitor a patient's response to therapy. The high titers present in untreated disease (eg, 1:32) traditionally decrease 4-fold within 6 to 12 months of treatment and become undetectable in 1 to 2 years.

The RPR test is a modification of the VDRL test and is commercially available as a reaction card. Serum from the patient is placed on the reaction card and observed for clumping. The RPR result is quantified by evaluating dilutions of the biologic specimen for reactivity, with the highest dilution that produces a fully reactive result being reported as the RPR titer (eg, 1:8 or 1:32). The RPR titer is also used to monitor a patient's response to therapy, where a 4-fold decline in titer 6 to 12 months after therapy would be suggestive of response. The RPR is easier to perform than the VDRL and is used by many laboratories and blood banks for routine syphilis screening. However, the RPR should not be used for the analysis of CSF specimens.

The nontreponemal antibody detection tests are nonspecific, so they are most useful for *screening* for the presence of syphilis.[46,81] Because it takes several weeks for the development of reagin antibodies after exposure to syphilis, false-negative results (up to 25% of patients with primary syphilis) can occur in the early stages of the disease. In addition, false-positive results (up to 1% to 2%) can also occur because of the numerous other conditions where reagin antibodies are produced.[3,46] Therefore, a positive RPR or VDRL test result should be confirmed with the fluorescent treponemal antibody absorption (FTA-ABS) or the microhemagglutination *T pallidum* (MHA-TP) test, both of which measure the presence of treponemal-specific antibodies.

The other type of serologic test measures the presence of *treponemal* antibodies and includes the FTA-ABS test and the MHA-TP test.[46,78,81] In the FTA-ABS test, the patient's serum or CSF is initially absorbed with non-*T pallidum* antigens to reduce cross-reactivity and then applied to a slide on which *T pallidum* organisms have been fixed followed by addition of a fluorescein-conjugated antihuman antibody for detection of specific antitreponemal antibodies. The amount of fluorescence is subjectively measured by the laboratory technician and reported as reactive, minimally reactive, or nonreactive. Therefore, this test is difficult to standardize among different laboratories. Because this test is also fairly expensive, it is primarily used to verify the results of a positive VDRL or RPR, rather than as a routine screening tool.[46,81] The FTA-ABS test can detect antibodies earlier in the course of syphilis than nontreponemal tests and, once positive, remains positive for the life of the patient.

The MHA-TP test is performed using erythrocytes from a turkey, sheep, or other mammal that have been coated with treponemal antigens. These erythrocytes are then mixed with the patient's serum and observed for agglutination, which signifies the presence of antibodies directed against *T pallidum*. The results are reported as reactive (positive) or nonreactive (negative). Lastly, EIA tests and PCR-based tests for the detection of *T pallidum* are being evaluated as screening or confirmatory tests for the diagnosis of syphilis, especially for patients in whom serologic testing is not reliable.[46,81]

### Trichomonas

Infection caused by the protozoan *T vaginalis* is the most common, nonviral STD in the United States, affecting 3.7 million people.[78] *T. vaginalis* is typically diagnosed through detection of actively motile organisms during microscopic examination of wet mount preparations of vaginal secretions, urethral discharge, prostatic fluid, or urine sediment.[61,78,81] Because the sensitivity of the wet mount preparation is 50% to 80%, other diagnostic tests have been developed for the detection of *T vaginalis* to enhance diagnostic yield, sensitivity, and specificity.[78,81] Culture using Diamond's medium is considered the diagnostic gold standard test because it is associated with >80% sensitivity; however, culture methods require proper collection and rapid inoculation for best results, so it is not routinely performed by most laboratories.[81] Several rapid antigen detection methods are commercially available for the diagnosis of infection caused by *T vaginalis* that are easy to perform and employ different assays (IFA and capillary flow ICA).[61] Lastly, NA detection methods are highly sensitive and specific tests for the detection of *Trichomonas* and include direct DNA probe Affirm VPIII (BD) and the APTIMA *T vaginalis* Assay (Hologic-GenProbe, San Diego, CA).[61,78]

## Assessing Sterile Body Fluids for Presence of Infection

Sterile body fluids such as pericardial fluid (pericarditis), pleural fluid (empyema), synovial fluid (septic arthritis), and peritoneal fluid (peritonitis) can be analyzed for the presence of infection. The specimens should be aseptically obtained by needle aspiration, placed in sterile collection tubes, and immediately transported to the laboratory for fluid analysis and culture. Approximately 1 to 5 mL of fluid should be obtained when analyzing pericardial, pleural, or synovial fluid, while up to 10 mL of peritoneal fluid is required for the diagnosis of peritonitis.[82] All sterile fluids should be processed for cell count (establishing the presence of WBCs with differential), chemistry (protein and glucose), direct microscopic examination including Gram stain (presence of bacteria), and culture. For pleural and synovial fluids, specific criteria are available to aid in the diagnosis of infection (**Tables 18-13** and **18-14**).[82-88] Peritoneal fluid characteristics that may be suggestive of peritonitis include a WBC of >250 cells/mm³, a lactate concentration >25 mg/dL, a pH <7.35, a fluid/blood glucose ratio of <0.7 (in TB peritonitis), and an elevated protein concentration (except in patients with cirrhosis).[89,90] The diagnosis of infection in each of these sites should be established based on the presence of WBCs and other characteristic chemistry abnormalities in the sterile fluid specimen, the growth of a pathogenic organism from the cultured material, and the characteristic signs and symptoms of infection at that site.

## ACUTE PHASE REACTANTS AND INFECTION

Chapters 16 and 20 provide information on the background, normal range, and clinical use of acute phase reactants such as the ESR, CRP, and procalcitonin in the diagnosis of inflammatory diseases. The ESR and CRP may also be elevated in the presence of infection.[91-96] Elevations in the ESR and CRP do not differentiate between inflammatory or infectious processes because they increase in response to tissue injury of any cause. However, the ESR and CRP are often elevated in the presence of infection, with increased levels reported in bacterial otitis media, osteomyelitis, endocarditis, PID, septic arthritis, prosthetic joint infections, and infections in transplant patients, and they may serve as an adjunctive modality to aid in the diagnosis

## TABLE 18-13. Pleural Fluid Findings and Interpretation

| | TRANSUDATIVE (SUGGESTIVE OF CONGESTIVE HEART FAILURE, CIRRHOSIS) | EXUDATIVE (SUGGESTIVE OF INFECTION SUCH AS EMPYEMA, MALIGNANCY, PANCREATITIS WITH ESOPHAGEAL PERFORATION, SLE) |
|---|---|---|
| Appearance | Clear, serous | Cloudy |
| pH | >7.2 | <7.2 |
| LDH (International Units/L) | <200 | ≥200 |
| Pleural fluid LDH to serum LDH ratio | <0.6 | >0.6 |
| Protein (g/dL) | <3 | >3 |
| Pleural fluid to serum protein ratio | <0.5 | >0.5 |
| Glucose (mg/dL) | >60 (same as serum) | <40–60 |
| WBCs (count/mm³) | <10,000 | >10,000 |
| WBC differential | <50% PMNs | If infectious, depends on pathogen |

LDH = lactate dehydrogenase; PMNs = polymorphonuclear leukocytes; SLE = systemic lupus erythematosus.
*Source:* References 82–85.

**TABLE 18-14.** Synovial Fluid Findings and Interpretation

| | NORMAL | NONINFLAMMATORY (OSTEOARTHRITIS, TRAUMA, AVASCULAR NECROSIS, SLE, EARLY RHEUMATOID ARTHRITIS) | INFLAMMATORY (RHEUMATOID ARTHRITIS, SPONDYLOARTHROPATHIES, VIRAL ARTHRITIS, CRYSTAL-INDUCED ARTHRITIS) | PURULENT (BACTERIAL INFECTION, TUBERCULOUS INFECTION, FUNGAL INFECTION) |
|---|---|---|---|---|
| WBCs (count/mm³) | <150–200 | <2,000 | 2,000–50,000 | >50,000 |
| WBC differential | No predominance | <25% PMNs | >70% PMNs, variable | >75% to 90% PMNs |
| Protein (g/dL) | 1.3–1.8 | 3–3.5 | >3.5 | >3.5 |
| Glucose (mg/dL) | Normal | Normal | 70–90 | <40–50 |

PMNs = polymorphonuclear leukocytes; SLE = systemic lupus erythematosus.
*Source:* References 86–88.

of these infections.[91-96] ESR levels of >100 mm/hr have a high specificity for the presence of infection, malignancy, or arteritis.[92] Serial measurement of the ESR, and especially the CRP, may also be useful in assessing the response to antibiotic therapy in the treatment of deep-seated infections such as endocarditis or osteomyelitis.[91-96]

Procalcitonin is the precursor of calcitonin, a calcium regulatory hormone, which is also an acute phase reactant that is produced in response to systemic inflammation.[91,97-99] During infection, the metabolism of procalcitonin is altered in response to toxins and cytokines from bacteria, malaria, and some fungi (not viruses).[97-100] As procalcitonin accumulates, its levels become detectable within 2 to 4 hours of infection and peak at 6 to 24 hours, with the extent of production correlating with bacterial load and severity of infection.[97,98] It was originally believed that procalcitonin levels increased in response to tissue injury or sepsis induced only by infection; however, levels of procalcitonin may be elevated in other inflammatory diseases or situations, such as autoimmune diseases, severe trauma, cirrhosis, pancreatitis, burns, cardiac surgery, cardiac arrest, certain types of cancer, receipt of some conditioning agents prior to stem cell transplantation, and hypotension during surgery.[91,92,97-100]

The use of procalcitonin in the diagnosis of infection has been evaluated in numerous studies involving different patient types, infections, and clinical settings, with several procalcitonin-based algorithms being developed to (1) determine the presence of infection/guide initiation of antibiotic therapy, (2) evaluate the efficacy of empiric antibiotic therapy, and (3) determine when antibiotic therapy can be deescalated or discontinued during the treatment of an infection.[97,98] Procalcitonin levels that correlate with the presence of infection have not been clearly defined for all infection types and clinical settings, but it does appear as if procalcitonin levels <0.1 mcg/L (eg, undetectable) exclude the presence of infection.[98] In the past decade, the role of procalcitonin has been studied in the context of sepsis and critically ill patients, lower respiratory tract infections, chronic obstructive pulmonary disease, acute infections

in the CNS, infectious complications of burns and pancreatitis, and polytrauma.[101] These studies demonstrate a wide variability in diagnostic accuracy, usefulness in guiding antibiotic discontinuation, and cost effectiveness. Additional research is needed to further define the role of procalcitonin in the diagnosis and management of different patient types, infections, and clinical settings.[97-99]

## SUMMARY

Although infectious disease is a rapidly changing field because of new challenges and technological advances, the diagnosis of infection is highly dependent on the proper performance and interpretation of numerous laboratory tests. For example, the Gram stain is a readily available, invaluable tool for examining clinical specimens for the presence of bacteria. Culture of clinical specimens using appropriate growth media allows for the cultivation and identification of many infecting bacteria, which often takes 24 to 48 hours. Numerous rapid diagnostic tests are now available for the identification of bacteria directly from clinical specimens, such as blood, stool, respiratory secretions, or body fluids, which substantially decrease the time to organism identification when compared with traditional bacterial culture and identification methods.[3] Susceptibility tests for rapidly growing aerobic bacteria are commonly performed using an automated microdilution or a manual disk diffusion method. Bacterial susceptibilities to various antimicrobial agents are reported as S, I, and R. National standards for susceptibility testing are available and help guide the performance of the tests, the choice of antimicrobial agents to evaluate for susceptibility, and the reporting procedures of susceptibility tests by the clinical microbiology laboratory. Empiric antimicrobial therapy is typically chosen based on the suspected site and subsequent potential causative organisms of infection (using local or regional susceptibility information). Once the results of bacterial culture and susceptibility testing are available, antimicrobial therapy is de-escalated, if possible, to a more targeted (directed) regimen based on the susceptibility profile of the infecting organism in conjunction with patient-specific (eg, clinical condition, site of infection, drug allergies, and renal function) and infection-specific information.

Lastly, several infection types (eg, meningitis, UTIs) and certain pathogens (eg, *B burgdorferi* and *L pneumophila*) often require specialized laboratory testing to aid in the identification of the infecting organism. The clinician should be aware of the diagnostic tests currently available for these infections.

## LEARNING POINTS

1.  **What methods for antimicrobial susceptibility testing are used by most microbiology laboratories in the United States, and how is this information conveyed to the clinician?**

    **ANSWER:** Microbiology laboratories often use several methods for antimicrobial susceptibility testing to accurately determine the activity of antibiotics against many different types of bacteria (eg, aerobic, anaerobic, and fastidious). However, most laboratories predominantly use automated broth microdilution methods (Vitek 2, MicroScan) that utilize commercially prepared, disposable microtiter trays or cassettes for antimicrobial susceptibility testing that can test the susceptibility of multiple antibiotics simultaneously while decreasing cost and labor. Although many microbiology laboratories perform rapid diagnostic tests for the identification of bacteria and the detection of pertinent resistant gene markers, antimicrobial susceptibility testing (using automated microdilution methods) is still being performed to determine the exact susceptibility and resistance profile of the infecting bacteria. The antimicrobial susceptibility results for each bacteria are compiled in a report that contains the following information: antibiotic tested, MIC or MIC range (especially with automated broth microdilution methods), and CLSI interpretive criteria (S, I, and R). These reports are usually located in the patient's medical chart (electronic or paper) and in the hospital laboratory information system. Refer to Minicase 2 for a specific example of an antimicrobial susceptibility report.

2.  **Is the antibiotic with the lowest MIC on an individual susceptibility report always the best antibiotic choice in the treatment of an infection?**

    **ANSWER:** No, the antibiotic with the lowest MIC on an individual susceptibility report may not always be the best choice for the treatment of a specific infection. While the MIC value is an indication of the in vitro activity of the antibiotic against an organism, other issues must be considered when choosing an antibiotic once susceptibility results have returned (these are the same considerations used to establish MIC breakpoints). Each antibiotic has its own unique pharmacokinetic profile and recommended dosage range, resulting in unique serum and site concentrations. An antibiotic might display potent in vitro active against a particular organism but may be ineffective in vivo because of poor penetration to the site of infection. Thus, both the site of infection and achievable serum/site concentrations should be considered. Other things that should also be considered when selecting an

antibiotic include the pharmacodynamic parameter that correlates with efficacy. The pharmacokinetic-pharmacodynamic relationship for each antibiotic-organism combination as well as the results of Monte Carlo simulations (analyses performed using population pharmacokinetic data of the antibiotic and bacteria MIC distribution data from susceptibility studies to evaluate the percentage of time the antibiotic will achieve adequate pharmacodynamic indices for the treatment of that organism in a simulated population), if available, should be reviewed to determine if optimal pharmacodynamic exposure will occur with the selected antibiotic based on the infecting organism's MIC value. The results from clinical efficacy studies should also be considered when selecting a specific antibiotic—has the antibiotic demonstrated efficacy in the treatment of the infection in controlled clinical trials/published studies and, if so, what MICs were observed in patients with clinical success versus clinical failure? Lastly, other factors, such as patient characteristics (eg, pregnancy, comorbidities, allergies), drug characteristics (eg, administration schedule, route of therapy, cost) and hospital/insurance company formulary, should also be considered when selecting an antibiotic.

3.  **What are the major laboratory tests that are used in the diagnosis of UTIs, meningitis, pneumonia, and septic arthritis?**

    **ANSWER:** In patients with signs and symptoms suggestive of a complicated UTI, a urine sample (clean-catch midstream, catheterized specimen, suprapubic aspiration) is usually sent to the laboratory for microscopic analysis (urinalysis) and culture. In patients with signs and symptoms suggestive of meningitis, a lumbar puncture is performed to obtain CSF that is evaluated for general appearance, glucose concentration, protein concentration, WBC count, WBC differential, Gram stain, and culture. In addition, depending on the medical history of the patient, specialized tests may also be performed on the CSF. In patients with signs and symptoms suggestive of pneumonia, a sputum sample (expectorated, BAL, PSB) is submitted to the laboratory for adequacy evaluation, Gram stain and culture, and, occasionally, *S. pneumoniae* urinary antigen. In patients with suspected septic arthritis, a synovial fluid aspirate is analyzed for cell count (presence of WBCs with differential), chemistry (protein and glucose), direct microscopic examination including Gram stain (presence of bacteria), and culture. Patients with septic arthritis may also have an elevated ESR or CRP. Also, in all infections discussed in this chapter, patients may also exhibit leukocytosis and a left shift, which would be demonstrated on a CBC.

## REFERENCES

1.  Specimen management. In: Tile PM, ed. *Bailey and Scott's Diagnostic Microbiology*. 14th ed. St Louis, MO: Elsevier Inc; 2017:56-71.

2.  Miller JM, Binnicker MJ, Campbell S, et al. A guide to utilization of the microbiology laboratory for diagnosis of infectious diseases: 2018 update by the Infectious Diseases Society of America (IDSA) and the American Society for Microbiology (ASM). *Clin Infect Dis*. 2018;67(6):e1-e94. PubMed

3.  Patel R. The clinician and the microbiology laboratory: test ordering, specimen collection, and result interpretation. In: Bennett JE, Dolin R, Blaser MJ, eds. *Principles and Practice of Infectious Diseases*. 9th ed. Philadelphia, PA: Elsevier, Inc.; 2020:194-210.

4. McElvania E, Singh K. Specimen collection, transport, and processing: Bacteriology. In: Carroll KC, Pfaller MA, Landry ML, et al., eds. *Manual of Clinical Microbiology*. 12th ed. Washington, DC: American Society for Microbiology Press; 2019:302-330.

5. Popescu A, Doyle RJ. The Gram stain after more than a century. *Biotech Histochem*. 1996;71(3):145-151.PubMed

6. Role of microscopy. In: Tile PM, ed. *Bailey and Scott's Diagnostic Microbiology*. 14th ed. St Louis, MO: Elsevier Inc; 2017:72-85.

7. Woods GL, Walker DH. Detection of infection or infectious agents by use of cytologic and histologic stains. *Clin Microbiol Rev*. 1996;9(3):382-404. PubMed

8. Atlas R, Snyder J. Reagents, stains, and media: bacteriology. In: Carroll KC, Pfaller MA, Landry ML, et al., eds. *Manual of Clinical Microbiology*. 12th ed. Washington, DC: American Society for Microbiology Press; 2019:331-361.

9. Graman PS, Menegus MA. Microbiology laboratory tests. In: Betts RF, Chapman SW, Penn RL, eds. *A Practical Approach to Infectious Diseases*. 5th ed. Philadelphia, PA: Lippincott, Williams and Wilkins; 2003:929-956.

10. Bacteria. In: Wilborn JW, ed. *Microbiology*. Springhouse, PA: Springhouse Corporation; 1993:36-50.

11. Werth BJ, Barber KE, Smith JR, Rybak MJ. Laboratory tests to direct antimicrobial pharmacotherapy. In: DiPiro JT, Yee GC, Posey L, et al., eds. *Pharmacotherapy: A Pathophysiologic Approach*. 11th ed. New York, NY: McGraw-Hill; 2020. https://accesspharmacy.mhmedical.com/content.aspx?bookid=2577&sectionid=219306547. Accessed June 29, 2020.

12. Traditional cultivation and identification. In: Tile PM, ed. *Bailey and Scott's Diagnostic Microbiology*. 14th ed. St Louis: Elsevier Inc; 2017:86-112.

13. Lagier JC, Edouard S, Pagnier I, et al. Current and past strategies for bacterial culture in clinical microbiology. *Clin Microbiol Rev*. 2015;28(1):208-236.PubMed

14. Nucleic acid-based analytical methods for microbial identification and characterization. In: Tile PM, ed. *Bailey and Scott's Diagnostic Microbiology*. 14th ed. St Louis, MO: Elsevier Inc; 2017:113-143.

15. Pliakos EE, Andreatos N, Shehadeh F, et al. The cost-effectiveness of rapid diagnostic testing for the diagnosis of bloodstream infections with or without antimicrobial stewardship. *Clin Microbiol Rev*. 2018;31(3): e1-e22 10.1128/CMR.00095-17.PubMed

16. Nolte FS. Molecular microbiology. In: Carroll KC, Pfaller MA, Landry ML, et al., eds. *Manual of Clinical Microbiology*. 12th ed. Washington, DC: American Society for Microbiology Press; 2019:86-123.

17. Versalovic J, Highlander SK, Ganesh BP, Petrosino JF. The human microbiome. Carroll KC, Pfaller MA, Landry ML, et al., eds. *Manual of Clinical Microbiology*. 12th ed. Washington, DC: American Society for Microbiology Press; 2019:254-267.

18. Reese RE, Betts RF. Principles of antibiotic use. In: Betts RF, Chapman SW, Penn RL, eds. *A Practical Approach to Infectious Diseases*. 5th ed. Philadelphia, PA: Lippincott, Williams and Wilkins; 2003:969-988.

19. Kalil AC, Metersky ML, Klompas M, et al. Management of adults with hospital-acquired and ventilator-associated pneumonia: 2016 Clinical Practice Guidelines by the Infectious Diseases Society of America and the American Thoracic Society. *Clin Infect Dis*. 2016;63:1-51.

20. Laboratory methods and strategies for antimicrobial susceptibility testing. In: Tile PM, ed. *Bailey and Scott's Diagnostic Microbiology*. 14th ed. St Louis, MO: Mosby Inc; 2017:177-204.

21. Clinical and Laboratory Standards Institute (CLSI). *Development of In Vitro Susceptibility Testing Criteria and Quality Control Parameters; Approved Guideline*. 5th ed. Wayne, PA: Clinical and Laboratory Standards Institute; 2018.

22. Peterson LR, Shanholtzer CJ. Tests for bactericidal effects of antimicrobial agents: technical performance and clinical relevance. *Clin Microbiol Rev*. 1992;5(4):420-432.PubMed

23. Simner PJ, Humphries R. Special phenotypic methods for detecting antibacterial resistance. In: Carroll KC, Pfaller MA, Landry ML, et al., eds. *Manual of Clinical Microbiology*. 12th ed. Washington, DC: American Society for Microbiology Press; 2019:1316-1347.

24. DeGirolami PC, Eliopoulos G. Antimicrobial susceptibility tests and their role in therapeutic drug monitoring. *Clin Lab Med*. 1987;7(3):499-512. PubMed

25. Jorgensen JH, Ferraro MJ. Antimicrobial susceptibility testing: a review of general principles and contemporary practices. *Clin Infect Dis*. 2009;49(11):1749-1755.PubMed

26. Clinical and Laboratory Standards Institute (CLSI). *Performance Standards for Antimicrobial Susceptibility Testing*. 30th ed. Wayne, PA: Clinical and Laboratory Standards Institute; 2020.

27. Clinical and Laboratory Standards Institute (CLSI). *Methods for Dilution Antimicrobial Susceptibility Tests for Bacteria That Grow Aerobically; Approved Standard*. 11th ed. Wayne, PA: Clinical and Laboratory Standards Institute; 2018.

28. Clinical and Laboratory Standards Institute (CLSI). *Performance Standards for Antimicrobial Disk Susceptibility Tests; Approved Standard*. 13th ed. Wayne, PA: Clinical and Laboratory Standards Institute; 2018.

29. Koeth LM, Miller LA. Antimicrobial susceptibility test methods: dilution and disk diffusion methods. In: Carroll KC, Pfaller MA, Landry ML, et al., eds. *Manual of Clinical Microbiology*. 12th ed. Washington, DC: American Society for Microbiology Press; 2019:1284-1299.

30. Pulidot MR, García-Quintanilla M, Martín-Peña R, et al. Progress on the development of rapid methods for antimicrobial susceptibility testing. *J Antimicrob Chemother*. 2013;68(12):2710-2717.PubMed

31. Clinical and Laboratory Standards Institute (CLSI)/National Committee for Clinical Laboratory Standards. *Methods for Determining Bactericidal Activity of Antimicrobial Agents*. Wayne, PA: Clinical and Laboratory Standards Institute; 1999.

32. Reller LB. The serum bactericidal test. *Rev Infect Dis*. 1986;8(5):803-808. PubMed

33. Clinical and Laboratory Standards Institute (CLSI)/National Committee for Clinical Laboratory Standards. *Methodology for the Serum Bactericidal Test*. Wayne, PA: Clinical and Laboratory Standards Institute; 1999.

34. Bush K. Past and present perspectives on β-lactamases. *Antimicrob Agents Chemother*. 2018;62(10):1-18.PubMed

35. Paterson DL, Bonomo RA. Extended-spectrum β-lactamases: a clinical update. *Clin Microbiol Rev*. 2005;18(4):657-686.PubMed

36. Humphries RM, Bard JD. Susceptibility test methods: fastidious bacteria. In: Carroll KC, Pfaller MA, Landry ML, et al., eds. *Manual of Clinical Microbiology*. 12th ed. Washington, DC: American Society for Microbiology Press; 2019:1348-1376.

37. Thomson KS. Extended-spectrum β-lactamases, AmpC, and carbapenemase issues. *J Clin Microbiol*. 2010;48(4):1019-1025.PubMed

38. Abbott AN, Fang FC. Molecular detection of antibacterial drug resistance. In: Carroll KC, Pfaller MA, Landry ML, et al., eds. *Manual of Clinical Microbiology*. 12th ed. Washington, DC: American Society for Microbiology Press; 2019:1420-1431.

39. van Belkum A, Rochas O. Laboratory-based and point-of-care testing for MSSA/MRSA detection in the age of whole genome sequencing. *Front Microbiol*. 2018;9:1-9.PubMed

40. Anaerobic bacteriology: overview and general laboratory considerations. In: Tile PM, ed. *Bailey and Scott's Diagnostic Microbiology*. 14th ed. St Louis, MO: Mosby Inc; 2017:499-512.

41. Schuetz AN, Carpenter DE. Susceptibility test methods: anaerobic bacteria. In: Carroll KC, Pfaller MA, Landry ML, et al., eds. *Manual of Clinical Microbiology*. 12th ed. Washington, DC: American Society for Microbiology Press; 2019:1377-1397.

42. Clinical and Laboratory Standards Institute (CLSI). *Methods for Antimicrobial Susceptibility Testing of Anaerobic Bacteria; Approved Standard*. 9th ed. Wayne, PA: Clinical and Laboratory Standards Institute; 2018.

43. Schuetz AN. Antimicrobial resistance and susceptibility testing of anaerobic bacteria. *Clin Infect Dis*. 2014;59(5):698-705.PubMed

44. *Bordetella pertussis, Bordetella parapertussis* and related species. In: Tile PM, ed. *Bailey and Scott's Diagnostic Microbiology*. 14th ed. St Louis, MO: Mosby Inc; 2017:475-479.

45. Sanchez E, Vannier E, Wormser GP, Hu LT. Diagnosis, treatment and prevention of Lyme disease, human granulocytic anaplasmosis, and babeiosis: a review. *JAMA.* 2016;315(16):1767-1777.PubMed

46. The spirochetes. In: Tile PM, ed. *Bailey and Scott's Diagnostic Microbiology.* 14th ed. St Louis, MO: Mosby Inc; 2017:578-589.

47. Brucella. In: Tile PM, ed. *Bailey and Scott's Diagnostic Microbiology.* 14th ed. St Louis, MO: Mosby Inc; 2017:470-474.

48. Obligate intracellular and nonculturable bacterial agents. In: Tile PM, ed. *Bailey and Scott's Diagnostic Microbiology.* 14th ed. St Louis, MO: Mosby Inc; 2017:555-669.

49. McDonald LC, Gerding DN, Johnson S, et al. Clinical practice guidelines for *Clostridium difficile* infection in adults and children: 2017 update by the Infectious Diseases Society of America (IDSA) and the Society for Healthcare Epidemiology of America (SHEA). *Clin Infect Dis.* 2018;66(7):e1-e48.PubMed

50. Intestinal protozoa. In: Tile PM, ed. *Bailey and Scott's Diagnostic Microbiology.* 14th ed. St Louis, MO: Mosby Inc; 2017:629-669.

51. Dumler JS, Madigan JE, Pusterla N, et al. Ehrlichioses in humans: epidemiology, clinical presentation, diagnosis, and treatment. *Clin Infect Dis.* 2007;45(suppl 1):S45-S51.PubMed

52. Biggs HM, Behravesh CB, Bradley KK, et al. Diagnosis and management of tickborne rickettsial diseases: Rocky Mountain spotted fever and other spotted fever group rickettsioses, ehrlichioses, and anaplasmosis, United States. *MMWR Recomm Rep.* 2016;65(2)(No. RR 2):1-44.PubMed

53. Makristathis A, Hirschl AM, Mégraud F, Bessède E. Review: diagnosis of *Helicobacter pylori* infection. *Helicobacter.* 2019;24(suppl 1):e12641.PubMed

54. Edelstein PH. Legionella. In: Carroll KC, Pfaller MA, Landry ML, et al., eds. *Manual of Clinical Microbiology.* 12th ed. Washington, DC: American Society for Microbiology Press; 2019:905-920.

55. Blood and tissue protozoa. In: Tile PM, ed. *Bailey and Scott's Diagnostic Microbiology.* 14th ed. St Louis, MO: Mosby Inc; 2017:670-690.

56. Waites KB, Bebear C. *Mycoplasma* and *Ureaplasma.* In: Carroll KC, Pfaller MA, Landry ML, et al., eds. *Manual of Clinical Microbiology.* 12th ed. Washington, DC: American Society for Microbiology Press; 2019:1117-1136.

57. Opportunistic atypical fungus: *Pneumocystic jirovecii.* In: Tile PM, ed. *Bailey and Scott's Diagnostic Microbiology.* 14th ed. St Louis, MO: Mosby Inc; 2017:822-824.

58. Mejia R, Weatherhead J, Hotez PJ. Intestinal nematodes (roundworms). In: Bennett JE, Dolin R, Blaser MJ, eds. *Principles and Practice of Infectious Diseases.* 9th ed. Philadelphia, PA: Elsevier, Inc.; 2020:3436-3442.

59. White AC Jr, Coyle CM, Rajshekhar V, et al. Diagnosis and Treatment of Neurocysticercosis: 2017 Clinical Practice Guidelines by the Infectious Diseases Society of America (IDSA) and the American Society of Tropical Medicine and Hygiene (ASTMH). *Clin Infect Dis.* 2018;66(8):e49-e75. PubMed

60. Murat JB, Hidalgo HF, Brenier-Pinchart MP, et al. Human toxoplasmosis: which biological diagnostic tests are best suited to which clinical situations? *Expert Rev Anti Infect Ther.* 2013;11(9):943-956.PubMed

61. Protozoa from other body sites. In: Tile PM, ed. *Bailey and Scott's Diagnostic Microbiology.* 14th ed. St Louis, MO: Mosby Inc; 2017:691-702.

62. Clinical and Laboratory Standards Institute (CLSI). *Analysis and Presentation of Cumulative Antimicrobial Susceptibility Test Data; Approved Guideline.* 4th ed. Wayne, PA: Clinical and Laboratory Standards Institute; 2014.

63. Tunkel AR, Hartman BJ, Kaplan SL, et al. Practice guidelines for the management of bacterial meningitis. *Clin Infect Dis.* 2004;39(9): 1267-1284.PubMed

64. Meningitis and other. infections of the central nervous system. In: Tile PM, ed. *Bailey and Scott's Diagnostic Microbiology.* 14th ed. St Louis, MO: Mosby Inc; 2017:965-975.

65. Koutsari C, Dilworth TJ, Holt J, et al. Central nervous system infections. In: DiPiro JT, Yee GC, Posey L, et al., eds. *Pharmacotherapy: A Pathophysiologic Approach.* 11th ed. New York, NY: McGraw-Hill; 2020. https://accesspharmacy.mhmedical.com/content.aspx?bookid =2577&sectionid=219306547. Accessed June 29, 2020.

66. Hasbun R, Tunkel AR. Approach to the patient with central nervous system infection. In: Bennett JE, Dolin R, Blaser MJ, eds. *Principles and Practice of Infectious Diseases.* 9th ed. Philadelphia, PA: Elsevier, Inc.; 2020:1176-1182.

67. Poplin V, Boulware DR, Bahr NC. Methods for rapid diagnosis of meningitis etiology in adults. *Biomarkers Med.* 2020;14(6):459-479. PubMed

68. Shulman ST, Bisno AL, Clegg HW, et al. Clinical practice guideline for the diagnosis and management of group A streptococcal pharyngitis: 2012 update by the Infectious Diseases Society of America. *Clin Infect Dis.* 2012;55(10):1279-1282.PubMed

69. Leung AK, Newman R, Kumar A, Davies HD. Rapid antigen detection testing in diagnosing group A β-hemolytic streptococcal pharyngitis. *Expert Rev Mol Diagn.* 2006;6(5):761-766.PubMed

70. Infections of the lower respiratory tract. In: Tile PM, ed. *Bailey and Scott's Diagnostic Microbiology.* 14th ed. St Louis, MO: Mosby Inc; 2017:942-956.

71. Metlay JP, Waterer GW, Long AC, et al. Diagnosis and treatment of adults with community-acquired pneumonia. An official clinical practice guideline of the American Thoracic Society and Infectious Diseases Society of America. *Am J Respir Crit Care Med.* 2019;200(7):e45-e67. PubMed

72. Graham JC, Galloway A. The laboratory diagnosis of urinary tract infections. *J Clin Pathol.* 2001;54:911-919.PubMed

73. Infections of the urinary tract. In: Tile PM, ed. *Bailey and Scott's Diagnostic Microbiology.* 14th ed. St Louis, MO: Mosby Inc; 2017:987-998.

74. Fernandez JM, Coyle EA. Urinary tract infections and prostatitis. In: DiPiro JT, Yee GC, Posey L, et al., eds. *Pharmacotherapy: A Pathophysiologic Approach*, 11th ed. New York, NY: McGraw-Hill; 2020. https://accesspharmacy.mhmedical.com/content.aspx?bookid =2577&sectionid=219306547. Accessed June 29, 2020.

75. Gupta K, Hooton TM, Naber KG, et al. International clinical practice guidelines for the treatment of acute uncomplicated cystitis and pyelonephritis in women: A 2010 update by the Infectious Diseases Society of America and the European Society for Microbiology and Infectious Diseases. *Clin Infect Dis.* 2011;52(5):103-120.PubMed

76. Hooton TM, Bradley SF, Cardenas DD, et al. Diagnosis, prevention, and treatment of catheter-associated urinary tract infection in adults: 2009 International Clinical Practice Guidelines from the Infectious Diseases Society of America. *Clin Infect Dis.* 2010;50(5):625-663.PubMed

77. Meares EM, Stamey TA. Bacteriologic localization patterns in bacterial prostatitis and urethritis. *Invest Urol.* 1968;5(5):492-518.PubMed

78. Centers for Disease Control and Prevention. Sexually transmitted diseases treatment guidelines, 2015. *MMWR Recomm Rep.* 2015;64(RR-03):1-137. PubMed

79. Centers for Disease Control and Prevention. Recommendations for the laboratory-based detection *Chlamydia trachomatis* and *Neisseria gonorrhoeae*—2014. *MMWR Recomm Rep.* 2014;63:1-19.

80. Genital tract infections. In: Tile PM, ed. *Bailey and Scott's Diagnostic Microbiology.* 14th ed. St Louis: Mosby Inc; 2017:999-1014.

81. Duhon B, Burnett Y. Sexually transmitted diseases. In: DiPiro JT, Yee GC, Posey L, et al., eds. *Pharmacotherapy: A Pathophysiologic Approach*, 11th ed. New York, NY: McGraw-Hill; 2020. https://accesspharmacy. mhmedical.com/content.aspx?bookid=2577&sectionid=219306547. Accessed June 29, 2020

82. Normally sterile body fluids, bone and bone marrow, and solid tissues. In: Tile PM, ed. *Bailey and Scott's Diagnostic Microbiology.* 14th ed. St Louis, MO: Mosby Inc; 2017:1046-1054.

83. Wilcox ME, Chong CAKY, Stanbrook MB, et al. Does this patient have an exudative pleural effusion? The Rational Clinical Examination systematic review. *JAMA.* 2014;311(23):2422-2431.PubMed

84. Penn RL, Betts RF. Lower respiratory tract infections (including tuberculosis). In: Betts RF, Chapman SW, Penn RL, eds. *A Practical Approach to Infectious Diseases.* 5th ed. Philadelphia: Lippincott, Williams and Wilkins; 2003:295-371.

85. Parta M. Pleural effusion and empyema. In: Bennett JE, Dolin R, Blaser MJ, eds. *Principles and Practice of Infectious Diseases*. 9th ed. Philadelphia, PA: Elsevier, Inc.; 2020:914-925.

86. Brannan SR, Jerrard DA. Synovial fluid analysis. *J Emerg Med*. 2006;30(3):331-339.PubMed

87. Ohl CA. Infectious arthritis of native joints. In: Bennett JE, Dolin R, Blaser MJ, eds. *Principles and Practice of Infectious Diseases*. 9th ed. Philadelphia, PA: Elsevier, Inc.; 2020:1400-1417.

88. Bergman SJ, Armstrong EP. Bone and joint infections. In: DiPiro JT, Yee GC, Posey L, et al., eds. *Pharmacotherapy: A Pathophysiologic Approach*, 11th ed. New York, NY: McGraw-Hill; 2020. https://accesspharmacy.mhmedical.com/content.aspx?bookid=2577&sectionid=219306547. Accessed June 29, 2020.

89. Bush LM, Levison ME. Peritonitis and intraperitoneal abscesses. In: Bennett JE, Dolin R, Blaser MJ, eds. *Principles and Practice of Infectious Diseases*. 9th ed. Philadelphia, PA: Elsevier, Inc.; 2020:1009-1036.

90. Riggio O, Angeloni S. Ascitic fluid analysis for diagnosis and monitoring of spontaneous bacterial peritonitis. *World J Gastroenterol*. 2009;15(31):3845-3850.PubMed

91. Dayer E, Dayer JM, Roux-Lombard P. Primer: the practical use of biological markers of rheumatic and systemic inflammatory diseases. *Nat Clin Pract Rheumatol*. 2007;3(9):512-520.PubMed

92. Markanday A. Acute phase reactants in infections: evidence-based review and a guide for clinicians. *Open Forum Infect Dis*. 2015;2(3):ofv098.PubMed

93. Young B, Gleeson M, Cripps AW. C-reactive protein: a critical review. *Pathology*. 1991;23(2):118-124.PubMed

94. Hogevik H, Olaison L, Andersson R, et al. C-reactive protein is more sensitive than erythrocyte sedimentation rate for diagnosis of infective endocarditis. *Infection*. 1997;25(2):82-85.PubMed

95. Olaison L, Hogevik H, Alestig K. Fever, C-reactive protein, and other acute-phase reactants during treatment of infective endocarditis. *Arch Intern Med*. 1997;157(8):885-892.PubMed

96. Heiro M, Helenius H, Sundell J, et al. Utility of serum C-reactive protein in assessing the outcome of infective endocarditis. *Eur Heart J*. 2005;26(18):1873-1881.PubMed

97. Davies J. Procalcitonin. *J Clin Pathol*. 2015;68:675-679.PubMed

98. Schuetz P, Albrich W, Mueller B. Procalcitonin for diagnosis of infection and guide to antibiotic decisions: past, present and future. *BMC Med*. 2011;9:107.PubMed

99. Gilbert DN. Use of plasma procalcitonin levels as an adjunct to clinical microbiology. *J Clin Microbiol*. 2010;48(7):2325-2329.PubMed

100. Vincent JL, Van Nuffelen M, Lelubre C. Host response biomarkers in sepsis: the role of procalcitonin. In: Mancini N, ed. *Sepsis: Diagnostic Methods and Protocols*. New York, NY: Humana Press; 2015:213-224.

101. Azzini AM, Dorizzi RM, Sette P, et al. A 2020 review on the role of procalcitonin in different clinical settings: an update conducted with the tools of the evidence based laboratory medicine. *Ann Transl Med*. 2020;8(9):610.PubMed

# 19

# Infectious Diseases: Fungi, Viruses, and Mycobacteria

*Rodrigo M. Burgos, Sharon M. Erdman, and Keith A. Rodvold*

## OBJECTIVES

*After completing this chapter, the reader should be able to*

- Describe the basic methods that may be used in the diagnosis of invasive fungal infections

- Discuss the laboratory tests that are commonly used in the diagnosis of common viral infections such as influenza, herpes simplex virus, cytomegalovirus, and respiratory syncytial virus

- Discuss the laboratory tests that are commonly used in the diagnosis of human immunodeficiency virus; describe the laboratory tests that are commonly used in the assessment and monitoring of patients with human immunodeficiency virus infection

- Discuss the laboratory tests that are commonly used in the diagnosis of infections due to *Mycobacterium tuberculosis* and nontuberculous mycobacteria

The assessment, diagnosis, and treatment of a patient with a fungal, viral, or mycobacterial infection can be challenging tasks for most clinicians. This may be partly due to the nonspecific presentation and clinical recognition of infectious processes; the continuously changing taxonomy and diagnostic procedures of infecting organisms; the emergence of multidrug resistant pathogens such as *Candida auris* and *Aspergillus tanneri*; the understanding of drug resistance mechanisms and interpretation of susceptibility characteristics; and the recognition of the potential role of older and newer therapeutic agents in the prevention and/or treatment of these infections.[1-8] It is important to note that diagnostic tests for many infectious diseases, particularly the diagnosis of COVID-19 caused by a coronavirus (ie, SARS-CoV-2) and human immunodeficiency virus (HIV) infection, are continuously evolving to reflect technological advances in laboratory procedures.[8,9] Nucleic acid amplification test (NAAT), sequencing-based identification methods, and/or proteomics (eg, matrix-assisted laser desorption/ionization-time-of-flight mass spectroscopy [MALDI-TOF MS]) are transforming diagnostic microbiology and becoming rapidly accepted detection techniques of fungal, viral, and mycobacterial pathogens.[10-13]

This chapter describes the laboratory tests commonly used in the diagnosis of common infections due to fungi, mycobacteria, and viruses. Laboratory tests used in the diagnosis of viral hepatitis are addressed in Chapter 15.

## FUNGI

*Fungi* are classified as one of the six kingdoms of life. There are approximately 500 named species of fungi that are known to cause infection in humans and other vertebrate animals.[14] Approximately 50 fungal species are associated with infections in healthy subjects and most fungal infections occur in immunocompromised or debilitated patients by organisms that are part of the normal human flora. However, an increasing number of serious and life-threatening opportunistic infections are being caused by ubiquitous environmental molds.

Some of the most challenging and frustrating aspects of diagnostic medical mycology are the terminology, taxonomy, classification, and nomenclature of fungi.[14,15] For example, the correct name for a species of fungi is that which was published earliest and met the requirements in the International Code of Botanical Nomenclature for algae, fungi, and plants (http://www.iapt-taxon.org/nomen/main.php). Since January 1, 2013, the concept of "One Fungus/One Name" has been applied, eliminating the use of dual names (eg, anamorph and teleomorph names of fungal species). All subsequent names are considered synonyms; however, exceptions do exist, particularly when a later name is more commonly used than the earlier name or if research requires a species to be transferred to a different genus. Changes have occurred within the kingdom fungi (eg, the phylum Zygomycota is no longer recommended because of polyphyletic characteristics). Because of these issues, the reader is referred to the latest editions of standard microbiology textbooks and reference manuals (eg, *Manual of Clinical Microbiology*, American Society for Microbiology Press) and the following links (http://www.mycobank.org/; https://mycology.adelaide.edu.au/; http://www.indexfungorum.org/names/names.asp; https://www.fungaltaxonomy.org/; http://www.clinicalfungi.org) for more detailed information and updates on taxonomy and classifications of fungi.[14,15] In addition, a glossary of common mycological terms is often included.

DOI 10.37573/9781585286423.019

Fungi are eukaryotic and can be either unicellular or multicellular organisms. Fungi have cell walls composed mainly of chitins, glucan, and mannam with a membrane-bound cell nucleus with chromosomes. The dominant sterol in the cytoplasmic membrane of fungi is ergosterol, compared with cholesterol in mammalian cells. These organisms are heterotropic (eg, require exogenous energy sources) and can reproduce by either asexual (involving mitosis) or sexual (involving meiosis) cell division. Fungi may exist in a morphologic form that results from sexual reproduction (teleomorph, or perfect state) and a form that results from asexual reproduction (anamorph,

or imperfect state), in which each of the forms has its own name (eg, the sexual form of *Scedosporium apiospermum* complex is *Pseudallescheria boydii*). The use of separate anamorph and teleomorph species names ended in January 2013, and all legitimate names for the species can be used. It will likely take a significant period (eg, a decade or more) before these nomenclatural changes of fungal organisms achieve stability and acceptance.

Fungi have traditionally been categorized into mold, yeast, or dimorphic fungi based on morphologic and structural features (**Table 19-1**).[14-18] *Molds* (or moulds) are long, cylindrical, and

## TABLE 19-1. Categorization of Selected Medically Important Fungi[a]

| YEASTS AND YEAST-LIKE ORGANISMS | | DIMORPHIC FUNGI[b] | |
|---|---|---|---|
| *Candida* spp.[c] | *Saccharomyces cerevisiae* | *Histoplasma capsulatum* | *Sporothrix schenckii* complex[e] |
| *Cryptococcus* spp. | *Trichosporon* spp. | *Blastomyces dermatitidis* | *Talaromyces marneffei* |
| *Rhodotorula* spp. | *Blastoschizomyces capitatus* | *Paracoccidioides brasiliensis* | |

### MOLDS

| Mucormycetes[d] | Dematiaceous Fungi | Dermatophytes | Hyaline Hyphomycetes |
|---|---|---|---|
| *Rhizopus* spp. | *Fonsecaea pedrosoi* | *Microsporum* spp. | *Coccidioides* spp.[b] |
| *Mucor* spp. | *Fonsecaea compacta* | *Trichophyton* spp. | *Hormographiella aspergillata* |
| *Rhizomucor* spp. | *Rhinocladiella* spp. | *Epidermophyton floccosum* | *Aspergillus* spp. |
| *Lichtheimia corymbifera* complex | *Phialophora verrucosa* | | *Penicillium* spp. |
| *Apophysomyces elegans* | *Pleurostomophora richardsiae* | | *Paecilomyces* spp. |
| *Saksenaea vasiformis* | *Phaeoacremonium parasiticum* | | *Purpureocillium lilacinum* |
| *Cunninghamella bertholletiae* | *Phialemonium* spp. | | *Scopulariopsis* spp. |
| *Basidiobolus* spp. | *Cladophialophora* spp. | | *Emmonsia* spp. |
| *Conidiobolus coronatus* | *Scedosporium* spp. complex | | *Acremonium* spp. |
| | *Lomenospora prolificans* | | *Fusarium* spp. |
| | *Verruconis gallopava* | | *Lecythophora* spp. |
| | *Exophiala jeanselmei* complex | | |
| | *Exophiala dermatitidis* | | |
| | *Hortaea werneckii* | | |
| | *Stachybotrys chartarum* | | |
| | *Curvularia* spp. | | |
| | *Bipolaris* spp. | | |
| | *Exserohilum* spp. | | |
| | *Alternaria* spp. | | |

[a]Refer to reference 15 for further details and other organisms not listed.
[b]*Coccidioides immitis* is often placed with dimorphic fungi (listed in this table under hyaline hyphomycetes because it does not produce yeast-like colonies or cells at 35°C to 37°C on routine mycology agar).
[c]Several *Candida* spp. have had a change in nomenclature to names of teleomorphs (in parenthesis): *C lusitaniae* (*Clavispora lusitaniae*); *C krusei* (*Pichia kudriavzevii*); *C kefyr* (*Kluveromyces marxianus*); *C guilliermondii* (*Meyerozyma guilliermondii*); *C lipolytica* (*Yarrowia lipolytica*). We have kept the original *Candida* spp. names because most laboratories and medical providers are more familiar with this nomenclature of fungi.
[d]The phylum Glomerulomycota (Mucormycetes) has replaced the former term Zygomycetes. Mucormycetes is divided into two subphylums, Mucormycotina and Entomophthoromycotina. The subphylum Mucormycotina contains the order Mucorales, which includes the genera *Rhizopus, Mucor, Rhizomucor*, and *Lichtheimia* (formerly *Absidia*). The subphylum Entomophthoromycotina contains the order Entomophthorales, which includes genera *Basidiobolus* and *Conidiobolus*.
[e]*Sporothrix schenckii* grows as a dematiaceous mold when incubated at 25°C to 30°C but is yeast like at 35°C to 37°C. It is commonly categorized among dimorphic fungi but is often considered a dematiaceous mold.

threadlike (filamentous) fungi that form multicellular mycelium or thallus, an intertwined mass of branching hyphae (tube-like extensions or filament-like cells), with septa (having cross walls; being septate) or pauciseptate. An asexual spore (conidium) is produced on conidiophores, a specialized hyphal structure that serves as a stalk, and macroconidia and microconidia may be present. Thermally, monomorphic molds can be divided into four groups: (1) Mucormycetes, (2) dematiaceous fungi, (3) dermatophytes, and (4) hyaline hyphomycetes. Mucormycetes have broad hyphae that are almost nonseptate, with asexual spores (sporangiospores) formed by cleavage in a saclike structure (sporangium). The most common Mucormycetes observed in the clinical laboratory are from the order Mucorales, which are associated with severe fungal infections referred to as *mucormycosis*. Two genera from the order Entomophthorales, *Basidiobolus* and *Conidiobolus*, are less commonly observed Mucormycetes but are responsible for subcutaneous infections in otherwise healthy individuals. Dematiaceous fungi produce dark-colored colonies of olive, brown, gray, or black due to melanin pigment in the cell walls. Some of the common infections associated with dematiaceous fungi include chromoblastomycosis, phaeohyphomycosis, and mycetoma. Dematiaceous fungi also cause tinea nigra and black piedra. Dermatophytes are most often associated with superficial fungal infections (tinea or ringworm) of the skin, hair, and nails. These filamentous fungi colonize the outermost layer of the skin and digest keratin as a source of nutrients. The three genera (*Microsporum*, *Trichophyton*, and *Epidermophyton*) are differentiated by their conidium formation (macroconidia or microconidia). Hyaline hyphomycetes are colorless, septate hyphae molds that produce conidia that may be either colorless or pigmented. *Coccidioides immitis* and *Coccidioides posadasii* are known pathogens from this group whereas most other organisms cause opportunistic infections in immunocompromised patients.

Yeasts (and yeast-like organisms) appear as round or oval cells that are unicellular and generally reproduce at their surface by budding (blastoconidia). Some produce pseudohyphae (an elongated chain of cells, like a chain of sausages, resembling hyphae; however, borders between cells are delineated by marked constrictions), whereas others have true hyphae (tend to be straighter and without constrictions at the septa), which may be septate or without septa (aseptate). Ascospores, a sexual spore in a saclike structure (ascus), are produced by only some yeast. Yeasts are the most frequently encountered fungi in the clinical microbiology laboratory and are considered opportunistic pathogens. *Candida* spp. and *Cryptococcus* spp. are among the most common yeasts causing fungal infections. Yeasts are not considered a formal taxonomic group but a growth form of unrelated fungi (members of the phyla Basidiomycota and Ascomycota).

Thermally, *dimorphic fungi* have two distinct morphologic forms in which their growth forms can change from a multicellular mold (in their natural environment or when cultured at 25°C to 30°C) to budding, unicellular yeasts (during tissue invasion or when cultured at 35°C to 37°C). Medically important dimorphic fungi include *Histoplasma capsulatum*, *Blastomyces dermatitidis*, and *Paracoccidioides brasiliensis*. Each of these fungi is considered pathogenic and must be handled with caution in the clinical laboratory.

## The Identification of Fungi

The following section provides a summary of the common methods currently used in diagnostic testing of medically important fungi.[15-18] Fungal identification has traditionally been based on morphologic characteristics, such as the color of the colonies, the size and shape of cells, the presence of a capsule, and the production of hyphae, pseudohyphae, or chlamydospores. Culture remains the "gold standard" in most clinical microbiology laboratories and is the only method that allows subsequent susceptibility testing. NAAT, molecular characteristics, and/or proteomics (MALDI-TOF MS) are rapidly gaining a larger routine role in fungal identification, particularly when morphology-based identification is atypical, confusing, or not helpful (eg, organisms that fail to sporulate) and in cases in which precise identification is required (eg, epidemiologic studies).[18-22] Because no one test is perfect, it is often necessary to perform several diagnostic tests (both morphologic and genotypic methodologies) to maximize the accuracy of fungal identification. Laboratory diagnosis of fungal infections includes direct microscopic examination, morphologic identification, isolation in culture, and use of non–culture-based methods, such as antigen and/or antibody detection, 1,3-β-D-glucan detection, molecular and nonmolecular diagnostic testing, and MALDI-TOF MS.[10,14,18-27] As with all types of infections, appropriate biological specimens need to be selected, collected, and transported to the laboratory for immediate processing.[16] Because different fungi are capable of causing infection at a number of anatomic sites, specimens from the site of infection and peripheral blood specimens should be considered and submitted for culture and microscopic examination. Communication with the laboratory regarding the clinical infection and suspected fungi is important and may be useful for determining how best to process specimens safely and efficiently, including pretreatment and staining procedures, selection and incubation of media, and choice of additional diagnostic testing. Early identification of the infecting fungal pathogen may have direct diagnostic, epidemiologic, prognostic, and therapeutic implications.

The first step is usually identifying yeast-like fungi (pasty, opaque colonies) from molds (large, filamentous colonies that vary in texture, color, and topography). Drawings, color plates, and brief descriptions found in standard textbooks can serve as guides and assist in the preliminary identification of fungi seen on direct microscopic examination of clinical specimens.[14-17] Microscopic examination of the clinical specimen can delineate morphologic features (**Table 19-2**) and often provides preliminary identification of many fungi (eg, *Aspergillus* spp., Mucormycetes, dematiaceous molds). Microscopic morphology can often provide definitive identification of a mold whereas the addition of biochemical tests, serology, nucleic acid-based molecular testing, and/or MALDI-TOF MS are usually needed for identifying the genus and species of most yeast and yeast-like fungi. Direct microscopic examination of properly stained clinical specimens and tissue sections is usually the most rapid (within a few minutes or hours) and cost-effective method for

**TABLE 19-2.** Laboratory Testing and Characteristic Features Used in the Diagnosis of Selected Opportunistic and Pathogenic Fungi

| FUNGAL ORGANISM | POTENTIAL CLINICAL SPECIMENS | MICROSCOPIC MORPHOLOGIC FEATURES OF CLINICAL SPECIMENS | MORPHOLOGIC FEATURES IN CULTURE MACROSCOPIC | MICROSCOPIC | SEROLOGIC TESTS ANTIGEN | ANTIBODY | ADDITIONAL TESTS FOR IDENTIFICATION |
|---|---|---|---|---|---|---|---|
| *Candida* spp. | Blood; bone marrow; catheter sites; eye; respiratory sites; skin, nails, mucous membrane; urine; vaginal, urethral, prostatic secretions or discharge; multiple systemic sites | Round to oval budding yeasts (3–6 µm in diameter), singly, in chains, or in small loose clusters; true hyphae (no or slight constrictions at the septa) and pseudohyphae (5–10 µm in diameter; chains of elongated blastoconidia) when invading tissues; blastoconidia develop along the sides of either type of hyphae  *Candida glabrata* slightly smaller (2–5 µm in diameter) than other species and does not produce any hyphal forms | Variable morphology; colonies usually pasty, white to tan, and opaque; may have smooth or wrinkled morphology | Clusters of blastoconidia, pseudohyphae and terminal chlamydospores in some species | Serum (1,3)-β-D-glucan (Fungitell Assay Reagent) indicated for presumptive diagnosis of invasive fungal infection and should be used in conjugation with other diagnostic procedures | EIA test for detection of *Candida* mannan antigen and antimannan antibody; both the antigen and antibody test should be performed together to maximize early diagnosis | Morphology on CHROMagar, corn meal agar, rapid trehalose test  Germ tube production by *Candida albicans*, *Candida dubliniensis*, and *Candida stellatoidea*  PNA-FISH  T2 *Candida* Panel  BioFire FilmArray  MALDI-TOF MS  Gene sequencing  Carbohydrate assimilation |
| *Cryptococcus neoformans* | Most commonly in CSF and blood; bone marrow; catheter sites; respiratory sites; skin, mucous membrane; urine; multiple systemic sites | Spherical (football shaped) or round, budding yeasts of variable size (2–15 µm) with thin dark walls; thick capsule may or may not be present; no hyphae or pseudohyphae | Colonies are shiny, mucoid, dome-shaped, and cream to tan in color | Budding spherical cells of varying size; capsule present; no pseudohyphae; cells may have multiple narrow-based buds | LFD, LA, or EIA test for polysaccharide antigen | | MALDI-TOF MS  Tests for urease (+), phenoloxidase (+), and nitrate reductase (−)  Mucicarmine and melanin stains in tissue  Differentiation from *C gattii* with CGB (L-canavanine, glycine, bromthymol blue) agar |

| Organism | Sources | Direct microscopy | Colony morphology | Microscopic morphology | Antigen detection | Serologic tests | Identification / Comments |
|---|---|---|---|---|---|---|---|
| | | | | | | | India ink can demonstrate capsule in ~50% of cases on smeared specimens; this low sensitivity has resulted in antigen testing or MALDI-TOF MS as primary laboratory techniques for identification |
| *Aspergillus* spp. | CSF; eye; respiratory sites; skin, mucous membrane; urine; multiple systemic sites | Septate with uniform diameter (3–6 µm); dichotomously branched hyphae at 45° angles; tend to grow in radial fashion (like spokes on a wheel) | Varies with species; *Aspergillus fumigates*: blue-green to gray; *Aspergillus flavus*: yellow to green; *Aspergillus niger*: black with white margins and yellow surface mycelium | Varies with species; conidiophores with enlarged vesicles covered with flask-shaped metulae or phialides; hyphae are hyaline and septate | Galactomannan detection (eg, ELISA assay; Platelia *Aspergillus* GM antigen kit) is useful tool in the diagnosis of invasive aspergillosis, especially in hematologic malignancy and stem cell transplantation patients; Serum $(1,3)$-$\beta$-D-glucan (Fungitell Assay Reagent) indicated for presumptive diagnosis of invasive fungal infection and should be used in conjugation with other diagnostic procedures (eg, PCR) | Useful for chronic and allergic aspergillosis | Identification based on colony characteristics and microscopic morphology features to identify *Aspergillus* Culture-based identification remains important Molecular techniques (eg, sequencing-based and non-sequence-based PCR methods) are attractive as alternative methods (eg, Luminex xMAP technology with *Aspergillus* species-specific assays) MALDI-TOF MS attractive as alternative method but requires adequate sample preparation procedure and supplementation with reference spectra |

(continued)

**TABLE 19-2.** Laboratory Testing and Characteristic Features Used in the Diagnosis of Selected Opportunistic and Pathogenic Fungi, cont'd

| FUNGAL ORGANISM | POTENTIAL CLINICAL SPECIMENS | MICROSCOPIC MORPHOLOGIC FEATURES OF CLINICAL SPECIMENS | MORPHOLOGIC FEATURES IN CULTURE MACROSCOPIC | MORPHOLOGIC FEATURES IN CULTURE MICROSCOPIC | SEROLOGIC TESTS ANTIGEN | SEROLOGIC TESTS ANTIBODY | ADDITIONAL TESTS FOR IDENTIFICATION |
|---|---|---|---|---|---|---|---|
| Mucormycetes | CSF; eye; respiratory sites; skin, mucous membrane; multiple systemic sites | Broad, thin-walled, pauciseptate hyphae (6–25 µm) with nonparallel sides and branching irregularly, nondichotomous, and at various angles; hyphae stain poorly with GMS stain and often stain well with H&E stain | Colonies are rapid growing, wooly, or fluffy (cotton candylike), and gray-black in color | Differentiation of various genera based on presence and location (or absence) of rhizoids, nature of sporangiophores, shape of columella, appearance of an apophysis, and size and shape of the sporangia | | | Identification based on microscopic morphologic features Culture results need to be evaluated along with the clinical presentation, examination of morphologic features, and/or histopathology |
| Dematiaceous molds | CSF; eye; respiratory sites; skin, mucous membrane; multiple systemic sites | Pigmented (brown; tan, or black) polymorphous hyphae (2–6 µm in diameter) with single septa and in chains of swollen rounded cells | Colonies are usually rapidly growing, wooly, and gray, olive, black, or brown in color | Varies depending on genus and species; hyphae are pigmented; conidia may be single or in chains, smooth, or rough, and dematiaceous | | | Colony characteristics and microscopic morphology features are used to identify dermatophytes NAAT (eg, PCR) and MALDI-TOF MS (included on some commercial systems [eg, Vitek MS system]) are available; however, they are not routinely used |
| *Histoplasma capsulatum* | Blood; bone marrow; CSF; eye; respiratory sites; skin, mucous membrane; urine; multiple systemic sites | Small (2–4 µm in diameter), oval to round budding cells; often clustered within histiocytes or intracellular (macrophages, monocytes) | Colonies are slow growing and white or buff brown in color (25°C); yeast phase colonies (37°C) are smooth, white, and pasty | Thin, septate hyphae that produce tuberculate macroconidia and smooth wall microconidia (25°C); small, oval, budding yeasts produced at 37°C | Various methods (eg, EIA, ELISA) for initial antigen detection in urine, serum, or CSF (useful in disseminated and acute pulmonary histoplasmosis; also monitoring therapy) | Various methods (eg, ID, CF, LA) for serologic testing (useful in rapid diagnosis of histoplasmosis, particularly disseminated, chronic pulmonary, and *Histoplasma* meningitis) | AccuProbe test may be useful for confirming identification Demonstration of thermal dimorphism conversion (mold to yeast) Exoantigen and nucleic acid probe tests allow identification without dimorphism testing |

| | | | | | | |
|---|---|---|---|---|---|---|
| | Can be difficult to differentiate Histoplasma from other small yeasts (eg, Candida spp.) or some parasites | | | Serum (1,3)-β-D-glucan (Fungitell Assay Reagent) indicated for presumptive diagnosis of invasive fungal infection and should be used in conjugation with Histoplasma-specific testing | Antigen screening test should be validated with antibody testing | NAAT (eg, PCR) may be useful |
| Blastomyces dermatitidis | CSF; respiratory sites; skin, mucous membrane; urine; multiple systemic sites | Large (8–15 μm in diameter) and spherical, thick-walled (commonly referred to as "double contoured") cell; each yeast cell produces a single bud, attached to parent cell on a broad base | At 25°C to 30°C, colonies vary from cottony or fluffy white with aerial mycelium (first 2–3 days) to a glabrous, tan, nonconidiating colony. When grown at 35°C to 37°C, cream to tan color, wrinkled, folded, and glabrous (waxy in appearance) | On a wet mount at 25°C to 30°C, septate hyphae with one-celled smooth conidia (lollipop-like appearance); at 37°C, large, thick walled and double contoured yeast-like cell, budded on a broad base | Sandwich EIA available to detect antigenuria and antigenemia in disseminated blastomycosis; can potentially be used to test antigen in other body fluids | Several methods available; however, they are not useful for a definitive diagnosis of blastomycosis because of low sensitivity and specificity | AccuProbe test may be useful for confirming identification. Demonstration of thermal dimorphism. Exoantigen and nucleic acid probe tests allow identification without dimorphism testing. NAAT (eg, real-time PCR) may be useful |
| Coccidioides immitis/ posadasii | Blood; bone marrow; CSF; eye; respiratory sites; skin, mucous membrane; urine; multiple systemic sites | Round, thick-walled spherules that vary in size (20–200 μm in length); mature spherules contain small (2–15 μm in diameter) endospores; septate hyphae, barrel-shaped arthroconidia may be seen in cavitary and necrotic lesions | Great variation in morphology; at 25°C or 37°C, colonies initially appear moist and glabrous, rapidly develops a white, cottony aerial mycelium, which becomes gray-white to a tan or brownish | Hyaline hyphae with rectangular (barrel-shaped) arthroconidia separated by empty disjunctor cells | EIA can be used with urine, serum, plasma, BAL, CSF, and other body fluid samples (uses antibodies against Coccidioides galactomannan) | Various methods (ID and CF most reliable) for initial antibody screening; EIA assays also available and more often used for screening with confirmation of positive results by ID and CF | Identification by direct microscopic visualization and histopathologic examination. AccuProbe may be useful for confirmation of unknown isolates as Coccidioides species (but does not distinguish between two species of Coccidioides) |

(continued)

**TABLE 19-2.** Laboratory Testing and Characteristic Features Used in the Diagnosis of Selected Opportunistic and Pathogenic Fungi, cont'd

| FUNGAL ORGANISM | POTENTIAL CLINICAL SPECIMENS | MICROSCOPIC MORPHOLOGIC FEATURES OF CLINICAL SPECIMENS | MORPHOLOGIC FEATURES IN CULTURE | | SEROLOGIC TESTS | | ADDITIONAL TESTS FOR IDENTIFICATION |
| | | | MACROSCOPIC | MICROSCOPIC | ANTIGEN | ANTIBODY | |
|---|---|---|---|---|---|---|---|
| | | | | | Serum (1,3)-β-D-glucan (Fungitell Assay Reagent) indicated for presumptive diagnosis of invasive fungal infection but has a limited role because of low sensitivity (44%) | | Exoantigen and nucleic acid probe tests PCR-based assay (Gene STAT.MDx *Coccidioides* test) for detection from clinical samples was recently approved by FDA |
| *Sporothrix schenckii* | Blood; CSF; respiratory sites; skin, mucous membrane; multiple systemic sites | Small (2–6 μm in diameter) yeast-like cells of varying sizes and shapes (oval or round or cigar shaped); single or multiple elongated "pipe stem;" bud is on a narrow base | At 25°C–30°C, colonies are initially small, moist smooth, moist and white to pale orange to orange-gray with no cottony aerial hyphae; later, colonies become moist, wrinkled, leathery, or velvety and darken to brown or black; at 35°C–37°C, colonies are white to tan, dry, smooth, and yeast-like | At 25°C–30°C, thin or narrow, septate, and branching, with slender, tapering conidiophores rising at right angles; conidia borne in rosette-shaped clusters at the end of the conidiophores; at 35°C–37°C, variable-sized round, oval, and fusiform budding yeasts (cigar bodies) | | LA test is commercially available (rarely used but could be helpful for disseminated cases, and potentially CNS sporotrichosis when culture-based diagnosis had failed) | Demonstration of thermal dimorphism |

| Organism | Specimen sources | Microscopic morphology | Colony morphology | Microscopic morphology in culture | Serology | Antigen detection | Molecular / other identification |
|---|---|---|---|---|---|---|---|
| *Talaromyces* (formerly *Penicillium*) *marneffei* | Blood; bone marrow; CSF; respiratory sites; skin, mucous membrane; urine; multiple systemic sites | Oval (2.5–5 µm in length) or elongated or cylindrical, curved yeast-like cells; found within histiocytes (intracellular); has visible septa and budding does not occur (reproduces by fission [arthroconidium-like]) | Colonies are flat, powdery to velvet, and tan, and then produce diffusible red-yellow pigment at 25°C–30°C; at 35°C–37°C, colony is soft, white to tan, dry, yeast-like | At 25°C–30°C, smooth conidiophores with four to five terminal metulae bearing phialides; chains of short, narrow extensions connect the round to oval conidia in a "paint brush" distribution; at 35°C–37°C, arthroconidial yeast cells divide by fission and may elongate | | Not applicable | Demonstration of thermal dimorphism. NAAT (eg, single-step or nested PCR) are attractive as alternative methods but are mainly in-house systems without standardization being available. MALDI-TOF MS attractive as alternative method requiring supplementation with reference spectra |
| *Pneumocystis jirovecii* | Respiratory sites; multiple systemic sites | Cysts are round, ovoid, or collapsed crescent shaped (4–7 µm in diameter); stains should be used to visualize cyst forms for diagnosis; trophozoites are small (1–4 µm in diameter), pleomorphic forms | Not applicable | Not applicable | Useful for epidemiology studies but not for diagnosis | Serum $(1,3)$-β-D-glucan (Fungitell Assay Reagent) indicated for presumptive diagnosis of invasive fungal infection and should be used in conjugation with other diagnostic procedures | Direct microscopic detection using stains: methenamine silver (Gomori/Grocott), Giemsa and rapid Giemsa-like, toluidine blue, direct and indirect immunofluorescence, calcofluor white, Gram-Weigert, and papanicolaou. Several nucleic acid detection techniques (eg, real-time PCR) have been successful and commercially available outside the United States |

EIA = enzyme immunoassay; MALDI-TOF MS = matrix-assisted laser desorption/ionization-time-of-flight mass spectroscopy; CSF = cerebrospinal fluid; LFD = lateral-flow device; LA = latex agglutination; ELISA = enzyme-linked immunosorbent assay; PCR = polymerase chain reaction; NAAT = nucleic acid amplification assay; ID = immunodiffusion; CF = complement fixation; BAL = bronchoalveolar lavage; CNS = central nervous system; FDA = Food and Drug Administration.

Table is modified from reference 24.

*Source:* Adapted with permission from Murray PR, Rosenthal KS, Pfaller MA. Serologic diagnosis. In: *Medical Microbiology.* 9th ed. Philadelphia, PA: Elsevier; 2020:30–35.

References 1,15,18,24,27

a preliminary diagnosis of fungal infection. In addition, microscopic detection of fungi can assist the laboratory in the selection of media and interpretation of culture results.

The Gram stain that is typically used for bacterial processing may also allow the detection of most fungi, especially *Candida* spp., because the size of the smallest fungi is similar in size to large bacteria; the presence of budding cells can also be observed. A wide range of stains is available (**Table 19-3**) to assist in the rapid detection of fungal elements.[10,14,17,18] A common approach to wet preparations of specimens or smeared dried material is to use a 10% solution of potassium hydroxide (KOH) with or without fluorescent calcofluor white stain. The strong alkaline KOH solution digests tissue elements to allow better visualization of the fungi, while the calcofluor white stain binds to chitin and polysaccharides in the fungal cell wall, allowing it to appear white under ultraviolet light. Specific staining techniques are often used to outline morphologic features that

are diagnostic and distinctive of the suspected fungal organism (eg, India ink stain for detection of a polysaccharide capsule of *Cryptococcus neoformans*). In suspected cases of histoplasmosis, the Giemsa or Wright stain is useful for detecting intracellular yeast cells within macrophages from blood or bone marrow specimens.

Histopathologic stains are extremely valuable for identifying fungal elements in tissues and host tissue reactions to fungal infection.[24,25] Histology laboratories commonly use stains such as hematoxylin and eosin for these general purposes. Periodic acid-Schiff and Gridley fungus stains can also assist in visualization of fungal elements, especially if debris is present in the tissue background. Special stains (eg, Gomori methenamine silver, mucicarmine, and Fontana-Masson) are useful for enhancing the detection of specific fungal elements (Table 19-3) for a histopathological diagnosis of fungal infections.[15,17,18]

## TABLE 19-3. Stains Used to Enhance the Direct Microscopic Detection of Fungi

| STAIN (ABBREVIATION) | DETECTION | CHARACTERISTICS/COMMENTS |
|---|---|---|
| Alcian blue | Polysaccharide capsule produced by *Cryptococcus neoformans* (in CSF) | Mucopolysaccharide stain showing clear halos against black background; often negative in many cases of meningitis |
| Calcofluor white (CFW) | Most fungi, including *Pneumocystis jirovecii* (cysts) | Binds to chitin in fungal cell wall and fluoresces bluish white against dark background; requires fluorescent microscope; mixed with KOH for easier and rapid observation of fungi |
| Fontana-Masson (FM) | Dematiaceous fungi, *Cryptococcus neoformans*, and *Cryptococcus gattii*; may also be useful for *Aspergillus fumigates*, *Aspergillus flavus*, *Trichosporon* spp., and some Mucormycetes | Stains fungi brown to black against reddish background; demonstration of melanin or melanin-like substances in the lightly pigmented agents of phaeohyphomycosis |
| Giemsa or Wright | Visualization of intracellular *Histoplasma capsulatum*; trophic forms of *Pneumocystis jirovecii*; fission yeast cells of *Talaromyces marneffei* | Stains blue-purple (fungi and bacteria); examination of bone marrow or peripheral blood smears for disseminated disease |
| Gomori methenamine silver (GMS) | Most fungi in histopathologic sections; *Pneumocystis jirovecii* (respiratory specimens) | Detects fungi elements; however, requires specialized staining method; stains hyphae and yeast forms gray to black against a pale green or yellow background |
| Gram | Yeast and pseudohyphae appear gram-positive and hyphae (septate and aseptate) appear gram-negative | Commonly performed on clinical specimens; some fungi stain poorly (eg, *Cryptococcus* spp., *Nocardia*) |
| Gridley fungus (GF) | Most fungi in histopathologic sections | Fungi stain purplish red; filaments of Actinomycetes are not stained |
| Hematoxylin and eosin (H&E) | General purpose histopathologic stain; best method for visualizing host tissue reactions to infecting fungus | Stains some fungal elements violet to bluish purple in contrast to lighter background; *Aspergillus* spp. and Zygomycetes stain well; some fungi difficult to differentiate from background |

**TABLE 19-3.** Stains Used to Enhance the Direct Microscopic Detection of Fungi, cont'd

| STAIN (ABBREVIATION) | DETECTION | CHARACTERISTICS/COMMENTS |
|---|---|---|
| Immunohistochemical | *Aspergillus* spp., *Candida albicans*, *Pneumocystis jirovecii* | Commercial antibodies used in the immunohistochemical diagnosis of fungal infections, especially to distinguish fungal elements on atypical appearing tissue sections |
| India ink, nigrosin | *Cryptococcus neoformans* (in CSF) | Sensitivity is <50% of meningitis cases |
| Modified acid-fast | *Nocardia* (filaments are partially acid-fast and stain pink) and some isolates of *Blastomyces dermatitidis* | *Actinomyces* and other actinomycetes are negative |
| Mucicarmine | *Cryptococcus neoformans* (capsular material) and *Cryptococcus gattii*; cell walls of *Blastomyces dermatitidis* and *Rhinosporidium seeberi* | Histopathologic stain for mucin; capsular material stains deep rose to red; tissue elements stain yellow |
| Periodic acid–Schiff | Histopathologic stain for fungi, especially yeast cells and hyphae in tissue; commonly used stain by dermatopathologists | Fungal elements stain bright pink–magenta or purple against orange background (picric acid counterstain) or green background (if light green used); hyphae of molds and yeast can be readily distinguished; demonstrates double-contoured refractile wall of *Blastomyces dermatitidis*; *Nocardia* do not stain well |
| Potassium hydroxide (KOH) | Most fungi (more readily visible); hyaline molds and yeast appear transparent; dematiaceous molds display golden brown hyphae | Used to dissolve tissue material, allowing more visible fungal elements; can be combined with calcofluor white for fluorescence detection |
| Toluidine blue | *Pneumocystis jirovecii* (respiratory specimens: biopsy or BAL) | Stains cysts of *Pneumocystis jirovecii* reddish blue or dark purple against light blue background |

*Source*: References 14,15,17,18.

Culture remains the gold standard for isolation and identification of fungi suspected of causing infection. Petri plates are preferred over screw-cap tubes because of the larger surface area and dilution of inhibitory substances in the specimens. However, for laboratory safety reasons, most thermally dimorphic fungi (eg, *Histoplasma*, *Blastomyces*, *Paracoccidioides*, *T marneffei*) and *Coccidioides* spp. are pathogenic and should be grown on slants (ie, avoid the use of Petri plates and slide culture). A variety of media are available for the isolation and cultivation of yeasts and molds (**Table 19-4**).[15-17] Sabouraud dextrose, brain heart infusion, and inhibitory mold agars are enriched media commonly recommended to permit the growth and isolation of yeasts and molds. Several media, with (selective) and without (nonselective) inhibitory agents, should be used because no one medium is adequate for all the different types of specimens or organisms. Antibiotics such as chloramphenicol or gentamicin are included as inhibitory substances of most bacterial contaminants, whereas cycloheximide is used to inhibit saprobes and prevent the overgrowth of contaminating molds. Nonselective media (without inhibitory agents) should be used with specimens from sterile sites, and when suspected, fungi are likely to

be inhibited by cycloheximide (eg, *Aspergillus fumigatus*, *C neoformans/gattii*, *Lomentospora prolificans*, *T* [*Penicillium*] *marneffei*, some *Candida* spp., most Mucormycetes) or by antibiotics (eg, *Nocardia* or other filamentous bacteria). Direct microbiological examination (outlined previously) of clinical specimens can assist in the selection of media based on specimen type and suspected pathogen. In addition, the choice of media will be influenced by the patient population, local endemic pathogens, cost, availability, and laboratory preferences.

Proper temperature and adequate time for incubation are necessary to optimize the recovery of medically important fungi from clinical specimens. Inoculated media should be incubated aerobically at 30°C. If an incubator at that temperature is not available, then 25°C (room temperature) can be considered. Other temperatures (eg, 35°C to 37°C for thermally dimorphic organisms) should be reserved for selected fungi that prefer a higher temperature. In general, yeasts are detected within 5 days or less, dermatophytes within 1 week, and dematiaceous and dimorphic fungi between 2 and 4 weeks. Cultures should be regularly reviewed (eg, every day the first week, every 2 to 3 days the second week, twice during the third week, once weekly thereafter) to account

**TABLE 19-4.** Examples of Various Media Used for the Recovery of Fungi from Clinical Specimens

| GROWTH MEDIUM | COMMENTS AND USES |
|---|---|
| **Primary Media Without Antibacterials or Antifungals** | |
| Brain heart infusion (BHI) agar | Enriched media used for cultivation and isolation of all fungi; designed to enhance the recovery of fastidious dimorphic fungi more than SDA does |
| Sabouraud dextrose agar (SDA) | General-purpose medium that supports primary growth or sporulation and provides classic pigment and morphology |
| SDA, Emmons modification | Compared with SDA, Emmons Modification contains 2% (versus 4%) glucose and has a pH of 6.9–7.0 (versus pH 5.6 [slightly acidic]) |
| SADHI medium | Enriched media using combined ingredients of BHI and SDA; supports growth of all fungi; designed for better recovery of fastidious dimorphic fungi than does SDA |
| **Primary Media with Antibacterials or Antifungals** | |
| Any of the above media | Usually with chloramphenicol (inhibits gram-negative and gram-positive bacteria) with or without gentamicin (inhibits gram-negative bacteria); penicillin and streptomycin have also been used; cycloheximide added to inhibit sensitive fast-growing saprophytic fungi |
| Inhibitory mold agar (IMA) | A selective and enriched media providing better recovery of fastidious fungi than SDA; usually contains chloramphenicol; some formulations contain gentamicin |
| Littman Oxgall agar | General purpose selective medium for isolation of all fungi. Oxgall restricts the spreading of fungal colonies; contains crystal violet and streptomycin to inhibit bacteria growth |
| Mycosel or mycobiotic agar | Selective medium containing chloramphenicol and cycloheximide primarily used for isolation of dermatophytes; can also be used for isolation of other pathogenic fungi from contaminant specimens |
| **Selective/Differential Media** | |
| Dermatophyte test medium (DTM) | Screening medium for the recovery, selection, and differentiation of dermatophytes (eg, *Microsporum, Trichophyton, Epidermophyton*) from hair, skin, and nail (keratinous) specimens; contains chloramphenicol, gentamicin, and cycloheximide; other saprophytic fungi and *Aspergillus* spp. can grow on this medium (thus, it is recommended only as a screening medium) |
| Yeast extract phosphate agar with ammonia (Smith's medium) | Used for isolation and sporulation of slowly growing dimorphic fungi (ie, *Histoplasma capsulatum* and *Blastomyces dermatitidis*) from contaminated specimens; contains chloramphenicol and ammonium hydroxide to suppress the growth of bacteria, molds, and yeasts |
| CHROMagar *Candida*[a] | Chromogenic media used for direct and rapid differentiation of many clinically important yeast spp; contains chloramphenicol to inhibit bacteria and is available with or without fluconazole (selection of fluconazole-resistant *Candida krusei*); CHROMagar differentiates more *Candida* spp. than CAN2; useful in identifying mixed cultures of yeasts |
| chromID *Candida* agar (CAN2)[a] | Chromogenic media used for direct and rapid identification of *Candida albicans* versus other species of yeasts; useful in identifying mixed cultures of yeasts |
| **Specialized Media** | |
| Canavanine glycine bromothymol blue (CGB) agar | Solid medium recommended for use in qualitative procedures for selective and differential isolation of *Cryptococcus gattii* (ie, *Cryptococcus* serotypes B and C) from *Cryptococcus neoformans* |
| Cornmeal agar (CMA) | CMA with 1% dextrose used for the cultivation of fungi and differentiation of *Trichophyton mentagrophytes* from *Trichophyton rubrum* (based on pigment production); CMA with Tween 80 used for the cultivation and differentiation of *Candida* spp. (based on mycelial characteristics); Tween 80 promotes growth and production of red pigment by *Trichophyton rubrum* |

**TABLE 19-4.** Examples of Various Media Used for the Recovery of Fungi from Clinical Specimens, cont'd

| GROWTH MEDIUM | COMMENTS AND USES |
|---|---|
| Potato dextrose agar (PDA) or potato flake agar (PFA) | PDA is used to stimulate conidium production by fungi and enhance pigment production by some dermatophytes; PDA is most commonly used with slide culture technique to view morphologic characteristics; PFA used for the simulation of conidia of fungi; PFA can be made selective by including cycloheximide and chloramphenicol |
| Rapid sporulation agar (RSA) | Used for isolation and identification of dermatophytes; contains chloramphenicol and chlortetracycline to inhibit bacteria and cycloheximide to inhibit saprobic fungi; similar to DTM but can increase the production of conidia and improve color visualization of the isolate (bromothymol blue in the formulation) |
| Niger seed or bird seed agar and esculin base medium (EBM) | Selective and differential medium for isolation of *Cryptococcus* spp., especially *C neoformans* and *C gattii*; chloramphenicol as a selective agent; creatinine to enhance melanization of some strains of *C. neoformans* |

[a]Several commercial sources of yeast chromogenic agar media are available.[17] CHROMagar *Candida* and chromID *Candida* agar are examples of selected chromogenic agar products that are approved by the FDA for use in U.S. laboratories. *Candida* spp. identified with chromogenic agar differs by medium and manufacturer. Further testing is required for final identification.
*Source*: References 15–17.

for the growth rates and identification of fungi. It is generally recommended that fungal cultures be incubated for 4 weeks before being considered negative (no growth for fungus). Several factors influence the length of incubation including the choice of media (eg, yeasts on chromogenic [48 hours] versus routine media [5 to 7 days]) and type of fungus suspected (eg, slow-growing dimorphic systemic fungi may need 8 weeks).

Once the organism has been cultured and isolated, the following approach has usually been conducted: (1) determine the morphology of the unknown fungus and determine if it is consistent with any of the groups listed in Table 19-1 or filamentous bacterium (some of the aerobic actinomycetes [eg, *Nocardia*] resemble fungi and must be ruled out) and (2) note the rate of growth, colony, and microscopic morphologies of the possible organism(s) (Table 19-2) and refer to necessary textbooks to compare descriptions, drawings, color plates, discussions of characteristics, and other test results to assist in differentiating the likely organism.[15,18] In the case of yeasts and yeast-like organisms, additional testing, such as the germ tube test, biochemical testing using commercially available systems, or the urease test, may allow species identification of isolates from various body sites. Both NAAT and MALDI-TOF MS are increasingly being used to modernize clinical microbiology laboratories. These rapid, inexpensive, and accurate methods for identification of fungal organisms allow less dependency on performing time-consuming biochemical procedures and/or needing visual expertise for detection of microscopic and colonial morphology.[10,18-24,26]

## Antigen Detection

Cell wall components of various invasive fungi have been used as diagnostic markers for antigen testing. Galactomannan is a polysaccharide component of the cell wall of *Aspergillus* and it is released by growing hyphae. A commercial enzyme-linked immunosorbent assay (ELISA) (Platelia *Aspergillus* Galactomannan Test [Bio-Rad Laboratories, Marens-La-Coquette,

France]) is available to detect circulating galactomannan antigen in serum or bronchoalveolar lavage (BAL) fluid and has been shown to be an earlier diagnostic marker for invasive aspergillosis in neutropenic patients with hematologic malignancies and hematopoietic stem cell transplantation.[18,27] The monitoring of antigen titers has also been shown to correlate with the response to antifungal therapy, patient survival, and autopsy findings in neutropenic patients. Other genera of fungi, including *Histoplasma*, *Penicillium*, *Alternaria*, *Geotrichum*, and *Paecilomyces*, have shown reactivity to the assay kit. Several causes of false-positive results have also been reported, including patients receiving specific antibiotics (eg, piperacillin-tazobactam, amoxicillin-clavulanic acid), certain foods (eg, pasta, vegetables, milk), and Plasma-Lyte A. The detection of galactomannan is also reduced in patients receiving antifungal agents active against molds and patients with chronic granulomatous disease. A nongalactomannan antigen method has recently been developed as a point-of-care (POC) test for rapid detection of invasive pulmonary aspergillosis. This rapid detection method uses a monoclonal antibody (JF5) and a lateral-flow device (LFD) (OLM Diagnostics, Newcastle upon Tyne, UK) to detect an extracellular glycoprotein antigen produced by *A. fumigatus*. This test has a high negative predictive value and good sensitivity and specificity, especially with BAL fluid. U.S. Food and Drug (FDA) approval of this test for diagnostic use is still pending.

Antigen testing is considered the primary diagnostic test in screening cerebrospinal fluid (CSF) for suspected cases of cryptococcal meningitis because the India ink procedure has a low sensitivity. The combination of antigen detection test and an India ink stain of the CSF are recommended for the primary evaluations of suspected cases of cryptococcal meningitis. Several commercial kits are available for the detection of cryptococcal antigen in serum and CSF.[18] Galactoxylomannan is a polysaccharide capsular component of *Cryptococcus* and is the antigen detected for infections caused by serotypes of

*C neoformans, C gattii,* and *C deneoformans.* Latex agglutination (LA) and enzyme immunoassay (EIA) methods are sensitive (93% to 100%) and specific (93% to 100%) diagnostic tests for the detection and quantitation of circulating cryptococcal antigen in serum and CSF. The reported titer determinations of the two testing methods (eg, LA versus EIA testing) or from different commercial latex kits are not numerically similar. Thus, the same testing method and latex kit should be used to monitor serial samples for a patient. Numerous causes have been responsible for false-positive results, with both testing methods including rheumatoid factor, soaps, disinfectants, hydroxyethyl starch, malignancy, and infections associated caused by bacteria, *Trichosporon, Capnocytophage, Rothia,* or *Geotrichum beigelii.* Both low and high antigen titers can result in false-negative results. Recently, LFD device has become available for measuring cryptococcal antigen from serum and CSF samples. The advantages of LFD include similar specificity and increased sensitivity as LA and EIA for testing serum samples, ease of use, lower costs compared with other test kits, and the similar accuracy between whole blood samples and blood obtained from finger pricks. False-positive results with LFD have been reported at low titers in patients without a history of cryptococcal infection.

Enzyme immunoassay can be used to detect a polysaccharide antigen from *H capsulatum* in body fluids (eg, serum or plasma, urine, CSF, or BAL fluid). It has been recommended that the antigen screening test be validated by antibody testing (eg, immunodiffusion [ID] and complement fixation [CF]).[18] The diagnosis of histoplasmosis should be based on a combination of diagnostic test results because antigen testing is associated with cross-reactivity to other fungal infections (eg, blastomycosis, coccidioidomycosis, paracoccidioidomycosis) and false-positive results (eg, rheumatoid factor, rabbit antithymocyte globulin). The test sensitivity varies with disease presentation (eg, 77% for acute pulmonary histoplasmosis, 34% for subacute pulmonary histoplasmosis, 21% for chronic pulmonary histoplasmosis, 92% for progressively disseminated histoplasmosis), patient groups (eg, HIV infection, immunocompromised, disseminated diseases), and specimen type (60% to 86% in serum, 80% to 95% in urine, 25% to 50% in CSF, 93.5% in BAL). A monoclonal antibody ELISA has also been developed and has improved sensitivity (98%) and specificity (97%).

Antigen detection tests for *H capsulatum, B dermatitidis,* and *Coccidioides* species are performed by the clinical reference laboratory, MiraVista Diagnostics (Indianapolis, IN), on a fee-for-service basis. Antigen detection is generally not used as a diagnostic tool and has a limited role for blastomycosis and coccidioidomycosis because of low levels of detection in antigenemia and antigenuria, false-positive reactions, and/or cross-reactions are common in patients with other mycoses.

Mannin, a major component of the *Candida* cell wall, has been the main diagnostic marker used in antigen detection tests of *Candida* species.[18] For serology testing, antimannin antibodies can be monitored because mannin can induce a strong antibody response toward oligomannose epitopes. A wide range in assay sensitivity and specificity has been reported when either antigen or antibody detection tests are used alone for the diagnosis of candidemia and disseminated candidiasis. The combined detection of circulating mannan and antimannan antibodies in serum or plasma by immunoenzymatic assays (Platelia *Candida* Ag Plus and Platelia *Candida* Ab Plus, Bio-Rad Laboratories, Marens-La-Coquette, France) has been recommended to maximize the early diagnosis of invasive candidiasis. Concomitant detection of mannan and antimannan antibodies for *Candida* species has a median sensitivity of >80%, particularly for *C albicans, C glabrata,* and *C tropicalis.*

## Serology

Several different *serology* methodologies (eg, ID, countercurrent immunoelectrophoresis, ELISA, CF tests, fluorescent-enzyme immunoassay) have been investigated for the detection of specific fungal pathogens.[18,24] Interpretation of results for most fungal infections requires knowledge of the laboratory technique used to perform the antibody testing. Serologic assays are most useful as diagnostic testing of fungal infections in the immunocompetent host because a poor antibody response is common in immunosuppressed patients, resulting in a false-negative result.

Serologic tests (ie, ID and CF) play an important role in the clinical diagnosis of infections caused by *H capsulatum.*[18,24,27] These tests have been the most useful in patients with chronic pulmonary or disseminated histoplasmosis. The ID test is more specific than CF test and can serve as a useful screening procedure with and without the CF test. The CF test is more sensitive than ID but has shown cross-reactivity and positive results in patients with various other types of infections, including bacterial, viral, mycobacterial, and fungal (eg, aspergillosis, blastomycosis, candidiasis, coccidioidomycosis, paracoccidioidomycosis). CF test can also have false-negative results in the presence of rheumatoid factor or cold agglutinins. Other serologic assays (eg, LA, EIA, ELISA) have also been evaluated and may be useful for the diagnosis of specific types of *H capsulatum* infections. The potential of cross-reactivity or lack of commercial availability limits the current use of these assays.

The ID and CF tests are reliable serologic methods for the diagnosis of invasive infections of coccidioidomycosis and paracoccidioidomycosis.[18,27] The ID test mainly detects immunoglobulin M (IgM) antibodies (heated coccidioidin) and is useful in the diagnosis of active disease. The ID has replaced the historical use of a tube precipitin test. The CF detects IgG antibodies (unheated coccidioidin) and is useful in diagnosing acute or chronic diseases and predictive for monitoring treatment response and a poor prognosis. LA and a highly sensitive EIA are also available; however, false-positive results have been noted. These tests should only be used as a screening tool, in which a positive result must be confirmed by another method.

Finally, serology testing methods (ie, immunoelectrophoresis, ELISA, and fluorescent-enzyme immunoassay) for Aspergillus-specific antibodies are useful for the diagnosis of noninvasive diseases such as allergic bronchopulmonary aspergillosis, aspergilloma, and chronic cavitary aspergillosis.[18] Low sensitivity and/or specificity currently limit the use of serology testing as definitive diagnosis of invasive fungal infections caused by species of *Blastomyces, Candida,* and *Cryptococcus.*

## (1,3)-β-D-Glucan Detection

Commercial assays for the detection of *(1,3)-β-D-glucan*, a polysaccharide present in cell wall of common pathogenic yeasts, have been used as a panfungal diagnostic tool for invasive fungal infections such as aspergillosis, *Fusarium* infection, trichosporonosis, and candidiasis.[18,27] This assay has also been used to detect (1,3)-β-D-glucan from *P jirovecii*, in both HIV-positive and HIV-negative patients. This diagnostic assay is not useful for mucoraceous molds (eg, Zygomycetes such as *Rhizopus*, *Mucor*, and *Absidia*), which do not produce (1,3)-β-D-glucan, or *Cryptococcus* species and *B dermatitidis*, because they produce only low levels of (1,3)-β-D-glucan. Limited evaluations have assessed this diagnostic assay for the detection of histoplasmosis and coccidioidomycosis.

In the United States, Fungitell assay (Associates of Cape Cod Inc., East Falmouth, MA) is widely available and the only FDA-approved screening test for detecting (1,3)-β-D-glucan in serum. The manufacturer's recommended guidelines for a positive serum (1,3)-β-D-glucan value is ≥80 pg/mL and a negative value <60 pg/mL; values between 60 and 79 are considered indeterminate (http://www.acciusa.com). Repeat testing (eg, twice weekly) is recommended to improve the predictive value and specificity of the test. False-positive results have been observed in patients receiving hemodialysis (with cellulose membranes), treated with certain blood products (eg, albumin, immunoglobulins), having bacterial bloodstream infections, mucositis, or graft-versus-host disease, and/or exposed to glucan-containing materials (eg, gauze or swabs). Concurrent β-lactam therapy, such as piperacillin–tazobactam or amoxicillin–clavulanate, and antitumoral polysaccharides have also been associated with false-positive results. Because of these potential risks of a false-positive result, the test may be more useful in excluding a diagnosis of invasive fungal infection when results are reported negative. Because this assay is nonspecific with varying levels of sensitivity and specificity, its use should be in conjunction with clinical examination of the patient and other diagnostic tests and procedures to make a conclusive diagnosis of invasive fungal infection.

## Molecular Diagnosis

Molecular diagnostic tests have a significant and increasing role in the detection and identification of fungi.[15,18-24] The advantages of these techniques include organisms being observed microscopically but not grown on culture; a more rapid and objective identification of molds with unrecognizable or unproductive structures or yeasts not included in commercial databases; the ability to differentiate fungi with similar characteristics; and the precise genotyping for epidemiology studies and updates to taxonomy, classification, and nomenclature of fungi.[18] The reader is referred to a glossary of common molecular terms for comprehending information in this rapidly evolving field.[15,18]

The ribosomal targets and internal transcribed spacer regions have been the main target used for molecular identification of fungi. Procedural steps that are commonly involved with molecular identification techniques include extraction of DNA, amplification of DNA segment of interest, and DNA analysis. Amplification is most often performed by polymerase chain reaction (PCR) with non–sequencing-based or sequencing-based identification methods. A wide variety of methodologies are available, including local and in-house laboratory-developed PCR tests. Clinicians need to contact their laboratory to determine which tests are available and which molecular diagnostic tests may need to be sent to a reference laboratory. In addition, selection of appropriate primers and/or probes for molecular testing often relies on the initial impressions and/or characteristics of the isolate, particularly for less robust molecular identification methods. In many situations, a combination of morphologic and molecular testing methods is best used for species identification.

Many evaluations have been ongoing for different PCR assays for invasive *Candida* spp. and *Aspergillus* infections.[15,19,27] Limited and variable sensitivity and specificity have been some of the main issues restricting the routine use of this method. Additional issues that need to be addressed include specimen type, sample volume, best method of DNA extraction, target range, and definitions of positive results. However, further evaluation with standardized methodology and decreased inconsistencies between tests should allow PCR to become a promising method for detection of *Candida* and *Aspergillus* spp. Like other fungal infections, nucleic acid detection has been extensively used as a research-based tool with a slower progression to routine use by clinical microbiology laboratories and/or commercial availability.[27]

Several molecular-based diagnostic assays have been cleared by the FDA and are commercially available for clinical use in the United States.[15,18-22,27] Even more devices have been marked Conformitè Europèene In Vitro Diagnostic (CE-IVD) and marketed for use in Europe.[19] These devices have incorporated detection technologies such as DNA amplification followed by magnetic resonance, peptide nucleic acid fluorescent in situ hybridization (PNA-FISH), chemiluminescent labeled with single-stranded DNA probes, nested multiplex PCR or real-time PCR with DNA melt-curve analysis, and a system platform involving PCR amplification, flow cytometry, and dual-lasers detection. Most of the available commercial devices have focused on the detection and identification of fungi species commonly associated in infections, such as *Aspergillus*, *Cryptococcus*, and several *Candida* spp. (ie, *C albicans*, *C glabrata*, *C krusei*, *C parapsilosis*, and *C tropicalis*). The following brief discussion highlights a few examples of molecular devices that have FDA clearance for clinical use in the United States.

The T2Candida Panel and automated T2Dx Instrument (T2Biosystems, Lexington, MA) uses novel technologies to allow rapid (eg, 3 to 5 hours) and accurate diagnosis of invasive candidiasis directly from whole blood samples (no need for blood culture and isolation of *Candida* spp.).[15,18-22,27] The instrument is a fully automated as a clinical multiplex benchtop diagnostic system using PCR and miniaturized magnetic resonance technology. The T2Candida panel can identify *C albicans*, *C tropicalis*, *C parapsilosis*, *C glabrata*, and *P kudriavzevii*. Other panels are in development, including T2Cauris panel (research use only) for the detection of the emerging multidrug-resistant *Candida auris*. A T2Bacteria panel has FDA clearance and is available for use on the same instrument.

PNA-FISH (Yeast Traffic Light PNA FISH, OpGen, Gaithersburg, MD) provides rapid identification of up to five *Candida* spp. directly from yeast-positive blood cultures.[15,18-22] This device has a fast turnaround time (eg, approximately 90 minutes) with high sensitivity (92% to 100%) and specificity (94% to 100%). The rapid identification methodology used is hybridization of fluorescent PNA probes to organism-specific rRNA, with detection via fluorescent microscopy. After the Gram stain and the hybridization process are completed, *C albicans* and *C parapsilosis* are identified microscopically as bright green fluorescing cells, while *Candida tropicalis* fluoresces bright yellow, and *C glabrata* and *C krusei* fluoresce bright red. Other yeasts do not fluoresce. The colors of the light probes also provide an indication about the potential use of fluconazole in these patients because *C albicans* and *C parapsilosis* are generally susceptible to fluconazole (green light for go), *C glabrata* can be resistant to fluconazole, and *C krusei* is intrinsically resistant to fluconazole (red light for stop). The yellow signal produced by *C tropicalis* indicates that caution should be used because fluconazole susceptibility is variable for this organism. This method has a significant impact over traditional identification methods, which could take up to 3 or more days for identification of *Candida* spp., as well as guiding the most effective antifungal drug therapy. The PNA-FISH methodology is also used for rapid identification of bacteria, including gram-positive (ie, *Staphylococcus aureus*, coagulase-negative staphylococci, enterococci) and gram-negative (ie, *Escherichia coli*, *Klebsiella pneumoniae*, *Pseudomonas aeruginosa*) organisms. A single automated system using FISH technology (Accelerate Pheno BC kit, Accelerate Diagnostics, Inc., Tucson, AZ) has also been developed and can identify *C albicans*, *C glabrata*, and gram-positive and gram-negative organisms.

Probe-based assays for culture identification of fungi have become commercially available.[15,18-22] AccuProbe (Hologic, Inc., Mississauga, ON, Canada) uses luminometer to detect hybridization of a chemiluminescent labeled, single-stranded DNA probe to target rRNA present in a fungal culture. Three separate probes have FDA clearance and are available for the culture identification of dimorphic fungi, including *Blastomyces dermatitidis*, *Coccidioides immitis*, and *Histoplasma capsulatum*. Performance data have demonstrated high sensitivity (>98%) and specificity (>99%) for each pathogen. The *B dermatitidis* probe has the potential to cross-react with other fungi, including *Emmonsia* species, *Paracoccidioides brasiliensis*, and *Gymnascella* spp. In addition, the *Coccidioides* probe is unable to distinguish between species, namely *Coccidioides immitis* and *Coccidioides posadasii*. AccuProbe tests are also available for culture identification of bacteria (ie, *Neisseria gonorrheae*, *S aureus*, *Listeria monocytogenes*, *Streptococcus pneumoniae*) and mycobacteria.

BioFire FilmArray (BioFire, Salt Lake City, UT) is an automated in vitro diagnostic device that detects multiple nucleic acid targets by using nested multiplex PCR with DNA melting curve analysis.[15,18-22] Six different identification panels are currently available, with yeast being included on two of these panels. The Blood Culture ID (BCID) Panel can test for 43 targets associated with bloodstream infections, including gram-positive and gram-negative bacteria, yeast, and 10 antimicrobial resistance genes. The yeast detected by the BCID Panel includes six *Candida* spp. (ie, *C albicans*, *C auris*, *C glabrata*, *C krusei*, *C parapsilosis*, and *C tropicalis*) and *Cryptococcus neoformans/gatti*. This panel requires a positive blood culture sample. The overall sensitivity and specificity for the BCID Panel are 99% and 99.8%, respectively. *Cryptococcus neoformans/gatti*, along with 13 common bacterial and viral pathogens, are included on the Meningitis/Encephalitis (ME) Panel. The ME Panel can directly detect pathogens from a 0.2 mL sample of CSF, and has also demonstrated a high sensitivity (94.2%) and specificity (99.8%).

Luminex (xMAP and xTAG, Luminex Molecular Diagnostics, Inc., Austin, TX) is a commercially available multianalyte profiling platform that can provide detection and identification of clinically important pathogens directly from positive blood culture bottles and other types of clinical samples.[15,18-22] The platform has combined PCR amplification, flow cytometry, and dual-laser detection system to provide multiplexed assay capabilities. The xMAP (x = analyte or unknown; MAP = Multi-Analyte Profiling) hybridization technology can detect an antigen (target) by using a capture antibody attached to the surface of a color-coded microbeads (microsphere) and a detection antibody that incorporates a fluorescent label. Luminex-based technology has allowed rapid and reliable identification of clinically important fungal pathogens, including up to 10 genus- and 29 species-specific diagnoses. xTAG (the TAG name is derived from three nucleic acid bases being used: T, A, G) consists of the MagPlex-TAG microsphere (that are precoupled with anti-TAG sequence) and the user designator primer and TAG sequence that complements the x-TAG sequence on the bead. The xTAG analyte-specific reagents can be combined with xMAP instruments for amplification and detection. Evaluations of the xTAG Fungal ASR assay have demonstrated that multiple yeast species could be identified with 100% sensitivity, 99% specificity, and 99% positive and 100% negative predictive values when compared with traditional fungal culture results.

## MALDI-TOF Mass Spectrometry

*Matrix-assisted laser desorption-ionization time-of-flight* (MALDI-TOF) *mass spectrometry* (MS) is ideal for genus and species identification and has the potential for accurate strain typing and identification for fungi, bacteria, and mycobacterium.[5,10,15,18-20,26] This technology is a rapid and accurate method for identifying yeasts and molds recovered on culture media and using sample preparation for MALDI-TOF MS. Reports on the use of MALDI-TOF MS for routine rapid identification have focused on clinically important yeasts (eg, *Candida* spp., including *Candida auris*, *C neoformans, and C gattii* spp.) and dermatophyte species (eg, *Neoscytalidium* spp., *Trichophyton*, *Microsporum*, *Epidermophyton*, and *Arthroderma*). Identification of dimorphic and filamentous fungi as well as molds (eg, *Aspergillus* spp., *Fusarium* spp., *Pseudallescheria–Scedosporium* complex, *Penicillium* spp., *Lichtheimia* spp.) have been more challenging because of different developmental forms on agar media and the influences of the phenotype. MALDI-TOF MS is becoming the primary diagnostic method for rapid identification of fungus isolates in the clinical microbiology laboratory.

However, its initial use for fungal identification has moved at a slower pace than the current use of MALDI-TOF MS for bacterial identification.

The advantages of the MALDI-TOF MS for fungal identification are low cost of materials (a few cents) for each organism identification, ease of performance, and rapid, accurate results (approximately 11 minutes if just one isolate is tested; 2.5 minutes per isolate in a batch of 96 isolates, with the average time per isolate in published reports being 4 to 6 minutes). The simplicity of MALDI-TOF MS removes the specific skills and ability to visually identify fungi macroscopic and microscopic characteristics. Current limitations include the initial costs of instrumentation for the system, lack of sample preparation techniques, and inadequate fungal spectra in commercial database and software of manufacturers (ie, two commercial systems currently exist in the United States: Bruker, Billerica, MA and Vitek MS, bioMérideux, Inc, Durham, NC). The expansion of database libraries and developments in sample preparation are rapidly evolving to establish validated and routine procedures for large numbers of clinically important fungal strains and species. MALDI-TOF MS is also becoming a reliable and reproducible method for antifungal susceptibility testing (eg, caspofungin for isolates of *Candida* spp.).[20,28] Finally, MALDI-TOF MS is also being investigated for epidemiologic testing of fungal isolates for outbreak investigations and as an early surveillance test and/or screening tool for antifungal drug resistance.[20]

## Antifungal Susceptibility Testing

The importance of *antifungal susceptibility testing* has become increasingly recognized as a useful component in the treatment optimization of invasive infections caused by *Candida* spp. because of the increasing number of available antifungal agents, emerging resistance issues to standard therapy, and the changing epidemiology of invasive fungal disease. Obtaining antifungal susceptibility testing is particularly important when azole-resistant isolate is suspected, when failure to respond to antifungal therapy has occurred, and in species in which acquired resistance often exists (ie, *Candida glabrata*, *Candida auris*, and *Aspergillus fumigatus*).

The CLSI and European Committee on Antimicrobial Susceptibility Testing (EUCAST) has developed standardized reference methods for macrodilution and microdilution susceptibility testing of yeasts and molds and broth microdilution method for dermatophyte.[28-30] Agar-based alternative methodologies, including agar dilution, disk diffusion, E-test methods, and semisolid agar, have also been applied to susceptibility tests of yeasts and molds. The commercial availability of simplified and/or automated testing methods (eg, E-test and other gradient strip testing; Vitek 2; Sensititre YeastOne) consistent with CLSI reference methods is allowing an increasing number of clinical laboratories to routinely perform antifungal susceptibility testing. Molecular testing methods for the detection of resistance have also been expanding.[28-30]

Interpretive MIC breakpoints based on CLSI- and EUCAST-recommended in vitro susceptibility testing methods have been recommended for *Candida* spp.[28-30] Comprehensive reviews regarding the microbiological, molecular,

pharmacokinetic-pharmacodynamic, and clinical antifungal data for *Candida* spp. provide species-specific interpretive clinical breakpoints for azole agents and the echinocandins (**Table 19-5**).[28] These data have been used to establish epidemiologic cutoff values, detect emerging resistance among *Candida* spp., and harmonize antifungal susceptibility testing standards by CLSI and EUCAST.[28-30] In addition, tentative breakpoints for the multidrug-resistant pathogen *Candida auris* have been proposed (https://www.cdc.gov/fungal/candida-auris/c-auris-antifungal.html).

Interpretive breakpoint criteria for amphotericin B and some of the triazole agents against selected *Aspergillus* spp. have been reported; other fungal pathogens remain to be standardized.[28-30] The recommended EUCAST clinical breakpoints for *Aspergillus fumigatus* include ≤1 mg/L (susceptible) and >2 mg/L (resistant) for amphotericin, itraconazole, and voriconazole, and ≤0.125 mg/L (susceptible) and >0.25 mg/L (resistant) for posaconazole (provided sufficient drug concentrations can be achieved).

# VIRUSES

More than 650 viruses are known to cause infection in humans and other vertebrate animals.[31] The three major properties that classify viruses into families include (1) the nucleic acid (NA) core (either DNA or RNA but not both); (2) whether the viral NA is single-stranded or double-stranded (https://viralzone.expasy.org/656); and (3) the presence or absence of a lipoprotein envelope (**Tables 19-6** and **19-7**).[13,31,32] Viruses also differ based on their genome topology (eg, linear, circular, single versus multiple segments). Virus families can be further categorized based on morphology (eg, size, shape, and substructure), mode of replication, and molecular and genomic characteristics. The most recent information on the rapidly changing classification and taxonomy of viruses can be obtained from the website database (http://ictv.global/report/) that has been established by The International Committee on Taxonomy of Viruses (ICTV). The 2019 ICTV report now recognizes five hierarchical ranks consisting of 55 orders, 168 families, 103 subfamilies, 1421 genera, and 6,590 species of viruses; however, a larger number of viruses remain unclassified.

## The Identification of Viruses

The ability to detect and accurately identify viruses in the clinical laboratory has increased during the last 30 years as a result of wider applicability of diagnostic laboratory techniques with increased sensitivity and decreased turnaround time, the availability of newer reagents and rapid commercial diagnostic kits, and the addition of new antiviral drugs for specific viral infections.[1,13,32-37] In addition, several NA amplification tests (NAATs), specifically PCR and real-time PCR, are allowing routine clinical laboratories to provide virology services for the increasing frequency of infectious diseases that depend on rapid viral diagnosis.[1,13,32]

It is important to note that all diagnostic tests for the identification of viruses are not available at each institution, and

**TABLE 19-5.** Species-Specific Breakpoints for *In Vitro* Susceptibility Testing of *Candida* spp. According to CLSI and EUCAS

| ANTIFUNGAL AGENT | CANDIDA spp. | CLSI S | CLSI R | EUCAST S | EUCAST R |
|---|---|---|---|---|---|
| Anidulafungin | C albicans | ≤0.25 | >0.5 | ≤0.03 | >0.03 |
| | C krusei, C tropicalis | ≤0.25 | >0.5 | ≤0.06 | >0.06 |
| | C parapsilosis[a] | ≤2 | >4 | ≤0.002 | >4 |
| | C glabrata | ≤0.125 | >0.25 | ≤0.06 | >0.06 |
| Micafungin | C albicans | ≤0.25 | >0.5 | ≤0.016 | >0.03 |
| | C krusei, C tropicalis | ≤0.25 | >0.5 | | |
| | C parapsilosis[a] | ≤2 | >4 | ≤0.002 | >2 |
| | C glabrata | ≤0.06 | >0.125 | ≤0.03 | >0.03 |
| Fluconazole | C albicans, C tropicalis, C parapsilosis | ≤2 | >4 | ≤2 | >4 |
| | C glabrata[a] | SDD[b]: ≤32 | SDD[b]: >32 | ≤0.02 | >32 |
| Posaconazole | C albicans, C tropicalis, C parapsilosis | | | ≤0.06 | >0.06 |
| Voriconazole | C albicans, C tropicalis, C parapsilosis | ≤0.125 | >0.5 | ≤0.125 | >0.125 |
| | C krusei | ≤0.5 | >1 | | |

CLSI = Clinical and Laboratory Standards Institute (revised breakpoints from M27-S4 document); EUCAST = European Committee for Antimicrobial Susceptibility Testing; S = susceptible; R = resistant.

[a]The wild-type populations of *C parapsilosis* to anidulafungin and micafungin and *C glabrata* to fluconazole are classified as intermediate (I) category (values between S and R) to accommodate use of these agents in some clinical situations.

[b]The wild-type population of *C glabrata* is classified by CLSI as susceptible dose-dependent (SDD) to fluconazole to accommodate use of fluconazole at higher doses in some clinical situations.

Notes: Clinical breakpoint of ≤1 mg/L for amphotericin has been set by EUCAST for *Candida albicans*. EUCAST breakpoints for caspofungin have not been established due to an unacceptable variation in MIC ranges.

*Source:* Adapted with permission from Johnson EM, Cavling-Arendrup M. Susceptibility test methods: yeast and filamentous fungi. In: Carroll KC, Pfaller MA, Landry ML, et al, eds. *Manual of Clinical Microbiology.* 12th ed. Washington, DC: American Society for Microbiology Press; 2019:2351–2375.

the clinician must establish a relationship with the laboratory that will be performing viral testing. In certain clinical situations, samples may need to be sent out for diagnostic testing at either large reference or public health laboratories because they are able to provide the necessary methods that are difficult or impossible to routinely perform in the clinical virology laboratory. In addition, certain viruses (eg, arboviruses, arenaviruses, filoviruses, Variola virus, and rabies virus) require testing at biosafety level (BSL) 3 or 4 facilities and are often sent to the Centers for Disease Control and Prevention (CDC) or the CDC's Division of Vector-Borne Infectious Diseases.[13,32,33]

The ability to accurately diagnose a viral infection is highly dependent on appropriate selection, timing, collection, and handling of biological specimens.[32-34] In general, the highest titers of viruses are present early in the course of illness and decrease as the duration of illness increases. Therefore, it is important

to collect specimens for the detection of viruses in the early course of an infection. In most cases, identification of viruses is a specimen-driven process. Because collection procedures are highly dependent on viruses being suspected, attention needs to be taken regarding collection containers and devices, and transport systems (eg, whether a viral transport medium is needed). The different types of clinical specimens that can be collected for viral culture and antigen detection include respiratory specimens (eg, nasopharyngeal swabs, aspirates, and washes; throat swabs; BAL and bronchial washes), blood, bone marrow, CSF, stool, biopsy tissue, urine, ocular specimens, vesicles and other skin lesions, and amniotic fluid. In addition, specimens for molecular diagnostic testing (eg, PCR and other nucleic amplification techniques) must be obtained following specific guidelines so that the stability and amplifiability of the NAs are ensured.

**TABLE 19-6.** Characteristics and Laboratory Diagnosis of Selected DNA Viruses of Medical Importance to Humans

| FAMILY | NATURE | ENVELOPE | SHAPE | NUCLEOCAPSID, SYMMETRY | EXAMPLES OF SPECIES COMMONLY INFECTING HUMANS | METHODS COMMONLY USED FOR DETECTION OF VIRUS[a] |
|---|---|---|---|---|---|---|
| Adenoviridae | dsDNA, linear | No | Isometric | Icosahedral | Human mastadenovirus A to G | NAAT is most sensitive for detection. Quantitative NAAT used to monitor viral load in compromised hosts. Rapid antigen assays used for ocular, enteric, or respiratory adenoviruses (less sensitive than NAAT or culture). |
| Hepadnaviridae | dsDNA, reverse transcribing (RT), circular | Yes | Spherical | Icosahedral | Hepatitis B virus | Specific viral antigens and serology NAAT used to monitor therapy and determine genotype. |
| Herpesviridae | dsDNA, linear | Yes | Spherical | Icosahedral | Herpes simplex virus type 1 and 2 (HSV-1, HSV-2); macacine herpesvirus 1 (B virus) | NAAT is test of choice (especially for CSF infections). IFA is for rapid detection in skin and mucous membrane lesions. Serology is used to determine immune status. |
| | | | | | Varicella-zoster virus (VZV) | NAAT (sensitive and increasingly used) IFA (skin lesions) Serology (useful to determine immunity and CNS vasculopathy) Cell culture (slow and not sensitive) |
| | | | | | Epstein-Barr virus (EBV) | NAAT is test of choice for diagnosis of primary infection; also useful in monitoring viral load in blood Histology (immunohistochemistry and in situ hybridization) |
| | | | | | Human cytomegalovirus (human CMV) | NAAT (sensitive and can determine viral load) pp65 antigemia (to determine viral load in blood; alternative to NAAT) Culture (nonblood specimens) |

(continued)

**TABLE 19-6.** Characteristics and Laboratory Diagnosis of Selected DNA Viruses of Medical Importance to Humans, cont'd

| FAMILY | NATURE | ENVELOPE | SHAPE | NUCLEOCAPSID, SYMMETRY | EXAMPLES OF SPECIES COMMONLY INFECTING HUMANS | METHODS COMMONLY USED FOR DETECTION OF VIRUS[a] |
|---|---|---|---|---|---|---|
| | | | | | | Serology (to determine immune status [IgG antibody]; screen for recent infection [IgM antibody]; measure cell-mediate immunity [CMV-specific γ interferon release]) |
| | | | | | Human betaherpesvirus 6 (HHV-6A and 6B) and 7 (HHV-7) | NAAT is test of choice (but not routinely available for HHV-7). Serology for documenting infection in children (parotitis) |
| | | | | | Kaposi's sarcoma–associated herpesvirus | Serology to identify infected patients NAAT (useful in diagnosis posttransplant and monitoring therapy) Tissue histology |
| *Papillomaviridae* | dsDNA, circular | No | Isometric | Icosahedral | Human papillomavirus (HPV 1, 4, 5, 32, 41) | NAAT is test of choice (for detection and genotype differentiation). Cytopathology useful for diagnosis. |
| *Parvoviridae* | ssDNA, linear | No | Isometric | Icosahedral | Human bocavirus 1 and 2a TU Adeno-associated virus 1–5 Human parvovirus B19 Human parvovirus 4 | NAAT (is only available for diagnosis of bocaviruses); bocaviruses included on some multiplex respiratory panels (clinical relevance needs further investigation). NAAT is most sensitive for detection for adenoviruses; quantitative NAAT is used to monitor viral load in compromised hosts. Rapid antigen assays are used for ocular, enteric, or respiratory adenoviruses (less sensitive than NAAT or culture). Serology is used for diagnosis of B19 (immunocompetent patients). |

**TABLE 19-6.** Characteristics and Laboratory Diagnosis of Selected DNA Viruses of Medical Importance to Humans, cont'd

| FAMILY | NATURE | ENVELOPE | SHAPE | NUCLEOCAPSID, SYMMETRY | EXAMPLES OF SPECIES COMMONLY INFECTING HUMANS | METHODS COMMONLY USED FOR DETECTION OF VIRUS[a] |
|---|---|---|---|---|---|---|
| | | | | | | NAAT is test of choice for B19 (immunocompromised patients, early diagnosis [before antibody], and exposed fetuses). |
| *Polyomaviridae* | dsDNA, circular | No | Isometric | Icosahedral | JC polyomavirus (JCV) BK polyomavirus (BKV) | NAAT is test of choice (genetic variability can lead to falsely low or negative results). JC Virus DNA detection: in CSF (for presumptive diagnosis of progressive multifocal leukoencephalopathy [PML]), and to predict risk of PML. BK virus DNA quantification (plasma or urine) used for preemptive diagnosis of polyomavirus-associated nephropathy. Histology/Cytology: immunochemistry and electron microscopy |
| *Poxviridae* | dsDNA, linear | Yes | Brick-shaped or oval | Complex | Variola virus (Smallpox virus); Vaccinia virus; Cowpox virus; Monkeypox virus; Molluscum contagiosum virus Orf virus Yaba monkey tumor virus | NAAT (allows virus inactivation and rapid detection) EM for rapid diagnosis but has limited availability Cell culture[b] |

CMV = cytomegalovirus; CNS = central nervous system; dsDNA, double-stranded DNA; ssDNA = single-stranded DNA.
[a]Commonly used methods in clinical laboratories: electron microscopy (EM); immunoassays (IA) including immunofluorescence assay (IFA) and NAATs.
[b]The isolation of some pathogens (eg, smallpox) requires biosafety level (BSL) 3 or 4 facilities, usually only in specialized centers collaborating with World Health Organization. The isolation of Vaccinia virus requires BSL-2 (grows readily in cell culture).
*Source:* References 1,13,31,32.

**TABLE 19-7.** Characteristics and Laboratory Diagnosis of Selected RNA Viruses of Medical Importance to Humans

| FAMILY | NATURE | ENVELOPE | SHAPE | NUCLEOCAPSID SYMMETRY | EXAMPLES OF SPECIES INFECTING HUMANS | METHODS COMMONLY USED FOR DETECTION OF VIRUS[a] |
|---|---|---|---|---|---|---|
| *Arenaviridae* | ssRNA, (+/−), circular | Yes | Spherical | Helical | Lassa mammarenavirus | NAAT is key to rapid diagnosis. BSL 4 facility needed for culture. |
| | | | | | Lymphocytic choriomeningitis mammarenavirus (LCMV) | Diagnosed primarily by serology (patients with severe disease may die without developing antibody). |
| | | | | | Guanarito mammarenavirus | NAAT is key to rapid diagnosis. BSL 4 facility needed for culture. |
| | | | | | Junin mammarenavirus | NAAT is key to rapid diagnosis. BSL 4 facility needed for culture. |
| | | | | | Machupo mammarenavirus | NAAT is key to rapid diagnosis. BSL 4 facility needed for culture. |
| | | | | | Sabia mammarenavirus | NAAT is key to rapid diagnosis. BSL 4 facility needed for culture. |
| *Astroviridae* | ssRNA, (+), linear | No | Isometric | Icosahedral | Human astrovirus | NAAT is method of choice for diagnosis of viruses causing gastroenteritis. Syndrome-specific molecular testing panel (eg, BioFire FilmArray GI Panel) |
| *Bunyaviridae* | ssRNA, linear | Yes | Spherical, pleomorphic | Helical | La Crosse virus | Serology of serum or CSF (eg, IFA, Arbovirus IgM and IgG, Focus Diagnosis) NAAT, histopathology, and culture (in fatal cases) at specialized laboratories |
| | | | | | Hemorrhagic fever virus | NAAT and serology equally useful. BSL 4 facility needed for culture. Histology (in fatal cases; immunohistochemistry) |
| | | | | | Hantavirus | NAAT and serology equally useful (reference laboratory may need to perform serology of orthohantavirus-specific IgM and IgG). BSL 4 facility needed for culture. Histology (in fatal cases; immunohistochemistry) |
| *Caliciviridae* | ssRNA, (+), linear | No | Isometric | Icosahedral | Norwalk virus | NAAT is method of choice for diagnosis of viruses causing gastroenteritis; strain variability. |

| Family | Genome | Envelope | Shape | Symmetry | Virus/species | Notes |
|---|---|---|---|---|---|---|
| | | | | | Sapporo virus | Syndrome-specific molecular testing panel (ie, BioFire FilmArray GI Panel, Luminex xTAG GI Pathogen Panel, or Verigene Enteric Pathogens test) NAAT is method of choice for diagnosis of viruses causing gastroenteritis. Syndrome-specific molecular testing panel (eg, BioFire FilmArray GI Panel) |
| Coronaviridae | ssRNA, (+), linear | Yes | Spherical, pleomorphic | Helical | Human coronavirus-229E Human coronavirus-NL63 Human coronavirus-OC43 Human coronavirus-HKU1 | NAAT is used for respiratory coronavirus as part of multiplex panels. |
| | | | | | Severe acute respiratory syndrome-related coronavirus (SARS-CoV) Middle East respiratory syndrome-related coronavirus (MERS-CoV) | NAAT and serology tests are available only in public health or research laboratories. |
| | | | | | Severe acute respiratory syndrome-related coronavirus (SARS-CoV-2; COVID-19) | Numerous NAAT, antigen, and serology/antibody tests became rapidly available during the COVID-19 pandemic in 2020. Updated testing information is available at CDC website: https://www.cdc.gov/coronavirus/2019-ncov/symptoms-testing/testing.html |
| Deltavirus[b] | ssRNA, (−), circular | Yes | Spherical | Helical | Hepatitis δ virus | Testing confined to reference laboratories. Diagnosis is relevant only in the presence of hepatitis B infection. Immunohistochemistry of biopsy tissue is useful for diagnosis. |
| Filoviridae | ssRNA, (−), linear | Yes | Filamentous, pleomorphic | Helical | Bundibugyo ebolavirus; Sudan ebolavirus; Tai Forest ebolavirus; Zaire ebolavirus | NAAT is key to rapid diagnosis. BSL 4 facility needed for culture. |
| | | | | | Marburg marburgvirus | NAAT is key to rapid diagnosis. BSL 4 facility needed for culture. |
| Flaviviridae | ssRNA, (+), linear | Yes | Spherical | Icosahedral | Tick-borne encephalitis virus | Testing confined to reference laboratories. Serology, antibody detection (CSF) Commercial diagnostic tests available. |
| | | | | | Dengue virus | Testing confined to reference laboratories. NAAT, serology, IFA Commercial diagnostic tests available. |

(continued)

**TABLE 19-7.** Characteristics and Laboratory Diagnosis of Selected RNA Viruses of Medical Importance to Humans, cont'd

| FAMILY | NATURE | ENVELOPE | SHAPE | NUCLEOCAPSID SYMMETRY | EXAMPLES OF SPECIES INFECTING HUMANS | METHODS COMMONLY USED FOR DETECTION OF VIRUS[a] |
|---|---|---|---|---|---|---|
| | | | | | Japanese encephalitis virus | NAAT, serology, antibody detection (CSF). Commercial diagnostic tests available. |
| | | | | | Murray Valley encephalitis virus | Testing confined to reference laboratories. NAAT, serology, antibody detection (CSF) |
| | | | | | St. Louis encephalitis virus | Testing confined to reference laboratories. NAAT, serology, antibody detection (CSF). Commercial diagnostic tests available. |
| | | | | | West Nile virus | Testing confined to reference laboratories. NAAT, serology, antibody detection (CSF). Commercial diagnostic tests available. |
| | | | | | Yellow fever virus | Testing confined to reference laboratories. NAAT, serology, IFA. |
| | | | | | Zika virus | Testing confined to reference laboratories. NAAT, Serology. Commercial diagnostic tests available. |
| | | | | | Hepatitis C virus | Serology for diagnosis. NAAT used to confirm active infection and monitor response to therapy. Genotyping for determining drug regimen and duration of therapy. Antigen testing as alternative in low-resource areas. |
| *Herpesviridae* | ssRNA, (+), linear | No | Isometric | Icosahedral | Hepatitis E virus | Serology is the standard diagnostic test (varying sensitivity and specificity). NAAT for accurate diagnosis in transplant patients. Genotyping (performed at CDC) for autochthonous cases |
| *Orthomyxoviridae* | ssRNA, (−), linear | Yes | Pleomorphic | Helical | Influenzavirus A, B, C | NAAT (most sensitive and can provide subtypes). Rapid antigen tests (lower sensitivity and specificity). IFA and rapid culture (more accurate). Serology (useful for epidemiologic studies or retrospective diagnosis) |

| Family | Genome | Envelope | Symmetry | Capsid | Virus | Diagnostics |
|---|---|---|---|---|---|---|
| *Paramyxoviridae* | ssRNA, (−), linear | Yes | Helical | Pleomorphic | Mumps rubulavirus | Serology (most commonly used for diagnosis and determination for immunity). NAAT (useful for diagnosing infection among vaccinated individuals). |
| | | | | | Measles morbillivirus | Serology (used for diagnosis and determination for immunity) NAAT (best for acute infection) |
| | | | | | Human parainfluenza virus 1,2,3,4 | NAAT (more sensitive than isolation) IFA is most common rapid detection method. |
| *Picobirnaviridae* | dsRNA, linear | No | Icosahedral | Isometric | Human picobirnavirus | NAAT is method of choice for diagnosis of viruses causing gastroenteritis (viral etiological role as a cause of diarrhea is elusive). |
| *Picornaviridae* | ssRNA, (+), linear | No | Icosahedral | Isometric | Enterovirus A, B, C, D | NAAT is more sensitive than cultures and strongly preferred (especially for CNS infections) |
| | | | | | Rhinovirus A, B, C | NAAT is more sensitive than cultures (can cross-react with enteroviruses) |
| | | | | | Hepatitis A | Serology (false-positive IgM is problematic in low-prevalence areas) |
| | | | | | Human parechovirus | NAAT |
| *Pneumoviridae* | ssRNA, (−), linear | Yes | Helical | Pleomorphic | Human RSV | NAAT (most sensitive) Rapid antigen test (especially IFA) is useful for pediatric patients. Serology (useful for epidemiologic studies) |
| | | | | | Human metapneumovirus | NAAT (test of choice for diagnosis) IFA and shell vial culture (less sensitive options) Conventional culture is difficult. |
| *Reoviridae* | dsRNA, linear | No | Icosahedral | Isometric | Rotavirus A, B, C, H | Direct antigen detection (IA) Rotavirus A is on NAAT gastroenteritis panels (ie, BioFire FilmArray GI Panel, Luminex xTAG GI Pathogen Panel, or Verigene Enteric Pathogens test). EM is useful. |

*(continued)*

**TABLE 19-7.** Characteristics and Laboratory Diagnosis of Selected RNA Viruses of Medical Importance to Humans, cont'd

| FAMILY | NATURE | ENVELOPE | SHAPE | NUCLEOCAPSID, SYMMETRY | EXAMPLES OF SPECIES INFECTING HUMANS | METHODS COMMONLY USED FOR DETECTION OF VIRUS[a] |
|---|---|---|---|---|---|---|
| *Retroviridae* | ssRNA reverse transcribing (RT), linear, dimer | Yes | Spherical | Icosahedral | Human immunodeficiency virus 1 (HIV-1) and 2 (HIV-2) | Serology is primary diagnostic method. Antigen-antibody combination tests reduce seronegative window in acute infection. Quantitative RNA tests are used to guide therapy and monitor response. Proviral DNA tests useful for neonatal infections |
| | | | | | Primate T-lymphotropic virus 1 and 2 | NAAT; serology |
| | | | | | Simian foamy virus | NAAT; serology |
| *Rhabdoviridae* | ssRNA, (−), linear | Yes | Bullet shaped | Helical | Rabies lyssavirus | For human rabies, testing done at CDC. NAAT and cell culture used for saliva, CSF, and tissues. IFA used for skin biopsy samples. Serology used for CSF and serum. Serology available in commercial laboratories and used for monitoring antibody titers in vaccinated subjects. |
| *Togaviridae* | ssRNA, (+), linear | Yes | Spherical | Icosahedral | Arboviruses including *Alphavirus* genus, containing ~25 viruses | NAAT and IgM are useful in acute infection, depending on day of illness and clinical diseases. Most viruses are readily cultured but isolation may require BSL3 or BSL4 facilities. Commercial diagnostic tests available for specific viruses (eg, Chikungunya, Ross River, Eastern, and Western encephalitis). |
| | | | | | Rubella virus | Serology is used for diagnosis and immune status. NAAT is used for acute infection. Cell culture is useful for postnatal rubella if attempted early (prodromal period to 4 days postrash). In congenital rubella syndrome, virus can be cultured for weeks to month after birth. |

(+) = positive stranded; (−) = negative stranded; BSL = biosafety level; CDC = Centers for Disease Control and Prevention; dsRNA = double-stranded RNA; GI = gastrointestinal; ssRNA = single-stranded RNA.
[a]Commonly used methods in clinical laboratories: electron microscopy (EM); immunoassays (IA) including immunofluorescence assay (IFA) and NAATs.
[b]Deltavirus is genus (higher classification) and family in unassigned.
*Source:* References 1,13,31,32.

Once the sample is collected, it should be promptly transported to the laboratory in a sterile, leak-proof container using the appropriate viral transport media to maximize viral recovery. Every effort should be made to prevent delay between the time of specimen collection and its arrival to the laboratory. When delays are expected, viral samples should be refrigerated at 4°C or frozen at −70°C. Subsequently, the laboratory will need to follow specific processing procedures for each specimen and the different diagnostic viral test methodologies.

The laboratory techniques used in the diagnosis of viral infections include cell culture, cytology and histology, electron microscopy (EM), antigen detection, NAATs, and serologic testing.[1,13,32-38] The choice of test(s) varies depending on the clinical syndrome or disease, virus(es) involved, patient characteristics, collection site, purposes of the test (eg, screening, diagnosis, confirmation or monitoring), time to result, laboratory capabilities/staff expertise, and cost. The following section, as well as Tables 19-6 and 19-7, provides a brief summary of the common methods currently used in diagnostic testing of common viruses.[1,13,31,32] For more detailed information, the reader is referred to current published literature, standard reference books, and the latest edition of reference manuals (eg, *Manual of Clinical Microbiology*). A list of virology services offered by the CDC can be found on the CDC website (https://www.cdc.gov/laboratory/specimen-submission/list.html).

## Cell Culture

The use of *cell culture* rapidly expanded the knowledge about the epidemiology, clinical characteristics, and diagnosis of common viral infections in the 1950s and 1960s. Subsequently, the use of cell cultures to isolate a virus became the gold standard method for the diagnosis of viral infections in most clinical virology laboratories for the next 50 years.[13,32-36] During that time, other technologies for viral detection were slowly introduced in the clinical laboratories, including enzyme immunoassays, IgM class capture assays, rapid centrifugation cultures, direct viral antigen detection from clinical specimens by immunofluorescence, and monoclonal antibodies for identification. However, rapid and accurate serology and molecular methodologies have become cornerstones for virus detection and identification in clinical laboratories during the past decade, resulting in a decline in the use and prominence of cell cultures in larger academic medical centers and tertiary-care facilities. Despite these changes in routine diagnostic virology, viral cultures play an important role in the discovery of new or unknown viruses, identification of variants of known viruses, detection of drug-resistant viruses, typing of serologic strains, detection of viruses in special patient populations (eg, immunocompromised patients), research and development of antiviral drugs and vaccines, and performance of viral susceptibilities.[34-36]

The advantages of cell culture include good specificity and sensitivity, the capability of detecting multiple viruses if present, and the cultivation of the virus for further laboratory testing (eg, susceptibility testing, serologic strain typing), if needed.[32,34-36] Cell cultures can be useful when combined with highly specific monoclonal antibodies or engineered cell lines (eg, to produce virus-induced enzymes), especially if the cost of other testing methods is greater than cell cultures or when the clinical laboratory does not have the ability and equipment to perform molecular detection methods. The disadvantages of cell culture include the long time needed for the detection of viruses using conventional cell culture (eg, days to weeks), the need for cell culture facilities, the expense of performing cell culture, and the fact that the methodology is not applicable to all viruses (eg, viruses that have not grown in conventional cell cultures [ie, Group C rhinovirus]). This greater demand for technical laboratory experience with cell cultures, need for comprehensive quality control program, and strict procedures for handling biohazardous materials in the clinical virology laboratory are being replaced by rapid and sensitive antigen screening assays and NAATs.[34]

Several different types of cell culture are available to grow clinically important viruses.[32,34-36] Each virus requires a predefined cell line, which is established once a cell culture has been subcultured in vitro (the reader is referred to a comprehensive list of available cell lines and virus susceptibility profiles[34]). The different types of cell lines can be divided into three categories: primary, diploid (also called *low passage cell lines*), and heteroploid. Primary cell lines (eg, rhesus monkey kidney [RhMK] cells or human amnion cells) are prepared from animal or human tissues and can withstand only one or two passages until the cells die. Diploid cell lines are usually derived from fetal or newborn cells (eg, human embryonic lung fibroblast lines such as WI-38 or MRC-5) and can undergo 20 to 50 passages before cells are unable to survive. Continuous cell lines can undergo an indefinite number of passages without reducing the sensitivity to virus infection. Heteroploid cell lines are characteristically derived from human or animal cancers (eg, human epidermoid lung carcinoma [HEp-2, HeLa]) or are cells transformed in vitro (eg, LLC-MK$_2$). Heteroploid cell lines can also include genetically engineered cells (eg, ELVIS cell mixture for the detection of herpes simplex virus [HSV] types 1 and 2). Most specimens are inoculated onto two or more cell lines (eg, RhMK, MRC-5, HEp-2) based on the most likely viruses associated with the type of clinical specimen that was submitted.

The growth of a virus from a clinical specimen provides direct evidence that the patient was infected with a virus. The main method for detecting growth from the cell culture method is by microscopic examination of the unstained cell cultured monolayers for morphologic changes or cytopathic effect (CPE).[32,34-36] The characteristics of the CPE (eg, which cell culture types were affected; what is the resultant shape of the cells; whether the effect is focal or diffuse; the time of its appearance and progression) can be used for primary and definitive identification of the virus. Subsequently, direct and indirect fluorescent antibody (DFA and IFA, respectively) staining of cells with virus-specific monoclonal antibodies harvested from the culture is often used to confirm the identification of the virus (the reader is referred to a comprehensive list of available DFA and IFA reagents and target virus to detect[34]). Molecular or ancillary traditional testing can alternatively be used for viral identification.

Some viruses, such as influenza, parainfluenza, and mumps virus, grow in cell cultures without producing CPE so that other methods are used to identify and detect these viruses, including hemadsorption and interference.[32,34-36] Hemadsorption involves the removal of the culture medium from the inoculated cell culture, adding a suspension of erythrocytes, and examining for hemadsorption with a low-power microscope as manifested by adherence of the red cells to the cell culture monolayer due to the presence of a hemadsorbing virus. Hemadsorption is used to detect these viruses, which can grow rapidly and reach high titers in cell cultures without producing CPE. Used to detect viruses such as rubella, interference involves growing a virus that yields a cell culture resistant to other viruses (to which it is normally susceptible). The viruses that produce hemadsorption or interference subsequently can be identified by staining with virus-specific monoclonal antibodies or antiserum.

Shell vial cultures with centrifugation and pre-CPE detection are used to decrease the amount of time required to grow a virus by conventional cell cultures.[32,34-36] This technique makes use of cells grown on microscope coverslips that are placed within shell vials and covered with culture media. After cultures are incubated for 1 to 3 days, FA staining is performed on the cells on the coverslips to recognize an antigen in the nucleus of infected cells. Shell vial cultures have been commonly applied for the detection of cytomegalovirus (CMV), HSV, varicella-zoster virus (VZV), enteroviruses, and the human respiratory viruses. Centrifugation-enhanced rapid cell cultures can also be used with cocultivated cells (eg, mixture of two cell lines together) or genetically engineered cells (eg, ELVIS [enzyme-linked virus-inducible system], BGMK-hDAF [buffalo green monkey kidney cell line]) for the rapid identification (eg, 16 to 72 hours) and blind staining of multiple viruses from a single shell vial or tray well.[32,34-36]

## Molecular Diagnosis

The detection of specific viral NAs by molecular diagnostic techniques is revolutionizing the field of diagnostic virology.[1,13,32,34,38] NAATs have become the "gold standard" in clinical virology laboratories and are replacing older techniques such as cell cultures for detecting clinically significant viruses. Many different techniques are used in viral NA detection, including direct hybridization assays, target (template) amplification (eg, PCR, self-sustained sequence replication method, strand displacement amplification), and signal amplification (eg, branched-chain DNA [bDNA] assay and hybrid capture assay). Among these, PCR has been the most important technique in diagnostic virology because of its versatility in detecting DNA or RNA and being able to provide qualitative and quantitative information on specific viral NAs.

The use of NA detection has become the standard of care (eg, hepatitis C virus [HCV] and HIV) or the test of choice for routine diagnosis of many viral infections (eg, bocaviruses, HSV central nervous system [CNS] infections, human HVS 6 and 7, human metapneumovirus, human papillomavirus [HPV]).[1,13,32] The FDA has cleared or approved commercial molecular detection assays; several viruses, including hepatitis B and C viruses (HBV, HCV); HIV; HSV; CMV; adenovirus; avian flu; enteroviruses; influenza; and HPV. An FDA-approved simple multiplex PCR test (eg, xTAG Respiratory Viral Panel) is also available for rapidly screening common respiratory viruses (eg, respiratory syncytial virus [RSV], influenza A and B, adenovirus) or subtypes.[1,13,38-41] In addition, FDA-approved, high-throughput, syndromic viral tests are also available for detection of GI and CSF pathogens (eg, BioFire FilmArray GI and Meningitis/ Encephalitis panels).[1,39-43] An up-to-date listing of cleared or approved nucleic acid diagnostics tests is available at the FDA website (https://www.fda.gov/medical-devices/vitro-diagnostics /nucleic-acid-based-tests).

The advantages of viral NA detection methods include the rapidity of results (eg, hours for real-time PCR and one to several days for other methods), maximal sensitivity for virus-specific detection and identification, adequate to excellent specificity, dramatic increase in availability of commercial assays, the ability to detect viruses that are difficult to culture, and the ability to detect NAs without viable virus present in the clinical specimen. Historically, equipment and reagents costs, service contracts, and technical expertise have been the major barriers to implementing molecular testing. However, NAAT has rapidly evolved and allows viruses such as influenza virus and RSV to be detected within 20 to 30 minutes at near POC and with sensitivity similar to other laboratory testing methodologies.[1,13,39-41,44] Several devices (eg, FilmArray Respiratory Panel EZ assay [Biofilm, Salt Lake City, UT]; ID NOW RSV [Abbott Diagnostics, Scarborough, ME]; the cobas Liat Influenza A/B & RSV [Roche Diagnostics, Indianapolis, IN]) have been waived by the Clinical Laboratory Improvement Amendments (CLIA).[13,40,41,44] Molecular assays have become the standard of care for diagnosing viral infections and monitoring antiviral therapy and patient outcomes.[1,13,32]

## Cytology and Histology

Cytopathologic effects (CPEs) on cells are produced by many viruses. Cytologic examination can be performed on smears prepared from samples that are applied to a microscope slide or "touch preps" of unfixed tissues.[32,34-36] Cytologic findings are suggestive of a viral infection and provide identification of cell morphologies (eg, "owl's eye" nuclear inclusions consistent with CMV), cell lysis, or other cell changes (eg, vacuolation, syncytia, inclusion bodies). The specific virus cannot be identified unless virus-specific immunostaining techniques are used. Applications of *cytology* to viral diagnosis include the Tzanck smear with Giemsa reagent for demonstrating the presence of HSV or VZV infection, Papanicolaou staining of cells obtained from the uterine cervix (Pap smear) for providing evidence of HPV infection, and cytologic staining of urinary sediments for screening the presence of either CMV or polyomaviruses JCV and BKV.

Similar to cytology, histologic examination of tissue provides evidence to suggest a group of viruses that may be causing infection, but it does not identify a specific virus.[32,34] Despite this shortcoming, histopathology has been useful in differentiating between asymptomatic viral shedding and clinically important infections of CMV and has been used for the diagnosis of CMV infections in tissue samples obtained from biopsy or at autopsy. In addition, detection of specific viral antigens by immunohistochemistry and detection of specific viral NAs by in situ hybridization (ISH) or PCR has allowed specific viruses to be identified by histopathology.

## Electron Microscopy

Viruses are the smallest infectious pathogens that range in diameter from 18 to 300 nm.[32,37] Direct visualization of a virus with a light microscope can be performed only on pathogens with a diameter >200 nm. *Electron microscopy* (EM) allows visualization of characteristic viral morphology and, unlike direct detection or molecular methodologies, is capable of detecting the distinctive appearances of multiple viruses, if present.[32,37] EM is considered the most useful routine test for poxviruses.[66] Diagnostic virology laboratories also commonly use EM for detection of viruses that are not detected with cell cultures or other methods (eg, gastroenteritis viruses such as noroviruses, coronaviruses, astroviruses, enteric adenovirus, and calicivirus).[13,32,34,37,43]

Several techniques have been incorporated to allow the visualization of viruses with EM from various types of clinical specimens. Negative staining is a technique for identification of viruses in fluid samples, stool samples, and blister fluid. Thin sectioning can be performed on tissue samples that have been fixed with specific fixatives for EM study, and it can be used to visualize herpesviruses, respiratory viruses, and rabies virus.

More sensitive methods are replacing the routine use of EM for detecting clinically significant viruses.[13,32,37] An advantage of EM is its economical, quick (eg, same day), adaptable, and straightforward approach for detecting viruses. The major disadvantages of EM include poor sensitivity, initial equipment expenses, and need for highly skilled laboratory staff.

## Direct Antigen Detection

Antigen detection methods involve the use of virus-specific antibodies directed toward viral antigens in a clinical specimen.[1,13,32,38] Examples of viruses that can be identified by *direct antigen detection* include RSV, influenza virus, parainfluenza virus, adenovirus, HSV, VZV, CMV, rotavirus, HBV, and measles virus.[1,13,32,39-41] The advantages of direct antigen detection include the rapidity of diagnosis (eg, several hours to 1 day), usefulness for the identification of viruses that are difficult to culture, and detection of viral specific antigens even if viable virus is not present in the clinical specimen. The disadvantages include the potential for false-positive and false-negative results, difficulty of performing batch testing, and lack of sensitivity necessary for diagnostic applications for all viruses (eg, not applicable for rhinoviruses because there are >90 serotypes and cross-reacting antibodies).

The techniques commonly used for antigen detection include immunofluorescence assay (IFA; direct and indirect), EIA (including ELISA), chemiluminescent and fluorescence-based immunoassay, and particle agglutination assays. Several membrane immunochromatographic assays (dipstick tests) are available as influenza diagnostic tests (eg, Directigen Flu A or A+B Test, QuickVue influenza).[13,32,39,40] These viral antigen tests have become simple to use, are low cost, and allow rapid detection (≤30 minutes) of specific antigens from a single specimen at POC (eg, outpatient facilities, physician offices, patient bedside) and in the clinical laboratory. Many of these RIDT kits are CLIA-waived because the methodologies are simple to use and accurate, and the likelihood of erroneous results is negligible.[13,39,45] Rapid influenza diagnostic tests (RIDTs) have lower specificity but variable sensitivity (higher in children and for detecting influenza A). The need for improved sensitivity of RIDTs was also observed during the 2009 pandemic of H1N1 influenza. These issues, in part, resulted in a medical device reclassification by the FDA in 2017 and additional compliance requirements of RIDTs for influenza.[13,39,45] Further details on RIDTs and NA detection-based tests for influenza virus can be found at the CDC website (https//www.cdc.gov/flu/professionals/diagnosis/rapidlab.htm).

## Serology

Serologic tests are designed to detect an antibody response in serum samples after exposure to viral antigens has occurred.[32] The major uses of *serology* for the detection of viral infections include the demonstration of immunity or exposure to a virus, the diagnosis of postinfectious sequelae, and the screening of blood products. In several clinical situations, serologic testing remains the primary means for the laboratory diagnosis of viruses that are difficult to culture or detect by direct methods (eg, rubella virus, Epstein-Barr virus, hepatitis viruses, HIV, arboviruses).[1,13,32] Serologic testing may also serve as a supportive or adjunctive role in clinical situations in which viral cultures or direct detection methods are available.

For viral infections, serologic testing can identify the virus, distinguish the strain or serotype, differentiate between primary infection and reinfection, and determine if the infection is in an acute or convalescent phase. Virus-specific immunoglobulin antibodies (eg, IgM or IgG) are produced during the time course of a viral infection. In general, virus-specific IgM is detected in serum sooner than virus-specific IgG. The results measure the relative concentration of antibody in the body as a titer, with the titer representing the lowest antibody concentration (or inverse of the greatest dilution; a dilution of 1:128 is expressed as a titer of 128) that demonstrates activity in a patient's serum. The exact value for a titer varies with each testing method, the specific virus involved, the timing of specimen collection, and the presence of active disease.

For most viral infections, virus-specific IgM can be detected as soon as 3 to 7 days after the onset of infection. The presence of virus-specific IgM in a single serum sample shortly after the onset of symptoms (acute phase) is usually indicative of a recent or current primary infection. Titers of virus-specific IgM usually decline to near undetectable amounts within 1 to 4 months after the onset of infection. Virus-specific IgG can be detected during the acute phase of infection (eg, 1 to 2 weeks) and continues to increase for several months before reaching a maximal titer. Thereafter, the IgG titer declines, but it usually remains detectable in serum for the remainder of a person's life. Seroconversion has occurred when at least a 4-fold increase in IgG titer has occurred between serum samples collected in the acute and convalescent (two to four weeks afterward) phases. The presence of virus-specific IgG is also indicative of a past infection.

Serologic tests are also used to assess the immunity or exposure to a virus. The presence of antibody can detect which patients have been previously infected by or vaccinated for a specific virus. For example, a positive result (presence of antibody) for rubella in a woman of childbearing age implies that congenital infection will not occur during subsequent pregnancies. A negative result (absence of antibody) implies susceptibility to infection, and the woman should receive rubella vaccination as a preventative measure if she is not pregnant. Some other examples of viruses for which serologic determination of immune status is useful include hepatitis A and B (HAV, HBV), measles, mumps, parvovirus B19, and VZV.[1,13,32]

The techniques commonly used for serologic assays include CF, EIA, IFA, anticomplement immunofluorescence, and western immunoblotting. In the diagnosis of certain viral syndromes (eg, CNS infections), a serology panel may be helpful so that a battery of antigens is tested for antibody to several viruses. The advantages of viral serology include the assessment of immunity or response of a virus isolated from a nonsterile site, serum specimens are easy to obtain and store, and it can be used to identify viruses that are difficult to culture or detect by immunoassay. The disadvantages include the time to results (eg, few days to weeks), the potential for cross-reactions between different viruses, and the need for both acute and convalescent specimens.

## Antiviral Susceptibility Testing

The emergence of drug-resistant strains of viruses to antiviral agents is an increasing problem, especially in immunocompromised hosts. Unlike antibiotics, in vitro susceptibility testing of viruses has not been routinely available. The major variables that have limited the standardization of antiviral susceptibility testing include cell lines, inoculums titer, incubation period, testing range of antiviral drug concentrations, reference strains, assay methodology, and criteria, calculation, and interpretation of end points.[46] However, emerging molecular technology and the phasing out of virus culture-based methods have permitted phenotypic and genotypic antiviral susceptibility testing vividly advance.

The FDA-cleared assays for viral susceptibility testing for the past decade have mainly been limited to phenotypic and genotypic assays for HIV. Antiviral resistance and cases of drug failure has led to increased interest in susceptibility testing of HSV, VZV, CMV, and influenza viruses.[46] Thus far, most susceptibility testing for these pathogens has been limited to research use only or laboratory user-developed tests. The CLSI has published an approved standard for phenotypic susceptibility testing of HSV.[47] This standard outlined the use of a plaque reduction assay and denotes resistance to acyclovir and foscarnet when inhibitory concentration 50% ($IC_{50}$) values are $\geq 2$ mcg/mL and $\geq 100$ mcg/mL, respectively. Proposed guidelines for antiviral susceptibility results of HSV, CMV, VZV, and influenza A and B viruses for various other phenotypic testing methods (ie, DNA hybridization, EIA, neuraminidase inhibition assay, late antigen reduction assay) and antiviral agents (ie, famciclovir, vidarabine, cidofovir, ganciclovir, neuraminidase inhibitors) have also been outlined.[46] Interpretation of these values must be carefully made in conjunction with the clinical response of the individual patient. Additional consensus documents and further standardization of phenotypic and genotypic assays for antiviral susceptibility testing are needed.

# HUMAN IMMUNODEFICIENCY VIRUS

Human immunodeficiency virus (HIV) is the causative agent of AIDS. The HIV virus is an enveloped, positively stranded RNA virus that belongs to the Retroviridae (retrovirus) family and Lentivirus genus.[48] The mature virus measures approximately 100 nm in diameter and has a characteristic conical core containing proteins, enzymes, and two identical copies of single-stranded RNA. Viral proteins within the core and the lipid envelope play a significant role in the detection, diagnosis, and treatment of HIV.[49,50] The replication process of HIV involves transcription of viral RNA into proviral DNA using the reverse transcriptase (RT) enzyme. The proviral DNA is then integrated into the host's genome using the integrase enzyme, resulting in lifelong latent infection. The virus is transmitted to humans by the exchange of blood or other body fluids containing the virus through sexual contact; exposure to contaminated blood; transfusion of contaminated blood and blood products; or via contaminated needles (eg, intravenous drug users or accidental needle sticks). In addition, infants can acquire HIV from an infected mother in utero, during labor or delivery, or during breastfeeding.[49,51]

There are two distinct serotypes of HIV, namely HIV-1 and HIV-2; while HIV-1 is the most prevalent serotype of HIV infections worldwide, HIV-2 infection is most commonly distributed in Western Africa and other limited geographic locations.[49-51] Routine diagnostic testing of HIV-2 is not recommended in the United States because its prevalence is extremely low. Thus, the following discussion focuses mainly on laboratory tests used for the diagnosis and management of HIV-1 infection. However, HIV-2 testing may be indicated in persons at risk for HIV-2 infection or for those who have symptoms suggestive of HIV infection with negative or indeterminate test results for HIV-1. In addition, all blood donations in the United States are tested for both HIV-1 and HIV-2.[49-51]

## Laboratory Tests for Human Immunodeficiency Virus-1 Infection

Several laboratory tests are available for the diagnosis and monitoring of patients with HIV-1 infection. The most common virologic testing methods include HIV-1 antibody assays, HIV-1 p24 antigen assays, DNA-PCR, plasma HIV-1 RNA (viral load) assays, and viral phenotypic and genotypic assays. In addition, the absolute number of CD4+ lymphocytes and the ratio of helper (CD4+) to suppressor (CD8+) lymphocytes (CD4+:CD8+ ratios) are routinely measured to evaluate the patient's immune status and response to antiretroviral therapy, because HIV primarily infects and depletes CD4+ T helper lymphocytes. Viral cultures for HIV are not typically performed beyond clinical research studies due to the labor-intensive nature of the testing methods as well as the extensive time required to obtain results.[33-35]

Laboratory tests for HIV-1 infection are clinically used for diagnosing HIV-1 infection, monitoring progression of HIV infection and the response to antiretroviral therapy, and screening blood donors. The selection of these tests is highly dependent on the clinical situation, the patient population, and the specified purpose for the testing, as described in **Table 19-8**.[8,51-54]

**TABLE 19-8.** Recommended Laboratory Tests for the Diagnosis, Monitoring, and Blood Donor Screening for HIV

| CLINICAL SITUATION | RECOMMENDED TEST(S) | COMMENTS |
|---|---|---|
| Diagnosis of HIV infection, including acute infection (excluding infants) | Initial fourth-generation antibody/antigen ELISA + supplemental antibody differentiation immunoassay | Only a reactive initial ELISA requires a supplemental HIV-1/HIV-2 antibody differentiation immunoassay<br><br>A nonreactive initial ELISA does not require further testing<br><br>An HIV RNA test may be necessary if initial testing is indeterminate |
| Diagnosis of HIV in infants (<18 months of age) born to HIV-infected mother | HIV DNA PCR or plasma HIV RNA viral load | Initial testing recommended between 14 and 21 days of life, 1–2 months, and 3–6 months; diagnosis of HIV by two positive virologic tests<br><br>HIV antibody testing not recommended due to persistence of maternal antibodies |
| Indeterminate supplemental antibody differentiation immunoassay | Nucleic acid test for HIV-1 | Only HIV-1 nucleic acid test available |
| Prognosis | Plasma HIV RNA viral load and CD4$^+$ T cell count | Risk of disease progression greater with HIV RNA >100,000 copies/mL |
| Response to antiretroviral therapy | Plasma HIV RNA viral load and CD4$^+$ T cell count | Decision to start therapy should be based on laboratory results as well as clinical findings, patient interests, adherence issues, and risks of toxicity and drug interactions |
| Antiretroviral drug resistance testing | Phenotypic and genotypic resistance assays | Recommended for acute and chronic HIV infection on entry into care, treatment naïve patients, pregnant patients, and cases of virologic failure (testing recommended within 4 weeks of treatment discontinuation)<br><br>Not recommended for patients with HIV RNA <1,000 copies/mL |
| Blood donor screening | Fourth-generation antibody/antigen ELISA + Supplemental antibody differentiation immunoassay; plasma HIV RNA viral load | In the United States, blood from all donors is tested for HIV-1 and HIV-2 antibodies as well as p24 antigen |

DNA = deoxyribonucleic acid; ELISA = enzyme-linked immunosorbent assay; HIV = human immunodeficiency virus; RNA = ribonucleic acid; PCR = polymerase chain reaction.
*Source:* References 8,51–54.

The following section briefly reviews each of the specific tests, but more comprehensive descriptions of the various commercial assays and their clinical applications can be found elsewhere.[49,51,52,55]

### Human Immunodeficiency Virus Antibody Tests

Infection with HIV affects both humoral and cell-mediated immune function. The humoral immune response results in the production of antibodies directed against HIV-specific proteins and glycoproteins. For most patients, antibodies to HIV-1 can be detected in the blood by 4 to 8 weeks after exposure to the virus. However, it may take up to 6 to 12 months in some patients. There are several tests currently available for the detection of HIV antibody in infected patients.

The methodology of EIA (commonly referred to as *ELISA*) is widely used as the *initial* screening test to detect HIV-specific antibodies.[49,51,52,56] Like all immunoassays, ELISA is based on the concept of antigen and antibody reaction to form a measurable precipitate. The ability of ELISA to detect HIV antibodies during earlier infection has improved over recent years. Although

## MINICASE 1

### Testing for Human Immunodeficiency Virus While on Pre-Exposure Prophylaxis

Brian W. is an HIV-negative partner in a serodiscordant relationship who is currently taking tenofovir/emtricitabine for HIV pre-exposure prophylaxis (PrEP). He reports taking PrEP regularly without missed doses and does note occasional unprotected intercourse with his HIV-positive partner. He routinely gets tested for HIV every 3 months but is wondering if he needs to wait that long to get tested if he has an HIV sexual exposure from his partner. He has heard that it takes several months before HIV can be detected after exposure, and he would rather know as soon as possible.

QUESTION: How soon after exposure can current HIV tests detect infection?

DISCUSSION: The current tests for diagnosing HIV infection include the fourth-generation ELISA (or EIA) and a supplemental antibody differentiation immunoassay. Because fourth-generation assays combine the detection of HIV-1 and HIV-2 antibodies as well as HIV-1 p24 antigen, they are able to detect both acute and established HIV infection. The detection of HIV-1 p24 antigen by third-generation and fourth-generation immune assays is estimated to be between 14 and 20 days after infection. Thus, this patient does not need to wait until his scheduled routine HIV test and could seek earlier testing for reassurance. Additionally, he should be counseled on the importance of condom use while taking PrEP and on the decreased likelihood of transmission if his partner has an undetectable HIV viral load.

## MINICASE 2

### Speciation of Mycobacteria

Eva J. is a 42-year-old woman with HIV/AIDS, cerebral toxoplasmosis, and disseminated MAC. She was admitted to the hospital 10 days ago with abdominal pain and found to have a psoas abscess, which was drained. A preliminary culture result of this abscess stained positive for AFB with pending speciation. She has been taking tenofovir alafenamide/emtricitabine/bictegravir, ethambutol and azithromycin, and atovaquone for the past 4 months since her diagnosis of HIV/AIDS, toxoplasmosis, and disseminated MAC, respectively. Although she is taking medications with activity against mycobacteria, it would be best to tailor her antimycobacterial regimen to address the organism causing her psoas abscess.

## MINICASE 2 (cont'd)

QUESTION: What laboratory could be used to determine the species of this AFB?

DISCUSSION: The staining methods can detect the presence of mycobacteria in a clinical specimen but cannot differentiate between species of mycobacteria. Molecular techniques that use NA amplification (PCR) to detect *M tuberculosis* complex in acid-fast smear positive or negative respiratory specimens have been commercially developed to augment identification. Because of their high specificity and faster results, the CDC recommends performing NA amplification tests on respiratory specimens of patients suspected of having pulmonary TB. However, none of these assays are currently FDA-approved for the detection of *Mycobacterium* from nonrespiratory specimens such as in our patient case. For optimal cultivation and identification of mycobacteria, a combination of culture media, including at least one solid growth medium and one liquid growth medium, should be used during specimen processing to facilitate growth and optimize pigment production of the organism. Cultures for mycobacteria typically require prolonged incubation periods, sometimes up to 8 weeks, because most of the more common pathogens grow rather slowly. Rapidly growing mycobacteria such as *M fortuitum*, *M chelonae*, and *M abscessus* typically grow within 7 days on solid media, while slow growing mycobacteria such as *M tuberculosis* complex, MAC, *M kansasii*, and *M marinum* require 7 days to 7 weeks for growth. Hence, culture tubes or plates are examined weekly during the incubation period for the presence of mycobacterial growth. Colonies grown in culture are examined microscopically for characteristic colonial morphologic features, pigmentation, and growth rate; are subjected to biochemical tests; and are evaluated using rapid molecular detection methods, such as PCR methods mentioned earlier, DNA hybridization using DNA probes, and chromatographic methods, such as high-performance liquid chromatography or gas liquid chromatography, to detect mycobacterial lipids for definitive identification. The DNA probes can be used only with mycobacteria grown in culture (not directly on patient specimens), are highly sensitive and specific, and are commercially available for the rapid identification of *M tuberculosis* complex, *M gordonae*, *M kansasii*, and MAC. The molecular methods have replaced the use of biochemical tests in many laboratories because they provide more accurate identification in a significantly shorter time frame, within 14 to 21 days of specimen receipt as compared with several weeks or months using traditional identification methods. Recently, the use of MALDI-TOF MS for the identification of mycobacteria and other organisms was approved by the FDA. Although more expensive and not widely available, MALDI-TOF can provide faster time to speciation. However, the speciation of certain mycobacteria such as MTBC remains mostly unavailable with this method.

less specific, first-generation ELISA tests introduced in 1985 were capable of detecting HIV-1 antibodies as soon as 40 days after exposure. Second-generation ELISA, introduced in 1987, incorporated recombinant antigens that increased specificity, sensitivity, and the ability to detect antibodies as soon as 34 days after infection. With the introduction of antigens from HIV-2, and the addition of antigens from HIV-1 groups M, N, and O and group M subtypes in the 1990s, specificity and sensitivity were improved. Third-generation ELISA, introduced in the mid-1990s, was redesigned as an antigen-antibody-antigen format, which dramatically improved sensitivity and specificity, and able to detect IgM and non-IgG antibodies as soon as 22 days after infection.

Fourth-generation ELISA detects the presence of both HIV-1 and HIV-2 antibodies and HIV-1 p24 antigen, which has reduced the detection period to approximately 15 days after infection, similar to the period of detection of p24 antigen.[51] The improved sensitivity of fourth-generation assays has led to current recommendations by the CDC for their use as initial test in the diagnosis of HIV (**Figure 19-1**).[51] Commercial fourth-generation ELISA kits used by most diagnostic laboratories can detect both HIV-1 and HIV-2 and have a sensitivity and specificity of >99%; however, false-positive and false-negative results can occur, particularly with previous generation assays. False-positive results have been reported with improper specimen handling (eg, heating) and in patients with autoimmune diseases, recent influenza vaccination, acute viral infection, alcoholic liver disease, chronic renal failure requiring hemodialysis, lymphoma, hematologic malignancies, and positive rapid plasma reagin (RPR) tests due to reactivity of the antibodies used for testing. Several causes have been identified for false-negative ELISA results and include the concomitant use of immunosuppressive therapy, the presence of severe hypogammaglobulinemia, and testing for HIV infection shortly after infection (acute HIV infection) or too late in the course of HIV infection.[49,51]

The results of a fourth-generation assay are reported as reactive (positive) or nonreactive (negative). If the initial result is nonreactive, no further testing for HIV antibodies is performed and the person is considered uninfected unless they are suspected of having acute HIV infection. When the initial result of a fourth-generation test is reported as reactive, a supplemental assay that differentiates between HIV-1 and HIV-2 antibodies must be performed. If the supplemental antibody differentiation test result is nonreactive or indeterminate, an HIV-1 nucleic acid test (NAT) must be performed to confirm the diagnosis of HIV-1 infection.[51] Currently, laboratories can routinely use only the APTIMA HIV-1 RNA Qualitative Assay (Gen-Probe, Inc., San Diego, CA) as an aid in diagnosing HIV-1 (including acute or primary infection), and quantitative (viral load) HIV-1 RNA assays require a written order by a physician.[57] As of this writing, no NAT has been approved for HIV-2 by the FDA, and

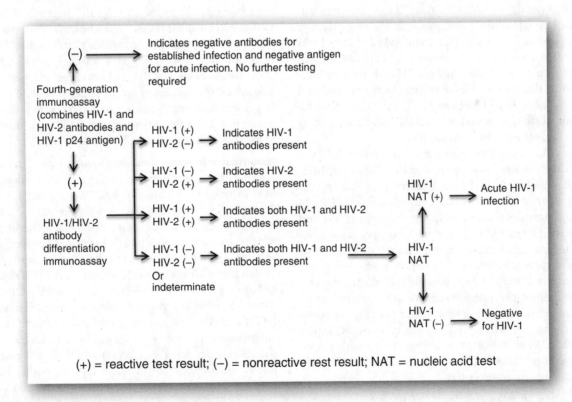

**FIGURE 19-1.** CDC-recommended HIV laboratory testing algorithm for serum/plasma samples. (*Source*: Adapted from Centers for Disease Control and Prevention, and Association of Public Health Laboratories. Laboratory testing for the diagnosis of HIV infection: updated recommendations. 2014:1–68. http://dx.doi.org/10.15620/cdc.23447.)

the CDC recommends consultation with an expert in suspected cases of HIV-2 infection.

The western blot (WB) was the confirmatory test of choice for detecting HIV-specific antibody for many years.[49,51,56,58] WB is a protein electrophoretic immunoblot technique that detects specific antibodies to HIV protein and glycoprotein antigens. The proteins and glycoproteins are detected by WB as "bands" and can be divided into Env (envelope) glycoproteins (gp41, gp120, gp160), Gag or nuclear proteins (p17, p24/25, p55), and Pol or endonuclease-polymerase proteins (p34, p40, p52, p68). Criteria for the interpretation of WB results have been published by different healthcare organizations and may vary depending on the issuing body. WB traditionally was considered to have a low level of sensitivity and high specificity, but newer data showed the WB misinterpreted most HIV-2 infections as being HIV-1.[51] The WB test is technically difficult to perform, expensive, and associated with a relatively high rate of indeterminate results (4% to 20%) and has a long turnaround time (results are available in 1 to 2 weeks).[49,51,52] Because of these limitations and the availability of more reliable assays, WB is no longer recommended for the diagnosis of HIV in the United States.[51]

Compared with WB, the use of an HIV-1/HIV-2 differentiation assay detects HIV-1 antibodies earlier, reduces indeterminate results, identifies HIV-2 infections, has a shorter turnaround for test results, and an overall lower cost.[51] To date, only the Geenius HIV 1/2 Supplemental Assay (Bio-Rad Laboratories, Redmond, WA) differentiation ELISA remains available as an FDA-approved supplemental test following a reactive fourth-generation HIV-1 and HIV-2 antibody and HIV-1 p24 antigen initial assay.[59] Differentiation assays are not without flaws, and an increase in the number of HIV-1–positive individuals with false-positive HIV-2 results (more than the total number of confirmed and probable HIV-2 cases) has called for the revision of the CDC-recommended HIV laboratory testing algorithm (Figure 19-1) by many experts.[60]

An assay that does not require supplemental HIV-1/HIV-2 antibody differentiation was approved by the FDA in July 2015. The Bio-Rad BioPlex 220 HIV Ag-Ab Assay (Bio-Rad Laboratories) simultaneously detects HIV antibodies and HIV-1 p24 antigen and provides separate antibody results for HIV-1 and HIV-2.[59] Considered a fifth-generation assay, specimens reactive only to HIV-1 p24 antigen do not require antibody confirmation, and specimens reactive only to HIV antibodies do not require antigen confirmation.[61] Because it eliminates supplemental antibody differentiation and antibody/antigen confirmatory procedures, broad implementation of this assay would require a change in the CDC HIV laboratory testing algorithm (Figure 19-1). As of June 2020, no changes in the testing algorithm have been announced or published by the CDC with regards to a fifth-generation assay.

***Rapid human immunodeficiency virus screening tests.*** Technological advances have allowed for the development of rapid (eg, 30 minute) screening tests for the detection of HIV antibodies. The methodology of the rapid HIV antibody assays involves typically either membrane EIA or immunocytochemical assays. Currently, only seven FDA-approved rapid HIV-1 screening tests remain available on the market in the United States: OraQuick ADVANCE Rapid HIV-1/2 Antibody Test (OraSure Technologies, Bethlehem, PA); Reveal Rapid HIV-1 Antibody Test (MedMira, Halifax, Nova Scotia); INSTI HIV-1/HIV-2 Antibody Test (bioLytical Laboratories, Richmond, BC); Alere Determine HIV-1/2 Ag/Ab Combo (Alere Scarborough, Scarborough, ME); (Clearview Complete) SURE CHECK HIV 1/2 Assay, (Clearview) HIV 1/2 STAT-PAK Assay, and Chembio DPP HIV 1/2 Assay (Chembio Diagnostic Systems, Medford, NY).[49,59] All currently approved tests display specificity and sensitivity similar to ELISA, require only basic training in test performance and interpretation, can be stored at room temperature, and require minimal specialized laboratory equipment.[49,55] All assays, except for the Reveal Rapid HIV-1 Antibody Test, have received waivers under CLIA, which allow POC testing where dedicated laboratories are not available. POC tests are less complex to perform than traditional diagnostic tests and have minimal chance for error.[49,55]

Rapid HIV testing has proven useful for the detection of HIV infection in a number of clinical settings, such as during labor and delivery of pregnant women at high risk for HIV infection with unknown serostatus for the purposes of preventing perinatal transmission, facilities where return rates for HIV test results are low, and following occupational exposure to potentially HIV-infected body fluids (eg, through a needlestick) in which immediate decisions regarding postexposure prophylaxis are needed.[49,55,58] It is important to note that rapid HIV tests are not recommended by the CDC for the diagnosis of HIV infection due to insufficient data, and a positive result from a rapid HIV test must be confirmed with a fourth-generation ELISA before the final diagnosis of HIV infection can be established. If the results of a rapid HIV test are negative, a person is considered uninfected. However, retesting should be considered in persons with possible exposure to HIV within the previous 3 months because the testing may have been performed too early in the infection to detect antibodies to the virus.[49,53,55]

***Noninvasive human immunodeficiency virus-1 tests.*** Several tests have been developed for testing HIV antibodies from oral fluid or urine.[49,51,58,59] The OraSure Western Blot Kit (OraSure Technologies, Bethlehem, PA) is a supplemental confirmatory test for the OraSure HIV-1 Oral Specimen Collection Device, which uses a cotton fiber pad that is placed between the cheek and lower gum for 2 minutes to collect oral mucosal transudate containing IgG. The OraSure HIV-1 oral device is FDA-approved and has a specificity of 99.4% (similar to EIA). The DPP HIV 1/2 Assay (Chembio Diagnostic Systems) detects antibodies against HIV-1 and HIV-2 by swabbing a flat pad against the upper and lower outer gums once and then inserting the sample collection pad into the developer solution vial. After 25 to 40 minutes, the results window indicates whether HIV antibodies have been detected. Two urine-based HIV-1 tests (ELISA and WB) have also been FDA-approved for use but are associated with lower sensitivity and specificity than the oral fluid testing. As with ELISA testing of blood samples, confirmatory testing is required for both types of tests if the initial results are positive. Noninvasive HIV-1 testing should be considered in persons who are unable to access healthcare facilities, have poor venous access, or are reluctant to have their blood drawn. The advantages of these tests include avoidance of blood drawing for sample collection, ease of use, low cost, and stability of samples for up to 3 weeks at room temperature.[49,51,57]

***Home sample collection tests.*** As of June 2020, the OraQuick In-Home HIV Test (OraSure Technologies) remains the only FDA-approved assay available over-the-counter for at-home use.[62] The test requires swabbing upper and lower gums with a collection stick that is inserted into a test solution for 20 minutes, after which time the results can be read. A line on the control and test areas indicates a positive result. The advantages of home sample collection tests include ready access to HIV-1 testing, convenience, lower costs, anonymity, and privacy.[51,57]

### p24 Antigen Tests

A main structural core protein of HIV is *p24,* with levels of p24 antigen being elevated during the early stages of HIV infection. Testing for p24 antigen has diagnostic use during early infection when low levels of HIV antibody are present.[49,52] The direct detection of HIV-1 p24 antigen can be performed using a plasma or serum EIA assay.[51,58] Similar to antibody testing, positive results of the initial testing for HIV-1 p24 antigen must be retested in duplicate using the same EIA method. In addition, these results need to be confirmed with a neutralization assay due to the potential for p24 antigen testing to produce false-positive reactions resulting from interfering substances.[49,51]

The p24 antigen test may be used for screening blood donors, detecting growth in viral cultures, and serving as an alternative diagnostic test for HIV-1 in patients suspected of having acute HIV infection or infants <18 months of age born to HIV-infected mothers (Table 19-8).[49,51,58] The advantages of the p24 antigen test include earlier detection of HIV infection compared with antibody testing (16 days versus 22 days), ease of performance, low cost, and specificity that approaches 100%. However, the DNA PCR assays and plasma HIV-RNA concentrations demonstrate greater sensitivity and have replaced the p24 antigen tests in many clinical situations.

### Human Immunodeficiency Virus DNA Polymerase Chain Reaction

*HIV DNA PCR is* used for early detection of proviral HIV-1 DNA in a patient's peripheral blood mononuclear cells. HIV DNA PCR is currently recommended for the diagnosis of HIV infection in infants (<18 months of age) born to HIV-infected mothers, and any clinical situations in which antibody tests are inconclusive or undetectable (Table 19-8).[49,53] Antibody tests are not useful for diagnosing HIV infection in infants because maternal HIV antibodies can persist in the infant for up to 18 months after birth. Therefore, infants should be tested with the HIV DNA PCR or HIV RNA viral load test initially between 14 and 21 days of age, then at 1 to 2 months, and age 3 to 6 months.[53] Negative tests at birth can be repeated at 14 days of life because the assay sensitivity is increased by 2 weeks of life. To confirm the diagnosis of HIV infection, a positive result at any sampling time needs to be confirmed by a second HIV virologic test. HIV infection may be excluded in infants with two or more negative HIV virologic results when initial testing occurred at age ≥1 month and the second testing occurred at age ≥4 months.[53]

The advantages of the HIV DNA PCR test include a high level of sensitivity and specificity (96% and 99% at ~1 month of age, respectively), the requirement for only a small volume of blood (eg, 200 μL), and the rapid turnaround time.[49] The disadvantages include the expense, the high level of interlaboratory variability, and the availability of only one commercial assay (COBAS AmpliPrep/COBAS TaqMan HIV-1 Test; Roche Diagnostics, Indianapolis, IN), which is not currently FDA-approved for proviral DNA quantitation.[49,53]

### Human Immunodeficiency Virus-RNA Concentration (Human Immunodeficiency Virus RNA Viral Load)

The accurate measurement of plasma *HIV-RNA concentrations* (also known as the *HIV viral load*) in conjunction with CD4+ T lymphocyte count has become an essential component in the management of patients with HIV-1 infection.[8,49,53] These two laboratory tests provide the clinician with information regarding a patient's virologic and immunologic status, which is needed to make decisions regarding the initiation or changing of antiretroviral therapy and to predict the risk of disease progression from HIV infection to AIDS. In addition, plasma HIV-RNA concentrations can assist in the diagnosis of HIV infection in selected clinical situations (Table 19-8).[8,53]

Methods that measure the amount of HIV-RNA in plasma include coupling reverse transcription to a DNA polymerase chain reaction (RT-PCR), identification of HIV-RNA with signal amplification by bDNA, and NA sequence-based amplification. Currently, there are five commercial assays approved by the FDA for clinical use: Amplicor HIV-1 Monitor version 1.5 (Roche Molecular Systems, Pleasanton, CA) in standard and ultrasensitive versions; Versant HIV-1 RNA 3.0 Assay (bDNA) (Siemens Healthcare Diagnostics, Tarrytown, NY); COBAS AmpliPrep/COBAS TaqMan HIV-1 versions 1 and 2 (Roche Diagnostics); and RealTime HIV-1 (Abbott Molecular, Des Plaines, IL).[8,49,59] The results of these tests are expressed as the number of HIV copies/mL. Higher HIV-RNA levels (eg, >100,000 copies/mL) represent a substantial risk for disease progression. These assays differ in their dynamic ranges and lower limits of detection of HIV viral copies/milliliter of plasma. For example, the Versant assay has a lower limit of detection of <75 copies/mL whereas the COBAS AmpliPrep/COBAS TaqMan version 2 assay detection limit is <20 copies/mL. Some of these assays have different versions according to the degree of automation and simplicity. For instance, the Amplicor HIV-1 Monitor version 1.5 is a manual test; the COBAS Amplicor HIV-1 Monitor is semiautomated, and the COBAS AmpliPrep/COBAS Amplicor HIV-1 Monitor is automated. Additionally, the Amplicor HIV-1 Monitor and its variants exist as two FDA-approved assays—standard and ultrasensitive—due to limited dynamic range. The standard assay has a lower limit of detection of 400 copies/mL compared with the ultrasensitive assay, which has a limit of 50 copies/mL. It is recommended to use both assays concurrently when testing samples that fall outside of the dynamic range. Therefore, if a viral load is reported as "undetectable," it signifies that the plasma HIV-RNA concentrations are below the lower limits of detection of the assay used.[8,49] When performing plasma HIV-RNA viral load levels for each patient, the same laboratory and method should be used to minimize variation.

Once the diagnosis of HIV-1 infection has been confirmed, a plasma HIV-RNA level should be measured to assist in assessing antiretroviral treatment efficacy. Ideally, a plasma HIV-RNA level (and CD4+ T lymphocyte count) is measured on two separate occasions as the baseline measurement. Although antiretroviral therapy is recommended for everyone regardless of HIV-RNA levels and CD4+ T lymphocyte count, these values along with clinical findings and symptoms, the willingness of the patient to adhere to therapy, and the potential complications associated with therapy help decide whether treatment can be temporarily deferred and for how long when patients cannot initiate therapy right away. When initiating antiretroviral therapy, current guidelines recommend monitoring plasma HIV-RNA levels at the following time intervals: immediately before treatment initiation and 2 to 8 weeks after starting or changing antiretroviral drug therapy; 3 to 4 months following therapy initiation and every 3 to 6 months while on therapy; and any time when clinically indicated, including for patients who experience a significant decline in CD4+ T lymphocyte count.[8] Testing HIV-RNA is not recommended during the period of an acute illness (eg, bacterial or *P jirovecii* pneumonia) or in patients who have been recently vaccinated because these circumstances may increase the viral load for 2 to 4 weeks. For patients receiving antiretroviral therapy, the goals of therapy include specific reductions in the HIV viral load measured in log reductions over a given time frame as well as achieving a viral load "below the limits of detection." Changes in the amount of plasma HIV-RNA are often reported in log base 10 values. For example, a change from 10,000 to 1,000 copies/mL in a patient on antiretroviral therapy would be considered a 1-log decrease in viral load. With optimal therapy, plasma HIV-RNA levels should decrease by $\geq 1 \log_{10}$ during the first 2 to 8 weeks after initiation of therapy and should continue to decline over subsequent weeks, with the ultimate goal of achieving an undetectable viral load (eg, <50 copies/mL) 16 to 24 weeks after initiation of therapy.[8] However, every patient responds differently. The reader is encouraged to review the most recent HIV diagnostic and treatment guidelines because recommendations for different patient populations are continuously being modified as newer data become available.[8,53,54]

## CD4+ T Lymphocyte Count

The cell-mediated immune function effects of HIV infection are demonstrated by reductions in the *CD4+ T lymphocyte count.* Flow cytometry can be used to identify the various subsets of lymphocytes by their cluster of differentiation (CD) of specific monoclonal antibodies to surface antigens. The CD4+ T lymphocytes are the helper-inducer T cells, whereas the CD8+ T lymphocytes are the cytotoxic-suppressor T cells. HIV infection causes a decrease in the total number of lymphocytes (particularly the CD4+ T lymphocytes) as well as changes in the ratios of the different types of lymphocytes. CD4+ T lymphocyte counts of <200 cells/mm³ (normal count 800 to 1,100 cells/mm³) or a CD4+ T lymphocyte percentage of <14% of the total lymphocyte count (normal 40% of total lymphocytes) are indicative

of severe immunosuppression, placing the patient at risk for development of opportunistic infections.[8] A CD4+/CD8+ ratio <1 is considered a hallmark of HIV infection, and lower ratios are indicative of immune senescence and associated with serious non-AIDS events and death.[63] This ratio is not commonly used in clinical practice as it may reflect immune activation and not immune reconstitution but is often used in research in trying to characterize immune activation or senescence. Because of its limited clinical utility, measurement of the CD4+/CD8+ ratio is not routinely recommended.[8]

Current HIV treatment guidelines recommend initiation of antiretroviral therapy in all HIV-infected patients regardless of the plasma HIV RNA viral load or CD4+ T lymphocyte count.[8] As stated earlier, the CD4+ T lymphocyte count is used in conjunction with the plasma HIV-RNA level to provide essential information regarding a patient's virologic and immunologic status and risk of disease progression from HIV infection to AIDS and to determine whether to modify antiretroviral therapy or initiate chemoprophylaxis against opportunistic infections.[8,53,54] Because of the significant impact on disease progression and survival, most guidelines recommend monitoring CD4+ T lymphocyte counts at baseline and every 3 to 6 months to assess the immunologic response to treatment in patients starting or modifying antiretroviral treatment, or even yearly or longer in people on stable therapy.[8]

## Phenotypic and Genotypic Assays for Antiretroviral Drug Resistance

Resistance of HIV-1 to antiretroviral drugs is an important cause for treatment failure. *Genotypic assays* use gene sequencing or probes to detect resistance mutations in genes of circulating RNA known to confer drug resistance in the RT, protease (PR), envelope, and integrase genes of HIV-1. Two genotypic assays have been approved by the FDA: TruGene (Siemens Healthcare Diagnostics, Tarrytown, NY) and ViroSeq (Celera Diagnostics, Alameda, CA).[50,59] *Phenotypic assays* measure the quantity of viral replication in the presence of various concentrations of antiretroviral agents. Sequences from the RT, PR, envelope, and integrase genes of the patient's HIV virus are inserted into a wild-type virus in the laboratory. The concentration of the drug needed to inhibit 50% of viral replication ($IC_{50}$) is reported. The ratio of IC values for the test and reference viruses is calculated and used to report the quantitative fold-increase in resistance of each antiretroviral agent. The interpretation of results from both assays is complex and requires expert knowledge and consultation.[8,49]

The current guidelines recommend drug resistance testing for patients with acute and chronic HIV infection when they enter into care, regardless of the decision to initiate antiretroviral therapy; pregnant women prior to antiretroviral therapy initiation; women contemplating or entering pregnancy with a detectable HIV-RNA level during treatment; patients with virologic failure while receiving antiretroviral therapy; and patients with suboptimal suppression of plasma HIV-RNA level after the initiation of antiretroviral therapy.[8,54]

*Genotypic assays* are typically recommended for resistance testing in the treatment of naïve patients and pregnant women.

In the setting of virologic failure, current guidelines recommend performing resistance testing immediately after or within 4 weeks of discontinuation of antiretroviral therapy for optimal results. Resistance testing is discouraged in patients with plasma HIV-RNA levels <1,000 copies/mL or patients who have been off antiretroviral therapy for extended periods of time because the population of mutant virus may not be sufficient for detection. A newer generation of *genotypic assays* that analyze proviral DNA and do not depend on detectable HIV-RNA can be considered in patients with undetectable HIV-RNA.[8]

The advantages and disadvantages of genotypic and phenotypic assays for the detection of HIV-1 resistance have been previously described.[51] The genotypic assay may be preferred over the phenotypic assay because of availability, clinical utility, faster turnaround time (1 to 2 weeks versus ≥2 weeks), and lower cost.[50] Because they are labor-intensive and more expensive than genotypic assays, phenotypic assays are generally reserved for cases in which antiretroviral resistance cannot be predicted based on known genetic mutations alone. However, both assays are complex, technically demanding, and expensive and are not routinely performed in most clinical laboratories. Proviral DNA *genotypic assays* may be useful in people with a history of multiple treatments, treatment failures, or no available genotypic resistance test results who are virally suppressed on a complex antiretroviral regimen, which they need to modify due to drug–drug interactions, pill fatigue, or toxicity.[8] Proviral DNA *genotypic assays* may not be useful in people on their first or second antiretroviral regimen without prior failures or with available prior genotypic testing results.

### Additional Laboratory Testing for Patients with Human Immunodeficiency Virus

***Coreceptor tropism assays.*** After attachment of HIV to the CD4[+] T lymphocytes, fusion of the virus and CD4[+] cell membranes involves binding to a coreceptor molecule. The two coreceptors used by HIV are chemokine coreceptor 5 (CCR5) and CXC coreceptor (CXCR4). The recently approved antiretroviral agent maraviroc is a CCR5-coreceptor antagonist that prevents the entry of HIV into the CD4[+] cell by binding to the CCR5 receptor. Most acutely or recently infected patients harbor the CCR5-tropic virus, while untreated patients with advanced disease and those with disease progression shift from CCR5-tropic to CXCR4-tropic or both (dual-tropic or mixed-tropic). Treatment-experienced patients with high levels of drug resistance are more likely to harbor dual-tropic or mixed-tropic virus. Current HIV treatment guidelines recommend performing a coreceptor tropism assay when considering the use of a CCR5-coreceptor antagonist or in the event of virologic failure during maraviroc therapy.[8] Currently, a phenotypic assay, Trofile (Monogram Biosciences, South San Francisco, CA), and a genotypic tropism assay, HIV-1 Coreceptor Tropism (Quest Diagnostics, Madison, NJ), are available in the United States.[84]

***HLA-B*5701 screening.*** Abacavir, a nucleoside reverse transcriptase inhibitor, is associated with a potentially life-threatening hypersensitivity reaction reported in 5% to 8% of patients in clinical trials. The hypersensitivity reaction appears to occur more frequently in white patients (5% to 8%) than black patients (2% to 3%) and is associated with the presence of MHC class I allele HLA-B*5701. Treatment guidelines recommend screening patients for the presence of HLA-B*5701 prior to the initiation of abacavir-containing regimens in areas in which the screening test is available, and patients with a positive result should not receive abacavir.[8] However, the initiation of abacavir therapy can be reasonably considered using clinical judgment with appropriate monitoring and extensive patient education about the signs and symptoms of the hypersensitivity reaction in settings in which the HLA-B*5701 screening test may not be available.

## MYCOBACTERIA

*Mycobacteria* are nonmotile, nonspore-forming, aerobic bacilli that continue to cause infection as well as significant morbidity and mortality, especially in developing countries.[64-72] Currently, >100 species of mycobacteria have been identified, with only a number of species causing infection in humans, including *M tuberculosis, M leprae, M avium complex, M kansasii, M fortuitum, M chelonae, M abscessus,* and *M marinum*.[11,64-66] Depending on the species, mycobacteria can be nonpathogenic, pathogenic, or opportunistic and, therefore, may cause infection in both immunocompetent and immunocompromised hosts. **Table 19-9** lists the most common pathogenic mycobacteria species with their typical associated infections and environmental sources.[11,64-69]

Mycobacteria are generally divided into two groups based on epidemiology and spectrum of disease: (1) the *M tuberculosis* complex (MTBC), including the species *M tuberculosis, M bovis, M bovis* bacille Calmette-Guerin (BCG), *M africanum,* and *M microti*; and (2) nontuberculous mycobacteria (NTM; also referred to as *mycobacteria other than tuberculosis*), which include all other species of mycobacteria.[11,64,66] *M tuberculosis* is the most clinically significant mycobacteria and is the causative organism of tuberculosis (TB). The incidence of TB in the United States declined between 1953 (when it became a notifiable disease) and 1985 as a result of improved diagnostic methods, enhanced public health efforts to isolate patients infected with TB, and the introduction of effective antimycobacterial agents.[65,66,70] This decline in TB cases led experts to predict the elimination of the disease by 2010. However, between 1986 and 1992, an increase in the incidence of TB was observed in the United States due to deterioration of the TB public health programs, emergence of the HIV epidemic, increase in immigration to the United States, and emergence of MDR-TB.[65,70] Since 1992, the number of cases of TB in the United States has steadily declined due to improved public health control strategies.[71] Despite advances in medical care and treatment, TB continues to be one of the most common infectious diseases worldwide. The World Health Organization estimated that approximately 10 million persons were afflicted with TB worldwide in 2018, and there were more than 1.4 million deaths that year.[72] Because TB can be transmitted from person to person, rapid diagnosis is necessary to decrease the spread of infection.[70]

**TABLE 19-9.** Pathogenic Mycobacteria and Associated Infections

| MYCOBACTERIUM SPECIES | ASSOCIATED INFECTIONS | ENVIRONMENTAL SOURCES |
|---|---|---|
| *Mycobacterium tuberculosis* complex (tuberculosis [TB]) | Pulmonary infection, lymphadenitis, musculoskeletal infection, gastrointestinal infection, peritonitis, hepatitis, pericarditis | Humans |
| *M bovis* | Soft tissue infection, gastrointestinal infection | Humans, cattle |
| *M leprae* (Leprosy, Hansen disease) | Skin and soft tissue infections | Humans, armadillos |
| *M avium* complex (MAC) | Pulmonary infection, cutaneous ulcers, lymphadenitis, disseminated infection | Soil, water, swine, cattle, birds |
| *M kansasii* | Pulmonary infection, musculoskeletal infection, disseminated infection, cervical lymphadenitis | Water, cattle |
| *M fortuitum* | Skin and soft tissue infections, disseminated infection | Soil, water, animals, marine life |
| *M chelonae* | Skin and soft tissue infections, osteomyelitis, disseminated infection | Soil, water, animals, marine life |
| *M abscessus* | Skin and soft tissue infections, osteomyelitis, disseminated infection | Soil, water, animals, marine life |
| *M marinum* | Skin and soft tissue infections, bacteremia | Fish, fresh water, salt water |
| *M ulcerans* | Skin and soft tissue infections, osteomyelitis | Soil, stagnant water |

*Source:* References 11,64–69.

## Identification of Mycobacteria

Mycobacteria possess several unique characteristics that contribute to the difficulties with the growth, identification, and treatment of these organisms. The cell wall of mycobacteria is complex and composed of peptidoglycan, polypeptides, and a lipid-rich hydrophobic layer.[11,66] This cell wall structure confers a number of distinguishing properties in the mycobacteria, including (1) resistance to disinfectants and detergents, (2) the inability to be stained by many common laboratory identification stains, (3) the inability of mycobacteria to be decolorized by acid solutions (a characteristic that has given them the name of acid-fast bacilli [AFB]), (4) the ability of mycobacteria to grow slowly, and (5) resistance to common anti-infective agents.[11,64,66] These characteristics have led to the continuous modification and improvement of laboratory practices used in the identification and diagnosis of mycobacterial infections. Many of these laboratory practices involve specialized staining techniques, growth media, identification techniques, environmental conditions (BSL-3 facilities for *M tuberculosis*), and susceptibility testing methods that may be unavailable in some clinical laboratories.[66,68]

The ability to accurately cultivate mycobacteria is highly dependent on the appropriate selection and collection of biologic specimens for staining and culture.[11,64-66] Because different mycobacteria are capable of causing a number of infections (Table 19-9), the following biologic specimens may be submitted for mycobacterial culture based on the site of infection:

respiratory tract secretions (eg, expectorated or induced-sputum and bronchial washings) or gastric lavage specimens for the diagnosis of pulmonary TB; CSF for the diagnosis of TB meningitis; blood for the diagnosis of disseminated *M avium* complex (MAC) infection; stool for the diagnosis of disseminated MAC infection; and urine, tissue, exudate, or wound drainage, bone marrow, sterile body fluids, lymph node tissue, and skin specimens for infection due to any mycobacteria.[65-68] For the diagnosis of pulmonary TB, several early morning expectorated or induced-sputum specimens are recommended to enhance diagnostic accuracy. Biologic specimens for mycobacterial culture should be immediately processed according to specified guidelines to prevent the overgrowth of bacteria that may also be present in the specimen and should be concentrated to enhance diagnostic capability.[65,66,68] Similar to the processing of specimens for bacterial culture, biologic specimens submitted for mycobacterial culture should be stained for microscopic examination and plated for culture. The staining techniques and culture media, however, are somewhat different because mycobacteria are poorly visualized in the Gram stain (they do not reliably take up the dyes and are referred to as *acid-fast*) and take longer to grow than conventional bacteria.

Staining with subsequent microscopic examination for mycobacteria is a rapid diagnostic test that involves the use of stains that are taken up by the lipid and mycolic acid components in the mycobacterial cell wall.[11,66] Several acid-fast stains are available for the microscopic examination of mycobacteria, including carbolfuchsin-based stains that are viewed using light microscopy (Ziehl-Neelsen or Kinyoun method) and fluorochrome stains (auramine-rhodamine) examined under fluorescence microscopy that are thought to be more sensitive tests, especially on direct specimens.[11,64-67,73] The sensitivity of the staining method is highly dependent on the type of clinical specimen, the species of mycobacteria present, the technique used in specimen processing, the thickness of the smear, and the experience of the laboratory technologist.[11,65,66] The staining methods can detect the presence of mycobacteria in a clinical specimen but cannot differentiate between species of mycobacteria. Therefore, several molecular techniques have been commercially developed to augment identification, which use NA amplification (PCR) to detect *M tuberculosis* complex in acid-fast smear–positive respiratory specimens (Amplicor *Mycobacterium tuberculosis* Test by Roche Diagnostics, and the Amplified *Mycobacterium tuberculosis* Direct Test by Gen-Probe) or acid-fast smear–negative respiratory samples (Amplified *M tuberculosis* Direct Test by Gen-Probe).[11,64,11,66,68,73] Both of these tests display high sensitivity in detecting the presence of *M tuberculosis* complex in smear-positive respiratory specimens (>97%).[11,66,73] Because of their high specificity and the rapid availability of results, the CDC recommends performing NA amplification tests on respiratory specimens of patients suspected of having pulmonary TB.[12,74] However, none of these assays are currently FDA-approved for the detection of *Mycobacterium* from non-respiratory specimens.[12,74,75]

For optimal cultivation and identification of mycobacteria, a combination of culture media, including at least one solid growth medium and one liquid growth medium, should be used during specimen processing to facilitate growth and optimize pigment production of the organism.[11,66,67,69,70,73] The preferred commercially available solid growth media for the cultivation of mycobacteria include an agar-based medium such as Middlebrook 7H10 or an egg-based medium such as Lowenstein-Jensen. Several liquid growth media systems are available for culture of mycobacteria, some of which use continuous automated monitoring systems for the detection of mycobacterial growth.[11,66,67,69] The liquid growth media systems often provide more rapid isolation of AFB compared with conventional solid media, with results within 10 days as compared with 17 days or longer using solid growth media.[65-68,73] The most commonly used semiautomated systems with liquid growth media include the MB Redox (Heipha Diagnostika Biotest, Heidelberg, Germany), BACTEC 460 TB system (BD), the Septi-Chek AFB System (BD), and the Mycobacteria Growth Indicator Tube (BD).[11,66,69,73] The most commonly used automated, continuous monitoring systems with liquid growth media include the ESP Culture System II (Trek Diagnostics, Westlake, OH), the BACTEC 9000 MB System (BD), the MB BacT/Alert System (bioMérieux, Marcy-l'Étoile, France), and the BACTEC MGIT 960 (BD Biosciences, Sparks, MD).[11,66,69,73] Once growth is detected in the liquid media systems, an acid-fast stain is performed on the specimen to confirm the presence of mycobacteria, with subsequent subculture onto solid media.

The optimal growth conditions of mycobacteria depend on the species; therefore, the clinical laboratory should follow a standardized procedure outlining the process that should be used to enhance cultivation of the suspected *Mycobacterium* from the submitted clinical specimen based on the suspected site of infection. The optimal conditions for incubation of mycobacterial cultures are 28°C to 37°C in 5% to 10% $CO_2$ for 6 to 8 weeks, depending on the organism.[11,66,68,69] Cultures for mycobacteria typically require prolonged incubation periods, sometimes up to 8 weeks, because most of the more common pathogens grow rather slowly. Rapidly growing mycobacteria such as *M fortuitum*, *M chelonae*, and *M abscessus* typically grow within seven days on solid media, while slow-growing mycobacteria such as *M tuberculosis* complex, MAC, *M kansasii*, and *M marinum* require 7 days to 7 weeks for growth.[11,67,69] Therefore, culture tubes or plates are examined weekly during the incubation period for the presence of mycobacterial growth.

Colonies grown in culture are examined microscopically for characteristic colonial morphologic features, pigmentation, and growth rate, are subjected to biochemical tests, and are evaluated using rapid molecular detection methods, such as PCR methods mentioned earlier, DNA hybridization using DNA probes, and chromatographic methods, such as high-performance liquid chromatography or gas liquid chromatography, to detect mycobacterial lipids for definitive identification.[11,66-69] The DNA probes can be used only with mycobacteria grown in culture (not directly on patient specimens), are highly sensitive and specific, and are commercially available for the rapid identification of *M tuberculosis* complex, *M gordonae*, *M kansasii*, and MAC.[11,66-69] The molecular methods have replaced the use of biochemical tests in many laboratories because they provide more accurate identification in a significantly shorter time frame, within 14 to 21 days of specimen receipt, as compared with several weeks or months using traditional identification methods.[11,65] For example, the Xpert MTB/RIF Assay (Cepheid, Sunnyvale, CA) was cleared by the FDA in 2013 for the identification of MTBC and rifampin resistance mutations via DNA RT-PCR from respiratory specimens, and was adopted by the CDC and WHO as part of the initial diagnostic tools.[76,77] Later in 2017, the FDA cleared the use of MALDI-TOF MS for the identification of mycobacteria and other organisms with the Vitek MS system (bioMérieux, Inc, Marcy-l'Étoile, France).[78] Although this method of identification is rapid, there are still significant disadvantages with respect to cumbersome extraction protocols, inability to identify MTBC species, and high initial set up and operation costs.[79]

## Susceptibility Testing of Mycobacteria

The choice of antibiotic or antimycobacterial agent to use in the treatment of mycobacterial infection depends on the species of mycobacteria involved. It is important for the clinician to have an understanding of the typical susceptibility patterns of specific mycobacterial species, the current treatment guidelines outlining which and how many drugs to use, and the methodology available for drug susceptibility testing for the particular mycobacterial species being treated.

Standardized guidelines have been published for the susceptibility testing of *M tuberculosis* complex.[80] Susceptibility testing is currently recommended on the initial isolate of all patients with *M tuberculosis* complex infection, on isolates from patients who remain culture positive after 3 months of appropriate therapy, and on isolates from patients who are not clinically responding to therapy.[11,66,70,80] Susceptibility testing of *M tuberculosis* complex is initially performed with primary antituberculous agents such as isoniazid (using two concentrations, 0.2 and 1 mcg/mL), rifampin, ethambutol, and pyrazinamide. However, if resistance to any of these first-line drugs is detected, susceptibility testing should be subsequently performed using second-line drugs, including streptomycin, a higher concentration of ethambutol (10 mcg/mL), ethionamide, capreomycin, ciprofloxacin, ofloxacin or levofloxacin, kanamycin, *p*-aminosalicylic acid, and rifabutin.[66,68,80]

Susceptibility testing of *M tuberculosis* complex can be performed directly using mycobacteria from a smear-positive specimen (direct method) or using mycobacteria isolated from culture (indirect method).[11,66,68] The direct method of mycobacterial susceptibility testing produces faster results but is less standardized so that susceptibility testing is usually performed using isolates grown in culture.[66,68] Four conventional methods are used worldwide for determining the susceptibility of *M tuberculosis* isolates to antituberculous agents, including the absolute concentration method, the resistance ratio method, the agar proportion method, and the agar proportion method using liquid medium (commercial radiometric, nonradiometric, or broth systems, including the BACTEC 460TB System [BD]; BACTEC MGIT 960 [BD]; ESP Culture System II [Trek Diagnostics, Westlake, OH]; and MB/BacT-Alert 3D [bioMérieux]). The agar proportion method and the commercial broth systems are the methods commonly used for mycobacterial susceptibility testing in the United States.

The agar proportion method is a modified agar dilution test that evaluates the extent of growth of a standardized inoculum of *M tuberculosis* in control and drug-containing agar medium. The organism is considered resistant if growth is >1% on the agar plate containing critical concentrations of the antituberculous drug.[80] The critical concentration for each drug represents the lowest concentration of the drug that inhibits 95% of wild-type *M tuberculosis* strains that have never been exposed to the drug.[66,80] Susceptibility results using the agar proportion method are typically available 21 days after the plates have been inoculated.

The commercial susceptibility testing systems use liquid growth medium in which the growth of the organism is measured in the presence and absence of antituberculous drugs.[65-69,73,80] These systems provide rapid susceptibility results for the primary antituberculous agents but cannot be used for susceptibility testing of second-line agents. Commercial susceptibility tests are recommended over agar proportion methods because the results are often available within 5 to 7 days after inoculation and can help guide appropriate therapy without the unnecessary delay of the agar proportion method.[65,68,69,80]

Several other susceptibility testing methods are currently being evaluated for drug susceptibility testing of *M tuberculosis*. Many antimycobacterial drugs are now available in E-test strips, including streptomycin, ethambutol, isoniazid, and ethionamide.[11,73,80] Several studies have evaluated their performance as compared with the commercial methods; however,

further studies are needed to validate the use of the E-test as a suitable, alternative susceptibility testing method. In addition, newer molecular methods for drug susceptibility testing of *M tuberculosis* are currently being evaluated that are easier to perform and produce more reliable results in a shorter period.[11,66-69] These methods include PCR amplification, DNA sequencing line probe assays, and reverse hybridization-based probe assays for the detection of specific drug-resistance mutations. As stated earlier, the use of the Xpert MTB/RIF Assay (Cepheid) for the identification of MTBC and the rifampin resistance mutations in the *rpoB* gene is recommended as part of initial diagnosis of MTBC but does not invalidate the need for additional molecular and traditional growth methods of susceptibility testing against other first- and second-line agents. Further study, however, is warranted before newer susceptibility testing methods can replace conventional methods.

Guidelines for susceptibility testing of NTM have recently been published by the CLSI, in which testing is recommended on the initial isolate for clinically significant isolates (blood, tissue) that display variability in susceptibility to antituberculous drugs or for organisms that may be associated with acquired resistance.[80] The guidelines contain protocols for the susceptibility testing of rapidly growing NTM (*M fortuitum, M chelonae,* and *M abscessus*) and slow-growing NTM (MAC, *M kansasii,* and *M marinum*), including the recommended methodology and drugs to be tested for each organism.[11,66,68,80] Standard broth microdilution should be used to evaluate the susceptibility of any clinically significant, rapidly growing NTM.[67,80] Drugs that may be considered for susceptibility testing include amikacin, cefoxitin, ciprofloxacin, clarithromycin, doxycycline, imipenem, sulfamethoxazole, trimethoprim–sulfamethoxazole, and tobramycin (for *M chelonae* only).[67,80] Susceptibility testing of MAC is recommended for clarithromycin only using a broth-based method (macrodilution or microdilution) for initial blood or tissue isolates in patients with disseminated infection, for clinically significant isolates from patients receiving previous or current macrolide therapy, for isolates from patients who develop bacteremia while receiving macrolide prophylaxis, and for isolates from patients who relapse while receiving macrolide therapy.[67,80] Regarding the other slow-growing NTMs, susceptibility testing of *M kansasii* should be routinely performed only on rifampin using the commercial radiometric systems, broth microdilution, or the modified proportion method, while routine susceptibility testing of *M marinum* is not recommended.[67,80] The integration of molecular and culture-based methods for both MTBC and NTM for better estimation of drug efficacy is also addressed in CLSI guidelines.

### Skin Testing

The *Mantoux test* or *tuberculin skin test* (TST) is one test available for the detection of latent TB (LTBI) and involves the intradermal injection of a purified protein derivative (PPD) of the tubercle bacilli, which is obtained from a culture filtrate derived by protein precipitation.[68,81] Injection of the PPD into individuals previously exposed to TB elicits a delayed hypersensitivity reaction involving T cells that migrate to the area of intradermal injection (usually the dorsal aspect of the forearm), inducing the release of lymphokines that produce induration and edema within 48 to 72 hours after injection. The diameter of induration is measured between 48 and 72 hours after injection by a healthcare professional.[68,81] Published guidelines are available for interpretation of the TST reaction based on the size of the induration and clinical and demographic characteristics of the patient. An induration of ≥5 mm is considered positive in persons at high risk of developing TB disease, including HIV infected patients; patients receiving immunosuppressive therapy including tumor necrosis factor blocking agents; patients who have been recently exposed to a person with TB; and patients with an abnormal chest radiographic consistent with prior TB.[64,68,81] An induration of ≥10 mm is considered positive in patients who are not immunocompromised but who are at high risk for having LTBI or for progressing from LTBI to TB, such as persons born in high TB burden countries; injection drug users; residents and employees of high-risk settings (eg, prisons, healthcare facilities, and mycobacteria laboratory personnel); persons with chronic medical conditions of high risk (eg, diabetes, silicosis, and chronic renal failure), and children younger than 5 years of age. An induration of ≥15 mm is considered positive in persons with no risk factors or at low risk for developing active infection with TB.

A two-step TST is recommended by the CDC in certain populations (*initial* skin testing of newly hired healthcare workers without a documented negative TST within the past 12 months and persons expected to undergo serial screening for TB, such as residents and staff of long-term care facilities) to identify individuals with past TB infection whose delayed-type hypersensitivity to tuberculin has diminished over time.[82,83] The first TST is administered as described previously, with a second TST administered following the same procedure 1 to 3 weeks later in persons with a negative initial test result.[82] The premise behind the administration of two TSTs in these settings is to delineate between past TB infection or BCG vaccination from recent conversion/infection. That is, the first injection stimulates (boost) the delayed hypersensitivity response in a patient with previous TB infection or BCG vaccination and the second TST then elicits a positive reaction.[82,83]

### Blood Assay for Mycobacterium *Tuberculosis*

Two in vitro diagnostic tests using whole blood have become recently available in the United States for the detection of latent *M tuberculosis* infection: (1) a blood assay for *M tuberculosis* (BAMT), the QuantiFERON-TB Gold In-Tube test (Cellestis, Chadstone, Victoria, Australia) and (2) T-SPOT.TB (Oxford Immunotec, Oxford, UK).[65,68] These tests use ELISA to measure the amount of interferon-γ released from sensitized lymphocytes from prior exposure to *M tuberculosis* following overnight incubation with PPD from *M tuberculosis* and control antigens.[68,84] Because the tests use peptide antigens from *M tuberculosis,* they have more specificity than the TST for the diagnosis of latent *M tuberculosis* infection and do not produce false-positive results in patients with previous BCG vaccination or infection due to NTM.[82,84] The results of BAMT testing are stratified according to risk for TB infection (like the TST) but are not influenced by the subjectivity of reader bias or error, as may be seen with the TST. Because these tests are unable to distinguish between active or latent infection, the exact role of the BAMT and the TST in the diagnosis of latent TB infection are unclear and currently under investigation. However, the BAMT test can be used to assist in the diagnosis of latent TB infection in high-risk populations, such as recent immigrants from high-prevalence countries, injection drug users, inmates, prison employees, and healthcare workers at high risk for exposure to TB.[82,84] The BAMT test can also be considered the initial and serial screening test for latent TB infection in healthcare workers and military personnel.[82,84] It is important to note that the FDA has approved these tests as aids in the diagnosis of *M tuberculosis* infection and are intended to be used in conjunction with other diagnostic techiques.[84]

## SUMMARY

New testing methodologies and diagnostic guidelines continue to become available for the recovery, identification, and susceptibility testing of fungi, viruses, and mycobacteria. These processes created new opportunities and challenges for clinical microbiology laboratories with regard to what diagnostic tests offer and for which pathogens. Introduction and rapid acceptance of MALDI-TOF MS has allowed proteomics to be applied for the rapid identification of fungi and mycobacterial pathogens. Rapid antigen tests, NAATs, and serology have revolutionized diagnostic microbiology and impacted the need for traditional staining and culturing procedures, particularly in viral infections. A variety of molecular diagnostic assays allowed laboratory testing of SARS-CoV-2 to expand and become rapidly available during the recent global pandemic. Accurate SARS-CoV-2 NAATs have been critical for viral detection, public health quarantine decisions for preventing transmission, infection control measures, and patient management and treatment guidelines. Multiplex NAAT tests have become commercially available with syndromic panels that include fungal, viral, and bacterial pathogens commonly associated with respiratory tract infections, gastrointestinal pathogen detection, and central nervous system infections. Rapid POC testing for viral infections such as RSV, influenza, and HIV are allowing the latest diagnostic technology to move from the clinical laboratory setting to outpatient clinics, emergency departments, and healthcare offices. Genotypic and phenotypic resistance testing is regularly performed for HIV infections. Susceptibility and resistance testing for mycobacterial, fungal, and other viral pathogens continue to expand. Not all laboratories have broad testing capabilities with the latest technologies. It is essential to consult your local laboratory and appreciate the current diagnostic methods being offered, which tests are referred to external reference and/or public health laboratories, and the likely turnaround times in reporting results.

## LEARNING POINTS

1. *Matrix-assisted laser desorption ionization-time of flight mass spectrometry (MALDI-TOF MS) has become a proteomic methodology for the identification of bacterial, fungal, and mycobacteria colonies on a variety of*

*laboratory media. How does MALDI-TOF MS work for identification of fungi? What advantages does MALDI-TOF MS offer compared with traditional identification methods of fungi? What are the limitations of using MALDI-TOF MS for identification of fungi?*

**ANSWER:** A pure colony of fungus is needed to produce a mass spectrum fingerprint characteristic of the organism. A colony of fungal cells is spread across the conductive metallic target plate ("spot") of the MALDI-TOF MS. The cells may or may not be treated (eg, with formic acid) on the target plate, and the spot is overlaid with a matrix and air dried. This plate is loaded into the ionization chamber of the mass spectrometer and ultraviolet laser pulses hit the target spot, causing the sample to be vaporized (forming ions). A cloud of desorbed and ionized molecules is released to be accelerated by a high-voltage electric charge and fly through the time-of-flight (TOF) tube (or field-free drift region). The ions strike the detector at the other end of the flight tube (smaller ions travel faster than larger ions) and masses of the ions are determined from the time it took them to travel the length of the flight tube. A mass spectral signature is determined by mass-to-charge ratio (essentially molecular weight given MALDI predominantly produces singly charged ions) and the number of ions with a particular size striking the detector (intensity). Mass spectrometry identifies the protein fingerprints and a direct comparison of the spectral pattern of the organism in question is made with commercial or supplemental database patterns of different microorganisms. Depending on the database, it may be possible to identify the genus, species, and/or strain levels of the detected microbe.

The MALDI-TOF MS approach offers multiple advantages, including fast results, affordability, ease of use, and a highly accurate identification of fungal colonies to allow earlier decision-making of optimal antifungal therapy. Turnaround time is approximately 3 to 5 minutes for batch runs (compared with 1.5 days for traditional methods). This method is technically simple to perform, has minimal waste disposition, and has low reagent cost per test (although acquisition of the initial instrumentation system is rather costly). The method is considered robust and reliable because of an extremely low level of false identification of yeast and several filamentous fungi. It can be particularly helpful when morphology-based identification is not possible (ie, atypical morphology, lack of sporulate, lengthy identification processes) or if the phenotypic result is confusing. MALDI-TOF MS can extend its use beyond organism identification to include the detection of drug resistance and biomarkers. It is also a reliable and reproducible method for growth-based antifungal susceptibility testing of yeast (eg, fluconazole and echinocandin susceptibility testing of *Candida*) although it is labor-intensive and time-consuming.

Some of the major limitations of MALDI-TOF MS for identification of fungi center around reference mass spectral databases, specimen requirement, possibilities of errors, and the updates of taxonomy that are regularly needed. Most databases for MALDI-TOF MS are proprietary (not publicly available) and differences exist between manufacturers, including identification algorithms and instrumentation. In addition, limited commercial databases, variability in the spectra because of structural features of mold colonies, and lack of standardized processes has constrained the routine use of mold identification (except *Aspergillus* spp.) in some clinical laboratories. Widely published user-developed or in-house fungal databases can be used; however, applying and/or creating such supplemental databases may be difficult for some clinical laboratories. Another disadvantage is the requirement of organism recovery on culture media before sample preparation can begin for MALDI-TOF MS. Ongoing evaluations have had inconsistent results for organism detection directly from clinical samples. Finally, there is a learning curve for users of this system, including colony testing (eg, homogeneity of the smear, amount of organism and placement on target plate location, minimizing the use impure colonies, cleanup procedures of reusable plates) and minimizing sources of errors.

2. *In vitro testing for circulating galactomannan can be used as a diagnostic tool for invasive aspergillosis. What is galactomannan? Which fungal pathogen is it most useful as a diagnostic aid? What type of assay is used to detect galactomannan in the United States? Outline the precautions to consider when interpreting the results from galactomannan testing.*

**ANSWER:** Galactomannan is a polysaccharide present as a major cell wall component of the mold *Aspergillus*. Concentrations of galactomannan are released during the growth phase of the infection, with the highest concentrations occurring during the terminal phases of aspergillosis.

The Platelia *Aspergillus* Ag is an EIA sandwich microplate assay cleared by the FDA for the detection of *Aspergillus* galactomannan antigen in serum and BAL fluid. The assay uses a rat monoclonal antibody (EBA-2) directed to bind *Aspergillus* galactomannan antigen. The antibody binds to the antigen and serves as the detector for the antigen in the conjugate reagent (peroxidase-linked monoclonal antibody). The performance of the galactomannan assay has been similar for adults and children.

Serum galactomannan can often be detected 7 to 14 days before other diagnostic tests become apparent. The test should be used in conjunction with other diagnostic procedures (eg, microbiological culture, histologic examination of biopsy samples, radiographic evidence) as an aid in the diagnosis of invasive aspergillosis. The combined use of galactomannan antigen testing and NAAT (ie, PCR) has been shown as a successful approach in the earlier diagnosis of invasive aspergillosis. A negative result does not rule out the diagnosis of invasive aspergillosis. Repeat testing is recommended if the result is negative but invasive aspergillosis is suspected. Patients at risk for invasive aspergillosis should have a baseline serum tested and should be monitored twice a week for increasing galactomannan antigen levels. Galactomannan antigen concentrations may be useful in the assessment of therapeutic response (eg, antigen concentrations decline in response to antifungal therapy).

Other genera of fungi such as *Penicillium* and *Paecilomyces* have shown reactivity with the monoclonal antibody used in the assay. Specimens containing *Histoplasma* antigen may cross-react in the *Aspergillus* galactomannan assay. The specificity of the assay for *Aspergillus* species cannot exclude the involvement of other fungal pathogens (eg, *Fusarium*, *Alternaria*, and *Mucorales*). The assay may exhibit reduced detection of galactomannan in patients with chronic granulomatous disease and Job syndrome.

Certain foods (eg, pasta, cereals, rice, cow's milk) contain galactomannan. It is thought that damage to the gut wall by cytotoxic therapy, irradiation, or graft-versus-host disease enables translocation of the galactomannan from the gut lumen into the blood, which may result in the high false-positive rate of this assay. Antibiotics such as piperacillin–tazobactam, amoxicillin, and/or amoxicillin–clavulanate (eg, drugs derived from the genus *Penicillium*) have been demonstrated to cross-react with monoclonal antibody in the assay. False-positive galactomannan results have occurred in patients receiving Plasma-Lyte, either for intravenous hydration or BAL. The concomitant use of antifungal therapy in some patients with invasive aspergillosis may result in reduced sensitivity of the assay or false-negative results.

**3.** *In vitro testing for circulating (1,3)-β-ᴅ-glucan can be used as a diagnostic tool for several invasive fungal pathogens. What is (1,3)-β-ᴅ-glucan? Briefly explain the type of assay used to detect (1,3)-β-ᴅ-glucan in the United States. Outline the pathogens this test can detect and what precautions need to be considered when interpreting the results from (1,3)-β-ᴅ-glucan testing.*

**ANSWER:** The unique composition of the fungal cell wall makes it particularly well suited to be a nonmolecular biomarker test. A broad range of pathogenic molds and yeasts have the polysaccharide (1,3)-β-ᴅ-glucan present in their cell wall. Concentrations of (1,3)-β-ᴅ-glucan are released into the blood of patients with several types of invasive fungal infections.

In the United States, Fungitell assay (Associates of Cape Cod Inc., East Falmouth, MA) is widely available and is the only FDA-approved screening test for detecting (1,3)-β-ᴅ-glucan in serum. There are several commercially available assays outside the United States. This test uses the coagulation pathway derived from the *Limulus* horseshoe crab as the detector method given (1,3)-β-ᴅ-glucan can activate factor G in this coagulation cascade. Optimal sensitivity is usually obtained by testing patients twice weekly. False-positive results have been associated with the administration of intravenous immunoglobulins or albumin, hemodialysis using cellulose membranes, the use of glucan-containing gauzes or swabs, bacteremia, mucositis or graft-versus-host disease, and the use of selected antibiotics and antitumoral polysaccharides.

(1,3)-β-ᴅ-glucan is associated with *Aspergillus*, *Candida*, and *Fusarium*. In addition, the (1,3)-β-ᴅ-glucan test has been shown to be a sensitive and specific diagnostic marker for *Pneumocystis jirovecii* in patients with and without HIV. Cryptococci and the mucoraceous molds (eg, Zygomycetes such as *Rhizopus*, *Mucor*, and *Absidia*) have little to no measurable amounts of (1,3)-β-ᴅ-glucan, so this test will not be positive in patients with these fungal infections. The test has also performed poorly in patients with infections caused by *Blastomyces* spp. The major limitation in a positive test result is the lack of evidence on the specific fungal etiology.

Guidelines from the Infectious Diseases Society of America (IDSA), the European Organization for Research and Treatment of Cancer. and the Mycosis Study Group Education and Research Consortium support the use of (1,3)-β-ᴅ-glucan to aid in the diagnosis of invasive aspergillosis. Guidelines from the European Society of Clinical Microbiology and Infectious Diseases (ESCMID) have recommended its use for the diagnosis of candidemia, invasive candidiasis, and chronic disseminated candidiasis. The results of (1,3)-β-ᴅ-glucan testing have been shown to be more sensitive for detecting invasive aspergillosis versus invasive candidiasis. Most studies support the use of (1,3)-β-ᴅ-glucan in hematology patients because a limited number of studies have been conducted in patients without cancer and concerns regarding test specificity have occurred in solid-organ transplant recipients.

**4.** *What laboratory tests are used in the diagnosis of HIV infection? What surrogate laboratory markers are used to assess the immunocompetence of patients infected with HIV? What laboratories are available to detect HIV resistance to available antiretrovirals?*

**ANSWER:** Current recommendations for the diagnosis of HIV infection include the initial use of a fourth-generation antibody/antigen combination ELISA (or EIA) followed by a supplemental HIV-1/HIV-2 antibody differentiation immunoassay when the initial test is reactive (positive), and the use of NA tests when the antibody differentiation immunoassay is nonreactive or indeterminate (Figure 19-1). The CD4 cell count and the plasma HIV viral load are the two surrogate laboratory markers that are routinely used throughout the course of HIV infection. A CD4⁺ T-cell count is used to assess the immunocompetence of patients infected with HIV. An absolute CD4⁺ T-cell value of <200 cells/mm³ or <14% is associated with significant immunocompromise and risk for different opportunistic infections. The CD4⁺/CD8⁺ T-cell ratio is sometimes used to assess immune senescence or activation in the research context, but it is not clinically useful, generally, and therefore not routinely recommended. Plasma HIV viral load is a marker of antiretroviral treatment efficacy. HIV genotypic assays sequence or probe genes in specific areas of the virus in which different classes of antiretrovirals exert their action. This type of assay is recommended after HIV diagnosis, before starting antiretroviral therapy, and when HIV resistance is suspected based on unresponsiveness of the viral load despite good adherence to therapy. Genotypic assays most commonly are performed on RNA when HIV-RNA viral load is detectable, ideally ≥1,000 copies/mL, but can be obtained from proviral DNA when HIV-RNA is undetectable. HIV phenotypic assays measure the quantity of viral replication in the presence of various concentration of antiretroviral agents. Because they are labor-intensive and more expensive than genotypic assays, phenotypic assays are generally reserved for cases in which antiretroviral resistance cannot be predicted based on known genetic mutations alone.

## REFERENCES

1. Miller JM, Binnicker MJ, Campbell S, et al. A guide to utilization of the microbiology laboratory for diagnosis of infectious diseases: 2018 update by the Infectious Diseases Society of America and the American Society for Microbiology. *Clin Infect Dis.* 2018;67(6):e1-e94.PubMed

2. Hage CA, Carmona EM, Epelbaum O, et al. Microbiological laboratory testing in the diagnosis of fungal infections in pulmonary and critical

care practice. An official American Thoracic Society clinical practice guideline. *Am J Respir Crit Care Med*. 2019;200(5):535-550.PubMed

3. Zaheen A, Bloom BR. Tuberculosis in 2020: new approaches to a continuing global health crisis. *N Engl J Med* 2020;38214:e26.

4. Brandt ME, Warnock DW. Taxonomy, classification, and nomenclature of fungi. In: Carroll KC, Pfaller MA, Landry ML, et al, eds. *Manual of Clinical Microbiology*. 12th ed. Washington, DC: ASM Press; 2019: 2007-2015.

5. Lone SA, Ahmad A. Candida auris: the growing menace to global health. *Mycoses*. 2019;62(8):620-637.PubMed

6. Seyedmousavi S, Lionakis MS, Parta M, et al. Emerging *Aspergillus* species almost exclusively associated with primary immunodeficiencies. *Open Forum Infect Dis*. 2018;5(9):ofy213.PubMed

7. Aruanno M, Glampedakis E, Lamoth F. Echinocandins for the treatment of invasive aspergillosis: from laboratory to bedside. *Antimicrob Agents Chemother*. 2019;63(8):e00399-e19.PubMed

8. Panel on Antiretroviral Guidelines for Adults and Adolescents. Guidelines for the Use of Antiretroviral Agents in Adults and Adolescents with HIV. Department of Health and Human Services. Available at http://www.aidsinfo.nih.gov/ContentFiles/AdultandAdolescentGL.pdf. Accessed Jun 28, 2020.

9. Hanson KE, Caliendo AM, Arias CA, et al. Infectious Diseases Society of America guidelines on the diagnosis of COVID-19: serologic testing. *Clin Infect Dis*. 2020;ciaa1343.PubMed

10. Carroll KC, Patel R. Systems for identification of bacteria and fungi. In: Carroll KC, Pfaller MA, Landry ML, et al, eds. *Manual of Clinical Microbiology*. 12th ed. Washington, DC: ASM Press; 2019:45-71.

11. Martin I, Pfyffer GE, Parrish N. *Mycobacterium*: general characteristics, laboratory detection, and staining procedures. In: Carroll KC, Pfaller MA, Landry ML, et al, eds. *Manual of Clinical Microbiology*. 12th ed. Washington, DC: ASM Press; 2019:558-575.

12. Caulfield AJ, Richter E, Brown-Elliott BA, et al. *Mycobacterium*: laboratory characteristics of slow growing mycobacteria other than *Mycobacterium tuberculosis*. In: Carroll KC, Pfaller MA, Landry ML, et al, eds. *Manual of Clinical Microbiology*. 12th ed. Washington, DC: ASM Press; 2019:595-611.

13. Landry ML, Caliendo AM, Ginocchio CC, et al. Algorithms for detection and identification of viruses. In: Carroll KC, Pfaller MA, Landry ML, et al, eds. *Manual of Clinical Microbiology*. 12th ed. Washington, DC: ASM Press; 2019:1472-1476.

14. Brandt ME, Warnock DW. Taxonomy, classification, and nomenclature of fungi. In: Carroll KC, Pfaller MA, Landry ML, et al, eds. *Manual of Clinical Microbiology*. 12th ed. Washington, DC: ASM Press; 2019: 2007-2015.

15. Walsh TJ, Hayden RT, Larone DH. *Larone's Medically Important Fungi: A Guide to Identification*. 6th ed. Washington, DC: ASM Press; 2018.

16. Berkow EL, McGowan KL. Specimen collection, transport, and processing: mycology. *In*: Carroll KC, Pfaller MA, Landry ML et al, eds. *Manual of Clinical Microbiology*. 12th ed. Washington, DC: ASM Press; 2019:2016-2024.

17. Lindsley MD. Reagents, stains, and media: mycology. In: Carroll KC, Pfaller MA, Landry ML, et al, eds. *Manual of Clinical Microbiology*. 12th ed. Washington, DC: ASM Press; 2019:2025-2034.

18. Ashbee HR. General approaches for direct detection and identification of fungi. In: Carroll KC, Pfaller MA, Landry ML, et al, eds. *Manual of Clinical Microbiology*. 12th ed. Washington, DC: American Society for Microbiology Press; 2015:2035-2055.

19. Wickes BL, Wiederhold NP. Molecular diagnostics in medical mycology. *Nat Commun*. 2018;9(1):5135.PubMed

20. Gabaldón T. Recent trends in molecular diagnostics of yeast infections: from PCR to NGS. *FEMS Microbiol Rev*. 2019;43(5):517-547.PubMed

21. White PL, Alanio A, Cruciani M, et al. Nucleic acid tools for invasive fungal disease diagnosis. *Curr Fungal Infect Rep*. 2020;14:76-88.

22. Kidd SE, Chen SC-A, Meyer W, Halliday CL. A new age in molecular diagnostics for invasive fungal disease: are we ready? *Front Microbiol*. 2020;10:2903.PubMed

23. Arvanitis M, Anagnostou T, Fuchs BB, et al. Molecular and nonmolecular diagnostic methods for invasive fungal infections. *Clin Microbiol Rev*. 2014;27(3):490-526.PubMed

24. Murray PR, Rosenthal KS, Pfaller MA. Serologic Diangosis. In: *Medical Microbiology*. 9th ed. Philadelphia, PA: Elsevier; 2020:30-35.

25. Guarner J, Brandt ME. Histopathologic diagnosis of fungal infections in the 21st century. *Clin Microbiol Rev*. 2011;24(2):247-280.PubMed

26. Patel R. A moldy application of MALDI-ToF mass spectrometry for fungal identification. *J Fungi (Basel)*. 2019;5(1):E4.PubMed

27. Donnelly JP, Chen SC, Kauffman CA, et al. Revision and update of the consensus definitions of invasive fungal disease from the European Organization for Research and Treatment of Cancer and the Mycoses Study Group Education and Research Consortium. *Clin Infect Dis*. 2020;71(6):1367-1376.PubMed

28. Johnson EM, Cavling-Arendrup M. Susceptibility test methods: yeast and filamentous fungi. In: Carroll KC, Pfaller MA, Landry ML et al. *Manual of Clinical Microbiology*. 12th ed. Washington, DC: American Society for Microbiology Press; 2019:2351-2375.

29. Ostrosky-Zeichner L, Andes D. The role of in vitro susceptibility testing in the management of *Candida* and *Aspergillus*. *J Infect Dis*. 2017;216(suppl 3):S452-S457.PubMed

30. Badali H, Wiederhold NP. Antifungal resistance testing and implications for management. *Curr Fungal Infect Rep*. 2019;13:274-283.

31. Lefkowitz EJ. Taxonomy and classification of viruses. In: Carroll KC, Pfaller MA, Landry ML, et al, eds. *Manual of Clinical Microbiology*. 12th ed. Washington, DC: ASM Press; 2019:1435-1445.

32. Murray PR, Rosenthal KS, Pfaller MA. Laboratory diagnosis of viral disease. In: *Medical Microbiology*. 9th ed. Philadelphia, PA: Elsevier Saunders; 2020:396-402.

33. Dunn JJ, Pinsky BA. Specimen collection, transport, and processing: virology. In: Carroll KC, Pfaller MA, Landry ML, et al, eds. *Manual of Clinical Microbiology*. 12th ed. Washington, DC: ASM Press; 2019: 1446-1461.

34. Capraro GA, Ginocchio CC. Reagents, stains, media, and cell cultures: virology. In: Carroll KC, Pfaller MA, Landry ML, et al, eds. *Manual of Clinical Microbiology*. 12th ed. Washington, DC: ASM Press; 2019: 1462-1471.

35. Hodinka RL, Kaiser L. Point: is the era of viral culture over in the clinical microbiology laboratory? *J Clin Microbiol*. 2013;51(1):2-4.PubMed

36. Leland DS, Ginocchio CC. Role of cell culture for virus detection in the age of technology. *Clin Microbiol Rev*. 2007;20(1):49-78.PubMed

37. Roingeard P, Raynal P-I, Eymieux S, et al. Virus detection by transmission electron microscopy: still useful for diagnosis and a plus for biosafety. *Rev Med Virol*. 2019;29(1):e2019.PubMed

38. Artika IM, Wiyatno A, Ma'roef CN. Pathogenic viruses: molecular detection and characterization. *Infect Genet Evol*. 2020;81:104215. PubMed

39. Uyeki TM, Bernstein HH, Bradley JS, et al. Clinical practice guidelines by the Infectious Diseases Society of America: 2018 update on diagnosis, treatment, chemoprophylaxis, and institutional outbreak management of seasonal influenza. *Clin Infect Dis*. 2019;68(6):e1-e47.PubMed

40. Atmar RL. Influenza viruses. In: Carroll KC, Pfaller MA, Landry ML, et al, eds. *Manual of Clinical Microbiology*. 12th ed. Washington, DC: ASM Press; 2019:1510-1527.

41. Babady NE, Tang Y-W. Respiratory syncytial virus and human metapneumovirus. In: Carroll KC, Pfaller MA, Landry ML, et al, eds. *Manual of Clinical Microbiology*. 12th ed. Washington, DC: ASM Press; 2019:1541-1559.

42. Amjad M. An overview of the molecular methods in the diagnosis of gastrointestinal infectious diseases. *Int J Microbiol*. 2020;2020:8135724. PubMed

43. Pang X, Smieja M. Gastroenteritis viruses. In: Carroll KC, Pfaller MA, Landry ML, et al, eds. *Manual of Clinical Microbiology*. 12th ed. Washington, DC: ASM Press; 2019:1656-1673.

44. Babady NE, Dunn JJ, Madej R. CLIA-waived molecular influenza testing in the emergency department and outpatient settings. *J Clin Virol*. 2019;116:44-48.PubMed

45. Green DA, StGeorge K. Rapid antigen test for influenza: rationale and significance of the FDA reclassification. *J Clin Microbiol*. 2018;56(10):e00711-e00718.PubMed

46. Huang DD, Pinsky BA, Bankowski MJ. Susceptibility test methods: viruses. In: Carroll KC, Pfaller MA, Landry ML, et al, eds. *Manual of Clinical Microbiology*. 12th ed. Washington, DC: ASM Press; 2019: 1985-2003.

47. Clinical and Laboratory Standards Institute (CLSI). *Antiviral Susceptibility Testing: Herpes Simplex Virus by Plaque Reduction Assay*. Wayne, PA: Clinical and Laboratory Standards Institute; 2004, CLSI document M33-A.

48. Fanales-Belasio E, Raimondo M, Suligoi B, Buttò S. HIV virology and pathogenetic mechanisms of infection: a brief overview. *Ann Ist Super Sanita*. 2010;46(1):5-14.PubMed

49. Owen SM. Human immunodeficiency viruses. In: Carroll KC, Pfaller MA, Landry ML, et al, eds. *Manual of Clinical Microbiology*. 12th ed. Washington, DC: ASM Press; 2019:1477-1497.

50. Scosyrev E. An overview of the human immunodeficiency virus featuring laboratory testing for drug resistance. *Clin Lab Sci*. 2006;19(4):231-249. PubMed

51. Centers for Disease Control and Prevention, and Association of Public Health Laboratories. Laboratory Testing for the Diagnosis of HIV Infection: Updated Recommendations. 2014:1-68. http://dx.doi.org/10.15620/cdc.23447. Accessed Jun 28, 2020.

52. Parekh BS, Ou C-Y, Fonjungo PN, et al. Diagnosis of human immunodeficiency virus infection. *Clin Microbiol Rev*. 2018;32(1):e00064-e18.PubMed

53. Panel on Antiretroviral Therapy and Medical Management of Children Living with HIV. Guidelines for the Use of Antiretroviral Agents in Pediatric HIV Infection. http://aidsinfo.nih.gov/contentfiles/lvguidelines/pediatricguidelines.pdf. Accessed Jun 28, 2020.

54. Panel on Treatment of Pregnant Women with HIV Infection and Prevention of Perinatal Transmission. Recommendations for the Use of Antiretroviral Drugs in Pregnant Women with HIV Infection and Interventions to Reduce Perinatal HIV Transmission in the United States. http://aidsinfo.nih.gov/contentfiles/lvguidelines/PerinatalGL.pdf. Accessed Jun 28, 2020.

55. Franco-Paredes C, Tellez I, del Rio C. Rapid HIV testing: a review of the literature and implications for the clinician. *Curr HIV/AIDS Rep*. 2006;3(4):169-175.PubMed

56. Buttò S, Suligoi B, Fanales-Belasio E, Raimondo M. Laboratory diagnostics for HIV infection. *Ann Ist Super Sanita*. 2010;46(1):24-33.PubMed

57. Centers for Diseases Control and Prevention. Advantages and disadvantages of FDA-approved HIV assays used for screening, by test category. https://www.cdc.gov/hiv/pdf/testing/hiv-tests-advantages-disadvantages_1.pdf. Accessed Jun 26, 2020.

58. Mylonakis E, Paliou M, Lally M, et al. Laboratory testing for infection with the human immunodeficiency virus: established and novel approaches. *Am J Med*. 2000;109(7):568-576.PubMed

59. US Food and Drug Administration. Complete list of donor screening assays for infectious agents and HIV diagnostic assays. 2020. https://www.fda.gov/vaccines-blood-biologics/complete-list-donor-screening-assays-infectious-agents-and-hiv-diagnostic-assays#Anti-HIV%20Specimen%20Collection%20Devices,%20Testing%20Services,%20and%20Home%20Test%20Kits. Accessed Jun 28, 2020.

60. Peruski AH, Wesolowski LG, Delaney KP, et al. Trends in HIV-2 diagnoses and use of the HIV-1/HIV-2 differentiation test - United States, 2010-2017. *MMWR Morb Mortal Wkly Rep*. 2020;69(3):63-66.PubMed

61. Alexander TS. Human immunodeficiency virus diagnostic testing: 30 years of evolution. *Clin Vaccine Immunol*. 2016;23(4):249-253.PubMed

62. U.S. Department of Health and Human Services. New FDA information on OraQuick In-Home HIV Test. https://www.hiv.gov/blog/new-fda-information-oraquick-home-hiv-test. Accessed Jun 25, 2020.

63. Bruno G, Saracino A, Monno L, Angarano G. The revival of an "old" marker: CD4/CD8 ratio. *AIDS Rev*. 2017;19(2):81-88.PubMed

64. Murray PR, Rosenthal KS, Pfaller MA. Mycobacterium and related acid-fast bacteria. In: *Medical Microbiology*. 9th ed. Philadelphia, PA: Elsevier; 2020:226-240.

65. Woods GL. Mycobacteria. In: McPherson RA, Pincus MR, eds. *Henry's Clinical Diagnosis and Management by Laboratory Methods*. 23rd ed. St. Louis, MO: Elsevier; 2017:1187-1197.

66. Tille PM, ed. *Bailey & Scott's Diagnostic Microbiology*. 14th ed. St Louis: Elsevier; 2017:524-554.

67. Griffith DE, Aksamit T, Brown-Elliott BA, et al. An official ATS/IDSA statement: diagnosis, treatment, and prevention of nontuberculous mycobacterial diseases. *Am J Respir Crit Care Med*. 2007;175(4):367-416. PubMed

68. Lewinsohn DM, Leonard MK, LoBue PA, et al. Official American Thoracic Society/Infectious Diseases Society of America/Centers for Disease Control and Prevention Clinical Practice Guidelines: Diagnosis of Tuberculosis in Adults and Children. *Clin Infect Dis*. 2017;64(2):e1-e33. PubMed

69. Hale YM, Pfyffer GE, Salfinger M. Laboratory diagnosis of mycobacterial infections: new tools and lessons learned. *Clin Infect Dis*. 2001;33(6): 834-846.PubMed

70. American Thoracic Society. Controlling tuberculosis in the United States. *Am J Respir Crit Care Med*. 2005;172(9):1169-1227.PubMed

71. Center for Disease Control and Prevention. Trends in Tuberculosis, 2018. https://www.cdc.gov/tb/publications/factsheets/statistics/tbtrends.htm. Accessed Jun 27, 2020.

72. World Health Organization. *Global Tuberculosis Report 2019*. Geneva, Switzerland: 2019.

73. Palomino JC. Nonconventional and new methods in the diagnosis of tuberculosis: feasibility and applicability in the field. *Eur Respir J*. 2005;26(2):339-350.PubMed

74. Centers for Disease Control and Prevention (CDC). Updated guidelines for the use of nucleic acid amplification tests in the diagnosis of tuberculosis. *MMWR Morb Mortal Wkly Rep*. 2009;58(1):7-10.PubMed

75. US Food and Drug Administration. Nucleic Acid Based Tests. 2020. https://www.fda.gov/medical-devices/vitro-diagnostics/nucleic-acid-based-tests. Accessed Jun 27, 2020.

76. Centers for Disease Control and Prevention (CDC). Availability of an assay for detecting *Mycobacterium tuberculosis*, including rifampin-resistant strains, and considerations for its use - United States, 2013. *MMWR Morb Mortal Wkly Rep*. 2013;62(41):821-827.PubMed

77. World Health Organization. Automated real-time nucleic acid amplification technology for rapid and simultaneous detection of tuberculosis and rifampicin resistance: Xpert MTB/RIF system: policy statement. 2011.

78. bioMérieux. bioMérieux receives FDA clearance for expanded pathogen identification capability on VITEK MS. https://www.biomerieux-usa.com/biomerieux-receives-fda-clearance-expanded-pathogen-identification-capability-vitek-ms. Accessed Jun 27, 2020.

79. Association of Public Health Laboratories. Best practices for identification of *Mycobaterium* species using matrix-assisted laser desorption ionization-time of flight mass spectrometry. 2019. https://www.aphl.org/aboutAPHL/publications/Documents/ID-2019Aug-MALDI-TOF-TB-Fact-Sheet.pdf. Accessed on Jun 28, 2020.

80. Clinical and Laboratory Standards Institute (CLSI). *Susceptibility Testing of Mycobacteria, Nocardia, and Other Aerobic Actinomycetes; Approved Standard*. 3rd ed. Wayne, PA: Clinical and Laboratory Standards Institute; 2018.

81. American Thoracic Society. Targeted tuberculin testing and treatment of latent tuberculosis infection. *MMWR Recomm Rep*. 2000;49(RR-6):1-51. PubMed

82. Centers for Disease Control and Prevention. Guidelines for preventing the transmission of *Mycobacterium tuberculosis* in healthcare settings, 2005. *MMWR*. 2005;. :RR-17.

83. Frenzel EC, Thomas GA, Hanna HA. The importance of two-step tuberculin skin testing for newly employed healthcare workers. *Infect Control Hosp Epidemiol*. 2006;27(5):512-514.PubMed

84. Mazurek GH, Jereb J, Vernon A, et al. Updated guidelines for using Interferon Gamma Release Assays to detect Mycobacterium tuberculosis infection – United States, 2010. *MMWR Recomm Rep*. 2010;59(RR-5):1-25.PubMed

# Rheumatic Diseases

*Susan P. Bruce*

## OBJECTIVES

*After completing this chapter, the reader should be able to*

- Describe the physiologic basis for rheumatic laboratory tests and the pathophysiologic processes that result in abnormal test results

- Describe the appropriate clinical applications for laboratory tests used to diagnose or assess the activity of select rheumatic diseases

- Interpret the results of laboratory tests used to diagnose or manage common rheumatic diseases

- Use the results of rheumatic laboratory tests to make decisions about the effectiveness of pharmacotherapy

- Employ laboratory tests to identify and prevent adverse reactions to drugs used to treat rheumatic diseases

The diagnosis and management of most rheumatic diseases depend primarily on patient medical history, symptoms, and physical examination findings. A variety of laboratory tests are used to assist in the diagnosis of rheumatic disorders, but many are nonspecific tests that are not pathognomonic for any single disease. However, the results of some specific laboratory tests may be essential for confirming the diagnosis of some diseases. Consequently, laboratory tests are important diagnostic tools when used in concert with the medical history and other subjective and objective findings. Some laboratory test results are also used to assess disease severity and to monitor the beneficial and adverse effects of pharmacotherapy.

The diagnostic utility of a laboratory test depends on its sensitivity, specificity, and predictive value (Chapter 1). Tests that are highly sensitive and specific for certain rheumatic diseases often have low predictive values because the prevalence of the suspected rheumatic disease is low. The most important determinant of a laboratory test's diagnostic usefulness is the pretest probability of disease, or a clinician's estimated likelihood that a certain disease is present based on history and clinical findings. As the number of disease-specific signs and symptoms increases and approaches diagnostic confirmation, the pretest probability also increases.

After briefly reviewing pertinent physiology of immunoglobulins, this chapter discusses various tests used to diagnose and assess rheumatic diseases, followed by interpretation of these test results in common rheumatic disorders. Tests used to monitor antirheumatic pharmacotherapy are also described.

## STRUCTURE AND PHYSIOLOGY OF IMMUNOGLOBULINS

Many rheumatic laboratory tests involve detection of immunoglobulins (antibodies) that are directed against normal cellular components. The structure and functions of immunoglobulins are reviewed briefly here to facilitate an understanding of these tests.

When the immune system is challenged by a foreign substance (antigen), activated B lymphocytes differentiate into immunoglobulin-producing plasma cells. Immunoglobulins are Y-shaped proteins with an identical antigen-binding site (called *Fab* or *fraction antigen-binding*) on each arm of the Y (**Figure 20-1**). Each arm is composed of a light (L) amino acid chain covalently linked to a heavy (H) amino acid chain. The terms *light* and *heavy* refer to the number of amino acids in each chain. Because the heavy chain has more amino acids than the light chain, it is longer and has a higher molecular weight.

Both types of chains have a variable region and a constant region. The variable regions contain the antigen-binding sites and vary in amino acid sequence. The sequences differ to allow immunoglobulins to recognize and bind specifically to thousands of different antigens. Within the variable regions, there are four framework regions and three complementary-determining regions; together these make up the antigen-binding pocket. The constant region of the light chain is a single section. Immunoglobulins that have identical constant regions in their heavy chains are of the same class.

DOI 10.37573/9781585286423.020

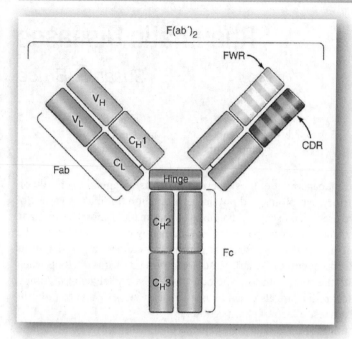

**FIGURE 20-1.** Schematic of the antibody molecule. (*Source*: Adapted with permission from Four Chain Structure of a Generic Antibody-IgG2 Structures by OpenStax College—Anatomy & Physiology, Connexions Website. http://cnx.org/content/col11496/1.6/, Jun 19, 2013. Licensed under CC BY 3.0 via Wikmedia Commons– https://commons.wikimedia.org/wiki/File:2220_Four_Chain _Structure_of_a_Generic_Antibody-IgG2_Structures.jpg.)

The five classes of immunoglobulins are IgA, IgD, IgE, IgG, and IgM. Depending on the immunoglobulin, the constant region of the heavy chain has either three domains and a hinge region (IgA, IgD, and IgG) that promotes flexibility, or four domains without a hinge region (IgE and IgM). Thus, the immunoglobulin's heavy chain determines its class ($\alpha$ heavy chains, IgA; $\delta$ heavy chains, IgD; $\epsilon$ heavy chains, IgE; $\gamma$ heavy chains, IgG; and $\mu$ heavy chains, IgM). Tests are available to measure the serum concentrations of the general types of immunoglobulins as well as immunoglobulins directed against specific antigens (viruses, other infectious agents, other allergens).

In Figure 20-1, the second and third domains of the heavy chain are part of the fraction crystallizable (Fn) portion of the immunoglobulin. This portion has two important functions: (1) activation of the complement cascade (discussed later) and (2) binding of immunoglobulins (which react with and bind antigen) to cell surface receptors of effector cells such as monocytes, macrophages, neutrophils, and natural killer cells.[1]

# TESTS TO DIAGNOSE AND ASSESS RHEUMATIC DISEASES

Blood tests that are relatively specific for certain rheumatic diseases include rheumatoid factors (RFs), anticitrullinated protein antibodies (ACPAs), antinuclear antibodies (ANAs),

antineutrophil cytoplasmic antibodies (ANCAs), and complement. Nonspecific blood and other types of tests include erythrocyte sedimentation rate (ESR), C-reactive protein (CRP), analysis of synovial fluid, and others. Where applicable, the sections that follow discuss quantitative assay results (where normal values are reported as a range of concentrations), qualitative assay results (where assay results are reported as only positive or negative), and their use in common rheumatic and nonrheumatic diseases.

## Rheumatoid Factor

*Rheumatoid factors* (RFs) are immunoglobulins (predominantly IgM but may also be IgG or IgA) that are abnormally directed against the Fc portion of IgG. These immunoglobulins do not recognize the IgG as being "self." Therefore, the presence of RFs in the blood indicates an autoimmune process. The RF measured in most laboratories is IgM-anti-IgG (an IgM antibody that specifically binds IgG). Like all IgM antibodies, IgM RF is composed of five subunits whose Fc portions are attached to the same base. The variable regions of each IgM antibody can bind up to five IgG molecules at its multiple binding sites, making IgM RF the most stable and easiest to quantify.

Rheumatoid factors are most commonly associated with rheumatoid arthritis (RA) but are not specific for that disease. Other rheumatic diseases in which circulating RFs have been identified include systemic lupus erythematosus (SLE), systemic sclerosis (scleroderma), mixed connective tissue disease (MCTD), and Sjögren syndrome.[3] The significance of RFs in these diseases is unknown.

The presence of RF is not conclusive evidence that a rheumatic disease exists. Patients with various acute and chronic inflammatory diseases as well as healthy individuals may be RF positive. Nonrheumatic diseases associated with RFs include mononucleosis, hepatitis, malaria, tuberculosis, syphilis, subacute bacterial endocarditis, cancers after chemotherapy or irradiation, chronic liver disease, hyperglobulinemia, and cryoglobulinemia.

The percentage of individuals with positive RF concentrations and the mean RF concentration of the population increase with advancing age but is 1% to 2% of the heathy population on average. Although RFs are associated with several rheumatic and many nonrheumatic diseases, the concentrations of RFs in these diseases are lower than those observed in patients with RA.

### Quantitative Assay Results

*Normal values: <1:16 or <15 International Units/mL*
When a quantitative RF test is performed, results are reported as either a dilutional titer or a concentration in International Units per milliliter. RF titers are reported positive as a specific serum dilution; the ability to detect RF is tested at each dilution. The greatest dilution that results in a positive test is reported as the endpoint. A titer of >1:16 or a concentration >15 International Units/mL is generally considered to be positive. However, reference ranges vary depending on the method used, so it is important to use the limits provided by the individual laboratory.

### Qualitative Assay Results

At a serum dilution at which 95% of the normal population is RF negative, 70% to 90% of RA patients will have a positive RF test. The remaining RA patients who have RF titers within the normal range may be described as seronegative.

## Anticitrullinated Protein Antibodies

Citrullination is the process by which susceptible genes exposed to environmental factors undergo an abnormal change. As a result, citrullinated proteins become antigens and lead to the formation of autoantibodies. ACPAs bind to the nonstandard amino acid citrulline that is formed from removal of amino groups from arginine. Nonstandard amino acids are generally not found in proteins and often occur as intermediates in the metabolic pathways of standard amino acids. In the joints of patients with RA, proteins may be transformed to citrulline during the pathogenesis that leads to joint inflammation. When these antibodies are present, there is a 90% to 95% likelihood that the patient has RA. The combination of both positive RF and positive ACPA has 99.5% specificity for RA. Positive ACPAs may occur in other diseases, including SLE, systemic sclerosis, psoriasis, and tuberculosis.

Anticitrullinated protein antibodies are important considerations in the context of RA for multiple reasons: (1) presence is associated with more erosive forms of RA, (2) presence is considered one of the clinical features of RA that is associated with a worse long-term prognosis, and (3) presence is a positive predictor of future RA diagnosis in patients with undifferentiated arthritis. Therefore, ACPA-positive patients should receive aggressive treatment early and be followed closely throughout the course of their disease to control systemic inflammation.

### Quantitative and Qualitative Assay Results

*Normal values: <20 EU/mL (assay dependent)*
Quantitative ACPAs are tested by enzyme-linked immunosorbent assay (ELISA) and are reported in ELISA units (EU). The relationship between these values and qualitative results are generally reported in the following way:

- <20 EU: negative
- 20 to 39 EU: weakly positive
- 40 to 59 EU: moderately positive
- >60 EU: strongly positive

## Antinuclear Antibodies

*Antinuclear antibodies* (ANAs) are a heterogeneous group of autoantibodies directed against nucleic acids and nucleoproteins within the nucleus and cytoplasm. Intracellular targets of these autoantibodies include DNA, RNA, individual nuclear histones, acidic nuclear proteins, and complexes of these molecular elements (**Table 20-1**).[4-7]

The ANA test is included in the diagnostic criteria for idiopathic SLE, drug-induced lupus, and MCTD because of

**TABLE 20-1.** Laboratory and Clinical Characteristics of Antibodies to Nuclear/Cytoplasmic Antigens

| ANA | TARGETED CELLULAR MATERIAL | SENSITIVITY | SPECIFICITY |
|---|---|---|---|
| dsDNA | dsDNA | SLE: 70%<br>RA: 1%<br>Systemic sclerosis: <1% | SLE: high (>95%)<br>Drug-induced lupus: low (1% to 5%)<br>RA: low (1%)<br>Systemic sclerosis: low (<1%)<br>Sjögren syndrome: low (1% to 5%) |
| ssDNA | ssDNA | SLE: 80%<br>Drug-induced lupus: 80%<br>RA: 60% | SLE: low<br>Drug-induced lupus: low<br>RA: moderate |
| Sm[a] | Nuclear ribonucleoproteins | SLE: 10% to 50%<br>Drug-induced lupus: 1%<br>RA: 1%<br>Systemic sclerosis: <1%<br>Sjögren syndrome: 1% to 5% | SLE: high (55% to 100%) |
| RNP (or U$_1$RNP) | Nuclear ribonucleoproteins | MCTD: 100%<br>SLE: 3% to 69%<br>Systemic sclerosis: <1%<br>RA: 25%<br>Polymyositis: <1% | MCTD: low<br>SLE: low<br>Systemic sclerosis: low<br>RA: low<br>Polymyositis: low |

*(continued)*

**TABLE 20-1.** Laboratory and Clinical Characteristics of Antibodies to Nuclear/Cytoplasmic Antigens, cont'd

| ANA | TARGETED CELLULAR MATERIAL | SENSITIVITY | SPECIFICITY |
|---|---|---|---|
| Histone | Chromatin and DNA-packing protein | SLE: 70%<br>Drug-induced lupus: 95%<br>RA: 15% to 20%<br>Systemic sclerosis: <1% | SLE: moderate<br>Drug-induced lupus: high<br>RA: low<br>Systemic sclerosis: low |
| Ro[a]/SSA[b] | Nuclear ribonucleoproteins | Sjögren syndrome: 10% to 60%<br>SLE: 40%<br>Polymyositis: 18%<br>RA: 5%<br>Systemic sclerosis: 5% | Sjögren syndrome: moderate<br>SLE: low<br>Polymyositis: low<br>RA: low<br>Systemic sclerosis: low |
| La[a]/SSB[b] | Nuclear ribonucleoproteins | Sjögren syndrome: 70% to 95%<br>SLE: 10% to 35% | Sjögren syndrome: high (94%)<br>SLE: low |
| Centromere (ACA) | Chromatin and centromere | Systemic sclerosis: 25% to 30%<br>CREST: 50% to 90%<br>Raynaud phenomenon: 15% to 30% | Systemic sclerosis: high<br>CREST, Raynaud phenomenon: high (>95%) |
| DNA topoisomerase I (Scl$_{70}$) | Chromatin and DNA-catalyzing protein | Systemic sclerosis: 15% to 20% | Systemic sclerosis: high (>95%) |
| Jo-1 | Cytoplasm and histidyl tRNA synthetase | SLE: low<br>Drug-induced lupus: low<br>RA: low<br>Systemic sclerosis: low<br>Sjögren syndrome: low<br>Polymyositis: 30%<br>Jo-1 syndrome: 50% | SLE: low<br>Drug-induced lupus: low<br>RA: low<br>Systemic sclerosis: low<br>Sjögren syndrome: low<br>Polymyositis with interstitial lung disease: high<br>Jo-1 syndrome: high |

ACA = anticentromere antibody; CREST = syndrome characterized by calcinosis, Raynaud phenomenon, esophageal motility disorder, sclerodactyly, and telangiectasias; La/SSB = La/Sjögren syndrome B antibody; RNP = ribonucleoprotein; Ro/SSA = Ro/Sjögren syndrome A antibody; Scl$_{70}$ = scleroderma-70 or DNA topoisomerase I antibody; U$_1$RNP = uridine-rich ribonuclear protein.
[a]Represents the first two letters of the surname of the patient whose serum was used to identify the reaction in agar diffusion.
[b]Sjögren syndrome A and B.
*Source:* From references 4–7.

its high rate of positivity in these disorders. However, its low specificity makes it unsuitable for use as a screening test for rheumatic or nonrheumatic diseases in asymptomatic individuals. A positive ANA can also be found in otherwise healthy individuals. ANAs are also associated with various genetic and environmental factors (eg, intravenous drug abuse), hormonal factors, and increased age. They also are associated with nonrheumatic diseases, both immunologically mediated (eg, Hashimoto thyroiditis, idiopathic pulmonary fibrosis, primary pulmonary hypertension, idiopathic thrombocytopenic purpura, and hemolytic anemia) and nonimmunologically mediated (eg, acute or chronic bacterial, viral, or parasitic infections and neoplasm).

Antibody tests that have clinical use for diagnosis of SLE, drug-induced lupus, and other diseases are as follows.

### Double-Stranded DNA (anti-dsDNA) Antibodies

*Normal values: negative (ELISA), <1:10 titer (FANA)*
These antibodies are relatively specific for SLE, which makes them useful for diagnosis. In some patients with SLE, the titers tend to rise with a disease flare and fall (usually into the normal range) when the flare subsides. Thus, anti–double-stranded DNA (dsDNA) titers may be helpful in managing disease activity in some patients with SLE. Anti-dsDNA antibodies have been found in low titers in many other autoimmune diseases (eg, RA, Sjögren syndrome, systemic sclerosis, Raynaud phenomenon,

MCTD, discoid lupus, juvenile idiopathic arthritis [JIA], and autoimmune hepatitis).[6] The presence of anti-dsDNA antibodies has also been reported in patients receiving some drugs used to treat rheumatic diseases (eg, minocycline, etanercept, infliximab, and penicillamine).

## Single-Stranded DNA (Anti-ssDNA) Antibodies

These antibodies identify and react primarily with purine and pyrimidine bases within the β-helix of dsDNA. They may also bind with nucleosides and nucleotides. They are much less specific for SLE than anti-dsDNA antibodies. They are of limited clinical use.

## Smith (Anti-Sm) Antibodies

*Normal values: negative*

These antibodies bind to a series of nuclear proteins complexed with small nuclear RNAs. These complexes are known as *small nuclear ribonucleoprotein particles* and are important in the processing of RNA transcribed from DNA.[6] The anti-Sm antibody test has low sensitivity (10% to 50% depending on assay methodology) but high specificity (55% to 100%) for SLE. Titers usually remain positive after disease activity has subsided and titers of anti-DNA antibodies have declined to the normal range. Thus, the anti-Sm antibody titer may be a useful diagnostic tool, especially when anti-DNA antibodies are undetectable. There is currently no evidence that monitoring anti-Sm antibodies is useful for following the disease course or predicting disease activity.[6]

## Ribonucleoprotein (Anti-RNP) or Uridine-Rich Ribonuclear Protein (Anti-U₁RNP) Antibodies

*Normal values: Negative*

This antibody system reacts to antigens that are related to Sm antigens. However, these antibodies bind only to the $U_1$ particle, which is involved in splicing nuclear RNA into messenger RNA. Ribonucleoprotein antibodies are found in many patients with SLE (3% to 69%), and low titers may be detected in other rheumatic diseases (eg, Raynaud phenomenon, RA, systemic sclerosis).[6] Importantly, anti-U₁RNP antibodies are a hallmark feature of MCTD. A positive test result in a patient with suspected MCTD increases the probability that this diagnosis is correct, even though the test is nonspecific. On the other hand, a negative anti-RNP result in a patient with possible MCTD virtually excludes this diagnosis.

## Anti-Histone (Nucleosome) Antibodies

*Normal values: Negative*

These antibodies target the protein portions of nucleosomes, which are DNA–protein complexes comprising part of chromatin. These antibodies are present in virtually all cases of drug-induced lupus. In fact, the diagnosis of drug-induced lupus should be questioned in their absence. Most cases of drug-induced lupus are readily diagnosed because a commonly implicated drug (eg, hydralazine, isoniazid, procainamide) is being taken or a strong temporal relationship exists between drug initiation and the onset of SLE signs and symptoms. However, in some cases of potential drug-induced lupus, histone autoantibody testing can be helpful. Histone antibodies appear less commonly in other diseases, including RA, JIA, autoimmune hepatitis, scleroderma, and others. There is some evidence that histone antibodies correlate with disease activity in SLE.

Two closely related ANA tests are detected frequently in patients with Sjögren syndrome, but they are nonspecific; they may also be helpful for diagnosis of SLE.

1. Ro/Sjögren Syndrome A (Anti-Ro/SSA) Antibody

   *Normal values: Negative*

   Autoantibodies directed against Ro/SSA recognize one of two cellular proteins, one in the nucleus (Ro60) and one in the cytoplasm (Ro52). The numbers represent the molecular weight of the protein in kilodalton.

2. La/Sjögren Syndrome B (Anti-La/SSB) Antibody

   *Normal values: Negative*

   Autoantibodies directed against La/SSB targets a protein found in the nucleus that goes back and forth between the cytoplans and the nucleus.

The presence of either antibody in patients with suspected Sjögren syndrome strongly supports the diagnosis. It is unusual to detect the anti-La/SSB antibody in patients with SLE or Sjögren syndrome in the absence of the anti-Ro/SSA antibody. In women of childbearing age who have a known connective-tissue disease (eg, SLE, MCTD), a positive anti-Ro/SSA antibody is associated with an infrequent (1% to 2%) but definite risk of bearing a child with neonatal SLE and congenital heart block. Presence of the anti-Ro/SSA antibody also correlates with late-onset SLE and secondary Sjögren syndrome. In patients who are ANA negative but have clinical signs of SLE, a positive anti-Ro/SSA antibody may be useful in establishing a diagnosis of SLE.

It has been recommended that the anti-Ro/SSA antibody test be ordered in the following situations[7]: (1) women with SLE or Sjögren syndrome who are planning to become pregnant, (2) women with a history of giving birth to children with heart block or myocarditis, (3) women known to be ANA positive who wish to become pregnant, (4) patients suspected of having a systemic connective tissue disease with a negative ANA screening test, and (5) patients with xerostomia, keratoconjunctivitis sicca, and salivary and lacrimal gland enlargement.

Two ANAs are highly specific for systemic sclerosis (scleroderma), but the tests have low sensitivity:

- Antikinetochore (centromere) antibody
- Antitopoisomerase I (Scl₇₀) antibody

In addition, these two antibodies are highly specific for CREST syndrome (associated with <u>c</u>alcinosis, <u>R</u>aynaud phenomenon, <u>e</u>sophageal dysmotility, <u>s</u>clerodactyly, and <u>t</u>elangiectasias), Raynaud phenomenon, and occasionally SLE. When systemic sclerosis is suspected on clinical grounds, antibody testing for antikinetochore and Scl₇₀ can be useful in making the diagnosis. However, negative results do not exclude the disease because of low test sensitivity.

The Jo-1 antibody (anti-Jo) is highly specific for idiopathic inflammatory myopathy, including polymyositis and dermatomyositis, or myositis associated with another rheumatic disease or interstitial lung disease. The titer or quantitative value should be considered when evaluating the clinical significance of ANA test results.

### Quantitative Antinuclear Antibody Assay Results

*Normal: Negative at 1:40 dilution (varies among laboratories)*
The indirect immunofluorescence antinuclear antibody test (FANA) is a rapid and highly sensitive method for detecting the presence of ANAs.[4] It is considered the gold standard for ANA testing. Although the FANA is positive in >95% of patients with SLE, it is also positive in some normal individuals and patients with drug-induced lupus and other autoimmune diseases. An ELISA also provides a rapid and highly sensitive method for detecting the presence of ANA; however, the sensitivity is lower than FANA. Many laboratories perform screening ANA tests by the ELISA technique because it can be automated and is less labor intensive; FANA testing is performed only in specimens testing positive by ELISA.[5] It is important for the clinician to know the technique used at a specific laboratory to interpret the results correctly.

Laboratories usually report the ANA titer, which is the highest serum dilution that remains positive for ANAs. A high concentration (titer >1:640) should raise suspicion for an auto-immune disorder but is not in itself diagnostic of any disease. In the absence of clinical findings, these individuals should be monitored closely for the overt development of an autoimmune disorder. On the other hand, a high ANA titer is less useful in a patient who already has definite clinical evidence of a systemic autoimmune disease. The finding of a low antibody titer (<1:80) in the absence of signs or symptoms of disease is not of great concern, and such patients require less frequent follow-up than those with high titers. False-positive ANAs are common in the normal population and tend to be associated with low titers (<1:40). The positive antibody titers in healthy persons tend to remain fairly constant over time; this finding can also be seen in patients with known disease.

### Qualitative Antinuclear Antibody Assay Results

The pattern of nuclear fluorescence after staining may reflect the presence of antibodies to one or more nuclear antigens. The nuclear staining pattern was used commonly in the past, but the pattern type is now recognized to have relatively low sensitivity and specificity for individual autoimmune diseases. For this reason, specific antibody tests have largely replaced use of patterns.[5] The common immunofluorescent patterns are as follows:

- **Homogeneous:** This pattern is seen most frequently in patients with SLE but can also be observed in patients with drug-induced lupus, RA, vasculitis, and polymyositis. This pattern reflects antibodies to the DNA-histone complex.

- **Speckled:** This pattern is also seen most frequently in patients with SLE but can appear in patients with MCTD, Sjögren syndrome, progressive systemic sclerosis, polymyositis, and RA. This pattern is produced by antibodies to Sm, Ro/SSA, La/SSB, DNA topoisomerase I (Scl$_{70}$), and other antigens.

- **Nucleolar:** This pattern is infrequently observed in patients with SLE but is more frequently seen in patients with poly-myositis, progressive systemic sclerosis, and vasculitis. It is

produced by antibodies to RNA polymerase I and several other antigens.

- **Peripheral or nuclear rim:** This is the only pattern that is highly specific for any rheumatic disease and is observed predominantly (98%) in SLE patients. It is produced by antibodies to DNA (dsDNA, ssDNA) and nuclear envelope antigens (antibodies to components of the nuclear envelope, such as certain glycoproteins).

Table 20-1 summarizes the most frequently identified ANAs, their corresponding targeted cellular material, and disease sensitivities and specificities.[4-7]

## Antineutrophil Cytoplasmic Antibodies

As the name implies, *antineutrophil cytoplasmic antibodies* (ANCAs) are antibodies directed against neutrophil cytoplasmic antigens. Testing for ANCAs is important for the diagnosis and classification of various forms of vasculitis. In these disorders, the target antigens are proteinase 3 (PR3) and myeloperoxidase (MPO). Both antigens are located in the azurophilic granules of neutrophils and the peroxidase-positive lysosomes of monocytes. Antibodies that target PR3 and MPO are known as *PR3-ANCA* and *MPO-ANCA*.[8] There is an association between ANCA and several major vasculitic syndromes: granulomatosis with polyangiitis (GPA), microscopic polyangiitis, eosinophilic granulomatosis with polyangiitis, and certain drug-induced vasculitis syndromes.[8]

GPA is a vasculitis of unknown origin that can damage organs by restricting blood flow and destroying normal tissue. Although any organ system may be involved, the disorder primarily affects the respiratory tract (sinuses, nose, trachea, and lungs) and the kidneys. Approximately 90% of patients with active GPA have ANCAs. In patients with limited disease presentations, typically limited to the respiratory tract, up to 40% may be ANCA-negative. Thus, although a positive ANCA test result is useful to support a suspected diagnosis, a negative ANCA test result does not exclude it. For this reason, the ANCA test is usually not used alone to diagnose GPA.

In patients with vasculitis, immunofluorescence after ethanol fixation reveals two characteristic patterns: cytoplasmic (cANCA) and perinuclear (pANCA). With cANCA, there is diffuse staining throughout the cytoplasm, which is usually caused by antibodies against PR3. The pANCA pattern is characterized by staining around the nucleus and perinuclear fluorescence. In patients with vasculitis, the antibody causing this pattern is generally directed against MPO.

Although detection and identification of ANCAs are most useful in diagnosing various vasculitides, ANCAs have been reported in connective tissue diseases (eg, RA, SLE, and myositis), chronic infections (eg, cystic fibrosis, endocarditis, and human immunodeficiency virus), and gastrointestinal diseases (eg, inflammatory bowel disease, sclerosing cholangitis, and autoimmune hepatitis). Some medications may induce vasculitis associated with positive ANCA (usually MPO-ANCA).[9] The drugs most strongly associated with ANCA-associated vasculitis are propylthiouracil, methimazole, carbimazole, hydralazine, and minocycline. Penicillamine, allopurinol, procainamide, thiamazole, clozapine, phenytoin, rifampin, cefotaxime, isoniazid, and indomethacin are less commonly associated with the disorder.[8]

### Quantitative Assay Results

*Normal value: Negative*

When used in the diagnosis of GPA, the specificity of PR3-ANCA is approximately 90%. The sensitivity of the test is about 90% when the disease is active and 40% when the disease is in remission. Thus, the sensitivity of PR3-ANCA is related to the extent, severity, and activity of the disease at the time of testing.

The use of obtaining serial PR3-ANCA tests in assessing disease activity is controversial. Some data suggest that a rise in titers predicts clinical exacerbations and justifies increasing immunosuppressive therapy. However, other studies have shown that disease flares cannot be predicted in a timely fashion by elevations in ANCA titers. Further, the immunosuppressive and cytotoxic therapies used are associated with substantial adverse effects. For these reasons, an elevation in ANCA should not be used as the sole justification for initiating immunosuppressive therapy. Rather, patients with rising ANCA titers should be monitored closely with therapy withheld unless there are clear clinical signs of active disease.[8]

### Qualitative Assay Results

The association of cANCA and pANCA tests for various antigens and diseases are listed in **Table 20-2**. The presence of cANCAs denotes a spectrum of diseases ranging from idiopathic glomerulonephritis to extended GPA.[10] In most cases of vasculitis, renal disorder, and granulomatous disease, patient sera are negative for cANCAs.

The pANCA test has limited diagnostic value. A positive pANCA test result should be followed by antigen-specific assays such as anti-MPO. In ulcerative colitis, the specificity of

the pANCA test has been reported to be as high as 94%. However, with only moderate sensitivity and inconsistent correlation between titers and disease activity, pANCA screening may be of little value. Although sensitivity can reach 85% in primary sclerosing cholangitis, the pANCA test lacks specificity in the differential diagnosis of autoimmune hepatic diseases. In RA, pANCA may be related to aggressive, erosive disease. The sensitivity of the test increases in RA complicated by vasculitis, but its specificity remains low.

## Complement

The *complement* system consists of approximately 60 different plasma and membrane proteins that provide a defense mechanism against microbial invaders and serve as an adjunct or "complement" to humoral immunity. The system works by depositing complement components on pathologic targets and by the interaction of plasma proteins in a cascading sequence to mediate inflammatory effects such as opsonization of particles for phagocytosis, leukocyte activation, and assembly of the membrane attack complex (MAC).[11] Six plasma control proteins and five integral membrane control proteins regulate this cascade. These proteins circulate normally in a precursor (inactive) form (eg, C3 and C4). When the initial protein of a given pathway is activated, it activates the next protein (eg, C3a and C4a) in a cascading fashion similar to that seen with coagulation factors.

Activation of this system can occur through any one of three proteolytic pathways:

1. **Classic pathway:** This pathway is activated when IgM or IgG antibodies bind to antigens such as viruses or bacteria.

2. **Alternative pathway:** This evolutionary surveillance system does not require the presence of specific antibodies.

3. **Lectin pathway:** This pathway is activated similarly to the classic pathway, but instead of antibody binding, mannose-binding protein binds to sugar residues on the surface of pathogens.

Activation by any of the three pathways generates enzymes that cleave the third and fifth complement components (C3 and C5). A final common (or terminal) sequence culminates in the assembly of the MAC. Five proteins (C5 through C9) interact to form the MAC, which creates transmembrane channels or pores that displace lipid molecules and other elements, resulting in disruption of cell membranes and cell lysis.

Because the complement system is an important part of immune system regulation, complement deficiency predisposes an individual to infections and autoimmune syndromes. In disorders associated with autoantibodies and the formation of immune complexes, the complement system can contribute to tissue damage.

Serum complement levels reflect a balance between synthesis and catabolism. Hypocomplementemia occurs when the C3 or C4 concentration falls below its reference range. Most cases of hypocomplementemia are associated with hypercatabolism (complement depletion) due to activation of the immune system rather than decreased production of complement components (hyposynthesis). Most diseases associated with the formation

**TABLE 20-2.** Rheumatic Disease Associations of Antinuclear Cytoplasmic Antibodies

| ANCA | DISEASE | PERCENT ANCA POSITIVE (%) |
|------|---------|---------------------------|
| cANCA | GPA | 70–90 |
| | MPA | 20–30 |
| | Pauci-immune crescentic glomerulonephritis | 10 |
| | EGPA | 10 |
| pANCA | MPA | 65–90 |
| | Pauci-immune crescentic glomerulonephritis | 80 |
| | EGPA | 30–40 |
| | GPA | 25 |

EGPA = eosinophil granulomatosis with polyangiitis; MPA = microscopic polyangiitis.
Adapted from references 8–10.

of IgG- or IgM-containing circulating immune complexes can cause hypocomplementemia. Rheumatic diseases included in this category are SLE, RA with extraarticular disease, Sjögren syndrome, and systemic vasculitis. Nonrheumatic diseases associated with hypocomplementemia include antiphospholipid syndrome, subacute bacterial endocarditis, hepatitis B surface antigenemia, pneumococcal infection, gram-negative sepsis, viral infections (eg, measles), recurrent parasitic infections (eg, malaria), and mixed cryoglobulinemia.[11,12]

Because errors in interpretation of complement study results can occur, three important aspects should be considered when interpreting these results:

1. **Reference ranges are relatively wide.** Therefore, new test results should be compared with previous test results rather than with a reference range. It is most useful to examine serial test results and correlate changes with a patient's clinical picture.

2. **Normal results should be compared with previous results, if available.** Inflammatory states may increase the rate of synthesis and elevate serum complement protein levels. For example, some patients with SLE have concentrations of specific complement components that are two to three times the upper limit of normal (ULN) when their disease is clinically inactive. When the disease activity increases to the point that increased catabolism of complement proteins occurs, levels may then fall into the reference range. It would be a misinterpretation to conclude that these "normal" concentrations represent an inactive complement system. Consequently, serial determinations of complement levels may be more informative than measurements at a single point.

3. **Complement responses do not correlate consistently with disease activity**. In some patients, the increase and decrease of the complement system should not be used to assess disease activity.

Assessment of the complement system should include measurement of the total hemolytic complement activity by the complement hemolytic 50% ($CH_{50}$) test and determination of the levels of C3 and C4.

### Total Hemolytic Complement

*Reference range: 150 to 250 International Units/mL*
The *total hemolytic complement* (THC or $CH_{50}$) measures the ability of a patient's serum to lyse 50% of a standard suspension of sheep erythrocytes coated with rabbit antibody. All nine components of the classic pathway are required to produce a normal reaction. The $CH_{50}$ screening test may be useful when a complement deficiency is suspected or a body fluid other than serum is involved. For patients with SLE and lupus nephritis, serial monitoring of $CH_{50}$ may be useful for guiding effectiveness of drug therapy.

### C3 and C4

*Reference ranges: C3, 80 to 160 mg/dL or 0.8 to 1.6 g/L; C4, 16 to 48 mg/dL or 0.16 to 0.48 g/L*
Because C3 is the most abundant complement protein, it was the first to be purified and measured by immunoassay. However, C4 concentrations appear to be more sensitive to smaller changes in complement activation and more specific for identifying complement activation by the classic pathway. Results of C3 and C4 testing are helpful in following patients who initially present with low levels and then undergo treatment, such as those with SLE.

## Acute-Phase Reactants

The concentration of a heterogeneous group of plasma proteins, called *acute-phase proteins* or *acute-phase reactants*, increases in response to inflammatory stimuli such as tissue injury and infection. Concentrations of CRP, serum amyloid A protein, $\alpha_1$-acid glycoprotein, $\alpha_1$-antitrypsin, fibrinogen, haptoglobin, ferritin, and complement characteristically increase, whereas serum transferrin, albumin, and prealbumin (transthyretin) concentrations decrease. Their collective change is referred to as the *acute-phase response*.

In general, if the inflammatory stimulus is acute and of short duration, these proteins return to normal within days to weeks. However, if tissue injury or infection is persistent, acute-phase changes may also persist. Additionally, white blood cell (WBC) and platelet counts may be elevated significantly.

Rheumatic diseases are chronic and associated with varying severities of inflammation. The ESR and CRP are two tests that can be helpful in three ways: (1) estimating the extent or severity of inflammation, (2) monitoring disease activity over time, and (3) assessing prognosis.[13] Unfortunately, both tests are nonspecific and cannot be used to confirm or exclude any particular diagnosis. However, the results may be helpful in RA, for example, for inclusion in an assessment of a patient's overall disease activity (ie, disease activity score - 28) and subsequent treatment modifications.

### Erythrocyte Sedimentation Rate

*Reference range (Westergren method): men, 0 to 15 mm/hr; women, 0 to 20 mm/hr*
For many years, the *erythrocyte sedimentation rate* (ESR) has been used widely as a reflection of the acute-phase response and inflammation. The test is performed by placing anticoagulated blood in a vertical tube and measuring the rate of fall of erythrocytes in millimeters/hour. In rheumatic diseases, the ESR is an indirect screen for elevated concentrations of acute-phase plasma proteins, especially fibrinogen.[13] An elevated ESR occurs when elevated protein concentrations (especially fibrinogen) cause aggregation of erythrocytes, resulting in a faster fall of those cells in the tube.

Several factors unrelated to inflammation may result in an increased ESR, such as obesity and increasing age. The ESR also responds slowly to an inflammatory stimulus. Despite these limitations, the test remains in wide use because it is inexpensive and easy to perform, and a tremendous amount of data are available about its clinical significance in numerous diseases. The Westergren method of performing an ESR test is preferred over the Wintrobe method because of the relative ease of performing the former method in clinical or laboratory settings.

Correlation of serial Westergren ESR results with patient data may influence therapeutic decisions. Two rheumatic diseases, polymyalgia rheumatica and temporal arteritis (giant cell arteritis), are almost always associated with an elevated Westergren ESR. The ESR is usually >60 mm/hr but can be markedly elevated >100 mm/hr in these disorders. During initial therapy or treatment initiated after a disease flare, a significant decrease or a return to a normal ESR usually indicates that systemic inflammation has decreased substantially. In the absence of clinical symptoms, an increased ESR may indicate that more aggressive therapy is needed. Disease activity can then be monitored by ESR results. Of course, if symptoms are present, they should be treated.

### C-Reactive Protein

*Reference range: 0 to 0.5 mg/dL or 0 to 0.005 g/L*
*C-reactive protein* (CRP) is a plasma protein of the acute-phase response. In response to a stimulus such as injury or infection, CRP can increase up to 1,000 times its baseline concentration. The precise physiologic function of CRP is unknown, but it is known to participate in activation of the classic complement pathway and interact with cells in the immune system.

Serum CRP levels can be quantitated accurately and inexpensively by immunoassay or laser nephelometry. Most healthy adults have concentrations of <0.3 mg/dL, although concentrations of 1 mg/dL are sometimes seen. Moderate increases range from 1 to 10 mg/dL, and marked increases are >10 mg/dL.[13] Values >15 to 20 mg/dL are usually associated with bacterial infections. In general, concentrations >1 mg/dL reflect the presence of a significant inflammatory process. As with the Westergren ESR, serial measurements of CRP are the most valuable, especially in chronic inflammatory diseases.

Currently, the routine use of CRP for the assessment of rheumatic diseases is limited. As with the ESR, CRP concentrations generally increase and decrease with worsening and improving signs and symptoms, respectively. Nevertheless, CRP concentrations are not specific for any disease.

Using an assay method called *high-sensitivity CRP (hs-CRP)*, several studies have shown a correlation between elevated levels and cardiovascular events, including myocardial infarction. The units of measurement for the hs-CRP (milligrams/liter) are different from those of the conventional CRP test (milligrams/deciliter). Because CRP levels fluctuate over time, when the hs-CRP is used for cardiovascular risk assessment, the test should be measured twice at least 2 weeks apart and the two values averaged.[14]

### Human Leukocyte Antigen B27

*Human leukocyte antigen B27* (HLA-B27) is an antigen on the surface of WBCs encoded by the B locus in the major histocompatibility complex on chromosome 6. The HLA-B27 test is qualitative and is either present or absent. Its presence is associated with autoimmune diseases known as *seronegative spondyloarthropathies*. An HLA-B27 test may be ordered when a patient has pain and inflammation in the spine, neck, chest, eyes, or joints and an autoimmune disorder associated with the presence of HLA-B27 is the suspected cause. The test may be obtained to confirm a suspected diagnosis of ankylosing spondylitis, Reiter syndrome, or anterior uveitis. However, a positive test result cannot distinguish among these diseases and cannot be used

to predict progression, severity, prognosis, or degree of organ involvement. Some patients with these disorders may have a negative HLA-B27 test. Further, the test cannot definitively diagnose or exclude any rheumatic disease. It is frequently ordered in concert with other rheumatic tests (eg, RF, ESR, CRP), based on the clinical presentation.

A positive HLA-B27 in a person without symptoms or a family history of HLA-B27–associated disease is not clinically significant and in this case does not predict the likelihood of developing an autoimmune disease. However, the presence or absence of HLA antigens can be genetic. For example, it does not help predict the likelihood of developing an autoimmune disease. The presence or absence of HLA antigens is genetically determined. If a family member has an HLA-B27–related rheumatic disease, other family members who share the HLA-B27 antigen have a higher risk of developing a similar disease. Individuals who already know they are HLA-B27 positive may wish to seek genetic counseling to understand the hereditary impact on their family.

New genetic testing methods permit separation of HLA-B27 into subtypes. Approximately 15 subtypes have been identified, the most common of which are HLA-B*2705 and HLA-B*2702. The precise clinical significance of individual subtypes is an area of continuing investigation.[15]

## Synovial Fluid Analysis

*Synovial fluid* is essentially an ultrafiltrate of plasma to which synovial lining cells add hyaluronate. This fluid lubricates and nourishes the avascular articular cartilage. Normally, synovial fluid is present in small amounts and is clear and acellular (<200 cells/mm³) with a high viscosity because of the hyaluronic acid concentration. Normal fluid does not clot because fibrinogen and clotting factors do not enter the joint space from the vascular space. Protein concentration is approximately one-third that of plasma, and glucose concentration is similar to that of plasma.

When performing arthrocentesis (joint aspiration), a needle is introduced into the joint space of a diarthrodial joint. With a syringe, all easily removed synovial fluid is drained from the joint space. Arthrocentesis is indicated as a diagnostic procedure when septic arthritis, hemarthrosis (bleeding into a joint space), or crystal-induced arthritis is suspected. Furthermore, arthrocentesis may be indicated in any clinical situation, rheumatic or nonrheumatic, if the cause of new or increased joint inflammation is unknown. Arthrocentesis is also performed to administer intraarticular corticosteroids.

When arthrocentesis is performed, the synovium may be inflamed, allowing fibrinogen, clotting factors, and other proteins to diffuse into the joint. Therefore, the collected synovial fluid should be placed in heparinized tubes to prevent clotting and allow determination of cell type and cell number. If diagnostic arthrocentesis is indicated, the aspirated joint fluid should be analyzed for volume, clarity, color, viscosity, cell count, culture, glucose, and protein. Synovial fluid is subsequently reported as normal, noninflammatory, inflammatory, or septic.[16] **Table 20-3** presents the characteristics of normal and three pathologic types of synovial fluid. The presence and type of crystals in the fluid

**TABLE 20-3.** Synovial Fluid Characteristics and Classification

| CHARACTERISTIC | NORMAL | NONINFLAMMATORY | INFLAMMATORY | SEPTIC |
|---|---|---|---|---|
| Viscosity | High | High | Low | Variable |
| Color | Colorless to straw | Straw to yellow | Yellow | Variable |
| Clarity | Translucent | Translucent | Translucent–opaque | Opaque |
| WBC (/mm³) | <200 | 200–3,000 | 2,000–50,000 | >50,000 |
| PMN | <10% | <10% | Often >50% | >75% |
| Culture | Negative | Negative | Negative | Often positive |
| Glucose (a.m. fasting) | ≅ blood | ≅ blood | >25 mg/dL but lower than blood | <25 mg/dL (much lower than blood) |
| Protein (g/dL) | 1–2 | 1–3 | 3–5 | 3–5 |

PMN = polymorphonuclear neutrophils; WBC = white blood cells.

**TABLE 20-4.** Morphology of Synovial Fluid Crystals Associated with Joint Disease

| CRYSTALS | SIZE (μm) | MORPHOLOGY | BIREFRINGENCE[a] | DISEASES |
|---|---|---|---|---|
| Monosodium urate | 2–10 | Needles, rods | Negative | Gout |
| CPPD | 2–10 | Rhomboids, rods | Positive (weak) | CPPD crystal deposition disease (pseudogout), OA |
| Calcium oxalate | 2–10 | Polymorphic, dipyramidal shapes | Positive | Renal failure |
| Cholesterol | 10–80 | Rectangles with notched corners; needles | Negative or positive | Chronic rheumatoid or osteoarthritic effusions |
| Depot corticosteroids | 4–15 | Irregular rods, rhomboids | Negative or positive | Iatrogenic postinjection flare |

CPPD = calcium pyrophosphate dihydrate.
[a]The property of birefringence is the ability of crystals to pass light in a particular plane. When viewed under polarized light, the crystals are brightly visible in one plane (birefringent) but are dark in a plane turned 90°. Birefringence observed under polarized light can be categorized as "positive" and "negative" based on the speed at which rays of light travel through the crystals in perpendicular planes (at right angles).

should be determined. The presence of crystals identified by polarized light microscopy with red compensation can be diagnostic (**Table 20-4**) (**Minicase 1**).

## Nonrheumatic Tests

The three most commonly performed groups of nonrheumatic tests performed in rheumatology are the *complete blood count* (CBC), *serum chemistry panel*, and *urinalysis*. These tests are not specific for any rheumatic disorder, and abnormal results may occur in association with many rheumatic and nonrheumatic diseases. These tests are discussed from a more general perspective in other chapters.

Chronic inflammatory diseases such as RA and SLE are commonly associated with anemia. Microcytic anemia may occur as a result of drug therapy for rheumatic diseases (eg, gastroduodenal hemorrhage from nonsteroidal anti-inflammatory drugs [NSAIDs]). Autoimmune hemolytic anemia may be seen in SLE and other rheumatic diseases and is associated with a rapid onset that may be life threatening. The platelet count may be elevated in some disorders (thrombocytosis) and decreased in others (thrombocytopenia). Leukopenia may be associated with Felty syndrome and may also be caused by therapy with immunosuppressive agents used to treat rheumatic diseases. For example, thrombocytopenia and leukopenia may be seen in cases of SLE.

Antiphospholipid syndrome may be seen with SLE and other disorders and is associated with abnormalities in coagulation. Patients with antiphospholipid antibodies should be evaluated further to determine thrombosis risk.

Systemic lupus erythematosus may be associated with hepatic dysfunction, which can be assessed by determination of hepatic lab tests. Some drugs used in the treatment of

## MINICASE 1

### Assessment of Synovial Fluid

A 45-year-old woman presents to her physician with reports of pain and swelling in her hands and feet over the last 8 weeks. Physical examination reveals swollen and tender joints bilaterally and limited ability to close a fist or move her thumbs. She reports that she wakes up with stiff joints and it usually takes 60 to 90 minutes until she can use her hands effectively, sometimes longer. The synovial fluid from one swollen joint is aspirated. The aspirate, noted to be thin, cloudy, and yellow, is sent in heparinized tubes to the laboratory for Gram stain, bacterial culture, cell count, and chemistry panel. After receiving the pathology report, the physician reviews the preliminary laboratory results of the aspirate (refer to Table 20-3 for reference values):

- 45,000 WBCs/mm$^3$
- 75% PMNs
- 23 mg/dL glucose
- 4.5 g/dL protein
- Culture, negative

QUESTION: What is the likely diagnosis in this patient? What additional laboratory studies should be performed?

DISCUSSION: Based on physician observations and the pathology report, the aspirate appears to be inflammatory because the viscosity is low, the clarity is not translucent, and an infection is not present. Considered with the patient's age, gender, joint presentation (bilateral, small joints), and stiffness that lasts for 60 minutes or more, the likely diagnosis is rheumatoid arthritis.

Additional testing should be considered to confirm a diagnosis of RA—specifically, ACPA, RF, and acute-phase reactants (ESR, CRP). Baseline CBC, chemistry panels, and assessment of renal and hepatic function should be conducted if recent results are not available. ACPA is especially helpful because it is the most specific for RA. In addition to confirming the diagnosis, a positive ACPA result, if present, is also indicative of more erosive disease and worse long-term prognosis. An early diagnosis allows aggressive treatment to be initiated with the goal of controlling systemic inflammation and slowing or stopping the erosions. RF alone is not specific enough to indicate a diagnosis of RA, but when combined with ACPA, the specificity of diagnosis, if both are positive, increases to 99.5%. The results of ESR and CRP are not specific to RA, but they provide information about the ongoing inflammation. The results are also helpful while the physician is evaluating the disease activity. The remaining test results are helpful for understanding the baseline status of the patient and determining treatment options that are safe for her to receive.

---

rheumatic disease may also cause hepatic injury. Renal function tests (usually the serum creatinine [SCr] and blood urea nitrogen [BUN]) may provide evidence of renal involvement in patients with lupus nephritis. Proteinuria, hematuria, and pyuria may be seen in cases of SLE and with use of drugs to treat rheumatic disorders.

## INTERPRETATION OF LABORATORY TESTS IN SELECT RHEUMATIC DISEASES

### Rheumatoid Arthritis in Adults

In 2010, the American College of Rheumatology (ACR) and the European League Against Rheumatism (EULAR) published new classification criteria for RA.[17] The criteria were developed to help define homogeneous treatment populations for research trials, not for clinical diagnosis. In practice, the clinician must establish the diagnosis for an individual patient using many more aspects (including perhaps some additional laboratory tests) based on the clinical presentation. Nevertheless, the formal classification criteria are useful as a general guide to making a clinical diagnosis. The 2010 criteria are aimed at diagnosing RA earlier in newly presenting patients so patients can be started on treatment sooner, with the goal of preventing erosive joint damage and improving long-term outcomes. Patients with erosive disease typical of RA and those with longstanding disease (including patients whose disease is inactive with or without treatment) should also be classified as having RA if they previously fulfilled the 2010 criteria.[17]

Two mandatory criteria must be met before the classification criteria can be applied to an individual patient. First, there must be evidence of definite clinical synovitis in at least one joint as determined by an expert assessor; the distal interphalangeal joints, first carpometacarpal joints, and first metatarsophalangeal joints are excluded from consideration because these joints are usually involved in osteoarthritis (OA). Second, the synovitis cannot be better explained by another disease such as SLE, psoriatic arthritis, or gout. When these two criteria are met, classification of definite RA is based on achieving a score of 6 or more out of 10 points in four domains:

1. Joint distribution

    1 large joint (shoulder, elbow, hip, knee, ankle) = 0 points

    2 to 10 large joints = 1 point

    1 to 3 small joints (metacarpophalangeal joints, proximal interphalangeal joints, second to fifth metatarsophalangeal joints, thumb interphalangeal joints, wrists) = 2 points

    4 to 10 small joints = 3 points

    – More than 10 joints (with at least 1 small joint) = 5 points

2. Serology

    Negative RF and ACPA = 0 points

    Low-positive RF or ACPA = 2 points

    High-positive RF or ACPA = 3 points

3. Acute-phase reactants
   Normal CRP and ESR = 0 points
   Elevated CRP or ESR = 1 point
4. Symptom duration (by patient report)
   Less than 6 weeks = 0 points
   6 weeks or more = 1 point

Patients who do not achieve a score of 6 or higher should be regularly reassessed because they may meet the classification criteria cumulatively over time.

### Anticitrullinated Protein Antibodies

Patients with a diagnosis of RA should be treated aggressively early in the disease course because in 90% of patients most damage from bone erosions occurs within the first 2 years. For this reason, a timely and accurate early diagnosis is critical. Many patients with early RA have mild, nonspecific symptoms; in these cases, the ability to detect a disease-specific antibody such as ACPA could be of crucial diagnostic and therapeutic importance.

The ACPA test has several useful characteristics as a marker for RA diagnosis and prognosis: (1) it is as sensitive as RF and more specific than RF for RA in patients with early as well as fully established disease; (2) it may be detectable in seemingly healthy persons years before the onset of clinical RA findings; (3) it may predict the future development of RA in patients with undifferentiated arthritis; and (4) it is a predictor for the eventual development of erosive disease. As stated previously, ACPAs can be detected in about 50% to 60% of patients with early RA, usually after having nonspecific symptoms for 3 to 6 months prior to seeing a physician.

In some patients with nonspecific arthritis, it is difficult to make a definitive diagnosis of RA because of the lack of disease-specific serum markers for other conditions in the differential diagnosis. In some situations, the presence of ACPAs may help differentiate RA from polymyalgia rheumatica or erosive forms of SLE.[3]

Several reports suggest that patients with early RA who are ACPA positive develop more erosive disease than those who are antibody-negative.[3] Early identification of patients who are at risk for a more severe disease course could lead to more rapid and aggressive institution of disease-modifying therapies. However, clinical trials are needed to determine whether this diagnostic and therapeutic approach is indeed beneficial.

### Rheumatoid Factor

In patients with RA, affected diarthrodial joints have an inflamed and proliferating synovium infiltrated with T lymphocytes and plasma cells. Plasma cells in the synovial fluid generate large amounts of IgG RF and abnormally low amounts of normal IgG. However, plasma cells in the bloodstream of patients with RA produce IgM RF predominantly.[2]

Approximately 75% to 80% of adults with RA have a positive RF titer, and most of those who are positive have titers of at least 1:320. A positive RF is not specific for the diagnosis of RA. Positive RF titers are also associated with some connective disease, such as SLE and Sjögren syndrome. RF levels may also be increased in some infections (eg, malaria, rubella, hepatitis C). Furthermore, up to 5% of the normal healthy population may be RF positive. Patients with RA generally have higher RF titers than individuals with other nonrheumatic conditions. In patients who have RA and a positive RF, the titer generally increases as disease activity (inflammation) increases. Consequently, as the serum RF titer increases, the specificity of the test for the diagnosis of RA also increases.[2] Higher titers or serum concentrations suggest the presence of more severe disease than lower levels and are associated with a worse prognosis.

Rheumatoid factor is one of the two serologic tests (along with ACPA) included in the 2010 ACR/EULAR classification criteria for RA.[17] Based on the reporting of RF levels in International Units/milliliter, a *negative* RF is considered to be less than or equal to the ULN for the laboratory and assay. A *low-positive* test is higher than the ULN but less than or equal to three times the ULN. A *high-positive* test is more than three times the ULN for the assay. When the RF is reported as only positive or negative by the laboratory, patients reported as having a positive RF should be scored as "low-positive" for RF scoring purposes.[17]

Although RFs are usually identified and quantified from serum samples, RA is a systemic, extravascular, autoimmune disease affecting the synovium. As a result, some RFs may be present in sites other than peripheral blood. IgG RFs are found in the synovial fluid of many patients with severe RA. IgA RF may be detected in the saliva of patients with RA or Sjögren syndrome. The presence of IgE RF is correlated with extraarticular findings of RA.[2]

Although most patients with RA are seropositive for RF, some patients have negative titers. However, some of these patients may have non-IgM RF, predominantly IgG RF. Also, some seronegative patients convert to seropositive on repeat testing. A small percentage of adult patients with RA (<10%) are considered to be truly seronegative. When compared with RF-positive patients, seronegative patients usually have milder arthritis and are less likely to develop extraarticular manifestations (eg, rheumatoid nodules, lung disease, and vasculitis).

Because current treatment guidelines call for aggressive early treatment of RA—before end-organ damage—clinicians must be aware of the relationship between disease onset and RF development. Unfortunately, the RF test is least likely to be positive at the onset of RA, when it might be of the most help. After RA has been diagnosed, RF titers are not routinely used to assess a patient's current clinical status or modify a therapeutic regimen. A specific titer or a change in titers for an individual does not correlate reliably with disease activity.

In summary, RF is not sensitive or specific enough to use as the sole laboratory test to diagnose or manage RA. Although it is present in msot patients with RA, it is negative in some patients with the disease. RF may be useful as a prognostic indicator, because patients with RA with high RF titers generally have a more severe disease course.

### Antinuclear Antibodies

Antinuclear antibodies are usually negative in patients with RA. The frequency of positive ANAs in patients with RA is highly variable. As determined by indirect immunofluorescence, this frequency varies from 10% to 70%, depending on the substrate used and the titer considered positive. In patients with a positive ANA, tests for dsDNA and Sm antibodies should be performed because these tests are highly specific for SLE.

### Complement

The serum complement level is usually normal or elevated in RA. Complement elevations often occur as part of the acute-phase response. These increases parallel changes in other acute-phase proteins (eg, CRP). Elevations of total hemolytic activity (CH$_{50}$), C3, and C4 are usually observed during active stages of most rheumatic diseases, including RA. The presence of circulating immune complexes in RA may lead to hypercatabolism of complement and acquired hypocomplementemia.

### Acute Phase Reactants

As in other inflammatory diseases, the nonspecific ESR test is usually elevated in active RA. The degree of elevation is directly related to the severity of inflammation; the Westergren ESR can be 50 to 80 mm/hr or more in patients with severely active RA. It usually decreases or normalizes when systemic inflammation decreases during initial treatment or after treatment for a disease flare. However, there is a large variability in response to treatment among individuals. Subsequent increases in disease activity will be mirrored by corresponding increases in ESR.

C-reactive protein levels may be elevated (approximately 2 to 3 mg/dL) in adult patients with RA with moderate disease activity. However, there is substantial individual variability, and 5% to 10% of such patients have normal values. Some patients with severe disease activity have levels of 14 mg/dL or higher.

Because of their nonspecificity, the ESR and CRP are of little use in distinguishing between RA and other rheumatic diseases, such as OA or mild SLE. The tests also are elevated in patients with vasculitis associated with RA and reflect the generalized systemic inflammatory state. These tests are more appropriate for monitoring disease activity in RA. Elevations of ESR and CRP are individually associated with radiologic damage in RA as assessed by the number of joint erosions. Elevation of both ESR and CRP is a stronger predictor of radiologic progression than an elevation in CRP alone.[18,19]

### Synovial Fluid Analysis

If a joint effusion is present and the diagnosis is uncertain, arthrocentesis and *synovial fluid analysis* are performed to exclude gout, pseudogout, or infectious arthritis.[18] Synovial fluid analysis should include WBC count with differential, analysis for crystals, and Gram stain and culture. In early RA, the analysis typically reveals straw-colored, turbid fluid with fibrin fragments. A clot forms if the fluid is left standing at room temperature. There are usually 5,000 to 25,000 WBC/mm$^3$, at least 85% of which are polymorphonuclear neutrophils (PMN). Complement C4 and C2 levels are usually slightly decreased, but the C3 level is generally normal. The glucose level is decreased, sometimes to <25 mg/dL. No crystals should be present, and cultures should be negative.

### Nonrheumatic Tests

The CBC may reveal an anemia that is either normochromic-normocytic or hypochromic-microcytic. Microcytic anemia

is due to iron deficiency that may result from gastrointestinal blood loss associated with drug use (eg, NSAIDs) or other causes. The WBC count may show a slight leukocytosis with a normal differential. Eosinophilia (>5% of the total WBC count) may be associated with RF-positive severe RA. Felty syndrome may be associated with granulocytopenia. Thrombocytosis may be present in clinically active RA as part of the acute-phase response. As the disease improves spontaneously or as a result of drug therapy, the platelet count returns toward normal.

## Osteoarthritis

*Osteoarthritis* (OA) results from the complex interplay of numerous factors, such as joint integrity, genetics, mechanical forces, local inflammation, and biochemical processes.[20,21] It is generally considered to be a noninflammatory arthritis; however, inflammation may be present. It is not considered an autoimmune disease. The synovium is normal, and the synovial fluid usually lacks inflammatory cells. Although affected joints are painful, they are frequently not inflamed. The primary use of laboratory tests when OA is suspected is to rule out other disorders in the differential diagnosis.

No clinical laboratory tests are specific for the diagnosis of OA. Laboratory tests that may be performed in patients suspected of having OA include ESR, RF titers, and evaluation of synovial fluid.[21] The ESR (and CRP) is usually normal but may be slightly increased if inflammation is present. The RF test is negative, and serum chemistries, hematology tests, and urinalysis are normal. Research is underway to determine if certain biomarkers (ie, CRP), if elevated, correlate with disease activity or radiographic progression.

Synovial fluid analysis may be undertaken, especially in patients with severe, acute joint pain. Findings generally reveal either a noninflammatory process or mild inflammation (WBC <2,000 cells/mm$^3$). Crystals are absent when the synovial fluid is examined using compensated polarized light microscopy (**Minicase 2**).

## Juvenile Idiopathic Arthritis

The term *juvenile idiopathic arthritis* (JIA) encompasses a heterogeneous group of childhood arthritis conditions of unknown cause. Because JIA includes a variety of arthritis categories that differ from adult-onset RA, the term JIA has replaced the name *juvenile rheumatoid arthritis*.[22] Juvenile idiopathic arthritis begins before 16 years of age and persists for at least 6 weeks; other known causes must be excluded before the diagnosis of JIA can be made. Juvenile idiopathic arthritis is divided into categories based on presenting clinical and laboratory findings: (1) systemic arthritis, (2) oligoarthritis, (3) polyarthritis (RF negative), (4) polyarthritis (RF positive), (5) psoriatic arthritis, (6) enthesitis-related arthritis, and (7) undifferentiated arthritis.[22-25]

The diagnosis of JIA is made primarily on clinical grounds. No single laboratory test or combination of tests can confirm the diagnosis. However, laboratory tests can be useful in providing evidence of inflammation, supporting the clinical diagnosis, and monitoring toxicity from therapy.

## MINICASE 2

### Evaluation of Arthritis

A 62-year-old postmenopausal woman presents to her family physician with reports of pain and stiffness in her knees for the last month. She notes the pain is worse in the morning when she wakes up and resolves about 20 minutes later. Her past medical history is significant for hypertension and dyslipidemia for approximately 5 years. She quit smoking 1 year ago following a 20 pack-per-year smoking history. She started a diet (low fat, low sodium) and exercise (walking 30 minutes daily) program about 2 months ago. On physical exam, no swelling or tenderness is found in her knees. Significant crepitus and decreased range of motion are noted. No additional joints appear to be affected. Current medications (stable for the past 6 months) include lisinopril, hydrochlorothiazide, atorvastatin, and one aspirin tablet a day. She is allergic to sulfa and intolerant to penicillin (stomach upset). She started taking ibuprofen about 1 month ago in response to the joint pain.

Laboratory results obtained at this visit:

- RF titer 10 International Units/mL
- ACPA 10 EU
- ANA 1:40

- ESR 15 mm/hr
- CRP 0.3 mg/dL

QUESTIONS: What are two likely diagnoses, which one is most likely, and what data support that diagnosis?

DISCUSSION: The two most common causes of joint pain and stiffness include OA and RA. Upon initial presentation, either may be a possibility. The physical exam findings are key to identifying joints that are typically affected by RA versus OA. Morning stiffness is a common symptom of either condition; however, morning stiffness associated with OA typically lasts for less than 30 minutes, whereas stiffness associated with RA lasts an hour or more. The laboratory results are also helpful in distinguishing between the two conditions. First, OA does not involve systemic inflammation, so it is unlikely to cause elevated acute-phase reactants (ESR and CRP). Second, RF is negative; however, the presence of positive RF is not specific for a diagnosis of RA. Finally, ACPA is sensitive and specific for RA, and the result is negative. The clinical presentation (ie, large joints, no inflammation, joint stiffness that resolves in less than 30 minutes) and the normal/negative lab results indicate the patient is experiencing OA.

### Rheumatoid Factor

Rheumatoid factor–positive polyarthritis constitutes 5% to 10% of JIA cases and is the childhood arthritis that is most similar to adult RA. It is defined as arthritis affecting five or more joints in the first 6 months of disease with a positive RF test on two occasions at least 3 months apart.[22] RF-positive polyarthritis is six to 12 times more common in girls than boys. As in adult RA, the RF test usually detects IgM-anti-IgG. RF-negative polyarthritis constitutes 20% to 30% of new JIA cases. It also includes arthritis in five or more joints during the first 6 months, but the RF test is negative. Although the presence of RF overall is low in JIA, its presence indicates more aggressive disease.

Oligoarthritis is the most common form of JIA; it is four times more common in girls than boys and has a peak onset before the age of 6 years. Oligoarthritis affects four or fewer joints in the first 6 months; the RF test is usually negative. The RF is negative in systemic arthritis, psoriatic arthritis, enthesitis-related arthritis, and undifferentiated arthritis.[22]

### Anticitrullinated Protein Antibodies

The APCA test alone is not helpful in diagnosing a subcategory of JIA. This is consistent with the fact that JIA is a heterogeneous group of disorders, most of which are different from adult RA. Similar to RA in adults, positive ACPA results in JIA have been associated with RF-positive disease and erosive arthritis.[22] Approximately 60% to 70% of patients with RF-positive polyarthritis are ACPA positive. Approximately 50% to 80% of patients with RF-negative polyarthritis are ACPA positive.[22]

### Antinuclear Antibodies

In oligoarthritis, 70% to 80% of children have positive (low to moderate titer) ANA tests, typically 1:40 to 1:320. ANA positivity is high in girls with an early onset of disease. Although ANA is not useful for monitoring or predicting a patient's disease or symptoms, it is helpful to determine risk for developing uveitis. Patients diagnosed with oligo- or polyarticular arthritis at an early age who are ANA positive are at a higher risk of uveitis. This is especially important because a patient may be asymptomatic and thereby undiagnosed and untreated, potentially leading to permanent vision loss. The ANA test is positive in 40% of patients with RF-negative polyarthritis and positive in up to 55% of patients with RF-positive polyarthritis. The ANA is positive in about 15% to 20% of children with psoriatic arthritis. It may be positive in some patients with enthesitis-related arthritis. The test result is seldom positive (<10%) in children with systemic JIA.

### Complement

As with adult-onset RA, serum complement components (especially C3) are usually elevated in systemic JIA.

### Acute-Phase Reactants

In systemic arthritis, the ESR and CRP are typically high during an acute flare. In oligoarthritis, there is little systemic inflammation, and the ESR and CRP are usually normal. Some cases of oligoarthritis may be associated with mildly or moderately elevated ESR or CRP; however, elevated acute-phase reactants in this category should raise suspicion for other conditions, such as subclinical inflammatory bowel disease associated with arthropathy. Acute-phase reactants may be elevated in either

RF-positive or RF-negative polyarthritis and in psoriatic arthritis. The ESR may be elevated in enthesitis-related arthritis, but this abnormality should raise suspicion for subclinical inflammatory bowel disease. Acute-phase reactants are typically mildly elevated in patients with the psoriatic arthritis subcategory of JIA.

### Synovial Fluid Analysis

Arthrocentesis in JIA is typically consistent with inflammatory fluid. As in adult RA, synovial fluid glucose levels are low.

### Nonrheumatic Tests

Children with systemic arthritis may have anemia, leukocytosis with neutrophilia, and thrombocytosis. The anemia is normochromic-normocytic (anemia of chronic disease); hemoglobin values may be in the range of 7 to 10 g/dL. WBC counts in the range of 20,000 to 30,000 cells/mm$^3$ are not uncommon, and counts may exceed 60,000 to 80,000 cells/mm$^3$. In severe cases, liver enzymes, ferritin, and coagulation screen also may be abnormal. Patients with enthesitis-related or psoriatic arthritis may have a mild anemia of chronic disease.

## Systemic Lupus Erythematosus

Criteria for the classification of *systemic lupus erythematosus* (SLE) were updated by the EULAR and ACR in 2019. The criteria were updated to address shortcomings of previous criteria, including a need to improve sensitivity and specificity of the criteria and earlier detection of patients with early disease for inclusion in research trials. The wide variety of manifestations and unpredictable course often make SLE difficult to diagnose.

According to the new classification criteria, the first criterion that must be met is a positive ANA at a titer of ≥ 1:80. This is a significant change from previous criteria and the expert panel recommends further research into the very small group of patients that are ANA-negative and displaying symptoms similar to SLE. The new criteria include clinical domains (ie, hematologic, mucocutaneous, musculoskeletal, renal) and immunology domains (ie, antiphospholipid antibodies, SLE-specific antibodies). The classification criteria now follow a weighed system whereby clinical and immunologic features are given higher weighting to align with their significance. The weighting ranges from 2 to 10. A patient's presentation is classified as SLE if 10 or more points are scored across all domains and at least one clinical criterion is present. When the criteria were applied to a cohort for validation purposes, the sensitivity slightly decreased to 96.1% and specificity increased to 93.4% when compared with previous criteria, 96.7% and 83.7%, respectively.[26,27]

### Antinuclear Antibodies

Antinuclear antibody testing is usually performed initially if SLE is suspected because of its high sensitivity and ease of use. To be considered in the classification criteria, a patient must pass the entry criterion, which is a positive ANA (titer ≥1:80). The ANA test has low specificity for SLE; many other conditions are associated with a positive test result (eg, systemic sclerosis, polymyositis, dermatomyositis, RA, autoimmune thyroiditis or hepatitis, infections, malignancies, and many drugs). Some healthy persons also may have a positive ANA test result. Consequently, results of an ANA test are always interpreted in light of a patient's clinical presentation.

***Anti-dsDNA and anti-ssDNA antibodies.*** The *anti–double-stranded DNA* (anti-dsDNA) test is positive in 50% to 60% of patients with SLE at some point in the disease course, and the test is 95% specific for SLE. In contrast, testing for antibodies to single-stranded DNA (anti-ssDNA) has poor specificity for SLE but is more sensitive (90%). Although the anti-ssDNA antibody appears to be important in the immunopathogenesis of SLE, the test has little diagnostic utility because of poor specificity. There is evidence that anti-dsDNA and anti-ssDNA antibodies are important in the pathogenesis of lupus nephritis because they appear to correlate with its presence and severity. Titers of these antibodies tend to fall with successful treatment, frequently becoming undetectable during sustained remission.

### Anti-Sm, Anti-Ro/SSA, and Anti-La/SSB Antibodies

The *anti-Sm* antibody is an immunoglobulin specific against Sm, a ribonucleoprotein found in the cell nucleus. The anti-Sm antibody test is positive in 20% to 30% of patients with SLE, and presence of these antibodies is pathognomonic for SLE.[26] *Anti-Ro/SSA* and *anti-La/SSB* antibodies are present in 30% and 20% of patients with SLE, respectively, but they are not specific for the disease.

### Complement

Total CH$_{50}$ levels are decreased at some point in most patients with SLE. Complement levels decrease in SLE because of deposition of immune complexes in active disease (hypercatabolism). Complement depletion has been associated with increased disease severity, particularly renal disease. Analysis of various complement components has revealed low levels of C1, C4, C2, and C3. Serial determinations have demonstrated that decreased levels may precede clinical exacerbations.[11] As acute episodes subside, levels return toward normal. Some experts consider it helpful to follow complement measurements in SLE patients receiving treatment, especially if C4 and C3 were low at the time of diagnosis.[11]

### Acute-Phase Reactants

Serum ESR and CRP concentrations are elevated in many patients with active SLE, but many individuals have normal CRP levels. Those with acute serositis or chronic synovitis are most likely to have markedly elevated CRP levels. Patients with other findings of SLE, such as lupus nephritis, may have modest or no elevations.

Several studies have examined the hypothesis that elevations in CRP during the course of SLE result from superimposed infection rather than activation of SLE. In hospitalized patients, substantially elevated serum CRP levels occur most frequently in the setting of bacterial infection. Consequently, CRP elevations >6 to 8 mg/dL in patients with SLE (as well as other diseases) should signal the need to exclude the possibility of infection. Such CRP increases should not be considered proof of infection because CRP elevation can be related to active SLE in the absence of infection.

### Nonrheumatic Tests

*Antiphospholipid antibodies* (ie, anticardiolipin antibodies and the lupus anticoagulant) can occur as an idiopathic disorder and in patients with autoimmune and connective tissue diseases such as SLE.[28,29] Anticardiolipin antibody and the lupus anticoagulant are closely related but are different antibodies. Consequently, an individual can have one antibody and not the other. The presence of these antibodies may increase the risk of future thrombotic events. This clinical situation is referred to as *antiphospholipid syndrome* (APS). When APS occurs in patients with no other diagnosis, it is referred to as *primary APS*. Patients who also have SLE or another rheumatic disease are said to have secondary APS.

Anemia is present in many patients with SLE. The CBC may reveal a normochromic-normocytic anemia (anemia of chronic disease) that is not associated with erythropoietin deficiency. Hemolytic anemia with a compensatory reticulocytosis also may occur due to antierythrocyte antibodies. Most patients also have a positive Coombs test result. Anemia in SLE also can result from blood loss, renal insufficiency, medications, infection, hypersplenism, and other reasons.[30]

Leukopenia is present in approximately 50% of patients but is usually mild. It results primarily from decreased numbers of lymphocytes, which may be caused by the disease or its treatment. If the patient is not being treated with corticosteroids or immunosuppressive agents, ongoing immunologic activity should be suspected. Neutropenia in SLE may occur from immune mechanisms, medications, bone marrow suppression, or hypersplenism.[30] Mild thrombocytopenia (100,000 to 150,000/mm$^3$) occurs in 25% to 50% of patients with SLE and is usually due to immune-mediated platelet destruction. Increased platelet consumption and impaired platelet production also may be contributing factors.[30]

Liver function tests may reveal increased hepatic aminotransferases (AST, ALT), lactate dehydrogenase, and alkaline phosphatase in patients with active SLE. These elevations usually decrease as the disease improves with treatment. Urinalysis is important to screen and monitor for lupus nephritis. The current recommendation for protein assessment is to use a 12- or 24-hour urine collection to calculate the protein/creatinine ratio. Hematuria and pyuria also may occur. If lupus nephritis is suspected, a renal biopsy should be conducted to confirm diagnosis and determine the level of disease activity.

## Fibromyalgia

*Fibromyalgia* is a common syndrome associated with chronic widespread pain, fatigue, sleep disturbances, and other medical problems lasting for at least 3 months without another medical diagnostic explanation.[31] It is a challenging syndrome to categorize and treat. It may be comorbid with other conditions, thereby making the differential diagnosis challenging.

Laboratory testing should be used prudently when evaluating patients with clinical features suggestive of fibromyalgia. A satisfactory patient assessment is usually obtained by a careful medical history and physical examination and perhaps performance of routine laboratory tests, such as CBC and serum chemistry, to rule out other disorders. Serologic tests such as ANA titers are not usually necessary unless there is strong evidence of an autoimmune disorder. Once a diagnosis is made, there is no evidence that repeatedly checking laboratory testing provides value.

If the results of laboratory testing suggest a diagnosis other than fibromyalgia, a more directed evaluation is required. Individuals who actually have fibromyalgia are sometimes misdiagnosed with autoimmune disorders. This may be due to the common complaints of arthralgias, myalgias, fatigue, morning joint stiffness, and a history of swelling of the hands and feet. Conversely, patients with existing autoimmune diseases may suffer from symptoms suggestive of fibromyalgia.

## TESTS TO MONITOR DRUG THERAPY FOR SELECT RHEUMATIC DISORDERS

Pharmacotherapy for rheumatic diseases can cause significant adverse reactions that are reflected in laboratory test results.[32-34] Abnormal test results may necessitate dose reduction, temporary discontinuation, or permanent withdrawal of the offending drug. The laboratory tests most commonly affected are the WBC count, platelet count, hepatic aminotransferases, total bilirubin, SCr, BUN, and urinalysis (**Table 20-5**). An important part of a patient care plan is regular evaluation of the associated laboratory tests to ensure safety of the medication regimen. In addition, patients should be counseled to report any signs or symptoms of adverse reactions so the healthcare provider can determine if they are related to the medication regimen.

A common approach in treatment of rheumatic diseases is "treat to target." Once a patient is diagnosed with a rheumatic condition and a treatment regimen is determined, a timeframe for follow-up (eg, 1 month) should be established. This timeframe should also consider the time to see evidence of efficacy from the medication regimen. At the point of follow-up, the current disease activity should be evaluated. If the patient has moderate or high disease activity, the medication regimen should be adjusted to bring the disease activity under control. The target for most conditions is remission or, at a minimum, low disease activity. The medication regimen should be continually reevaluated and adjusted if the patient has not yet achieved the target of treatment.

For example, if a patient with RA is started on a regimen of methotrexate and etanercept, prior to initiating therapy, the following lab tests should be conducted: CBC with differential and platelet count, hepatic transferases, bilirubin, and serum albumin. A tuberculin skin test should be placed. Assuming all tests come back normal, the healthcare provider should follow up with the patient in 1 month to assess safety (repeat lab tests) and efficacy (assess disease activity) to determine if the treatment regimen of methotrexate and etanercept is still appropriate or if adjustment should be made. The patient should be counseled upon initiation of the medications to monitor for signs and symptoms of infection and contact the healthcare provider if they occur.

**TABLE 20-5.** Routine Laboratory Tests to Monitor Patients Receiving Select Drugs for Common Rheumatic Diseases

| DRUG | DISEASE | LABORATORY TEST | ADVERSE DRUG REACTION |
|---|---|---|---|
| Abatacept | RA | Baseline tuberculin skin test<br>CBC with differential and platelet count<br>Monitor for infection | Infection, sepsis |
| Allopurinol | Gout and hyperuricemia | CBC with differential and platelet count<br>Serum uric acid<br>Hepatic aminotransferases<br>BUN, SCr | Myelosuppression<br>Gout flare (monitor uric acid)<br>Hepatotoxicity<br>Nephrotoxicity |
| Anakinra | RA | CBC with differential and platelet count<br>Monitor for infection | Neutropenia<br>Infection, sepsis |
| Belimumab | SLE | Monitor for infection | Infection, sepsis |
| Colchicine | Gout and hyperuricemia | CBC with differential and platelet count<br>Hepatic aminotransferases<br>BUN, SCr | Myelosuppression<br>Elevated aminotransferases |
| Corticosteroids | RA, OA, SLE, gout flares | CBC with differential and platelet count<br>Serum sodium, potassium, bicarbonate<br>Serum calcium<br>Blood glucose<br>Fasting lipid panel<br>Urinalysis | Anemia due to peptic ulceration and blood loss<br>Electrolyte disturbances<br>Osteoporosis<br>Hyperglycemia<br>Dyslipidemia<br>Glycosuria |
| Febuxostat | Gout and hyperuricemia | Serum uric acid<br>Hepatic aminotransferases | Gout flare (monitor uric acid)<br>Elevated aminotransferases |
| Hydroxychloroquine | RA | CBC with differential and platelet count<br>Urinalysis | Thrombocytopenia<br>Proteinuria |
| JAK inhibitors (baricitinib, tofacitinib, upadacitinib) | RA | Baseline tuberculin skin test<br>CBC with differential and platelet count<br>Monitor for infection<br>Fasting lipid panel | Infection, sepsis<br>Hepatic enzyme elevations<br>Dyslipidemia |
| Leflunomide | RA | CBC with differential and platelet count<br>Hepatic aminotransferases, bilirubin | Pancytopenia<br>Elevated aminotransferases<br>Hepatic necrosis |
| Lesinurad | Gout and hyperuricemia | Serum uric acid<br>BUN, SCr | Gout flare (monitor uric acid) |
| Methotrexate | RA | CBC with differential and platelet count<br>Hepatic aminotransferases, bilirubin, serum albumin<br>Monitor for infection | Leukopenia<br>Pancytopenia<br>Hepatotoxicity<br>Infection, sepsis |
| Mycophenolate mofetil | SLE | CBC with differential and platelet count<br>Monitor for infection | Neutropenia, red cell aplasia<br>Opportunistic infections, sepsis |

*(continued)*

**TABLE 20-5.** Routine Laboratory Tests to Monitor Patients Receiving Select Drugs for Common Rheumatic Diseases, cont'd

| DRUG | DISEASE | LABORATORY TEST | ADVERSE DRUG REACTION |
|---|---|---|---|
| NSAIDs, including aspirin | RA, OA, SLE, gout flares | CBC with differential and platelet count<br>Hepatic aminotransferases<br>BUN, SCr<br>Sodium, potassium<br>Urinalysis | Anemia (due to gastroduodenal ulceration and blood loss)<br>Hepatotoxicity<br>Nephrotoxicity<br>Electrolyte disturbances<br>Proteinuria, hematuria, pyuria |
| Pegloticase | Gout and hyperuricemia | Serum uric acid | Gout flare (monitor uric acid) |
| Probenecid | Gout and hyperuricemia | Serum uric acid<br>BUN, SCr | Gout flare (monitor uric acid) |
| Rituximab | RA | CBC with differential and platelet count<br>Monitor for infection | Infection, sepsis |
| Sulfasalazine | RA | CBC with differential and platelet count<br>Hepatic aminotransferases | Leukopenia<br>Hepatotoxicity |
| TNF antagonists (adalimumab, certolizumab, etanercept, golimumab, infliximab) | RA | Baseline tuberculin skin test<br>CBC with differential and platelet count<br>Monitor for infection | Activation of tuberculosis<br>Infection, sepsis |
| Tocilizumab | RA | CBC with differential and platelet count<br>Monitor for infection<br>Hepatic transaminases<br>Fasting lipid panel | Infection, sepsis<br>Hepatic enzyme elevations<br>Dyslipidemia |

# TESTS TO GUIDE MANAGEMENT OF GOUT AND HYPERURICEMIA

The serum uric acid and urine uric acid concentrations are the two most commonly used tests to diagnose gout and assess the effectiveness of its treatment. The BUN and SCr also should be monitored as appropriate.

## Serum Uric Acid

*Reference range: 4 to 8.5 mg/dL (237 to 506 µmol/L) for males >17 years old; 2.7 to 7.3 mg/dL (161 to 434 µmol/L) for females >17 years old*

Uric acid is the metabolic end-product of the purine bases of DNA. In humans, uric acid is not metabolized further and is eliminated unchanged by renal excretion. It is completely filtered at the renal glomerulus and is almost completely reabsorbed. Most excreted uric acid (80% to 86%) is the result of active tubular secretion at the distal end of the proximal convoluted tubule.[35-37]

As urine becomes more alkaline, more uric acid is excreted because the percentage of ionized uric acid molecules increases.

Conversely, reabsorption of uric acid within the proximal tubule is enhanced and uric acid excretion is suppressed as urine becomes more acidic.

In plasma at normal body temperature, the physicochemical saturation concentration for urate is 7 mg/dL. However, plasma can become supersaturated, with the concentration exceeding 12 mg/dL. In nongouty subjects with normal renal function, urine uric acid excretion abruptly increases when the *serum uric acid* concentration approaches or exceeds 11 mg/dL. At this concentration, urine uric acid excretion usually exceeds 1,000 mg/24 hr.

### Hyperuricemia

When serum uric acid exceeds the upper limit of the reference range, the biochemical diagnosis of *hyperuricemia* can be made. Hyperuricemia can result from an overproduction of purines and reduced renal clearance of uric acid. When specific factors affecting the normal disposition of uric acid cannot be identified, the problem is diagnosed as *primary* hyperuricemia. When specific factors can be identified (eg, another disease or drug therapy), the problem is referred to as *secondary* hyperuricemia.

As the serum urate concentration increases above the upper limit of the reference range, the risk of developing clinical signs and symptoms of gouty arthritis, renal stones, uric acid nephropathy, and subcutaneous tophaceous deposits increases. However, many hyperuricemic patients are asymptomatic. If a patient is hyperuricemic, it is important to determine if there are potential causes of false laboratory test elevation and contributing extrinsic factors. In general, clinical studies have not shown that impaired renal function is caused by chronic hyperuricemia (unless there are other renal risk factors and excluding acute uric acid nephropathy resulting from tumor lysis syndrome). However, long-term, high serum uric acid levels (eg, ≥13 mg/dL in men or 10 mg/dL in women) may predispose individuals to renal dysfunction. This level of hyperuricemia is uncommon, and a conclusive link to renal insufficiency has not been established. Recent studies suggest reducing serum urate levels may slow progression of renal failure, risk of myocardial infarction, and improve insulin resistance. Further exploration is needed to fully appreciate the effects of hyperuricemia independent of a gout diagnosis.

*Exogenous causes.* Medications are the most common exogenous causes of hyperuricemia. The two primary mechanisms whereby drugs increase serum uric acid concentrations are (1) decreased renal excretion resulting from drug-induced renal dysfunction or competition with uric acid for secretion within the kidney tubules and (2) rapid destruction of large numbers of cells from antineoplastic therapy for leukemias and lymphomas.

The reduction in glomerular filtration rate accompanying renal impairment decreases the filtered load of uric acid and causes hyperuricemia. Several drugs cause hyperuricemia by renal mechanisms that may include interference with renal clearance of uric acid. These agents include low-dose aspirin, pyrazinamide, nicotinic acid, ethambutol, ethanol, cyclosporine, acetazolamide, hydralazine, ethacrynic acid, furosemide, and thiazide diuretics. Diuretic-induced volume depletion results in enhanced tubular reabsorption of uric acid and a decreased filtered load of uric acid. Salicylates, including aspirin, taken in low doses (1 to 2 g/day) may decrease urate renal excretion. Moderate doses (2 to 3 g/day) usually do not alter urate excretion. Large doses (>3 g/day) generally increase urate renal excretion, thereby lowering serum urate concentrations.

Many cancer chemotherapeutic agents (eg, methotrexate, nitrogen mustards, vincristine, 6-mercaptopurine, and azathioprine) increase the turnover rate of nucleic acids and the production of uric acid. Drug-induced hyperuricemia after cancer chemotherapy, especially high-dose regimens, can lead to acute renal failure. Allopurinol is routinely administered prophylactically to decrease uric acid formation. In other clinical situations, drug-induced hyperuricemia may not be clinically significant.

The decision to continue or discontinue a drug that may be causing hyperuricemia depends on three factors: (1) the risk of precipitating gouty symptoms, based on the patient's past history and current clinical status, (2) the feasibility of substituting another drug that is less likely to affect uric acid disposition, and (3) the plausibility of temporarily or permanently discontinuing the drug. If the regimen of the causative drug must remain unchanged, pharmacologic treatment of hyperuricemia may be instituted.

Diet is another exogenous cause of hyperuricemia. High-protein, weight-reduction programs can greatly increase the amount of ingested purines and subsequent uric acid production. If the average daily diet contains a high proportion of meats, the excess nucleoprotein intake can lead to increased uric acid production. Fasting or starvation also can cause hyperuricemia because of increased muscle catabolism. Furthermore, lead poisoning from paint, batteries, or "moonshine," in addition to recent alcohol ingestion, obesity, diabetes mellitus, and hypertriglyceridemia, are associated with increases in serum uric acid concentration (**Minicase 3**).

*Endogenous causes.* Endogenous causes of hyperuricemia include diseases, abnormal physiologic conditions that may or may not be disease related, and genetic abnormalities. Diseases include (1) renal diseases (eg, renal failure), (2) disorders associated with increased destruction of nucleoproteins (eg, leukemia, lymphoma, polycythemia, hemolytic anemia, sickle cell anemia, toxemia of pregnancy, and psoriasis), and (3) endocrine abnormalities (eg, hypothyroidism, hypoparathyroidism, pseudohypoparathyroidism, nephrogenic diabetes insipidus, and Addison disease).

Predisposing abnormal physiologic conditions include shock, hypoxia, lactic acidosis, diabetic ketoacidosis, alcoholic ketosis, and strenuous muscular exercise. In addition, men and women are at risk for developing asymptomatic hyperuricemia at puberty and menopause, respectively. Genetic abnormalities include Lesch-Nyhan syndrome, gout with partial absence of the enzyme hypoxanthine guanine phosphoribosyltransferase, increased phosphoribosyl pyrophosphate P-ribose-PP synthetase, and glycogen storage disease type I.

### Hypouricemia

*Hypouricemia* is not important pathophysiologically, but it may be associated with low-protein diets, renal tubular defects, xanthine oxidase deficiency, and drugs (eg, high-dose aspirin, allopurinol, probenecid, and megadose vitamin C).

### Assays and Interferences with Serum Uric Acid Measurements

In the laboratory, the concentration of uric acid is measured by either the phosphotungstate colorimetric method or the more specific uricase method. With the colorimetric method, ascorbic acid, caffeine, theophylline, levodopa, propylthiouracil, and methyldopa can all falsely elevate uric acid concentrations. With the uricase method, purines and total bilirubin >10 mg/dL can cause a false depression of uric acid concentrations. False elevations may occur if ascorbic acid concentrations exceed 5 mg/dL or if plasma hemoglobin exceeds 300 mg/dL (in hemolysis).

## Urine Uric Acid Concentration

*Reference range: 250 to 750 mg/24 hr (1.48 to 4.46 mmol/24 hr)*

In hyperuricemic individuals who excrete an abnormal amount of uric acid in the urine (hyperuricaciduria), the risk of uric acid and calcium oxalate nephrolithiasis increases. However,

## MINICASE 3

## Hyperuricemia and Gout

A 45-year-old obese man began a daily exercise program 2 weeks ago in an attempt to lose 50 lb. In addition, he has begun a high-protein liquid diet because he knows that "fatty foods are not healthy." He sees his family physician for his first complete physical examination in approximately 7 years. He tells his physician he has recently started walking briskly for 1 hour three times a week and is watching his diet carefully. The only abnormal finding on physical examination is a BP of 150/95 mm Hg. After drawing blood for a CBC with differential and a full chemistry panel and obtaining a urine sample for urinalysis, the physician prescribes hydrochlorothiazide 25 mg once daily for hypertension. Three days later, he is notified that his laboratory results, including serum uric acid, are normal.

Two weeks later, he returns on crutches to see his physician. He explains that he injured his right foot 3 days prior when taking his daily walk before sunrise, and he accidentally stubbed his right foot on a rock. He also says he woke up 2 days prior with a fever and felt as if his right great toe was "in a vise while an ice-cold knife was being pushed into the joint."

Examination of his right foot reveals abrasions on all five toes. The skin of the great toe appears shiny, the toe is swollen and warm to the touch, and he is in obvious pain. Whitish fluid oozes from a small wound on the dorsal aspect of the great toe. After anesthetizing the joint, the physician aspirates several drops of the whitish fluid. The physician then performs a Gram stain and examines the fluid on a slide, finding needle-shaped crystals but no bacteria. He also orders a serum uric acid level.

QUESTION: What is this patient's likely diagnosis and prognosis?

DISCUSSION: He probably has experienced his first acute gout attack. Although his previous serum uric acid concentration was described as normal, one endogenous and two exogenous factors may have precipitated this attack. Hypertension is frequently associated with hyperuricemia. Also, the sudden change to a high-protein diet greatly increased his ingestion of purines, which are metabolized to uric acid. Finally, he also was started on hydrochlorothiazide, which is an inhibitor of the renal clearance of uric acid. The abrupt change in physical exertion probably did not contribute to the attack because it was low in intensity.

Although he attributes the condition to his traumatic toe-stubbing event, his physician notes that none of his other abraded toes appear to be "infected." Examination of the synovial fluid using a polarizing-light microscope reveals monosodium urate crystals without bacteria (Table 20-4). An elevated serum uric acid level would be consistent with a diagnosis of gout, but some patients can have acute gout attacks with a serum urate level that is within the reference range.

With appropriate treatment for acute gout, discontinuation of hydrochlorothiazide, and adequate follow-up monitoring, the patient's symptoms should improve substantially within 24 to 48 hours. Some patients never have a second gout attack, whereas others experience frequent and severe episodes. If the serum uric acid concentration that was ordered is reported as highly elevated (>10 mg/dL), initiating therapy to reduce hyperuricemia may be considered after resolution of the acute attack. According to the 2020 ACR guidelines for treating hyperuricemia, patients should be evaluated on a case-by-case basis to determine causes for elevated uric acid and need for urate-lowering therapy.[38] Any patient with frequent attacks (defined as two or more per year), tophi, radiographic damage due to gout, chronic kidney disease stage 3 or greater, or a history of urolithiasis should receive urate-lowering therapy.[38] The results of a 24-hour urine collection would be useful in determining whether the patient is an overproducer or underexcretor of uric acid and help to guide therapy with either allopurinol or probenecid, respectively.

---

the prevalence of stone formation is only twice that observed in the normouricemic population. When a stone does form, it rarely produces serious complications. Furthermore, treatment can reverse stone disease related to hyperuricemia and hyperuricaciduria.

Pathologically, uric acid nephropathy—a form of acute renal failure—is a direct result of uric acid precipitation in the lumen of collecting ducts and ureters. Uric acid nephropathy most commonly occurs in two clinical situations: (1) patients with marked overproduction of uric acid secondary to chemotherapy-induced tumor lysis (leukemia or lymphoma) and (2) patients with gout and profound hyperuricaciduria. Uric acid nephropathy also has developed after strenuous exercise or convulsions.

In hyperuricemia unrelated to increased uric acid production, quantification of urine uric acid excreted in 24 hours can help to direct prophylaxis or treatment. Patients at higher risk of developing renal calculi or uric acid nephropathy (patients with gout or malignancies) excrete ≥1,100 mg of uric acid per 24 hours. Prophylaxis may be recommended for these patients; allopurinol should be used instead of uricosuric agents (eg, probenecid) to minimize the risk of nephrolithiasis. Prophylactic therapy may be started at the onset of gout-like symptoms.

## SUMMARY

Diagnosing and managing rheumatic diseases rely heavily on a thorough medical history and physical exam. Clinicians can use laboratory tests to help confirm or rule out specific diagnoses. Every laboratory test ordered must be carefully evaluated to determine the next steps in an individual patient's care.

When used alone, no single test is diagnostic for any particular disease. However, positive RF, ACPA, and ANA tests are commonly observed in patients with RA and SLE, respectively.

The cANCA antibody is highly specific for the disease spectrum of GPA, and anti-MPO antibodies are highly specific for systemic vasculitis and idiopathic crescentic glomerulonephritis. The most complete screen of complement activation includes measurements of C3, C4, and $CH_{50}$. The Westergren ESR and CRP tests are nonspecific markers of systemic inflammation and must be interpreted in light of the clinical presentation and other laboratory tests.

Patients with hyperuricemia are usually asymptomatic. After treatment of an episode of acute gout, the decision to initiate antihyperuricemic therapy depends on the frequency and severity of acute attacks. Allopurinol or febuxostat therapy is recommended for patients at risk for forming renal calculi.

## LEARNING POINTS

### 1. How are laboratory tests used in patients with RA and OA?

**ANSWER:** A carefully collected history and physical can help to distinguish between RA and OA in a patient who reports joint pain. Identifying which joints are affected and inquiring about morning joint stiffness and the duration of time necessary to resume normal function of the affected joint provide important information. Laboratory tests can be conducted once the history and physical are completed to rule in or rule out diagnoses. ACPA and RF, if positive, can rule in a diagnosis of RA with 99.5% specificity. ESR and CRP, if positive, indicate the presence of systemic inflammation, though they are not specific to RA. If ACPA, RF, ESR, and CRP are negative or normal, a diagnosis of OA is more likely.

### 2. How important are the sensitivity and specificity of laboratory tests for diagnosing or assessing rheumatic diseases?

**ANSWER:** With many rheumatic diseases, significant information can be gathered through a patient's medical history and physical exam to narrow down the potential causes of the patient's signs and symptoms. Then and only then should lab tests be considered to rule in or rule out specific diseases. Lab tests should not be ordered arbitrarily. Understanding the sensitivity and specificity of the tests available is critical to understanding their association with diagnosis. For example, if a new test to diagnose RA is only 75% sensitive, this means that 25% of patients who actually have the disease will show a negative result. If a new test to diagnose RA is only 75% specific, 25% of people tested who have a positive result do not actually have RA. For some laboratory tests, poor specificity is due to substances not associated with the disease that cross-react with the target compound.

### 3. What issues should be considered before ordering a laboratory test for a patient with a rheumatic disorder?

**ANSWER:** Laboratory testing can be expensive and may be inconvenient to perform. Consequently, several questions should be posed before ordering another test.

1. Are the results of other tests already available that provide the same information?

2. If a test was performed previously, are there important reasons to repeat the test now?

3. Has enough time elapsed since the previous test to make new results meaningful?

4. Will the results of this test change the diagnosis, prognosis, or therapeutic interventions I might make? In other words, will knowing this result change what I do?

5. Are the benefits to the patient worth the possible discomfort, inconvenience, and extra cost?

The results of laboratory tests should always be interpreted in light of the clinical picture (ie, the patient's signs and symptoms).

## REFERENCES

1. Zou YR, Grimaldi C, Diamond B. B cells. In: Firestein GS, Budd RC, Gabriel SE, et al, eds. *Kelley's Textbook of Rheumatology*. 10th ed. Philadelphia, PA: Saunders Elsevier; 2017:207-230.

2. Andrade F, Darrah E, Rosen A. Autoantibodies in rheumatoid arthritis. In: Firestein GS, Budd RC, Gabriel SE, et al, eds. *Kelley's Textbook of Rheumatology*. 10th ed. Philadelphia, PA: Saunders Elsevier; 2017: 831-845.

3. Taylor PC. Biologic markers in the diagnosis and assessment of rheumatoid arthritis. In: Post TW, ed. *UpToDate*. Waltham, MA. https://www.uptodate.com/contents/biologic-markers-in-the-diagnosis-and-assessment-of-rheumatoid-arthritis?search=biologic%20markers%20in%20the%20diagnosis%20and%20assessment%20of%20rheumatoid%20arthritis&source=search_result&selectedTitle=1~150&usage_type=default&display_rank=1. Accessed June 22, 2020.

4. Peng ST, Craft JE. Anti-nuclear antibodies. In: Firestein GS, Budd RC, Gabriel SE, et al, eds. *Kelley's Textbook of Rheumatology*. 10th ed. Philadelphia, PA: Saunders Elsevier; 2017:817-830.

5. Bloch DB. Measurement and clinical significance of antinuclear antibodies. In: Post TW, ed. *UpToDate*. Waltham, MA. https://www.uptodate.com/contents/measurement-and-clinical-significance-of-antinuclear-antibodies?search=measurement%20and%20clinical%20significance%20of%20antinuclear%20antibodies&source=search_result&selectedTitle=1~150&usage_type=default&display_rank=1. Accessed June 22, 2020.

6. Bloch DB. Antibodies to double-stranded (ds)DNA, Sm, and U1 RNP. In: Post TW, ed. *UpToDate*. Waltham, MA. https://www.uptodate.com/contents/antibodies-to-double-stranded-ds-dna-sm-and-u1-rnp?search=antibodies%20to%20double-stranded%20(ds)DNA&source=search_result&selectedTitle=1~150&usage_type=default&display_rank=1. Accessed June 22, 2020.

7. Bloch DB. The anti-Ro/SSA and anti-La/SSB antigen-antibody systems. In: Post TW, ed. *UpToDate*. Waltham, MA. https://www.uptodate.com/contents/the-anti-ro-ssa-and-anti-la-ssb-antigen-antibody-systems?search=the%20anti%20ro%20ssa%20and%20anti%20la%20ssb&source=search_result&selectedTitle=1~150&usage_type=default&display_rank=1. Accessed June 22, 2020.

8. Falk RJ. Clinical spectrum of antineutrophil cytoplasmic antibodies. In: Post TW, ed. *UpToDate*. Waltham, MA. https://www.uptodate.com/contents/clinical-spectrum-of-antineutrophil-cytoplasmic-autoantibodies?search=clinical%20spectrum%20of%20antineutrophil&source=search_result&selectedTitle=1~150&usage_type=default&display_rank=1. Accessed June 22, 2020.

9. Chung S. Monach. Anti-neutrophil cytoplasmic antibody-associated vasculitis. In: Firestein GS, Budd RC, Gabriel SE, et al, eds. *Kelley's Textbook of Rheumatology*. 10th ed. Philadelphia, PA: Saunders Elsevier; 2017:1541-1558.

10. Suwanchote S, Rachayon M, Rodsaward P, et al. Anti-neutrophil cytoplasmic antibodies and their clinical significance. *Clin Rheum*; 2018:875-884.

11. Trouw LA. Complement system. In: Firestein GS, Budd RC, Gabriel SE, et al, eds. *Kelley's Textbook of Rheumatology*. 10th ed. Philadelphia, PA: Saunders Elsevier; 2017:355-365.

12. Liszewski MK, Atkinson JP. Overview and clinical assessment of the complement system. In: Post TW, ed. *UpToDate*. Waltham, MA. https://www.uptodate.com/contents/overview-and-clinical-assessment-of-the-complement-system?search=overview%20and%20clinical%20assessment%20of%20the%20complement%20system&source=search_result&selectedTitle=1~150&usage_type=default&display_rank=1. Accessed June 22, 2020.

13. Fors Nieves C, Bronstein BN, Saxena A. Acute phase reactants and the concept of inflammation. In: Firestein GS, Budd RC, Harris ED Jr, et al, eds. *Kelley's Textbook of Rheumatology*. 10th ed. Philadelphia, PA: Saunders Elsevier; 2017:846-857.

14. Castro AR, Silva SO, Soares SC. The use of high sensitivity c-reactive protein in cardiovascular disease detection. *J Pharm Furs Sci*. 2018;21(1):496-503.PubMed

15. Van der Linden S, Brown M, Kenna T, et al. Ankylosing Spondylitis. In: Firestein GS, Budd RC, Harris ED Jr, et al, eds. *Kelley's Textbook of Rheumatology*. 10th ed. Philadelphia, PA: Saunders Elsevier; 2017:1256-1279.

16. El-Gabalawy HS. Synovial fluid analyses, synovial biopsy, and synovial pathology. In: Firestein GS, Budd RC, Gabriel SE, et al, eds. *Kelley's Textbook of Rheumatology*. 10th ed. Philadelphia, PA: Saunders Elsevier; 2017:784-801.

17. Aletaha D, Neogi T, Silman AJ, et al. 2010 Rheumatoid arthritis classification criteria: an American College of Rheumatology/European League Against Rheumatism collaborative initiative. *Arthritis Rheum*. 2010;62(9):2569-2581.PubMed

18. Venables PJW. Diagnosis and differential diagnosis of rheumatoid arthritis. In: Post TW, ed. *UpToDate*. Waltham, MA. https://www.uptodate.com/contents/diagnosis-and-differential-diagnosis-of-rheumatoid-arthritis?search=diagnosis%20and%20differential%20diagnosis%20of%20rheumatoid%20arthritis&source=search_result&selectedTitle=1~150&usage_type=default&display_rank=1. Accessed June 22, 2020.

19. Taylor PC, Maini RN. Biologic markers in the diagnosis and assessment of rheumatoid arthritis. In: Post TW, ed. *UpToDate*. Waltham, MA. https://www.uptodate.com/contents/biologic-markers-in-the-diagnosis-and-assessment-of-rheumatoid-arthritis?search=Biologic%20markers%20in%20the%20diagnosis%20and%20assessment%20of%20rheumatoid%20arthritis&source=search_result&selectedTitle=1~150&usage_type=default&display_rank=1. Accessed June 22, 2020.

20. Di Cesare PE, Haudenschild DR, Samuels J, Abramson SB. Pathogenesis of osteoarthritis. In: Firestein GS, Budd RC, Gabriel SE, et al, eds. *Kelley's Textbook of Rheumatology*. 10th ed. Philadelphia, PA: Saunders Elsevier; 2017:1685-1704.

21. Doherty M, Abhishek A. Clinical manifestations and diagnosis of osteoarthritis. In: Post TW, ed. *UpToDate*. Waltham, MA. https://www.uptodate.com/contents/clinical-manifestations-and-diagnosis-of-osteoarthritis?search=clinical%20manifestations%20and%20diagnosis%20of%20osteoarthritis&source=search_result&selectedTitle=1~150&usage_type=default&display_rank=1. Accessed June 22, 2020.

22. Hsu JJ, Lee TC. Clinical features and treatment of juvenile idiopathic arthritis. In: Firestein GS, Budd RC, Gabriel SE, et al, eds. *Kelley's Textbook of Rheumatology*. 10th ed. Philadelphia, PA: Saunders Elsevier; 2017:1826-1843.

23. Petty RE, Southwood TR, Manners P, et al. International League of Associations for Rheumatology classification of juvenile idiopathic arthritis: second revision, Edmonton, 2001. *J Rheumatol*. 2004;31(2):390-392.PubMed

24. Mahmud SA, Binstadt BA. Autoantibodies in the pathogenesis, diagnosis, and prognosis of juvenile idiopathic arthritis. *Front Immunol*. 2019;9:3168.PubMed

25. Kimura Y. Systemic juvenile idiopathic arthritis: clinical manifestations and diagnosis. In: Post TW, ed. *UpToDate*. Waltham, MA. https://www.uptodate.com/contents/systemic-juvenile-idiopathic-arthritis-clinical-manifestations-and-diagnosis?search=autoantibodies%20in%20the%20pathogenesis,%20diagnosis,%20and%20prognosis%20of%20juvenile%20idiopathic%20arthritis&source=search_result&selectedTitle=4~150&usage_type=default&display_rank=4. Accessed June 22, 2020.

26. Aringer M, Costenbader K, Daikh D, et al. European League Against Rheumatism/American College of Rheumatology classification criteria for systemic lupus erythematosus. *Arthritis Rheumatol*. 2019;71(9):1400-1412.PubMed

27. Petri M, Orbai AM, Alarcón GS, et al. Derivation and validation of the Systemic Lupus International Collaborating Clinics classification criteria for systemic lupus erythematosus. *Arthritis Rheum*. 2012;64(8):2677-2686.PubMed

28. Wallace DJ, Gladman DD. Clinical manifestations and diagnosis of systemic lupus erythematosus in adults. In: Post TW, ed. *UpToDate*. Waltham, MA. https://www.uptodate.com/contents/clinical-manifestations-and-diagnosis-of-systemic-lupus-erythematosus-in-adults?search=Clinical%20manifestations%20and%20diagnosis%20of%20systemic%20lupus&source=search_result&selectedTitle=1~150&usage_type=default&display_rank=1. Acessed; June 22, 2020.

29. Erkan D, Salmon JE, Lockshin MD. Antiphospholipid syndrome. In: Firestein GS, Budd RC, Gabriel SE, et al, eds. *Kelley's Textbook of Rheumatology*. 10th ed. Philadelphia, PA: Saunders Elsevier; 2017:1389-1399.

30. Dall'Era M, Wofsy D. Clinical features of systemic lupus erythematosus. In: Firestein GS, Budd RC, Gabriel SE, et al, eds. *Kelley's Textbook of Rheumatology*. 10th ed. Philadelphia, PA: Saunders Elsevier; 2017:1345-1367.

31. Crofford LJ. Fibromyalgia. In: Firestein GS, Budd RC, Gabriel SE, et al, eds. *Kelley's Textbook of Rheumatology*. 10th ed. Philadelphia, PA: Saunders Elsevier; 2017:768-783.

32. Buys LM, Wiedenfeld SA. Osteoarthritis. In: DiPiro JT, Yee GC, Posey L, et al, eds. *Pharmacotherapy: A Pathophysiologic Approach*. 11th ed. McGraw-Hill. New York, NY. https://accesspharmacy.mhmedical.com/content.aspx?bookid=2577&sectionid=223397868. Accessed June 26, 2020.

33. Gruber S, Lezcano B, Hylland S. Rheumatoid arthritis. In: DiPiro JT, Yee GC, Posey L, et al, eds. *Pharmacotherapy: A Pathophysiologic Approach*. 11th ed. McGraw-Hill. New York, NY. https://accesspharmacy.mhmedical.com/content.aspx?bookid=2577&sectionid=238237911. Accessed June 26, 2020.

34. Resman-Targoff BH. Systemic Lupus Erythematosus. In: DiPiro JT, Yee GC, Posey L, et al, eds. *Pharmacotherapy: A Pathophysiologic Approach,* 11th ed. McGraw-Hill. New York, NY. https://accesspharmacy.mhmedical.com/content.aspx?bookid=2577&sectionid=233055227. Accessed June 26, 2020.

35. Fravel MA, Ernst ME. Gout and Hyperuricemia. In: DiPiro JT, Yee GC, Posey L, et al, eds. *Pharmacotherapy: A Pathophysiologic Approach,* 11th ed. McGraw-Hill. New York, NY. https://accesspharmacy.mhmedical.com/content.aspx?bookid=2577&sectionid=237232322. Accessed June 26, 2020.

36. Keenan RT, Krasnokkutsky S, Pillinger MH. Etiology and pathogenesis of hyperuricemia and gout. In: Firestein GS, Budd RC, Gabriel SE, et al, eds. *Kelley's Textbook of Rheumatology*. 10th ed. Philadelphia, PA: Saunders Elsevier; 2017:1597-1619.

37. Burns CM, Wortmann RL. Clinical features and treatment of gout. In: Firestein GS, Budd RC, Gabriel SE, et al, eds. *Kelley's Textbook of Rheumatology*. 10th ed. Philadelphia, PA: Saunders Elsevier; 2017:1620-1644.

38. FitzGerald JD, Dalbeth N, Mikuls T, et al. American College of Rheumatology guideline for the management of gout. *Arthritis Care Res (Hoboken)*. 2020;72(6):744-760.PubMed

# 21

# Cancers and Tumor Markers

*Sarah A. Schmidt*

## OBJECTIVES

*After completing this chapter, the reader should be able to*

- Define tumor markers, describe the characteristics of an ideal tumor marker, and discuss the usefulness of tumor markers in the diagnosis, staging, and treatment of malignant diseases

- List malignant and nonmalignant conditions that may increase carcinoembryonic antigen levels and define the role of carcinoembryonic antigen in the management of colon cancer

- Describe how cancer antigen 125 may be used to diagnose and monitor ovarian cancer

- Describe how human chorionic gonadotropin and α-fetoprotein are used to diagnose and monitor germ cell tumors

- Discuss the role of estrogen and progesterone receptors and human epidermal growth factor receptor 2 in determining treatment decisions for breast cancer

- Outline the role of the *BCR-ABL* gene in the diagnosis and as a target for treatment in patients with chronic myelogenous leukemia

- Describe how mutations in epidermal growth factor receptor, V-Ki-ras2 Kirsten rat sarcoma viral oncogene homolog, v-Raf murine sarcoma viral oncogene homolog B1, or anaplastic lymphoma kinase are used in determining treatment decisions for melanoma, lung cancer, and colorectal cancer

*(continued on page 514)*

DOI 10.37573/9781585286423.021

For most types of cancer, treatment is likely to be most successful if the diagnosis is made while the tumor mass is relatively small. Unfortunately, many common types of cancer (eg, carcinomas of the lung, breast, and colon) are frequently not diagnosed until the tumor burden is relatively large and the patient has developed symptoms related to the disease. As the search for more effective treatments for cancer has intensified, much effort and many resources have been dedicated to elucidating new methods of detecting cancers earlier while the tumor burden is low and the patient is asymptomatic. These efforts have led to improved radiologic and other diagnostic imaging and identification of biologic substances, which occur in relation to the tumor and can be detected even at low concentrations in the blood or other body fluids.

The term *tumor marker* is used to describe a wide range of proteins that are associated with various malignancies. Typically, these markers are either proteins that are produced by or in response to a specific type of tumor or other physiologic proteins that are produced by malignant cells in excess of the normal concentrations. In either case, the concentration of the marker usually correlates with the volume of tumor cells (eg, as the tumor grows or the number of malignant cells increases, the concentration of the marker also increases). In other cases, the presence of a biologic marker may be used to predict response to treatment (eg, the estrogen receptor [*ER*] or progesterone receptor [*PR*] in breast cancer) or monitor the effects of treatment. More recently, some tumor markers have been shown to be essential to the viability of tumor cells, and specific therapies have been developed that target these markers of disease. These tumor markers are often identified by genetic mutations, translocations, or amplification of genetic material.

This chapter describes tumor markers that are used clinically to detect cancers, monitor cancer burden, and help choose drug therapy as well as the laboratory methods used to measure them. In addition, the sensitivity, specificity, and factors that may interfere with evaluation of these tests are briefly discussed. For tumor markers that are widely used to screen for cancers, confirm a cancer diagnosis, or assess response to treatment, the clinical applications are described. More commonly, molecular markers are being discovered and driving therapy.

## TUMOR MARKERS

*Tumor markers* may be found in the blood or other body fluids or may be measured directly in tumor tissues or lymph nodes. They can be grouped into three broad categories: (1) tumor-specific proteins, markers that are produced only by tumor cells, usually in response to genetic changes such as translocation of an oncogene, that contribute to the proliferation of the tumor, (2) protein expression typically isolated to embryonic development that can be expressed by cancer cells, and (3) proteins that are normally found in the body but are expressed or secreted at a much higher rate by malignant cells than normal cells.[1] In addition to the laboratory tests described in this chapter, it also should be remembered that abnormalities in other commonly used laboratory tests may provide some evidence that a malignancy exists. However, they are not related to specific tumors. For example, suppression of blood counts may represent infiltration of the bone marrow by tumor cells. Increased uric acid and lactate dehydrogenase are frequently associated with large

## OBJECTIVES

- Review biomarkers for immunotherapy, including programmed death-ligand 1 and tumor mutation burden, and their role in treatment for various cancers

tumor burdens. Alkaline phosphatase is frequently elevated in patients with tumors of the biliary tract or bone. Occasionally, tumors may also produce hormones in excessive amounts, such as calcitonin or adrenocorticotropin. Common tumor markers are reviewed in this chapter, but many are not covered, including B-cell immunoglobulin gene rearrangement, bladder tumor antigen, chromogranin A, *C-kit*, gastrin, *ROS1* gene rearrangement, thyroblobulin, and others. The intent of this chapter is to introduce common tumor markers; however, not every tumor marker is covered in detail, and progress in this field is rapidly moving forward.

## Clinical Uses

Tumor markers are used for several purposes, including detection of occult cancers in asymptomatic individuals (eg, cancer screening and early detection), determining the relative extent or volume of disease (staging), estimating prognosis, predicting and assessing responsiveness to treatment, and monitoring for disease recurrence or progression.[1] **Table 21-1** lists many of the commonly used tumor markers that are used most often for screening and monitoring of response to a variety of treatments. **Table 21-2** lists tumor markers with their clinical applications. The characteristics of an ideal tumor marker are somewhat dependent on the specific application. Normal values are provided, although laboratory reference ranges (normal values) may slightly differ, as will the interpretation of the laboratory value in individual patients. For example, rising levels of a tumor marker that are still in the normal range may indicate early tumor recurrence.

### Sensitivity and Specificity

For a tumor marker to be clinically useful in screening for cancer, it must have a high degree of *sensitivity* and *specificity*. That is, the presence of the marker should correlate with the presence of the tumor, and a negative test result should indicate, with some certainty, that the patient does not have the cancer. Chapter 1 describes the methodology in determining sensitivity and specificity and should be reviewed before reading this chapter. Knowledge of the sensitivity, specificity, and predictive values of tumor marker tests is particularly important when they are used to screen asymptomatic patients. If a tumor marker test is positive only in a portion of patients who actually have cancer or if a test result is negative in patients who do have the disease, then diagnoses would be missed. In the case of malignant diseases, delay of the diagnosis until symptoms or other clinical findings appear may mean the difference between curable and incurable disease.

Outcomes studies evaluating the usefulness of tumor marker testing in asymptomatic individuals must result in decreased mortality rates due to the disease, not just establishment of a diagnosis. On the other hand, false-positive test results not only cause a high level of anxiety but also typically result in the performance of costly and sometimes invasive additional diagnostic tests. Because of these limitations, the only tumor marker routinely used to screen for malignancies is prostate-specific antigen (PSA). Although this is the single example, the use of PSA alone for prostate cancer screening is declining because it does not appear to reduce mortality.[2]

Sensitivity and specificity are also important when tumor marker tests are used to monitor for recurrent disease in patients who have previously been treated for the cancer. A negative tumor marker test that is known to have a high degree of specificity gives the patient, the family, and clinicians a great deal of comfort and sense of security that the disease has been eliminated. If the test has a lower degree of sensitivity, then it is likely that other screening and diagnostic tests will need to be performed at regular intervals to monitor for disease recurrence. In some cases, the presence of a positive tumor marker may be indication enough to resume cancer treatment. A decision to initiate or resume treatment should be made when there is a high degree of certainty that actual disease is present because most cancer treatments are associated with significant toxicity and a small, but appreciable, mortality risk. When tumor markers are used to assess the extent of disease or the presence of specific tumor characteristics (eg, HER2/neu), the quantitative sensitivity may also be important in determining prognosis, appropriate diagnostic tests, and treatment options. Genetic mutational testing is a dichotomous endpoint that is present or not present; however, depending on the quality of tissue and type of testing, the sensitivity (false-negative results) can be affected.

### Accessibility

If a tumor marker test is to be used to screen asymptomatic individuals for cancer, both patients and clinicians are more likely to include them if they do not necessitate painful, risky, or lengthy procedures to obtain the necessary fluid or tissue. Most clinicians request—and patients willingly provide—samples of blood, urine, or sputum in the course of regular physical examinations. However, if a test requires biopsy of other tissues or involves procedures that are associated with a significant risk of morbidity, patients and clinicians are likely only to consent to or include them in physical examinations if there is a high likelihood—or other evidence that supports the presence—of the disease. Tumor markers that are obtained from tumor tissue directly are obtained at the time of diagnosis with the original tissue.

### Cost-Effectiveness

Widespread screening of asymptomatic individuals with a tumor marker test can be expensive. It is not surprising that insurance companies, health plans, and health policy decision-makers are also more likely to support the inclusion of these tests during routine physical examinations or other screening programs if health economic evaluations demonstrate that they may result in lower overall treatment costs and a positive benefit to society, such as prolongation of a patient's productivity.

**TABLE 21-1.** Serum Tumor Markers in Clinical Use

| TUMOR MARKER | MALIGNANT DISEASE | SCREENING | DIAGNOSIS | STAGING OR PROGNOSIS | MONITORING TREATMENT OUTCOME OR DISEASE RECURRENCE | COMMENTS |
|---|---|---|---|---|---|---|
| PSA | Prostate carcinoma | X | | X | X | Usually combined with digital rectal examination of the prostate for screening<br><br>Inflammatory disorders of the prostate, instrumentation of the genitourinary tract, and mechanical manipulation of the prostate by biopsy, transurethral resection of the prostate or prostatectomy may increase PSA<br><br>Certain medications may decrease PSA, including 5-α reductase inhibitors, NSAIDs, statins, and thiazide diuretics<br><br>Herbal products (eg, saw palmetto) may also decrease PSA |
| CEA | Colon, breast carcinoma, ovarian, pancreatic, and others | | | X (in colon) | X | Hepatic cirrhosis, hepatitis, pancreatitis, peptic ulcer disease, hypothyroidism, ulcerative colitis, or Crohn disease may elevate CEA |
| CA 15-3, CA 27.29 | Breast carcinoma | | | X | X Metastatic disease only | Other cancers (eg, gastric, colorectal, lung), benign breast disease, and liver disease may all elevate levels |
| CA-125 | Ovarian carcinoma | | | X | X | Endometriosis, ovarian cysts, liver disease, or pregnancy may elevate CA-125; in certain high-risk groups (strong family history) CA-125 in combination with ultrasound technology may be used to screen asymptomatic patients |
| hCG | Germ cell tumors of ovaries and testes; hydatidiform mole; trophoblastic tumors | | X | X | X | Pregnancy, other types of cancer, or marijuana use may elevate hCG |
| CA 19-9 | Pancreatic carcinoma | | | X | X | Pancreatitis, cirrhosis, gastric, and colon cancer may elevate CA 19-9 |

*(continued)*

**TABLE 21-1.** Serum Tumor Markers in Clinical Use, cont'd

| TUMOR MARKER | MALIGNANT DISEASE | SCREENING | DIAGNOSIS | STAGING OR PROGNOSIS | MONITORING TREATMENT OUTCOME OR DISEASE RECURRENCE | COMMENTS |
|---|---|---|---|---|---|---|
| AFP | Hepatocellular carcinoma; testicular (nonseminomatous germ cell tumors) | X (hepatocellular carcinoma) | X | X | X | Pregnancy; hepatitis; cirrhosis; and pancreatic, gastric, lung, and colon cancers all can elevate AFP; some non-U.S. countries, which have a high incidence of hepatocellular cancer, use AFP to screen for hepatocellular cancer |
| $B_2M$ | Multiple (plasma cell) myeloma; chronic lymphocytic leukemia | | | X | X | Lymphomas, chronic lymphocytic leukemia, and renal failure may elevate |

NSAIDs = nonsteroidal antiinflammatory drugs.

**TABLE 21-2.** Tumor Markers Used to Personalize Treatment

| TUMOR MARKER | MALIGNANT DISEASE | TEST OUTCOME OF INTEREST | IMPACT ON DRUG SELECTION |
|---|---|---|---|
| ALK | Lung | ALK rearrangement | ALK rearrangement predicts response to ALK-inhibitors (crizotinib, ceritinib, lorlatinib, alectinib, and brigatinib) |
| BCR-ABL translocation | CML or Ph+ ALL | BCR-ABL translocation | TKI therapy used in treatment (imatinib, bosutinib, dasatinib, nilotinib, ponatinib) |
| BRAF | Melanoma Lung Thyroid | BRAF V600E and V600K mutation | BRAF mutation predicts response to vemurafenib, dabrafenib, and trametinib |
| EGFR | Lung | Mutation in exon 19 or 21 | Mutation predictive of response to EGFR TK inhibitors predicts response to afatinib, erlotinib, gefitinib, osimertinib, dacomitinib |
| ER/PR | Breast carcinoma | ER or PR positive disease | Hormonal therapy indicated in treatment (tamoxifen, fulvestrant, exemestane, letrozole) |
| KRas | Colorectal cancer | Mutation versus wild type (nonmutated) | EGFR monoclonal antibodies (cetuximab and panitumumab) only effective against wild-type |
| HER2 | Breast carcinoma, gastric cancer | HER2 overexpression | HER2 monoclonal antibodies or TKI therapy may be indicated (ado-trastuzumab emtansine, fam-trastuzumab deruxtecan, lapatinib, neratininb, pertuzumab, trastuzumab, and tucatinib) |

BRAF = v-Raf murine sarcoma viral oncogene homolog B1; EGFR = epidermal growth factor receptor; KRas = V-Ki-ras2 Kirsten rat sarcoma viral oncogene homolog.

## Prostate-Specific Antigen

*Standard reference range: 0 to 4 ng/mL (4 mcg/L)*
*Prostate-specific antigen* (PSA) is a protein produced by both normal (benign) and malignant prostate tissue that is secreted into the blood. The role of PSA in the screening, diagnosis, and monitoring of treatment response of patients with prostate cancer is reviewed in Chapter 25.

## Carcinoembryonic Antigen

*Normal range: <2.5 ng/mL nonsmokers (<2.5 mcg/L); <5 ng/mL smokers (5 mcg/L)*

*Carcinoembryonic antigen* (CEA) is a protein that is found in fetal intestine, pancreas, and liver. In healthy adults, the level of this protein is usually <2.5 ng/mL. CEA is a protein generally found in a fetus, and the protein diminishes at birth. Serum CEA levels are frequently elevated in patients with colon, breast, gastric, thyroid, or pancreatic carcinomas and a variety of nonmalignant conditions, including hepatic cirrhosis, hepatitis, pancreatitis, peptic ulcer disease, hypothyroidism, ulcerative colitis, and Crohn disease. Occasionally, CEA also is elevated in patients with lung cancer. CEA levels are usually modestly increased in individuals who smoke; the normal serum level in these individuals is usually considered to be <5 ng/mL. Nonmalignant conditions are usually not associated with CEA levels >10 ng/mL. However, many patients with malignant conditions have CEA levels that greatly exceed 10 ng/mL.

Blood samples for CEA testing preferably should be obtained in a red top tube. Following separation of the serum (or plasma), the specimen can be refrigerated if it is to be assayed within 24 hours or frozen at −20°C if the specimen is to be assayed later. Immunoassays from different manufacturers may provide different values; therefore, the same laboratory and assay method should be used whenever possible for repeat testing in an individual patient.

Carcinoembryonic antigen is most commonly used in the assessment of colon cancer. Unfortunately, this test does not have adequate sensitivity or specificity to make it a useful screening test for asymptomatic individuals. It may be elevated in a wide variety of conditions as noted previously and may be negative in patients with widely metastatic disease. It is most commonly used in monitoring patients with a known history of colon cancer.[2] Following detection of early-stage colon cancer by screening tests and further diagnostic workup, a baseline serum CEA level is usually measured to determine if the tumor produces excessive amounts of CEA. If the CEA level is grossly increased, then the CEA level may be used to monitor the success of treatment or for evidence of tumor recurrence after successful treatment.

The CEA level also may provide some information on a patient's prognosis.[3,4] The elevation of CEA level may relate to the extent of disease (stage), which often correlates with overall survival. After surgical removal of colon cancer, the CEA level should return to normal (<2.5 ng/mL) within 4 to 6 weeks.[5] If the CEA level remains elevated beyond this point, it may indicate that either residual primary tumor or metastatic disease is present.

In early-stage colon cancer (stages II and III), CEA levels should be followed every 3 to 6 months for 5 years after the completion of all cycles of adjuvant chemotherapy.[6] Rising CEA levels mandate evaluation of the patient for metastatic disease. In patients with metastatic disease, CEA levels should be monitored at the start of therapy and then every 1 to 3 months during therapy.[6] Rising levels may indicate therapy failure, although increasing levels may result from chemotherapy at the beginning of treatment and require careful evaluation.[6,7] When CEA levels are monitored in conjunction with other follow-up tests, including computed tomography scans of the liver and colonoscopy, several studies have reported improved overall survival and other benefits, including cost-effectiveness, that are attributable to earlier detection of recurrent disease.[6,8]

Carcinoembryonic antigen may also be used to monitor patients with metastatic breast cancer. The American Society of Clinical Oncology guidelines for use of tumor markers in breast cancer state that CEA levels in combination with imaging, medical history, and physical exam may indicate treatment failure and prompt evaluation for worsening of disease.[9] Rising CEA levels alone should not be used to monitor treatment efficacy. Unlike colon cancer, monitoring of CEA levels in early-stage breast cancer (stages I to III) is not recommended after a patient has received primary therapy (**Minicase 1**).

## CA 15-3

*Normal range: <30 units/mL*

*Cancer antigen 15-3* (CA 15-3) is defined by an assay using monoclonal antibodies directed against circulating mucin antigen shed from human breast cancer. In addition to elevation in the serum of many women with breast cancer, it may also be elevated in lung cancer and other nonmalignant conditions, including liver and breast disorders. Elevated *CA 15-3* has been demonstrated to be a poor prognostic factor in early-stage breast cancer, but the test is not sensitive enough to use as a screening test for early-stage breast cancer.[10] This test is used in combination with imaging studies, physical examination, and medical history to monitor response to treatment in women with metastatic disease in whom no other reasonable measure of disease is feasible[11,12] (**Minicase 2**).

## CA 27.29

*Normal range: <38 units/mL*

*Cancer antigen 27.29* (CA 27.29) is also defined by an assay using a monoclonal antibody that detects circulating mucin antigen in blood.[9] It is a newer test than CA 15-3 but has the same clinical indications. *CA 27.29* is used only in combination with other clinical factors, such as imaging studies, physical examination, and medical history, to monitor response to treatment in patients with metastatic breast cancer, but it is not useful as a screening test or for detection of recurrence after primary therapy in early-stage disease.[9]

## CA-125

*Normal range: <35 units/mL*

*Cancer antigen 125* (CA-125 antigen) is a protein usually found on cells that line the pelvic organs and peritoneum. It may also be detected in the blood of women with ovarian cancer and adenocarcinoma of the cervix or fallopian tubes. It may be elevated in nonmalignant conditions, including endometriosis,

## MINICASE 1

## A Case of Elevated Carcinoembryonic Antigen Levels

Phil L., a 64-year-old white man, presents to the clinic with a 6-week history of worsening diarrhea (five to six stools a day), pain in his right upper quadrant, and general gastrointestinal discomfort. Patient has a history of stage I colon cancer, following resection, and no further treatment 2 years ago. Additional past medical history includes hypercholesterolemia for the past 5 years. Medications include simvastatin 20 mg daily. He drinks one to two glasses of wine a day and has a 30 pack/year history of smoking.

A review of systems reveals lethargy and slight confusion but no apparent distress. Vital signs show a sitting blood pressure of 125/75 mm Hg (standing blood pressure not measured), a regular heart rate of 86 beats/min, and a rapid and shallow respiration rate of 36 breaths/min. His physical examination is pertinent for signs of dehydration (poor skin turgor). Laboratory values are drawn. They are unremarkable except for serum sodium (153 mEq/L), serum creatinine (1.7 mg/dL), and blood urea nitrogen (45 mg/dL). The decision is made to admit him based on his dehydration and worsening diarrhea. Additional laboratory values are drawn in the hospital, including a CEA level of 27 ng/mL.

QUESTION: What is the most likely cause of this patient's fluid status? How is the CEA level interpreted in relation to colon cancer?

Should any other laboratory or imaging tests be obtained to further assess if he has a malignant tumor?

DISCUSSION: This patient most likely has a malignant tumor in his colon that has relapsed. Common signs and symptoms of colon cancer include pain and a change in bowel habits, which result from the tumor blocking part of the colonic lumen and interfering with normal colonic function. This can lead to the severe diarrhea and dehydration as seen in this patient.

Although other nonmalignant conditions and smoking also are associated with increased CEA levels, levels >10 ng/mL indicate a high likelihood of cancer. An elevated CEA level alone is not enough to make a diagnosis of colon cancer; a complete workup, including computed tomography scan and a tissue diagnosis, need to be obtained prior to therapy. Additional laboratory values that may be useful are *CA 19-9* levels and a complete hepatic panel to assess for metastatic disease.

The CEA level may be used to monitor the success of treatment, check for evidence of tumor recurrence following primary treatment, and provide some indication of his prognosis.

## MINICASE 2

## A Case of Using Tumor Markers for Breast Cancer

Sarah H., a 41-year-old white woman, was recently diagnosed with breast cancer. She presents for her first scheduled routine mammogram, and a small lump is detected in her left breast. A fine-needle biopsy is performed, and the lump is found to be positive for breast cancer. A complete workup determines that this is local disease, and she is diagnosed with stage II breast cancer. Additional medical history is unremarkable; she only takes seasonal allergy medicine and drospirenone/ethinyl estradiol oral contraceptives.

A review of systems is noncontributory. Her physical examination is pertinent for a small lump palpable on the left breast near her nipple. Her cancer is evaluated for the presence of tumor markers, and the pathology shows ER/PR = positive and HER2 = 2+ on IHC.

QUESTION: How will these markers be evaluated and used to make treatment decisions in this patient? Are there any other tumor markers or tests you would recommend be performed on her?

DISCUSSION: The two most important tumor markers in determining prognosis and treatment decisions are ER/PR status and HER2 status, and both were performed on this patient. Her ER/PR receptors were found to be positive. There are many ways to report ER/PR status, with most being determined by IHC. Because the presence of even small amounts of ER/PR has been correlated with prognosis and the need for hormonal therapy, ER/PR status is

commonly reported as either positive or negative. Because her ER/PR status is positive, she will benefit from hormonal therapy that targets the ER receptor. The use of RT-PCR in determining ER/PR status could be done to confirm her ER/PR status.

She also has her HER2 status reported. Her value is 2+ as determined by IHC. This value is in the inconclusive range. Because HER2 status is critical in determining the benefit from anti-HER2 therapies (eg, trastuzumab and lapatinib), inconclusive values require further workup. The confirmatory test that should be performed is a FISH assay. This test measures the number of HER2 gene copies and provides a ratio of HER2/CEP 17 (also called *FISH ratio*). A positive test for HER2 gene amplification is a gene copy number >6 or a FISH ratio >2.2.

She should have this test performed. If positive, she will be offered trastuzumab as part of her adjuvant therapy. If she has a negative FISH test result for HER2, then she will not receive adjuvant therapy with trastuzumab and will instead receive a standard adjuvant chemotherapy regimen followed by hormonal therapy.

Additional markers, such as CEA, CA 15-3, and CA 27.29, would not be useful in following this patient because she does not have metastatic disease, and these markers only are useful for determining progressive disease during treatment for metastatic breast cancer.

ovarian cysts, liver disease, and pregnancy and occasionally in many other types of cancer.[11] It is not, however, elevated by mucinous epithelial carcinomas of the ovaries. Levels of *CA-125* also increase during menstruation and are lower at the luteal phase of the cycle. Levels are lower in women who use systemic contraceptives and decline after menopause.[11]

*CA-125* is assessed using a blood sample collected in a red top tube. The sample should be refrigerated within 2 hours of collection. The level of *CA-125* in the serum has been reported to correlate with the likelihood of malignancy, with levels >65 units/ mL strongly associated with the presence of a malignancy. However, such levels should not be considered diagnostic.[11,13] Several studies evaluating serial levels of *CA-125* in healthy women have shown that serum levels may start to rise 1 to 5 years before the detection of ovarian cancer.[11] It does not, however, have sufficient sensitivity to be recommended as a routine screening test for ovarian cancer in asymptomatic women. The sensitivity in early-stage ovarian cancer (before symptoms are usually evident) is believed to be <60%; thus, many cases would not be detected. Using *CA-125* levels with other tests, such as transvaginal ultrasound, has been investigated to increase the use of *CA-125*. However, using transvaginal ultrasound in patients with elevated *CA-125* levels does not appear to increase the detection of early tumors and the routine use of the combination is not recommended.[11,14] However, recent data of the largest published prospective screening trial conducted to date demonstrated that using serial biomarker measurements doubled the number of screen-detected ovarian cancers.[15] This study used serial *CA-125* levels in conjunction with a risk algorithm and compared this to serial *CA-125* levels alone. The investigators concluded that using the algorithm in combination with serial *CA-125* levels increased the number of cancers detected at screening.[15] The impact of this on ovarian cancer mortality is still unknown. Some advocate that rising serial *CA-125* levels could be used as a trigger to do more extensive (and often costly) screening tests in high-risk women; however, this approach has not proven beneficial and may result in unacceptable morbidity in women at average risk for ovarian cancer.

Most often, *CA-125* is measured to monitor for evidence of disease recurrence or residual disease in women who have undergone surgical resection of ovarian cancer.[11] This indication is useful in women whose tumors expressed *CA-125* prior to surgery. For women who have undergone a tumor debulking operation before chemotherapy, a level measured approximately 3 weeks after surgery correlates with the amount of residual tumor mass and is predictive of overall survival.[16] Serial levels during and after chemotherapy are used to monitor response to treatment, disease progression, and prognosis. However, many women with *CA-125* levels that have returned to the normal reference range during treatment still have residual disease as determined by a second-look laparotomy to pathologically evaluate the disease.[17] A more rapid decline of serum *CA-125* during treatment has been associated with a more favorable prognosis.[11,18,19] Nadir values <10 units/mL predict improved survival, and increases in *CA-125* from the nadir (even when <35 units/mL) may be used to predict disease progression.[17,20] Failure of *CA-125* level to decline may also be used to identify

tumors that are not responding to chemotherapy; an increase usually indicates progression.[20] However, a large European trial involving >1,400 women failed to demonstrate an improvement in survival in treating women based on rising *CA-125* levels alone.[21] Additional trials are ongoing to confirm these results. Subsequently, rising *CA-125* levels without any other evidence of disease require careful clinical interpretation to determine if patients require treatment interventions.

## Human Chorionic Gonadotropin

*Normal range: serum <5 milli-International Units/mL (<5 International Units/L)*

*Human chorionic gonadotropin* (hCG) is a glycoprotein consisting of $\alpha$ and $\beta$ subunits that is normally produced by the placenta during pregnancy.[22,23] Elevations in nonpregnant women and in men requires evaluation for malignant conditions. The $\beta$ subunit is most commonly used as the determinant in both serum as a tumor marker and in urine tests for pregnancy. hCG is also commonly produced by tumors of germ cell origin, including mixed germ cell or pure choriocarcinoma, tumors of the ovaries and testis, extragonadal tumors of germ cell origin, and gestational trophoblastic disease (eg, hydatidiform mole). Occasionally, islet cell tumors and gastric, colon, pancreas, liver, and breast carcinomas also produce hCG. Patients with trophoblastic disease often produce irregular forms of hCG that may or may not be recognized by various automated assays, and false-positive hCG immunoreactivity also has been reported. Newer highly specific and highly sensitive immunoassays have improved the reliability of this test. Radioimmunoassays and the DPC Immulite hCG test have been reported to have the greatest accuracy.

In patients with testicular cancer, elevated levels of hCG may be present with either seminomatous (1% to 25%) or nonseminomatous disease (10% to 70%) depending on the stage of disease, so the test is not sensitive enough to be used as a screening tool for asymptomatic patients.[22] hCG has an important prognostic role, with levels >50,000 milli-International Units/mL indicating a poor prognosis in nonseminomatous disease.[23] Most frequently, hCG is used to monitor response to therapy (ie, an elevated level is evidence of residual disease following surgery) and monitor for evidence of disease progression or recurrence during or after treatment.[22,23] hCG has a half-life of only 18 to 36 hours, so serum levels decline rapidly after therapeutic interventions; failure to do so may indicate residual disease.[22-24]

## CA 19-9

*Normal range: <37 units/mL*

*Cancer antigen 19-9 (CA 19-9)* is an oncofetal antigen expressed by several cancers, including pancreatic (71% to 93% of cases), gastric (21% to 42% of cases), and colon (20% to 40% of cases) carcinomas. Serum for this test is collected in a red top tube, and the sample is frozen for shipping for analysis. The sensitivity of the test is insufficient to be useful as a screening test for early-stage diseases. It was originally developed for colon cancer monitoring but is no longer recommended for this indication.[6] It is primarily used in pancreatic cancer to help discriminate benign pancreatic disease from cancer, monitor for disease recurrence, and assess response to treatment interventions.[6,25] *CA 19-9* levels have been used to evaluate the effectiveness of a chemotherapy regimen, with rising values indicating a shorter patient survival and the possible need to change chemotherapy regimens.[26] An elevated CA 19-9 level is a poor prognostic factor in patients with inoperable pancreatic cancer.[27]

## α-Fetoprotein

*Normal range: <20 ng/mL*

*α-Fetoprotein* (AFP) is a glycoprotein made in the liver, gastrointestinal tract, and fetal yolk sac. It is found in high concentrations in serum during fetal development (~3 mg/mL); following birth, it declines rapidly to <20 ng/mL. Serum for AFP evaluation should be collected in a red top tube and refrigerated until assayed using radioimmunoassay. It is elevated in 70% of patients with hepatocellular carcinoma, 50% to 70% of patients with testicular nonseminomatous germ cell tumors, and occasionally in patients with other tumors such as ovarian germ cell, pancreatic, gastric, lung, and colon cancers.[23] Nonmalignant conditions that may be associated with increased levels of AFP include pregnancy, hepatitis, and cirrhosis. In patients with nonseminomatous germ cell tumors, the level of AFP serum concentrations seems to correlate with the stage of the disease.[23] In some parts of the world, AFP is used as a screening test for hepatocellular carcinoma in patients who are positive for HBsAg, and are at increased risk for hepatocellular carcinoma. In the United States, however, AFP is used primarily to assist in the diagnosis of hepatocellular carcinoma. AFP levels >1,000 ng/mL are common in patients with hepatocellular carcinoma.[28,29]

These AFP levels also are used to monitor patients with hepatocellular carcinoma or ovarian and testicular germ cell tumors for disease progression or recurrence and to assess the impact of treatment interventions. The serum half-life of AFP is 5 to 7 days, and usually an elevation of the serum level for more than 7 days following surgery is an indication that residual disease was left behind.[25] After successful treatment for nonseminomatous germ cell tumors of the testis, hCG and AFP tests are repeated every 1 or 2 months during the first year, every 2 or 3 months during the second year, and less frequently thereafter, along with physical exams and chest radiographs.[25] Increases in these serum tests are considered an indication for further treatment, such as chemotherapy. Rising levels in patients receiving chemotherapy indicate that therapy should be changed, whereas declining levels predict a more favorable outcome.[23]

## β2-Microglobulin

*Normal range: <2.5 mcg/mL*

*β2-microglobulin* ($B_2M$) is a protein found on the surface of lymphocytes as well as in small quantities in the blood and urine. Elevations of $B_2M$ may be seen in lymphoproliferative disorders, including multiple (plasma cell) myeloma and chronic lymphocytic leukemia lymphoma. $B_2M$ is renally excreted and may be elevated in nonmalignant conditions such as renal failure.[30]

$B_2M$ is a reflection of tumor mass in multiple myeloma and is considered standard for the measurement of tumor burden. Measurement of serum $B_2M$ is most commonly done in the evaluation of multiple myeloma and is an important part of the staging and prognosis for that disease. Additionally, $B_2M$

is used to follow patients with multiple myeloma for treatment efficacy, with increases in $B_2M$ potentially indicating progressive disease.[30-32]

## Estrogen and Progesterone Receptor Assays

The levels of *estrogen receptor* (ER) and *progesterone receptor* (PR) in biopsy tissue from breast cancers predict both the natural history of the disease and the likelihood that the tumor will respond to hormonal manipulations. This test is not a blood test but requires tissue from the cancer obtained by biopsy. ER status is also a prognostic factor, with ER-negative tumors having a worse prognosis than ER-positive ones. For >30 years, it has been the standard of practice to evaluate breast cancer tissue for these protein receptors and use that information in directing therapeutic interventions. The relative expression of hormone receptors can be determined using small amounts of tumor tissue.

The current standard of practice is to measure each protein using immunohistochemistry (IHC) to determine if patients will benefit from endocrine therapy; this method detects protein expression through an antibody–antigen interaction.[33] Although the method (eg, antibody) used can vary, the biopsy is read by pathologists with the results reported as a percent positive cells. If ≥1% of cells is positive, one is considered to have ER-positive or PR-positive disease.[31] Biopsies scored 1% to 10% may be considered "weakly" positive, and risks and benefits of hormonal therapy should be discussed with patients, but the patient is still considered to have ER-positive or PR-positive disease. This category is now described as "ER Low Positive."[34] Because of the variety of methods to evaluate IHC staining and intraobserver/interobserver variability, newer methods of measuring ER and PR status are under investigation, including the use of reverse-transcriptase polymerase chain reaction (RT-PCR), which measures gene expression of ERs in tissue. Classification of ER- and PR-positive tumors are based on cutoff points of 6.5 and 5.5 units, respectively.[34] This test demonstrated statistically significant superiority over IHC in predicting relapse in tamoxifen-treated, ER-positive patients in one retrospective trial.[34] Further validation of the test is needed before it becomes routinely used in clinical practice.[34]

Positive ER/PR levels correlate with response to hormonal therapies, including removal of the ovaries in premenopausal women or administration of an antiestrogen, such as tamoxifen, or an aromatase inhibitor such as anastrozole.[33] In addition, ER/PR content in tumor biopsies correlates with benefit from adjuvant hormonal therapy after surgical removal of the tumor. After 15 years of follow-up in ER/PR-positive breast cancer patients, adjuvant tamoxifen decreased mortality by 9% in women who received 5 years of therapy.[35]

## Human Epidermal Growth Factor Receptor 2

*Human epidermal growth factor receptor 2* (HER2) is a transmembrane glycoprotein member of the epidermal growth factor receptor (EGFR) family with intracellular tyrosine kinase (TK) activity.[36] This group of receptors functions in the growth and control of many normal cells as well as malignant cells. The gene that encodes for HER2 is *c-erb B2*.[37] About 20% of samples from human breast cancers exhibit amplification of *c-erb B2* or overexpression of HER2.[35]

There are many potential clinical applications based on HER2 status in breast cancer. (1) Studies have described the role of HER2 in the prognosis of patients with breast cancer, with poor prognosis seen in overexpressers. (2) HER2 status may predict responsiveness to certain chemotherapy (eg, anthracyclines, taxanes). (3) HER2 status may be used to predict resistance to other therapies (eg, tamoxifen). (4) HER2 status predicts benefit from anti-HER2 therapies, such as monoclonal antibodies (eg, trastuzumab, ado-trastuzumab emtansine, and pertuzumab) and TK inhibitors (eg, lapatinib).[38-43]

However, the considerable variability in study design and the well-recognized heterogeneity of the disease itself have made interpretation difficult, and HER status alone should not determine whether a woman should receive specific adjuvant therapy or whether endocrine therapy should be used.[10]

It is well-established that HER2 overexpression is predictive of a response to treatment with trastuzumab, ado-trastuzumab, and pertuzumab, which are all monoclonal antibodies against HER2; lapatinib, a TK inhibitor of human epidermal growth factor receptor 1 (HER1) and HER2; and neratinib and tucatinib, a TK inhibitor of HER2.[39,40,44-48] Therefore, it is necessary to evaluate all invasive breast cancers for HER2 status to select appropriate patients for these anti-HER2 therapies.[43,49]

Although a portion of the HER2 receptor can dissociate from the cell and be detected in the serum, biopsies of the tumor are routinely used to evaluate HER2 status. It can be measured for overexpression of the protein by IHC or by gene amplification, most commonly by using fluorescence in situ hybridization (FISH) assays.[43] Several commercial assays have been recommended to aid in the selection of patients for anti-HER2 therapy. Immunohistochemistry assays assess for the overexpression of the HER2 protein, and a score of 0, 1+, 2+, or 3+ is reported. Clinical trials have demonstrated that women with a score of 0 or 1+ should be considered HER2 negative and do not benefit from anti-HER2 therapy, and women who have a score of 3+ are HER2 positive and benefit from therapy.[39,43] A score of 2+ should be considered inconclusive and requires further evaluation with a FISH assay.

The FISH assay can be used as the initial test for HER2 positivity and is preferred by some groups because of decreased variability and increased ability to predict efficacy of therapies aimed at the HER2 receptor.[43] The FISH assay measures both the number of gene copies of HER2 gene and provides a ratio of HER2/CEP 17 (also called *FISH ratio*). Tumors are measured by the ratio of HER2 signals divided by the number of signals determined by the centromeric portion of chromosome 17 (CEP 17). A positive test for HER2 gene amplification is a gene copy number >4 or a FISH ratio >2. HER2-negative tumors are defined as a gene copy number <4 or FISH ratio <2, and FISH ratios between 1.8 to 2.2 are inconclusive. Additional cells should be scored and the results compared.[41] Only patients with FISH-positive tumors derive benefit from anti-HER2 therapy.[43]

In summary, routine testing for HER2 with either IHC or FISH is recommended in all patients with invasive breast cancer, with FISH as the preferred method.[10,43] Patients who are HER2 positive benefit from HER2-targeted therapy in neoadjuvant, adjuvant, and metastatic settings.[37,38,44] The use of HER2 testing to determine benefit of additional therapies (eg, tamoxifen, anthracyclines, taxanes) is inconclusive at this time[10,43] (Minicase 2).

## BCR-ABL

The identification of tumor markers in the pathogenesis of malignancy has led to the development of therapeutic strategies that specifically target the cause of the malignancy. By definition, patients with chronic myelogenous leukemia (CML) possess the Philadelphia (Ph) chromosome that indicates the presence of the *BCR-ABL* fusion gene.[50,51] The *BCR-ABL* fusion gene also can be found in acute lymphoblastic leukemia and rarely in acute myeloid leukemia. *ABL* and *BCR* are normally found on chromosomes 9 and 22, respectively. The translocation of *ABL* and *BCR* t(9;22), in which both genes are truncated and form the characteristic *BCR-ABL* fusion gene on the Ph chromosome, is diagnostic for CML and is present in almost all patients with the disease by definition.[50,51] The *BCR-ABL* gene encodes a protein with deregulated, constitutively active TK activity that has become the primary target for treating CML.

The Ph chromosome can be tested by the following three methods[50,51]: (1) conventional cytogenetic testing, in which bone marrow cells are aspirated and the individual chromosomes are examined for the presence of the Ph chromosome (the term *cytogenetic remission* has been developed to describe the elimination of the Ph chromosome on testing by this method after treatment); (2) FISH testing, which can be done on either blood or bone marrow cells (genetic probes are used to look for abnormal cells that contain the *BCR-ABL* gene); and (3) RT-PCR testing, which is the most sensitive test for monitoring response to therapy and counts the number of cells that contain the *BCR-ABL* gene (it can be done on either blood or bone marrow cells). Testing with RT-PCR is referred to as *molecular monitoring* and responses are called *molecular responses*. The quantitative PCR is typically drawn every 3 months; labs can use their own assay, but *BCR-ABL1* transcripts obtained should be converted to the international scale (IS) by applying a lab-specific conversion factor. Bone marrow cytogenetics are obtained at diagnosis and if patient does not achieve the expected response or if there is a loss of response. There is a strong correlation between results obtained from peripheral blood using quantitative PCR and bone marrow cytogenetics, allowing for molecular monitoring without bone marrow aspirations. **Table 21-3** lists the response criteria for CML using cytogenetic and molecular monitoring.[50,51]

Therapies (eg, imatinib, nilotinib, dasatinib, bosutinib, and ponatinib) have been developed that target the abnormal TK activity of the *BCR-ABL* gene.[4,52] As mentioned, efficacy is monitored by the elimination of the Ph chromosome (cytogenetic or molecular), and detection of increasing amounts of the *BCR-ABL* fusion gene often require adjustments in therapy.

Several mutations in the *BCR-ABL* gene have been identified that may predict resistance to the currently available TK inhibitors. Patients who present in advanced-phase disease or have an inadequate or loss of response to TK inhibitors should

**TABLE 21-3.** Criteria for Cytogenetic and Molecular Response in Patients with Chronic Myelogenous Leukemia

| CYTOGENETIC RESPONSE | MOLECULAR RESPONSE |
|---|---|
| Complete: Ph +0% | Early molecular response: BCR-ABL1 (IS) ≤10% at 3 and 6 mo |
| Major: Ph +0% to 35% Partial: Ph +1% to 35% | Major molecular response: BCR-ABL1 (IS) ≤0.1% or a ≥3-long reduction in BCR-ABL1 mRNA from the standardized baseline, if qPCR (IS) is not available |
| Minor: Ph +36% to 65% | Complete molecular response: variably described, but best defined by the assay's level of sensitivity |

undergo mutational analysis, so that the appropriate therapy may be selected. Patients with threonine-to-isoleucine mutation at codon 315 (T315I) were previously referred for stem cell transplantation because of a lack activity of the available TK inhibitors to this mutation. Ponatinib is a U.S. Food and Drug Administration (FDA)-approved TK inhibitor that is active against this mutation, and patients who have the T315I mutation should be considered for this therapy. Failure with multiple therapies may lead to a referral for stem cell transplantation.[53]

## Epidermal Growth Factor Receptor

*Epidermal growth factor receptor* (EGFR) (human epidermal growth factor receptor, HER1, c-erb B1) is a transmembrane glycoprotein member of the EGFR family with intracellular TK activity (same family as HER2). When EGFR receptors are activated, they support tumor growth by influencing cell motility, adhesion, invasion, survival, and angiogenesis. The gene that encodes for EGFR can have activating mutations in exon 18 through 21, but the ones of most interest influence the sensitivity or resistance to erlotinib, gefitinib, afatinib, dacomitinib, and osimertinib (EGFR TK inhibitors [TKi]) that are used in non–small cell lung (NSCL) cancer. Class I mutations in exon 19 account for approximately 44% of all EGFR TK-activating mutations, and a point mutation in exon 21 accounts for approximately 41% of EGFR TK-activating mutations. These mutations are most commonly found in adenocarcinoma of the lung from nonsmokers. They are also more common in Asians and women, which matches patient subset analysis from clinical trials with erlotinib. Approximately 15% of all U.S. patients with adenocarcinoma of the lung have one of these activating mutations. A secondary mutation in exon 20 (T790M) has been found to convey resistance EGFR TKi drugs except for osimertinib. Recent recommendations state that all patients who are being considered for first-line therapy with an EGFR TKi should have mutational analysis run on their tumor tissue.[54] For patients with NSCL

cancer, it is recommended that next-generation sequencing (NGS) or another broad, panel-based approach be performed to identify oncologic drivers, including EGFR mutational analysis and would many EGFR variants, including rare variants and variants of unknown significance. In contrast, a RT-PCR can also be used but would only detect the common EGFR variants, such as exon 18 through 21.[55,56] RT-PCR detects overexpressed protein caused by the underlying fusion transcript, and target break-apart FISH probes can detect a rearrangement regardless of the fusion partner but is not able to screen for large samples for other rearrangements (such as *ALK, ROS1,* and *RET*) that occur at a low frequency.[57] Some EGFR mutations show a decreased response from TKI inhibitors, such as EGFR exon 20 insertions and p.T790M. Osimertinib was FDA-approved for metastatic patients with EGFR T790M mutation positive NSCL cancer in patients who have progressed with EGFR TKIs. It was approved with a companion diagnostic test, Guardant360 CDx assay, that uses a tumor or plasma specimen. This was the first liquid biopsy companion diagnostic to use NGS technology to guide treatment decisions.[58]

## V-Ki-Ras2 Kirsten Rat Sarcoma Viral Oncogene Homolog

*V-Ki-ras2 Kirsten rat sarcoma viral oncogene homolog* (KRas) is an intracellular GTPase that plays an important role in signal transduction. Functionally, it works like an on/off switch that is downstream of many cell surface receptors, including EGFR. When activated it conveys proliferative, growth, and survival signals; in the normal setting it turns off after conveying the activation signal. Mutated or oncogenic Ras performs the same function, but mutations in exon 1 (codons 12 and 13) lead to a permanently active Ras. Oncogenic Ras is found in 20% to 25% of all human tumors and in up to 90% of pancreatic cancers. This is obviously a target for drug development, but currently, no therapy has reached the market that inhibits this signal. Mutated KRas is present in approximately 40% of colorectal tumors, where it conveys resistance to cetuximab and panitumumab. Current national guidelines and many payers require KRas mutational testing before giving either of these anti-EGFR monoclonal antibodies for colorectal cancer. Real-time PCR methods with fluorescent probes to common mutations in codon 12 and 13 are commonly used to determine if a KRas mutation exists; however, other methods, including direct gene sequencing, can be used, but this is typically part of a larger panel.[59,60]

## V-Raf Murine Sarcoma Viral Oncogene Homolog B1

*V-Raf murine sarcoma viral oncogene homolog B1* (BRAF) is a serine/threonine-specific protein kinase that plays an important role in signal transduction. It has activating mutations in 7% to 8% of all cancers and 40% to 60% of melanomas. The two most common mutations are V600E mutation (glutamic acid for valine substitution at amino acid 600) and V600K mutation (valine to lysine substitution at amino acid 600).[61] This mutation means that the kinase is always turned on, signaling downstream partners in the mitogen-activated protein kinase pathway, such as mitogen-activated extracellular kinase (MEK).[62] Vemurafenib was the first *BRAF* inhibitor approved to treat melanoma in patients whose tumor contains this mutation. Concurrent with the approval of vemurafenib, the CobasC 4800 *BRAF* V600 mutation test was introduced, which uses real-time PCR to identify the V600E mutation in tumors; now other tests are available to detect V600E and V600K mutations, including NGS technology. An NGS companion test was approved in patients with NSCL cancer, Oncomine Dx Target Test (Thermo Fischer Scientific, Waltham, MA) for dabrafenib, a *BRAF* inhibitor, in combination with trametinib, a *MEK* 1 and 2 inhibitor; this test can also detect other markers such as ROS1 fusion positivity and EGFR L858R and exon 19 deletion positive patients, which would be indications for other therapies. The prescribing information requires that the test be performed and the result be positive for the mutation before using the drug.[63] Encorafenib is another *BRAF* inhibitor approved to treat metastatic colorectal cancer in combination with cetuximab in patients with the V600E mutation and t iis indicated in metastatic melanoma in combination with binimetinib in patients with the V600E or V600K mutation.[64] BRAF inhibitors are approved for various malignancies, including melanoma, NSCL cancer, thyroid cancer, and colorectal cancer.

## Anaplastic Lymphoma Kinase

*Anaplastic lymphoma kinase* (*ALK*) is a fusion gene formed when the echinoderm microtubule-associated, protein-like 4 (EML4) is fused to *ALK*. The abnormal fusion protein promotes malignant cancer cell growth. Multiple *ALK* inhibitors are available that are highly effective for patients with lung cancer whose tumors contain this translocation; these agents are crizotinib, alectinib, brigatinib, ceritinib, and lorlatinib. The mutation most commonly occurs in nonsmokers with lung adenocarcinoma, and it rarely occurs in combination with *KRas* or EGFR mutations. Although the mutation is found only in 2% to 7% of patients with non–small cell lung cancer, it should be routinely tested for because of significant improvement in outcomes with *ALK* inhibitors that target this mutation. As stated in the EGFR section, NGS technology, such as FoundationOne CDx, should be performed on these patients to detect the possible tumor markers and direct therapy. *ALK* can also be detected by PCR, FISH, or IHC.[65,66]

## Programmed Death-Ligand 1

*Programmed death-ligand 1* (PD-L1) is a ligand of programmed death 1 (PD-1). In some cancers, PD-L1 can be overexpressed, which is an oncologic driver and inhibits the proliferation and differentiation of T cells.[67] The PD-1/PD-L1, also known as a checkpoint pathway, is important for immune tolerance, and tumor cells can turn off the function of normal immune response, causing loss of T-cell activity. Expression of PD-L1 can be detected by IHC.[68] Targeting this pathway has played important role in advancement of treatment for many cancers, such as lung cancer, breast cancer, bladder cancer, melanoma, ovarian cancer, gastrointestinal malignancies, and many others. PD-1 inhibitors (nivolumab, pembrolizumab,

avelumab, and cemiplimab) and PD-L1 inibitors (atezolizumab and durvalumab) bind to PD-1 and PD-L1, respectively, blocking the interaction between PD-1 with PD-L1 on tumor cells and reactivating the immune system, allowing T cells to destroy the tumor. PD-L1 can be tested on tumor cells and is reported as a tumor proportion score. Tumor and inflammatory cells can also be reported and resulted as a combined positive score. PD-L1 expression has shown to be predictive for PD-1/PD-L1 inhibitors; however, some tumors show benefit with low or no expression. Companion tests have been approved for various indications but are not required for all indications.[69]

Genomic alterations of the mismatch repair (MMR) system can also predict efficacy PD-1 and PD-L1 inhibitors. MMR recognizes and repairs errors arising during DNA replication. It is made up of four major genes: MLH1, PMS2, MSH2, and MSH6. If a patient has a germline or somatic mutation or a deletion of any these four genes, the patient would have deficient MMR (dMMR). MMR deficiency may induce microsatellite instability (MSI). Microsatellites are small repeating segments of a consistent length. Instability is considered if the length of the microsatellite repeat in tumor DNA is different from the length in corresponding germline DNA. Five standard sites are tested, and a patient is considered MSI-high (MSI-H) if two or more sites are altered.[70] MSI-H and dMMR are considered interchangeable terms because there is a high level of consistency between them in tumors. These tumors contain increased neoantigen formation, which can be a target for the immune system; also these tumors can upregulate immune checkpoints, such as PD-L1 in infiltrating lymphocytes, making them susceptible PD-L1 inhibitors. The FDA has approved a tumor agnostic indication for pembrolizumab in solid tumors that are MSI-H or dMMR that have progressed following prior treatment and have no satisfactory treatment options as well as for colon cancer. Pembrolizumab can be used in the first-line setting for unresectable or metastatic MSI-H or dMMR disease that has progressed with a fluoropyrimidine, oxaliplatin, and irinotecan.[71] MSI-H can be found in endometrial carcinoma, colon adenocarcinoma, stomach adenocarcinoma, rectal adenocarcinoma, adrenocortical carcinoma, and many more malignancies. Sensitive standardized detection of MSI status is necessary with tests such as NGS; older methods include PCR.[70] NGS is a massively parallel DNA sequencing method that allows the simultaneous analysis of millions of fragments of DNA. A sample from the patient's tumor is sequenced alongside a sample of normal tissue from the patient, which allows genetic variants to be identified. The results show somatic mutations, which are found only in the tumor, or germline mutations that are inherited and found in both the tumor sample and the normal tissue.[72]

Another biomarker that shows promise in predicting the use of PD-1/PD-L1 inhibitors is tumor mutation burden (TMB). Currently there is no consensus on how to measure this. Nivolumab in combination with ipilumumab has been evaluated in patients with NSCL cancer. Patients with high TMB had increased PFS with nivolumab and ipilumuab compared with chemotherapy.[73]

# SUMMARY

To be clinically useful as a screening tool in asymptomatic individuals, tumor markers should be both sensitive and specific. Unfortunately, most of the tumor markers identified to date lack the sensitivity to be used in this capacity. In addition, many nonmalignant conditions cause elevations of these markers. Currently, only PSA is in widespread use as a screening tool when used along with the results of a digital rectal exam. Tumor markers are valuable to monitor for disease recurrence in patients who have undergone definitive surgery for cancers or to assess a patient's response to chemotherapy or other treatment interventions. In these situations, serial measurements of tests such as PSA for prostate cancer, CEA for colon cancer, hCG and AFP for testicular cancer, and *CA-125* for ovarian cancer are considered standards in the follow-up care of patients with these malignancies. Increasingly tumor markers are being used to choose appropriate therapeutic strategies. Some tumor markers, such as HER2 and ER, are used as indicators of tumor sensitivity to therapies that target those receptors. Others such as the *BCR-ABL* fusion gene found in CML patients, *BRAF* V600E and V600K mutations found in melanoma, and EGFR mutations found in lung cancer provide a specific target in which therapeutic strategies have been developed to inhibit the actual pathogenesis of the cancer. Molecular targets detected by NGS technology have become a mainstay of treatment for many patients with cancer.

# LEARNING POINTS

1. *If a patient with CML has a complete cytogenetic response, is the patient considered to be cured of leukemia and thus can stop therapy?*

   ANSWER: Obtaining a complete cytogenetic response to therapies demonstrates that the patient is responding to treatment. However, molecular responses, particularly complete molecular responses, are the most sensitive test to determine if the Ph chromosome is still present. Unfortunately, reaching undetectable levels of *BCR-ABL* transcripts in a patient is not common and does not indicate cure; therefore, the patient should continue therapy.

2. *A patient with testicular cancer has serum AFP level drawn 2 days after his surgery and it is still elevated (250 ng/mL). Is this cause for concern?*

   ANSWER: Using serum tumor markers after surgery in testicular cancer is common, and the rate by which they decline has prognostic implications. However, because the serum half-life of AFP is 5 to 7 days, a level drawn so close to surgery is of little value. In contrast, hCG has a half-life of only 18 to 36 hours. If hCG does not decrease within 2 days after surgery, this should be cause for concern.

3. *In a patient is diagnosed with metastatic melanoma, which pathway mutations should be checked prior to initiating therapy?*

   ANSWER: The two most common mutations in metastatic melanoma are the BRAF V600E and the V600K mutations. This results in the constitutive activation of the mitogen-activated protein kinase

pathway. Currently, we have therapies that inhibit the components BRAF and MEK in these mutation-positive patients. Trials show that the combination of BRAF and MEK inhibitors is synergistic and may be used in combination if the patient is mutation-positive.

# REFERENCES

1. Duffy MJ. Role of tumor markers in patients with solid cancers: a critical review. *Eur J Intern Med.* 2007;18(3):175-184.PubMed

2. Slomski A. USPSTF finds little evidence to support advising PSA screening in any man. *JAMA.* 2011;306(23):2549-2551.PubMed

3. Harrison LE, Guillem JG, Paty P, et al. Preoperative carcinoembryonic antigen predicts outcomes in node-negative colon cancer patients: a multivariate analysis of 572 patients. *J Am Coll Surg.* 1997;185(1):55-59. PubMed

4. Wiratkapun S, Kraemer M, Seow-Choen F, et al. High preoperative serum carcinoembryonic antigen predicts metastatic recurrence in potentially curative colonic cancer: results of a five-year study. *Dis Colon Rectum.* 2001;44(2):231-235.PubMed

5. Minton JP, Martin EW Jr. The use of serial CEA determinations to predict recurrence of colon cancer and when to do a second-look operation. *Cancer.* 1978;42(3 suppl):1422-1427.PubMed

6. Meyerhardt JA, Mangu PB, Flynn PJ, et al. Follow-up care, surveillance protocol, and secondary prevention measures for survivors of colorectal cancer: American Society of Clinical Oncology clinical practice guideline endorsement. *J Clin Oncol.* 2013;31(35):4465-4470.PubMed

7. Hine KR, Dykes PW. Prospective randomised trial of early cytotoxic therapy for recurrent colorectal carcinoma detected by serum CEA. *Gut.* 1984;25(6):682-688.PubMed

8. Barillari P, Ramacciato G, Manetti G, et al. Surveillance of colorectal cancer: effectiveness of early detection of intraluminal recurrences on prognosis and survival of patients treated for cure. *Dis Colon Rectum.* 1996;39(4):388-393.PubMed

9. Harris L, Fritsche H, Mennel R, et al. American Society of Clinical Oncology 2007 update of recommendations for the use of tumor markers in breast cancer. *J Clin Oncol.* 2007;25(33):5287-5312.PubMed

10. Martín A, Corte MD, Alvarez AM, et al. Prognostic value of pre-operative serum CA 15.3 levels in breast cancer. *Anticancer Res.* 2006;26(5B): 3965-3971.PubMed

11. Felder M, Kapur A, Gonzalez-Bosquet J, et al. MUC16 (CA125): tumor biomarker to cancer therapy, a work in progress. *Mol Cancer.* 2014;13:129.PubMed

12. Van Poznak C, Somerfield MR, Bast RC, et al. Use of biomarkers to guide decisions on systemic therapy for women with metastatic breast cancer: American Society of Clinical Oncology Clinical Practice Guideline. *J Clin Oncol.* 2015;33(24):2695-2704.PubMed

13. Eltabbakh GH, Belinson JL, Kennedy AW, et al. Serum CA-125 measurements >65 U/mL: clinical value. *J Reprod Med.* 1997;42(10): 617-624.PubMed

14. Buys SS, Partridge E, Black A, et al. Effect of screening on ovarian cancer mortality: the Prostate, Lung, Colorectal and Ovarian (PLCO) Cancer Screening Randomized Controlled Trial. *JAMA.* 2011;305(22):2295-2303. PubMed

15. Menon U, Ryan A, Kalsi J, et al. Risk algorithm using serial biomarker measurements doubles the number of screen-detected cancers compared with a single-threshold rule in the United Kingdom collaborative trial of ovarian cancer screening. *J Clin Oncol.* 2015;33(18):2062-2071.PubMed

16. Markman M, Liu PY, Rothenberg ML, et al. Pretreatment CA-125 and risk of relapse in advanced ovarian cancer. *J Clin Oncol.* 2006;24(9): 1454-1458.PubMed

17. Prat A, Parera M, Peralta S, et al. Nadir CA-125 concentration in the normal range as an independent prognostic factor for optimally treated advanced epithelial ovarian cancer. *Ann Oncol.* 2008;19(2):327-331. PubMed

18. Juretzka MM, Barakat RR, Chi DS, et al. CA125 level as a predictor of progression-free survival and overall survival in ovarian cancer patients with surgically defined disease status prior to the initiation of intraperitoneal consolidation therapy. *Gynecol Oncol.* 2007;104(1): 176-180.PubMed

19. Markmann S, Gerber B, Briese V. Prognostic value of Ca 125 levels during primary therapy. *Anticancer Res.* 2007;27(4 A):1837-1839.PubMed

20. Liu PY, Alberts DS, Monk BJ, et al. An early signal of CA-125 progression for ovarian cancer patients receiving maintenance treatment after complete clinical response to primary therapy. *J Clin Oncol.* 2007;25(24):3615-3620.PubMed

21. Rustin GJ, van der Burg ME, Griffin CL, et al. Early versus delayed treatment of relapsed ovarian cancer (MRC OV05/EORTC 55955): a randomised trial. *Lancet.* 2010;376(9747):1155-1163.PubMed

22. Cole LA, Shahabi S, Butler SA, et al. Utility of commonly used commercial human chorionic gonadotropin immunoassays in the diagnosis and management of trophoblastic diseases. *Clin Chem.* 2001;47(2):308-315.PubMed

23. Gilligan TD, Seidenfeld J, Basch EM, et al. American Society of Clinical Oncology Clinical Practice Guideline on uses of serum tumor markers in adult males with germ cell tumors. *J Clin Oncol.* 2010;28(20):3388-3404. PubMed

24. Toner GC, Geller NL, Tan C, et al. Serum tumor marker half-life during chemotherapy allows early prediction of complete response and survival in nonseminomatous germ cell tumors. *Cancer Res.* 1990;50(18): 5904-5910.PubMed

25. Safi F, Schlosser W, Falkenreck S, et al. CA 19-9 serum course and prognosis of pancreatic cancer. *Int J Pancreatol.* 1996;20(3):155-161. PubMed

26. Ziske C, Schlie C, Gorschlüter M, et al. Prognostic value of CA 19-9 levels in patients with inoperable adenocarcinoma of the pancreas treated with gemcitabine. *Br J Cancer.* 2003;89(8):1413-1417.PubMed

27. Maisey NR, Norman AR, Hill A, et al. CA19-9 as a prognostic factor in inoperable pancreatic cancer: the implication for clinical trials. *Br J Cancer.* 2005;93(7):740-743.PubMed

28. Soresi M, Magliarisi C, Campagna P, et al. Usefulness of alpha-fetoprotein in the diagnosis of hepatocellular carcinoma. *Anticancer Res.* 2003;23(2 C):1747-1753.PubMed

29. Zhang BH, Yang BH, Tang ZY. Randomized controlled trial of screening for hepatocellular carcinoma. *J Cancer Res Clin Oncol.* 2004;130(7): 417-422.PubMed

30. Munshi NC, Anderson KC. Plasma cell neoplasms. In: DeVita VT, Lawrence TS, Rosenberg SA, eds. *Cancer: Principles and practice of Oncology.* 9th ed. Philadelphia, PA: Lippincott Williams & Wilkins; 2011;107:1819-1855.

31. Mikhael J, Ismaila N, Cheung MC, et al. Treatment of multiple myeloma: ASCO and CCO joint clinical practice guideline. *J Clin Oncol.* 2019;37(14):1228-1263.PubMed

32. Greipp PR, San Miguel J, Durie BG, et al. International staging system for multiple myeloma. *J Clin Oncol.* 2005;23(15):3412-3420.PubMed

33. Hammond ME, Hayes DF, Dowsett M, et al. American Society of Clinical Oncology/College of American Pathologists guideline recommendations for immunohistochemical testing of estrogen and progesterone receptors in breast cancer. *J Clin Oncol.* 2010;28(16):2784-2795.PubMed

34. Allison KH, Hammond MEH, Dowsett M, et al. Estrogen and progesterone receptor testing in breast cancer: ASCO/CAP guideline update. *J Clin Oncol.* 2020;38(12):1346-1366.PubMed

35. Early Breast Cancer Trialists' Collaborative Group (EBCTCG). Effects of chemotherapy and hormonal therapy for early breast cancer on recurrence and 15-year survival: an overview of the randomised trials. *Lancet.* 2005;365(9472):1687-1717.PubMed

36. Citri A, Yarden Y. EGF-ERBB signalling: towards the systems level. *Nat Rev Mol Cell Biol.* 2006;7(7):505-516.PubMed

37. Slamon DJ, Clark GM, Wong SG, et al. Human breast cancer: correlation of relapse and survival with amplification of the HER-2/neu oncogene. *Science.* 1987;235(4785):177-182.PubMed

38. Carlomagno C, Perrone F, Gallo C, et al. c-erb B2 overexpression decreases the benefit of adjuvant tamoxifen in early-stage breast cancer without axillary lymph node metastases. *J Clin Oncol.* 1996;14(10): 2702-2708.PubMed

39. Cobleigh MA, Vogel CL, Tripathy D, et al. Multinational study of the efficacy and safety of humanized anti-HER2 monoclonal antibody in women who have HER2-overexpressing metastatic breast cancer that has progressed after chemotherapy for metastatic disease. *J Clin Oncol.* 1999;17(9):2639-2648.PubMed

40. Geyer CE, Forster J, Lindquist D, et al. Lapatinib plus capecitabine for HER2-positive advanced breast cancer. *N Engl J Med.* 2006;355(26): 2733-2743.PubMed

41. Hayes DF, Thor AD, Dressler LG, et al. HER2 and response to paclitaxel in node-positive breast cancer. *N Engl J Med.* 2007;357(15):1496-1506. PubMed

42. Pritchard KI, Shepherd LE, O'Malley FP, et al. HER2 and responsiveness of breast cancer to adjuvant chemotherapy. *N Engl J Med.* 2006;354(20): 2103-2111.PubMed

43. Wolff AC, Hammond ME, Hicks DG, et al. Recommendations for human epidermal growth factor receptor 2 testing in breast cancer: American Society of Clinical Oncology/College of American Pathologists clinical practice guideline update. *J Clin Oncol.* 2013;31(31):3997-4013.PubMed

44. Baselga J, Cortés J, Kim SB, et al. Pertuzumab plus trastuzumab plus docetaxel for metastatic breast cancer. *N Engl J Med.* 2012;366(2):109-119. PubMed

45. Verma S, Miles D, Gianni L, et al. Trastuzumab emtansine for HER2-positive advanced breast cancer. *N Engl J Med.* 2012;367(19):1783-1791.PubMed

46. Chan A, Delaloge S, Holmes FA, et al. Neratinib after trastuzumab-based adjuvant therapy in patients with HER2-positive breast cancer (ExteNET): a multicentre, randomised, double-blind, placebo-controlled, phase 3 trial. *Lancet Oncol.* 2016;17(3):367-377.PubMed

47. Murthy RK, Loi S, Okines A, et al. Tucatinib, trastuzumab, and capecitabine for HER2-positive metastatic breast cancer. *N Engl J Med.* 2020;382(7):597-609.PubMed

48. Wolff AC, Hammond MEH, Allison KH, et al. Human epidermal growth factor receptor 2 testing in breast cancer: American Society of Clinical Oncology/College of American Pathologists clinical practice guideline focused update. *J Clin Oncol.* 2018;36(20):2105-2122.PubMed

49. Romond EH, Perez EA, Bryant J, et al. Trastuzumab plus adjuvant chemotherapy for operable HER2-positive breast cancer. *N Engl J Med.* 2005;353(16):1673-1684.PubMed

50. Baccarani M, Cortes J, Pane F, et al. Chronic myeloid leukemia: an update of concepts and management recommendations of European LeukemiaNet. *J Clin Oncol.* 2009;27(35):6041-6051.PubMed

51. Radich JP. Measuring response to BCR-ABL inhibitors in chronic myeloid leukemia. *Cancer.* 2012;118(2):300-311.PubMed

52. Shami PJ, Deininger M. Evolving treatment strategies for patients newly diagnosed with chronic myeloid leukemia: the role of second-generation BCR-ABL inhibitors as first-line therapy. *Leukemia.* 2012;26(2):214-224. PubMed

53. Hochhaus A, Baccarani M, Silver RT, et al. European LeukemiaNet 2020 recommendations for treating chronic myeloid leukemia. *Leukemia.* 2020;34:966-984.

54. Lipton JH, Bryden P, Sidhu MK, et al. Comparative efficacy of tyrosine kinase inhibitor treatments in the third-line setting, for chronic-phase chronic myelogenous leukemia after failure of second-generation tyrosine kinase inhibitors. *Leuk Res.* 2015;39(1):58-64.PubMed

55. Khoo C, Rogers TM, Fellowes A, et al. Molecular methods for somatic mutation testing in lung adenocarcinoma: EGFR and beyond. *Transl Lung Cancer Res.* 2015;4(2):126-141.PubMed

56. Keedy VL, Temin S, Somerfield MR, et al. American Society of Clinical Oncology provisional clinical opinion: epidermal growth factor receptor (EGFR) mutation testing for patients with advanced non-small-cell lung cancer considering first-line EGFR tyrosine kinase inhibitor therapy. *J Clin Oncol.* 2011;29(15):2121-2127.PubMed

57. Raman G, Wallace B, Patel K et al. Update on Horizon scans of genetic tests currently available for clinical use in cancers. *AHRQ Technology Assessment Program.* 2011 Apr.

58. Guardant Health Guardant360 CDx. First FDA-approved liquid biopsy for comprehensive tumor mutation profiling across all solid cancers. https://bit.ly/3aclIdI. Accessed September 22, 2020.

59. Allegra CJ, Jessup JM, Somerfield MR, et al. American Society of Clinical Oncology provisional clinical opinion: testing for KRAS gene mutations in patients with metastatic colorectal carcinoma to predict response to anti-epidermal growth factor receptor monoclonal antibody therapy. *J Clin Oncol.* 2009;27(12):2091-2096.PubMed

60. Sepulueda AR, Hamilton SR, Allegra CJ, et al. Molecular biomarkers for the evaluation of colorectal cancer: Guideline from the American Society for Clinical Pathology, College of American Pathologist, Association for Molecular Pathology, and the American Society of Clinical Oncology. *J Clin Oncol.* 2017;25:1453-1486.

61. Long GV, Menzies AM, Nagrial AM, et al. Prognostic and clinicopathologic associations of oncogenic BRAF in metastatic melanoma. *J Clin Oncol.* 2011;29(10):1239-1246.PubMed

62. Arkenau HT, Kefford R, Long GV. Targeting BRAF for patients with melanoma. *Br J Cancer.* 2011;104(3):392-398.PubMed

63. Tafinlar (dabrafenib) [package insert]. Research Triangle Park, NC: GlaxoSmithKline; 2014.

64. Braftovi (encorafenib) [package insert]. Boulder, CO: Array BioPharm; 2018.

65. Just PA, Cazes A, Audebourg A, et al. Histologic subtypes, immuno-histochemistry, FISH or molecular screening for the accurate diagnosis of ALK-rearrangement in lung cancer: a comprehensive study of Caucasian non-smokers. *Lung Cancer.* 2012;76(3):309-315.PubMed

66. Shaw AT, Solomon B, Kenudson MM. Crizotinib and testing for ALK. *J Natl Compr Canc Netw.* 2011;9(12):1335-1341.PubMed

67. Yi M, Jiao D, Xu H, et al. Biomarkers for predicting efficacy of PD-1/PD-L1 inhibitors. *Mol Cancer.* 2018;17(1):129.PubMed

68. Kythreotou A, Siddique A, Mauri FA, et al. PD-L1. *J Clin Pathol.* 2018;71(3):189-194.PubMed

69. Udall M, Rizzo M, Kenny J, et al. PD-L1 diagnostic tests: a systematic literature review of scoring algorithms and test-validation metrics. *Diagn Pathol.* 2018;13(1):12.PubMed

70. Zhao P, Li L, Jiang X, Li Q. Mismatch repair deficiency/microsatellite instability: high as a predictor for anti-PD-1/PD-L1 immunotherapy efficacy. *J Hematol Oncol.* 2019;12(1):54.PubMed

71. Lemery S, Keegan P, Pazdur R. First FDA approval agnostic of cancer site: when a biomarker defines the indication. *N Engl J Med.* 2017;377(15):1409-1412.PubMed

72. Nangalia J, Campbell PJ. Genome sequencing during a patient's journey through cancer. *N Engl J Med.* 2019;381(22):2145-2156.PubMed

73. Hellmann MD, Ciuleanu TE, Pluzanski A, et al. Nivolumab plus ipilumumab in lung cancer with high tumor mutation burden. *N Engl J Med.* 2018;378(22):2093-2104.PubMed

## QUICKVIEW | Carcinoembryonic Antigen

| PARAMETER | DESCRIPTION | COMMENTS |
|---|---|---|
| **Common reference range** | | |
| Adults | <2.5 ng/mL (<2.5 mcg/L) | |
| Children | Unknown | |
| **Critical value** | Yes, levels >10 ng/mL (>10 mcg/L) generally indicate cancerous process | |
| **Inherent activity** | Unknown | |
| **Location** | | |
| Production | Intestine, pancreas, liver | Normally found during fetal development only; detected in serum of patients |
| Storage | Unknown | |
| Secretion/excretion | Unknown | |
| **Causes of abnormal values** | | |
| High | Cancer (mainly colon), smoking, hepatitis, pancreatitis, peptic ulcer disease, hypothyroidism, ulcerative colitis, Crohn disease | Usually <10 ng/mL in nonmalignant conditions |
| Low | Not applicable | |
| **Signs and symptoms** | | |
| High level | Not applicable | |
| Low level | Not applicable | |
| **After event, time to....** | | |
| Initial elevation | Not applicable | |
| Peak values | | |
| Normalization | | |
| **Causes of spurious results** | Not applicable | |
| **Additional info** | Not reliable to screen for cancers because elevated in other conditions; can be used to monitor effectiveness of therapy in patients with cancer | |

## QUICKVIEW | CA-125

| PARAMETER | DESCRIPTION | COMMENTS |
|---|---|---|
| **Common reference range** | | |
| Adults | <35 units/mL | |
| Children | Unknown | |
| **Critical value** | Not applicable | |
| **Inherent activity** | Unknown | |
| **Location** | | |
| Production | | Detected in serum of patients |
| Storage | Unknown | |
| Secretion/excretion | Unknown | |
| **Causes of abnormal values** | | |
| High | Cancer (mainly ovarian, cervical, and fallopian tube carcinomas), endometriosis, ovarian cysts, liver disease, pregnancy, menstruation | |
| Low | Luteal phase of cycle, patients on oral contraceptives, menopausal women | |
| **Signs and symptoms** | | |
| High level | Not applicable | |
| Low level | Not applicable | |
| **After event, time to....** | | |
| Initial elevation | Not applicable | |
| Peak values | | |
| Normalization | | |
| **Causes of spurious results** | Not applicable | |
| **Additional info** | Not reliable to screen for cancers because elevated in other conditions; can be used to monitor effectiveness of therapy in patients with ovarian cancer; rate of rise and fall of levels may indicate disease recurrence or residual disease | |

## QUICKVIEW | CA 15-3

| PARAMETER | DESCRIPTION | COMMENTS |
|---|---|---|
| **Common reference range** | | |
| Adults | <30 units/mL | |
| Children | Unknown | |
| **Critical value** | Not applicable | |
| **Inherent activity** | Unknown | |
| **Location** | Serum | |
| Production | Unknown | Antibody detects circulating mucin antigen secreted |
| Storage | Unknown | |
| Secretion/excretion | Secreted from breast tissue | |
| **Causes of abnormal values** | | |
| High | Breast cancer, may be elevated in other cancers of lung, colon, ovary, and pancreas origin and benign breast and liver disorders | |
| Low | Not applicable | |
| **Signs and symptoms** | | |
| High level | Not applicable | |
| Low level | Not applicable | |
| **After event, time to....** | | |
| Initial elevation | Not applicable | |
| Peak values | | |
| Normalization | | |
| **Causes of spurious results** | Not applicable | |
| **Additional info** | Mainly used in combination with other markers or in clinical trials | |

## QUICKVIEW | CA 27.29

| PARAMETER | DESCRIPTION | COMMENTS |
|---|---|---|
| **Common reference range** | | |
| Adults | <38 units/mL | |
| Children | Unknown | |
| **Critical value** | Not applicable | |
| **Inherent activity** | Unknown | |
| **Location** | Serum | |
| Production | Unknown | Antibody detects circulating mucin antigen secreted |
| Storage | Unknown | |
| Secretion/excretion | Secreted from breast tissue | |
| **Causes of abnormal values** | | |
| High | Breast carcinoma, may be elevated in benign breast disorders | |
| Low | Not applicable | |
| **Signs and symptoms** | | |
| High level | Not applicable | |
| Low level | Not applicable | |
| **After event, time to....** | | |
| Initial elevation | Not applicable | |
| Peak values | | |
| Normalization | | |
| **Causes of spurious results** | Not applicable | |
| **Additional info** | Mainly used in combination with other markers or in clinical trials | |

## QUICKVIEW | Human Chorionic Gonadotropin

| PARAMETER | DESCRIPTION | COMMENTS |
|---|---|---|
| **Common reference range** | | |
| Adults | <5 milli-International Units/mL (<5 International Units/L) | β subunit commonly measured, serum levels drawn when used as a tumor marker |
| Children | Unknown | |
| **Critical value** | Not applicable | |
| **Inherent activity** | Unknown | |
| **Location** | | |
| Production | Made by cells of the placenta | Detected in patient serum and urine |
| Storage | Unknown | |
| Secretion/excretion | Secreted from the placenta or malignant germ cells | |
| **Causes of abnormal values** | | |
| High | Pregnancy, mixed germ cell tumors, or choriocarcinoma of the testes or ovary, increased in other rare tumors | If elevated in men or in nonpregnant women, cancer is suspected |
| Low | Not applicable | |
| **Signs and symptoms** | | |
| High level | Not applicable | |
| Low level | Not applicable | |
| **After event, time to....** | | |
| Initial elevation | Not applicable | |
| Peak values | | |
| Normalization | | |
| **Causes of spurious results** | Not applicable | |
| **Additional info** | Most commonly used in testicular cancer as a prognostic factor as well as to monitor effects of treatment; levels >50 milli-International Units/mL indicate a poor prognosis | |

## QUICKVIEW | CA 19-9

| PARAMETER | DESCRIPTION | COMMENTS |
|---|---|---|
| **Common reference range** | | |
| Adults | <37 units/mL | |
| Children | Unknown | |
| **Critical value** | Not applicable | |
| **Inherent activity** | Unknown | |
| **Location** | | |
| Production | Pancreas, gastric cells, colon | Detected in patient serum |
| Storage | Unknown | |
| Secretion/excretion | Secreted from breast tissue | |
| **Causes of abnormal values** | | |
| High | Pancreatic, gastric, and colon carcinomas; also in benign pancreatic disorders | |
| Low | Not applicable | |
| **Signs and symptoms** | | |
| High level | Not applicable | |
| Low level | Not applicable | |
| **After event, time to....** | | |
| Initial elevation | Not applicable | |
| Peak values | | |
| Normalization | | |
| **Causes of spurious results** | Not applicable | |
| **Additional info** | Only recommended to evaluate treatment response and recurrence in patients with pancreatic cancer | |

## QUICKVIEW | α-Fetoprotein

| PARAMETER | DESCRIPTION | COMMENTS |
|---|---|---|
| **Common reference range** | | |
| Adults | <20 ng/mL | |
| Children | Unknown | |
| **Critical value** | Not applicable | |
| **Inherent activity** | Unknown | |
| **Location** | | |
| Production | Protein made normally during fetal and neonatal stages by liver, gastrointestinal tract, and yolk sac cells | Detected in patient serum; levels should decline after birth |
| Storage | Unknown | |
| Secretion/excretion | Unknown | |
| **Causes of abnormal values** | | |
| High | Cancer (mainly liver and testicular); can be elevated in other cancers, such as pancreatic, gastric, lung, and colon carcinomas; elevated in nonmalignant conditions, including pregnancy, hepatitis, and cirrhosis | High results may be used to screen for liver cancer in parts of the world at increased risk for this malignancy |
| Low | Not applicable | |
| **Signs and symptoms** | | |
| High level | Not applicable | |
| Low level | Not applicable | |
| **After event, time to....** | | |
| Initial elevation | Not applicable | |
| Peak values | | |
| Normalization | | |
| **Causes of spurious results** | Not applicable | |
| **Additional info** | Only recommended to evaluate treatment response and recurrence in patients with testicular cancer | |

## QUICKVIEW | β2-Microglobulin

| PARAMETER | DESCRIPTION | COMMENTS |
|---|---|---|
| **Common reference range** | | |
| Adults | <2.5 mcg/mL | |
| Children | Unknown | |
| **Critical value** | Not applicable | |
| **Inherent activity** | Unknown | |
| **Location** | Protein found on surface of lymphocytes and other MHC I molecules | Also present in small amounts in urine and blood; level should decline after birth |
| Production | Unknown | |
| Storage | Unknown | |
| Secretion/excretion | Unknown | |
| **Causes of abnormal values** | | |
| High | Multiple (plasma cell) myeloma, lymphoma, and in patients with renal failure | Renally excreted so elevated levels may indicate renal failure |
| Low | Not applicable | |
| **Signs and symptoms** | | |
| High level | May see signs of renal failure | |
| Low level | Not applicable | |
| **After event, time to....** | | |
| Initial elevation | Not applicable | |
| Peak values | | |
| Normalization | | |
| **Causes of spurious results** | Not applicable | |
| **Additional info** | Used in patients with multiple myeloma to assist in determining disease stage, prognosis, and response to treatment | |

MHC = major histocompatibility complex.

## QUICKVIEW | Estrogen and Progesterone Receptors

| PARAMETER | DESCRIPTION | COMMENTS |
|---|---|---|
| **Common reference range** | | |
| Adults | Not applicable | Not a normal serum laboratory value, only determined in breast biopsies; if >1% of cells are positive for the receptor, it is considered ER-positive or PR-positive |
| Children | Not applicable | |
| **Critical value** | Not applicable | |
| **Inherent activity** | Growth of breast and other hormone sensitive cells | |
| **Location** | Throughout the body (eg, breast tissue, ovaries, bone) | Also present in small amounts in urine and blood; level should decline after birth |
| Production | Unknown | |
| Storage | Not applicable | |
| Secretion/excretion | Not applicable | |
| **Causes of abnormal values** | | |
| High | Not applicable | It is unknown if the levels are higher in cancer, but they are checked to determine if blocking them with hormonal therapy will be useful |
| Low | Not applicable | |
| **Signs and symptoms** | | |
| High level | May see signs of renal failure | |
| Low level | Not applicable | |
| **After event, time to....** | | |
| Initial elevation | Not applicable | |
| Peak values | | |
| Normalization | | |
| **Causes of spurious results** | Not applicable | |
| **Additional info** | Antiestrogens (eg, tamoxifen) and aromatase inhibitors (eg, anastrozole) often given if these receptors are positive in women with breast cancer | |

## QUICKVIEW | Human Epidermal Growth Factor Receptor 2

| PARAMETER | DESCRIPTION | COMMENTS |
| --- | --- | --- |
| **Common reference range** | | |
| Adults | Considered positive by IHC if 3+ cells stain for HER2 or by FISH if *HER2* gene copy number >4 or FISH ratio >2 | Not a normal serum laboratory value, only determined in breast biopsies; FISH preferred |
| Children | Not applicable | |
| **Critical value** | Not applicable | |
| **Inherent activity** | Protein involved in normal growth and development of cells by activating intracellular pathways that send growth signals to the nucleus | In cancer the growth signal is abnormal and amplified, leading to uncontrolled proliferation of the cancerous cells |
| **Location** | Surface of many epidermal cells | Also present in small amounts in urine and blood; level should decline after birth |
| Production | Not applicable | |
| Storage | Not applicable | |
| Secretion/excretion | Not applicable | |
| **Causes of abnormal values** | | |
| High | Cancer | Either number of receptors may be higher or there may be an increase in *HER2* gene copies indicating increased function of the gene |
| Low | Not applicable | |
| **Signs and symptoms** | | |
| High level | Not applicable | |
| Low level | Not applicable | |
| **After event, time to....** | | |
| Initial elevation | Not applicable | |
| Peak values | | |
| Normalization | | |
| **Causes of spurious results** | Not applicable | |
| **Additional info** | Anti-HER2 therapies (eg, trastuzumab, ado-trastuzumab, fam-trastuzumab deruxtecan, pertuzumab, lapatinib, neratinib, and tucatinib) often given if positive | |

## QUICKVIEW | BCR-ABL

| PARAMETER | DESCRIPTION | COMMENTS |
|---|---|---|
| **Common reference range** | | |
| Adults | Not applicable | This is an abnormal fusion gene that results from a genetic translocation producing a fusion; mRNA normally not present in any significant amount unless a malignancy is present |
| Children | Not applicable | |
| **Critical value** | Not applicable | |
| **Inherent activity** | When present, causes abnormal growth of cells | Translocation results in an abnormal fusion protein with increased TK activity, which continually signals cells to grow |
| **Location** | Chromosome 22 resulting from t(9;22) translocation | Also present in small amounts in urine and blood; level should decline after birth |
| Production | Not applicable | |
| Storage | Not applicable | |
| Secretion/excretion | Not applicable | |
| **Causes of abnormal values** | | |
| High | Cancer | |
| Low | Not applicable | |
| **Signs and symptoms** | | |
| High level | Not applicable | |
| Low level | Not applicable | |
| **After event, time to....** | | |
| Initial elevation | Not applicable | Rising levels of BCR-ABL mRNA correlate with increasing disease activity whereas falling levels are consistent with response to therapy |
| Peak values | | |
| Normalization | | |
| **Causes of spurious results** | Not applicable | |
| **Additional info** | Called the Philadelphia chromosome; levels of BCR-ABL mRNA should decrease with therapy, and failure to do so indicates treatment failure | |

## QUICKVIEW | EGFR Mutation (Exon 19 and 21)

| PARAMETER | DESCRIPTION | COMMENTS |
|---|---|---|
| **Common reference range** | | |
| Adults | Not applicable | This is a gene that codes for a transmembrane receptor; it does not normally contain any mutations |
| Children | Not applicable | |
| **Critical value** | Not applicable | |
| **Inherent activity** | When present, causes abnormal growth of cells | Mutation in lung cancer cells leads to perpetual signaling |
| **Location** | Located on chromosome 7p12; region of interest is exon 19 and 21h | |
| Production | Not applicable | |
| Storage | Not applicable | |
| Secretion/excretion | Not applicable | |
| **Causes of abnormal values** | | |
| High | Not applicable | |
| Low | Not applicable | |
| **Signs and symptoms** | | |
| High level | Not applicable | |
| Low level | Not applicable | |
| **After event, time to....** | | |
| Initial elevation | Not applicable | |
| Peak values | | |
| Normalization | | |
| **Causes of spurious results** | Not applicable | |
| **Additional info** | The presence of a mutation in exon 19 or 21 in lung cancer indicates a higher likelihood of response to erlotinib, afatinib, gefitinib, dacomitnib, and osimertinib | |

## QUICKVIEW | KRas Mutation

| PARAMETER | DESCRIPTION | COMMENTS |
|---|---|---|
| **Common reference range** | | |
| Adults | Not applicable | This is a gene that codes for a GTPase that is a binary switch in cell signaling; it does not normally contain any mutations; when mutations are not present it is referred to as WT |
| Children | Not applicable | |
| **Critical value** | Not applicable | |
| **Inherent activity** | When present, causes abnormal growth of cells | Mutation in colorectal cancer cells leads to perpetual signaling and resistance to monoclonal antibodies targeting EGFR |
| **Location** | Chromosome 12p12; region of interest is exon 1 (codon 12 and 13) | |
| Production | Not applicable | |
| Storage | Not applicable | |
| Secretion/excretion | Not applicable | |
| **Causes of abnormal values** | | |
| High | Mutation common in lung adenocarcinoma, mucinous adenoma, ductal carcinoma of the pancreas, and colorectal carcinoma | |
| Low | Not applicable | |
| **Signs and symptoms** | | |
| High level | Not applicable | |
| Low level | Not applicable | |
| **After event, time to....** | | |
| Initial elevation | Not applicable | |
| Peak values | | |
| Normalization | | |
| **Causes of spurious results** | Not applicable | |
| **Additional info** | Cetuximab and panitumumab only should be used for patients with colorectal cancer with WT KRas tumors | |

WT = wild-type.

## QUICKVIEW | BRAF Mutation

| PARAMETER | DESCRIPTION | COMMENTS |
|---|---|---|
| **Common reference range** | | |
| Adults | Not applicable | This is a gene that codes for a kinase involved in cell signaling through the MAP kinase pathway; it does not normally contain any mutations |
| Children | Not applicable | |
| **Critical value** | Not applicable | |
| **Inherent activity** | When present, causes abnormal growth of cells | Mutation in cancer cells leads to perpetual signaling |
| **Location** | Chromosome 7q34; mutation of interest is at amino acid 600 (BRAF V600E or V600K) | |
| Production | Not applicable | |
| Storage | Not applicable | |
| Secretion/excretion | Not applicable | |
| **Causes of abnormal values** | | |
| High | Mutation common in non-Hodgkin lymphoma, colorectal cancer, malignant melanoma, thyroid carcinoma, non–small cell lung carcinoma, and adenocarcinoma of lung | |
| Low | Not applicable | |
| **Signs and symptoms** | | |
| High level | Not applicable | |
| Low level | Not applicable | |
| **After event, time to....** | | |
| Initial elevation | Not applicable | |
| Peak values | | |
| Normalization | | |
| **Causes of spurious results** | Not applicable | |
| **Additional info** | Patients with malignant melanoma should receive only vemurafenib and dabrafenib if they have a tumor with the V600E mutation; or if the combination of dabrafenib and trametinib, vemurafenib and cobimetinib, or encorafenib and binimetinib is used, a V600E or V600k mutation should be present | |

MAP = mitogen-activated protein.

## QUICKVIEW | Anaplastic Lymphoma Kinase Mutation

| PARAMETER | DESCRIPTION | COMMENTS |
|---|---|---|
| **Common reference range** | | |
| Adults | Not applicable | This is a fusion gene between EML4- and ALK; the resulting protein promotes cancer growth through increased kinase signaling activity; cells do not normally contain this gene fusion |
| Children | Not applicable | |
| **Critical value** | Not applicable | |
| **Inherent activity** | When present, causes abnormal growth of cells | Mutation in cancer cells leads to increased signaling |
| **Location** | Chromosome 2 contains the genes for EML4 and ALK; mutation of interest is translocation/fusion gene EML4-ALK | |
| Production | Not applicable | |
| Storage | Not applicable | |
| Secretion/excretion | Not applicable | |
| **Causes of abnormal values** | | |
| High | Mutation most commonly found in adenocarcinoma of the lung in nonsmokers | |
| Low | Not applicable | |
| **Signs and symptoms** | | |
| High level | Not applicable | |
| Low level | Not applicable | |
| **After event, time to....** | | |
| Initial elevation | Not applicable | |
| Peak values | | |
| Normalization | | |
| **Causes of spurious results** | Not applicable | |
| **Additional info** | Patients with metastatic non–small cell lung cancer should receive only crizotinib, alectinib, brigatinib, ceritinib, or lorlatinib if they have a tumor with the ALK rearrangement | |

# 22

# Drug Screens and Toxicological Tests

*Peter A. Chyka*

DOI 10.37573/9781585286423.022

## OBJECTIVES

*After completing this chapter, the reader should be able to*

- List the general analytical techniques used in substance abuse and toxicological screening and discuss their limitations

- Compare the uses of preliminary and confirmatory urine drug tests

- Discuss the considerations in interpreting a positive and negative drug screen result

- Discuss why interfering substances can cause false-negative and false-positive results of screening tests

- Describe how the characteristics of urine, serum, saliva, and hair specimen affect the drug testing process

- Discuss how toxicologic analyses may be helpful in medicolegal situations, postmortem applications, athletic competition, and substance use disorder

## SUBSTANCE ABUSE, POISONING, AND OVERDOSE

When substance abuse, poisoning, or overdose is suspected, the testing of biological specimens is crucial for characterizing usage or exposure, monitoring therapy or abstinence, or aiding in diagnosis or treatment. Millions of Americans are potentially subject to these types of tests. According to the 2018 National Survey on Drug Use and Health (NSDUH), 31.9 million Americans aged 12 years and older (11.7% of the population) reported using an illicit drug in the past month, and 53.2 million (19.4%) reported illicit drug use during the past year (**Table 22-1**).[1]

Poison control centers document approximately 2 million unintentional and intentional poison exposures each year, with one-half occurring in children <6 years of age. Ninety percent of cases occur in homes and two-thirds are managed onsite in a non-healthcare facility. Drugs are responsible for approximately 60% of poison exposures (**Table 22-2**).[2]

In the 2018 NSDUH report, 20.4 million part-time and full-time workers aged ≥18 years reported use of an illicit drug in the past month, and 12.4 million claimed heavy alcohol use (five or more drinks per occasion on ≥5 days) in the past month.[1] Based on 9 million urine drug screens performed by a nationwide laboratory service in 2018 for the combined U.S. workforce, 4.4% had positive test results (**Table 22-3**).[3]

Driving under the influence of alcohol at least once during the past year was reported by 20.8 million persons (8.0% of people aged ≥16 years) with 12.6 million (4.9%) driving under the influence of illicit drugs. Drugged driving was reported for 28.1 million people (11.0% of people ≥16 years) under the influence of alcohol or selected illicit drugs (marijuana, cocaine, heroin, hallucinogens, inhalants, methamphetamine) in 2018.[1]

For eighth-grade, tenth-grade, and twelfth-grade students, the lifetime prevalence of the use of illicit drugs during 2018 was 19%, 34%, and 48%, respectively (**Table 22-4**).[4] Substance use disorder involves dependence or abuse of illicit drugs or alcohol. The 2018 NSDUH reported 20.3 million people (7.4% of people ≥12 years) had a substance use disorder in the past year.[5]

During 2018, 72,473 people died of poisoning or overdose, with 85 deaths (0.1%) occurring in children <5 years of age.[6] Poisoning became the leading cause of injury-related death in the United States in 2008; 93% of these deaths in 2018 were caused by drugs. The rate of drug-related, age-adjusted overdose deaths has increased from 6.2 per 100,000 (*n* = 17,415) in 2000 to 20.7 per 100,000 (*n* = 67,367) in 2018—a 236% increase in 19 years.[6,7] The 67,367 overdose deaths involved opioids in 69.5% of cases, which included prescription opioids, heroin, illicitly manufactured fentanyl, and fentanyl analogs.[8]

There is no comprehensive tabulation of all incidents of substance abuse or poisoning, and the available databases have strengths and weaknesses.[9] Nevertheless, substance abuse and poisoning are common problems facing healthcare professionals, law enforcement officials, employers, teachers, family members, and individuals throughout society. The detection and management of these incidents often involves laboratory testing and interpretation of the results. On a personal basis, healthcare professionals are asked by family members, acquaintances, and patients about drug testing and the potential impact on their lives. It is often prudent to refer the person to the testing laboratory or physician who ordered the test in question when pertinent facts are not available or when they are unable to

**TABLE 22-1.** Americans Aged 12 Years or Older Reporting Use of Illicit Drugs During 2018

| SUBSTANCE | PERCENTAGE OF THE TOTAL POPULATION | |
| --- | --- | --- |
| | PAST YEAR (%) | PAST MONTH (%) |
| Any illicit drug | 19.4 | 11.7 |
| Marijuana and hashish | 15.9 | 10.1 |
| Cocaine | 2.0 | 0.7 |
| Crack cocaine | 0.3 | 0.2 |
| Heroin | 0.3 | 0.1 |
| Hallucinogens | 2.0 | 0.6 |
| LSD | 0.8 | 0.2 |
| MDMA, Ecstasy | 0.9 | 0.3 |
| Methamphetamine | 0.7 | 0.4 |
| Inhalants | 0.7 | 0.2 |
| Any illicit drug other than marijuana | 8.5 | 3.2 |
| Nonmedical use of any of the following | | |
| Psychotherapeutic drug | 6.2 | 2.0 |
| Pain reliever | 3.6 | 1.0 |
| Tranquilizer | 2.1 | 0.7 |
| Stimulant | 1.9 | 0.6 |
| Sedative | 0.4 | 0.1 |

LSD = lysergic acid diethylamide; MDMA = 3,4-methylenedioxy-*N*-methamphetamine.
*Source:* Adapted from Center for Behavioral Health Statistics and Quality. Results from the 2018 national survey on drug use and health: detailed tables. Rockville, MD: Substance Abuse and Mental Health Services Administration; 2019. https://www.samhsa.gov/data/report/2018-nsduh-detailed-tables.

be properly assessed. This chapter focuses on urine drug testing and serum drug concentration determinations as a means to aid in the management of substance abuse and poisoning.

# URINE DRUG SCREENS

## Objectives of Analysis

A *drug screen* provides a qualitative result based on the presence of a specific substance or group of substances. This determination is also called a *toxicology screen* or *tox screen*. Urine is the specimen of choice, and it is widely used for most situations requiring a drug screen. The collection of urine is generally noninvasive and can be collected in unresponsive patients after urinary catheterization. Adequate urine samples of 20 to 100 mL are easily collected. Most drugs and their metabolites are excreted and concentrated in urine. They are also stable in frozen urine, allowing long-term storage for batched analyses or reanalysis. Urine is a relatively clean matrix for analysis due to the usual absence of protein and cellular components, thereby eliminating preparatory steps for analysis.[10-14]

A urine drug screen result does not provide an exact determination of how much of the substance is present in the urine. The concentration of the substance is actually measured by urine drug screen assays in the process of determining whether the drug is present in a significant amount to render the test result as positive. For each substance, the test has performance standards established by the intrinsic specificity and sensitivity of the analytical process that are linked to regulatory or clinical thresholds, commonly called *cutoff values*. These thresholds are a balance of the actual analytical performance, likelihood for interfering substances, and the potential for false positives, which together suggest that the substance is actually present in the urine. Cutoff values may be set by an individual laboratory to meet regulatory or clinical needs or by purchasing immunoassay kits with the desired cutoff values.

Regulatory cutoff values are typically used to monitor people in the workplace or patients undergoing therapy for substance use disorder. The Substance Abuse and Mental Health Services Administration (SAMHSA) in the Department of Health and Human Services specifies cutoff values for the drug categories that should be routinely included in urine screens for federal requirements (**Table 22-5**).[15] (See the SAMHSA website for updated rules at www.samhsa.gov/workplace/drug-testing.) In hospital and forensic settings, cutoff values are sometimes lowered relative to workplace values to detect more positive results, which can serve as an aid in verifying or detecting an overdose or poisoning.[13,15] Reports of urine drug screen results typically list the cutoff value for a substance and whether the substance was detected at the specified value.

## General Analytical Techniques

There is no standardized urine drug screen that uses the same panel of tested drugs, analytical techniques, or turnaround times. Although there is some commonality among laboratories, tests differ by individual laboratory. Generally, urine drug screens are categorized by level of sensitivity and specificity of the analytical technique (preliminary versus confirmatory) and by the variety of drugs tested.[11,16] *Preliminary tests*, also known as *initial, provisional,* or *stat urine drug screens,* typically use one of six currently available immunoassays (EMIT, KIMS, CEDIA, RIA, FPIA, or ELISA). (See Chapter 2 for more in-depth discussion.)

Immunoassays can be performed on auto-analyzers that are available in most hospitals. These assays are available for many substances of abuse, and results can be reported within 1 to 2 hours.[13,16] Many point-of-care tests (POCTs) also use an immunoassay technique, and results can be available within 5 to 15 minutes. Unfortunately, the result of an immunoassay

**TABLE 22-2.** Ranking of Twelve Most Frequent Poison Exposure Categories Reported to U.S. Poison Control Centers During 2018[a,b]

| ALL EXPOSURES | CHILDREN (<6 YEARS) | ADULTS (>19 YEARS) |
|---|---|---|
| Analgesics | Cosmetics, personal care products | Analgesics |
| Cleaning substances | Cleaning substances | Sedatives, antipsychotics |
| Cosmetics, personal care products | Analgesics | Antidepressant drugs |
| Sedatives, antipsychotics | Foreign bodies | Cardiovascular drugs |
| Antidepressant drugs | Topical medicines | Cleaning substances |
| Cardiovascular drugs | Antihistamines | Alcohols |
| Antihistamines | Vitamins | Anticonvulsants |
| Foreign bodies | Dietary supplements | Stimulants, street drugs |
| Pesticides | Pesticides | Pesticides |
| Alcohols | Gastrointestinal drugs | Antihistamines |
| Stimulants, street drugs | Plants | Hormones and antagonists |
| Anticonvulsants | Antimicrobial drugs | Cosmetics, personal care products |

[a]In decreasing order of frequency and based on 2,541,958 substances reported in 2,099,751 cases.
*Source*: Adapted from Gummin DD, Mowry JB, Spyker DA, et al. 2018 Annual Report of the American Association of Poison Control Centers' National Poison Data System (NPDS): 36th Annual Report. *Clin Toxicol (Phila)*. 2019;57(12):1220–1413.

**TABLE 22-3.** Rate of Positive Urine Drug Screens for the Combined U.S. Workforce During 2018 as Reported by a Nationwide Laboratory Service for 9 Million Tests

| SUBSTANCE | POSITIVE URINE DRUG SCREENS (%)[a] |
|---|---|
| Marijuana | 2.30 |
| Amphetamines | 1.10 |
| Opiates | 0.73 |
| Benzodiazepines | 0.52 |
| Oxycodones | 0.38 |
| Cocaine | 0.28 |
| Barbiturates | 0.22 |
| Methadone | 0.18 |
| 6-acetylmorphine (heroin) | 0.02 |
| PCP | 0.01 |

PCP = phencyclidine.
[a]Some samples had multiple drugs identified.
*Source*: Adapted with permission from Quest Diagnostics. Drug testing index: employer solutions annual report Spring 2019. Lyndhurst, NJ: Quest Diagnostics Inc; 2019. https://www .questdiagnostics.com/dms/Documents/Employer-Solutions /DTI-2019/quest-drug-testing-index-brochure-2019.pdf.

is preliminary due to compromises in specificity that lead to cross-reactivity, particularly with amphetamines and opioids. A preliminary urine drug screen result cannot stand alone for medicolegal purposes and must be confirmed with another type of analysis that is more specific.[10,14] For clinical purposes, some laboratories routinely confirm the results of preliminary drug screens, but others do so only on request of the physician. The need for confirming preliminary test results is based on several factors: whether the result would affect the patient's care, whether the patient is expected to be discharged by the time the results are known, whether any legal actions are anticipated, and whether the cost justifies the possible outcome.

Confirmatory techniques are more specific than preliminary tests and use another analytical technique.[11,16] These tests include high-performance liquid chromatography, gas chromatography, or mass spectrometry, depending on the substances being confirmed. The "gold standards" of confirmatory tests are *gas chromatography* with *mass spectrometry*, often referred to as *GC mass spec* or *GC-MS* and *liquid chromatography* with *tandem mass spectrometry*. Compared with preliminary tests, these techniques are more time-consuming and more costly, require greater technical expertise, and require greater time for analysis—often several hours to days. Most hospital clinical laboratories do not have the capability to perform confirmatory tests and must send the specimen to a local reference laboratory or a regional laboratory. Transportation of the specimen adds to the delay in obtaining results. Confirmatory tests are routinely performed for workplace settings and forensic and medicolegal purposes, and the delay is often less critical than in clinical settings (**Minicase 1**).[10]

**TABLE 22-4.** Categories of Substances Abused as Claimed by High School Seniors During 2018

| SUBSTANCE | PERCENTAGE OF SURVEY RESPONDENTS | |
| --- | --- | --- |
| | PAST YEAR (%) | EVER (%) |
| Alcohol | 53.3 | 58.5 |
| Any illicit drug | 38.8 | 47.8 |
| Marijuana and hashish | 35.1 | 43.6 |
| Any prescription drug | 9.9 | – |
| Sedatives | 6.1 | 4.2 |
| Amphetamines | 5.5 | 8.6 |
| Hallucinogens | 4.3 | 6.6 |
| Tranquilizers | 3.9 | 6.6 |
| Synthetic cannabinoids | 3.5 | – |
| Opioids (excluding heroin) | 3.4 | 6.0 |
| LSD | 3.2 | 5.1 |
| Cocaine | 2.3 | 3.9 |
| 3,4-methylenedioxy-N-methamphetamine (MDMA, Ecstasy) | 2.2 | 4.1 |
| Inhalants | 1.6 | 4.4 |
| Androgenic anabolic steroids | 1.1 | 1.6 |
| Ketamine | 0.7 | – |
| Methamphetamine | 0.5 | 0.7 |
| Heroin | 0.4 | 0.8 |

*Source*: Adapted with permission from Miech RA, Johnston LD, O'Malley PM, et al. Secondary school students, Vol. I: Monitoring the Future national results on drug use 1975–2018. Ann Arbor, MI: Institute for Social Research, The University of Michigan; 2019. http://monitoringthefuture.org/pubs/monographs/mtf-vol1_2018.pdf.

## Common Applications

The purpose of a urine drug screen depends on the circumstances for its use, the condition of the patient, and the setting of the test. In an emergency department (ED) where a patient is being evaluated for a poisoning or overdose, the primary purposes are to verify substances claimed to be taken by the patient and to identify other toxins that could be likely causes of the poisoning or symptoms.[13] This is particularly important when the patient has an altered mental status and cannot give a clear history or is experiencing nondrug causes of coma, such

**TABLE 22-5.** Federal Cutoff Concentrations for Urine Drug Tests[a]

| DRUG | INITIAL TEST (ng/mL) | CONFIRMATORY TEST (ng/mL) |
| --- | --- | --- |
| Amphetamine/methamphetamine | 500 | 250 |
| MDMA/MDA | 500 | 250 |
| Cocaine metabolite[b] | 150 | 100 |
| Marijuana metabolite[c] | 50 | 15 |
| Codeine/morphine | 2,000 | 2,000 |
| Hydrocodone/hydromorphone | 300 | 100 |
| Oxycodone/oxymorphone | 100 | 100 |
| 6-acetylmorphine[d] | 10 | 10 |
| PCP | 25 | 25 |

MDA = 3,4-methylenedioxyamphetamine.
[a]Standards issued by Substance Abuse Mental Health Services Administration for urine specimens collected by federal agencies and by employers regulated by the Department of Transportation effective October 2017; see website for changes (https://www.samhsa.gov/workplace/drug-testing).
[b]Metabolite as benzoylecgonine.
[c]Metabolite as δ-9-tetrahydrocannabinol-9-carboxylic acid.
[d]A metabolite specific to heroin.
*Source*: Adapted from Department of Health and Human Services, Substance Abuse and Mental Health Services Administration. Mandatory guidelines for federal workplace drug testing programs. Fed Regist. 2017; 82:7920–7970. https://www.samhsa.gov/workplace/drug-testing.

as traumatic head injury or stroke. The value of routinely performing urine drug screens in the ED for patients who overdose has been questioned.[17] The benefits include having objective evidence of the toxin's presence to confirm the exposure, suggesting alternative toxins in the diagnosis, ruling out a toxin as a cause of symptoms of unknown etiology, and providing medicolegal documentation. The disadvantages include being misled by false-positive results, impractical delays in receiving the results that do not influence therapy, and limited practical value because many poisonings can be recognized by a collection of signs and symptoms.[18,19]

The American College of Emergency Physicians states in a clinical policy on the immediate treatment of poisonings that "qualitative toxicologic screening tests rarely assist the emergency physician in patient management."[20] Urine drug testing can be important, with substances exhibiting delayed onset of toxic symptoms, such as sustained-release products, when patients ingest multiple agents, or when patients are found with multiple agents at the scene. Some trauma centers routinely

## MINICASE 1

### Reliability of Amphetamine Results

Kisha T., a 21-year-old college student, is brought to the ED by her family because of bizarre behavior. She is having visual hallucinations and is paranoid and jittery. She is clinically dehydrated, tachycardic, and delirious. A stat preliminary urine drug screen is positive for amphetamines.

**QUESTION:** Is this patient abusing amphetamine?

**DISCUSSION:** Amphetamine abuse is possible, but alternative causes should be considered. Her parents report that she has just completed a week of final exams, is taking a full course load, and is working two part-time jobs. She is described as studious and a compulsive achiever. After 6 hours of supportive therapy, rest, and intravenous (IV) fluids, she is lucid and confesses to drinking more than a dozen energy drinks to stay awake in the past 2 days and taking two loratadine with pseudoephedrine 12-hour tablets 6 hours ago for allergy symptoms. A targeted confirmatory assay for amphetamines was negative for amphetamines and methamphetamine. Urine drug screens by immunoassay for amphetamines are subject to cross-reactivity with several sympathomimetic amine-type drugs (eg, ephedrine and pseudoephedrine and their variants are often found in dietary supplements marketed for energy and weight loss and as decongestants), which would cause a false-positive result for amphetamines by immunoassay. Caffeine found in many energy drinks and dietary supplements for weight loss and energy are likely the principal causes of her symptoms. Caffeine was not detected in the urine screen because it was not on the testing panel of screened drugs.

The inclusion of a substance on a drug screen is also subject to individual laboratory discretion. Workplace and substance abuse monitoring programs are required to test for five categories of substances (marijuana metabolites, cocaine metabolites, opiate metabolites, PCP, and amphetamines) as specified by the "Fed 5" (Table 22-5). Most immunoassay manufacturers design the range of assays to meet this need and offer additional categories that a laboratory may choose to include.[13,24] The expense of developing an immunoassay is balanced with the promise of economic recovery with widespread use. This economic reality precludes the development of a test for emerging substances of abuse, such as synthetic cathinones, synthetic cannabinoids, designer fentanyl analogs, and life-threatening overdoses, such as calcium channel antagonists and β-adrenergic blockers. Techniques used for confirmatory tests would be required to detect many of the substances not included in the panel of the preliminary drug screen.

perform urine drug screens on newly admitted patients, although the value of this practice has been questioned.[21] People who are experiencing suicidal thoughts or with substance use disorder can be poor or misleading historians, whereby the amounts, number of substances, and routes of exposure may be exaggerated or downplayed. A urine drug screen may assist in identifying potential substances involved in these cases and lead to specific monitoring or treatment (**Minicase 2**).

In the workplace, the purpose of a urine drug screen may include pre-employment tests, monitoring during work, postaccident evaluation, and substance abuse treatment monitoring.[10] Employers who conduct pre-employment urine drug tests generally make hiring contingent on a negative test result. Many positions in the healthcare industry require pre-employment drug tests, and some employers perform random tests for employees in positions requiring safety or security as a means to deter drug use and abuse that could affect performance. In addition to random tests, some employers test individuals based on a reasonable suspicion of substance abuse, such as evidence of use or possession, unusual or erratic behavior, or arrests for drug-related crimes. For employees involved in a serious accident, employers may test for substances when there is suspicion of use—to determine whether substance abuse was a factor—or as a necessity for legal or insurance purposes. Employees who return to work after treatment for substance abuse are often randomly tested as one of their conditions for continued employment or licensure. In the workplace setting, specific procedures must be followed to ensure that the rights of employees and employers are observed.

The Division of Workplace Programs of SAMHSA specifies guidelines for procedures, due process, and the appeals process and lists certified laboratories.[10] Two critical elements of workplace drug testing include establishing a chain-of-custody and control for the specimen and involving a medical review officer (MRO) to interpret positive test results. The chain-of-custody starts with close observation of urine collection. Patients are required to empty their pockets, and they are placed in a collection room without running water and where blue dye has been added to the toilet water. These measures minimize the risk of adulteration or dilution of the urine sample. After urine is placed in the container, the temperature is taken, the container is sealed, and the chain-of-custody documentation is completed. After the chain-of-custody form is completed by everyone in possession of the specimen, it reaches the laboratory, where the seal is broken and further procedures are observed. Positive specimens are often frozen for 1 year or longer if requested by the client or if the results are contested by a court. Chain-of-custody procedures are time-consuming and are not typically considered in the clinical management of poisonings and overdoses, but they are important to sustain the validity of the sample and its result in a court of law.[10]

An MRO is typically a physician trained in this specialty who has responsibility to determine whether the result of the drug test is related to substance abuse.[10,22] Duties involve interviewing the donor; reviewing his or her therapeutic drug regimen; reviewing possible extraneous causes of a positive result, such as a false-positive result from a prescribed medication or substance

## MINICASE 2

### Drug Screens and Emergent Care

Bob C., a 26-year-old man, is dropped off at an ED in the late evening after he becomes progressively more unresponsive in a hotel room. His acquaintances do not know his medical history but eventually admit that he had swallowed some drugs. They promptly leave the area. Bob C. is unconscious with some response to painful stimuli, and he exhibits pinpoint pupils and depressed respirations at 12 breaths/min. His other vital signs are satisfactory. Oxygen administration and IV fluids are started. A bedside stat glucose determination yields a result of 60 mg/dL. A 50-mL IV bolus of dextrose 50% is administered with no change in his level of consciousness. Naloxone 0.8 mg is given IV push, and within minutes Bob C. awakens, begins talking, and exhibits an improved respiratory rate. He admits to drinking some whiskey and taking a handful of several combination tablets of hydrocodone and acetaminophen shortly before he was dropped off at the ED.

In addition to routine laboratory assessment, a serum acetaminophen concentration is determined. During the next 24 hours, he receives supportive care in the critical care unit and requires two additional doses of naloxone. He is scheduled for a psychiatric evaluation to assess treatment options for his substance abuse, but he walks out of the hospital against medical advice on the second day. A urine drug screen by immunoassay that was obtained in the ED is reported as positive for opiates and marijuana on the morning of his second day of hospitalization. The serum acetaminophen concentration reported 2 hours after ED arrival was 60 mcg/mL, which was obtained approximately 6 hours after drug ingestion. Ethanol was not included in the drug screen panel.

QUESTION: Was a urine drug screen necessary for the immediate care of this patient? How is a urine drug screen helpful in this type of situation?

DISCUSSION: In emergent situations like this one, which involves an apparent acute opiate overdose, the results of a urine drug screen are not necessary for immediate evaluation and effective treatment. The symptoms and history clearly indicate that an opiate overdose is likely.[18,19] The response to naloxone confirms that an opiate is responsible for the CNS depressant effects. Because immediate treatment was necessary, waiting for the results of the preliminary drug screen—even if it was reported within hours—would not change the use of supportive care, glucose, and naloxone. The urine drug screen may be helpful to confirm the diagnosis for the record and assist in guiding substance abuse treatment. Obtaining a serum acetaminophen concentration is important in cases of intentional drug use (ie, suicide attempt and substance abuse). This practice is particularly important in situations of multiple drug exposure, unknown drug exposure, or when acetaminophen may be contained in multiple-ingredient, oral drug products (eg, analgesics, cough and cold medicines, sleep aids, and nonprescription allergy medicines). A serum specimen is needed because acetaminophen is not part of routine urine drug screens, and serum assays on acetaminophen generally have a quick turnaround time so they can be used clinically to assess the potential severity of the exposure. In this patient's case, the serum acetaminophen concentration did not indicate a risk for hepatotoxicity (Figure 22-1). Another benefit of obtaining a serum acetaminophen concentration in this case is that it indirectly confirms that an opioid combination product was involved and is consistent with his response to naloxone.

interfering with the analytical test; rendering an opinion on the validity of the test result; considering a retest of the donor or the same specimen; reporting the result to the employer; and maintaining confidential records. This individualized interpretation is critical not only because people's careers, reputations, livelihood, and legal status can be affected but also because it is a regulatory requirement.

Drug screening is also used in the criminal justice system for several purposes, such as informing judges for setting bail and sentencing, monitoring whether specified drug abstinence is being observed, and identifying individuals in need of treatment. For example, a positive drug test result at the time of arrest may identify substance abusers who need medical treatment prior to incarceration, which may result in a pretrial release condition that incorporates periodic drug testing. If a defendant is being monitored while on parole or work release, a drug screen can verify that he or she is remaining drug free. Drug tests in prisons can also assist in monitoring substance use in jail.

The impact of a drug screen result can be profound if it affects decisions of medical care, employment, legal importance, and

a person's reputation. In addition, several factors can affect the reliability and interpretation of drug screen results. These issues should be considered when evaluating a drug screen and are described in the following section.

### Unique Considerations

When a urine drug screen is reported as negative, it does not mean that the drug was not present or not taken—it means that it was not detected. The drug in question may not be part of a testing panel of the particular drug screen (Table 22-6). For example, methadone, meperidine, and fentanyl are not detected on opiate immunoassays.[13,23] Illicitly synthesized and manufactured analogs or homologs of drugs or substances, also called *designer drugs*, are not detected by routine drug screens because the chemical structure is often unknown, a reference standard and assay have yet to be developed, and variations of a chemical structure are frequently introduced into the illicit drug marketplace. At this time, there are no commercial immunoassays for the increasing number of illicit fentanyl analogs. Another factor may involve urine that is too dilute for detection of the substance. This may be due to renal

**TABLE 22-6.** Categories of Drugs and Chemicals Often Not Detected by Routine Drug Screens[a]

Androgenic anabolic steroids

Anesthetics (eg, ketamine, lidocaine)

Angiotensin-converting enzyme inhibitors

Animal venoms

Antidysrhythmic drugs

Anticoagulant drugs

β-adrenergic agonists

β-adrenergic antagonists

Calcium channel antagonists

Chemical terrorism agents

Dietary supplements[b]

Designer cannabinoids

Designer cathinones (eg, bath salts, flakka)

Designer phenethylamines (eg, 2Cs, N-BOMe drugs)

Heavy metals (eg, lead, arsenic, and mercury)[c]

Hydrocarbon solvents and inhalants

Nonbenzodiazepine hypnotics (eg, zolpidem, eszopiclone, zaleplon)

Pesticides

Plant toxins

Selective serotonin reuptake inhibitors

Synthetic opioids (eg, fentanyl, meperidine, methadone)

[a]See Quickviews for more examples.
[b]Those without chemically similar drug counterparts are not detected on a drug screen.
[c]Heavy metals require a special collection container, collection duration, and assay.

disease, intentional dilution to avoid detection, or administration of large volumes of IV fluids as part of a critically ill patient's care. The urine may have been collected before the drug was excreted, but this is unlikely in most symptomatic acute overdoses or poisonings. The time that an individual tests positive (ie, the drug detection time) depends on pharmacologic factors, including dose, route of administration, rates of metabolism and elimination, and analytical factors (eg, sensitivity, specificity, and accuracy). In some cases, the urine sample may have been intentionally adulterated to mask or avoid detection.

Adulteration of a urine sample either intentionally or unintentionally can lead to negative or false-positive results through several means.[10,23,24] A freshly voided urine sample may be replaced with a drug-free sample when urine collection is not directly observed. The ingestion of large volumes of water with or without a diuretic may dilute a drug in the urine, thereby reducing the concentration of the urine below

the assay detection limit. Urine specimens for workplace testing and substance abuse monitoring are tested for temperature within 4 to 5 minutes after collection and later tested for creatinine concentration, pH, specific gravity, and the presence of oxidizing adulterants (eg, chromates, nitrites) as part of routine specimen validity testing.

Adding a chemical to a urine sample may invalidate some test results. Adulteration products that are available through the Internet contain chemicals such as soaps, glutaraldehyde, nitrites, other oxidants, and hydrochloric acid. Depending on the assay method and test, these substances may interfere with absorbance rates or enzyme activity, produce false-positive or false-negative results, or oxidize metabolites that are measured in the immunoassay. For example, some chromate-based and peroxidase-based oxidizers degrade 9-carboxy-tetrahydrocannabinol, a principal metabolite of tetrahydrocannabinol, and lead to a negative result for marijuana.[23,24] Taking large amounts of sustained-release niacin (2.5 to 5.5 g over 36 to 48 hours) has been promoted on the Internet as a means to rid the body of cocaine and marijuana and interfere with urine drug screens. Niacin may also darken diluted urine to seem "normal" in appearance. This practice is unlikely to produce the desired outcome, but it has produced niacin poisonings ranging from skin flushing to life-threatening symptoms that required hospitalization.[25] The effects of adulterants vary with the immunoassay technique and the specific test used by the laboratory; they are not reliable ways to mask drug use. Most adulterants do not affect the GC-MS or liquid chromatography with tandem mass spectrometry analysis for drugs in urine, but such a confirmatory step would be ordered only if there was a high suspicion of adulteration. A positive immunoassay result is typically used to justify the use of a confirmatory GC-MS or liquid chromatography with tandem mass spectrometry analysis.

A positive drug test can show the presence of specific drugs in urine at the detectable level of the test. It does not indicate the dosage, when the drug was administered, how it was administered, or the degree of impairment. Many drugs can be detected in urine for up to 3 days after being taken and some up to 2 weeks or more (**Table 22-7**).[11,13,23,24] It is possible for a legitimate substance in the urine to interact with the immunoassay and produce a false-positive result.[13,24,26,27]

Exposure to interfering substances can affect the results of an immunoassay urine drug screen (Table 22-7). A positive immunoassay result for opiates may result from the ingestion of pastries containing poppy seeds because they contain codeine and morphine in small, but sufficient, amounts to render the test positive. The result is a true positive but not a positive indicator of drug abuse. The immunoassay for amphetamines is prone to false-positive results from drugs with similar structures such as ephedrine, pseudoephedrine, and bupropion.[13,24,26] Also, drugs seemingly dissimilar from the target of an immunoassay can cause false-positive results. For example, naproxen can produce false-positive results for marijuana and barbiturates and was found to do so in 1 of 14 volunteers tested.[28] Most fluoroquinolone antibiotics can produce false-positive opiate

**TABLE 22-7.** Detection Times and Interfering Substances for Immunoassay Urine Drug Screens[a,b]

| DRUG | DETECTION TIME | POTENTIAL FALSE-POSITIVE AGENTS AND COMMENTS |
|---|---|---|
| Amphetamines | 2–4 days; up to 7–10 days with prolonged or heavy use | Ephedrine, pseudoephedrine, ephedra (ma huang), phenylephrine, selegiline, chlorpromazine, promethazine, trazodone, bupropion, desipramine, trimipramine, ritodrine, amantadine, ranitidine, phenylpropanolamine, brompheniramine, 3,4-methylenedioxy-*N*-methamphetamine (MDMA, Ecstasy), isometheptene, labetalol, phentermine, methylphenidate, isoxsuprine, trimethobenzamide |
| Barbiturates | Short-acting, 1–7 days; intermediate-acting, 1–3 wk; chronic use, up to 4 wks | Ibuprofen, naproxen |
| Benzodiazepines | Up to 1 wk; up to 4 wk with chronic use of some agents | Oxaprozin, sertraline; benzodiazepines vary in cross-reactivity, persistence, and detectability; flunitrazepam may not be detected |
| Cocaine metabolite (benzoylecgonine) | 12–72 hr; up to 1–2 wk with prolonged or heavy use | Cross-reactivity with cocaethylene varies with the assay because assay is directed to benzoylecgonine; false positives from -caine anesthetics and other drugs are unlikely |
| LSD | 1–2 days typically; up to 5 days possible | |
| Marijuana metabolite (δ 9-tetrahydrocannabinol -9-carboxylic acid) | 1–5 days; 1 mo or more with prolonged or heavy use | Efavirenz, pantoprazole; ibuprofen, naproxen, tolmetin are possible but uncommon; patients taking dronabinol also have positive test results; designer cannabinoids are not detected |
| Methadone | 3–14 days | Diphenhydramine, doxylamine, clomipramine, chlorpromazine, thioridazine, quetiapine, verapamil |
| Opioids | 2–3 days typically; up to 6 days with sustained-release formulations; up to 1 wk with prolonged or heavy use | Rifampin, some fluoroquinolones, poppy seeds, quinine in tonic water; the assay is directed toward morphine with varying cross-reactivity for codeine, oxycodone, hydrocodone, and other semisynthetic opioids; synthetic opioids (eg, fentanyl, meperidine, methadone, pentazocine, propoxyphene, tramadol, buprenorphine, loperamide) have minimal cross-reactivity and may not be detected |
| Phencyclidine (PCP) | 2–10 days; 1 mo or more with prolonged or heavy use | Ketamine, dextromethorphan, diphenhydramine, imipramine, mesoridazine, thioridazine, venlafaxine, ibuprofen, meperidine, tramadol |

[a]Time after which a drug screen remains positive after last use.
[b]Because performance characteristics may vary with the type of immunoassay, manufacturer, and lot; consult the laboratory technician and package insert for the particular test.
*Source*: Data from references 11, 23, 24, 26, 27.

results, but this interference varies with the fluoroquinolone and immunoassay.[29] The immunoassay manufacturer's package insert should be consulted for information on known interfering substances. In workplace settings, the MRO is obligated to assess whether a person's legitimate drug therapy could interfere with the result (**Minicase 3**).

The persistence of the substance in the urine is an important factor in the interpretation of the results (Table 22-7).[26] For laboratory results reported as negative, it may indicate that the specimen was obtained too early or too late after exposure to a chemical, thereby producing a urine specimen with insufficient concentration of the drug to lead to a positive result.

## MINICASE 3

### Workplace Drug Screen Interpretations

Beau G., a 45-year-old pharmacist, applies for a position at a hospital pharmacy. As part of his pre-employment evaluation, he is asked to provide a urine specimen in a specially designed room for drug testing. His urine sample is positive for opiates and marijuana by immunoassay. His case is referred to the hospital's MRO for a review of the findings. The physician orders a confirmatory test on the same urine specimen. The human resources department of the hospital learns from his current employer that he is an above average worker with no history of substance abuse. A criminal background check is negative for any criminal record. The MRO contacts Beau G. and learns that he was taking acetaminophen and codeine prescribed for pain from suturing of a laceration of his hand for 2 days prior to drug testing. He also routinely takes pantoprazole (Protonix) for gastroesophageal reflux. He had forgotten to list the recent use of these drugs on his employment application because his injured hand began to ache while writing.

QUESTION: Has this patient used any drugs or substances that should prevent him from being considered for employment?

DISCUSSION: Consideration of several factors is important in interpreting the urine drug screen result in this case. The patient has no obvious symptoms of intoxication and has a good employment record. It is likely that the codeine prescribed for pain control produced the positive opiate result. This drug is being used for a legitimate purpose with a valid prescription. The positive test for marijuana is likely from his use of pantoprazole causing a false-positive result. The confirmatory test by GC-MS was negative for marijuana, but it was positive for codeine and morphine. Codeine is metabolized in part to morphine. The MRO reviewing this case would likely conclude that the test results are not indicative of opioid abuse and the marijuana immunoassay result was a false positive. If there are concerns about his suitability for employment, he may be subjected to an unannounced drug test during his probationary employment period. Acetaminophen and pantoprazole were not reported as a result because they were not on the routine assay panel.

Drugs with short half-lives, such as amphetamines, may not be detectable several hours after use. A common concern for individuals undergoing workplace testing is the length of time after use that the drug is still detectable. This varies with the sensitivity of the assay, whether the assay is directed to the parent drug or the metabolite, whether the drug or its metabolites exhibits extensive distribution to tissues that will affect its half-life, the dose of the drug taken, and whether the drug was used chronically or only once. For example, cocaine is rarely detected in a urine specimen because of its rapid metabolism. Immunoassays are directed to cocaine metabolites, such as benzoylecgonine, which are detected for up to 2 to 3 days after use and up to 1 to 2 weeks with heavy use. The major active component of marijuana, δ-9-tetrahydrocannabinol, is converted to several metabolites of which δ-9-tetrahydrocannabinol-9-carboxylic acid is the agent to which antibodies are directed in many immunoassays. This metabolite is distributed to tissues and can be detected for days to weeks after use.[13,26] Chronic or heavy use can lead to detection up to a month or more after stopping use (**Minicase 4**). Immunoassays may lead to false-negative reports in part due to incomplete cross-reactivity across a drug class. For example, the benzodiazepine immunoassay is designed to detect oxazepam, nordiazepam, and temazepam, which are metabolites of diazepam, but the assay does not react with alprazolam, clonazepam, or lorazepam.[30]

## MINICASE 4

### Evidence of Heroin

Danny W., a 23-year-old assembly line worker at a computer manufacturing facility, is examined by the company's physician within an hour of being involved in a workplace accident. She observes a laceration on his left arm, pupil size of 1 to 2 mm (normal, 2 to 5 mm), bilateral ptosis, and recent punctate lesions on the left antecubital fossa. The rest of the physical exam is unremarkable. Danny W. denies eating poppy seeds, taking any medication or dietary supplement, or having a neurologic condition. He has no history of substance abuse in his files. The physician suspects heroin use and orders a focused urine drug test for opiates. Several days later, the laboratory report indicates positive results for morphine, codeine, and 6-acetylmorphine.

QUESTION: Has this patient used a drug or substance that would impair his ability to work? What, if any, substance is likely?

DISCUSSION: This patient has likely used heroin several hours before the accident and several symptoms are consistent with opiate intoxication. Heroin may not be present in sufficient amounts to be detected, in part, because it is metabolized to several compounds such as morphine and 6-acetylmorphine, which can be detected in the urine of heroin users. Because 6-acetylmorphine is only found in urine following heroin use, its presence confirms heroin but other opioids could also contribute to his symptoms. The presence of small amounts of codeine in heroin abusers is likely from contamination of the heroin with codeine and is not because codeine is a metabolic byproduct of heroin or because he had consumed codeine.

## MINICASE 5

### Interpreting Cocaine Results

Shelly N., a 56-year-old supervisor for a large utility company, had recently conducted an inspection at a nuclear power plant. She then left for a 2-week vacation with a friend. After returning to work, she was asked to submit a urine sample for drug testing because the company performs random drug tests for compliance with regulatory, insurance, and contractual requirements. A week later, the results of the immunoassay are reported as positive for the cocaine metabolite, benzoylecgonine. A confirmatory test by GC-MS confirms the immunoassay result. Shelly N. is asked to report to the company's medical office. During the interview with the physician, she denies illicit drug use but states that she had dental work performed immediately before returning to work from her vacation and that she had received procaine hydrochloride (Novocaine) for local anesthesia.

**QUESTION:** What caused the positive test result for cocaine?

**DISCUSSION:** This patient apparently believed that any substance with a name ending in -*caine* must share chemical similarity with cocaine and could be a probable cause of a false-positive result. Although interference with immunoassays is possible, a false positive for cocaine with local anesthetics is unlikely unless the anesthetic preparation contains cocaine. The positive result was confirmed by a confirmatory test that is not subject to this type of interference. In this patient's case, use of cocaine is the most likely explanation for the positive result.

For clinical applications, the time it takes for the test result to be reported to the clinician after specimen collection, also known as *turnaround time*, can affect the use of the drug screen. Many hospital laboratories can perform preliminary immunoassay urine drug screens using mechanized analytical technology, which is used for common clinical tests or using dedicated desktop analyzers. Results from in-hospital laboratories can often be returned within 2 hours of collection. For many urgent situations, such as an acute overdose or poisoning, this delay is unlikely to influence the immediate therapy of the victim. The results may lead to later consideration of alternative or additional diagnoses. Most clinics, small hospitals, or specimen collection sites do not possess such capability and must rely on making the specimen a "send out" that is performed at a nearby or regional reference laboratory. The turnaround time from a reference laboratory varies with the laboratory and the need for urgency. Most results for clinical applications are reported within 24 to 48 hours. However, some results may take up to 3 to 7 days. In some situations, such as pre-employment workplace testing, this delay is acceptable. The turnaround time for confirmatory testing depends on the laboratory, transportation time from the collection site to the laboratory, the tests being performed or requested, and the need for urgency. The delay could be as short as 24 hours or as long as a month or more, particularly for postmortem samples (**Minicase 5**).

## SERUM CONCENTRATIONS

### Objectives of Analysis

Quantitative assays determine the concentration of a substance in a biological specimen; typically this involves serum. The availability of serum concentrations for toxins is based on considerations of whether the concentration correlates with an effect, the outcome or need for therapy, the existing use of the assay for another application such as therapeutic drug monitoring, and technical ease of performing the assay. Serum is typically not used for drug screening purposes in clinical or workplace settings.

Many poisonings and overdoses can be adequately managed without quantitative analysis.[9,19] A history of the exposure, signs and symptoms, and routinely available clinical tests—such as full blood count, electrolytes, glucose, International Normalized Ratio, liver function tests, blood urea nitrogen, serum creatinine, anion gap, serum osmolality and osmolal gap, arterial blood gases, and creatinine kinase—can guide patient management decisions. Intravenous lipid emulsion (ILE) therapy (eg, infusing bolus doses of Intralipid) is an increasingly used rescue therapy for toxicity and poisoning from local anesthetics and highly lipophilic drugs. There is mounting evidence that the resulting lipemia from ILE may affect common clinical laboratory tests and drug concentration assays, leading to spurious results when the blood sample is drawn during or close to the administration of ILE.[31]

Serum concentrations of potential toxins can be complementary to clinical tests or become essential in several situations (**Table 22-8**).[16] A serum concentration can confirm the diagnosis of a poisoning when in doubt or when a quantitative assessment in the serum is important to interpret a qualitative urine drug screen. When there is a relationship between serum concentration and toxicity, a serum concentration can assist in patient evaluation or for medicolegal purposes. When sustained-release drug formulations have been ingested, serial serum concentrations can indicate when peak serum concentrations have occurred and whether efforts to decontaminate the gastrointestinal tract with activated charcoal or whole bowel irrigation have been achieved. A serum concentration can also be useful in determining when to reinitiate drug therapy after the drug has caused toxicity. For some agents, serum concentrations can guide the decision to use therapies that are often risky, invasive, or expensive such as antidotes (eg, acetylcysteine, digoxin immune antibody, and fomepizole) or special treatments (eg, hemodialysis and hyperbaric oxygen).

**TABLE 22-8.** Examples of the Use of Therapies to Treat Toxicity Guided by Serum Concentrations

| THERAPY | DRUG OR TOXIN |
|---|---|
| Antidote | Acetaminophen, ethylene glycol, methanol |
| Chelation | Iron, lead |
| Hemodialysis | Ethylene glycol, lithium, methanol, salicylate, theophylline, valproic acid |
| Multiple-dose activated charcoal | Carbamazepine, phenobarbital, theophylline, valproic acid |
| Toxin-specific antibody | Digoxin |
| Urine alkalinization | Phenobarbital, salicylate |

**TABLE 22-9.** Relationship of Blood Ethanol Concentration and Toxic Effects

| BLOOD ETHANOL CONCENTRATION (mg/dL) | TOXIC EFFECT OR CONSEQUENCE |
|---|---|
| 0.08% (80) | Legal definition for driving impairment |
| 0.15% (150) | Euphoria, loss of critical judgment, slurred speech, incoordination, drowsiness |
| 0.2% (200) | Increased incoordination, staggering gait, slurred speech, lethargy, disorientation, visual disturbances (diplopia, reduced acuity, and perception) |
| 0.3% (300) | Loss of motor functions, marked decreased response to stimuli, impaired consciousness, marked incoordination and inability to stand or walk, vomiting and incontinence, possible amnesia of the event |
| 0.4% (≥400) | Comatose, unresponsive to physical stimuli, absent reflexes, unstable vital signs, shallow and decreased respirations, hypotension, hypothermia, potentially lethal |

*Source*: Adapted from National Highway Traffic Safety Administration. The ABCs of BAC: a guide to understanding blood alcohol concentration and alcohol impairment. https://www.nhtsa.gov/sites/nhtsa.dot.gov/files/809844-theabcsofbac.pdf.

## General Analytical Techniques

There is no standardized panel of quantitative serum assays for toxicologic use, and the availability of tests differs by individual laboratory. Generally, serum concentrations use existing technologies (eg, immunoassay, spectrophotometry, gas chromatography, high-performance liquid chromatography, and atomic absorption spectrometry) that are commonly used for therapeutic drug monitoring (see Chapter 2). Assays for carboxyhemoglobin, methemoglobinemia, and serum cholinesterase activity are available in many hospitals.[16] In most toxicological applications, the specimen is usually 5 to 10 mL of blood in adults (1 to 5 mL in children depending on the assay) that has been allowed to clot for several minutes. It is then centrifuged, and the clear serum, which is devoid of red blood cells and coagulants, is aspirated and subjected to analysis or frozen for later analysis. The type of test tube, test tube additive, and quantity of blood necessary should be verified with the laboratory prior to blood collection.

## Common Applications

Serum concentrations of several drugs and chemicals can be helpful in the assessment of patients who may be poisoned or overdosed and arrive at a hospital for evaluation and treatment. Although general treatment approaches—such as supportive care, resuscitation, symptomatic care, and decontamination—are performed without the need of serum concentrations, the severity of several toxicities are related to serum concentrations (Table 22-8). The examples of ethanol, salicylates, acetaminophen, and digoxin demonstrate important principles in the application of serum concentrations to toxicity and therapy.

One of the most widely studied and used toxicologic tests involves blood, serum, or breath ethanol concentrations. Because of the absence of protein binding and small volume of ethanol distribution, the serum concentration generally correlates with many of the acute toxic effects of ethanol, as shown

in **Table 22-9**.[32] Regular ethanol use can lead to tolerance, and ethanol concentrations in excess of 0.4% (400 mg/dL) can easily be tolerated by some patients (eg, they can converse and exhibit stable vital signs).[33,34] Conversely, uninitiated drinkers, such as small children who ingest household products containing ethanol (eg, cologne and mouthwash) and those who concurrently ingest other central nervous system (CNS) depressants, may have an exaggerated effect. Most acute poisonings can be managed with supportive and symptomatic care; an unstable patient with exceedingly high ethanol concentrations may be the rare candidate for hemodialysis.

Ethanol concentrations also have medicolegal applications involving driving or work performance and ethanol intake. In 2005, the minimum legal threshold for driving under the influence of ethanol intoxication was set by all states of the United States at blood ethanol concentrations of 0.08% (equivalent to 0.08 g/dL or 80 mg/dL).[32] This value can be determined at the scene or at bedside by a breath alcohol test.[35] The breath alcohol test is based on the assumption that equilibrium exists between ethanol in the blood supply of the lung and the alveolar air at a relatively uniform partition ratio. A number of variables can affect this relationship, such as temperature, hematocrit, and sampling technique. The National Highway Traffic and Safety Administration publishes a list of breath alcohol testing devices that conform to their standards (www.nhtsa.gov).

Because ethanol concentrations are reported in several different units for either serum or blood, verification of the unit of measure is important.[16,36] Further, many hospital-based laboratories perform ethanol determinations on serum and use the units of milligrams/deciliter versus forensic situations that typically use blood and report the value as %, g%, or grams/deciliter (all of which are equivalent expressions except milligrams/deciliter). Serum concentrations of ethanol are greater than blood concentrations by a median factor of 1.2, which varies with the hematocrit value because of the greater water content of serum compared with whole blood.[16,36] Although legal standards are written in terms of whole blood concentrations, this difference is without clinical significance.

Ethanol is also used as a drug to treat poisonings by methanol (blindness, acidosis, and death) and ethylene glycol (acidosis, renal failure, and death). To achieve a consistent concentration near 100 mg/dL, serial serum ethanol concentrations are obtained to ensure that sufficient quantities have been administered to prevent severe toxicities of methanol and ethylene glycol (during therapy, hemodialysis removes ethanol while also removing methanol and ethylene glycol). Fomepizole, which blocks the metabolism of methanol and ethylene glycol to prevent the formation of toxic metabolites, was U.S. Food and Drug Administration (FDA)-approved for use in 1997, and the use of ethanol for these poisonings has decreased.

An early attempt to correlate serum drug concentrations with acute toxicity over time involved the Done nomogram for salicylate poisoning.[37] Categories of toxicity (mild, moderate, and severe) were demarcated on a semilogarithmic plot of serum salicylate versus time after ingestion as an aid to interpreting serum concentrations. Given the limited knowledge available at the time, the nomogram was based on several assumptions (zero-order kinetics and back extrapolation of single concentrations to time zero) that were later proven to be false. The nomogram did not guide therapy to any great extent and was not confirmed to be clinically useful in subsequent studies.[38]

Clinical findings such as vital signs, electrolytes, anion gap, and arterial blood gases, which have quick turnaround times in most hospitals, are more direct indicators of salicylate toxicity and are now preferred to the Done nomogram. A patient, with exceedingly high serum salicylate concentrations (> 90 mg/dL) who is unresponsive to supportive and symptomatic therapy, may benefit from hemodialysis to remove salicylate from the body.[39] Elderly and very young patients with unexplained changes in consciousness, acid–base balance, and respiratory rate who present to an ED could be suffering from unrecognized acute or chronic salicylate poisoning.[39,40] A routine serum salicylate concentration in such patients could determine the contribution of excessive salicylate to their symptoms.

Serum acetaminophen concentrations after acute overdoses are essential in assessing the potential severity of poisoning and determining the need for antidotal therapy with acetylcysteine.[41,42] Acetaminophen toxicity differs from many other poisonings in that there is delay of significant symptoms by 1 to 3 days after ingestion, whereas most other poisonings have definite symptoms within 6 hours of exposure. This delay in onset makes it difficult to use signs, symptoms, and clinical diagnostic tests (such as serum transaminase, bilirubin, or International Normalized Ratio) as an early means to assess the risk of acetaminophen toxicity.[9] A serum concentration of acetaminophen obtained at least 4 hours after an acute ingestion (**Figure 22-1**) can be used to assess whether a patient is at risk for developing acetaminophen hepatotoxicity.[41,42] The acetaminophen nomogram is intended to be used only for an acute, single-episode ingestion of immediate-release acetaminophen and not in situations when acetaminophen is ingested in supratherapeutic doses over several hours or days.

The semilogarithmic plot of serum acetaminophen concentration versus time, also called the *Rumack-Matthew nomogram* or *acetaminophen nomogram*, is also used to determine whether there is a need to administer acetylcysteine to reduce the risk of toxicity.[41,42] If the results are not expected to be available within 10 hours of ingestion, acetylcysteine is typically administered provisionally and then continued or discontinued based on the serum acetaminophen concentration. In situations when the specimen is sent to a reference laboratory, the results may take several days to be reported, and, consequently, the patient may receive the entire course of therapy that may last for 72 hours with the oral regimen or 21 hours with the IV regimen. Because of the widespread availability of acetaminophen, it is commonly ingested in suicide attempts. Several professional groups have advocated that all patients who are suspected of intentionally taking drugs should have a serum acetaminophen concentration determined as part of their evaluation in the ED.[19] In the case of acetaminophen

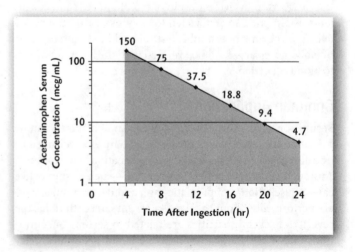

**FIGURE 22-1.** Risk of hepatotoxicity after an acute ingestion of acetaminophen. Acetaminophen serum concentrations in the shaded area are not associated with hepatotoxicity, whereas those above the line are at risk for developing hepatotoxicity and acetylcysteine therapy should be considered.

## MINICASE 6

### Value of Acetaminophen Concentrations

A mother calls a poison control center about her 16-year-old daughter, Kelly A., who has acutely ingested approximately 30 acetaminophen 500-mg tablets 1 hour ago. She thinks that her daughter was "trying to hurt herself." The pharmacist at the poison center refers Kelly A. to the nearest hospital for evaluation due to the amount of acetaminophen and the intent of the ingestion. The mother is asked to bring any medicine to which Kelly A. may have had access. At the ED, Kelly A. vomits several times but has no other physical complaints or symptoms. A physical exam is unremarkable except for the vomiting. Baseline electrolytes, complete blood count, liver function tests, urine drug screen, and a pregnancy test are ordered. An IV line is placed and maintenance IV fluids are started. At 4 hours after the acetaminophen ingestion, a blood specimen is drawn to determine the serum acetaminophen concentration. Ninety minutes later, the result is reported as 234 mcg/mL.

QUESTION: Is this patient at risk for acetaminophen hepatotoxicity? Should she be treated with acetylcysteine?

DISCUSSION: When the serum acetaminophen concentration of 234 mcg/mL is plotted on the acetaminophen nomogram at 4 hours (Figure 22-1), it is clearly above the treatment line. This indicates that this patient is at risk for developing hepatotoxicity and that treatment with acetylcysteine should be initiated immediately.[41] The dose of acetaminophen that she ingested is also associated with a risk of developing hepatotoxicity, but patients with intentional overdoses (substance abuse or attempted suicide) do not always provide accurate histories. If the results of the acetaminophen assay would not have been available within 2 hours of sampling or within 8 to 10 hours of ingestion, acetylcysteine therapy would have been started provisionally. After learning the acetaminophen concentration, the physician would have decided to continue or stop acetylcysteine. Because most patients do not exhibit signs and symptoms of acute hepatic injury until 1 to 3 days after acute acetaminophen overdose, serum transaminase and bilirubin values would not be expected to be abnormal at the time of this patient's assessment in the ED.

poisoning, the serum concentration becomes a valuable determinant of recognition, therapy, and disposition (**Minicase 6**).

A serum concentration can also guide the use or dosage determination of antidotes that are in short supply or are expensive, such as digoxin immune fragment antibody (DigiFab). Life-threatening acute or chronic digoxin toxicity may require the administration of digoxin immune fragment antibody to quickly reverse the toxic effects of digoxin. The dose of digoxin immune fragment antibody can be determined empirically, based on the amount ingested, or by a steady-state serum concentration (consult current prescribing information).[43,44]

Number of vials of digoxin immune fragment antibody
= serum concentration of digoxin (ng/mL)
× patient weight (kg)/100

Once the digoxin immune fragment antibody is administered, the serum concentration of digoxin precipitously rises and has no correlation to the degree of toxicity (**Figure 22-2**).[43,44] This sharp increase of digoxin reflects total digoxin (protein-bound and unbound) in the serum that has been redistributed from tissue sites. The digoxin bound to digoxin immune fragment antibody is not pharmacologically active, and it is eventually excreted in the urine.

### Unique Considerations

The timing of sample collection for poisoned or overdosed patients is variable due to the varying times of arrival at an ED after the exposure and the delay in the recognition of poisoning (unless it is obvious from the history or symptoms).[45] Most specimens are collected at the time of admission to the ED except when specified times are important, such as acetaminophen or when adequate absorption has yet to occur. This variability of serum

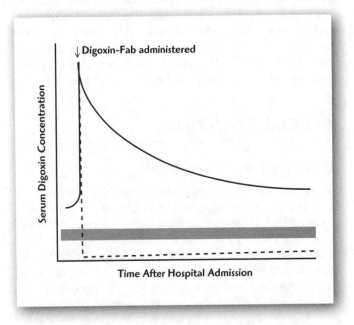

**FIGURE 22-2.** Simulated serum digoxin concentrations before and after administration of digoxin fragment antibodies (Fab). Total digoxin concentrations (*solid line*) rapidly rise to often dramatically high concentrations after administration of digoxin-Fab. Total digoxin concentrations fall with the excretion of digoxin bound to Fab. Free digoxin concentrations (*dashed line*) are associated with pharmacologic activity and rapidly drop to low or unmeasurable concentrations within one hour of digoxin-Fab administration. The shaded area represents the range of therapeutic serum digoxin concentrations.

concentrations among patients makes it difficult to clearly establish a relationship with the concentration and toxicity.

The pharmacokinetics of drugs and chemicals on overdose, sometimes termed *toxicokinetics*, can affect interpretation of a serum concentration.[9] Few studies have compared the pharmacokinetics of drugs in therapeutic and toxic doses because toxic doses cannot be administered to human volunteers and overdosed patients are too heterogeneous to make clear assessments. Nevertheless, there are several examples in which the absorption, distribution, metabolism, and elimination of drugs are significantly different on overdose.[46,47] It is generally inappropriate to apply pharmacokinetic parameters derived from therapeutic doses to situations when massive overdoses are involved. Many patients who are poisoned or have overdosed are critically ill, and multiple samples of blood have been obtained for a variety of tests to monitor their condition. When the toxic agent is recognized late in the course of therapy or when serial determinations could be helpful in understanding some aspect of therapy or toxicity, scavenging aliquots of existing serum samples may be helpful for retrospective toxicological analysis. Laboratories often retain serum samples for several days in case a retest is needed so immediate consultation with the clinical laboratory technician is essential to save the specimen for testing. Another sample collection technique involves collecting a blood or urine specimen at presentation to the ED but not performing the assay. This approach, sometimes called *toxicology hold*, allows collection of a specimen at a time when concentrations may be highest even if the need for the assay may not be clear.[13] The blood specimen can be refrigerated or the serum or urine can be frozen and assayed on request.

# SPECIAL SITUATIONS

## Other Biological Specimens

There is great interest in using other biological specimen—such as hair, saliva, perspiration, and expired breath—and the application of POCTs for quantitative or qualitative analysis.[46] These are typically less invasive than venipuncture, and some provide unique markers of long-term exposure or use (**Table 22-10**). Once a technology has been fully validated and sampling techniques refined to minimize interference, POCTs can be useful for drug screens at the bedside and worksite or longitudinal evaluation of chronic use (eg, cocaine and marijuana in hair samples). The FDA has approved several types of POCTs for clinical use. Although POCT results are typically available within 5 to 10 minutes, the test may be less accurate than laboratory-based analysis when the operator is not sufficiently trained and experienced with the particular POCT device.[14] A common and accepted application of POCTs is breath alcohol determination to assess driving impairment from ethanol use at the scene of an accident or arrest.[35]

## Forensic and Legal Issues

In addition to clinical and regulatory applications for urine drug screens and serum drug concentrations, toxicological analysis

has an important role in providing evidence for suspected cases of homicide, suicide, child abuse, drug-facilitated sexual assault ("drugged date rape"), environmental contamination, malpractice, workers' compensation, insurance claims, and product liability litigation. Chemical exposure monitoring of workers or the work environment requires specialized approaches such as long-term, onsite monitoring by an industrial hygiene specialist. Toxicological tests are also important in establishing brain death in patients being considered for organ donation or to remove life support. It is essential to establish that the apparent vegetative or unresponsive state is not due to drugs. Whenever legal action is anticipated, it is necessary to maintain a specimen chain-of-custody that can be documented as part of the evidence presentation.[10,13]

Postmortem analysis of biological specimens, such as gastric contents, organs, vitreous humor, bile, blood, and urine, can assist in determining the cause of death. These specimens are often collected at the time of autopsy, which may be days to weeks after death. The study of the changes that occur in drug distribution and metabolism after death has been called *postmortem toxicology* or *necrokinetics*. In addition to diffusion of some drugs to or from tissues and blood after death, the effects of putrefaction, fluid shifts on drug concentrations, and chemical stability need to be considered. This is an evolving field of study, which has already demonstrated that postmortem drug concentrations from various biological specimens may not always be appropriately referenced to drug concentration results derived from living humans.[49,50]

When unknown powders, tablets, liquids, plant material, or animal material are found at the scene of a suspected life-threatening poisoning or overdose, specialized analysis is required, such as GC-MS and liquid chromatography with tandem mass spectrometry. At times the specimen is sent to a specialized laboratory for analysis, such as the Federal Bureau of Investigation Laboratory. This situation typically involves the local medical examiner, who would oversee the analysis and report the findings to law enforcement officials and prosecuting attorneys.

## Pediatrics

The toxicological testing of newborn babies, preschool-age poisoning victims, and adolescents involves several unique ethical, technical, and societal concerns. Intrauterine drug exposure can lead to medical complications of newborns; such abuse may be confirmed by drug screens. When mothers do not admit to prepartal drug use, the routine screening of a newborn's urine or meconium poses economic and practical challenges, such as the cost of a generalized screening policy, difficulty in obtaining an adequate urine sample from a neonate, and the preanalytical processing of meconium to make it suitable for analysis. Toxicological analysis of the mother's urine and the neonate's urine and meconium is helpful for identifying substances that would lead to neonatal abstinence syndrome and informing clinicians of its anticipated onset and duration.[51,52]

The use of urine drug screens in the pediatric ED provides minimally useful information because the offending agent is typically known and attempts at concealment are infrequent.[53]

**TABLE 22-10.** Characteristics of Selected Specimens for Toxicological Analysis

| SPECIMEN | STRENGTHS | WEAKNESSES | DETECTION TIMES |
|---|---|---|---|
| Urine | Available in sufficient quantities<br><br>Higher concentrations of drugs or metabolites in urine than in blood<br><br>Well-researched testing techniques<br><br>Relatively inexpensive<br><br>Availability of POCTs | Specimen can be adulterated, substituted, or diluted<br><br>May require observed collection<br><br>Some individuals experience "shy bladder" syndrome and cannot produce a specimen<br><br>Biological hazard for specimen handling and shipping to laboratory | Limited window of detection after drug use<br><br>Typically 1–5 days, some substances are detected for 1–4 wk |
| Hair | Observed and noninvasive specimen collection<br><br>Good specimen stability (does not deteriorate)<br><br>Convenient shipping and storage (no need to refrigerate)<br><br>Difficult to adulterate or substitute | Few labs perform testing<br><br>Costly and time-consuming to prepare specimen for testing<br><br>Difficult to interpret results<br><br>Cannot detect alcohol use<br><br>Does not detect recent drug use (ie, 7–10 days prior to test)<br><br>Difficult to detect low-level use (eg, single-episode)<br><br>Costly | Longest window of detection; best suited for chronic drug use<br><br>Depends on hair length in the sample<br><br>1.5-in specimen reflects a 3-mo history; hair grows about 0.5 in per month |
| Saliva | Observed and noninvasive specimen collection<br><br>Minimal risk of tampering<br><br>Samples can be collected easily in virtually any setting<br><br>Availability of POCTs | Drugs and metabolites do not remain in oral fluids as long as they do in urine<br><br>Limited specimen volume<br><br>Requires supervision for 10–30 min before sampling<br><br>Oral fluids contaminated by marijuana do not reflect presence in saliva and blood | Reflects recent drug use (ie, approximately 10–24 hr prior to test) |
| Sweat | Observed and noninvasive specimen collection<br><br>Simple application and removal of skin patch<br><br>Variable application time of 1–2 wk<br><br>Difficult to adulterate | Few labs perform testing<br><br>Risk of accidental or deliberate removal of patch<br><br>External contamination of the patch may affect results<br><br>Requires two visits (application and removal of patch) | Patch retains evidence of drug use for at least 7 days<br><br>Detects low levels of some drugs 2–5 hr after last use |

*Source*: Adapted with permission from references 14,24,48.

However, a broad or focused drug screen may be helpful for cases of suspected child abuse by poisoning or when the history of the poisoning is unclear.[51]

Prerequisite drug testing of adolescents for participation in school activities and routine screening by school officials, concerned parents, and pediatricians present several ethical dilemmas. Parents and school officials want assurance that substance abuse is not occurring, but the confidentiality and consent of the adolescent should be recognized. The American Academy of Pediatrics states that it "has strong reservations about testing adolescents at school or at home and believes that more research is needed on both safety and efficacy before school-based testing programs are implemented."[54] This policy statement is at odds with the desire of some parent groups to perform such tests without the adolescent's consent and with court rulings upholding a school's ability to perform mass or random drug tests of its students.[55] Drug use in school-age children has been associated with a variety of risk-taking behaviors, such as carrying a gun, engaging in unprotected sexual intercourse with multiple partners, and suffering injury from a physical fight.[56] These behaviors may indicate the need for monitoring drug abuse with appropriate behavioral and health counseling. Many drug testing products are promoted for home use on the Internet, but their reliability and benefits are questionable.[57]

## Sports and Drugs

Drugs are used by some amateur and professional athletes in hopes of enhancing athletic performance and by nonathletes to improve physical appearance. In 2017, an estimated 2.9% (range by 21 states = 2.1% to 9.2%) of high school seniors (3.3% boys and 2.4% girls) have used androgenic anabolic steroids; of these students, nearly one-third do not participate in sports but use steroids to change their appearance.[56,58] The types and variety of substances are typically different from those encountered in poisonings or substance abuse. Most workplace or clinical drug screens do not detect athletic performance-enhancing drugs such as anabolic androgenic steroids, growth hormone, and erythroid-stimulating agents (**Table 22-11**).[59] The international term for drug use in sports is *doping*, and efforts to combat this practice are referred to as *doping control* or *antidoping*.

Governing athletic organizations, such as the International Olympic Committee, the United States Olympic Committee, and the National Collegiate Athletic Association, have established

## TABLE 22-11. Some Purported Athletic Performance-Enhancing Substances

Amino acids (eg, arginine, ornithine, lysine, aspartate, glutamine, leucine, tryptophan, carnitine)

Amphetamines[a]

Androgenic anabolic steroids

Androstenedione

Antiestrogenic agents (eg, anastrozole, tamoxifen, clomiphene, fulvestrant)

Antioxidants (eg, megadoses of ascorbic acid [vitamin C], tocopherol [vitamin E], β-carotene)

β-adrenergic blockers

β-2 agonists

Caffeine

Clenbuterol

Cocaine[a]

Corticotropin (ACTH)

Creatine

Designer anabolic steroids

Dehydroepiandrostenedione (DHEA)

Diuretics

Erythropoietin

Ethanol

γ-hydroxybutyrate (GHB)

Human chorionic gonadotropin

Human growth hormone

Selective androgen receptor modulators

Theophylline

[a]Can be detected on most routine immunoassay urine drug screens. The other substances are typically not detected in routine clinical drug screens.

policies and analytical procedures for testing athletes as well as lists of banned substances. Most organized sports observe the World Antidoping Agency's guidelines for analytical tests, banned substances, and screening procedures.[60] The technical and scientific challenges in detecting many of these substances are unique to this field. Using banned drugs can result in an unfair, artificial advantage for competitive athletes and physical injury or permanent disability from the drug's effects, such as those from anabolic steroids.[58,59]

## Substance Use Disorders

During the past two decades, the abuse of prescription and illicit drugs has risen dramatically and has increased in adolescent and adult age groups.[7] This trend has been recognized as a national epidemic.[24,61] A consequence of drug and substance abuse is the escalation of a chronic condition—substance abuse disorder. "Substance use disorders are characterized by impairment caused by the recurrent use of alcohol or other drugs (or both), including health problems, disability, and failure to meet major responsibilities at work, school, or home."[5] Virtually any one or more illicit drugs or alcohol can lead to substance use disorder. In 2018, 20.3 million people aged 12 years or older developed substance abuse disorder during the past year. There were 12.2 million people only with alcohol use disorder, 5.4 million people with only illicit drug use disorder, and 2.7 million with alcohol use disorder and illicit drug use disorder.[5]

Guidelines for the management of chronic pain have been developed or adopted by professional societies, governmental agencies, and medical practices that typically provide guidance for monitoring pain medication with urine drug screening. The frequency and type of drug testing varies with the patient's history, behavior, adherence, and response. An example of a three-tier approach (**Table 22-12**) takes these factors in consideration.[14]

In evaluating patients who may be abusing prescription drugs, a careful history, physical examination, review of a prescription drug monitoring program, and use of behavioral screening tools are important elements that can be supported by drug screens.[41,48,62,63] A urine drug screen can assist in the detection of inappropriate use when there is sufficient suspicion. If a patient is on a methadone treatment program or is regularly receiving opioids for the relief of chronic pain, the urine drug screen should produce positive results. A negative finding could suggest poor adherence and possible diversion (**Minicase 7**). Characteristics of the drug (eg, short duration of action) and the assay (eg, ability to detect some synthetic opioids) should be considered before discussing the issue with the patient. Knowledge and training at primary care settings on urine drug screening would enhance the ability to detect and help patients who are abusing prescription drugs and help stem the rise in substance use disorder, diversion, and deaths.[48] Differences in federal workplace testing and the clinical setting, such as specimen type, collection procedures, drug testing panel, cutoff concentrations, and MRO involvement, should be recognized.[10,14,24,48]

**TABLE 22-12.** Example of Three-Tier Approach to Drug Testing for Chronic Pain Medicine

| WHEN TO ORDER | DRUG CLASS TO TEST |
|---|---|
| Tier 1<br><br>Routine Monitoring | Amphetamines, barbiturates, benzodiazepines, cannabinoids, cocaine, opiates/opioids |
| Tier 2<br><br>High-risk patients with a known history of abuse for a medication, prevalence of drug abuse locally, risky polypharmacy, multiple providers, or lack of efficacy or toxicity for a prescribed drug | Alcohol, anticonvulsants, antidepressants, synthetic cathinones, hallucinogens, muscle relaxants, dextromethorphan, ketamine, propoxyphene |
| Tier 3<br><br>As clinically indicated | Nonprescription analgesics, antihistamines, antipsychotics, synthetic cannabinoids |

*Source*: Adapted with permission from Langman LJ, Jannetto PJ. Laboratory medicine practice guideline: using clinical data to monitor drug therapy in pain management patients. American Association of Clinical Chemistry Academy, 2018. https://www.aacc.org/-/media/Files/Science-and-Practice/Practice-Guidelines/Pain-Management/LMPGPain-Management20171220.pdf?la=en&hash=19670524407619F78999AB60731A24CB4901939D.

## SUMMARY

Testing for substance abuse, poisonings, and overdose affects society at several levels. Knowledge of assay limitations, sampling procedures, interfering substances, patient factors, and regulatory requirements aids in the interpretation of the value of the test and its clinical relevance. In this chapter, several approaches and applications are discussed, but other situations that involve potential toxins—such as environmental contamination, chemical terrorism, and product safety testing—call for different approaches and pose unique challenges.

## Sources of Information

Because test characteristics vary with the type of test, manufacturer, assay kit, setting, and application, information about a specific test is critical for proper use and interpretation. Good communication with laboratory technicians is an important first step in ensuring proper testing. Laboratory technicians can provide guidance on sample collection, cutoff values, interfering substances, and other technical aspects. The package insert for immunoassays or other commercial assay kits is an important and specific guide to assay performance and known interfering substances with the specific assay. There are several textbooks that can be helpful in understanding techniques, values, and interfering substances.[64-68] Clinical toxicologists in poison control centers (list at www.aapcc.org or contact the local program at 1-800-222-1222 nationwide) can also provide useful information on laboratory tests particularly as they relate to poisonings. Several relevant publications are available at Internet websites of governmental agencies, such as the SAMHSA (www.samhsa.gov) and the U.S. Drug Enforcement Administration (www.dea.gov).

# MINICASE 7

## Monitoring Chronic Therapy with Opioid Analgesics

Alex P., a 32-year-old construction worker, developed chronic pain after a lower back injury. He currently has a prescription for a long-acting morphine preparation. Alex P. has had a history of anxiety and substance abuse of a variety of illicit and prescription drugs. He is otherwise healthy. During the past 24 months on this medication, he has lost his prescription twice and asked for a replacement. His physician has also written additional prescriptions at times when he complained that the dosage was inadequate to provide pain relief. His current daily total dose of morphine is 120 mg. He was recently arrested for forging a prescription to obtain additional opioid medication. Alex P. has had several random urine drug screens during the past 18 months that have been positive for morphine. On one occasion, the test result was positive for oxycodone for which he had a prescription from another physician.

QUESTION: How can urine drug screens be helpful in assessing adherence to an opioid analgesic regimen and identifying potential abuse of opioids?

DISCUSSION: The opioid drug treatment of non cancer-related chronic pain can be complicated by many factors, such as the need for escalating doses for adequate pain relief, potential for diversion of the drugs by selling or giving the drugs to others, abuse of the drugs to get high or satisfy a drug craving, and the risks of overdose and death. One of the approaches to monitor chronic therapy with opioids is to perform random drug screens. A positive drug screen can support that the person is taking the drug, whereas a negative result should raise the question of whether the person is diverting it to others or has stopped taking it for some reason. A drug screen that shows illicit, nonprescribed drugs or prescriptions from multiple or other prescribers, such as oxycodone in this case, strongly suggests that abuse of other medications is taking place or his current pain medicine is inadequate, which raise the risks for addiction, overdose, and death. The physician is faced with several significant signals in this case that need attention to provide safe and effective care. If the physician is not a pain specialist, referral to one for this patient's chronic pain care should be considered.

## MINICASE 8

### Where's the LSD?

In a backyard with two friends, Jacob C., an 18-year-old man, began exhibiting bizarre, agitated, hyperactive behavior 30 minutes after putting two paper blotters on his tongue, which were believed to contain lysergic acid diethylamide (LSD). When he soon exhibited seizure activity lasting 15 to 20 minutes, an ambulance was called to the scene. Tonic-clonic seizures continued during transport and hospitalization for another hour, despite aggressive therapy to stop the seizures. During the next 36 hours, Jacob C. exhibited tachycardia, hyperthermia, acidosis, hypertension, renal failure, and minimal responsiveness. A computed tomography scan of his head indicated cerebral edema. A urine drug screen on admission was positive for marijuana and benzodiazepines, the latter from drugs used to manage his seizures. After a complicated hospital course, his pupils became pinpoint and minimally responsive. Magnetic resonance imaging indicated anoxic brain injury. He expired on the fifth day of hospitalization. At autopsy, anoxic brain injury was confirmed, and a sophisticated analysis of his blood, urine, and tissues revealed the presence of a designer hallucinogenic amphetamine, 2C-1NBOMe.

QUESTION: Why was the designer amphetamine not detected in the initial urine drug screen?

DISCUSSION: Only drugs or substances that are part of the drug screen analysis can be detected when considering all potential limitations of a false-negative or false-positive result. In this case, an immunoassay was used for a stat urine drug screen that only included the substances required by SAMHSA (Table 22-5). Marijuana and benzodiazepines are included in this panel, but LSD is not. In this case, knowing the identity of the substance would not have changed the symptomatic and resuscitative treatment he appropriately received. When the medical examiner pursued a more extensive analysis at autopsy, the designer drug was identified. No LSD was detected. This patient's friends had purchased the 2C-1NBOMe as a "research chemical" on the Internet thinking it was a form of LSD.

---

These websites can also increase awareness of persistent or emerging drugs of abuse (**Minicase 8**). Quickviews of eight common urine drug screens by immunoassay include information on the signs and symptoms of these agents after abuse and overdose.[9,11,14,23,67,68]

## LEARNING POINTS

1. **How long does it take for a drug to clear the body and result in a negative urine drug screen?**

   **ANSWER:** It depends on several factors. Length of time for detection varies with the sensitivity of the assay, whether the assay is directed to the parent drug or the metabolite, whether the drug or its metabolites exhibit extensive distribution to tissues, whether the drug is a sustained release dosage form or is known to form pharmacobezoars (concretions), the drug's elimination rate (with therapeutic doses and overdoses) from the body, the dose of the drug taken, and whether the drug was used chronically or only once.

2. **What does a negative test result from a drug screen mean?**

   **ANSWER:** A negative test result does not mean that the drug was not present or not taken; it means that it was not detected. Some reasons include that the drug may not have been part of the testing panel, the concentration of the drug is below the assay's detection level, the urine may have been too dilute for detection, the urine may have been collected before the drug was excreted in the urine, the urine sample may have been adulterated after collection to mask or avoid detection, or the specimen was obtained too late after the exposure.

3. **How can serum concentrations be useful in the treatment of poisoned patients?**

   **ANSWER:** When a poisoning or overdose is suspected, a serum concentration is obtained to confirm the diagnosis of a poisoning when in doubt, aid the interpretation of a qualitative urine drug screen, determine whether antidotal therapy is indicated, or determine the effectiveness of a therapy. For assays not primarily intended for overdoses or poisonings (eg, digoxin, iron, phenytoin), drug concentrations occasionally are measured when the assay is used for another application such as therapeutic drug monitoring. In clinical settings, serum is typically not used for drug screening.

4. **What should you do if the results do not make sense?**

   **ANSWER:** Consider actions that include checking the report and units of measure, talking with the laboratory technician, checking the package insert of the assay, searching the literature, seeking alternative causes of symptoms, and repeating the assay at the same or different laboratory.

5. **Why are there so few drugs and substances on drug screens?**

   **ANSWER:** Whether a drug or substance is on a drug screen depends on several factors, as follows. The entity paying or requiring the drug screen can include as many drugs on the panel as financially and technically feasible. The SAMHSA panel (Table 22-5) reflects several common drugs of abuse and has been updated periodically through the federal regulatory process. Employers can and do add other drugs of concern for pre-employment, random monitoring, and accident investigation situations. Clinicians can often request or choose from a menu of drug panels to meet the needs of the patient situation or purpose, such as monitoring specific opioid analgesic use, misuse, and adherence. Assays beyond the routine menu are typically performed at a reference laboratory and require a longer turnaround time. In forensic settings, more extensive and sophisticated analytical techniques are often used to identify substances that are compared with an analytical library of known substances. A novel substance, such as a designer drug, poses significant analytical challenges when developing a procedure specific for the substance to identify its chemical composition. The decision to pursue analysis of a specific drug or substance is based on the consideration of the need for analysis, assay availability, timeliness, and cost. A key question to ask is "How will the results be useful for the particular circumstance?"

# REFERENCES

1. Center for Behavioral Health Statistics and Quality. Results from the 2018 national survey on drug use and health: detailed tables. Rockville, MD: Substance Abuse and Mental Health Services Administration; 2019. https://www.samhsa.gov/data/report/2018-nsduh-detailed-tables. Accessed Jun 4, 2019.

2. Gummin DD, Mowry JB, Spyker DA, et al. 2018 Annual Report of the American Association of Poison Control Centers' National Poison Data System (NPDS): 36th Annual Report. *Clin Toxicol (Phila)*. 2019;57(12):1220-1413.PubMed

3. Quest Diagnostics. Drug testing index: employer solutions annual report Spring 2019. Lyndhurst, NJ: Quest Diagnostics Inc; 2019. https://www.questdiagnostics.com/dms/Documents/Employer-Solutions/DTI-2019/quest-drug-testing-index-brochure-2019.pdf. (accessed 2019 Dec 20).

4. Miech RA, Johnston LD, O'Malley PM, et al. *Secondary school students*, Vol. I: *Monitoring the Future national results on drug use 1975-2018*. Ann Arbor, MI: Institute for Social Research, The University of Michigan; 2019. http://monitoringthefuture.org/pubs/monographs/mtf-vol1_2018.pdf. Accessed Jun 4, 2020.

5. Center for Behavioral Health Statistics and Quality. Key substance use and mental health indicators in the United States: Results from the 2018 National Survey on Drug Use and Health. Rockville, MD: Substance Abuse and Mental Health Services Administration; 2019. https://www.samhsa.gov/data/sites/default/files/cbhsq-reports/NSDUHNationalFindingsReport2018/ NSDUHNationalFindingsReport2018.pdf. Accessed Jun 4, 2020.

6. Centers for Disease Control and Prevention. Web-based injury statistics query and reporting system (WISQARS). https://webappa.cdc.gov/sasweb/ncipc/mortrate.html. Accessed Jun 2, 2020.

7. Hedegaard H, Miniño AM, Warner M. *Drug overdose deaths in the United States, 1999-2018. NCHS data brief, no 356.* Hyattsville, MD: US Department of Health and Human Services, CDC, National Center for Health Statistics; 2020. https://www.cdc.gov/nchs/data/databriefs/db356-h.pdf. Accessed Jun 2, 2020.

8. Wilson N, Kariisa M, Seth P, et al. Drug and opioid-involved overdose deaths: United States, 2017-2018. *MMWR Morb Mortal Wkly Rep.* 2020;69(11):290-297.PubMed

9. Chyka PA. Clinical toxicology. In: DiPiro JT, Talbert RL, Yee GC, et al, eds. *Pharmacotherapy: A Pathophysiologic Approach.* 10th ed. New York, NY: McGraw-Hill; 2017:e115-e137.

10. Substance Abuse and Mental Health Services Administration. Drug-free workplace programs. https://www.samhsa.gov/workplace/drug-testing. Accessed May 15, 2020.

11. Tests for drugs of abuse. *Med Lett Drugs Ther.* 2002;44(1137):71-73.PubMed

12. DePriest AZ, Black DL, Robert TA. Immunoassay in healthcare testing applications. *J Opioid Manag.* 2015;11(1):13-25.PubMed

13. Grunbaum AM. Laboratory principles. In: Nelson LS, Howland MA, Lewin NA, et al, eds. *Goldfrank's Toxicologic Emergencies.* 11th ed. New York, NY: McGraw-Hill; 2019:101-113.

14. Langman Lj, Jannetto PJ. Laboratory Medicine Practice Guideline: Using clinical data to monitor drug therapy in pain management patients. American Association of Clinical Chemistry Academy, 2018 https://www.aacc.org/-/media/Files/Science-and-Practice/Practice-Guidelines/Pain-Management/LMPGPain-Management20171220.pdf?la=en&hash=19670524407619F78999AB60731A24CB4901939D. Accessed Jun 10, 2019.

15. Department of Health and Human Services, Substance Abuse and Mental Health Services Administration. Mandatory guidelines for federal workplace drug testing programs. *Fed Regist.* 2017; 82:7920-7970. https://www.samhsa.gov/workplace/drug-testing#HHS. Accessed Feb 20, 2017.

16. Wu AH, McKay C, Broussard LA, et al. National academy of clinical biochemistry laboratory medicine practice guidelines: recommendations for the use of laboratory tests to support poisoned patients who present to the emergency department. *Clin Chem.* 2003;49(3):357-379.PubMed

17. Tenenbein M. Do you really need that emergency drug screen? *Clin Toxicol (Phila).* 2009;47(4):286-291.PubMed

18. Nice A, Leikin JB, Maturen A, et al. Toxidrome recognition to improve efficiency of emergency urine drug screens. *Ann Emerg Med.* 1988;17(7):676-680.PubMed

19. Holstege CP, Borek HA. Toxidromes. *Crit Care Clin.* 2012;28(4):479-498. PubMed

20. American College of Emergency Physicians. Clinical policy for the initial approach to patients presenting with acute toxic ingestion or dermal or inhalation exposure. *Ann Emerg Med.* 1999;33(6):735-761.PubMed

21. Carrigan TD, Field H, Illingworth RN, et al. Toxicological screening in trauma. *J Accid Emerg Med.* 2000;17(1):33-37.PubMed

22. Substance Abuse and Mental Health Services Administration. Medical review officer manual for federal workplace drug testing programs, effective October 1, 2017. https://www.samhsa.gov/sites/default/files/workplace/mro-guidance-manual-oct2017_2.pdf. Accessed Jun 2, 2020.

23. Hoffman RJ. Testing for drugs of abuse. In: Traub SJ, Grayzel J, eds. *UpToDate.* New York, NY: Wolters Kluwer; 2020.

24. Mahajan G. Role of urine drug testing in the current opioid epidemic. *Anesth Analg.* 2017;125(6):2094-2104.PubMed

25. Mittal MK, Florin T, Perrone J, et al. Toxicity from the use of niacin to beat urine drug screening. *Ann Emerg Med.* 2007;50(5):587-590.PubMed

26. Moeller KE, Lee KC, Kissack JC. Urine drug screening: practical guide for clinicians. *Mayo Clin Proc.* 2008;83(1):66-76.PubMed

27. Brahm NC, Yeager LL, Fox MD, et al. Commonly prescribed medications and potential false-positive urine drug screens. *Am J Health Syst Pharm.* 2010;67(16):1344-1350.PubMed

28. Rollins DE, Jennison TA, Jones G. Investigation of interference by nonsteroidal anti-inflammatory drugs in urine tests for abused drugs. *Clin Chem.* 1990;36(4):602-606.PubMed

29. Zacher JL, Givone DM. False-positive urine opiate screening associated with fluoroquinolone use. *Ann Pharmacother.* 2004;38(9):1525-1528. PubMed

30. Mayo Medical Laboratories. Benzodiazepines. http://www.mayomedicallaboratories.com/test-info/drug-book/benzodiazepines.html. Accessed Dec 21, 2015).

31. Grunbaum AM, Gilfix BM, Hoffman RS, et al. Review of the effect of intravenous lipid emulsion on laboratory analyses. *Clin Toxicol (Phila).* 2016;54(2):92-102.PubMed

32. National Highway Traffic Safety Administration. The ABCs of BAC: a guide to understanding blood alcohol concentration and alcohol impairment. https://www.nhtsa.gov/sites/nhtsa.dot.gov/files/809844-theabcsofbac.pdf. Accessed Mar 31, 2017.

33. Hammond KB, Rumack BH, Rodgerson DO. Blood ethanol: a report of unusually high levels in a living patient. *JAMA.* 1973;226(1):63-64. PubMed

34. van Heyningen C, Watson ID. Survival after very high blood alcohol concentrations. *Ann Clin Biochem.* 2002;39(Pt 4):416-417.PubMed

35. Kwong TC. Point-of-care testing for alcohol. In: Shaw LM, Kwong TC, Rosana TG, et al, eds. *The Clinical Toxicology Laboratory: Contemporary*

*Practice of Poisoning Evaluation.* Washington, DC: American Association of Clinical Chemistry Press; 2001:190-196.

36. Kurt TL, Doan-Wiggins L. Serum alcohol is not the same as blood alcohol concentration. *Ann Emerg Med.* 1995;25(3):430-431.PubMed

37. Done AK. Salicylate intoxication: significance of measurements of salicylate in blood in cases of acute ingestion. *Pediatrics.* 1960;26: 800-807.PubMed

38. Dugandzic RM, Tierney MG, Dickinson GE, et al. Evaluation of the validity of the Done nomogram in the management of acute salicylate intoxication. *Ann Emerg Med.* 1989;18(11):1186-1190.PubMed

39. Palmer BF, Clegg DJ. Salicylate toxicity. *N Engl J Med.* 2020;382(26): 2544-2555.PubMed

40. Sporer KA, Khayam-Bashi H. Acetaminophen and salicylate serum levels in patients with suicidal ingestion or altered mental status. *Am J Emerg Med.* 1996;14(5):443-446.PubMed

41. Heard KJ. Acetylcysteine for acetaminophen poisoning. *N Engl J Med.* 2008;359(3):285-292.PubMed

42. Smilkstein MJ, Knapp GL, Kulig KW, et al. Efficacy of oral N-acetylcysteine in the treatment of acetaminophen overdose: analysis of the national multicenter study (1976 to 1985). *N Engl J Med.* 1988;319(24):1557-1562.PubMed

43. Zucker AR, Lacina SJ, DasGupta DS, et al. Fab fragments of digoxin-specific antibodies used to reverse ventricular fibrillation induced by digoxin ingestion in a child. *Pediatrics.* 1982;70(3):468-471.PubMed

44. Antman EM, Wenger TL, Butler VP Jr, et al. Treatment of 150 cases of life-threatening digitalis intoxication with digoxin-specific Fab antibody fragments: final report of a multicenter study. *Circulation.* 1990;81(6):1744-1752.PubMed

45. Bosse GM, Matyunas NJ. Delayed toxidromes. *J Emerg Med.* 1999;17(4):679-690.PubMed

46. Sue YJ, Shannon M. Pharmacokinetics of drugs in overdose. *Clin Pharmacokinet.* 1992;23(2):93-105.PubMed

47. Roberts DM, Buckley NA. Pharmacokinetic considerations in clinical toxicology: clinical applications. *Clin Pharmacokinet.* 2007;46(11): 897-939.PubMed

48. Substance Abuse and Mental Health Services Administration. Clinical drug testing in primary care. Technical Assistance Publication (TAP) 32. HHS Publication No. SMA 12-4668. https://store.samhsa.gov/product /TAP-32-Clinical-Drug-Testing-Primary-Care/SMA12-4668. Accessed Aug 17, 2012.

49. Ferner RE. Post-mortem clinical pharmacology. *Br J Clin Pharmacol.* 2008;66(4):430-443.PubMed

50. Rao RB, Flomenbaum M. Postmortem toxicology. In: Nelson LS, Howland MA, Lewin NA, et al, eds. *Goldfrank's Toxicologic Emergencies.* 11th ed. New York, NY: McGraw-Hill; 2019:1884-1891.

51. Chang G. Screening for alcohol and drug use during pregnancy. *Obstet Gynecol Clin North Am.* 2014;41(2):205-212.PubMed

52. Kocherlakota P. Neonatal abstinence syndrome. *Pediatrics.* 2014;134(2):e547-e561.PubMed

53. Belson MG, Simon HK, Sullivan K, et al. The utility of toxicologic analysis in children with suspected ingestions. *Pediatr Emerg Care.* 1999;15(6):383-387.PubMed

54. Knight JR, Mears CJ. Testing for drugs of abuse in children and adolescents: addendum: testing in schools and at home. *Pediatrics.* 2007;119(3):627-630.PubMed

55. Schwartz RH, Silber TJ, Heyman RB, et al. Urine testing for drugs of abuse: a survey of suburban parent-adolescent dyads. *Arch Pediatr Adolesc Med.* 2003;157(2):158-161.PubMed

56. Kann L, McManus T, Harris WA, et al. Youth risk behavior surveillance: United States, 2017. *MMWR Surveill Summ.* 2018;67(8):1-114. PubMed

57. Levy S, Van Hook S, Knight J. A review of Internet-based home drug-testing products for parents. *Pediatrics.* 2004;113(4):720-726. PubMed

58. Calfee R, Fadale P. Popular ergogenic drugs and supplements in young athletes. *Pediatrics.* 2006;117(3):e577-e589.PubMed

59. De Rose EH. Doping in athletes: an update. *Clin Sports Med.* 2008;27(1):107-130.PubMed

60. World Anti-doping Agency. World anti-doping code. 2015 with 2019 amendments. https://www.wada-ama.org/sites/default/files/resources /files/wada_anti-doping_code_2019_english_final_revised_v1_linked .pdf. Accessed Aug 9, 2020.

61. Paulozzi L, Baldwin G, Franklin G, et al. CDC grand rounds: prescription drug overdoses. A U.S. epidemic. *MMWR Morb Mortal Wkly Rep.* 2012;61(1):10-13.PubMed

62. Peppin JF, Passik SD, Couto JE, et al. Recommendations for urine drug monitoring as a component of opioid therapy in the treatment of chronic pain. *Pain Med.* 2012;13(7):886-896.PubMed

63. Passik SD. Issues in long-term opioid therapy: unmet needs, risks, and solutions. *Mayo Clin Proc.* 2009;84(7):593-601.PubMed

64. Baselt RC. *Disposition of Toxic Drugs and Chemicals in Man.* 12th ed. Foster City, CA: Biomedical Publications; 2020.

65. Kwong TC, Barbarajean M, Rosana TG, et al, eds. *The Clinical Toxicology Laboratory: Contemporary Practice of Poisoning Evaluation.* 2nd ed. Washington, DC: American Association of Clinical Chemistry Press; 2013.

66. Levine BS, and Kerrigan S, eds. *Principles of Forensic Toxicology.* 5th ed. New York, NY: Springer; 2020.

67. National Institute on Drug Abuse. Drug topics. https://www.drugabuse .gov/drug-topics. Accessed Aug 9, 2020.

68. Drug Enforcement Administration, US Department of Justice. Drugs of abuse, 2020 edition: a DEA resource guide. https://www.dea.gov /sites/default/files/2020-04/Drugs%20of%20Abuse%202020-Web%20 Version-508%20compliant-4-24-20_0.pdf. Accessed Aug 9, 2020.

## QUICKVIEW | Urine Drug Screen, Amphetamines, and Methamphetamine

| PARAMETER | DESCRIPTION | COMMENTS |
|---|---|---|
| Critical value | Positive | Check for possible interferents; confirm result with confirmatory test |
| **Major causes of...** | | |
| Positive results | Following ingestion, intranasal application, injection, smoking (methamphetamine) | |
| Associated signs and symptoms | None may be evident at time of specimen collection; may involve exposure to illicit substances; may be used for legitimate purposes; abuse may involve exposure to illicit forms | Typical symptoms include CNS stimulation, euphoria, irritability, insomnia, tremors, seizures, paranoia, and aggressiveness; overdoses cause hypertension, tachycardia, stroke, arrhythmias, cardiovascular collapse, rhabdomyolysis, and hyperthermia |
| **After use, time to...** | | |
| Negative result from light, sporadic use | 2–5 days; clearance is faster in acidic urine | Methylphenidate typically will not be detected |
| Negative result from chronic use | Up to 2 wk | |
| Possible spurious positive results with immunoassays | Ephedrine, pseudoephedrine, ephedra (ma huang), phenylephrine, selegiline, chlorpromazine, promethazine, trazodone, bupropion, desipramine, trimipramine, ritodrine, amantadine, ranitidine, phenylpropanolamine, brompheniramine, isometheptene, labetalol, phentermine, methylphenidate, isoxsuprine, trimethobenzamide, 3,4-methylenedioxy-*N*-methamphetamine (MDMA, Ecstasy) | A false-positive result may be caused by patient's use of drugs and dietary supplements; verify possible false-positive with laboratory and assay package insert |

## QUICKVIEW | Urine Drug Screen, Barbiturates

| PARAMETER | DESCRIPTION | COMMENTS |
|---|---|---|
| Critical value | Positive | Check for possible interferents; confirm result with confirmatory test |
| **Major causes of...** | | |
| Positive results | Following ingestion; rarely injected or used as a suppository | |
| Associated signs and symptoms | None may be evident at time of specimen collection; may involve exposure to medicines used for legitimate purposes or abuse | Typical symptoms include sedation; overdoses cause coma, ataxia, nystagmus, depressed reflexes, hypotension, and respiratory depression; increased sedation with ethanol or other sedatives; primidone is metabolized to phenobarbital |
| **After use, time to...** | | |
| Negative result from light, sporadic use | 1–7 days | Depends on drug and extent and duration of use |
| Negative result from chronic use | 1–3 wk | Phenobarbital may be detected up to 4 wk after stopping use |
| **Possible spurious positive results with immunoassays** | Ibuprofen, naproxen | Verify possible false positive with laboratory and assay package insert |

## QUICKVIEW | Urine Drug Screen, Benzodiazepines

| PARAMETER | DESCRIPTION | COMMENTS |
| --- | --- | --- |
| Critical value | Positive | Check for possible interferents; confirm result with confirmatory test |
| **Major causes of...** | | |
| Positive results | Following ingestion or injection | Benzodiazepines vary in cross-reactivity and detectability |
| Associated signs and symptoms | None may be evident at time of specimen collection; may involve exposure to medicines used for legitimate purposes or abuse; may involve exposure to illicit forms | Typical symptoms include drowsiness, ataxia, slurred speech, sedation; oral overdoses can cause tachycardia and coma with rare severe respiratory or cardiovascular depression; rapid IV use can cause severe respiratory depression; increased sedation with ethanol or other sedatives |
| **After use, time to...** | | |
| Negative result | Typically up to 2 wk; up to 6 wk with chronic use of some agents | Some benzodiazepines may persist for a longer period of time and some have an active metabolite that may or may not be detected; flunitrazepam may not be detected; not all benzodiazepines will be detected by all immunoassays |
| Possible spurious positive results with immunoassays | Oxaprozin, sertraline | Verify possible false positive with laboratory and assay package insert |

## QUICKVIEW | Urine Drug Screen, Benzoylecgonine (Cocaine Metabolite)

| PARAMETER | DESCRIPTION | COMMENTS |
|---|---|---|
| Critical value | Positive | Check for possible interferents; confirm result with confirmatory test |
| **Major causes of...** | | |
| Positive results | Following snorting, smoking, injection, topical application (vagina, penis) or rectal insertion; ingestion | |
| Associated signs and symptoms | None may be evident at time of specimen collection with heavy or chronic use; may involve exposure to illicit forms | Typical symptoms include CNS stimulation that produces euphoric effects and hyperstimulation such as dilated pupils, increased temperature, tachycardia and hypertension; overdoses cause stroke, myocardial infarction, seizures, coma, respiratory depression, arrhythmias |
| **After use, time to...** | | |
| Negative result from light, sporadic use | 12–72 hr | Cross-reactivity with cocaethylene (metabolic product of concurrent cocaine and ethanol abuse) varies with the assay |
| Negative result from chronic use | Up to 1–2 wk | |
| Possible spurious positive results with immunoassays | Topical anesthetics containing cocaine; coca leaf tea | False positives from -caine anesthetics (eg, lidocaine, procaine, benzocaine) are unlikely; verify possible false positive with laboratory and assay package insert |

## QUICKVIEW | Urine Drug Screen, Δ-9-tetrahydrocannabinol-9-carboxylic Acid

| PARAMETER | DESCRIPTION | COMMENTS |
| --- | --- | --- |
| **Critical value** | Positive | Check for possible interferents; confirm result with confirmatory test |
| **Major causes of...** | | |
| **Positive results** | Following smoking, ingestion, possible passive inhalation | Patients taking dronabinol will have positive test results |
| Associated signs and symptoms | None may be evident at time of specimen collection with heavy or chronic use; may involve exposure to illicit substances; may involve exposure to medicine used for legitimate purposes or abuse | Typical symptoms include delirium, conjunctivitis, food craving; other effects include problems with memory, thinking, problem solving, distorted perception, loss of coordination, sedation, tachycardia, hyperemesis syndrome |
| **After use, time to...** | | |
| Negative result from light, sporadic use | 5–7 days | |
| Negative result from chronic use | 6–8 wk typically, up to 3 mo possible | May persist for a longer period of time with heavy, long-term use |
| **Possible spurious positive results with immunoassays** | Efavirenz, pantoprazole; ibuprofen, naproxen, tolmetin are possible but uncommon | False-positive result |
| | | False positive for abuse; verify possible false positive with laboratory and assay package insert |

## QUICKVIEW | Urine Drug Screen, LSD

| PARAMETER | DESCRIPTION | COMMENTS |
|---|---|---|
| Critical value | Positive | Check for possible interferents; confirm result with confirmatory test |
| **Major causes of...** | | |
| Positive results | Following ingestion, placement in buccal cavity or ocular instillation | Not well-absorbed topically |
| Associated signs and symptoms | May involve exposure to illicit substances | Typical symptoms include unpredictable hallucinogenic effects; physical effects include mydriasis, elevated temperature, tachycardia, hypertension, sweating, loss of appetite, sleeplessness, dry mouth, and tremors; flash-backs months later are possible |
| **After use, time to...** | | |
| Negative result | 24–48 hr typically, up to 5 days possible with heavy use | |
| Possible spurious positive results with immunoassays | | LSD is a schedule I drug with no legitimate routine medical use; verify possible false positive with laboratory and assay package insert |

## QUICKVIEW | Urine Drug Screen, Opioids

| PARAMETER | DESCRIPTION | COMMENTS |
|---|---|---|
| **Critical value** | Positive | Check for possible interferents; confirm result with confirmatory test |
| **Major causes of...** | | |
| **Positive results** | Following ingestion, injection, dermal application of drug-containing patches, rectal insertion | Synthetic opioids (eg, fentanyl, fentanyl analogs, meperidine, methadone, tramadol, buprenorphine, loperamide) have minimal cross-reactivity and may not be detected |
| Associated signs and symptoms | None may be evident at time of specimen collection; may involve exposure to illicit substances; may involve exposure to medicines used for legitimate purposes or abuse; ingestion of large amounts of food products made with poppy seeds | Typical symptoms include CNS depression, drowsiness, miosis, constipation; overdoses cause coma, hypotension, respiratory depression, pulmonary edema, seizures; increased sedation with ethanol or other sedatives |
| | | Heroin use is confirmed by the presence of 6-acetylmorphine (6-AM) |
| **After use, time to...** | | |
| Negative result | 2–3 days typically, up to 6 days with sustained-release formulations, up to 1 wk with prolonged or heavy use | |
| **Possible spurious positive results with immunoassays** | Poppy seeds | False positive for drug abuse |
| | Rifampin, some fluoroquinolones, quinine | False-positive result; consider patient's legitimate use of opioid analgesics, including long-term pain management and opioid withdrawal treatment with methadone, or buprenorphine; verify possible false positive with laboratory and assay package insert |

## QUICKVIEW | Urine Drug Screen, PCP

| PARAMETER | DESCRIPTION | COMMENTS |
|---|---|---|
| Critical value | Positive | Check for possible interferents; confirm result with confirmatory test such as GC-MS |
| Major causes of... | | |
| Positive results | Following ingestion, smoking, snorting, or injection | |
| Associated signs and symptoms | None may be evident at time of specimen collection; may involve exposure to illicit substances; may involve exposure to medicines containing dextromethorphan or diphenhydramine used for legitimate purposes or abuse | Typical symptoms include hallucinations, schizophrenia-like behavior, hypertension, elevated temperature, diaphoresis, tachycardia; high doses cause nystagmus, ataxia, hypotension, bradycardia, depressed respirations, seizures, and coma |
| After use, time to... | | |
| Negative result from light, sporadic use | 2–5 days | May persist for a longer period of time with heavy, long-term use or massive overdose preceded by chronic use |
| Negative result from chronic use | Weeks or months | |
| Possible spurious positive results with immunoassays | Ketamine, dextromethorphan, diphenhydramine, imipramine, mesoridazine, thioridazine, venlafaxine, ibuprofen, meperidine, tramadol | False-positive result; verify possible false positive with laboratory and assay package insert |

# PART III

## TESTS FOR SPECIAL POPULATIONS

# 23 Interpreting Pediatric Laboratory Data

*Jessica L. Jacobson, Beth S. Shields, and Donna M. Kraus*

## OBJECTIVES

*After completing this chapter, the reader should be able to*

- Define the various pediatric age group terminology

- Discuss general pediatric considerations as they relate to blood sampling

- Describe how pediatric reference ranges are determined

- Discuss the age-related physiologic differences that account for variations by age in the normal reference ranges for serum sodium, potassium, bicarbonate, calcium, phosphorus, and magnesium

- List common pediatric causes of abnormalities in the electrolytes and minerals listed above

- Explain why age-related differences in serum creatinine and kidney function tests occur

- Discuss the age-related differences that occur in serum albumin, liver enzyme tests, and bilirubin

- Describe what is meant by the physiologic anemia of infancy and explain how it occurs

The interpretation of laboratory data in the pediatric patient population can be complex. Compared with adults, the pediatric population is much more dynamic. Alterations in body composition, organ function, and physiologic activity accompany the normal processes of maturation and growth that occur from birth through adolescence. These alterations can result in different normal reference ranges in pediatric patients for various laboratory tests. Pediatric patients have not only different normal laboratory values compared with adults but also normal laboratory values may differ in various pediatric age groups. It is important for the clinician to understand the reasons for these different, commonly accepted reference ranges and to use age-appropriate reference ranges when providing pharmaceutical care to pediatric patients.

The measurement of substances in neonates, infants, and young children is further complicated by a patient's smaller physical size and difficulty in obtaining blood and urine samples. The smaller blood volume in these patients requires blood samples to be smaller; thus, special microanalytical techniques must be used. Additionally, in the neonate, substances that normally occur in higher amounts in the blood—such as bilirubin, lipids, and hemoglobin—may interfere with certain assays. This chapter briefly reviews pertinent general pediatric principles and focuses on the different age-related factors that must be considered when interpreting commonly used laboratory data in pediatric patients.

## GENERAL PEDIATRIC CONSIDERATIONS

Knowledge of pediatric age group terminology is important to better understand age-related physiologic differences and other factors that may influence the interpretation of pediatric laboratory data. These terms are defined in **Table 23-1** and are used throughout this chapter.[1,2]

The interpretation of any patient's laboratory data must be viewed in light of the patient's clinical status. This includes the patient's symptoms, physical signs of disease, and physiologic parameters such as respiratory rate, heart rate, and blood pressure. For example, an elevated $PaCO_2$ from an arterial blood gas may be clinically more significant in a patient who is extremely tachypneic (perhaps indicating impending respiratory failure) compared with a patient whose respiratory rate is mildly elevated. Thus, it is important to know the relative differences in physiologic norms that occur in the various pediatric age groups.

Normal respiratory rates are higher in neonates and young infants compared with children, adolescents, and adults. The average respiratory rate of a newborn is 60 breaths/min at 1 hour after birth but 30 to 40 breaths/min at >6 hours after birth. Mean respiratory rates of infants and young children <2 years of age (25 to 30 breaths/min) continue to be higher than in children 3 to 9 years of age (20 to 25 breaths/min) and adolescents (16 to 20 breaths/min).[1]

Normal heart rates follow a similar pattern, with higher heart rates in neonates and young infants, which then slowly decrease with increasing age through adolescence. For example, the mean heart rate of a newborn in the first week of life is 125 beats/min, with a normal high of 160 beats/min. The mean heart rate of a 1-month-old infant is 145 beats/min, while that of a 1-year-old child is 120 beats/min and that of a 12-year-old child is 85 beats/min.[3]

DOI 10.37573/9781585286423.023

**TABLE 23-1.** Definition of Age Group Terminology

| | |
|---|---|
| Gestational age (GA) | The time from conception until birth; more specifically, GA is defined as the number of weeks from the first day of the mother's LMP until the birth of the baby; GA at birth is assessed by the date of the LMP and by physical and neuromuscular examination (eg, New Ballard Score) |
| Postnatal age (PNA) | Chronological age since birth |
| Postmenstrual age (PMA)[a] | Postmenstrual age is calculated as gestational age plus postnatal age (PMA = GA + PNA) |
| Neonate | A full-term newborn 0–28 days PNA; some experts may also apply this terminology to a premature neonate who is >28 days PNA but whose PMA is ≤ 42–46 wk |
| Premature neonate | Neonate born at <37 wk GA |
| Full-term neonate | Neonate born at 37 wk 0 days to 41 wk 6 days (average ~40 wk) GA |
| Infant | 1 mo (>28 days) to 12 mo of age |
| Child/children | 1–12 yr |
| Adolescent | 13–18 yr |
| Adult | >18 yr |

LMP = last menstrual period.

[a]The term *postconceptional age* (PCA; age since conception) is no longer recommended for use in clinical pediatrics.[2] However, this term may be found in pediatric literature. Traditionally, PCA was defined as GA + PNA. Because the exact time of conception is not generally known (except in cases of assisted reproductive technology) and GA is calculated as above (according to the mother's LMP), PMA is considered a more accurate term to use. When PCA is used in the pediatric literature, it should be defined within the article where it is used. *Source*: Adapted with permission from Taketomo CK, Hodding JH, Kraus DM. *Pediatric and Neonatal Dosage Handbook*. 26th ed. Hudson, OH: Lexi-Comp Inc; 2019.

In pediatric patients, normal blood pressure values vary according to age, sex, and percentile height of the patient.[4,5] Blood pressures are lower in neonates and increase throughout infancy and childhood. For example, typical blood pressures for a full-term newborn would be in the range of 65 to 95 mm Hg systolic and 30 to 60 mm Hg diastolic. The normal blood pressure (blood pressure <90th percentile) for a 1-year-old girl of average height (50th percentile height) would be <100/54 mm Hg, whereas that of a 15-year-old girl of average height would be <123/79 mm Hg. Blood pressures are slightly different for girls compared with boys and are higher in taller children. Appropriate references should be consulted to obtain normal blood pressure values when providing clinical care to pediatric patients.[3-5]

In addition to age-related physiologic differences in respiratory rates, heart rates, and blood pressures, age-related changes in body composition (eg, fluid compartments), cardiac output, organ perfusion, and organ function also exist. These age-related changes may result in different normal laboratory values for pediatric patients compared with adults. For example, age-related changes in fluid compartments affect normal laboratory values for serum electrolytes, as discussed in the Serum Electrolytes and Minerals section. Being aware of the normal laboratory values for age is important for proper monitoring of efficacy and toxicity of pediatric drug therapy.

## Pediatric Blood Sampling

The smaller physical size of pediatric patients makes it more difficult to obtain blood samples. In general, venipuncture techniques used in adults can be used in older children and adolescents. However, vacuum containers used for blood sampling may collapse the small veins of younger children and are not recommended in these patients.[6] Capillary puncture (also called *microcapillary puncture* or *skin puncture*) is used in patients with small or inaccessible veins. Thus, it is the blood sampling method of choice for premature neonates, neonates, and young infants. Because this method also helps preserve total blood volume, it may also be beneficial to use in infants and small children who require multiple blood tests.[7]

The physical sites that are used for capillary puncture include the heel, finger, and great toe.[6,7] The preferred site in neonates and younger infants is the medial or lateral portion of the plantar surface of the heel. The central area of the foot is avoided because of the risk of damage to the calcaneus bone, tendons, nerves, and cartilage. Automatic lancet devices are recommended when performing heel stick capillary blood sampling as they have been associated with less pain, fewer complications, and higher precision (lower resampling rate) when compared with manual lancets. The automatic devices are available in different needle lengths and incision depths for use in premature neonates, term neonates, and younger infants and have automatic retractable needles for user safety.[8] Fingersticks may be used in older infants (generally >6 months of age and weighing >10 kg) and children, whereas capillary puncture of the great toe (which is rarely used) should be reserved for nonambulatory patients >1 year of age.[8,9] Once children begin to walk, heel stick and great toe capillary puncture are used less frequently because bruising from sampling may result in pain upon walking and callus formation on feet may preclude vascular access and the ability to successfully obtain a sample.

Because capillary and venous blood are similar in composition, the capillary puncture method may be used to obtain samples for most chemistry and hematology tests.[7] However, differences may occur between venous and capillary blood for certain substances, such as glucose, calcium, potassium, and total protein. For example, glucose concentrations may be 10% higher when the sample is collected by capillary puncture compared with venipuncture.[6] In addition, improper capillary puncture sample collection may result in hemolysis or introduction of interstitial fluid into the specimen. This may result in higher concentrations for potassium, magnesium, lactate dehydrogenase, and other substances. Therefore, using the proper procedure to collect blood by the capillary puncture method is essential. It is also important that the site of capillary puncture be warmed prior to sample collection, especially for blood gas determinations.[6] Complications of capillary puncture include infection, hematoma, and bruising.

The size of the blood sample is an important issue to the pediatric clinician. Compared with adults, pediatric patients have a much smaller total blood volume (**Table 23-2**). For example, a full-term newborn of average weight (3.4 kg) has an approximate total blood volume of 78 to 86 mL/kg, or about 265 to 292 mL total.[10] However, a 70-kg adult has an estimated total blood volume of 68 to 88 mL/kg or 4,760 to 6,160 mL total. If a standard 10-mL blood sample were to be drawn from a pediatric patient, it would represent a much higher percent of total blood volume compared with an adult. Therefore, the smaller total blood volume in pediatric patients requires blood sample sizes to be smaller. This issue is further complicated in newborns because their relatively high hematocrit (approximately 60% or higher) decreases the yield of serum or plasma from the amount of blood collected. Microanalytical techniques have reduced the required size of blood samples. However, critically ill pediatric patients may require multiple or frequent blood sample determinations. Thus, it is essential to plan pediatric laboratory tests, especially in the neonate and premature neonate, to avoid precipitating iatrogenic anemia from excessive blood drawing.

Substances that normally occur in higher amounts in the blood of neonates, such as bilirubin, lipids, and hemoglobin, may interfere with certain assays. Hyperbilirubinemia may occur in premature and term neonates. High bilirubin concentrations may produce falsely low creatinine or cholesterol values when measured by certain analytical instruments.[6] Neonates, especially those who are born prematurely, may have lipemia when receiving intravenous (IV) fat emulsions. Lipemia may interfere with spectrophotometric determinations of any substance or with flame photometer determinations of potassium and sodium. Newborns have higher hemoglobin values, and hemoglobin may interfere with certain assays. For example, hemolysis and the presence of hemoglobin may interfere with bilirubin measurements. Therefore, it is important to ensure that the assay methodology selected for measurement of substances in neonatal serum or plasma is not subject to interference from bilirubin, lipids, or hemoglobin.

## Pediatric Reference Ranges

Various methods can be used to determine reference ranges, and each method has its own advantages and disadvantages. In adults, reference ranges are usually determined by obtaining samples directly from known healthy individuals (direct method). The frequency distribution of the obtained values are assessed and the extreme outliers (eg, 0 to 2.5th percentile and 97.5 to 100th percentile) are excluded. This leaves the values of the 2.5 to 97.5th percentiles to define the reference range.[11] However, it also labels the 0 to 2.5th percentile and 97.5 to 100th percentile values from the healthy individuals as being outside of the reference range. If the frequency distribution of the obtained values fall in a bell-shaped or Gaussian distribution, then the mean (or average) value plus or minus two standard deviations (SDs) can then be used to define the reference range. The mean value plus or minus two SDs includes 95% of

**TABLE 23-2.** Total Blood Volume by Age Group

| AGE | EXAMPLE WEIGHT (kg), AGE | APPROXIMATE TOTAL BLOOD VOLUME (mL/kg)[a] | ESTIMATED TOTAL BLOOD VOLUME (mL) |
|---|---|---|---|
| Premature neonate | 1.5 | 89–105 | 134–158 |
| Full-term neonate | 3.4 | 78–86 | 265–292 |
| 1–12 mo | 7.6 (6 mo) | 73–78 | 555–593 |
| 1–3 yr | 12.4 (2 yr) | 74–82 | 918–1,017 |
| 4–6 yr | 18.2 (5 yr) | 80–86 | 1,456–1,565 |
| 7–18 yr | 45.5 (13 yr) | 83–90 | 3,777–4,095 |
| Adult | 70.0 | 68–88 | 4,760–6,160 |

[a]Approximate total blood volume information compiled from Nathan DG, Orkin SH, eds. *Nathan and Oski's Hematology of Infancy and Childhood.* 5th ed. Philadelphia, PA: WB Saunders; 1998.
*Source*: Adapted with permission from Taketomo CK, Hodding JH, Kraus DM. *Pediatric and Neonatal Dosage Handbook.* 22nd ed. Hudson, OH: Lexi-Comp Inc; 2015.

the sample. This method labels 5% of the healthy individuals as having values that fall outside of the reference range.

In the pediatric population, however, one cannot easily obtain blood samples directly from known healthy individuals. Large sample sizes of healthy pediatric individuals that include an appropriate age distribution from birth to 18 years of age would be required. Furthermore, it may be difficult to obtain blood samples from healthy pediatric patients when these individuals cannot legally give informed consent and there is no direct benefit to these individuals of obtaining the blood sample. Therefore, many pediatric reference ranges have traditionally been determined via an indirect method: by using results of tests from hospitalized sick pediatric patients and applying special statistical methods.[11] The statistical methods are designed to remove outliers and distinguish the normal values from the values found in the sick patients. Obviously, problems in determining the true reference range may arise, especially when overlap between values from the diseased and nondiseased population occurs.

More recently, the Canadian Laboratory Initiative on Pediatric Reference Intervals (CALIPER) has attempted to address the limitations of using indirect methods to establish pediatric reference ranges.[12] Over the course of more than a decade, the CALIPER project has developed age- and sex-specific normal pediatric reference ranges for >100 laboratory tests using blood samples obtained directly from >9,700 known healthy children and adolescents from various communities and ethnic backgrounds in Canada. The CALIPER extensive database also includes neonates and infants; however, blood samples for these individuals (<1 year of age) were obtained largely from outpatient clinics. Current applicability of reference ranges for this age group to healthy individuals may be limited, but further studies by CALIPER are underway to address this limitation.

As in adults, many factors can influence the pediatric reference range, including the specific assay methodology used, type of specimen analyzed, specific population studied, nutritional status of the individual, time of day the sample is obtained, timing of meals, medications taken, and specific patient demographics (age, sex, height, weight, body surface area [BSA], and ethnicity). These factors, if not properly identified, may also influence the determination of reference ranges. In addition, because many pediatric reference ranges are typically established in hospitalized patients, concomitant diseases may also influence the determination of the specific reference range being studied. These factors, plus the greater heterogeneity (variance) observed in the pediatric population, make determination of pediatric reference ranges more complex.

Pediatric studies that define reference ranges may not always give detailed information about factors that may have influenced the determination of the specific pediatric reference range. Furthermore, due to the variation in influencing factors, most published pediatric reference ranges are not in exact agreement with each other.[1,3,11-17] Some studies report reference ranges by age for each year, others by various age groups, and others only by graphic display. This makes it difficult to ascertain standard values for pediatric reference ranges and to apply published pediatric reference ranges to one's own patient population.

The reference ranges listed in this chapter reflect a compilation from various sources and are meant to be general guidelines. Clinicians should consult with their institution's laboratory to determine specific age-appropriate pediatric reference ranges to be used in their patient population.

## Pediatric Clinical Presentation

In general, the clinical symptoms of laboratory abnormalities in pediatric patients are similar to symptoms observed in adults. However, certain manifestations of symptoms may be different in pediatric patients. For example, central nervous system (CNS) irritability due to electrolyte imbalances (such as hypernatremia) may manifest as a high-pitched cry in infants. Hypocalcemia is more likely to manifest as seizures in neonates and young infants (compared with adults) due to the immaturity of the CNS. Neonates may also have nonspecific or vague symptoms for many disorders. For example, neonates with sepsis, meningitis, or hypocalcemia may have poor feedings, lethargy, and vomiting. In addition, young pediatric patients are unable to communicate symptoms they may be experiencing. Thus, although symptoms of laboratory abnormalities in pediatric patients are important, often a correct diagnosis relies on the physical exam and appropriate laboratory tests.

# SERUM ELECTROLYTES AND MINERALS

The homeostatic mechanisms that regulate fluid, electrolyte, and mineral balance in adults also apply to the pediatric patient. However, several important age-related differences exist. Compared with adults, neonates and young infants have alterations in body composition and fluid compartments; increased insensible water loss; immature (decreased) renal function; and variations in the neuroendocrine control of fluid, electrolyte, and mineral balance.[18] In addition, fluid, electrolyte, and mineral intake are not controlled by the individual (ie, the neonate or young infant) but are controlled by the individual's caregiver. These age-related physiologic differences can result in alterations in the pediatric reference range for several electrolytes and minerals and can influence the interpretation of pediatric laboratory data.

A large percent of the human body is comprised of water. Total body water (TBW) can be divided into two major compartments: intracellular water (ICW) and extracellular water (ECW). The ECW compartment consists of the interstitial water and the intravascular water (or plasma volume) (**Figure 23-1**). Both TBW and ECW, when expressed as a percentage of body weight, are increased in the fetus and the newborn (especially the premature neonate) and decrease during childhood with increasing age (**Figure 23-2**).[19,20] The TBW of a fetus is 94% during the first month of gestation and decreases to 75% in a full-term newborn. The TBW of a preterm newborn may be 80%. The TBW decreases to approximately 60% by 6 to 12 months of age and to 55% in an adult. ECW is about 44% in a full-term newborn, 30% in a 3- to 6-month-old infant, 25% in a 1-year-old child, and 19% in an adult.[19,20] The decrease in TBW that is

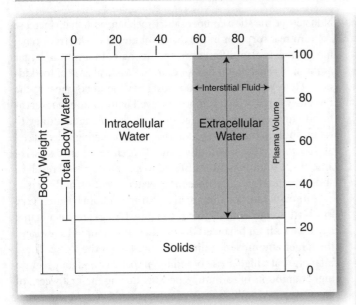

**FIGURE 23-1.** Distribution of body water in a term newborn infant expressed as a percentage of body weight. (*Source*: Reproduced with permission from Bell EF, Oh W. Fluid and electrolyte management. In: MacDonald MG, Seshia MMK, Mullett MD, eds. *Avery's Neonatology: Pathophysiology and Management of the Newborn*. 6th ed. Philadelphia, PA: Lippincott Williams & Wilkins; 2005:363.)

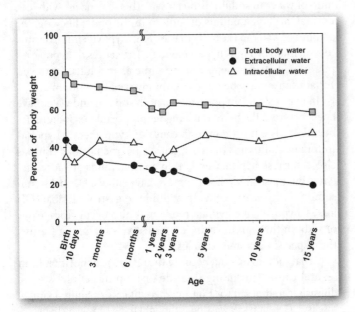

**FIGURE 23-2.** Changes in body water from birth to 15 years. (*Source*: Data from Friis-Hansen B. Changes in body water compartments during growth. *Acta Paediatr Suppl*. 1957;46(suppl 110):1–68.)

seen after birth is largely due to a contraction (or mobilization) of the ECW compartment. This mobilization is, most likely, the result of an increase in renal function that is seen after birth. The ICW compartment is lower at birth, increases slowly after

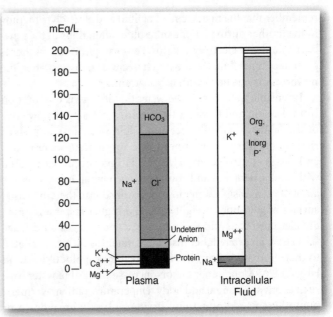

**FIGURE 23-3.** Ion distribution in the blood plasma, which represents extracellular fluid, and in the intracellular fluid compartment. (*Source*: Reproduced with permission from Bell EF, Oh W. Fluid and electrolyte management. In: MacDonald MG, Seshia MMK, Mullett MD, eds. *Avery's Neonatology: Pathophysiology and Management of the Newborn*. 6th ed. Philadelphia, PA: Lippincott Williams & Wilkins; 2005:364.)

birth, and is greater than ECW by about 3 months of age. It is important to note that the intake of water and electrolytes can influence these postnatal changes in TBW and the distribution between ECW and ICW.[18]

The electrolyte composition of ECW versus ICW is different (**Figure 23-3**). Sodium is the major cation found in intravascular water (plasma volume) of the ECW. Potassium, calcium, and magnesium make up a much smaller amount of the intravascular cations. Chloride is the primary intravascular anion and bicarbonate, protein, and other anions comprise the balance. The electrolyte composition of the interstitial component of ECW is similar to the intravascular composition, but protein content is lower. Potassium and magnesium are the major cations found in ICW. Phosphate (organic and inorganic) is the primary intracellular anion, and bicarbonate makes up a smaller amount.[18]

These compositional differences in ECW and ICW, along with the age-related differences in the amounts of these water compartments, can result in maturational differences in the amount of electrolytes per kilogram of body weight. For example, because premature neonates have a larger ECW compartment and ECW contains a higher amount of sodium and chloride, premature neonates contain a higher amount of sodium and chloride per kilogram of body weight compared with term neonates.[18] These principles are important to keep in mind when managing neonatal fluid and electrolyte therapy. One must also remember that the management of fluid and electrolyte therapy in the mother during labor can result in alterations in the newborn's fluid and electrolyte status. For example, if the mother is given too much fluid (ie, too much free water) during labor, the newborn may be born with hyponatremia.[21]

Insensible water loss is the water that is lost via evaporation from the skin and through the respiratory tract.[18] Knowledge of the factors that influence insensible water loss in pediatric patients is important to estimate appropriate water intake and assess electrolyte imbalances that may occur. Compared with adults, neonates and young infants have an increase in the amount of insensible water loss, primarily due to their increased surface area to body weight ratio and higher respiratory rate. Smaller newborns and those born at a younger gestational age (GA) have an even higher insensible water loss, which is related to their immature (thinner) skin, greater skin blood flow, and larger TBW. Many other factors increase insensible water loss, such as environmental and body temperature, radiant warmers, phototherapy, motor activity, crying, and skin breakdown or injury. Congenital skin defects, such as gastroschisis, omphalocele, or neural tube defects will also increase insensible water loss. The use of high inspired or ambient humidity, plastic heat shields or blankets, occlusive dressings, and topical waterproof agents decreases insensible water loss.

The primary functions of the kidney (glomerular filtration, tubular secretion, and tubular reabsorption) are all decreased in the newborn, especially in the premature newborn, compared with adults. These functions increase with GA at birth and with postnatal age (PNA). The decreased glomerular and tubular functions in the neonatal kidney result in differences in how the neonate handles various electrolyte loads and differences in the normal reference ranges for several electrolytes, as described later.

# Sodium

*Normal ranges are as follows:*[22]
*premature neonates (at 48 hours of life): 128 to 148 mEq/L (128 to 148 mmol/L)*
*neonates: 133 to 146 mEq/L (133 to 146 mmol/L)*
*infants: 139 to 146 mEq/L (139 to 146 mmol/L)*
*children: 138 to 145 mEq/L (138 to 145 mmol/L)*
*adults: 136 to 142 mEq/L (136 to 142 mmol/L)*

Sodium is primarily excreted via the kidneys, but it also is excreted via stool and sweat.[23] Usually, unless diarrhea occurs, sodium loss in the stool is minimal. In children with cystic fibrosis, aldosterone deficiency, or pseudohypoaldosteronism, the sodium concentration in sweat is increased and higher sweat losses may contribute to or cause sodium depletion.

In neonates and young infants, the renal handling of sodium is altered compared with adults.[24,25] Differences in tubular reabsorption, aldosterone concentrations, and patterns of renal blood flow help to maintain a positive sodium balance, which is required for growth. In the neonate, sodium reabsorption is decreased in the proximal tubule but increased in the distal tubule. Aldosterone increases sodium reabsorption in the distal tubules, and plasma concentrations of renin, angiotensin II, and aldosterone are all increased in neonates. This increase in

aldosterone may be a compensatory mechanism to help increase sodium reabsorption in the distal tubule. The pattern of renal blood flow is also different in the neonate. In adults, a larger amount of renal blood flow goes to the cortical area of the kidneys. However, in the neonate, most renal blood flow goes to the medullary area, which is more involved with sodium conservation than excretion. These factors help the neonatal kidney to retain sodium but also result in the neonate having a decreased ability to excrete a sodium load. Therefore, if an excessive amount of sodium is administered to a neonate, it will result in sodium retention with subsequent water retention and edema.

Although most infants are in a positive sodium balance, very low birth weight infants (birth weight <1.5 kg) are usually in a negative sodium balance[24] due to their immature kidneys and the larger amounts of sodium that are lost in the urine. These infants are at a higher risk of sodium imbalance and may require higher amounts of sodium, especially during the first weeks of life. Compared with adults, pediatric patients may be more susceptible to imbalances of sodium and water. This may be due to their higher amount of TBW and the common pediatric occurrence of causative factors, such as diarrhea and dehydration.

## Hyponatremia

In infants and children, *hyponatremia* is defined as a serum sodium <135 mEq/L, although slightly lower values would be considered acceptable for premature neonates and newborns.[22,23] As in adults, hyponatremia occurs in pediatric patients when the ratio of water to sodium is increased. This may occur with low, normal, or high amounts of sodium in the body; likewise, the amount of water in the body may be low (hypovolemic), normal (euvolemic), or high (hypervolemic). The causes of hyponatremia in pediatric patients are the same as in adults. However, certain causes may be more commonly seen in children.

In hypovolemic hyponatremia, both sodium and water have been lost from the body, but a higher proportion of sodium has been lost. The most common cause of hypovolemic hyponatremia in children is diarrhea due to gastroenteritis.[23] Emesis also can cause hyponatremia if hypotonic fluids are administered, but most children with emesis have either a normal serum sodium or hypernatremia. In addition to gastrointestinal (GI) losses, hypovolemic hyponatremia may also occur from losses of sodium through the skin (eg, excessive sweating or burns), third space losses, and renal losses.

Renal sodium loss can occur in the pediatric population from several causes, including thiazide or loop diuretics, osmotic diuresis, cerebral salt wasting, and hereditary or acquired kidney diseases. Cerebral salt wasting is thought to be caused by hypersecretion of atrial natriuretic peptide, which causes renal salt wasting. This condition is usually seen in patients with CNS disorders such as head trauma, brain tumors, hydrocephalus, cerebral vascular accidents, neurosurgery, and brain death.[26] Hereditary kidney diseases that can cause hypovolemic hyponatremia include juvenile nephronophthisis, autosomal recessive polycystic kidney disease, proximal (type II) renal tubular acidosis, 21-hydroxylase deficiency, and pseudohypoaldosteronism type I. Patients with congenital adrenal hyperplasia due to 21-hydroxylase deficiency have an absence of aldosterone. Aldosterone is needed for sodium retention and potassium and acid excretion in the kidneys. The lack of aldosterone in these patients produces hyponatremia, hyperkalemia, and metabolic acidosis. Patients with pseudohypoaldosteronism have elevated aldosterone serum concentrations, but the kidneys do not respond properly to aldosterone. A lack of response to aldosterone by the renal tubules may also occur in children with urinary tract obstruction and acute urinary tract infection and result in hyponatremia.[23]

In euvolemic hyponatremia, patients have no real evidence of volume depletion or volume overload.[23] Usually, these patients have a slight decrease in total body sodium with an excess of TBW. Although some patients may have an increase in body weight (indicating volume overload), they often appear clinically normal or have subtle signs of fluid overload. Causes of euvolemic hyponatremia include the syndrome of inappropriate antidiuretic hormone (SIADH), glucocorticoid deficiency, hypothyroidism, and water intoxication. Although SIADH is not common in children, it may occur in patients with CNS disorders or lung disease and tumors. Certain medications can cause an increase in antidiuretic hormone (ADH) secretion, as reviewed in Chapter 11.

Dilutional hyponatremia may commonly occur in hospitalized children who receive relatively large amounts of free water (eg, hypotonic IV solutions). This may even occur when medications are diluted in 5% dextrose in water, for example, and administered as 50- or 100-mL IV rider bags or piggyback riders. Neonates and young infants are more prone to this water overload (due to their lower glomerular filtration rate [GFR] and limited ability to excrete water), and should receive medications diluted in smaller volumes of IV fluid (which are usually administered via IV syringe pump). Other causes of hyponatremia due to water intoxication in pediatric patients include administration of diluted infant formula, tap water enemas, infant swimming lessons, forced water intake (child abuse), and psychogenic polydipsia[23] (**Minicase 1**).

## MINICASE 1

## A Case of Hyponatremia and Seizures

Peter P., a 3-day-old male, is currently in the neonatal intensive care unit being treated with antibiotics for suspected sepsis. He was born at 39 weeks' gestation to a mother with prolonged rupture of membranes (>72 hours). On the day of his birth, he was admitted to the neonatal intensive care unit with an elevated temperature, tachycardia (heart rate [HR] 166), and a low WBC count ($3.2 \times 10^3$ cells/mm$^3$). Blood and urine cultures were obtained, and antibiotics were started to treat his possible sepsis. Culture results are still pending. Medications include ampicillin 175 mg IV in 25 mL D5W administered as IV piggyback (IV rider bag) q 8 h (150 mg/kg/day) and gentamicin 14 mg IV in 50 mL D5W administered as IV piggyback q 24 h (4 mg/kg/day). This morning he began having rhythmic clonic twitching of his lower extremities, fluttering of his eyelids, and repetitive chewing movements, which are consistent with seizure activity.

His vital signs include blood pressure (BP) 77/50 mm Hg, HR 150 beats/min, respiratory rate (RR) 34 breaths/min, and temperature 99.1°F. Length is 51 cm (50th percentile for age), and weight is 3.5 kg (50th percentile for age). Laboratory data include sodium 119 mEq/L, potassium 4.5 mEq/L, chloride 100 mEq/L, total $CO_2$ 21 mEq/L, BUN 9 mg/dL, SCr 0.4 mg/dL, and glucose 88 mg/dL.

QUESTION: What is the most likely cause of this patient's seizure activity and electrolyte imbalance? What other laboratory tests should be obtained to further assess his seizure disorder?

DISCUSSION: Electrolyte imbalance is a common cause of neonatal seizures. As in adults, hyponatremia may cause seizure activity in neonates and occurs when the ratio of water to sodium is increased. The total body content of sodium in patients with hyponatremia may be low, normal, or high, and the volume status may be hypovolemic, euvolemic, or hypervolemic. There are many causes of hyponatremia, but the most likely cause in this patient is the extra D5W that he received with his antibiotics. Dilutional hyponatremia may occur in neonates and young infants when medications are administered in excess fluids, such as IV piggybacks or IV riders of 5% dextrose in water. These patients are more prone to water overload due to their lower GFR and their limited ability to excrete water. Medications for these patients should be diluted in smaller amounts of IV fluid and typically administered via an IV syringe pump (or slow IV push when appropriate) so that excess fluid is not administered. The neonate in this case received 125 mL/day (~36 mL/kg/day) of exogenous IV fluid from the antibiotic administration alone (ampicillin [25 mL × 3 doses/day = 75 mL] + gentamicin [50 mL × 1 dose/day = 50 mL] = 125 mL/day). An excess fluid amount of 36 mL/kg/day of D5W would be considered very large for this neonatal patient, who would typically have a normal daily fluid requirement of 100 mL/kg/day. Standard parenteral preparation and concentrations should be followed in neonatal and pediatric patients to avoid volume overload. In a neonate with a central line, ampicillin is typically diluted to a final concentration of 100 mg/mL and administered via slow IV push. For this case, the total volume per dose of ampicillin should be 1.75 mL (175 mg) IV push q 8 h. IV gentamicin is typically diluted with normal saline to a concentration of 2 mg/mL, or a total volume of 7 mL (14 mg), and would be administered via IV syringe pump q 24 h for this patient. This would have provided a total IV fluid volume from the antibiotics of only 12.25 mL/day (3.5 mL/kg/day), a reduction of approximately 113 mL/day.

To better define this patient's sodium and volume status, his total fluid intake and output, type of IV fluids administered, changes in body weight, and other laboratory data need to be assessed. In addition, other causes of hyponatremia, such as meningitis and SIADH, should be ruled out. A low WBC count, as observed in Peter P., often occurs in neonates with a serious bacterial infection (see section on White Blood Cell Count). Although the most likely cause of his seizure activity is his low serum sodium, his serum calcium, phosphorous, and magnesium levels also should be assessed because other electrolyte abnormalities can cause seizure activity.

In hypervolemic hyponatremia, both sodium and water are increased in the body, but there is a greater increase in water than sodium. Hypervolemic hyponatremia is typically observed in patients with congestive heart failure, cirrhosis, nephrotic syndrome, and chronic renal failure. It may also occur in patients with hypoalbuminemia or capillary leak syndrome due to sepsis.[23] These conditions decrease the patient's effective blood volume, either due to poor cardiac function or third spacing of fluid. The compensatory mechanisms in the body sense this decrease in blood volume; ADH and aldosterone are secreted and cause retention of water and sodium in the kidneys. A decrease in serum sodium occurs because the intake of water in these patients is greater than their sodium intake and ADH decreases water excretion.

Hyponatremia may also be caused by hyperosmolality (due to hyperglycemia or iatrogenic substances such as mannitol, sucrose, or glycine). For example, in pediatric patients with hyperglycemia during diabetic ketoacidosis, the high serum glucose concentration results in a high serum osmolality, which causes a shift of water from the intracellular space into the extracellular (intravascular) space. This shift of water has a dilutional effect on the serum sodium concentration, resulting in hyponatremia.[23] The decrease in serum sodium is proportional to the increased serum glucose concentration; for every 100 mg/dL increase in serum glucose above normal (ie, 100 mg/dL), the measured serum sodium declines by 1.6 mEq/L. The following equation can be used in pediatric patients with hyponatremia due to hyperglycemia to correct the measured (low) serum sodium concentration.

$$\text{Corrected serum sodium} = \text{Measured serum sodium} + \left[1.6 \times (\text{serum glucose} - 100 \text{ mg/dL})/100\right] \quad (1)$$

The calculated corrected serum sodium concentration better reflects the patient's true ratio of total body sodium to TBW; however, it should be remembered that the calculated value is only an estimate.

Pseudohyponatremia (falsely measured low serum sodium) may occur when serum contains high concentrations of lipids (hyperlipidemia) or proteins (hyperproteinemia), for example, in patients with hypertriglyceridemia or multiple myeloma.[23] This laboratory artifact may also occur in neonatal and pediatric patients who are receiving IV lipids for nutrition or IV immunoglobulin therapy.

### Hypernatremia

In general for pediatric patients, *hypernatremia* is defined as a serum sodium concentration >145 mEq/L. As in adults, hypernatremia occurs in pediatric patients when the ratio of sodium to water is increased. This may occur with low, normal, or high amounts of sodium in the body. Hypernatremia may occur with excessive sodium intake, excess water loss, or a combination of water and sodium loss when the water loss exceeds the sodium loss.[23]

Excessive sodium intake or sodium intoxication may occur due to improperly mixed infant formulas, excess sodium bicarbonate administration, IV hypertonic saline solutions, intentional salt poisoning (eg, child abuse), and ingestion of sodium chloride or seawater.[23] Neonates, especially premature newborns and young infants, can develop hypernatremia from excessive sodium due to the decreased ability of immature kidneys to excrete a sodium load. This becomes a problem, especially in the premature neonate when IV sodium bicarbonate is used to correct a metabolic acidosis. Excess water loss resulting in hypernatremia may occur in pediatric patients due to diabetes insipidus, increased insensible water losses, or inadequate intake. Diabetes insipidus can be of central or nephrogenic origin and either type can be acquired or congenital. Also, certain drugs may cause diabetes insipidus (see Chapter 11).

Neonates may be predisposed to hypernatremia from increased insensible water losses, especially during the first few days of life. A normal physiologic contraction of the ECW occurs after birth, resulting in a net loss of water and sodium. In term infants, this may result in a weight loss of 5% to 10% during the first week of life. In premature newborns, the weight loss may be 10% to 20%. This water loss, plus the relatively large and variable insensible water loss in neonates, can complicate the assessment of fluid and sodium balance. More premature newborns may be at higher risk for hypernatremia, as they have a more pronounced contraction of ECW and higher insensible water loss.[27] The use of radiant warmers and phototherapy (used to treat hyperbilirubinemia) further increases insensible water loss.

Inadequate water intake also can cause hypernatremia in pediatric patients. This may be due to the caregiver not administering enough fluids (eg, child neglect or abuse or ineffective breastfeeding). Ineffective breastfeeding may result in severe hypernatremic dehydration. Rarely, inadequate intake may be due to adipsia (absence of thirst).[23]

Hypernatremia due to water losses greater than sodium losses occurs in patients with water and sodium losses through the GI tract (eg, diarrhea, emesis, nasogastric suctioning, and osmotic cathartics), skin (eg, burns and excessive sweating), and kidneys (eg, diabetes mellitus, chronic kidney disease, osmotic diuretics, and acute tubular necrosis [polyuric phase]). Hypernatremia is most likely to occur in infants or children with diarrhea who also have inadequate fluid intake due to anorexia, emesis, or lack of access to water.

It should be noted that due to the immaturity of the blood vessels in their CNS, premature neonates are especially vulnerable to the adverse effects of hypernatremia (eg, intracranial hemorrhage). These patients are also at greater risk of adverse CNS effects (eg, cerebral edema) if an elevated serum sodium is corrected too rapidly. Thus, maintaining a proper sodium balance in these patients is extremely important.

## Potassium

*Normal ranges are as follows[14,22]:*
*premature neonates (at 48 hours of life): 3 to 6 mEq/L (3 to 6 mmol/L)*
*neonates: 3.7 to 5.9 mEq/L (3.7 to 5.9 mmol/L)*
*infants: 4.1 to 5.3 mEq/L (4.1 to 5.3 mmol/L)*
*children: 3.4 to 4.7 mEq/L (3.4 to 4.7 mmol/L)*
*adults: 3.8 to 5 mEq/L (3.8 to 5 mmol/L)*

Potassium is the major intracellular cation, and <1% of total body potassium is found in the plasma.[23] However, small changes in serum potassium can have large effects on cardiac, neuro-muscular, and neural function. Thus, appropriate homeostasis of extracellular potassium is extremely important. Insulin, aldosterone, acid–base balance, catecholamines, and renal function all play important roles in the regulation of serum potassium. Serum potassium can be lowered quickly when potassium shifts intracellularly or more slowly via elimination by the kidneys.

The kidney is the primary organ that regulates potassium balance and elimination. Potassium undergoes glomerular filtration and almost all filtered potassium is then reabsorbed in the proximal tubule. Urinary excretion of potassium, therefore, is dependent on distal potassium secretion by the collecting tubules. Neonates and young infants, however, have a decreased ability to secrete potassium via the collecting tubules. Thus, immature kidneys tend to retain potassium. This results in a positive potassium balance, which is required for growth (potassium is incorporated intracellularly into new tissues).[24,25] Potassium retention by the immature kidneys also results in higher serum potassium concentrations compared with the adult.[25]

## Hypokalemia

*Hypokalemia* is defined as a serum potassium concentration <3.5 mEq/L. As in adults, a low serum potassium may occur in pediatric patients due to an intracellular shift of potassium, decreased intake, or increased output (from renal or extrarenal losses). An intracellular shift of potassium may be seen with alkalosis, β-adrenergic stimulation, or insulin treatment. Endogenous β-adrenergic agonists (such as epinephrine released during stress) and exogenously administered β-agonists (such as albuterol) stimulate the cellular uptake of potassium. Other causes of an intracellular shift of potassium seen in pediatric patients include overdoses of theophylline, barium intoxication, and glue sniffing (toluene intoxication). A falsely low potassium concentration can be reported in a patient with an elevated white blood cell (WBC) count (eg, a patient with leukemia) if the plasma sample is inappropriately stored at room temperature. This allows the WBCs to uptake potassium from the plasma, resulting in a falsely low measurement.[23]

Most cases of hypokalemia in children are related to extrarenal losses of potassium due to gastroenteritis and diarrhea.[23] Hypokalemia caused by diarrhea is usually associated with a metabolic acidosis, because bicarbonate is also lost in the stool. Adolescent patients with eating disorders may be hypokalemic due to inadequate intake of potassium, such as patients with anorexia nervosa. Adolescents with bulimia or laxative abuse may also have significant extrarenal losses of potassium.

Many causes of hypokalemia resulting from renal potassium loss exist. Medications commonly used in the pediatric population that are associated with hypokalemia due to renal potassium loss include loop and thiazide diuretics, corticosteroids, amphotericin B, and cisplatin (see Chapter 11). Cushing syndrome, hyperaldosteronism, and ingestion of natural licorice (containing glycyrrhizic acid) may also cause hypokalemia via this mechanism.

In the pediatric population, other causes of increased renal potassium loss, such as hereditary diseases, must be considered. Remember that many hereditary diseases are first diagnosed during infancy and childhood. Renal tubular acidosis (both distal and proximal types) may present with hypokalemia and metabolic acidosis. Patients with cystic fibrosis have greater losses of chloride in sweat, which may lead to metabolic alkalosis, low urine chloride, and hypokalemia. Certain forms of congenital adrenal hyperplasia may also lead to increased renal potassium excretion and hypokalemia. Other inherited renal diseases that are due to defects in renal tubular transporters, such as Bartter syndrome, may result in metabolic alkalosis, hypokalemia, and high urine chloride. Thus, unlike the adult population, hereditary diseases need to be considered when certain electrolyte abnormalities are not explained by common causes.

## Hyperkalemia

In infants, children, and adults, *hyperkalemia* is defined as a serum potassium >5 mEq/L. Because a normal serum potassium is slightly higher in neonates and preterm infants, hyperkalemia is defined as a serum potassium >6 mEq/L in these patients. Hyperkalemia is one of the most alarming electrolyte imbalances because it has the potential to cause lethal cardiac arrhythmias.

As in adults, hyperkalemia in pediatric patients may be due to increased intake, an extracellular shift of potassium, or decreased renal excretion. Factitious hyperkalemia is common in pediatric patients because of the difficulty in obtaining blood samples. Hemolysis often occurs during blood sampling and potassium is released from red blood cells (RBCs) in sufficient amounts to cause falsely elevated test results. This may especially happen with improperly performed heel sticks (see section on Pediatric Blood Sampling). Potassium may also be released locally from muscles after prolonged tourniquet application or from fist clenching, which may also result in false elevations of measured potassium. A falsely elevated serum potassium also can be observed in patients with leukemia or extremely elevated WBC counts (usually >200,000/mm³) caused by the release of potassium from WBCs. Prompt analysis with measurement of a plasma sample usually avoids this problem.[23]

Hyperkalemia may occur as a result of extracellular shifts of potassium. During metabolic acidosis, hydrogen ions move into the cells (down a concentration gradient); in exchange, potassium ions move out of the cells into the extracellular (intravascular) space. This shift leads to a significant increase in serum potassium.

In older patients with fully developed (normal) renal function, hyperkalemia rarely results from increased intake alone. However, it may occur in patients receiving large amounts of oral or IV potassium or rapid or frequent blood transfusions (due to the potassium content of blood).[23] In patients with immature renal function or renal failure, increased intake of potassium can also lead to hyperkalemia due to decreased potassium excretion.

Decreased renal excretion of potassium is the most common cause of hyperkalemia. Decreased potassium excretion occurs in patients with immature renal function, renal failure, primary adrenal disease, hyporeninemic hypoaldosteronism, renal tubular disease, and with certain medications.[23] Hyperkalemia is the most common life-threatening electrolyte imbalance seen in neonates. Because of the decreased ability of immature kidneys to excrete potassium, neonates, particularly premature neonates, may be predisposed to hyperkalemia. These patients also cannot tolerate receiving extra potassium. Hyperkalemia can be seen in premature infants during the first 3 days of life, even when exogenous potassium is not given and when renal dysfunction is absent.[27] A rapid elevation in serum potassium is seen within the first day of life in more immature newborns. This hyperkalemia, which can be life-threatening, may be due to a shift of potassium from the intracellular space to the extracellular (intravascular) space, immaturity of the distal renal tubules, and a relative hypoaldosteronism.[28]

Acute or chronic renal failure in pediatric patients decreases potassium excretion and may result in hyperkalemia. Several inherited disorders may also cause decreased potassium excretion and hyperkalemia in pediatric patients, including certain types of congenital adrenal hyperplasia (eg, 21-hydroxylase deficiency), aldosterone synthase deficiency, sickle cell disease, and pseudohypoaldosteronism (types I and II).[23] Medications used in pediatric patients that may also cause hyperkalemia include angiotensin-converting enzyme inhibitors, $\beta_2$-adrenergic antagonists, potassium-sparing diuretics, nonsteroidal anti-inflammatory agents, heparin, trimethoprim, and cyclosporine.

## Serum Bicarbonate (Total Carbon Dioxide)

*Normal ranges are as follows[22,25]:*
*preterm infants: 16 to 20 mEq/L (16 to 20 mmol/L)*
*full-term infants: 19 to 21 mEq/L (19 to 21 mmol/L)*
*Infants–children 2 years: 18 to 28 mEq/L (18 to 28 mmol/L)*
*children >2 years and adults: 21 to 28 mEq/L (21 to 28 mmol/L)*

The *total carbon dioxide concentration* actually represents *serum bicarbonate*, the basic form of the carbonic acid–bicarbonate buffer system (ie, a low serum bicarbonate may indicate acidosis). In addition to the buffer systems, the kidneys also play an important role in acid–base balance. The proximal tubule reabsorbs 85% to 90% of filtered bicarbonate. The distal tubule is responsible for the net secretion of hydrogen ions and urinary acidification.[29] Compared with adults, neonates have a decreased capacity to reabsorb bicarbonate in the proximal tubule and, therefore, a decreased renal threshold for bicarbonate (the renal threshold is the serum concentration at which bicarbonate appears in the urine). The mean renal threshold for bicarbonate in adults is 24 to 26 mEq/L but only 18 mEq/L in the premature infant and 21 mEq/L in the term neonate. The renal threshold for bicarbonate increases during the first year of life and reaches adult values by about 1 year of age. Neonates also have decreased function of the distal tubules to secrete hydrogen ions and to acidify urine. The ability to acidify urine increases to adult values by about 1 to 2 months of age.[25,29] The neonate's decreased renal capacity to reabsorb bicarbonate and excrete hydrogen ions results in lower normal values for serum bicarbonate and blood pH. In addition, the neonate is less able to handle an acid load or to compensate for acid–base abnormalities.

It should be noted that for multiple reasons, the full-term newborn is in a state of metabolic acidosis immediately after birth (arterial pH 7.11 to 7.36).[3] The blood pH increases to more normal values within 24 hours, mostly due to increased excretion of carbon dioxide via the lungs.

## Calcium

Total serum calcium—*normal ranges are as follows[15]:*
*neonates 3 to 24 hours: 9 to 10.6 mg/dL (2.25 to 2.65 mmol/L)*
*neonates 24 to 48 hours: 7 to 12 mg/dL (1.75 to 3 mmol/L)*
*neonates 4 to 7 days: 9 to 10.9 mg/dL (2.25 to 2.73 mmol/L)*
*children: 8.8 to 10.8 mg/dL (2.2 to 2.7 mmol/L)*
*adolescents: 8.4 to 10.2 mg/dL (2.1 to 2.55 mmol/L)*
*adults: 8.7 to 10.2 mg/dL (2.2 to 2.6 mmol/L)*

Ionized calcium—*normal ranges are as follows:*
*neonates 3 to 24 hours: 4.3 to 5.1 mg/dL (1.08 to 1.28 mmol/L)*
*neonates 24 to 48 hours: 4 to 4.7 mg/dL (1 to 1.18 mmol/L)*
*infants, children, and adolescents: 4.5 to 4.92 mg/dL (1.13 to 1.23 mmol/L)*
*adults: 4.5 to 5.3 mg/dL (1.13 to 1.33 mmol/L)*

Calcium plays an integral role in many physiologic functions, including muscle contraction, neuromuscular transmission, blood coagulation, bone metabolism, and regulation of endocrine functions. Most calcium in the body (99%) is found in the bone, primarily as hydroxyapatite. Because of the growth that occurs during infancy and childhood, bone mass increases faster than body weight.[30] This increase in bone mass requires a significant increase in total body calcium. The increased calcium requirement is reflected in the higher recommended daily allowances (per kilogram of body weight) for pediatric patients compared with adults.

Calcium regulation in the body has two main goals.[30] First, serum calcium must be tightly regulated to permit the normal physiologic functions in which calcium plays a role. Second, calcium intake must be adequate to permit appropriate bone mineralization and skeletal growth. It is important to remember that bone mineralization may be sacrificed (ie, calcium may be released from the bone) to allow maintenance of a normal serum calcium concentration.

As in adults, serum calcium in pediatric patients is regulated by a complex hormonal system that involves vitamin D, serum phosphate, parathyroid hormone (PTH), and calcitonin. Briefly, calcium is absorbed in the GI tract, primarily via the duodenum and jejunum.[30] Although some passive calcium absorption occurs when dietary intake is high, most GI absorption of calcium occurs via active transport that is stimulated by 1,25-dihydroxyvitamin D. This occurs especially when dietary intake is low. Calcium excretion is controlled by the kidneys and influenced by multiple hormonal mediators (eg, PTH, 1,25-dihydroxyvitamin D, and calcitonin). In mature kidneys, approximately 99% of filtered calcium is reabsorbed by the tubules, with most (>50%) absorbed by the proximal tubules. Calcium also is absorbed in the loop of Henle, distal tubule, and collecting ducts.

During the first week of life, urinary calcium excretion is inversely related to GA (ie, more premature infants have a greater urinary calcium excretion).[25] Compared with adults, urinary calcium excretion is higher in neonates and preterm infants. The urinary calcium-to-creatinine ratio is about 0.2 in adults but may be >2 in premature neonates and up to 1.2 in full-term neonates during the first week of life. This high rate of calcium excretion may be related to the immaturity of the renal tubules and may contribute (along with other factors) to neonatal hypocalcemia. In addition, certain medications that are commonly administered to neonates and premature infants, such as furosemide, dexamethasone, and methylxanthines, further increase urinary calcium excretion. These medications may also increase the risk for hypocalcemia as well as nephrocalcinosis and nephrolithiasis.[25]

### Measurement of Calcium

Total serum calcium measures all three forms of extracellular calcium: complex bound, protein bound, and ionized. However, ionized calcium is the physiologically active form. Usually a parallel relationship exists between the ionized and total serum calcium concentrations. However, in patients with alterations in acid–base balance or serum proteins, the ionized serum calcium and total serum calcium are affected, respectively, and measurements of total serum calcium may no longer reflect the ionized serum concentration. Neonates have lower serum concentrations of protein (including albumin) and may be acidotic. This results in a lower total serum calcium concentration for a given ionized plasma concentration.[27] Although equations exist to adjust total serum calcium measurements for low concentrations of serum albumin, these equations have limitations and may not be precise. Therefore, ionized calcium should be measured in neonates (if microtechniques are available) and other pediatric patients with hypoalbuminemia or acid–base disorders.

### Hypocalcemia

As in adults, *hypocalcemia* may occur in pediatric patients for various reasons, including inadequate calcium intake, hypoparathyroidism, vitamin D deficiency, renal failure, redistribution of plasma calcium (eg, hyperphosphatemia and citrated blood transfusions), and hypomagnesemia. Hypocalcemia may also occur due to lack of organ response to PTH (eg, pseudohypoparathyroidism) and in the neonate because of other specific causes. The exact mechanism of how hypomagnesemia causes hypocalcemia is not clearly delineated. Magnesium can affect calcium balance, and significant hypomagnesemia can result in hypocalcemia due to intracellular cationic shifts. It is also thought that hypomagnesemia impairs the release of PTH and induces resistance to PTH effects. Because hypomagnesemia can result in hypocalcemia, a serum magnesium concentration is generally obtained in patients with hypocalcemia.

In the pediatric population, hypocalcemia most commonly occurs in neonates. *Early neonatal hypocalcemia* occurs during the first 72 hours of life and may be due to several factors. During fetal development, a transplacental active transport process maintains a higher calcium concentration in the fetus compared with the mother. After birth, this transplacental process suddenly stops. Serum calcium concentrations then decrease, even in healthy full-term newborns, reaching a nadir at 24 hours.[30] The high serum calcium concentrations in utero may also suppress the fetus' parathyroid gland. Thus, early neonatal hypocalcemia may also be caused by a relative hypoparathyroidism

in the newborn. In addition, newborns may have a decreased response to PTH. Early neonatal hypocalcemia is more likely to occur in premature and low birth weight newborns. It also occurs more commonly in infants of diabetic mothers, infants with intrauterine growth retardation, and newborns who have undergone prolonged, difficult deliveries. Inadequate calcium intake in critically ill newborns also contributes to hypocalcemia.

*Late neonatal hypocalcemia,* which usually presents during the first 5 to 10 days of life, is caused by high phosphate intake. It is much less common than early neonatal hypocalcemia, especially because the phosphorus content of infant formulas was decreased. It may, however, still occur if neonates are inappropriately given whole cow's milk. Cow's milk has a high phosphate load, which can cause hyperphosphatemia and secondary hypocalcemia in the neonate. To receive appropriate amounts of calcium and phosphorous to meet specific nutritional needs, neonates who are not breastfed should be given the proper infant formula according to their level of maturity (eg, special premature infant formula or infant formula for term infants). In general, cow's milk should not be introduced until 9 to 12 months of age.

Hypocalcemia may also occur in neonates born to mothers with hypercalcemia. Maternal hypercalcemia is usually due to hyperparathyroidism. In utero suppression of the fetal parathyroid gland can lead to hypoparathyroidism and hypocalcemia in the neonate. Hypocalcemia due to inadequate dietary calcium intake rarely occurs in the United States but can occur if infant formula or breast milk is replaced with liquids that contain lower amounts of calcium. Hypocalcemia may be iatrogenically induced if inadequate amounts of calcium are administered in hyperalimentation solutions. Adequate amounts of calcium and phosphorus may be difficult to deliver to preterm neonates because of their high daily requirements and limitations of calcium and phosphorus solubility in hyperalimentation solutions. Certain pediatric malabsorption disorders, such as celiac disease, may also cause inadequate absorption of calcium and vitamin D.

Hypoparathyroidism can be caused by many genetically inherited disorders, such as DiGeorge syndrome, X-linked hypoparathyroidism, and PTH gene mutations.[30] These and other syndromes must be considered when pediatric patients present with hypoparathyroidism.

In pediatric patients with vitamin D deficiency, hypocalcemia occurs primarily due to decreased intestinal absorption of calcium. The lower amounts of calcium in the blood stimulate the release of PTH from the parathyroid gland. PTH then prevents significant hypocalcemia via several different mechanisms. It causes bone to release calcium, increases urinary calcium reabsorption, and increases the activity of 1α-hydroxylase in the kidneys (the enzyme that converts 25-hydroxyvitamin D into 1,25-dihydroxyvitamin D, the active form of vitamin D). Hypocalcemia only develops after these compensatory mechanisms fail. In fact, most children with vitamin D deficiency present with rickets before they develop hypocalcemia.[30] In addition to elevated PTH concentrations, children with vitamin D deficiency have an elevated serum alkaline phosphatase concentration (due to increased osteoclast activity) and a low serum phosphorus (secondary to decreased intestinal absorption and decreased reabsorption in the kidneys), all as a result of the effects of PTH.

Vitamin D deficiency may be caused by several factors, including inadequate intake, lack of exposure to sunlight, malabsorption, or increased metabolism of vitamin D (eg, from medications such as phenobarbital and phenytoin). Generally, patients may have more than one of these factors. For example, institutionalized children who are not exposed to sunlight and receive chronic anticonvulsant therapy may be at a greater risk for developing vitamin D deficiency and rickets. Vitamin D deficiency may also occur with liver disease (failure to form 25-hydroxyvitamin D in the liver) and with renal failure (failure to form the active moiety, 1,25-dihydroxyvitamin D, due to a loss of activity of 1α-hydroxylase in the kidneys).

Genetic disorders, such as vitamin D-dependent rickets, may also cause hypocalcemia. The absence of the enzyme, 1-α-hydroxylase, in the kidneys occurs in children with vitamin D-dependent rickets type 1. Therefore, these children cannot convert 25-hydroxyvitamin D to its active form. Children with vitamin D-dependent rickets type 2 have a defective vitamin D receptor, which prevents the normal response to 1,25-dihydroxyvitamin D[30] (**Minicase 2**).

Hypocalcemia also occurs when patients receive citrated blood transfusions or exchange transfusions (citrate is used to anticoagulate blood). Citrate forms a complex with calcium and decreases the ionized calcium concentration. Pediatric patients at highest risk include those receiving multiple blood transfusions or exchange transfusions, such as neonates treated for hyperbilirubinemia and older children treated for sickle cell crisis. These patients may develop symptoms of hypocalcemia, such as tetany or seizures, due to the lower ionized calcium levels. It should be noted that the total serum calcium concentration in these patients can be normal or even elevated because the calcium-citrate complex is included in the measurement.[30]

### Hypercalcemia

*Hypercalcemia* is an uncommon pediatric electrolyte disorder. As in adults, it may be caused by excess PTH, excess vitamin D, excess calcium intake, excess renal reabsorption of calcium, increased calcium released from the bone, and miscellaneous factors, such as hypophosphatemia or adrenal insufficiency.[30] Causes of hypercalcemia that are of particular interest in pediatric patients include neonatal hyperparathyroidism, hypervitaminosis D, excessive calcium intake, malignancy associated hypercalcemia, and immobilization. Also, several genetic syndromes and disorders may cause hypercalcemia.

Neonatal hyperparathyroidism, an autosomal recessive disorder, can be severe and life-threatening.[30] Typically, these patients have defective calcium-sensing receptors in the parathyroid gland. Normally, high serum calcium concentrations would be sensed by the parathyroid gland and PTH levels would then decrease. In these patients, however, the parathyroid gland cannot sense the high serum calcium concentrations, and PTH continues to be released, which further increases serum calcium concentrations. Transient secondary neonatal hyperparathyroidism occurs in neonates born to mothers with hypocalcemia. Maternal hypocalcemia leads to hypocalcemia in the fetus

with secondary hyperparathyroidism. These neonates may be born with skeletal demineralization and bone fractures. Hypercalcemia in these patients usually takes days to weeks to resolve.

Excessive intake of vitamin D or calcium may also cause hypercalcemia. Typically, it may occur in children who are being treated with vitamin D and calcium with excessive doses. Excess calcium in hyperalimentation solutions commonly results in hypercalcemia.

Compared with adults, hypercalcemia from immobilization occurs more frequently in children, especially adolescents,[30] because of a higher rate of bone remodeling in these patients. Immobilization of children and adolescents may be required due to specific injuries, such as leg fractures, spinal cord paralysis, burns, or other severe medical conditions. In children with leg fractures that require traction, hypercalcemia usually occurs within 1 to 3 weeks. Immobilization may also result in isolated hypercalciuria, which may result in nephrocalcinosis, kidney stones, or renal insufficiency.

## Phosphorus

*Normal ranges are as follows[23]:*
*neonates 0 to 5 days: 4.8 to 8.2 mg/dL (1.55 to 2.65 mmol/L)*
*children 1 to 3 years: 3.8 to 6.5 mg/dL (1.23 to 2.1 mmol/L)*
*children 4 to 11 years: 3.7 to 5.6 mg/dL (1.2 to 1.8 mmol/L)*
*adolescents 12 to 15 years: 2.9 to 5.4 mg/dL (0.94 to 1.74 mmol/L)*
*adolescents 16 to 19 years: 2.7 to 4.7 mg/dL (0.87 to 1.52 mmol/L)*
*adults: 2.3 to 4.7 mg/dL (0.74 to 1.52 mmol/L)*

Phosphorus is the primary intracellular anion and plays an integral role in cellular energy and intracellular metabolism. It is also a component of phospholipid membranes and other cell structures. Most phosphorus in the body (85%) is found in bone, whereas <1% of phosphorus is found in the plasma. Like calcium, phosphorus is essential for bone mineralization and skeletal growth. During infancy and childhood, a positive phosphorus balance is required for proper growth to allow adequate amounts of phosphorus to be incorporated into bone and new cells. The higher phosphorus requirement that is needed to facilitate growth may help explain the higher serum concentrations seen in the pediatric population compared with adults.

The kidney is the primary organ that regulates phosphorus balance. Approximately 90% of plasma phosphate is filtered by the glomerulus, with most being actively reabsorbed at the proximal tubule. Some reabsorption also occurs more distally, but phosphate is not significantly secreted along the nephron.[23] Unlike other active transport systems, phosphate reabsorption, both proximal and distal, is greater in the neonatal kidney compared with adults.[25,29] Thus, the neonatal kidney tends to retain phosphate, perhaps as a physiologic adaptation to the high demands for phosphate that are required for growth. Neonatal renal phosphate reabsorption may be regulated by growth hormone.[29]

### Hypophosphatemia

As in adults, *hypophosphatemia* may occur in pediatric patients for several reasons, including increased renal excretion, decreased phosphate or vitamin D intake, or intracellular

# MINICASE 2

## Rickets in a Child

Raymond D., a 10-year-old male, is admitted to the emergency department from a local pediatric long-term care facility with pain, tenderness, and decreased movement to his right leg. He sustained a fall at the long-term care facility when he was being moved from his bed to his wheelchair. Born at term, he suffered a traumatic birth with severe perinatal asphyxia. He subsequently developed seizures that were controlled by the combined anticonvulsant therapy of phenobarbital and phenytoin. As a result of his asphyxia at birth, he developed spastic cerebral palsy and severe neurodevelopmental delay. He was transferred to the long-term care facility at 4 months of age and has remained on phenobarbital and phenytoin since that time. Two years ago, he was diagnosed with gastroesophageal reflux disease, which has been controlled with antacids. Medications include phenobarbital elixir 60 mg (15 mL) PO BID; phenytoin suspension 75 mg (3 mL) PO BID; and aluminum hydroxide suspension 10 mL PO QID.

His vital signs include BP 102/70 mm Hg; HR 92 beats/min; RR 24 breaths/min; and temperature 98.6°F. His height is 125 cm (<3rd percentile for age), and weight is 24 kg (<5th percentile for age). Physical exam of his chest is significant for a pigeon breast deformity and slightly palpable enlargement of costochondral junctions. He has redness in his right leg, 10 cm below the knee, and pain on movement. The preliminary radiographic findings reveal a fracture of his right tibia with osteomalacia and bone changes consistent with rickets.

Significant laboratory data are as follows:

  calcium: 8.2 mg/dL (normal for children: 8.8 to 10.8 mg/dL)

  ionized calcium: 4 mg/dL (normal for infants to adults: 4.5 to 4.92 mg/dL)

  phosphorus: 2.5 mg/dL (normal for 4 to 11 years: 3.7 to 5.6 mg/dL)

  magnesium: 1.6 mg/dL (normal for 2 to 14 years: 1.5 to 2.3 mg/dL)

  albumin 2.9 g/dL (normal for children 7 to 19 years: 3.7 to 5.6 g/dL)

  ALT: 55 units/L (normal for 1 to 19 years: 5 to 45 units/L)

  AST: 65 units/L (normal for children 10 to 15 years: 10 to 40 units/L)

  alkaline phosphatase: 863 units/L (normal for children 2 to 10 years: 100 to 320 units/L)

QUESTION: What evidence exists that this patient has rickets? How did his medications affect his serum phosphorus, calcium, and liver enzymes, and how would you modify his drug therapy?

DISCUSSION: Rickets is diagnosed by both radiologic and laboratory findings. The preliminary radiographic findings and the physical findings of the pigeon breast deformity (ie, the sternum and adjacent cartilage appear to be projected forward) and the palpable enlargement of costochondral junctions (rachitic rosary sign) are compatible with the diagnosis of rickets. Serum calcium may be low or normal in patients with rickets, depending on the etiology. The primary causes of rickets in the United States are vitamin D

deficiency (with secondary hyperparathyroidism), primary phosphate deficiency, and end-organ resistance to 1,25-dihydroxyvitamin D. In patients with vitamin D deficiency, serum calcium concentrations can be normal or low, phosphorus concentrations are usually low, and serum alkaline phosphatase is elevated. In patients with primary phosphate deficiency, serum calcium is normal, serum phosphorus is low, and serum alkaline phosphatase is elevated. In patients with end-organ resistance to 1,25-dihydroxyvitamin D, serum calcium is low, serum phosphorus may be low or normal, and serum alkaline phosphatase is elevated.

In this patient, ionized calcium and serum phosphorus are both low and serum alkaline phosphatase is high, all of which are consistent with a diagnosis of rickets. Serum magnesium is normal for age; ALT and AST are slightly elevated. The serum magnesium was obtained because hypomagnesemia may also cause hypocalcemia. He also has hypoalbuminemia. A total serum calcium measures all three forms of extracellular calcium: complex bound, protein bound, and ionized. In patients with low albumin, the concentration of ionized calcium will be increased for a given total serum calcium concentration. Equations can be used to "correct" total serum calcium measurements for low concentrations of serum albumin, but these equations have limitations and may not be precise. Thus, in patients with low albumin (like this patient), an ionized serum calcium should be obtained.

His medications affected his laboratory tests. He is receiving an aluminum-containing antacid, which binds phosphorus in the GI tract. This resulted in decreased absorption of phosphorus and contributed to his low serum phosphorus. Enzyme-inducing anticonvulsants, such as phenobarbital and phenytoin, increase the metabolism of vitamin D and may result in a deficiency of vitamin D with resultant anticonvulsant-induced osteomalacia and rickets. Both the aluminum-containing antacid and the anticonvulsants contributed to him developing rickets, and thus, to the elevated serum alkaline phosphatase. In addition, due to his other medical conditions, he is nonambulatory and resides at a long-term care facility. Thus, he may have a lack of exposure to sunlight and, therefore, a lack of vitamin D. This lack of vitamin D also would contribute to the development of rickets.

For treatment of his rickets, he should be started on oral supplements of calcium, phosphorous, and vitamin D. However, modifications in his preadmission medications should be made. The aluminum-containing antacid (aluminum hydroxide suspension) should be discontinued and replaced with a calcium-containing antacid (eg, calcium carbonate). The amount of calcium in this new antacid should then be subtracted from any calcium supplement that would be started in the hospital, so that the total daily dose of calcium stays the same. Alternatively, the total dose of calcium supplement can be given as calcium carbonate. Discontinuing the aluminum-containing antacid will result in a greater amount of phosphorus absorbed enterally, which will then require a decrease in the oral supplement of phosphate (depending on serum phosphorus concentrations). Once he is stable, his neurologist should be consulted to see if other anticonvulsants that have less of an enzyme-inducing effect could be used to treat his seizures.

shifting. Causes of excessive renal phosphorus excretion in pediatric patients include hyperparathyroidism, metabolic acidosis, diuretics, glucocorticoids, glycosuria, IV fluids and volume expansion, kidney transplantation, and inherited disorders such as hypophosphatemic rickets.

Inadequate dietary phosphate intake is an unusual cause of hypophosphatemia in adults. However, infants are more predisposed to nutritional hypophosphatemia due to their higher phosphorus requirements.[23] The phosphorus requirements of premature infants are even higher due to their rapid skeletal growth. If premature infants are fed regular infant formula (instead of premature infant formula that contains additional calcium and phosphorus), phosphorus deficiency and rickets may occur. Phosphorous deficiency and rickets also can occur in pediatric patients who receive aluminum hydroxide–containing antacids, which bind dietary and secreted phosphorous and prevent its absorption from the GI tract. Inadequate vitamin D intake and genetic causes of vitamin D deficiency (eg, vitamin D-dependent rickets type 1) also can result in hypophosphatemia in pediatric patients.

Hypophosphatemia caused by intracellular shifting of phosphorus occurs with processes that stimulate intracellular phosphorus use. For example, high serum levels of glucose stimulate insulin. Insulin then enables glucose and phosphorus to move into the cell, where phosphorus is used during glycolysis. Intracellular shifting of phosphorus also occurs during anabolism, such as in patients receiving hyperalimentation and during refeeding in patients with protein-calorie malnutrition (eg, severe anorexia nervosa). The high anabolic (growth) rate in infants (especially premature infants) and children make them more susceptible to hypophosphatemia when adequate amounts of phosphate are not supplied in the hyperalimentation solution. Hypophosphatemia as a result of refeeding malnourished children usually occurs within 5 days of refeeding. It may be prevented by a more gradual increase in nutrition and phosphate supplementation.[23]

## Hyperphosphatemia

*Hyperphosphatemia* in pediatric patients may be caused by decreased excretion of phosphorus, increased intake of phosphate or vitamin D, or a shift of intracellular phosphate to extracellular fluid. The most common cause of hyperphosphatemia in the pediatric population is decreased excretion of phosphorus due to renal failure. Excessive phosphorus intake in pediatric patients (especially in those with renal dysfunction or in neonates whose renal function is normally decreased due to immaturity) is a common cause of hyperphosphatemia.[23] Hyperphosphatemia may also occur if neonates are inappropriately given whole cow's milk. As previously mentioned, cow's milk contains a high phosphate load, which can cause hyperphosphatemia and secondary hypocalcemia in the neonate. Administration of sodium phosphorus laxatives or enemas to infants and children may also result in excessive phosphate intake. In addition, the pediatric dosing of phosphate supplements may be confusing to some because of the multiple salts available and multiple units of measure. This may result in unintentional overdoses with resultant hyperphosphatemia.

# Magnesium

*Normal ranges are as follows[15,16]:*
*neonates 0 to 6 days: 1.2 to 2.6 mg/dL (0.49 to 1.07 mmol/L)*
*neonates 7 days to children 2 years: 1.6 to 2.6 mg/dL (0.66 to 1.07 mmol/L)*
*children 2 years to adolescents 18 years: 1.5 to 2.3 mg/dL (0.62 to 0.95 mmol/L)*
*adults: 1.3 to 2.1 mEq/L (0.65 to 1.05 mmol/L)*

Magnesium plays an important role in neuromuscular function and is a required cofactor for many enzymatic systems in the body. Approximately 50% to 60% of magnesium is located in bone, with one-third being slowly exchangeable with extracellular fluid. About 45% of magnesium is found in the intracellular fluid, with only 1% in extracellular fluid. The kidney is the primary organ responsible for magnesium excretion. Approximately 95% to 97% of filtered magnesium is reabsorbed: 15% in the proximal tubule, 70% in the thick ascending limb of Henle, and 5% to 10% in the distal tubule.[23] In the neonate, reabsorption of magnesium may be increased in the proximal tubule. Thus, the immature neonatal kidney tends to retain magnesium compared with adults.[25] This results in slightly higher normal values for serum magnesium in neonates and infants compared with older children and adults. In fact, serum magnesium concentrations in the newborn have been shown to be inversely related to GA at birth and postmenstrual age (PMA). In other words, more immature neonates have slightly higher serum magnesium concentrations.[31,32]

## Hypomagnesemia

*Hypomagnesemia* occurs in pediatric patients because of excessive renal or GI losses, decreased GI absorption, decreased intake, and specific neonatal causes.[23] Hypomagnesemia may occur in neonates due to several maternal causes. Maternal diuretic use, laxative overuse or abuse, diabetes mellitus, or decreased intake due to vomiting during pregnancy may cause maternal hypomagnesemia and lead to hypomagnesemia in the newborn.[33] Hypomagnesemia also commonly occurs in neonates with intrauterine growth retardation (due to deficient placental transfer of magnesium) and in neonates who receive exchange transfusions with citrated blood.

Excessive renal losses of magnesium may be caused by various reasons. Of particular pediatric concern is the use of medications (eg, diuretics, amphotericin, proton pump inhibitors, aminoglycosides, and cisplatin) that may cause magnesium wasting. Hypomagnesemia may also occur due to rare hereditary renal magnesium-losing syndromes, such as Bartter syndrome and autosomal recessive renal magnesium–wasting syndrome. Excessive GI losses of magnesium may occur in pediatric patients with diarrhea or large losses of gastric contents (eg, emesis or nasogastric suction). Decreased GI absorption of magnesium may occur in patients with short gut syndrome. These patients have had a portion of their small bowel removed, which results in poor intestinal absorption. Other important pediatric GI diseases that may result in hypomagnesemia include cystic fibrosis, inflammatory bowel disease, and celiac disease.[23]

Poor magnesium intake may also result in hypomagnesemia. Although this rarely occurs in children fed orally, it may occur in hospitalized children receiving inadequate amounts of magnesium in IV fluids or parenteral nutrition solutions. Hypomagnesemia also can occur during the refeeding of children with protein-calorie malnutrition (eg, severe anorexia nervosa). These patients have low magnesium reserves but a high requirement of magnesium because of cellular growth.[23]

### Hypermagnesemia

As in adults, the most common cause of *hypermagnesemia* in pediatric patients is renal dysfunction. However, in neonates, the most common cause is the IV infusion of magnesium sulfate in the mother for the prevention and treatment of eclampsia or for fetal neuroprotection.[23,33] The high levels of magnesium in the mother are delivered transplacentally to the fetus. Neonates and young infants are also more prone to hypermagnesemia because of their immature renal function. Thus, these patients cannot easily tolerate a magnesium load. Other common pediatric causes of hypermagnesemia include excessive intake due to magnesium-containing antacids, laxatives, or enemas.

## AGE-RELATED DIFFERENCES IN KIDNEY FUNCTION TESTS

### Serum Creatinine

Jaffe Method—*normal ranges are as follows*[34]:
*neonates: 0.3 to 1 mg/dL (27 to 88 μmol/L)*
*infants: 0.2 to 0.4 mg/dL (18 to 35 μmol/L)*
*children: 0.3 to 0.7 mg/dL (27 to 62 μmol/L)*
*adolescents: 0.5 to 1 mg/dL (44 to 88 μmol/L)*
*adult males: 0.6 to 1.2 mg/dL (53 to 106 μmol/L)*
*adult females: 0.5 to 1.1 mg/dL (44 to 97 μmol/L)*

Isotope Dilution Mass Spectrometry (IDMS)–Traceable Enzymatic Method—*normal ranges are as follows*[15]:
*neonates to children 4 years: 0.03 to 0.5 mg/dL (2.65 to 44.2 μmol/L)*
*children 4 to 7 years: 0.03 to 0.59 mg/dL (2.65 to 52.2 μmol/L)*
*children 7 to 10 years: 0.22 to 0.59 mg/dL (19.4 to 52.2 μmol/L)*
*children and adolescents 10 to 14 years: 0.31 to 0.88 mg/dL (27.4 to 77.8 μmol/L)*
*adolescents >14 years: 0.5 to 1.06 mg/dL (44.2 to 93.7 μmol/L)*
Serum creatinine (SCr) is a useful indicator of renal function and can be used to estimate GFR. Creatinine is generated from the metabolism of creatine and creatine phosphate, a high-energy biochemical important in muscle activity. Creatinine is produced in muscles, released into the extracellular fluid, and excreted by the kidneys. Excretion of creatinine is primarily via glomerular filtration, but a smaller amount undergoes tubular secretion. The amount of creatinine that is secreted by the tubules increases in patients as GFR decreases. Thus, creatinine clearance (CrCl) overestimates the actual GFR in patients with renal insufficiency.[35,36]

In pediatric patients, three major factors influence the SCr concentration: muscle mass per unit of body size, GFR, and (in newborns) the exogenous (maternal) creatinine load.[36] At birth, the newborn's SCr reflects the maternal SCr because SCr crosses the placenta. If a pregnant woman has an elevated SCr, then the concentration of creatinine in the fetus also will be elevated. In fact, the plasma creatinine concentration of umbilical cord blood is almost equal to the creatinine concentration in the mother.[27] In full-term newborns, SCr may increase slightly shortly after birth because of the contraction of the ECW compartment.[36] SCr then decreases over the first few days of life and usually reaches 0.4 mg/dL (Jaffe method) by about 10 days of age.[36] The apparent half-life of this postnatal decrease in SCr is about 2.1 days in normal full-term infants and is due to the ongoing maturation of the kidneys and progressive increase in GFR. SCr is higher at birth in premature newborns compared with full-term newborns, and the postnatal decrease in SCr may occur more slowly. This is due to the preterm newborn's more immature kidneys and lower GFR.[27,37]

Compared with adults, pediatric patients have a lower muscle mass per unit of body size. Because the production of creatinine depends on muscle mass, this results in significantly lower normal values for SCr for neonates, infants, and children. The percentage of muscle mass differs with various pediatric age groups and increases with age from birth through young adulthood.[36] This increase in muscle mass accounts for the increase in the normal values for SCr with increasing age (see normal values for SCr above).

Creatinine excretion depends on GFR and, as in adults, SCr becomes elevated in pediatric patients with renal dysfunction. For example, an infant with an SCr as measured by the Jaffe method of 0.8 mg/dL (twice the normal value for age) has approximately a 50% decrease in GFR. Using age-appropriate normal values to interpret SCr is essential. In the previous example, an SCr of 0.8 mg/dL (which would be considered normal in an adult) denotes significant renal dysfunction in younger patients. Correct interpretation of SCr values is extremely important because the doses of fluids, many electrolytes, and medications that are renally eliminated need to be adjusted. Misinterpretation of SCr (eg, not recognizing renal dysfunction) can result in serious and potentially fatal fluid and electrolyte imbalances and overdosing of medications.

Reliable and accurate measurement of SCr is clinically important to properly assess renal function. Historically, SCr was measured by the alkaline picrate-based method, also known as the *Jaffe method*. However, substances that interfere with the measurement of creatinine by this method (ie, noncreatinine chromogens such as uric acid, glucose, fructose, and acetone) can cause an overestimation of SCr and, thus, an underestimation of kidney function. In addition, certain medications, endogenous substances, and medical conditions (eg, bilirubin, lipemia, and hemolysis) may interfere with the determination of SCr by this method.[6,14] This interference may be a problem in the neonatal population because neonates often have hyperbilirubinemia or lipemia, and blood sampling methods in neonates often results in hemolysis.

Inaccuracies of the Jaffe method and other methodologies have led the National Kidney Disease Education Program to recommend a recalibration and standardization of SCr measurements.[38] This has resulted in implementation of improved methods of SCr determinations, such as an enzymatic assay with an isotope dilution mass spectrometry (IDMS)–traceable international standard. It is important to know what methodology a laboratory is using because measurement by newer assays results in lower SCr determinations. Thus, the normal value of SCr for a specific patient depends on the assay method being used and the age of the patient (see normal values for SCr above). Further information about laboratory measurement and reporting of SCr can be found in Chapter 10.

## Age-Related Physiologic Development of Renal Function

Compared with adults, a newborn's kidneys are anatomically and functionally immature. The primary functions of the kidney (glomerular filtration, tubular secretion, and tubular reabsorption) are all decreased in the full-term newborn. These renal functions are even further decreased in the premature infant. After birth, glomerular and tubular renal function increase (ie, mature) with PNA. During the first 2 years of life, kidney function matures to adult levels in the following order: (1) glomerular filtration, (2) tubular secretion, and (3) tubular reabsorption. The interpretation of pediatric kidney functions tests can be better understood if one knows how each function of the kidneys matures during the first 2 years.

*Glomerular filtration.* In the fetus, nephrogenesis (ie, the formation of new nephrons) begins at 7 to 8 weeks of gestation and continues until 34 to 36 weeks of gestation.[35,39,40] Although the number of adult nephrons (~1 million) is reached at this time, the nephrons are smaller and not as functionally mature as the nephrons found in an adult kidney.[24] After 36 weeks of gestation, no new nephrons are formed. However, renal mass continues to increase due to the increase in renal tubular growth. GFR is very low in the young fetus but gradually increases during gestation (**Figure 23-4**). Before 36 weeks of gestation, the increase in GFR is primarily due to nephrogenesis and the increase in the number of new glomeruli.[39] From 36 weeks of gestation until birth, a much smaller increase in GFR occurs as renal mass and kidney function increase.

At birth, GFR increases dramatically compared with what it was in utero (Figure 23-4). This dramatic increase in GFR, which occurs at birth and continues during the early postnatal period, is the result of several important hemodynamic and physiologic changes. Cardiac output and systemic blood pressure increase at birth and a significant decrease in renal vascular resistance occurs. These changes result in an increase in renal blood flow and effective glomerular filtration pressure. In addition, alterations in the pattern of renal blood flow distribution occur and the permeability of the glomerular membrane and surface area available for filtration increase.[24,39,40] All of these changes help to increase GFR.

Despite the increase in GFR that occurs during this time, GFR is still very much decreased in comparison with adults. As determined by creatinine or inulin clearance, the GFR in a full-term newborn is only 10 to 15 mL/min/m² (2 to 4 mL/min). GFR then doubles by 1 to 2 weeks of age to 20 to 30 mL/min/m² (8 to 20 mL/min).[39] Adult values of GFR are approached by about 6 to 12 months of age (70 to 90 mL/min/m²). Compared

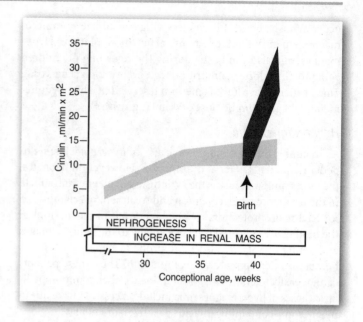

**FIGURE 23-4.** Maturation of GFR in relation to conceptional age. (*Source*: Reproduced with permission from Guignard JP. The neonatal stressed kidney. In: Gruskin AB, Norman ME, eds. *Pediatric Nephrology*. Philadelphia, PA: Martinus Nijhoff Publishers; 1981:507.)

with full-term newborns, GFR in premature newborns is much lower at birth (5 to 10 mL/min/m² or 0.7 to 2 mL/min) and increases at a less dramatic rate during the first 1 to 2 weeks after birth (10 to 12 mL/min/m² or 2 to 4 mL/min).[39] After the first postnatal week, the rate of increase in GFR is comparable in preterm and full-term infants, but the actual GFR value is still lower in preterm infants than full-term infants.

*Renal tubular function.* Tubular secretion and reabsorption are both decreased in the full-term newborn because of the small size and mass of the renal tubules, decreased peritubular blood flow, and immature biochemical processes that supply energy for active transport. In addition, full-term newborns have a limited ability to concentrate urine and have lower urinary pH values.[39] In the preterm newborn, renal tubular functions are further decreased. Limitations of the newborn's tubular function with respect to the renal handling of serum electrolytes are listed above in the discussion section of each serum electrolyte.

Tubular secretion transports certain electrolytes and medications from the peritubular capillaries into the lumen of the renal tubule. At birth, tubular secretion is only 20% to 30% of adult values and slowly matures by about 8 months of age. Tubular reabsorption, which also is decreased at birth, may not fully mature until 1 to 2 years of age. Thus, during infancy, a glomerulotubular imbalance occurs, with GFR maturing at a faster rate than renal tubular function.

The decreased renal function in newborns and the maturational changes in GFR and tubular function that occur throughout early infancy have important implications for the interpretation of laboratory data. For example, one must remember that even with a normal SCr for age, neonates and infants still have decreased renal function compared with adults. This decreased renal function must be taken into account, especially in the very young, when dosing electrolytes or medications that are eliminated by the kidneys. In addition, as in adults, certain medications, diseases, and medical conditions (such as hypoxic events that may occur in newborns) may cause further decreases in renal function.

### Standardization of Creatinine Clearance

Creatinine clearance (CrCl) can be expressed using several different units of measure, including mL/min, mL/min/m², or mL/min/1.73 m². To better compare the CrCl of patients of different body sizes, CrCl is most commonly standardized to the BSA of an average-sized adult (1.73 m²). Thus, CrCl is most commonly measured as mL/min/1.73 m². Using these units is especially helpful in pediatric patients, in whom a large range of body sizes occurs. For example, the average BSA ranges from 0.22 m² in a full-term newborn to 1.32 m² in a 12-year-old female and 1.77 m² in a 17-year-old male.[1] Expressing CrCl in mL/min or even mL/min/m² over this wide of a range of BSAs would give an extremely wide range of values.

### Estimating Body Surface Area in Pediatric Patients

Body surface area (BSA) can be estimated using several different methods. In pediatric patients, BSA is most commonly estimated using standard nomograms or equations and the patient's measured height and weight. Two equations are commonly used in pediatric practice, an older equation (the DuBois formula)[41]:

$$BSA\ (m^2) = Wt\ (kg)^{0.425} \times Ht\ (cm)^{0.725} \times 0.007184 \qquad (2)$$

and a more simplified equation (the Mosteller formula)[42]:

$$BSA\ (m^2) = \text{the square root of } ([Ht\ (cm) \times Wt\ (kg)]/3{,}600) \quad (3)$$

Estimation of the patient's BSA is required to calculate CrCl from a urinary collection.

### Determination of Creatinine Clearance from a Urinary Creatinine Collection

The same equation that is used in adults can be used in pediatric patients to calculate CrCl from a timed urine collection. The following equation is used:

$$CrCl = (UV/P) \times (1.73/BSA) \qquad (4)$$

where *CrCl* is in units of mL/min/1.73 m²; *U* is the urinary creatinine concentration in mg/dL; *V* (mL/min) is the total urine volume collected in milliliters divided by the duration of the collection in minutes; *P* is the SCr concentration in mg/dL; and *BSA* is the patient's BSA in m².

Ideally, urine should be collected over a 24-hour period. However, a full 24-hour collection period is difficult in pediatric patients, especially in those who do not have full control over their bladder and do not have a urinary catheter in place. Thus, shorter collection periods (eg, 8 or 12 hours) are sometimes used. Urinary specimen bags can be placed to collect urine in neonates and infants, but incomplete collection because of urine

leakage often occurs. The incomplete collection of urine results in an inaccurate calculation of CrCl.

With any urine collection for creatinine determination, it is important to have the patient empty the bladder and discard this specimen before beginning urine collection. All urine during the time period should be collected, including the urine that would be voided at the end of the collection period. An SCr is usually obtained once during the urinary collection period (ideally at the midpoint) if the patient has stable renal function. If the patient's renal function is changing, then two SCr samples (one at the beginning of the urine collection and one at the end of the urine collection) may be obtained. The average SCr can then be used in the above equation.[3]

Because of the inherent problems of collecting a 24-hour urine sample from pediatric patients and receiving inaccurate calculations, CrCl (or GFR) is often estimated using prediction equations that consider the patient's age, height, sex, and SCr (see below). In fact, using a 24-hour timed urine specimen to calculate CrCl has been shown to be no more reliable (and often less reliable) than using equations based on SCr.[43] Therefore, the National Kidney Foundation recommends that GFR should be estimated in children and adolescents using prediction equations, such as the one by Schwartz et al.[36] A timed urine collection (eg, 24-hour sample) may be useful for (1) estimations of GFR in patients with decreased muscle mass (eg, muscle wasting, malnutrition, or amputation) or patients receiving special diets (eg, vegetarian diets or creatine supplements); (2) assessments of nutritional status or diets; and (3) evaluations for the need to start dialysis.[43]

### Estimating Creatinine Clearance and Glomerular Filtration Rate from Serum Creatinine

In adults, several methods are used to estimate CrCl and GFR from an SCr. For example, the Cockcroft-Gault equation is used to estimate CrCl and the Chronic Kidney Disease Epidemiology Collaboration (CKD-EPI) equation can be used to estimate GFR. These equations cannot be used for pediatric patients because they have a different ratio of muscle mass to SCr. In addition, the amount of pediatric muscle mass per body weight changes over time. Adult equations are based on adult muscle mass and adult urinary creatinine excretion rates. Thus, the use of adult equations in pediatric patients results in erroneous calculations.

Several predictive equations have been developed to estimate CrCl in pediatric patients. One simple equation was developed for use in children 1 to 18 years of age with stable SCr[44]:

$$CrCl\ (mL/min/1.73\ m^2) = 0.48 \times Ht\ (cm)/SCr\ (mg/dL) \quad (5)$$

This equation was found to be clinically useful in predicting CrCl in children. However, it may be less accurate in children with a height <107 cm.[45]

Another equation, developed by Schwartz et al, is more commonly used to estimate GFR in pediatric patients:

$$GFR\ (mL/min/1.73\ m^2) = k \times Length\ (cm)/SCr\ (mg/dL) \quad (6)$$

where *k* is a constant of proportionality.[36] In patients with stable renal function, k is directly related to the muscle component of body weight, which correlates well with the daily rates of urinary creatinine excretion. Because the percentage of muscle mass per body weight varies for different age groups, a different value for k must be used for different age groups. In addition to age, the value of k is affected by body composition; thus, the values for k listed in **Table 23-3** should be used in pediatric patients with average build.

## TABLE 23-3. Mean Values of k by Age Group

| AGE GROUP | MEAN k VALUE |
|---|---|
| Low birth weight infants ≤1 yr[a] | 0.33 |
| Full-term infants ≤1 yr | 0.45 |
| Children 1–12 yr | 0.55 |
| Females 13–21 yr | 0.55 |
| Males 13–21 yr | 0.70 |

[a] Low birth weight infant is defined as an infant with a birthweight ≤2,500 g.
*Source*: Modified from Schwartz GJ, Brion LP, Spitzer A. The use of plasma creatinine concentration for estimating glomerular filtration rate in infants, children, and adolescents. *Pediatr Clin North Am*. 1987;34(3):571–590.

It is important to remember that these two equations were developed using the Jaffe method to assay SCr. Values for SCr as measured by newer methods (eg, the IDMS-traceable enzymatic method) are lower than those measured by the Jaffe method (especially at low concentrations of SCr). This results in an overestimation of GFR if these equations and constants are used when SCr is measured by the newer assays. In fact, use of the Schwartz equation and constants may overestimate GFR by approximately 20% to 30%.[46,47] Therefore, revised age-group constants for the Schwartz equation should be determined to better estimate GFR when SCr is measured by newer assays using IDMS-based reference standards (**Minicase 3**).

In 2009, an "updated" Schwartz bedside equation, based on SCr measured by an IDMS-traceable enzymatic method, was developed in children 1 to 16 years of age.[48]

$$\text{GFR (mL/min/1.73 m}^2) = 0.413 \times \text{Ht (cm)/SCr (mg/dL)} \quad (7)$$

The pediatric patients in whom this equation was developed had mild-to-moderate chronic kidney disease (95% of measured GFR values were between 21 and 76 mL/min/1.73 m²) and were short for their age and sex. Further studies of this equation in children with higher GFRs and a more normal body habitus are needed before it can be widely applied to the pediatric population.[48] However, in general, for children with chronic kidney disease, this equation provides a relatively

## MINICASE 3

## Part I: Piperacillin–Tazobactam Dose Determination Based on Estimated Glomerular Filtration Rate in a Child

Mary M., a 5-year-old female, presents to the emergency department with a 4-day history of irritability, diffuse abdominal pain, and inability to tolerate oral intake. Mary's parents report that in the past few hours, she has appeared more lethargic, had one episode of rectal bleeding, and has been febrile with a $T_{max}$ of 102.2°F. In the emergency department, the patient has signs of sepsis, including hypotension (BP 78/49 mm Hg) and tachycardia (HR 140 beats/min). Fluid resuscitation is initiated with a 20 mL/kg bolus of 0.9% sodium chloride, and a dose of ceftriaxone and metronidazole is administered. An abdominal radiograph is concerning for volvulus, a condition in which a part of the small intestine twists around itself, causing an obstruction that may impact blood flow to the intestinal tissue. The patient is taken immediately to the operating room for exploratory laparotomy with pediatric surgery. Her weight is 16 kg (25th percentile for age) and height is 107 cm (50th percentile for age); BSA is 0.69 m².

The patient arrives to the pediatric intensive care unit postoperatively after reduction of the volvulus. The surgery was complicated by need for an 8-cm bowel resection of necrotic intestinal tissue. The patient is intubated and sedated and remains hypotensive despite fluid resuscitation. Laboratory data include sodium 143 mEq/L, potassium 4.8 mEq/L, chloride 110 mEq/L, total $CO_2$ 21 mEq/L, BUN 31 mg/dL, SCr 2.3 mg/dL (Jaffe method), and glucose 109 mg/dL. Intraabdominal tissue cultures were obtained

during surgery; however, results are pending. The pediatric surgeon is recommending initiation of postoperative piperacillin–tazobactam for coverage of enteric gram-negative pathogens and anaerobes.

QUESTION: Knowing the following information, what dose of piperacillin–tazobactam would you recommend for this patient?

The normal dose of piperacillin–tazobactam used at this hospital for a complicated intra-abdominal infection is 300 mg piperacillin/kg/day divided q 6 h. The recommended dosing adjustment for patients with renal dysfunction is as follows[1]:

- GFR >50 mL/min/1.73 m²: no adjustment required
- GFR 30 to 50 mL/min/1.73 m²: 35 to 50 mg piperacillin/kg/dose q 6 h
- GFR <30 mL/min/1.73 m²: 35 to 50 mg piperacillin/kg/dose q 8 h

DISCUSSION: Piperacillin–tazobactam is a combination product of two antimicrobial agents. Dosing recommendations are based on the piperacillin component of this combination product. It is primarily excreted renally with 68% of piperacillin and 80% of tazobactam excreted as unchanged drug in the urine. Mary's BUN and SCr are elevated, indicating that she has some degree of renal impairment likely secondary to hypovolemia and septic shock. Thus, the dose of piperacillin–tazobactam must be adjusted for her renal dysfunction. To recommend an appropriate dose, her GFR needs to be calculated.

## MINICASE 3 (cont'd)

Because this laboratory used the Jaffe method to measure SCr, an estimation of GFR from her SCr and height can be obtained by using Equation 6 and the k value of 0.55 for children 2 to 12 years of age (Table 23-3). Her estimated GFR is ~26 mL/min/1.73 $m^2$. Because she weighs 16 kg, the normal dose of piperacillin–tazobactam for this patient would be 1,200 mg piperacillin IV q 6 h (300 mg piperacillin/kg/day divided q 6 h). Because her GFR is 26 mL/min/1.73 $m^2$, she should receive a dose of 35 to 50 mg piperacillin/kg/dose q 8 h. The higher end of this dosing range would be appropriate for this patient given her severity of illness. Therefore, a dose of 800 mg piperacillin IV q 8 h (150 mg piperacillin/kg/day divided q 8 h) should be recommended. The patient's clinical response to antimicrobial therapy and changes in renal function should be evaluated daily

to ensure appropriate response and/or toxicity. It should be noted that if SCr were measured by a newer enzymatic assay using IDMS-based reference standards, then Equation 7 should be used to estimate GFR. If Equation 6 and the constants from Table 23-3 were used, it would result in an overestimation of GFR by approximately 20% to 30%. Additionally, almost all drug dosage guidelines for patients with renal impairment (including those recommended by pharmaceutical manufacturers) were developed using SCr as measured by older assay methodologies. Thus, estimated GFR values may not correlate well with these dosage guidelines. These limitations further emphasize the need for appropriate follow-up and monitoring of laboratory parameters and clinical response to determine if dosage adjustments are required.

## Part II: Piperacillin–Tazobactam Dose Determination Based on Estimated Glomerular Filtration Rate in a Child

A few days later, Mary is extubated, is hemodynamically stable (BP 98/62 mm Hg), and appears to be clinically improving. This morning, the hospital instituted the newer assay using IDMS-traceable enzymatic reference standards for SCr measurement. Mary's SCr is now 1.1 mg/dL (IDMS-traceable method) and the medical resident suggests increasing the piperacillin–tazobactam dose to the normal dose of 300 mg piperacillin/kg/day divided q 6 h given the patient's GFR has "normalized."

QUESTION: Should Mary's piperacillin–tazobactam dose be adjusted to the normal dose of 300 mg piperacillin/kg/day divided q 6 h?

DISCUSSION: To answer this question and recommend an appropriate antibiotic dose, Mary's GFR needs to be calculated using the appropriate equation based on the laboratory assay utilized. Because the laboratory has switched to the IDMS method to measure SCr, an estimation of GFR from her SCr and height should be obtained by using Equation 7. Her estimated GFR is now ~40 mL/min/1.73 $m^2$ (= 0.413 × 107 cm/1.1 mg/dL). Although her GFR has improved from 26 mL/min/1.73 $m^2$, it has not completely normalized for her age. Her SCr of 1.1 mg/dL remains elevated with a normal SCr (IDMS method) for a child this age being 0.03 to 0.59 mg/dL. This shows that Mary is still experiencing some renal dysfunction or acute kidney injury. Although it is appropriate to increase her piperacillin–tazobactam dose for her improvement in

renal function, a dose of 35 to 50 mg piperacillin/kg/dose IV q 6 h should be used. A calculated dose of 800 mg piperacillin IV q 6 h (200 mg piperacillin/kg/day divided q 6 h) would be recommended based on the renal dose adjustments provided above and her illness severity. It should be noted that if Equation 6 and the constants from Table 23-3 had been used, the patient's GFR would have been calculated as 53.5 mL/min/1.73 $m^2$ (0.55 × 107 cm/1.1 mg/dL). This would be approximately a 30% overestimation of GFR. The medical resident's recommendation of increasing the piperacillin–tazobactam dose to 300 mg piperacillin/kg/day divided q 6 h was likely a result of using the wrong equation for estimating GFR. Utilization of this higher piperacillin-tazobactam dose, based on the GFR estimation by Equation 6 would have resulted in too high of a dosage for this patient's renal function, ultimately placing her at a higher risk of toxicity. Daily monitoring of laboratories is required because multiple dose adjustments may need to occur as her renal function continues to improve. An alternate approach to estimating GFR would have been to use cystatin C and Equation 8. The benefit of using the cystatin C method of GFR estimation is the lack of influence of other factors, such as muscle mass, sex, body composition, and age on GFR estimation. At this time, cystatin C is not widely utilized in clinical practice. Some hospital laboratories may not have the ability to process this test, requiring transfer of the sample to an offsite laboratory (with a delay in receiving results) and making the use of a cystatin C level in the acute setting limited.

accurate clinical estimate of GFR (when SCr is measured by an IDMS-traceable assay) and its use is recommended by the Kidney Disease Improving Global Outcomes (KDIGO) clinical practice guidelines for the evaluation and management of chronic kidney disease.[49,50] Use of this equation (Equation 7) is clinically recommended whenever SCr is measured by an IDMS-traceable assay because it results in a more accurate estimation of GFR, as compared with using the original Schwartz equation (Equation 6).

These equations may not be accurate in certain pediatric populations, including patients with unstable renal function (eg, acute kidney injury), abnormal body habitus (eg, obesity or malnutrition), decreased muscle mass (eg, cardiac patients),

severe chronic renal failure, or insulin-dependent diabetes.[36,51] If clinically indicated, CrCl should be determined by a timed urine collection in these patients.

### Estimating Glomerular Filtration Rate from Serum Cystatin C

To improve calculated estimations of GFR, other endogenous markers of renal function have been investigated. Cystatin C is a cysteine protease inhibitor that is produced by all nucleated cells at a relatively constant rate; it is freely filtered by the kidneys. Its rate of production is so constant that serum cystatin C levels are not thought to be influenced by muscle mass, sex, body composition, and age (after 12 months).

Reciprocal values of serum cystatin C have been correlated to measured GFR values in adults and children.[46] However, serum cystatin C alone may not accurately estimate GFR in renal transplant patients, patients with high C-reactive protein, diabetes with ketonuria, or thyroid dysfunction. Thus, other equations have been developed which incorporate multiple patient parameters and endogenous markers of renal function. One such pediatric equation includes terms for the ratio of height to SCr, the reciprocals of serum cystatin C and BUN, a factor for sex, and a separate factor for height alone.[48,49] This complex equation is not clinically friendly but is being further investigated in the National Institutes of Health–sponsored Chronic Kidney Disease in Children study. Results of this investigation may yield a more accurate equation to estimate GFR in pediatric patients.

Recently, a user-friendly, simplified single variate serum cystatin C equation for clinical use in children (1 to 18 years) with chronic kidney disease has been developed.[49]

$$\text{GFR (mL/min/1.73m}^2) = 70.69 \times [\text{serum cystatin C (mg/L)}]^{-0.931} \quad (8)$$

This equation is recommended by current KDIGO guidelines to estimate GFR in pediatric patients, if a serum cystatin C is measured.[50] Unfortunately at this time, serum cystatin C assays are not readily available at many institutions.

# AGE-RELATED DIFFERENCES IN LIVER FUNCTION TESTS

## Serum Albumin

*Normal ranges are as follows*[11]:

*neonates 0 to 5 days, body weight <2.5 kg: 2 to 3.6 g/dL (20 to 36 g/L)*

*neonates 0 to 5 days, body weight >2.5 kg: 2.6 to 3.6 g/dL (26 to 36 g/L)*

*children 1 to 3 years: 3.4 to 4.2 g/dL (34 to 42 g/L)*

*children 4 to 6 years: 3.5 to 5.2 g/dL (35 to 52 g/L)*

*children and adolescents 7 to 19 years: 3.7 to 5.6 g/dL (37 to 56 g/L)*

*adults: 4 to 5 g/dL (40 to 50 g/L)*

Serum proteins, including albumin, are synthesized by the liver. Thus, measurements of serum total protein, albumin, and other specific proteins are primarily a test of the liver's synthetic capability. Maturational differences in the liver's ability to synthesize protein help determine the normal range for serum albumin concentrations. The liver of the fetus is able to synthesize albumin beginning at approximately 7 to 8 weeks of gestation. However, the predominant serum protein in early fetal life is α-fetoprotein. As gestation continues, the concentration of albumin increases, whereas α-fetoprotein decreases. At approximately 3 to 4 months of gestation, the fetal liver is able to produce each of the major serum protein classes. However, serum concentrations are much lower than those found at maturity.[52]

At birth, the newborn liver is anatomically and functionally immature. Because of immature liver function and a decreased ability to synthesize protein, full-term neonates have decreased concentrations of total plasma proteins, including albumin, γ-globulin, and lipoproteins. Concentrations in premature newborns are even lower, with serum albumin levels as low as 1.8 g/dL.[15] Adult serum concentrations of serum albumin (~3.5 g/dL) are reached only after several months of age. Conditions that cause abnormalities in serum albumin in pediatric patients are the same as in adults and can be reviewed in Chapter 15.

## Liver Enzymes

Alanine aminotransferase (ALT, also called SGPT)—*normal ranges are as follows*[12,15]:

*neonates 0 to 7 days: 6 to 40 units/L (0.1 to 0.67 μkat/L)*

*neonatal males 8 to 30 days: 10 to 40 units/L (0.17 to 0.67 μkat/L)*

*neonatal females 8 to 30 days: 8 to 32 units/L (0.13 to 0.53 μkat/L)*

*infants: 12 to 45 units/L (0.2 to 0.75 μkat/L)*

*children and adolescents 1 to 19 years: 5 to 45 units/L (0.08 to 0.75 μkat/L)*

*adults: 7 to 41 units/L (0.12 to 0.68 μkat/L)*

Aspartate aminotransferase (AST, also called SGOT)—*normal ranges are as follows:*

*neonatal males 0 to 7 days: 30 to 100 units/L (0.5 to 1.67 μkat/L)*

*neonatal females 0 to 7 days: 24 to 95 units/L (0.4 to 1.59 μkat/L)*

*neonates 8 to 30 days: 22 to 71 units/L (0.37 to 1.19 μkat/L)*

*infants: 22 to 63 units/L (0.37 to 1.05 μkat/L)*

*children 1 to 3 years: 20 to 60 units/L (0.33 to 1 μkat/L)*

*children 3 to 9 years: 15 to 50 units/L (0.25 to 0.84 μkat/L)*

*children and adolescents 10 to 15 years: 10 to 40 units/L (0.17 to 0.67 μkat/L)*

*adolescent males 16 to 19 years: 15 to 45 units/L (0.25 to 0.75 μkat/L)*

*adolescent females 16 to 19 years: 5 to 30 units/L (0.08 to 0.5 μkat/L)*

*adults: 12 to 38 units/L (0.2 to 0.63 μkat/L)*

Alkaline phosphatase—*normal ranges are as follows:*

*neonates 0 to 14 days: 90 to 273 units/L (1.5 to 4.56 μkat/L)*

*neonates 15 days to infants: 134 to 518 units/L (2.24 to 8.65 μkat/L)*

*children 1 to <10 years: 156 to 369 units/L (2.61 to 6.16 μkat/L)*

*children 10 years to adolescents <13 years: 141 to 460 units/L (2.35 to 7.68 μkat/L)*

*adolescent males 13 to <15 years: 127 to 517 units/L (2.12 to 8.63 μkat/L)*

*adolescent females 13 to <15 years: 62 to 280 units/L (1.04 to 4.68 μkat/L)*

*adolescent males 15 to <17 years: 89 to 365 units/L (1.49 to 6.1 μkat/L)*

*adolescent females 15 to <17 years: 54 to 128 units/L (0.9 to 2.14 μkat/L)*

*adolescent males 17 to <19 years: 59 to 164 units/L (0.99 to 2.74 μkat/L)*

*adolescent females 17 to <19 years: 48 to 95 units/L (0.8 to 1.59 μkat/L)*

*adults: 33 to 96 units/L (0.55 to 1.6 μkat/L)*

Lactate dehydrogenase—*normal ranges are as follows:*

*neonates 0 to 14 days: 309 to 1,222 units/L (5.16 to 20.41 µkat/L)*

*neonates 15 days to infants: 163 to 452 units/L (2.72 to 7.55 µkat/L)*

*children 1 to <10 years: 192 to 321 units/L (3.21 to 5.36 µkat/L)*

*adolescent males 10 to <15 years: 170 to 283 units/L (2.84 to 4.73 µkat/L)*

*adolescent females 10 to <15 years: 157 to 272 units/L (2.62 to 4.54 µkat/L)*

*adolescents 15 to <19 years: 130 to 250 units/L (2.17 to 4.18 µkat/L)*

*adults: 115 to 221 units/L (1.92 to 3.69 µkat/L)*

The normal reference ranges for liver enzymes are higher in pediatric patients compared with adults. This may be due to the fact that the liver makes up a larger percentage of total body weight in infants and children compared with adults. For certain enzymes, such as alkaline phosphatase, the higher normal concentrations in childhood represent higher serum concentrations of an isoenzyme from other sources, specifically bone. Approximately 80% of alkaline phosphatase originates from liver and bone. Smaller amounts come from the intestines, kidneys, and placenta. Normally, growing children have higher osteoblastic activity during the bone growth period and an influx into serum of the alkaline phosphatase isoenzyme from bone.[14] Thus, the higher normal concentrations of alkaline phosphatase in childhood primarily represent a higher rate of bone growth. After puberty, the liver is the primary source of serum alkaline phosphatase. Differences in normal values for liver enzymes also exist between male and female patients at certain ages. For example, during adolescence, males have higher alkaline phosphatase compared with females.

One must keep these sex and age-related differences in mind when interpreting liver enzyme test results. For example, an isolated increase in alkaline phosphatase in a rapidly growing male adolescent—whose other liver function tests are normal—would not indicate hepatic or biliary disease but merely a rapid increase in bone growth. As in adults, increases in AST and ALT in pediatric patients are associated with hepatocellular injury whereas elevations of alkaline phosphatase are associated with cholestatic disease. Cholestasis and bone disorders (such as osteomalacia and rickets) are common causes of elevated serum alkaline phosphatase concentrations in pediatric patients.

## Bilirubin

Total bilirubin, premature neonates—*normal ranges are as follows*[53]:

*0 to 1 day: <8 mg/dL (<137 µmol/L)*

*1 to 2 days: <12 mg/dL (<205 µmol/L)*

*3 to 5 days: <16 mg/dL (<274 µmol/L)*

*>5 days: <2 mg/dL (<34 µmol/L)*

Total bilirubin, full-term neonates—*normal ranges are as follows:*

*0 to 1 day: <8 mg/dL (<137 µmol/L)*

*1 to 2 days: <11.5 mg/dL (<197 µmol/L)*

*3 to 5 days: <12 mg/dL (<205 µmol/L)*

*>5 days: <1.2 mg/dL (<21 µmol/L)*

Total bilirubin, adults—*normal range is as follows:*

*adults: 0.3 to 1.3 mg/dL (5.1 to 22 µmol/L)*

Conjugated bilirubin—*normal ranges are as follows:*

*neonates: <0.6 mg/dL (<10 µmol/L)*

*infants and children: <0.2 mg/dL (<3.4 µmol/L)*

*adults: 0.1 to 0.4 mg/dL (1.7 to 6.8 µmol/L)*

To better understand the age-related differences in serum bilirubin concentrations, a brief review of bilirubin metabolism is needed. A detailed discussion of bilirubin metabolism and abnormalities can be found in Chapter 15. Bilirubin is a breakdown product of hemoglobin. Hemoglobin, which is released from senescent or hemolyzed RBCs, is degraded by heme oxygenase into iron, carbon monoxide, and biliverdin. Biliverdin undergoes reduction by biliverdin reductase to bilirubin. Unconjugated bilirubin then enters the liver and is conjugated with glucuronic acid to form conjugated bilirubin, which is water soluble. Conjugated bilirubin is excreted in the bile and enters the intestines, where it is broken down by bacterial flora to urobilinogen. However, conjugated bilirubin also can be deconjugated by bacteria in the intestines or by β-glucuronidase in intestinal tissue and reabsorbed into the circulation.[54]

Compared with adults, newborns have higher concentrations of bilirubin. This results from a higher production of bilirubin in the neonate and a decreased ability to excrete it. A higher rate of production of bilirubin occurs in newborns due to the shorter life span of neonatal RBCs and the higher initial neonatal hematocrit. The average RBC life span is only 65 days in very premature neonates and 90 days in full-term neonates, compared with 120 days in adults.[55] In addition, full-term neonates have a mean hematocrit of about 50%, compared with adult values of approximately 44%. The shorter RBC life span plus the higher hematocrit both increase the load of unconjugated bilirubin to the liver. Newborn infants, however, have a decreased ability to eliminate bilirubin. The activity of neonatal uridine diphosphate glucuronosyltransferase, the enzyme responsible for conjugating bilirubin in the liver, is decreased. In addition, newborns lack the intestinal bacteria needed to break down conjugated bilirubin into urobilinogen. However, the newborn's intestine does contain glucuronidase, which can deconjugate bilirubin and allow unconjugated bilirubin to be reabsorbed back into the circulation (enterohepatic circulation). This enterohepatically reabsorbed bilirubin further increases the unconjugated bilirubin load to the liver.

Because of these limitations in bilirubin metabolism and the resultant unconjugated (indirect) hyperbilirubinemia, a "physiologic jaundice" commonly occurs in newborns. Typically in full-term neonates, high serum bilirubin concentrations occur in the first few days of life, with a decrease over the next several weeks to values seen in adults. High bilirubin concentrations may occur later in premature newborns, up to the first week of life, and are usually higher and persist longer than in full-term newborns. Physiologic jaundice is usually transient and benign; however, sometimes hyperbilirubinemia and jaundice in a neonate can be a symptom of an underlying medical condition.[54]

Pathological (or nonphysiological) jaundice due to unconjugated hyperbilirubinemia may occur in newborns for many reasons, including increased production of bilirubin, decreased uptake of unconjugated bilirubin into the liver, decreased conjugation of bilirubin in the liver, and increased enterohepatic circulation of bilirubin.[54] Increased production of bilirubin may occur with RBC hemolysis because of blood group incompatibilities (eg, Rh and ABO incompatibility), enzyme deficiencies of the erythrocytes (eg, glucose-6-phosphate dehydrogenase deficiency), erythrocyte structural defects (eg, hereditary spherocytosis), or certain racial or ethnic makeup (eg, Asian and Native American). Certain genetic disorders may cause neonatal hyperbilirubinemia. For example, patients with Gilbert syndrome have decreased activity of bilirubin uridine diphosphate glucuronosyltransferase, the enzyme that is responsible for conjugation of bilirubin in the liver. Infants with Crigler-Najjar syndrome may have absent (type I) or decreased (type II) activity of uridine diphosphate glucuronosyltransferase. Breastfeeding also is associated with neonatal hyperbilirubinemia and jaundice. Newborns who are exclusively breastfed, not feeding well, or not being enterally fed (ie, newborns who are not taking anything by mouth) may have increased intestinal reabsorption of bilirubin that can cause or worsen hyperbilirubinemia. Breastfeeding may also increase bilirubin concentrations by other mechanisms. Breast milk may contain substances that decrease the conjugation of bilirubin by inhibiting the enzyme uridine diphosphate glucuronosyltransferase. Some medications (eg, sulfonamides and certain cephalosporins, such as ceftriaxone) can displace unconjugated bilirubin from albumin-binding sites and may worsen unconjugated hyperbilirubinemia.[1,54] Use of these medications in neonates, especially those with or at risk for hyperbilirubinemia, is not recommended. For example, sulfonamides are not indicated for use in infants <2 months of age (unless as a last drug option to treat a life-threatening infection), and ceftriaxone is contraindicated for use in hyperbilirubinemic neonates and in premature neonates <41 weeks' postmenstrual age.[1]

Appropriate monitoring of serum bilirubin is important in neonates because high concentrations of unconjugated bilirubin can cause acute bilirubin encephalopathy or chronic bilirubin encephalopathy, also termed kernicterus (ie, deposits of unconjugated bilirubin in the brain). The neurotoxic effects of bilirubin are serious and potentially lethal. Clinical features of acute kernicterus include poor sucking, stupor, seizures, fever, hypotonia, hypertonia, opisthotonus, and retrocollis. Neonates who survive may develop mental retardation, cerebral palsy, delayed motor skills, movement disorders, and sensorineural hearing loss.[54,56] Phototherapy (which converts unconjugated bilirubin to a more water-soluble isomer for easier excretion) and exchange transfusion (which removes bilirubin from the bloodstream) are common treatments for neonatal unconjugated hyperbilirubinemia. IV immunoglobulin may be used in patients with isoimmune hemolytic disease (RBC hemolysis due to Rh and ABO incompatibility) to decrease the need for exchange transfusions.[54,56]

Pathologic jaundice due to conjugated (direct) hyperbilirubinemia (also termed cholestasis) may also occur in newborns. Etiological factors may include obstruction of the biliary system (eg, biliary atresia), defects of bile acid transport or synthesis, metabolic liver diseases (eg, $\alpha_1$-antitrypsin deficiency), or systemic conditions such as infection (eg, (t)oxoplasmosis, (o)ther agents, (r)ubella, (c)ytomegalovirus, and (h)erpes simplex [TORCH] infections), parenteral nutrition-associated cholestasis, or acute liver injury from hypoxia or liver ischemia.[54]

# AGE-RELATED DIFFERENCES IN HEMATOLOGIC TESTS

## Erythrocytes

Mean values and lower limit of normal (minus 2 standard deviations) for red blood cell count, hemoglobin and hematocrit are as follows.[57]

### Red Blood Cell Count

*birth (cord blood): 4.7 (3.9) × 10¹² cells/L (4.7 (3.9) × 10⁶ cells/µL)*
*1 to 3 days: 5.3 (4) × 10¹² cells/L (5.3 (4) × 10⁶ cells/µL)*
*1 week: 5.1 (3.9) × 10¹² cells/L (5.1 (3.9) × 10⁶ cells/µL)*
*2 weeks: 4.9 (3.6) × 10¹² cells/L (4.9 (3.6) × 10⁶ cells/µL)*
*1 month: 4.2 (3) × 10¹² cells/L (4.2 (3) × 10⁶ cells/µL)*
*2 months: 3.8 (2.7) × 10¹² cells/L (3.8 (2.7) × 10⁶ cells/µL)*
*3 to 6 months: 3.8 (3.1) × 10¹² cells/L (3.8 (3.1) × 10⁶ cells/µL)*
*0.5 to 2 years: 4.5 (3.7) × 10¹² cells/L (4.5 (3.7) × 10⁶ cells/µL)*
*2 to 6 years: 4.6 (3.9) × 10¹² cells/L (4.6 (3.9) × 10⁶ cells/µL)*
*6 to 12 years: 4.6 (4) × 10¹² cells/L (4.6 (4) × 10⁶ cells/µL)*
*12 to 18 years, female: 4.6 (4.1) × 10¹² cells/L (4.6 (4.1) × 10⁶ cells/µL)*
*12 to 18 years, male: 4.9 (4.5) × 10¹² cells/L (4.9 (4.5) × 10⁶ cells/µL)*
*18 to 49 years, female: 4.6 (4) × 10¹² cells/L (4.6 (4) × 10⁶ cells/µL)*
*18 to 49 years, male: 5.2 (4.5) × 10¹² cells/L (5.2 (4.5) × 10⁶ cells/µL)*

### Hemoglobin

*birth (cord blood): 16.5 (13.5) g/dL (10.2 (8.4) mmol/L)*
*1 to 3 days: 18.5 (14.5) g/dL (11.5 (9) mmol/L)*
*1 week: 17.5 (13.5) g/dL (10.9 (8.4) mmol/L)*
*2 weeks: 16.5 (12.5) g/dL (10.2 (7.8) mmol/L)*
*1 month: 14 (10) g/dL (8.7 (6.2) mmol/L)*
*2 months: 11.5 (9) g/dL (7.1 (5.6) mmol/L)*
*3 to 6 months: 11.5 (9.5) g/dL (7.1 (5.9) mmol/L)*
*0.5 to 2 years: 12 (10.5) g/dL (7.4 (6.5) mmol/L)*
*2 to 6 years: 12.5 (11.5) g/dL (7.8 (7.1) mmol/L)*
*6 to 12 years: 13.5 (11.5) g/dL (8.4 (7.1) mmol/L)*
*12 to 18 years, female: 14 (12) g/dL (8.7 (7.4) mmol/L)*
*12 to 18 years, male: 14.5 (13) g/dL (9 (8.1) mmol/L)*
*18 to 49 years, female: 14 (12) g/dL (8.7 (7.4) mmol/L)*
*18 to 49 years, male: 15.5 (13.5) g/dL (9.6 (8.4) mmol/L)*

### Hematocrit

*birth (cord blood): 51 (42)% (0.51 (0.42))*
*1 to 3 days: 56 (45)% (0.56 (0.45))*
*1 week: 54 (42)% (0.54 (0.42))*

*2 weeks: 51 (39)% (0.51 (0.39))*
*1 month: 43 (31)% (0.43 (0.31))*
*2 months: 35 (28)% (0.35 (0.28))*
*3 to 6 months: 35 (29)% (0.35 (0.29))*
*0.5 to 2 years: 36 (33)% (0.36 (0.33))*
*2 to 6 years: 37 (34)% (0.37 (0.34))*
*6 to 12 years: 40 (35)% (0.40 (0.35))*
*12 to 18 years, female: 41 (36)% (0.41 (0.36))*
*12 to 18 years, male: 43 (37)% (0.43 (0.37))*
*18 to 49 years, female: 41 (36)% (0.41 (0.36))*
*18 to 49 years, male: 47 (41)% (0.47 (0.41))*

Compared with adults, normal newborn infants have higher hemoglobin and hematocrit values. For example, the mean hemoglobin value in a full-term newborn on the first day of life is 18.5 g/dL, compared with 15.5 g/dL in adult males. Hemoglobin and hematocrit start to decrease within the first week of life and reach a minimum level at 8 to 12 weeks in term infants.[58] This normal decrease in hemoglobin and hematocrit is called the *physiologic anemia of infancy*. This physiologic anemia is normochromic and microcytic and is accompanied by a low reticulocyte count. Physiologic anemia of infancy (in term infants) does not require medical treatment.

Age-related changes in hemoglobin that occur during the first few months of life are due to several reasons. In utero, a low arterial $pO_2$ exists, which stimulates the production of erythropoietin in the fetus. This results in a high rate of erythropoiesis and accounts for the high levels of hemoglobin and hematocrit that exist at birth. At birth, $pO_2$ and oxygen content of blood significantly increase with the newborn's first breaths. The higher amount of oxygen that is available to the tissues downregulates erythropoietin production and decreases the rate of erythropoiesis.[59] Without the stimulation of erythropoietin to produce new RBCs, hemoglobin concentrations decrease as aged RBCs are removed from the circulation. The shorter life span of neonatal RBCs (90 days versus 120 days in adults) also contributes to the decline in hemoglobin.

Hemoglobin continues to decline in full-term infants until 8 to 12 weeks of age, when values reach 9 to 11 g/dL. These levels of hemoglobin result in lower amounts of oxygen delivery to tissues. Usually at this point, oxygen requirements exceed oxygen delivery and the relative hypoxia stimulates the production of erythropoietin. Erythropoiesis then increases and the reticulocyte count and hemoglobin concentrations begin to rise. It is important to remember that the iron from the aged RBCs that were previously removed from the circulation has been stored. The amount of this stored iron is usually adequate to meet the requirements of hemoglobin synthesis.

In premature infants, physiologic anemia occurs at 3 to 6 weeks of age (sooner than in full-term infants) and the nadir of the hemoglobin concentrations is lower (eg, 7 to 9 g/dL).[59] This can be explained by the even shorter life span of a premature infant's RBCs (65 days versus 90 days in full-term newborns) and inadequate synthesis of erythropoietin in response to anemia.[55,59] In addition, total body iron stores in premature infants are smaller and are depleted sooner. Thus, anemia of prematurity requires treatment with iron and may require blood transfusions or the use of recombinant human erythropoietin.[58,59]

Differences in RBC indices also exist for different pediatric ages. For example, compared with adults, newborns have larger erythrocytes (mean corpuscular volume of 108 fL compared with an adult value of 90 fL). Mean values and the lower limits of normal for RBC indices according to different ages are listed in **Table 23-4**.

Causes of the various types of anemias in pediatric patients are similar to the causes in adults. Of particular note is the iron deficiency anemia that occurs in infants who are fed whole cow's milk. The iron in whole cow's milk is less bioavailable and may cause inadequate iron intake. Typically infants with iron deficiency anemia from whole cow's milk have chronically consumed large amounts of cow's milk (>24 oz per day) and foods that are not supplemented with iron. Some infants receiving whole cow's milk develop severe iron deficiency due to chronic intestinal blood loss. The blood loss is thought to be due to intestinal exposure to a specific heat-labile protein found in whole cow's milk. Breast feeding, delaying introduction of whole cow's milk until 12 months of age, and decreasing the amount of whole cow's milk to <24 oz per day have been recommended to decrease the loss of blood.[60]

**TABLE 23-4.** Red Blood Cell Indices by Age: Mean Values and Lower Limits of Normal (–2 SD)

| | MCV fL | MCH pg/cell | MCHC g/dL |
|---|---|---|---|
| Birth (cord blood) | 108 (98) | 34 (31) | 33 (30) |
| 1–3 days | 108 (95) | 34 (31) | 33 (29) |
| 1 wk | 107 (88) | 34 (28) | 33 (28) |
| 2 wk | 105 (86) | 34 (28) | 33 (28) |
| 1 mo | 104 (85) | 34 (28) | 33 (29) |
| 2 mo | 96 (77) | 30 (26) | 33 (29) |
| 3–6 mo | 91 (74) | 30 (25) | 33 (30) |
| 0.5–2 yr | 78 (70) | 27 (23) | 33 (30) |
| 2–6 yr | 81 (75) | 27 (24) | 34 (31) |
| 6–12 yr | 86 (77) | 29 (25) | 34 (31) |
| 12–18 yr | | | |
| Female | 90 (78) | 30 (25) | 34 (31) |
| Male | 88 (78) | 30 (25) | 34 (31) |
| 18–49 yr | 90 (80) | 30 (26) | 34 (31) |

MCV = mean corpuscular volume; MCH = mean corpuscular hemoglobin; MCHC = mean corpuscular hemoglobin concentration. *Source*: Adapted from Osberg IM. Chemistry and hematology reference (normal) ranges. In: *Current Pediatric Diagnosis and Treatment*. 16th ed. New York, NY: Lange Medical Books/McGraw-Hill; 2003.

In pediatric patients with anemia, genetic disorders that produce inadequate RBC production (eg, Diamond-Blackfan anemia), hemolytic anemias (eg, hereditary spherocytosis), or hemoglobin disorders (eg, sickle cell disease) also must be considered.

## Leukocytes

### White Blood Cell Count

*Normal ranges are as follows[61]:*
*neonates 1 day: 9 to 30 × 10³ cells/mm³ (9 to 30 × 10⁹/L)*
*neonates 2 weeks: 5 to 21 × 10³ cells/mm³ (5 to 21 × 10⁹/L)*
*infants 3 months: 6 to 18 × 10³ cells/mm³ (6 to 18 × 10⁹/L)*
*children 0.5 to 6 years: 6 to 15 × 10³ cells/mm³ (6 to 15 × 10⁹/L)*
*children 7 to 12 years: 4.5 to 13.5 × 10³ cells/mm³ (4.5 to 13.5 × 10⁹/L)*
*adults: 4.4 to 11 × 10³ cells/mm³ (4.4 to 11 × 10⁹/L)*

Normal WBC counts are higher in neonates and infants compared with adults. Usually in adults with systemic bacterial infections, the WBC becomes elevated. However, in neonates and infants with a systemic bacterial infection, the WBC count is typically decreased; but it may sometimes be increased or within the normal range.[58] Neonates have a lower storage pool of neutrophils, and an overwhelming infection (eg, neonatal sepsis) may deplete this pool and cause neutropenia. Therefore, although an increase in WBCs is a nonspecific finding in neonates (ie, it may occur in many conditions other than sepsis), neutropenia is a highly significant finding and may be the first abnormal laboratory result that indicates neonatal bacterial infection. Not recognizing that neutropenia in neonates indicates a serious infection could result in a delay in treatment and significant morbidity or even mortality for the patient.

In addition to the age-related differences in total WBC count, the age-related differences in WBC differential also need to be taken into consideration when interpreting laboratory results (**Table 23-5**). After the newborn period and up until 5 to 6 years of age, lymphocytes represent the most prevalent circulating WBC type. Subsequent to this, neutrophils predominate in the blood for the remainder of life.

## Platelets

### Platelet Count

*Normal ranges are as follows[15]:*
*newborn ≤ 1 week: 84,000 to 478,000/mm³ (84 to 478 × 10⁹/L)*
*neonate >1 week, infants, children, adolescents, and adults: 150,000 to 400,000/mm³ (150 to 400 × 10⁹/L)*

Compared with adults, the normal platelet count in the newborn may be lower. Adult values are reached after 1 week of age, although platelet counts may range higher in children (up to 600,000/mm³) than in adults. Platelet counts are discussed in detail in Chapter 17.

## SUMMARY

Interpreting pediatric laboratory data can be complex. Age-related differences in normal reference ranges occur for many common laboratory tests. These differences may be the result of changes in body composition and the normal anatomic and physiologic maturation that occurs throughout childhood. Changes in various body compartments, the immature function of the neonatal kidney, and the increased electrolyte and mineral requirements necessary for proper growth help to explain many age-related differences in serum electrolytes and minerals. Alterations in skeletal muscle mass and the pattern of kidney function maturation account for the various age-related differences in SCr and kidney function tests. Neonatal hepatic immaturity and subsequent maturation help to explain the age-related differences in serum albumin, liver enzymes, and bilirubin. Likewise, the immature hematopoietic system of the newborn and its maturation account for the age-related differences in various hematologic tests.

This chapter also reviews several general pediatric considerations, including differences in physiologic parameters, pediatric blood sampling considerations, and the determination of pediatric reference ranges. Interpretation of pediatric laboratory data must take into account the various age-related differences in normal values. If these differences are not taken into consideration, inappropriate diagnoses and treatment may result.

**TABLE 23-5.** White Blood Cell Differential by Age

| | MEAN VALUES | | | |
|---|---|---|---|---|
| | NEUTROPHILS (%) | LYMPHOCYTES (%) | EOSINOPHILS (%) | MONOCYTES (%) |
| Birth | 61 | 31 | 2 | 6 |
| 2 wk | 40 | 63 | 3 | 9 |
| 3 mo | 30 | 48 | 2 | 5 |
| 0.5–6 yr | 45 | 48 | 2 | 5 |
| 7–12 yr | 55 | 38 | 2 | 5 |
| Adult | 55 | 35 | 3 | 7 |

*Source:* Adapted from Glader B. The anemias. In: Kliegman RM, Behrman RE, Jenson HB, et al, eds. *Nelson Textbook of Pediatrics.* 18th ed. Philadelphia, PA: Saunders Elsevier; 2007.

# LEARNING POINTS

1. *Would the dose of a medication that is primarily excreted by the kidney ever have to be adjusted in a patient with an SCr of 0.8 mg/dL?*

   **ANSWER:** The age of the patient must be taken into consideration when interpreting laboratory tests, especially SCr. In addition, the methodology used to assay SCr needs to be considered. For the Jaffe method, an SCr of 0.8 mg/dL indicates significant renal dysfunction in an infant whose normal SCr should be 0.2 to 0.4 mg/dL and mild or moderate renal dysfunction in a child whose normal SCr should be 0.3 to 0.7 mg/dL. However, an SCr of 0.8 mg/dL in an adolescent or adult would be considered within the normal range. Thus, medications that are primarily excreted by the kidney would need to have a dosage adjustment in infants and children with an SCr of 0.8 mg/dL as measured by the Jaffe method. For the IDMS-traceable enzymatic method, measured SCr values and normal values for age are lower than with the Jaffe method. An SCr of 0.8 mg/dL indicates significant renal dysfunction in an infant or young child (newborn to 4 years of age) whose normal SCr should be 0.03 to 0.5 mg/dL and mild-to-moderate renal dysfunction in a child 4 to 7 years of age whose normal SCr should be 0.03 to 0.59 mg/dL or in a child 7 to 10 years of age whose normal SCr should be 0.22 to 0.59 mg/dL. However, an SCr of 0.8 mg/dL in an adolescent or adult would be considered within the normal range.

2. *Are there any concerns with using ceftriaxone in a neonate?*

   **ANSWER:** Ceftriaxone has been shown in vitro to displace bilirubin from its albumin binding sites. Thus, ceftriaxone should not be used in hyperbilirubinemic neonates, especially premature neonates, because displacement of bilirubin from albumin-binding sites may lead to bilirubin encephalopathy. These concerns are so significant that current labeled contraindications to the use of ceftriaxone include premature neonates <41 weeks' postmenstrual age and hyperbilirubinemic neonates.[62] In addition, if ceftriaxone is used in a neonate, it should be administered slowly, over 60 minutes, to reduce the risk of bilirubin encephalopathy. Ceftriaxone may also cause sludging in the gallbladder and pseudolithiasis. Fatal reactions have been reported in neonates due to ceftriaxone–calcium precipitates in the lungs and kidneys when ceftriaxone and calcium-containing IV solutions were coadministered. In some cases, the ceftriaxone and calcium-containing solutions were administered through the same IV infusion line and a precipitate was sometimes observed. In at least one fatal case, the ceftriaxone and calcium-containing solutions were administered in different infusion lines and at different times. Therefore, ceftriaxone must not be administered to neonates who also are receiving (or who are expected to receive) calcium-containing IV solutions, including continuous infusions of parenteral nutrition that contain calcium.[62] This is also a labeled contraindication.

3. *Would a hemoglobin of 9.5 g/dL in a 10-week-old infant who was born at full-term require initiation of iron therapy?*

   **ANSWER:** No. Iron therapy would not be required because this anemia would be considered a normal physiologic anemia of infancy. In full-term infants, hemoglobin values of 9 to 11 g/dL normally occur at 8 to 12 weeks of age. After this time, the reticulocyte count and hemoglobin concentration should begin to rise. If an infant's hemoglobin concentration remained at 9.5 g/dL after 12 weeks of age, a further workup of the infant's anemia would be required. If the anemia was found to be the result of iron deficiency, then iron therapy would be required. Dietary causes of iron deficiency, such as consuming large amounts of whole cow's milk, also would need to be considered.

4. *Differences in TBW, ECW, and ICW occur in neonates (compared with older pediatric patients and adults) and are described in the beginning of this chapter. Could the differences in TBW, ECW, and ICW that occur in neonates have an impact on drug distribution?*

   **ANSWER:** Yes. Both TBW and ECW, when expressed as a percentage of body weight, are increased in the newborn (especially the premature neonate). The increase in TBW and ECW help explain why water-soluble drugs have an increased volume of distribution in these patients. In fact, the volume of distribution for gentamicin, a water-soluble drug that primarily distributes to the ECW compartment, correlates well with the volume of ECW. In the neonate, ECW is about 44% of body weight and the volume of distribution for gentamicin is approximately 0.45 L/kg.[1,19,20] Thus, the total amount of body water at birth, distribution between ECW and ICW, and the age-related changes that occur with time not only impact electrolyte composition and their respective normal laboratory values but also affect the distribution of medications and required doses.

5. *Why would a pediatric patient presenting with diabetic ketoacidosis (DKA) have low serum sodium?*

   **ANSWER:** The three key criteria in the diagnosis of DKA are the presence of hyperglycemia (blood glucose level >200 mg/dL [>11.1 mmol/L]), acidosis (venous pH <7.3 or serum bicarbonate <15 mmol/L), and accumulation of ketoacids (ketonemia and/or ketonuria).[63] In the setting of hyperglycemia, the plasma osmolarity rises and results in an osmotic shift of water from the intracellular to the extracellular (intravascular) space. This expanded extracellular volume results in measured serum sodium levels that appear low. This is referred to as dilutional hyponatremia, an excess of water relative to the amount of solute. In general, serum sodium concentrations decrease by 1.6 mmol/L for every 100 mg/dL increase in glucose concentration over normal (ie, normal value of 100 mg/dL). To account for this, sodium levels should be corrected for the degree of hyperglycemia using Equation 1. The corrected sodium value is an estimate of what the expected serum sodium would be in the absence of hyperglycemia. Because the calculated value is only an estimate, careful monitoring of serum sodium and other electrolytes is recommended. In most pediatric patients with DKA, corrected sodium levels are higher than the measured serum sodium levels. As a patient's hyperglycemia is treated with fluid resuscitation and insulin administration, the dilutional hyponatremia reverses and a rise in the measured serum sodium and corrected sodium levels should occur. In addition to the dilutional hyponatremia, a low serum sodium in patients with DKA may be caused by an increase in renal sodium loss. The hyperglycemia-associated increase in plasma osmolarity also results in an osmotic diuresis, leading to water loss (dehydration) and electrolyte losses, including sodium, potassium, chloride, and phosphate.[63,64] Failure of sodium levels to increase with correction of hyperglycemia may indicate a need to increase the sodium concentration of IV fluids.

# REFERENCES

1. Taketomo CK, Hodding JH, Kraus DM. *Pediatric and Neonatal Dosage Handbook*. 26th ed. Hudson, OH: Lexi-Comp Inc; 2019.

2. Engle WA, American Academy of Pediatrics Committee on Fetus and Newborn. Age terminology during the perinatal period. *Pediatrics*. 2004;114(5):1362-1364.PubMed

3. Kleinman K, McDaniel L, Molloy M, eds. *The Harriet Lane Handbook*. 22nd ed. Philadelphia, PA: Elsevier; 2021.

4. Task Force on Blood Pressure Control in Children. Report of the second task force on blood pressure control in children—1987. *Pediatrics*. 1987;79(1):1-25.PubMed

5. National High Blood Pressure Education Program Working Group on High Blood Pressure in Children and Adolescents. The fourth report on the diagnosis, evaluation, and treatment of high blood pressure in children and adolescents. *Pediatrics*. 2004;114(2)(Suppl 4th Report):555-576.PubMed

6. Hicks JM. Pediatric clinical biochemistry: why is it different? In: Soldin SJ, Rifai N, Hicks JM, eds. *Biochemical Basis of Pediatric Disease*. 2nd ed. Washington, DC: AACC Press; 1995:1-17.

7. Malarkey LM, McMorrow ME. Specimen collection procedures. In: *Saunders Nursing Guide to Laboratory and Diagnostic Tests*. 2nd ed. Philadelphia, PA: Elsevier Saunders; 2012:18-38.

8. Heelstick (Capillary Blood Sampling). In: Gomella T, Cunningham M, Eyal FG, et al, eds. *Neonatology: Management, Procedures, On-Call Problems, Diseases, and Drugs*. 7th ed. New York, NY: McGraw-Hill; 2013.

9. World Health Organization. *WHO Guidelines on Drawing Blood: Best Practices in Phlebotomy*. Geneva: World Health Organization; 2010.

10. Nathan DG, Orkin SH, eds. *Nathan and Oski's Hematology of Infancy and Childhood*. 5th ed. Philadelphia, PA: WB Saunders; 1998.

11. Soldin SJ, Brugnara C, Wong EC, eds. *Pediatric Reference Intervals*. 5th ed. Washington, DC: AACC Press; 2005.

12. Adeli K, Higgins V, Trajcevski K, White-Al Habeeb N. The Canadian laboratory initiative on pediatric reference intervals: A CALIPER white paper. *Crit Rev Clin Lab Sci*. 2017;54(6):358-413.PubMed

13. Malarkey LM, McMorrow ME. *Saunders Nursing Guide to Laboratory and Diagnostic Tests*. 2nd ed. Philadelphia, PA: Elsevier Saunders; 2012.

14. Jacobs DS, DeMott WR, Oxley DK. *Laboratory Test Handbook*. 5th ed. Hudson, OH: Lexi-Comp Inc; 2001.

15. Lo SF. Reference intervals for laboratory tests and procedures. In: Kliegman RM, St Geme JW, et al, eds. *Nelson Textbook of Pediatrics*. 21st ed. Philadelphia, PA: Elsevier; 2020.

16. Hoppe JE, Snyder R, Accurso FJ, et al. Chemistry and hematology reference intervals. In: Hay WW, Levin MJ, Deterding RR, et al, eds. *Current Diagnosis and Treatment: Pediatrics*. 24th ed. New York, NY: McGraw-Hill Education; 2018.

17. Jagarinec N, Flegar-Mestrić Z, Surina B, et al. Pediatric reference intervals for 34 biochemical analytes in urban school children and adolescents. *Clin Chem Lab Med*. 1998;36(5):327-337.PubMed

18. Bell EF, Segar JL, Oh W. Fluid and electrolyte management. In: MacDonald MG, Seshia MMK, eds. *Avery's Neonatology: Pathophysiology and Management of the Newborn*. 7th ed. Philadelphia, PA: Lippincott Williams & Wilkins; 2016.

19. Friis-Hansen B. Water distribution in the foetus and newborn infant. *Acta Paediatr Scand Suppl*. 1983;305:7-11.PubMed

20. Friis-Hansen B. Changes in body water compartments during growth. *Acta Paediatr Suppl*. 1957;46(suppl 110):1-68.PubMed

21. Tarnow-Mordi WO, Shaw JC, Liu D, et al. Iatrogenic hyponatraemia of the newborn due to maternal fluid overload: a prospective study. *Br Med J (Clin Res Ed)*. 1981;283(6292):639-642.PubMed

22. Malarkey LM, McMorrow ME. Serum electrolytes. In: *Nurses Manual of Laboratory Tests and Diagnostic Procedures*. 2nd ed. Philadelphia, PA: WB Saunders; 2000:82-103.

23. Greenbaum LA. Electrolyte and acid-base disorders. In: Kliegman RM, St Geme JW, et al, eds. *Nelson Textbook of Pediatrics*. 21st ed. Philadelphia, PA: Elsevier; 2020.

24. Blackburn ST. Renal function in the neonate. *J Perinat Neonatal Nurs*. 1994;8(1):37-47.PubMed

25. Nafday SM, Woda CB, Saland JM, et al. Renal disease. In: MacDonald MG, Seshia MMK, eds. *Avery's Neonatology: Pathophysiology and Management of the Newborn*. 7th ed. Philadelphia, PA: Lippincott Williams & Wilkins; 2016.

26. Breault DT, Majzoub JA. Other abnormalities of arginine vasopressin metabolism and action. In: Kliegman RM, St Geme JW, et al, eds. *Nelson Textbook of Pediatrics*. 21st ed. Philadelphia, PA: Elsevier; 2020.

27. Lorenz JM. Assessing fluid and electrolyte status in the newborn. *Clin Chem*. 1997;43(1):205-210.PubMed

28. Papageorgiou A, Pelausa E, Kovacs L. The extremely low birth weight infant. In: MacDonald MG, Seshia MMK, eds. *Avery's Neonatology: Pathophysiology and Management of the Newborn*. 7th ed. Philadelphia, PA: Lippincott Williams & Wilkins; 2016.

29. Jones DP, Chesney RW. Development of tubular function. *Clin Perinatol*. 1992;19(1):33-57.PubMed

30. Greenbaum LA. Electrolytes and acid-base disorders. In: Behrman RE, Kliegman RM, Jenson HB, eds. *Nelson Textbook of Pediatrics*. 17th ed. Philadelphia, PA: WB Saunders; 2004.

31. Stigson L, Kjellmer I. Serum levels of magnesium at birth related to complications of immaturity. *Acta Paediatr*. 1997;86(9):991-994.PubMed

32. Ariceta G, Rodríguez-Soriano J, Vallo A. Magnesium homeostasis in premature and full-term neonates. *Pediatr Nephrol*. 1995;9(4):423-427. PubMed

33. Geven WB, Monnens LA, Willems JL. Magnesium metabolism in childhood. *Miner Electrolyte Metab*. 1993;19(4-5):308-313.PubMed

34. Pesce MA. Reference ranges for laboratory tests and procedures. In: Kliegman RM, Behrman RE, et al, eds. *Nelson Textbook of Pediatrics*. 18th ed. Philadelphia, PA: Saunders Elsevier; 2007.

35. Nehus EJ. Introduction to glomerular diseases. In: Kliegman RM, St Geme JW, et al, eds. *Nelson Textbook of Pediatrics*. 21st ed. Philadelphia, PA: Elsevier; 2020.

36. Schwartz GJ, Brion LP, Spitzer A. The use of plasma creatinine concentration for estimating glomerular filtration rate in infants, children, and adolescents. *Pediatr Clin North Am*. 1987;34(3):571-590. PubMed

37. Bueva A, Guignard JP. Renal function in preterm neonates. *Pediatr Res*. 1994;36(5):572-577.PubMed

38. Myers GL, Miller WG, Coresh J, et al. Recommendations for improving serum creatinine measurement: a report from the Laboratory Working Group of the National Kidney Disease Education Program. *Clin Chem*. 2006;52(1):5-18.PubMed

39. Alcorn J, McNamara PJ. Ontogeny of hepatic and renal systemic clearance pathways in infants: part I. *Clin Pharmacokinet*. 2002;41(12):959-998. PubMed

40. Botwinski CA, Falco GA. Transition to postnatal renal function. *J Perinat Neonatal Nurs*. 2014;28(2):150-154. PubMed

41. DuBois D, Dubois EF. A formula to estimate the approximate surface area if height and weight be known. *Arch Intern Med (Chic)*. 1916;17:863-871.

42. Mosteller RD. Simplified calculation of body-surface area. *N Engl J Med*. 1987;317(17):1098.PubMed

43. Hogg RJ, Furth S, Lemley KV, et al. National Kidney Foundation's Kidney Disease Outcomes Quality Initiative clinical practice guidelines for chronic kidney disease in children and adolescents: evaluation, classification, and stratification. *Pediatrics*. 2003;111(6 Pt 1):1416-1421. PubMed

44. Traub SL, Johnson CE. Comparison of methods of estimating creatinine clearance in children. *Am J Hosp Pharm*. 1980;37(2):195-201.PubMed

45. Hernandez de Acevedo L, Johnson CE. Estimation of creatinine clearance in children: comparison of six methods. *Clin Pharm*. 1982;1(2):158-161. PubMed

46. Schwartz GJ, Work DF. Measurement and estimation of GFR in children and adolescents. *Clin J Am Soc Nephrol*. 2009;4(11):1832-1843.PubMed

47. Mian AN, Schwartz GJ. Measurement and estimation of glomerular filtration rate in children. *Adv Chronic Kidney Dis*. 2017;24(6):348-356. PubMed

48. Schwartz GJ, Muñoz A, Schneider MF, et al. New equations to estimate GFR in children with CKD. *J Am Soc Nephrol*. 2009;20(3):629-637. PubMed

49. Schwartz GJ, Schneider MF, Maier PS, et al. Improved equations estimating GFR in children with chronic kidney disease using an immunonephelometric determination of cystatin C. *Kidney Int*. 2012;82(4):445-453.PubMed

50. CKD Work Group, KDIGO. Kidney Disease: Improving Global Outcomes (KDIGO) 2012 clinical practice guideline for the evaluation and management of chronic kidney disease. *Kidney Int Suppl*. 2013;3:1-150.

51. Waz WR, Quattrin T, Feld LG. Serum creatinine, height, and weight do not predict glomerular filtration rate in children with IDDM. *Diabetes Care*. 1993;16(8):1067-1070.PubMed

52. Huppert SS, Balistreri WF. Morphogenesis of the liver and biliary system. In: Kliegman RM, St Geme JW, et al, eds. *Nelson Textbook of Pediatrics*. 21st ed. Philadelphia, PA: Elsevier; 2020.

53. Hughes HK, Kahl LK, eds. *The Harriet Lane Handbook*. 21st ed. Philadelphia, PA: Elsevier; 2018.

54. Pan DH, Rivas Y. Jaundice: Newborn to age 2 months. *Pediatr Rev*. 2017;38(11):499-510.PubMed

55. Lockitch G. Beyond the umbilical cord: interpreting laboratory tests in the neonate. *Clin Biochem*. 1994;27(1):1-6.PubMed

56. Gurria JP, Brown RL. Digestive system disorders. In: Kliegman RM, St Geme JW, et al, eds. *Nelson Textbook of Pediatrics*. 21st ed. Philadelphia, PA: Elsevier; 2020.

57. Osberg IM. Chemistry and hematology reference (normal) ranges. In: *Current Pediatric Diagnosis and Treatment*. 16th ed. New York, NY: Lange Medical Books/McGraw-Hill; 2003.

58. Dror Y, Chan A, Backer JM, et al. Hematology. In: MacDonald MG, Seshia MMK, eds. *Avery's Neonatology: Pathophysiology and Management of the Newborn*. 7th ed. Philadelphia, PA: Lippincott Williams & Wilkins; 2016.

59. Thornburg CD. Physiologic anemia of infancy. In: Kliegman RM, St Geme JW, et al, eds. *Nelson Textbook of Pediatrics*. 21st ed. Philadelphia, PA: Elsevier; 2020.

60. Rothman JA. Iron-deficiency anemia. In: Kliegman RM, St Geme JW, et al, eds. *Nelson textbook of Pediatrics*. 21st ed. Philadelphia, PA: Elsevier; 2020.

61. Glader B. The anemias. In: Kliegman RM, Behrman RE, Jenson HB, et al, eds. *Nelson Textbook of Pediatrics*. 18th ed. Philadelphia, PA: Saunders Elsevier; 2007.

62. Rocephin [package insert]. South San Francisco, CA: Genentech USA Inc; 2018.

63. Wolfsdorf J, Craig ME, Daneman D, et al. Diabetic ketoacidosis in children and adolescents with diabetes. *Pediatr Diabetes*. 2009;10(suppl 12):118-133.PubMed

64. Castellanos L, Tuffaha M, Koren D et al. Management of diabetic ketoacidosis in children and adolescents with type 1 diabetes mellitus. *Pediatric Drugs* Published ahead of print May 25, 2020 10.1007/s40272 -020-00397-0.

# 24

# Women's Health

*Candi C. Bachour*

DOI 10.37573/9781585286423.024

## OBJECTIVES

*After completing this chapter, the reader should be able to*

- Understand the reproductive cycle and recognize normal ranges for follicle-stimulating hormone, luteinizing hormone, estradiol, and progesterone and how they differ in premenopausal women, postmenopausal women, and women after oophorectomy

- Describe clinical symptoms, physical findings, and accompanying laboratory abnormalities in women with secondary amenorrhea

- Describe proposed diagnostic criteria, physical and radiologic findings, and accompanying laboratory abnormalities in women with polycystic ovary syndrome

- Describe signs of virilization, causes of hirsutism, and associated laboratory abnormalities

- Describe pertinent medical history, physical examination findings, and laboratory and gynecologic procedures to determine causes of infertility in women

- List and describe how drugs interfere with laboratory values of follicle-stimulating hormone, luteinizing hormone, progesterone, prolactin, and testosterone

## ANATOMY AND PHYSIOLOGY

The reproductive cycle depends on the complex cyclic interactions between hypothalamic gonadotropin-releasing hormone (GnRH), the pituitary gonadotropins follicle-stimulating hormone (FSH), and luteinizing hormone (LH) and the ovarian sex steroid hormones estradiol ($E_2$) and progesterone.[1] Feedback loops between the hypothalamus, pituitary gland, and ovaries are depicted in **Figure 24-1**. If the levels or relationship of any one (or more) of these hormones become altered, the reproductive cycle becomes disrupted, and ovulation and menstruation cease.

## MENSTRUAL CYCLE

The reproductive cycle is divided into three phases: menstruation and the follicular phase, ovulation, and the luteal phase.[1,2] These three phases, which refer to the status of the ovary during the reproductive cycle, are depicted in **Figure 24-2**.

### Phase I. Menstruation and the Follicular Phase

The first day of menstrual bleeding is considered day 1 of the typical 28-day menstrual cycle. Women usually menstruate for 3 to 5 days. Menstruation marks the beginning of the follicular phase of the cycle. With the beginning of menstruation, plasma concentrations of $E_2$, progesterone, and LH reach their lowest point (normal range of 1.8 to 2.4 ng/dL, 37 to 57 ng/dL, and 5 to 25 milli-International Units/mL, respectively).[1,2] An increase in FSH begins approximately 2 days before the onset of menstruation and continues in response to the reduction in negative feedback at the pituitary gland. Under the influence of FSH, the granulosa cells in the ovarian follicle begin to secrete $E_2$.

By the fourth day of the cycle, $E_2$ begins to rise in plasma. $E_2$ stimulates LH receptors on the theca cells in the ovarian follicle, further increasing secretion of androgen precursors, which are converted by aromatase to $E_2$ in granulosa cells. The upregulation of LH receptors and hormone production prepares the granulosa and theca cells for progesterone synthesis after ovulation.

With rising $E_2$ levels, there is negative feedback to the pituitary gland to decrease the release of FSH and positive feedback to the pituitary gland to increase the release of LH.

### Phase II. Ovulation

As the dominant follicle secretes more and more $E_2$ (normal range of 16.6 to 23.2 ng/dL), there is marked positive feedback to the pituitary gland to secrete LH. By days 11 to 13 of the normal cycle, an LH surge occurs (normal range of 40 to 80 milli-International Units/mL), which triggers ovulation. Ovulation occurs within 24 to 36 hours of the LH surge, causing the oocyte to be expelled from the follicle and the follicle to be converted into corpus luteum to facilitate progesterone production during the remainder of the cycle. In addition, there is a slight increase in the basal body temperature (BBT) after ovulation.

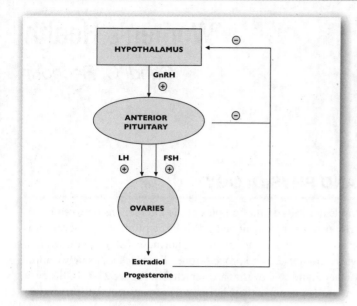

**FIGURE 24-1.** Hypothalamic-pituitary-ovarian axis. GnRH = gonadotropin-releasing hormone; LH = luteinizing hormone; FSH = follicle-stimulating hormone; (+) = stimulation of hormone secretion; (-) = inhibition of hormone secretion.

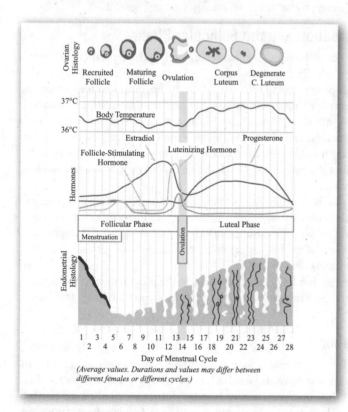

**FIGURE 24-2.** The menstrual cycle.

## Phase III. Luteal Phase

The luteal phase of the menstrual cycle is characterized by a change in secretion of sex steroid hormones from $E_2$ predominance to progesterone predominance. As FSH rises early in the cycle, stimulating production of $E_2$, additional LH receptors are created in the granulosa cells and then theca cells. With the LH surge at the time of ovulation, LH facilitates production of progesterone.

Production of progesterone begins approximately 24 hours before ovulation and rises rapidly thereafter. A maximum production of progesterone occurs 3 to 4 days after ovulation and is maintained for approximately 11 days after ovulation (normal range of 332 to 1,198 ng/dL). If fertilization and implantation do not occur, progesterone production diminishes rapidly, initiating events leading to the beginning of a new cycle.

Adequate progesterone production is necessary to facilitate implantation of the fertilized oocyte into the endometrium and sustain pregnancy into the early first trimester. If the initial rise in FSH is inadequate and the LH surge does not achieve maximal amplitude, an "inadequate luteal phase" can occur, resulting in progesterone production that is inadequate to facilitate implantation of a fertilized oocyte or sustain pregnancy.

Physiologic plasma levels of progesterone exert negative feedback on pituitary secretion of both FSH and LH. During the luteal phase of the cycle, both FSH and LH are suppressed to low levels (5 to 25 milli-International Units/mL). As the corpus luteum fails and progesterone secretion diminishes, FSH begins to rise to prepare a woman for the next reproductive cycle.

# LABORATORY TESTS

## Follicle-Stimulating Hormone[23]

*Normal ranges are as follows:*
*Children: 5 to 10 milli-International Units/mL (5 to 10 International Units/L)*
*Adult women, follicular phase: 5 to 25 milli-International Units/mL (5 to 25 International Units/L)*
*Adult women, midcycle: 20 to 30 milli-International Units/mL (20 to 30 International Units/L)*
*Adult women, luteal phase: 5 to 25 milli-International Units/mL (5 to 25 International Units/L)*
*Menopausal women: 40 to 250 milli-International Units/mL (40 to 250 International Units/L)*

*Follicle-stimulating hormone* (FSH)[23] is a glycoprotein pituitary hormone produced and stored in the anterior pituitary. It is under complex regulation by hypothalamic GnRH and by the gonadal sex hormones estrogen and progesterone. Normally, FSH increases occur at earlier stages of puberty, 2 to 4 years before LH reaches comparable levels. In females, FSH stimulates follicular formation in the early stages of the menstrual cycle and then the midcycle surge of LH causes ovulation of the FSH-ripened ovarian follicle.

This test may be helpful in determining whether a gonadal deficiency is of primary origin or is secondary to insufficient stimulation by the pituitary hormones. Decreased FSH levels may occur in feminizing and masculinizing ovarian tumors (when FSH production is inhibited because of increased estrogen secretion), pituitary adenomas, neoplasm of the adrenal glands (which influences secretion of estrogen or androgens), and polycystic ovary syndrome (PCOS).[56] Increased FSH levels occur in premature ovarian failure and in menopause.[56]

The date of the last menstrual period (LMP) should be considered when interpreting FSH in premenopausal women. Sometimes multiple blood specimens are necessary because of episodic releases of FSH from the pituitary gland. An isolated sample may not indicate the actual activity; therefore, multiple single blood specimens may be required.

Interfering factors include recently administered radioisotopes, hemolysis of the blood sample, pregnancy, and drugs, such as estrogens or oral contraceptives or testosterone. **Table 24-1** provides a detailed list of drugs affecting plasma laboratory test values of FSH.[56]

## Luteinizing Hormone[23]

*Normal ranges are as follows:*
*Children: 5 to 10 milli-International Units/mL (5 to 10 IU/L)*
*Adult women, follicular phase: 5 to 25 milli-International Units/mL (5 to 25 IU/L)*
*Adult women, midcycle: 40 to 80 milli-International Units/mL (40 to 80 IU/L)*
*Adult women, luteal phase: 5 to 25 milli-International Units/mL (5 to 25 IU/L)*
*Menopausal women: >75 milli-International Units/mL (> 75 IU/L)*

**TABLE 24-1.** Drugs Affecting Plasma Laboratory Test Values of FSH

| INCREASE FSH (OR CAUSE FALSE-POSITIVE VALUES) | DECREASE FSH (OR CAUSE FALSE-NEGATIVE VALUES) |
| --- | --- |
| Phenytoin | Anabolic steroids (eg, danazol) |
| Dopamine agonists (bromocriptine, levodopa) | Carbamazepine |
| Cimetidine | Diethylstilbestrol |
| GnRH agonists | Digoxin |
| Growth hormone-releasing hormone antagonists | Estrogen/oral contraceptives |
| Ketoconazole | Megestrol |
| Naloxone | Phenothiazines (eg, promethazine) |
| Pravastatin | Pravastatin |
| Spironolactone | Tamoxifen |
| Tamoxifen | Testosterone |

*Source:* Adapted with permission from Fischbach F. Chemistry studies. In: *A Manual of Laboratory and Diagnostic Tests.* 6th ed. Philadelphia, PA: Lippincott, Williams & Wilkins; 2000:418–449.

Like FSH, *luteinizing hormone* (LH)[23] is a glycoprotein pituitary hormone produced and stored in the anterior pituitary that is under complex regulation by hypothalamic-releasing hormone and by estrogen and progesterone. The midcycle surge of LH causes ovulation. Decreased LH and FSH occur in pituitary adenomas and eating disorders, whereas elevated levels are found in ovarian failure and menopause.[56] Elevated basal LH with an LH/FSH ratio of 3 or more and some increase of ovarian androgen in an essentially anovulatory adult woman are presumptive evidence of PCOS.[56]

The date of the LMP should be considered in premenopausal females. Interfering factors include recently administered radioisotopes, hemolysis of the blood sample, pregnancy, and estrogens or oral contraceptives or testosterone.[56] A detailed list of drugs that affect plasma laboratory test values of LH is shown in **Table 24-2**.[56]

## Estradiol[23]

*Normal ranges are as follows:*
*Children: <2 ng/dL*
*Adult women, follicular phase: 1.8 to 2.4 ng/dL (66 to 88 pmol/L)*

**TABLE 24-2.** Drugs Affecting Plasma Laboratory Test Values of LH

| INCREASE LH (OR CAUSE FALSE-POSITIVE VALUES) | DECREASE LH (OR CAUSE FALSE-NEGATIVE VALUES) |
| --- | --- |
| Anticonvulsants (eg, phenytoin) | Anabolic steroids (eg, danazol) |
| Dopamine agonists (bromocriptine) | Anticonvulsants (eg, carbamazepine) |
| Clomiphene | Corticotropin-releasing hormone |
| GnRH agonists | Diethylstilbestrol |
| Growth hormone-releasing hormone antagonists | Digoxin |
| Ketoconazole | Dopamine agonists |
| Mestranol | Estrogen/oral contraceptives |
| Spironolactone | Megestrol |
| | Phenothiazines (eg, thioridazine) |
| | Pravastatin |
| | Progesterone |
| | Tamoxifen |
| | Testosterone |

*Source:* Adapted with permission from Fischbach F. Chemistry studies. In: *A Manual of Laboratory and Diagnostic Tests.* 6th ed. Philadelphia, PA: Lippincott, Williams & Wilkins; 2000:418–449.

*Adult women, midcycle: 16.6 to 23.2 ng/dL (609 to 852 pmol/L)*

*Adult women, luteal phase: 6.3 to 7.3 ng/dL (231 to 268 pmol/L)*

Together with the FSH levels, *estradiol* ($E_2$)[23] is useful in evaluating menstrual and fertility problems as well as estrogen-producing tumors. $E_2$ is the most active of the endogenous estrogens. *Estriol* ($E_3$) levels in both plasma and urine rise as pregnancy advances; significant amounts are produced in the third trimester. $E_3$ is no longer considered useful for detection of fetal distress.[56]

$E_2$ levels are increased by estrogen-producing tumors, during menstruation, before ovulation, and during the weeks 23 to 41 of pregnancy. $E_2$ levels are decreased in premature ovarian failure and in menopause. Normal $E_2$ values vary widely between women and in the presence of pregnancy, the menopausal state, or follicular, ovulatory, or luteal stages of the menstrual cycle.

The number of weeks of gestation should be considered if the patient is pregnant when interpreting $E_2$ levels. The number of days into the menstrual cycle must be documented and considered for a nonpregnant woman. Interfering factors include radioactive pharmaceuticals and oral contraceptives.

## Progesterone[23]

*Normal ranges are as follows:*

*Adult women, early in cycle: 37 to 57 ng/dL (1.2 to 1.8 nmol/L)*

*Adult women, midcycle: rising*

*Adult women, luteal phase: 332 to 1,198 ng/dL (10.6 to 38.1 nmol/L)*

*Menopausal women: 10 to 22 ng/dL (0.3 to 0.7 nmol/L)*

*Progesterone*[23] is primarily involved in the preparation of the uterus for pregnancy and its maintenance during pregnancy. The placenta begins producing progesterone at 12 weeks of gestation. Progesterone level peaks in the midluteal phase of the menstrual cycle. In nonpregnant women, progesterone is produced by the corpus luteum. Progesterone on day 21 is the single best test to determine whether ovulation has occurred.

This test is part of a fertility evaluation to confirm ovulation, evaluate corpus luteum function, and assess risk for early spontaneous abortion. Testing of several samples during the cycle is necessary. Ovarian production of progesterone is low during the follicular (first) phase of the menstrual cycle. After ovulation, progesterone levels rise for 2 to 5 days and then fall. During pregnancy, there is a gradual increase from week 9 to week 32 of gestation, often to 100 times the level in the nonpregnant woman. Levels of progesterone in twin pregnancy are higher than in a single pregnancy.

Increased progesterone levels are associated with congenital adrenal hyperplasia (CAH) and some ovarian tumors. Decreased progesterone levels are associated with threatened spontaneous abortion and hyperprolactinemia.

The date of the LMP and length of gestation should be recorded. No radioisotopes should be administered within 1 week before the test. Drugs that affect plasma laboratory test values of progesterone are listed in **Table 24-3**.[56]

## Prolactin[23]

*Normal ranges are as follows:*

*Children: 1 to 20 ng/mL (1 to 20 mcg/L)*

**TABLE 24-3.** Drugs Affecting Plasma Laboratory Test Values of Progesterone

| INCREASE PROGESTERONE (OR CAUSE FALSE-POSITIVE VALUES) | DECREASE PROGESTERONE (OR CAUSE FALSE-NEGATIVE VALUES) |
|---|---|
| Valproic acid | Ampicillin |
| Clomiphene | Anticonvulsants (carbamazepine, phenytoin) |
| Corticotropin | Danazol |
| Ketoconazole | GnRH agonists (eg, leuprolide) |
| Progesterone | Oral contraceptives |
| Tamoxifen | Pravastatin |

*Source*: Adapted with permission from Fischbach F. Chemistry studies. In: *A Manual of Laboratory and Diagnostic Tests*. 6th ed. Philadelphia, PA: Lippincott, Williams & Wilkins; 2000:418–449.

*Adult women: 1 to 25 ng/mL (1 to 25 mcg/L)*

*Menopausal women: 1 to 20 ng/mL (1 to 20 mcg/L)*

*Prolactin*[23] is a pituitary hormone essential for initiating and maintaining lactation. The gender difference in prolactin does not occur until puberty, when increased estrogen production results in higher prolactin levels in females. A circadian change in prolactin concentration in adults is marked by episodic fluctuation and a sleep-induced peak in the early morning hours.[56]

This test may be helpful in the diagnosis, management, and follow-up of prolactin-secreting tumors, including the effectiveness of surgery, chemotherapy, and radiation treatment. Levels >100 ng/mL in a nonlactating female indicate a prolactin-secreting tumor; however, a normal prolactin level does not rule out pituitary tumor. In addition to pituitary adenomas, increased prolactin levels are associated with hypothyroidism (primary), PCOS, and anorexia nervosa; these increased levels are helpful in the differential diagnosis of infertility.

The patient should fast for 12 hours before testing. Specimens should be procured in the morning, 3 to 4 hours after awakening. Interfering factors occur in a number of circumstances. Increased values are associated with newborns, pregnancy, the postpartum period, stress, exercise, sleep, nipple stimulation, and lactation. Drugs such as estrogens, methyldopa, phenothiazines, and opiates may increase values. Dopaminergic drugs inhibit prolactin. Administration of dopaminergic agents can normalize prolactin levels in patients with galactorrhea, hyperprolactinemia, and pituitary tumor. **Table 24-4** provides a comprehensive list of drugs affecting plasma laboratory test values of prolactin.[56,57]

## Testosterone[23]

*Normal ranges are as follows:*

*Children: 0.12 to 0.16 ng/mL (0.4 to 0.6 nmol/L)*

*Adult women: 0.2 to 0.6 ng/mL (0.7 to 2.1 nmol/L)*

*Menopausal women: 0.21 to 0.37 ng/mL (0.7 to 1.3 nmol/L)*

**TABLE 24-4.** Drugs Affecting Plasma Laboratory Test Values of Prolactin

| INCREASE PROLACTIN (OR CAUSE FALSE-POSITIVE VALUES) | DECREASE PROLACTIN (OR CAUSE FALSE-NEGATIVE VALUES) |
| --- | --- |
| Antihistamines | Calcitonin |
| Antipsychotics (AP) (eg, Typical AP haloperidol) | Carbamazepine |
| Antipsychotics (AP) (eg, Atypical AP aripiprazole) | Clonidine |
| Calcitonin | Cyclosporin A |
| Cimetidine | Dexamethasone |
| Danazol | Dopamine agonists (apomorphine, bromocriptine, levodopa) |
| Diethylstilbestrol | Ergot alkaloid derivatives |
| Estrogens/oral contraceptives | Nifedipine |
| Fenfluramine | Opiates (morphine) |
| Furosemide | Pergolide |
| GnRH agonists | Ranitidine |
| Growth hormone-releasing hormone antagonists | Rifampin |
| Histamine antagonists | Secretin |
| Insulin | Tamoxifen |
| Interferon | |
| Labetalol | |
| Loxapine | |
| Megestrol | |
| Methyldopa | |
| Metoclopramide | |
| Monoamine oxidase inhibitors | |
| Molindone | |
| Nitrous oxide | |
| Opiates (eg, morphine) | |
| Parathyroid hormone | |
| Pentagastrin | |
| Phenothiazines (eg, chlorpromazine) | |
| Phenytoin | |
| Ranitidine | |
| Reserpine | |
| SNRIs (eg, venlafaxine) | |

**TABLE 24-4.** Drugs Affecting Plasma Laboratory Test Values of Prolactin, cont'd

| INCREASE PROLACTIN (OR CAUSE FALSE-POSITIVE VALUES) | DECREASE PROLACTIN (OR CAUSE FALSE-NEGATIVE VALUES) |
| --- | --- |
| SSRIs (eg, sertraline) Thiothixene | |
| Thyrotropin-releasing hormone | |
| Tumor necrosis factor | |
| Verapamil | |

SNRIs = serotonin-norepinephrine reuptake inhibitors; SSRIs = selective serotonin reuptake inhibitors.
*Source*: Adapted with permission from references 56, 57.

The adrenal glands and ovaries in women secrete *testosterone*.[23] Excessive production virilizes women. Testosterone exists in serum as both unbound (free) fractions and fractions bound to albumin, sex hormone–binding globulin (SHBG), and testosterone-binding globulin. Unbound (free) testosterone is the active portion. Testosterone serum levels undergo large and rapid fluctuations; levels peak in early morning.[56]

This test is useful in the detection of ovarian tumors and virilizing conditions in women. It also may be part of a fertility evaluation. Increased total testosterone levels occur in adrenal neoplasms, CAH, and ovarian tumors (benign or malignant). Increased free testosterone levels are associated with female hirsutism, PCOS, and virilization.

Blood should be drawn in the early morning (between 6:00 a.m. and 10:00 a.m.) to obtain the highest levels. Multiple pooled samples drawn at different times throughout the day may be necessary for more reliable results. No radioisotopes should be administered within 1 week before the test. Several drugs interfere with test results, including estrogen, androgens, and steroids, which decrease testosterone levels. Other drugs that interfere with interpretation of laboratory values of testosterone are provided in **Table 24-5**.[52,57]

# AMENORRHEA

*Amenorrhea* is the absence or abnormal cessation of the menses.[3] Primary and secondary amenorrhea describe the occurrence of amenorrhea before and after menarche, respectively. Primary amenorrhea can be diagnosed if a patient has normal secondary sexual characteristics but no menarche by 16 years of age.[4] Secondary amenorrhea is the absence of menses for 3 months in women with previously normal menstruation and for 9 months in women with previous oligomenorrhea (scant menses). Secondary amenorrhea is more common than primary amenorrhea.[5] The reader is referred to other texts for the evaluation of primary amenorrhea.

**TABLE 24-5.** Drugs Affecting Plasma Laboratory Test Values of Testosterone

| INCREASE TESTOSTERONE (OR CAUSE FALSE-POSITIVE VALUES) | DECREASE TESTOSTERONE (OR CAUSE FALSE-NEGATIVE VALUES) |
| --- | --- |
| Anabolic steroids (eg, danazol) | Alcohol |
| Anticonvulsants (eg, phenytoin, barbiturates, rifampin) | Anticonvulsants (eg, carbamazepine) |
| Cimetidine | Androgens |
| Clomiphene | Cimetidine |
| Dopamine agonists (eg, bromocriptine) | Corticosteroids (eg, dexamethasone) |
| Gonadotropin | Cyclophosphamide |
| Pravastatin | Diazoxide |
| Tamoxifen | Diethylstilbestrol |
| | Digoxin |
| | Estrogens/oral contraceptives |
| | Ketoconazole |
| | GnRH agonists (eg, leuprolide) |
| | Magnesium sulfate |
| | Medroxyprogesterone |
| | Phenothiazines (eg, thioridazine) |
| | Pravastatin |
| | Spironolactone |
| | Tetracycline |

*Source*: Adapted with permission from Fischbach F. Chemistry studies. In: *A Manual of Laboratory and Diagnostic Tests*. 6th ed. Philadelphia, PA: Lippincott, Williams & Wilkins; 2000:418–449.

The prevalence of amenorrhea not due to pregnancy, lactation, or menopause is ~3% to 4%.[3,5] History, physical examination, and measurement of FSH, thyroid-stimulating hormone (TSH), and prolactin identify the most common causes of amenorrhea. **Table 24-6** illustrates how symptoms elicited from a patient history assist in diagnosing the cause of amenorrhea.[4,6]

During the physical examination, the clinician should note the presence of galactorrhea, thyromegaly, or other evidence of hypothyroidism or hyperthyroidism, hirsutism, acne, or signs of virilization.[7] In addition, the patient's body mass index (BMI)

**TABLE 24-6.** Medical History Associated with Amenorrhea

| PATIENT HISTORY | ASSOCIATIONS |
| --- | --- |
| Acne, greasy or oily skin, hirsutism, obesity | PCOS |
| History of chemotherapy | Ovarian failure |
| History of radiation therapy | Ovarian failure |
| History of diabetes mellitus, Addison disease, or thyroid disease | Ovarian failure (autoimmune etiology) |
| Galactorrhea | Hyperprolactinemia |
| Weight loss, excessive exercise, severe dieting | Functional amenorrhea |
| Sexual activity | Pregnancy |
| Cessation of menstruation followed by hot flashes, vaginal dryness, dyspareunia, or mood swings | Menopause |
| Rapid progression of hirsutism | Adrenal or ovarian androgen-secreting tumor |
| Bodybuilder | Exogenous androgen use |
| Medication history | Amenorrhea secondary to medication use (eg, danazol, medroxyprogesterone [Depo-Provera], LHRH agonists, LHRH antagonists, oral contraceptives) |
| Constipation, hoarseness, loss of hair, memory impairment, sensation of cold, weakness, weight gain | Hypothyroidism |
| Headache, neurologic symptoms, visual field defect | CNS lesion (hypothalamic or pituitary) |
| History of PID, endometriosis, or D&C | Asherman syndrome |
| History of cautery for cervical intraepithelial neoplasia or obstructive cervical malignancy | Cervical stenosis |
| Debilitating illness | Functional amenorrhea |

CNS = central nervous system; D&C = dilation and curettage; LHRH = luteinizing hormone-releasing hormone; PID = pelvic inflammatory disease.
*Source*: Adapted with permission from references 4 and 6.

**TABLE 24-7.** Physical Examination Findings Associated with Amenorrhea

| FINDINGS | ASSOCIATIONS |
|---|---|
| Bradycardia | Hypothyroidism, physical or nutritional stress |
| Coarse skin, coarseness of hair, dry skin, edema of the eyelids, weight gain | Hypothyroidism |
| Galactorrhea | Hyperprolactinemia |
| Bradycardia, cold extremities, dry skin with lanugo hair, hypotension, hypothermia, minimum of body fat, orange discoloration of skin (hypercarotenemia) | Anorexia nervosa |
| Painless enlargement of parotid glands, ulcers or calluses on skin of dorsum of fingers or hands | Bulimia |
| Signs of virilization: clitoromegaly, frontal balding, increased muscle bulk, severe hirsutism | Adrenal or ovarian androgen-secreting tumor |
| Centripetal obesity, hirsutism, hypertension, proximal muscle weakness, striae | Cushing syndrome |
| Increased BMI, hirsutism, acne | PCOS |
| Transverse vaginal septum, imperforate hymen | Uterine outflow tract obstruction |

BMI = body mass index.
*Source:* Adapted with permission from references 4 and 6.

should be calculated. A BMI <20 kg/m$^2$ may indicate hypothalamic ovulatory dysfunction, such as occurs with anorexia or other eating disorders. The presence of breast development suggests there has been previous estrogen activity. Excessive testosterone secretion is suggested most often by hirsutism and rarely by increased muscle mass or signs of virilization. The combination of amenorrhea and galactorrhea strongly correlates with hyperprolactinemia and not virilization. The history and physical examination should include a thorough assessment of the external and internal genitalia. **Table 24-7** illustrates how physical examination findings assist in diagnosing the cause of amenorrhea.[4,6]

## Hypothyroidism

Although other clinical signs of thyroid disease are usually noted before amenorrhea presents, abnormal thyroid hormone levels can affect prolactin levels. Treatment of hypothyroidism should restore menses, but this may take several months.[8] **Table 24-8** provides differential diagnoses of anovulatory disorders and associated serum laboratory findings.[9]

## Hyperprolactinemia

A patient with markedly elevated prolactin levels, galactorrhea, headaches, or visual disturbances should receive imaging tests to rule out a pituitary tumor. Adenomas are the most common cause of anterior pituitary dysfunction.[10] A prolactin level >100 ng/mL suggests a prolactinoma, and magnetic resonance imaging should be performed. If tumor is excluded as the cause, medications (eg, oral contraceptive pills, antipsychotics, antidepressants, antihypertensives, histamine blockers, and opiates) are the next most common cause of hyperprolactinemia. Medications usually increase prolactin levels to >100 ng/mL.[10]

In most amenorrheic women with hyperprolactinemia, prolactin levels do not decline without treatment, and the amenorrhea does not resolve as long as the prolactin levels remain elevated.[10] In the absence of another organic condition, dopamine agonists (eg, bromocriptine) are the preferred treatment of hyperprolactinemia with or without a pituitary tumor.[3,11,12]

## Uterine Outflow Obstruction

The most common cause of outflow obstruction in secondary amenorrhea is Asherman syndrome (intrauterine scarring usually from curettage or infection).[4] Certain gynecological procedures can help diagnose Asherman syndrome. Other causes of outflow tract obstruction include cervical stenosis and obstructive fibroids or polyps.

## Functional (Hypothalamic) Amenorrhea

Functional disorders of the hypothalamus or higher centers are the most common reason for chronic anovulation. Psychogenic stress, weight changes, undernutrition, and excessive exercise are frequently associated with functional hypothalamic amenorrhea, but the pathophysiologic mechanisms are unclear. More cases of amenorrhea are associated with weight loss than with anorexia, but amenorrhea with anorexia nervosa is more severe.[11,13] Women involved in competitive sports activities have a 3-fold higher risk of primary or secondary amenorrhea than others, and the highest prevalence is among long-distance runners[14] (**Minicase 1**).

## Ovarian Failure

Approximately 1% to 5% of women have premature ovarian failure, a condition in which persistent estrogen deficiency and elevated FSH levels occur prior to the age of 40 years, resulting in amenorrhea.[17] Ovarian failure is confirmed by documenting an FSH level persistently in the menopausal range (40 to 250 milli-International Units/mL).[3] Iatrogenic causes of premature ovarian failure, such as chemotherapy and radiation therapy for malignancy, have a potential for recovery. Ovarian function may fluctuate, with an increasingly irregular menstrual cycle before permanent ovarian failure. The resulting fluctuations in gonadotropin levels account for the lack of accuracy associated

**TABLE 24-8.** Differential Diagnosis of Amenorrhea and Associated Serum Laboratory Findings[a]

| CONDITION | FSH | LH | PROLACTIN | TESTOSTERONE |
|---|---|---|---|---|
| Functional amenorrhea secondary to extreme exertion or rapid weight changes | ↔ | ↔ | ↔ | ↔ |
| Premature ovarian failure | ↑↑↑ | ↑↑↑ | ↔ | ↔ |
| Pituitary adenoma | ↓ | ↓ | ↑↑ | ↔ |
| Use of progestational agents | ↓ | ↓ | ↔ | ↔ |
| Hypothyroidism | ↔ | ↔ | ↔/↑ | ↔ |
| Eating disorders | ↓↓ | ↓↓ | ↔ | ↔ |
| PCOS | ↔/↓ | ↑↑ | ↔/↑ | ↔/↑↑ |
| CAH | ↔ | ↔ | ↔ | ↔/↑ |

[a]normal = ↔; mildly reduced = ↓; moderately reduced = ↓↓; significantly reduced = ↓↓↓; mildly elevated = ↑; moderately elevated = ↑↑; significantly elevated = ↑↑↑.
*Source*: Adapted with permission from Hunter MH, Sterrett JJ. Polycystic ovary syndrome: it's not just infertility. *Am Fam Physician*. 2000;62(5):1079–1088.

with a single FSH value.[18] Women with ovarian failure should be offered estrogen and progestin treatment to promote and maintain secondary sexual characteristics and reduce the risk of developing osteoporosis.

Menopause represents a type of "physiologic" ovarian failure, which is defined as the cessation of menses for at least 12 months. The climacteric and perimenopause are the periods of waning ovarian function before menopause (ie, the transition from the reproductive to the nonreproductive years).[1] The average age for menopause in the United States is between 50 and 52 years of age (median 51.5), with 95% of women experiencing this event between the ages of 44 and 55.[1] (**Minicase 2**.)

During perimenopause, the ovarian follicles diminish in number and become less sensitive to FSH.[1] The process of ovulation becomes increasingly inefficient, less regular, and less predictable than in earlier years. Initially, a woman may notice

# MINICASE 1

## Amenorrhea Secondary to Intense Exercise and Weight Loss

Tonya W., a 34-year-old woman, sees her doctor for a urine pregnancy test due to no menses for about 2 months. Tonya W. has no significant past medical history. Further questioning reveals she has lost a total of 28 lb over the past 4 months and complains of recent acne. Tonya W.'s vital signs include blood pressure (BP) 105/70 mm Hg, heart rate (HR) 55 beats/min, temperature 98.8°F, and weight 112 lb. Laboratory tests are as follows:

   urine human chorionic gonadotropin (hCG), negative

   FSH, 6 milli-International Units/mL

   LH 3, milli-International Units/mL,

   prolactin 20 ng/mL

   testosterone, 20 ng/dL

She also reports heavy exercise for the past year and a decreased appetite over the past 6 months.

QUESTION: What is the most likely diagnosis?

DISCUSSION: This patient reports amenorrhea. Pregnancy is not a cause of amenorrhea because her urine hCG is negative. Laboratory tests fall within normal range, and she has decreased appetite, bradycardia, and reports heavy exercise over an extended period of time—all indicative of a functional disorder. The combination of heavy exercise along with nutritional changes such as decreased appetite may contribute to functional amenorrhea.

Treatment of functional amenorrhea depends on the etiology, and it is important to encourage the patient to decrease the intensity of exercise and increase caloric intake. Women with excessive weight loss should be screened for eating disorders and treated if anorexia nervosa or bulimia nervosa is diagnosed. Menses usually will return after a healthy body weight is achieved.[15] With young athletes, menses may return after a modest increase in caloric intake or a decrease in athletic training. Women with amenorrhea also are susceptible to the development of osteoporosis.[16] In the athletic population, this is significant as these women are at an increased risk for stress fractures.[14] Diagnosis is one of exclusion, and the patient should be monitored for improvement before initiating other therapies.

## MINICASE 2

### Perimenopause

Fiona S., a 51-year-old woman, returns for further testing due to reports of irregular menses over the past 7 months, loss of sexual desire, vaginal dryness, and episodes of warmth and sweating throughout the day. Her past medical history includes breast cancer, for which she underwent chemotherapy and radiation. On examination, her BP is 120/68 mm Hg, her HR is 90 beats/min, and her temperature is 100°F. The thyroid gland is normal to palpation. Cardiac and lung examinations are unremarkable. Breast examination reveals symmetrical breasts, without masses or discharge. Examination of the external genitalia does not reveal any masses. Laboratory values are obtained on day 3 of menses and are as follows:

FSH, 34 milli-International Units/mL

LH, 39 milli-International Units/mL

QUESTION: What is the most likely diagnosis?

DISCUSSION: This patient complains of irregular menses, vaginal dryness, and intermittent sensations of warmth and sweating. This constellation of symptoms is consistent with perimenopause. Elevated FSH and LH levels confirm the diagnosis. Due to this woman's age and medical history, it is likely she is in the perimenopausal period. However, even when gonadotropins are in the menopausal range, as in this case, ovulation can still be occurring, albeit irregularly and unpredictably. Thus, it is best to draw FSH and LH levels during the follicular phase because they reach their lowest point during this phase. Hot flashes, which are typical vasomotor changes caused by decreasing estrogen levels, are associated with skin temperature elevation and sweating lasting for 2 to 4 minutes. The low estrogen concentration also decreases epithelial thickness of the vagina, leading to atrophy and dryness. Although her estradiol level would mostly likely be low, it is not a reliable indicator of menopausal transition because estradiol levels are prone to cyclical fluctuations, as shown in Figure 24-2. Thus, it is not necessary to draw an estradiol level.

Treatment for hot flashes includes hormone therapy with estrogen. Certain antidepressants, such as venlafaxine, can help with vasomotor symptoms as well, and paroxetine (Brisdelle) has been recently approved for the treatment of hot flashes in menopause.[19,20] When a woman still has her uterus, the addition of progestin to estrogen replacement is important for preventing endometrial cancer. Because significant increased risks of breast cancer, heart disease, pulmonary embolism, and stroke are associated with hormone therapy, estrogens are not the best treatment for vasomotor symptoms for this patient.[21,22]

---

a shortening of the cycle length. With increasing inefficiency of the reproductive cycle, the follicular phase shortens, but the luteal phase is maintained at normal length. With the passing of time, some cycles become anovulatory. As menopause approaches, the remaining follicles become almost totally resistant to FSH. The process of ovulation ceases entirely, and cyclic hormone production ends with menopause.

Serum FSH levels begin to rise with diminishing ovarian function; the elevation is first detected in the follicular phase. This early follicular phase rise in FSH has been developed into an endocrine test of ovarian functional reserve in which one draws an FSH level on cycle day 3. With a further decrease in ovarian function, the FSH level is elevated consistently throughout the menstrual cycle in perimenopausal women and in women after oophorectomy. **Table 24-9** depicts serum hormones according to age.[23]

The postmenopausal ovary is not quiescent. Under the stimulation of LH, androgens (ie, testosterone and androstenedione) are secreted. Testosterone concentrations decline after menopause but remain two times higher in menopausal women with intact ovaries than in those with ovaries removed (oophorectomy). Estrone is the predominant endogenous estrogen in postmenopausal women and is termed *extragonadal estrogen* because the concentration is directly related to body weight and androstenedione is converted to estrone in adipose tissue. **Table 24-10** compares concentrations of androgens and estrogens in premenopausal women, postmenopausal women, and women after oophorectomy.[9]

### Polycystic Ovary Syndrome

Polycystic ovary syndrome affects approximately 6% of women of reproductive age and is the most frequent cause of anovulatory infertility.[24,25] Clinical signs include those associated with a hyperandrogenic anovulatory state, including hirsutism and acne. Approximately 70% of affected women manifest growth of coarse hair in androgen-dependent body regions (eg, sideburn area, chin, upper lip, periareolar area, chest, lower abdominal midline and thigh) as well as upper-body obesity with a waist-to-hip ratio of >0.85.[9] Patients usually retain normal secondary sexual characteristics and rarely exhibit virilizing signs such as clitoromegaly, deepening of the voice, temporal balding, or masculinization of body habitus. Suggested diagnostic criteria for PCOS are provided in **Table 24-11**.[9]

Women with PCOS often develop polycystic ovaries as a function of a prolonged anovulatory state. Follicular cysts are observed on ultrasound in >90% of women with PCOS, but they also are present in up to 25% of normal women.[25-28] Although PCOS is primarily a clinical diagnosis, some debate exists about whether the diagnosis should be based on assays of circulating androgens rather than clinical signs and symptoms of hirsutism and acne as well as glucose abnormality. This is because a substantial number of women with PCOS have no overt clinical signs of androgen excess.[9]

Laboratory abnormalities in PCOS include elevated levels of testosterone and LH or an elevated LH/FSH ratio, an increased LH pulse frequency, and altered diurnal rhythm of LH secretion.

**TABLE 24-9.** Reference Ranges for Serum Hormones According to Age

| CATEGORY | FSH (mIU/mL) | LH (mIU/mL) | ESTRADIOL (ng/dL) | PROGESTERONE (ng/dL) |
|---|---|---|---|---|
| Children | 5–10 | 5–10 | <2 | |
| Adult women | | | | |
| Follicular phase | 5–25 | 5–25 | 1.8–2.4 | 37–57 |
| Midcycle | 20–30 | 40–80 | 16.6–23.2 | Rising |
| Luteal phase | 5–25 | 5–25 | 6.3–7.3 | 332–1198 |
| Menopausal women | 40–250 | >75 | <1.5 | 10–22 |

mIU = milli-International Unit.
*Source*: Adapted with permission from Sacher R, McPherson RA, Campos J. Reproductive, endocrinology. In: Sacher R, McPherson RA, Campos J, eds. *Widman's Clinical Interpretation of Laboratory Tests*. 11th ed. Philadelphia, PA: FA Davis Co; 2000:825–870.

**TABLE 24-10.** Steroid Hormone Serum Concentrations in Premenopausal Women, Postmenopausal Women, and Women After Oophorectomy

| HORMONE | PREMENOPAUSAL (NORMAL RANGE) | POSTMENOPAUSAL | POSTOOPHORECTOMY |
|---|---|---|---|
| Testosterone (ng/dL) | 32 (20–60) | 23 | 11 |
| Androstenedione (ng/dL) | 150 (50–300) | 80–90 | 80–90 |
| Estrone (pg/mL) | 30–200 | 25–30 | 30 |
| Estradiol (pg/mL) | 35–500 | 10–15 | 15–20 |

*Source*: Adapted with permission from Hunter MH, Sterrett JJ. Polycystic ovary syndrome: it's not just infertility. *Am Fam Physician*. 2000;62(5):1079–1088.

The LH/FSH ratio is used to facilitate diagnosis, and many researchers consider an LH/FSH ratio of ≥3:1 diagnostic of the syndrome.[29,30] Although serum testosterone levels are mildly-to-moderately elevated in women with PCOS, testosterone levels also are measured to rule out virilizing tumors. Prolactin levels are usually measured to exclude a possible prolactinoma. Suggested laboratory and radiologic evaluation for PCOS is provided in **Table 24-12**.[9]

Women with PCOS also should be screened for abnormal glucose metabolism because of an association with glucose intolerance. To aid in the possible prevention of cardiovascular disease, lipid abnormalities and blood pressure should be monitored annually.

The primary treatment for PCOS is weight loss through diet and exercise. Modest weight loss can lower androgen levels, improve hirsutism, normalize menses, and decrease insulin resistance.[30] Use of oral contraceptive pills or cyclic progestational agents can help maintain a normal endometrium. The optimal cyclic progestin regimen to prevent endometrial cancer is unknown, but a monthly 10-day to 14-day regimen is recommended.[30] Insulin-sensitizing agents such as metformin can reduce insulin resistance and improve ovulatory function.[30,31]

## Hyperandrogenism

Significantly elevated testosterone or dehydroepiandrosterone sulfate (DHEA-S) levels also may indicate an androgen-secreting tumor (ovarian or adrenal). DHEA-S is an androgen that arises almost exclusively from the adrenal gland. Levels of 17 α-hydroxyprogesterone (17-OHP) can help diagnose adult-onset CAH.[30] Cushing syndrome is rare; therefore, patients should be screened only when characteristic signs and symptoms (eg, striae, buffalo hump, significant central obesity, easy bruising, hypertension, proximal muscle weakness) are present.[30]

## Estrogen Status

If TSH and prolactin levels are normal, a progesterone challenge test can help detect endogenous estrogen that is affecting the endometrium. A withdrawal bleed usually occurs 2 to 7 days after the challenge test.[4] A negative progesterone challenge test signifies inadequate estrogenization and requires further follow-up for other underlying causes.

## TABLE 24-11. Suggested Diagnostic Criteria for PCOS

### CLINICAL FEATURES

Amenorrhea, oligomenorrhea, or dysfunctional uterine bleeding

Anovulatory infertility

Centripetal obesity

Hirsutism, acne

### ENDOCRINE ABNORMALITIES ON LABORATORY TESTS

Elevated androgen (ie, testosterone) levels

Elevated LH

Insulin resistance with hyperinsulinemia

LH-to-FSH ratio >3

Decreased FSH

### RADIOLOGIC ABNORMALITIES ON ULTRASOUND EXAMINATION

Increased ovarian stromal density and volume

Multiple (nine or more) subcortical follicular cysts

### EXCLUSION OF OTHER ETIOLOGIES

CAH

Cushing syndrome

Prolactinoma

Virilizing adrenal or ovarian tumors

*Source*: Adapted with permission from Hunter MH, Sterrett JJ. Polycystic ovary syndrome: it's not just infertility. *Am Fam Physician*. 2000;62(5):1079–1088.

## TABLE 24-12. Suggested Laboratory and Radiologic Evaluation of PCOS

17-OHP level[a]

DHEA-S level[a]

Dexamethasone suppression test[a]

Fasting glucose level

FSH level

Lipid profile (total, low-density and high-density lipoproteins)

LH level

Pelvic ultrasound examination[a]

Prolactin level

Testosterone level

hCG level

[a]Suggested only in selected patients.
*Source*: Adapted with permission from Hunter MH, Sterrett JJ. Polycystic ovary syndrome: it's not just infertility. *Am Fam Physician*. 2000;62(5):1079–1088.

# HIRSUTISM AND VIRILIZATION

*Hirsutism* is defined as the presence of excess terminal hair in androgen-dependent areas of a woman's body and occurs in up to 8% of women.[32-34] The disorder is a sign of increased androgen action on hair follicles from increased circulating levels of androgens (endogenous or exogenous) or increased sensitivity of hair follicles to normal levels of circulating androgens. Infrequently, hirsutism may signal more serious pathology, and clinical evaluation should differentiate benign causes from tumors or other conditions that require specific treatment. Hair growth varies widely among women, and distinguishing normal variations of hair growth from true hirsutism is important.

Although 60% to 80% of women with hirsutism have increased levels of circulating androgens, degrees of hirsutism correlate poorly with androgen levels.[35] DHEA-S is an uncommon cause of hirsutism. The ovary is the major source of increased levels of testosterone in women who have hirsutism.[32] Nearly all circulating testosterone is bound to SHBG and albumin, with free testosterone being the most biologically active form. When elevated insulin levels are present, SHBG levels decrease whereas free testosterone levels increase (**Minicase 3**).

When evaluating hirsutism, it is important to remember that it is only one sign of hyperandrogenism. Other abnormalities associated with excessive levels of androgen include acne, alopecia, android obesity, cardiovascular disease, and dyslipidemia, glucose intolerance/insulin resistance.[32] There are several causes of hirsutism. **Table 24-13** lists the causes of hirsutism according to diagnosis and the associated laboratory findings.[32]

Medications that may cause hirsutism include anabolic steroids (eg, oxymetholone), danazol, metoclopramide, methyldopa, phenothiazines, and progestins.[32] Increased androgen effect that results in hirsutism can be familial; idiopathic; or caused by excess androgen secretion by the ovary (eg, tumors, PCOS), excess secretion of androgens by adrenal glands (eg, CAH, Cushing syndrome, tumor), or exogenous pharmacologic sources of androgens.

Idiopathic hirsutism is common and often familial.[32] It is a diagnosis of exclusion and thought to be related to disorders in peripheral androgen activity. Onset occurs shortly after puberty with slow progression. Patients with idiopathic hirsutism generally have normal menses and normal levels of testosterone, 17-OHP, and DHEA-S.

As mentioned previously, PCOS is represented by chronic anovulation and hyperandrogenemia. Patients often report menstrual irregularities, infertility, obesity, and symptoms associated with androgen excess, and diagnosis usually is based on clinical rather than laboratory findings. Up to 70% of patients with PCOS have signs of hyperandrogenism.[32]

CAH is a spectrum of inherited disorders of adrenal steroidogenesis, with decreased cortisol production resulting in overproduction of androgenic steroids.[32,36] The serum 17-OHP measurement is a screening test for adult-onset CAH. Common signs in postadolescent women with adult-onset CAH are hirsutism, acne, and menstrual irregularity. As many as 25% of women with adult-onset CAH also exhibit LH hypersecretion.

## MINICASE 3

## Hirsutism Secondary to Adnexal Tumor

Vivian R., a 45-year-old parous woman, has noticed increasing hair growth on her face and abdomen over the past 8 months. She denies using steroid medications, weight change, or a family history of hirsutism. Her menses has been monthly with the exception of the past 3 months. Her past medical and surgical histories are unremarkable. On examination, her thyroid is normal to palpation. She has excess facial hair and male pattern hair on her abdomen. Acne is noted on her face. She also notes increased sweating and some thinning of her hair. Cardiac and pulmonary examinations are normal. Abdominal examination reveals no masses or tenderness. Examination of the external genitalia reveals possible clitoromegaly. Pelvic examination shows a normal uterus and cervix and an 8-cm, right adnexal mass. Her laboratory values obtained on the fourth day of her menstrual cycle are as follows:

LH, 10 milli-International Units/mL

FSH, 6 milli-International Units/mL

total testosterone, 72 ng/dL

prolactin, 13 ng/mL

QUESTION: What is the mostly likely diagnosis?

DISCUSSION: This patient has onset of excess male-pattern hair over the past 6 months as well as features of virilism (clitoromegaly). The patient has an elevated testosterone and other lab results are within normal range, so adrenal or ovarian tumors are possibilities. PCOS may be ruled out because she does not have an elevated LH or an LH/FSH ratio >3. This excess of androgens and the rapid onset suggests a tumor. She has a large adnexal mass, so the diagnosis is straightforward. Such tumors are normally of low malignant potential and are slow growing.[32] Surgical treatment may be warranted. She has irregular menses because of an inhibition of ovulation by androgens. She does not have the presentation of Cushing syndrome, such as hypertension, buffalo hump, abdominal striae, and central obesity. Likewise, she does not take any medications containing anabolic steroids (eg, oxymetholone). Although PCOS is probably the most common cause of hyperandrogenism, it does not fit her clinical presentation because it usually presents with a gradual onset of hirsutism and irregular menses since menarche.

**TABLE 24-13.** Causes of Hirsutism and Associated Laboratory Findings[a]

| DIAGNOSIS | TESTOSTERONE | 17-OHP | LH/FSH | PROLACTIN | DHEA-S | CORTISOL |
|---|---|---|---|---|---|---|
| CAH | ↔/↑ | ↑ | ↔ | ↔ | ↔/↑ | ↔/↓ |
| PCOS | ↔/↑ | ↔ | ↔/↑ LH | ↔/↑ | ↔/↑ | ↔ |
| | | | ↔/↓ FSH | | | |
| Ovarian tumor | ↑ | ↔ | ↔ | ↔ | ↔ | ↔ |
| Adrenal tumor | ↑ | ↔ | ↔ | ↔ | ↑ | ↔/↑ |
| Pharmacologic agents[b] | ↔ | ↔ | ↔ | ↔ | ↔ | ↔ |
| Idiopathic | ↔ | ↔ | ↔ | ↔ | ↔ | ↔ |
| Familial | ↔ | ↔ | ↔ | ↔ | ↔ | ↔ |

[a]Normal = ↔; decreased = ↓; increased = ↑.
[b]Pharmacologic agents: androgens (eg, testosterone, danazol), anabolic steroids (eg, oxymetholone), metoclopramide, methyldopa, phenothiazines (eg, prochlorperazine), progestins (eg, medroxyprogesterone).
*Source:* Adapted with permission from Hunter MH, Carek PJ. Evaluation and treatment of women with hirsutism. *Am Fam Physician.* 2003;67(12):2565–2572.

Serum levels of 17-OHP should be drawn at 8:00 a.m. when concentrations peak. Basal follicular-phase serum 17-OHP levels >5 ng/mL suggest adult-onset CAH caused by 21-hydroxylase deficiency. In contrast, serum 17-OHP levels are normal in women with PCOS.[37]

Hirsutism may result from use of exogenous pharmacologic agents, including danazol, anabolic steroids (eg, oxymetholone), and testosterone. Oral contraceptives containing levonorgestrel, norethindrone, and norgestrel tend to have stronger androgen

effects whereas those with ethynodiol diacetate, norgestimate, drospirenone, and desogestrel are less androgenic.[32]

Androgen-secreting tumors of the ovary or adrenal gland are usually heralded by virilization (eg, development of male characteristics in women) and rapid progression of hirsutism and cessation of menses. Androgen-secreting ovarian tumors are more common than adrenal tumors and are associated with a better prognosis.[32] Virilization occurs in >1% of patients with hirsutism. Signs of virilization are shown in **Table 24-14**.[32]

## TABLE 24-14. Signs of Virilization

Acne

Clitoromegaly

Deepening of voice

Hirsutism

Increased libido

Increased muscle mass

Infrequent/absent menses

Loss of breast tissue or normal female body contour

Malodorous perspiration

Temporal hair recession/balding

*Source*: Adapted with permission from Hunter MH, Carek PJ. Evaluation and treatment of women with hirsutism. *Am Fam Physician*. 2003;67(12):2565–2572.

A thorough history and physical examination are essential to evaluate women with hirsutism to determine which patients need additional diagnostic testing. Family history is important because 50% of women with hirsutism have a positive family history of the disorder.[32] Physical examination should distinguish normal amounts of hair growth from hirsutism. Diagnosis often can be made on clinical assessment alone or by limited laboratory testing. Virilization should be noted and abdominal and pelvic examinations should be performed to exclude any masses.

Identification of serious underlying disorders is the primary purpose of laboratory testing and should be individualized. Approximately 95% of these patients have PCOS or idiopathic hirsutism.[38] History and physical examination can exclude most underlying disorders, and full hormonal investigation is usually warranted only in patients with rapid progression of hirsutism, abrupt symptom onset, or virilization.

In patients with hirsutism of peripubertal onset and slow progression, regular menses, otherwise normal physical examination, and no virilization, the likelihood of an underlying neoplasm is small. Whether laboratory investigation in these patients is warranted is controversial; however, some experts recommend routine testing to exclude underlying ovarian and adrenal tumors and adult-onset adrenal hyperplasia.[34] For diagnostic purposes, serum levels of testosterone and 17-OHP are usually sufficient.[32]

For patients with irregular menses, anovulation, PCOS, late-onset adrenal hyperplasia, and idiopathic hirsutism, prolactin levels and thyroid function tests are suggested to identify thyroid dysfunction and pituitary tumors. Testing of glucose, testosterone, and 17-OHP levels should be considered, along with careful breast examination to rule out galactorrhea.

Hirsutism outside of the perimenarchal period, rapid progression of hirsutism, or signs of Cushing syndrome or virilization should indicate the possibility of an ovarian or adrenal neoplasm. Diagnostic testing should examine levels of serum testosterone, 17-OHP, and dehydroepiandrosterone sulfate (DHEA-S). Levels of serum testosterone >200 ng/dL and DHEA-S >700 ng/mL are strongly indicative of virilizing

tumors.[39] For patients with this degree of hormonal elevation or those whose history suggests a neoplasm, additional diagnostic imaging, including abdominal computed tomography to assess the adrenal glands, should be performed.

Pharmacologic treatment for hirsutism aims at blocking androgen action at hair follicles or suppression of androgen production. Classes of pharmacologic agents used include oral contraceptives, antiandrogens (eg, cyproterone), glucocorticoids, GnRH agonists (eg, leuprolide), antifungal agents (eg, ketoconazole), topical hair growth retardants (eg, depilatory agents), and insulin sensitizing agents (eg, metformin). Other options include spironolactone and drospirenone-containing contraceptives. Response to pharmacologic agents is slow, occurring over many months.

## INFERTILITY

*Infertility*, occurring in 10% to 15% of couples in the United States, is defined as 1 year of frequent, unprotected intercourse during which pregnancy has not occurred or 6 months for those other than 35 years of age.[7,40] Many of these couples present first to their primary care clinician, who may initiate evaluation and treatment. Infertility can be attributed to any abnormality in the female or male reproductive system and is distributed fairly equally among male factors, ovarian dysfunction, and tubal factors. A smaller percentage of cases is attributed to endometriosis, uterine or cervical factors, or other causes. In approximately one-fourth of couples, the cause is uncertain, and the etiology is multifactorial for some couples. Laboratory testing may include serum inhibin b and serum antimuellerian hormone collection. Serum antimuellerian hormone has been shown to be associated with fertility.[41] The reader is referred to other texts for the evaluation of male infertility (**Minicase 4**).

The medical history should include details of the menstrual cycle to determine whether the cycles are ovulatory or anovulatory. A menstrual cycle length of 22 to 35 days suggests ovulatory cycles, as does the presence of mittelschmerz and premenstrual symptoms.[44] During review of the woman's substance use history, caffeine intake should be assessed because high levels have been associated with lower fertility rates.[44] **Table 24-15** describes important elements in obtaining a medical history and performing a physical examination in women with infertility.[44]

Basal body temperature charting is a simple and inexpensive means of documenting ovulation.[45] In recent years, BBT charting for documentation of ovulation has largely been replaced by use of the less cumbersome urinary LH prediction kit. During ovulatory cycles, an LH surge can be detected in the urine 14 to 48 hours before ovulation.[46] Additionally, a single midluteal progesterone level, measured at the midpoint between ovulation and the start of the next menstrual cycle, can provide further confirmation as well as information about the adequacy of the luteal phase. A level >6 ng/mL implies ovulation and normal corpus luteal production of progesterone.[47] Of the three tests, the urinary LH kit provides the greatest accuracy in predicting ovulation.[47]

If ovulatory dysfunction is suspected based on the results of initial evaluation, focused laboratory investigation and other testing can help determine the underlying cause. Testing in patients with amenorrhea, irregular menses, or galactorrhea

# MINICASE 4

## Infertility Secondary to the Male Factor

Beatrice W., a 38-year-old woman, presents with a 3-year history of infertility. She states that her menses began at age 14 years and cycles occur at 28-day intervals. A biphasic BBT chart is recorded. She denies any history of smoking, illicit drug use, or sexually transmitted infection. A hysterosalpingogram (HSG) shows patent tubes and a normal uterine cavity. Labs tested on day 3 of her menstrual cycle include FSH 12 milli-International Units/mL and $E_2$ 122 pg/mL. Her husband is 37 years old, and they have been actively trying to conceive for the past 3 years.

QUESTION: What is the most likely etiology?

DISCUSSION: This patient has secondary infertility. In approaching infertility, there are five basic factors to examine: (1) ovulatory, (2) uterine, (3) tubal, (4) male factor, and (5) peritoneal. She has regular monthly menses, which argues strongly for regular ovulation; the biphasic BBT chart is further evidence for regular ovulation.

Uterine and tubal factors are normal based on the normal HSG. Laboratory testing showed FSH and $E_2$ levels favorable for follicular potential. If she had prior cryotherapy to the cervix, an examiner might consider cervical factor (rare).[42] Similarly, if she has symptoms of endometriosis (eg, dysmenorrhea, dyspareunia), then the examiner would focus on the peritoneal factor. For this patient, neither of these are likely, and there is no evidence of a past sexually transmitted disease or potential for pelvic inflammatory disease.

In general, an infertility evaluation is initiated after 12 months of unprotected intercourse during which pregnancy has not been achieved.[43] Because there are no hints favoring one factor over the other for this patient, the clinician should consider evaluation of the male factor. Causes of infertility are fairly equal among male and female reproductive abnormalities.[43] A semen analysis would be recommended for her male partner.

## TABLE 24-15. Medical History and Physical Examination in Women with Infertility

| HISTORY | PHYSICAL EXAMINATION |
|---|---|
| Coital practices | Breast formation |
| Medical history (eg, genetic disorders, endocrine disorders, PID) | Galactorrhea Genitalia (eg, patency, masses, tenderness, discharge) |
| Medications (eg, hormone therapy) | Hyperandrogenism (eg, hirsutism, acne, clitoromegaly) |
| Menstrual history | |
| Sexually transmitted diseases, genital inflammation (eg, vaginal discharge, dysuria, abdominal pain, fever) | |
| Previous fertility | |
| Substance abuse, including caffeine | |
| Surgical history (eg, genitourinary surgery) | |
| Toxin exposure | |

*Source*: Adapted with permission from Jose-Miller AB, Boyden JW, Frey KA. Infertility. *Am Fam Physician*. 2007;75(6):849–858.

should involve checking FSH, prolactin, and TSH levels.[43,48] Low or normal FSH levels are most common in patients with PCOS and hypothalamic amenorrhea.[43] The presence or absence of obesity and androgenization, generally occurring in women with PCOS, can be used to distinguish between the two disorders.[43] A high FSH level suggests possible ovarian failure.[43] Evaluation of a prolactin level is useful to rule out pituitary tumor, and measurement of TSH is necessary to rule out hypothyroidism.[43] Measurement of 17-OHP and serum testosterone levels is helpful in evaluating patients with hyperandrogenism or late-onset CAH and androgen-secreting tumors.[49] **Table 24-16** describes the key laboratory evaluations and specialized tests that should be performed in a woman with infertility.[44]

Women older than 35 years may benefit from testing of FSH and $E_2$ levels on day 3 of their menstrual cycle to assess ovarian reserve.[50] An FSH level of >10 milli-International Units/mL, combined with $E_2$ level of >80 pg/mL, suggests favorable follicular potential.[50] The clomiphene citrate challenge test—in which the FSH level is obtained on day 3 of the cycle and then again on day 10 after administration of clomiphene citrate 100 mg/day on days 5 to 9—also can be helpful in assessing ovarian reserve.[50] Normal and abnormal values vary by laboratory.

If the initial history and physical examination suggest tubal dysfunction or a uterine abnormality or if other testing has failed to reveal an etiology, hysterosalpingography, a radiologic study in which dye is placed into the uterine cavity via a transcervical catheter, is indicated.[43,48] The contour of the uterine cavity, including the presence or absence of any abnormalities, as well as tubal patency, can be assessed. Other gynecologic procedures can be performed to further detect tubal or uterine abnormalities.

**TABLE 24-16.** Laboratory Evaluation in Women with Infertility

| DOCUMENT OVULATION |
| --- |
| Measurement of midluteal progesterone level |
| Urinary LH using home prediction kit |
| BBT charting |

| DETERMINE ETIOLOGY IF OVULATORY DYSFUNCTION SUSPECTED |
| --- |
| Measurement of FSH, prolactin, TSH, 17-OHP, and testosterone (if hyperandrogenism suspected) |

| ASSESS OVARIAN RESERVE (WOMEN >35 YR OLD) |
| --- |
| Measurement of FSH and estradiol levels on day 3 of the menstrual cycle |
| Clomiphene citrate (Clomid) challenge test |

*Source*: Adapted with permission from Jose-Miller AB, Boyden JW, Frey KA. Infertility. *Am Fam Physician*. 2007;75(6):849–858.

Management of infertility involves treating the couple, treating the male partner (if infertile), and treating the female partner (if infertile). Couple management includes reviewing coital frequency, the "fertile window," use of ovulation kits, and emotional support. Men should be referred to a fertility specialist for evaluation of possible semen abnormalities. Women should be treated according to the underlying etiology, whether it is ovulatory dysfunction, tubal/uterine/pelvic disease, or unexplained infertility.

In women with anovulation resulting from a specific condition such as thyroid dysfunction, the underlying cause should be corrected if possible.[43] Women with hyperprolactinemia can be treated with dopaminergic agents (eg, bromocriptine), which may restore ovulation.[51] Insulin-sensitizing agents, such as metformin, have been shown to increase ovulation and pregnancy rates in patients with PCOS.[52] In other women with ovulatory dysfunction without evident cause or not otherwise correctable, the condition can be managed with the use of oral ovulation-inducing agents such as clomiphene citrate and aromatase inhibitors such as letrozole.[53] Tubal disease may be treated with tubal reparative surgery or with in vitro fertilization.[44,54] Patients with endometriosis may benefit from laparoscopic ablation or ovulation induction with or without in vitro fertilization.[55]

## SUMMARY

Knowledge of the normal reproductive cycle throughout a woman's lifespan, including pubertal development, menstruation, pregnancy, and menopause, helps understand related laboratory values. Monitoring changes in the gonadotrophic hormones FSH and LH and the ovarian steroid hormones $E_2$ and progesterone is essential in identifying underlying causes of conditions such as amenorrhea, hirsutism, and infertility. Moreover, pharmacologic treatments are often based on laboratory abnormalities of these hormones.

## LEARNING POINTS

1.  *What laboratory abnormalities are useful in the differential diagnosis of secondary amenorrhea?*

    **ANSWER:** In addition to history and physical examination, FSH, TSH, and prolactin levels identify the most common causes of amenorrhea.[3] When the physical examination is normal, the initial investigations should exclude pregnancy. When FSH values are normal or low, the problem is most often PCOS or functional (hypothalamic) amenorrhea due to anorexia or extreme exercise. Conversely, an elevated FSH would indicate premature ovarian failure or menopause. Measurement of TSH is useful to rule out subclinical hypothyroidism, even in the absence of thyroid-related symptoms. If the serum prolactin is persistently elevated and there is no history of medication or drug use that may elevate prolactin, a pituitary tumor should be considered.

2.  *What laboratory evaluations can be performed to confirm if patient symptoms are related to the perimenopausal period?*

    **ANSWER:** A history and physical examination are helpful when evaluating women who may be in the perimenopausal period. Women often present with a triad of symptoms, including irregular menses, feelings of inadequacy, and sensations of warmth and sweating. In the United States, 95% of women experience perimenopause between the ages of 44 and 55.[1] FSH and LH levels can be drawn to confirm diagnosis; however, it is important to draw the levels during the follicular phase because they are lowest during this time. $E_2$ levels are not reliable indicators of menopausal transition because they fluctuate over time.[23]

3.  *What laboratory evaluations can be done to detect ovulatory infertility in women?*

    **ANSWER:** Ovulation disorders constitute 40% of cases of female infertility.[44] To document ovulation, midluteal progesterone levels can be obtained in addition to urinary LH using home prediction kits and BBT charting. If ovulatory dysfunction is suspected based on results of initial evaluations, focused laboratory investigation can help determine the underlying cause. FSH, prolactin, TSH, and testosterone levels can help identify functional (hypothalamic) amenorrhea, pituitary tumor, thyroid disease, and adrenal disease. Low or normal FSH levels are most common in patients with PCOS and hypothalamic amenorrhea, such as occurs with extreme exertion or in eating disorders. Elevated FSH can identify premature ovarian failure. To assess ovarian reserve, measurement of FSH and $E_2$ levels on day 3 of the menstrual cycle or the clomiphene citrate challenge test may be done.

## REFERENCES

1.  Beckmann CRB, Ling FW, Smith RP, et al. *Obstetrics and Gynecology*. 5th ed. Philadelphia, PA: Lippincott Williams & Wilkins; 2006.

2.  Mesen TB, Young SL. Progesterone and the luteal phase: a requisite to reproduction. *Obstet Gynecol Clin North Am*. 2015;42(1):135-151. PubMed

3. Practice Committee of the American Society for Reproductive Medicine. Current evaluation of amenorrhea. *Fertil Steril.* 2006;86(5 suppl 1): S148-S155.PubMed

4. Master-Hunter T, Heiman DL. Amenorrhea: evaluation and treatment. *Am Fam Physician.* 2006;73(8):1374-1387.PubMed

5. Pettersson F, Fries H, Nillius SJ. Epidemiology of secondary amenorrhea. I. Incidence and prevalence rates. *Am J Obstet Gynecol.* 1973;117(1): 80-86.PubMed

6. Desai SP. *Clinician's Guide to Laboratory Medicine.* 3rd ed. Hudson, OH: Lexi-Comp Inc; 2004.

7. American College of Obstetricians and Gynecologists. *Management of Infertility Caused by Ovulatory Dysfunction (Practice Bulletin 34).* Washington, DC: ACOG; 2002.

8. Kalro BN. Impaired fertility caused by endocrine dysfunction in women. *Endocrinol Metab Clin North Am.* 2003;32(3):573-592.PubMed

9. Hunter MH, Sterrett JJ. Polycystic ovary syndrome: it's not just infertility. *Am Fam Physician.* 2000;62(5):1079-1090.PubMed

10. Pickett CA. Diagnosis and management of pituitary tumors: recent advances. *Prim Care.* 2003;30(4):765-789.PubMed

11. American College of Obstetrician and Gynecologists. *Management of Anovulatory Bleeding (Practice Bulletin 14).* Washington, DC: ACOG; 2000.

12. Schlechte J, Dolan K, Sherman B, et al. The natural history of untreated hyperprolactinemia: a prospective analysis. *J Clin Endocrinol Metab.* 1989;68(2):412-418.PubMed

13. Lucas AR, Crowson CS, O'Fallon WM, et al. The ups and downs of anorexia nervosa. *Int J Eat Disord.* 1999;26(4):397-405.PubMed

14. Warren MP, Goodman LR. Exercise-induced endocrine pathologies. *J Endocrinol Invest.* 2003;26(9):873-878.PubMed

15. Mitan LA. Menstrual dysfunction in anorexia nervosa. *J Pediatr Adolesc Gynecol.* 2004;17(2):81-85.PubMed

16. Davies MC, Hall ML, Jacobs HS. Bone mineral loss in young women with amenorrhoea. *BMJ.* 1990;301(6755):790-793.PubMed

17. Van Campenhout J, Vauclair R, Maraghi K. Gonadotropin-resistant ovaries in primary amenorrhea. *Obstet Gynecol.* 1972;40(1):6-12.PubMed

18. Conway GS, Kaltsas G, Patel A, et al. Characterization of idiopathic premature ovarian failure. *Fertil Steril.* 1996;65(2):337-341.PubMed

19. Ruddy KJ, Loprinzi CL. Antidepressants decrease hot flashes and improve life quality. *Menopause.* 2015;22(6):587-588.PubMed

20. Slaton RM, Champion MN, Palmore KB. A review of paroxetine for the treatment of vasomotor symptoms. *J Pharm Pract.* 2015;28(3):266-274. PubMed

21. Dehn B. Care of the menopausal patient: a nurse practitioner's view. *J Am Acad Nurse Pract.* 2007;19(8):427-437.PubMed

22. Rossouw JE, Anderson GL, Prentice RL, et al. Risks and benefits of estrogen plus progestin in healthy postmenopausal women: principal results from the Women's Health Initiative randomized controlled trial. *JAMA.* 2002;288(3):321-333.PubMed

23. Sacher R, McPherson RA, Campos J. Reproductive, endocrinology. In: Sacher R, McPherson RA, Campos J, eds. *Widman's Clinical Interpretation of Laboratory Tests.* 11th ed. Philadelphia, PA: FA Davis Co; 2000:825-870.

24. Franks S. Polycystic ovary syndrome [erratum published in *N Engl J Med.* 1995;333:1435]. *N Engl J Med.* 1995; 333:853-861.

25. Stein IF, Leventhal ML. Amenorrhea associated with bilateral polycystic ovaries. *Am J Obstet Gynecol.* 1935;29:181-191.

26. Guzick D. Polycystic ovary syndrome: symptomatology, pathophysiology, and epidemiology. *Am J Obstet Gynecol.* 1998;179(6 Pt 2):S89-S93. PubMed

27. Adams J, Franks S, Polson DW, et al. Multifollicular ovaries: clinical and endocrine features and response to pulsatile gonadotropin releasing hormone. *Lancet.* 1985;2(8469-70):1375-1379.PubMed

28. Fauser BCJM, Tarlatzis BC, Rebar RW, et al. Consensus on women's health aspects of polycystic ovary syndrome (PCOS): the Amsterdam ESHRE/ASRM-Sponsored 3rd PCOS Consensus Workshop Group. *Fertil Steril.* 2012;97(1):28-38.e25.PubMed

29. Lobo RA, Granger L, Goebelsmann U, et al. Elevations in unbound serum estradiol as a possible mechanism for inappropriate gonadotropin secretion in women with PCO. *J Clin Endocrinol Metab.* 1981;52(1): 156-158.PubMed

30. American College of Obstetricians and Gynecologists. *Polycystic Ovary Syndrome (Practice Bulletin 41).* Washington, DC: ACOG; 2002.

31. Kolodziejczyk B, Duleba AJ, Spaczynski RZ, et al. Metformin therapy decreases hyperandrogenism and hyperinsulinemia in women with polycystic ovary syndrome. *Fertil Steril.* 2000;73(6):1149-1154.PubMed

32. Hunter MH, Carek PJ. Evaluation and treatment of women with hirsutism. *Am Fam Physician.* 2003;67(12):2565-2572.PubMed

33. Knochenhauer ES, Key TJ, Kahsar-Miller M, et al. Prevalence of the polycystic ovary syndrome in unselected black and white women of the southeastern United States: a prospective study. *J Clin Endocrinol Metab.* 1998;83(9):3078-3082.PubMed

34. Redmond GP, Bergfeld WF. Diagnostic approach to androgen disorders in women: acne, hirsutism, and alopecia. *Cleve Clin J Med.* 1990;57(5):423-427.PubMed

35. Carmina E, Lobo RA. Peripheral androgen blockade versus glandular androgen suppression in the treatment of hirsutism. *Obstet Gynecol.* 1991;78(5 Pt 1):845-849.PubMed

36. Deaton MA, Glorioso JE, McLean DB. Congenital adrenal hyperplasia: not really a zebra. *Am Fam Physician.* 1999;59(5):1190-1196, 1172. PubMed

37. Ecklund LC, Usadi RS. Endocrine and reproductive effects of polycystic ovarian syndrome. *Obstet Gynecol Clin North Am.* 2015;42(1):55-65. PubMed

38. Rittmaster RS. Clinical relevance of testosterone and dihydrotestosterone metabolism in women. *Am J Med.* 1995;98(1A):17S-21S.PubMed

39. American College of Obstetricians and Gynecologists. *Evaluation and Treatment of Hirsute Women (Technical Bulletin 203).* Washington, DC: ACOG; 1995.</other>

40. Mosher WD, Bachrach CA. Understanding U.S. fertility: continuity and change in the National Survey of Family Growth, 1988-1995. *Fam Plann Perspect.* 1996;28(1):4-12.PubMed

41. Steiner AZ, Herring AH, Kesner JS, et al. Antimüllerian hormone as a predictor of natural fecundability in women aged 30-42 years. *Obstet Gynecol.* 2011;117(4):798-804.PubMed

42. Toy EC, Baker B, Ross J, et al, eds. *Case files: Obstetrics and Gynecology.* 2nd ed. New York, NY: Lange Medical Books/McGraw-Hill; 2007.

43. Practice Committee of the American Society for Reproductive Medicine. Optimal evaluation of the infertile female. *Fertil Steril.* 2004;82(suppl 1): S169-S172.PubMed

44. Jose-Miller AB, Boyden JW, Frey KA. Infertility. *Am Fam Physician.* 2007;75(6):849-858.PubMed

45. McCarthy JJ Jr, Rockette HE. Prediction of ovulation with basal body temperature. *J Reprod Med.* 1986;31(8 suppl):742-747.PubMed

46. Miller PB, Soules MR. The usefulness of a urinary LH kit for ovulation prediction during menstrual cycles of normal women. *Obstet Gynecol.* 1996;87(1):13-17.PubMed

47. Guermandi E, Vegetti W, Bianchi MM, et al. Reliability of ovulation tests in infertile women. *Obstet Gynecol.* 2001;97(1):92-96.PubMed

48. Marshburn PB. Counseling and diagnostic evaluation for the infertile couple. *Obstet Gynecol Clin North Am.* 2015;42(1):1-14.PubMed

49. Azziz R, Zacur HA. 21-Hydroxylase deficiency in female hyperandrogenism: screening and diagnosis. *J Clin Endocrinol Metab.* 1989;69(3): 577-584.PubMed

50. Practice Committee of the American Society for Reproductive Medicine. Aging and infertility in women. *Fertil Steril.* 2004;82(suppl 1):S102-S106. PubMed

51. Crosignani PG. Management of hyperprolactinemia in infertility. *J Reprod Med.* 1999;44(12 suppl):1116-1120.PubMed

52. Nestler JE, Stovall D, Akhter N, et al. Strategies for the use of insulin-sensitizing drugs to treat infertility in women with polycystic ovary syndrome. *Fertil Steril.* 2002;77(2):209-215.PubMed

53. Practice Committee of the American Society for Reproductive Medicine. Use of clomiphene citrate in infertile women: a committee opinion. *Fertil Steril.* 2013;100(2):341-348.PubMed

54. Lavy G, Diamond MP, DeCherney AH. Ectopic pregnancy: its relationship to tubal reconstructive surgery. *Fertil Steril.* 1987;47(4):543-556.PubMed

55. Practice Committee of the American Society for Reproductive Medicine. Endometriosis and infertility. *Fertil Steril.* 2004;82(suppl 1):S40-S45. PubMed

56. Fischbach F. Chemistry studies. In: Fischbach, F, ed. *A Manual of Laboratory and Diagnostic Tests.* 6th ed. Philadelphia, PA: Lippincott, Williams & Wilkins; 2000:418-498.

57. Ajmal A, Joffe H, Nachtigall LB. Psychotropic-induced hyperprolactinemia: a clinical review. *Psychosomatics.* 2014;55(1):29-36.PubMed

## QUICKVIEW | Follicle-Stimulating Hormone

| PARAMETER | DESCRIPTION | COMMENTS |
|---|---|---|
| **Reference range** | | |
| Children | 5–10 mIU/mL (5–10 IU/L) | Sometimes multiple blood specimens are necessary because of episodic increases of FSH |
| Adult women, follicular phase | 5–25 mIU/mL (5–25 IU/L) | |
| Adult women, midcycle | 20–30 mIU/mL (20–30 IU/L) | Document date of LMP |
| Adult women, luteal phase | 5–25 mIU/mL (5–25 IU/L) | |
| Menopausal women | 40–250 mIU/mL (40–250 IU/L) | |
| **Critical values** | Not established | Extremely high or low values should be reported quickly |
| **Natural substance?** | Yes | |
| **Inherent action?** | Yes | |
| **Major causes of...** | | |
| **High results** | | |
| Associated signs and symptoms | Premature ovarian failure | Hot flashes/night sweats |
| | Menopause | Hot flashes/night sweats |
| **Low results** | | |
| Associated signs and symptoms | Ovarian tumors | Virilization |
| | Pituitary adenoma | Galactorrhea/visual change |
| | Adrenal tumors | Virilization |
| | PCOS | Hirsutism/acne/obesity |
| | Eating disorders | Cachectic/decreased BMI |
| **After insult, time to...** | Not applicable | |
| Initial evaluation | | |
| Peak values | | |
| Normalization | | |
| **Diseases monitored with test** | Infertility | FSH >10 mIU/mL on day 3 of the menstrual cycle suggests normal ovarian reserve |
| **Drugs monitored with the test** | Clomiphene challenge test | Compares FSH before and after clomiphene administration to determine ovarian reserve |
| **Significant interferences with laboratory tests** | Recently administered radioisotopes | |
| | Hemolysis of blood sample | |
| | Estrogens, oral contraceptives, testosterone, progestational agents (Table 24-1) | |
| | Pregnancy | |

## QUICKVIEW | Leutinizing Hormone

| PARAMETER | DESCRIPTION | COMMENTS |
|---|---|---|
| **Reference range** | | |
| Children | 5–10 mIU/mL (5–10 IU/L) | Often measured with FSH to determine hormonally related functions/disorders |
| Adult women, follicular phase | 5–25 mIU/mL (5–25 IU/L) | |
| Adult women, midcycle | 40–80 mIU/mL (40–80 IU/L) | Document date of LMP |
| Adult women, luteal phase | 5–25 mIU/mL (5–25 IU/L) | |
| Menopausal women | >75 mIU/mL (7–75 IU/L) | |
| **Critical values** | Not established | Extremely high or low values should be reported quickly |
| **Natural substance?** | Yes | |
| **Inherent action?** | Yes | |
| **Major causes of...** | | |
| **High results** | | |
| Associated signs and symptoms | Premature ovarian failure | Hot flashes/night sweats |
| | Menopause | Hot flashes/night sweats |
| | PCOS | Hirsutism/acne/obesity |
| **Low results** | | |
| Associated signs and symptoms | Pituitary adenoma | Galactorrhea/visual changes |
| | Eating disorders | Cachectic/low BMI |
| **After insult, time to...** | | |
| Initial evaluation | Not applicable | |
| Peak values | | |
| Normalization | | |
| **Diseases monitored with test** | None | |
| **Drugs monitored with the test** | None | |
| **Significant interferences with laboratory tests** | Recently administered radioisotopes | |
| | Hemolysis of blood sample | |
| | Estrogens or oral contraceptives | |
| | Progestational agents, testosterone (Table 24-2) | |
| | Pregnancy | |

## QUICKVIEW | Estradiol (E$_2$)

| PARAMETER | DESCRIPTION | COMMENTS |
|---|---|---|
| **Reference range** | | |
| Children | <2 ng/dL | Estradiol is most active of endogenous estrogens |
| Adult women, early cycle | 1.8–2.4 ng/dL | |
| Adult women, midcycle | 16.6–23.2 ng/dL | Document date of LMP and length of gestation |
| Adult women, luteal phase | 6.3–7.3 ng/dL | |
| **Critical values** | Not established | Extremely high or low values should be reported quickly |
| **Natural substance?** | Yes | |
| **Inherent action?** | Yes | |
| **Major causes of…** | | |
| **High results** | | |
| Associated signs and symptoms | Estrogen-producing tumors | |
| | Menstruation/preovulatory weeks 23–41 of pregnancy | |
| **Low results** | | |
| Associated signs and symptoms | Menopause | Hot flashes/night sweats |
| | Premature ovarian failure | Hot flashes/night sweats |
| **After insult, time to…** | Not applicable | |
| Initial evaluation | | |
| Peak values | | |
| Normalization | | |
| **Diseases monitored with test** | Fertility | Estradiol >8 ng/dL on day 3 suggests adequate ovarian reserve |
| **Drugs monitored with the test** | None | |
| **Significant interferences with laboratory tests** | Radioactive pharmaceuticals and oral contraceptives | |

## QUICKVIEW | Progesterone

| PARAMETER | DESCRIPTION | COMMENTS |
|---|---|---|
| **Reference range** | | |
| Adult women, early cycle | 37–57 ng/dL (1.2–1.8 nmol/L) | Document LMP and length of gestation |
| Adult women, midcycle | Rising | |
| Adult women, luteal phase | 332–1198 ng/dL (10.6–38.1 nmol/L) | |
| Menopausal women | 10–22 ng/dL (0.3–0.7 nmol/L) | |
| **Critical values** | Not established | Extremely high or low values should be reported quickly |
| **Natural substance?** | Yes | |
| **Inherent action?** | Yes | |
| **Major causes of...** | | |
| **High results** | | |
| Associated signs and symptoms | CAH | ↑17-OHP, ↑DHEA-S, ↓cortisol, hirsutism/acne |
| | Ovarian tumor | Virilization, rapid progression of symptoms |
| **Low results** | | |
| Associated signs and symptoms | Spontaneous abortion | Vaginal bleeding |
| **After insult, time to...** | Not applicable | |
| Initial evaluation | | |
| Peak values | | |
| Normalization | | |
| **Diseases monitored with test** | Infertility | Midluteal progesterone >6 ng/mL suggests ovulation |
| **Drugs monitored with the test** | None | |
| **Significant interferences with laboratory tests** | Drugs may affect test outcome (Table 24-3) | |

## QUICKVIEW | Prolactin

| PARAMETER | DESCRIPTION | COMMENTS |
|---|---|---|
| **Reference range** | | |
| Children | 1–20 ng/mL (1–20 mcg/L) | Obtain 12-hr fasting samples in the morning |
| Adult women | 1–25 ng/mL (1–25 mcg/L) | |
| Menopausal women | 1–20 ng/mL (1–20 mcg/L) | |
| **Critical values** | Levels >100 ng/mL in nonlactating female may indicate a prolactin-secreting tumor | Extremely high or low values should be reported quickly |
| **Natural substance?** | Yes | |
| **Inherent action?** | Yes | |
| **Major causes of...** | | |
| **High results** | | |
| Associated signs and symptoms | Pituitary adenoma | Galactorrhea/visual changes |
| | Hypothyroidism (primary) | Coarse skin and hair |
| | PCOS | Hirsutism/acne/obesity |
| | Anorexia nervosa | Cachectic/low BMI |
| **Low results** | | |
| Associated signs and symptoms | No common disorders | |
| **After insult, time to...** | Not applicable | |
| Initial evaluation | | |
| Peak values | | |
| Normalization | | |
| **Diseases monitored with test** | Pituitary adenoma | |
| **Drugs monitored with the test** | Dopaminergic drugs | To monitor effect on prolactin levels in pituitary adenoma |
| **Significant interferences with laboratory tests** | Increased values are associated with newborns, pregnancy, postpartum period, stress, exercise, sleep, nipple stimulation, and lactation | |
| | Drugs (estrogens, methyldopa, phenothiazines, opiates) may increase values (Table 24-4) | |

## QUICKVIEW | Testosterone

| PARAMETER | DESCRIPTION | COMMENTS |
|---|---|---|
| **Reference range** | | |
| Children | 0.12–0.16 ng/mL (0.4–0.6 nmol/L) | Unbound (free) testosterone is active form |
| Adult women | 0.2–0.6 ng/mL (0.7–2.1 nmol/L) | Draw levels between 6:00 a.m. and 10:00 a.m |
| Menopausal women | 0.21–0.37 ng/mL (0.7–1.3 nmol/L) | |
| **Critical values** | Testosterone >200 ng/dL indicates virilizing tumor | Extremely high or low values should be reported quickly |
| **Natural substance?** | Yes | |
| **Inherent action?** | Yes | |
| **Major causes of...** | | |
| **High results** | | |
| Associated signs and symptoms | Adrenal neoplasms | Virilization, ↑DHEA-S, ↑cortisol, rapid progression of symptoms |
| | CAH | ↑17-OHP, ↑DHEA-S, ↓cortisol, hirsutism |
| | Ovarian tumors | Virilization, rapid progression of symptoms |
| | PCOS | Hirsutism/acne/obesity, ↑DHEA-S |
| | Cushing syndrome | Buffalo hump/obesity/striae |
| **Low results** | | |
| Associated signs and symptoms | No common disorders | |
| **After insult, time to...** | Not applicable | |
| Initial evaluation | Rapid progression of symptoms indicative of ovarian or adrenal tumor | |
| Peak values | | |
| Normalization | | |
| **Diseases monitored with test** | None | |
| **Drugs monitored with the test** | None | |
| **Significant interferences with laboratory tests** | Estrogen therapy increases testosterone levels (Table 24-5) | |
| | Many drugs, including androgens and steroids, decrease testosterone levels (Table 24-5) | |

*Source:* Adapted with permission from references 23 and 56.

# 25

# Men's Health

*Mary Lee and Roohollah Sharifi*

## OBJECTIVES

*After completing this chapter, the reader should be able to*

- Distinguish when serum free testosterone levels are preferred over serum total testosterone levels in selected patients

- Develop a laboratory monitoring plan for testosterone supplementation for the treatment of late-onset hypogonadism

- Explain why minimal laboratory testing is used to evaluate a patient with new-onset erectile dysfunction

- Explain the expected impact of benign prostatic hyperplasia on peak urinary flow rate and postvoid residual urinary volume

- Argue for and against the use of prostate-specific antigen screening for prostate cancer

- Describe the alteration of prostate-specific antigen levels in patients being treated with 5α-reductase inhibitors

- Describe the rationale for using age-related normal value ranges for prostate-specific antigen, percent free prostate-specific antigen, prostate-specific antigen doubling time, and prostate-specific antigen density levels in evaluating patients with prostate cancer

- Explain the advantages and disadvantages of using PCA3, PHI, and the 4K score over prostate-specific antigen for a patient with a prostate-specific antigen value of 4 to 10 ng/mL

*(continued on page 626)*

DOI 10.37573/9781585286423.025

This chapter focuses on laboratory and clinical tests used to evaluate several common medical disorders in aging men—hypogonadism, erectile dysfunction, benign prostatic hyperplasia (BPH), prostate cancer, and prostatitis. Tumor markers for assessing testicular cancer and lab tests for diagnosis of urinary tract infection and venereal diseases are discussed in other chapters.

## HYPOGONADISM

*Hypogonadism* refers to medical conditions in which the testes or ovaries fail to produce adequate amounts of testosterone or estrogen in men or women, respectively, to meet the physiologic needs of the patient. For the purposes of this chapter on men's health disorders, hypogonadism refers to conditions in which testicular production of testosterone is inadequate. Increasing patient age is associated with a greater percentage of men with serum testosterone levels that are below the normal range. Out of approximately 900 men in the Baltimore Longitudinal Study, the calculated incidence of hypogonadism was 12%, 19%, 28%, and 49% in men in their fifth, sixth, seventh, and eighth decade of life, respectively.[1]

### Testosterone Production and Physiologic Effects

Testosterone secretion is principally regulated by the hypothalamic-pituitary gonadal axis. The hypothalamus secretes gonadotropin-releasing hormone (GnRH). This hormone acts on anterior pituitary receptors to stimulate the release of follicle-stimulating hormone (FSH) and luteinizing hormone (LH). FSH acts on testicular Sertoli cells to stimulate spermatogenesis, whereas LH stimulates testicular Leydig cells to produce testosterone. Once the serum level of testosterone increases to within the normal physiologic range, it triggers a negative feedback loop, which inhibits GnRH release from the hypothalamus. Pituitary LH release is inhibited, too, but generally less so than GnRH. The testes secrete 95% of all androgens in men.[2]

In young men, 4 to 10 mg of testosterone is produced each day. Testosterone secretion follows a circadian pattern, such that the highest secretion occurs at 7:00 a.m. and the lowest secretion occurs at 8:00 p.m.

Testosterone is responsible for various age-related physiologic effects in men, but most notably, it is responsible for development of secondary sexual characteristics in men. The physiologic effects of testosterone and dihydrotestosterone (DHT) during the stages of life are included in (**Table 25-1**).

In nontarget tissue, including the liver and adipose tissue, aromatase enzyme can convert excess androgen to estrone and estradiol. In men, excess estrogen or a higher ratio of serum estrogen to androgen can result in gynecomastia or decreased libido and cause negative feedback to the hypothalamus and pituitary, which further suppresses serum testosterone production.[5]

Adrenocorticotrophin stimulates the adrenal gland to produce three androgens: dehydroepiandrosterone (DHEA), dehydroepiandrosterone sulfate (DHEA-S), and androstenedione. DHEA and DHEA-S are secreted at a daily rate of 15 to 30 mg, whereas androstenedione is secreted at a daily rate of 1.4 mg. All three adrenal androgens are weak androgens compared with testosterone. DHEA and DHEA-S combined

## OBJECTIVES

- Explain the role of histologic Gleason scoring in managing patients with prostate cancer
- Contrast the four-glass versus the two-glass method for diagnosis of prostatitis

only contribute to 1% of circulating androgens, so the clinical effect of adrenal androgens is considered minor in healthy men.

Testosterone comprises approximately 90% to 95% of circulating androgens. Of circulating testosterone, 55% (range, 44% to 60%) is bound tightly to sex hormone binding globulin (SHBG); 30% (range, 38% to 54%) is bound loosely to albumin, corticosteroid-binding globulin, and orosomucoid; and 1% to 3% is free and physiologically active.[2-4] At its targets in skeletal muscle, bone, brain, and Sertoli cells, testosterone itself appears to be physiologically active.[4] However, in the prostate and hair follicles of the scalp, where 5α-reductase enzyme is expressed, testosterone must be activated intracellularly by 5α-reductase to DHT, an androgen with at least twice the potency of testosterone. Two separate forms of 5α-reductase enzymes exist: type I and type II. Each enzyme type tends to predominate in a particular tissue. Type I enzyme concentrates in the skin, liver, and sebaceous glands of the scalp. Type II 5α-reductase predominates in the prostate and hair follicles of the scalp, and DHT in these tissues contributes to the development of BPH and alopecia, respectively.[3]

The level of physiologically active testosterone is directly related to multiple factors that affect SHBG production and serum levels. Factors that alter SHBG concentrations are included in **Table 25-2**. Measurement of free testosterone levels is essential in patients when the serum total testosterone level

### TABLE 25-1. Physiologic Effects of Testosterone and DHT[3,5]

| STAGE OF LIFE OF MALE | PHYSIOLOGIC EFFECT |
| --- | --- |
| In utero | Differentiation of male internal and external genitalia |
| At puberty | Male body habitus; deepening of voice; male hair distribution; enlargement of testes, penis, scrotum, and prostate; increased sexual drive and bone growth |
| Adulthood | Sexual drive, muscle strength and mass, bone mass, prostate enlargement, male hair growth and distribution, spermatogenesis |

DHT = dihydrotestosterone

### TABLE 25-2. Medical Conditions and Drugs That Alter SHBG Concentrations

| | INCREASED SHBG | DECREASED SHBG |
| --- | --- | --- |
| Medical conditions that produce an alteration of SHBG concentration | Hepatic cirrhosis<br>Hepatitis C<br>HIV disease<br>Anorexia nervosa<br>Hyperthyroidism<br>Aging men<br>Prolonged stress | Hypothyroidism<br>Nephrotic syndrome<br>Obesity<br>Acromegaly<br>Cushing syndrome<br>Diabetes mellitus |
| Drugs that produce an alteration of SHBG concentration | Estrogens<br>Phenytoin and other anticonvulsants<br>Thiazolidinediones (eg, pioglitazone, rosiglitazone)<br>Ethanol, chronic use | Testosterone supplements, excessive doses<br>Corticosteroids<br>Progestins<br>Tyrosine kinase inhibitors (eg, imatinib) |

HIV = human immunodeficiency virus.
*Source*: Adapted with permission from references 4,6.

is inconsistent with the clinical symptoms of the patient and the patient has a concurrent medical illness that can alter the level of SHBG.

## Hormonal Changes Associated with Primary, Secondary, and Tertiary Hypogonadism

*Primary hypogonadism* occurs when the testicles are absent or surgically removed or when they are nonfunctional secondary to an acquired disease (eg, mumps orchitis). *Secondary hypogonadism* occurs when the pituitary fails to release adequate amounts of LH; thus, the testes are not stimulated to produce adequate amounts of testosterone. *Tertiary hypogonadism* refers to a disorder of the hypothalamus such that there is inadequate release of GnRH, and a subsequent decrease in release of LH from the pituitary and testosterone from the testes. **Table 25-3** contrasts serum testosterone, LH, and GnRH levels in patients with primary, secondary, and tertiary hypogonadism.

## Late-Onset Hypogonadism

*Late-onset hypogonadism*, also known as *andropause* or *androgen deficiency in aging men* (ADAM), refers to the biochemical changes associated with age-related alterations in the hypothalamic-pituitary-gonadal axis, which may or may not be associated with clinically significant signs and symptoms.[7-9] Some men with decreased testosterone levels do not complain of their symptoms or have vague, nonspecific symptoms (eg, malaise or decreased energy) for which they do not seek medical treatment.[5,7,9] Although late-onset hypogonadism is often compared with menopause in aging women, these conditions are

**TABLE 25-3.** Etiology of and Laboratory Test Results in Patients with Primary, Secondary, and Tertiary Hypogonadism

|  | PRIMARY | SECONDARY | TERTIARY |
|---|---|---|---|
| Common causes | Klinefelter syndrome<br><br>Cryptorchidism<br><br>Mumps orchitis<br><br>Orchiectomy<br><br>Irradiation of testes<br><br>Traumatic injury to the testes<br><br>5α-reductase deficiency<br><br>Noonan syndrome<br><br>Autoimmune disorders (eg, Hashimoto thyroiditis or Addison disease)<br><br>Systemic disorders: HIV, hemochromatosis, cancer, liver cirrhosis<br><br>High-dose radiation therapy<br><br>Medications: high-dose ketoconazole, cytotoxins | Kallmann syndrome<br><br>Pituitary adenoma or infarction<br><br>Prolactinoma<br><br>Sleep apnea<br><br>Obesity<br><br>Metabolic syndrome<br><br>Type 2 diabetes mellitus<br><br>Chronic renal failure<br><br>Hepatic cirrhosis<br><br>Hypothyroidism<br><br>Anorexia nervosa<br><br>Medications: estrogens, LHRH agonists (eg, leuprolide, goserelin), LHRH antagonists (eg, degarelix), abiraterone, digoxin, prolonged course of high-dose corticosteroids, megestrol acetate, medroxyprogesterone, long-acting opioids | Infectious or infiltrative diseases of the hypothalamus (eg, tuberculosis, sarcoidosis, infectious abscess)<br><br>Isolated gonadotropin deficiency<br><br>Chronic opioid abuse |
| Serum testosterone level | Decreased | Decreased | Decreased |
| LH level | Increased | Decreased | Decreased |
| GnRH level | Increased | Increased | Decreased |

HIV = human immunodeficiency virus; LHRH = luteinizing hormone–releasing hormone.
*Source*: Adapted with permission from references 3,5,6.

different. In men, gonadal function decreases over decades, and symptoms develop slowly and often are not attributed to decreasing hormone levels. In women, gonadal function decreases over a comparatively shorter time period of 4 to 6 years, and symptoms are closely associated with decreasing hormone levels. **Table 25-4** contrasts physiologic changes associated with late-onset hypogonadism in men versus menopause in aging women.

Late-onset hypogonadism was once thought to be a type of primary hypogonadism. However, multiple alterations in the hypothalamic pituitary gonadal axis suggest that late-onset hypogonadism is a mixed type of hypogonadism. This phenomenon occurs in the face of a wide range of serum (total) testosterone and bioavailable testosterone levels among elderly men.[7] Whereas some symptomatic elderly men have serum testosterone levels that are below the normal physiologic range, others have levels that are decreased but are still within the normal range.[8,9]

## Hormonal Changes Associated with Late-Onset Hypogonadism

Starting at age 40, serum testosterone levels decrease by 1% to 2% annually. At age 80, the mean serum testosterone declines by approximately 40% of that typically observed in men at

age 40[7,8]; however, the serum testosterone level may remain in the normal range in elderly men because the normal range is wide. The symptoms of late-onset hypogonadism include physical weakness, decreased muscle mass, obesity, fatigue, psychologic depression, decreased libido, and erectile dysfunction. The incidence of clinically symptomatic hypogonadism is low and approximates 2.1% to 5.6% in men aged 40 to 70 years.[5] Low serum testosterone levels in patients with late-onset hypogonadism are due to multiple physiologic changes:

- Increased sensitivity of the hypothalamus and pituitary gland to negative feedback; thus, low circulating testosterone levels stimulate the negative feedback loop[9]
- Irregular, nonpulsatile secretion pattern of LH[10]
- Increased production of SHBG resulting in higher concentrations of physiologically inactive SHBG-bound testosterone and a reduced concentration of free active testosterone in plasma[7]
- Fewer functioning Leydig cells, which results in an age-related decrease in testicular production of testosterone[7]

A male patient age ≥50 years who presents with symptoms or signs of hypogonadism should undergo laboratory evaluation for late-onset hypogonadism. However, this is a diagnosis

**TABLE 25-4.** Characteristics of Late-Onset Hypogonadism in Aging Men Versus Menopause in Aging Women

| | LATE-ONSET HYPOGONADISM | MENOPAUSE |
|---|---|---|
| Time period over which gonadal function decreases | Decades, beginning at age 30–40 yr | 4–6 yr, beginning approximately at 50–52 yr |
| Fertility is maintained | Yes | No |
| Signs and symptoms | Decreased libido, erectile dysfunction, gynecomastia, weight gain, visceral obesity, moodiness, decreased sense of well-being, muscle aches, decreased muscle mass and strength (sarcopenia), weight gain, osteopenia, osteoporosis, hot flashes, reduced body hair, decreased testicular size, infertility | Menstrual cycles become progressively heavier and lighter, shorter and longer, and then stop; hot flashes, weight gain, vaginal dryness, dyspareunia, and hair loss |
| Symptoms and signs are linked to serum level of gonadal hormone | No | Yes |

*Source*: Adapted with permission from references 7,8.

of exclusion that is made after all other causes of low serum concentrations of testosterone have been ruled out. To assess symptom severity, the patient is commonly asked to complete a validated self-assessment questionnaire at baseline and at regular intervals after treatment is started. Because of the lack of specificity, these questionnaires are used to monitor a patient's treatment response, as opposed to diagnosing disease. For example, the St. Louis University ADAM questionnaire includes 10 questions that can be categorized into three symptom domains (psychologic, somato-vegetative, and sexual), and to which the patient responds either "yes" or "no."[11,12] An affirmative response to at least three questions on the survey is considered significant. The ADAM questionnaire has a sensitivity of 88% and a specificity of 60% and is considered to have the greatest reliability of the currently available questionnaires.

A similar alternative self-assessment instrument is the Aging Males' Symptoms (AMS) scale, which comprises 17 questions focused on symptoms associated with low testosterone. The patient rates the severity of each symptom on a scale of 1 (none) to 5 (extremely severe). It has a sensitivity of 83% and a low specificity of 39%.[13] Finally, a third tool, the Massachusetts Male Aging Survey comprises eight multiple-choice questions. Each response is assigned a certain number of points. Once all of the points are tallied, the total score has implications about the likelihood that the patient has hypogonadism. For example, a total score of 10 or higher suggests that the patient has a 50-50 chance of having hypogonadism, whereas a score of 4 or below suggests that the patient probably does not have hypogonadism. The Massachusetts Male Aging Survey is considered the least sensitive of the three tools. It has a sensitivity of 60% and a specificity of 59%.[11]

## Testosterone, Total

*Normal range, adult men: 280 to 1,100 ng/dL (9.7 to 38.17 nmol/L)*

*Normal range, age-related: boys, 6 to 9 years old: 3 to 30 ng/dL (0.1 to 1.04 nmol/L)*

*Boys, pubertal, 10 to 18 years old: 265 to 800 ng/dL (9.2 to 27.76 nmol/L)*

*Men, 19 to 39 years old: 264 to 916 ng/dL (9.2 to 31.8 nmol/L)*

A routine serum testosterone level reflects the total concentration of testosterone in the bloodstream in all three of its forms: free; loosely bound to albumin, corticosteroid-binding globulin, and orosomucoid; and tightly bound to SHBG.[4] Testosterone secretion follows a circadian pattern in younger men such that morning levels are approximately 15% to 20% (but can range up to 50%) higher than evening levels, which is a difference of approximately 140 ng/dL between the peak and nadir serum levels.[2] In addition, variability in measured testosterone levels is characteristic from day to day, from week to week, and seasonally.[2] This can result in a 20% to 25% difference in measured serum testosterone levels from the same patient.[2] Thus, when obtaining serum testosterone levels, it is recommended that blood samples be obtained between 7:00 a.m. and 11:00 a.m. in a patient who has fasted.[2,7,14] Furthermore, a single low serum testosterone level should be confirmed with a second sample usually at least 1 week later.[5,15] This is necessary because 30% of men with initial serum testosterone levels that are in the hypogonadal range have levels in the normal range when the laboratory test is repeated.[2] If the patient has a medical disorder or is taking medication that can alter serum testosterone levels, it is recommended that testing for serum testosterone levels be deferred until the medical disorder resolves or the medication is discontinued.[15] Common causes of decreased (Table 25-3) and increased serum testosterone levels are listed in **Table 25-5**.

The normal range is wide for serum testosterone levels and is based on laboratory results for young adult men. Although this normal range is applied to interpretation of serum testosterone levels in elderly men, no single threshold serum testosterone value has been identified to be pathognomonic for hypogonadism or low serum testosterone in this age group.[16,17] As an example, the U.S. Food and Drug Administration uses a serum testosterone of <300 ng/dL as an inclusion criterion for patients

**TABLE 25-5.** Common Causes of Increased Total Testosterone Levels

| |
|---|
| Hyperthyroidism |
| Adrenal tumors |
| Adrenal hyperplasia |
| Testicular tumors |
| Precocious puberty |
| Excessive exogenous testosterone use (usually seen with parenteral, but not transdermal use) |
| Anabolic steroids |

*Source*: Adapted with permission from Qaseem A, Horwitch CA, Vijan S, et al. Testosterone treatment in adult men with age-related low testosterone: a clinical guideline from the American College of Physicians. *Ann Intern Med*. 2020;172(2):126–133.

with hypogonadism in controlled clinical trials. However, some clinicians view that using a threshold serum testosterone value of <300 ng/dL results in excessive or unnecessary treatment of hypogonadism in asymptomatic men. As a result, the International Society for the Study of the Aging Male, the International Society of Andrology, the European Association of Urology, the European Association of Andrology, and the American Society of Andrology collectively have taken the position that a serum testosterone level of <230 ng/dL may be treated if the patient is symptomatic with decreased libido or inadequate response to type 5 phosphodiesterase inhibitor.[18] Furthermore, a serum testosterone level >350 ng/dL generally should not be associated with symptoms, nor should it be treated.[19] Generally, the following interpretation of serum testosterone levels is used:

- Serum testosterone <230 ng/dL: Most likely the patient has symptomatic hypogonadism and requires testosterone replacement.

- Serum testosterone 250 to 360 ng/dL: This level is equivocal for hypogonadism. The patient should be treated only if a low serum testosterone, free testosterone, or bioavailable testosterone level is confirmed and if the patient is symptomatic.[19]

- Serum testosterone >600 ng/dL: The patient does not have hypogonadism and requires no testosterone replacement.

- After instituting a testosterone replacement regimen, the goal of treatment is to increase the serum testosterone level between 400 and 700 ng/dL.[19] The onset of symptomatic improvement after initiating a testosterone replacement regimen is variable. An increase in libido and an improved perception of quality of life is evident in 3 weeks; signs of decreased mental depression may first appear at 3 to 6 weeks; increased muscle strength and decreased fat mass are observable at 12 to 16 weeks; and improved erectile dysfunction and bone density occur at 6 months.[20] Patients should be monitored for the effectiveness and safety of testosterone supplementation every 3 to 4 months for the first year of treatment and then annually thereafter.

- When treating patients with prostate cancer with luteinizing hormone–releasing hormone (LHRH) agonists or antagonists,

medical castration is induced. The target serum testosterone level is ≤50 ng/dL.

Testosterone levels are commonly determined using radioimmunoassay, nonradioactive immunoassays, or chemiluminescent detection methods, which are relatively easy to perform and inexpensive. However, these methods exhibit significant performance variability in the normal range and are limited in detecting serum testosterone levels <300 ng/dL.[21] That is, these assays may produce results that are significantly different than the true value. Thus, it is recommended that a physician try to ensure that a single patient's serum testosterone levels be assayed by the same clinical laboratory over time and that a normal range of serum testosterone be determined for each clinical laboratory that runs the assay.[21] The latter determination would require measurement of serum testosterone in approximately 40 normal, healthy men, age 20 to 40 years.[7] The Centers for Disease Control and Prevention initiated a program to standardize testosterone assays, which involves providing reference material to calibrate immunoassays. This reduces the variability of testosterone laboratory results among laboratories.[21] Despite the availability of more sensitive and specific antibodies for radioimmunoassays, stable isotope dilution liquid chromatography using benchtop tandem mass spectrometry (LC-MS) is generally considered the gold standard method for assaying serum testosterone.[22] Although both assays detect serum testosterone levels <300 ng/dL, LC-MS has greater accuracy and precision than radioimmunoassay[22] (**Minicase 1**).

## Free Testosterone

*Normal age-related ranges are as follows for adult men:*
*20 to 29 years, 10 to 15 ng/dL*
*30 to 39 years, 9 to 13 ng/dL*
*40 to 49 years, 7 to 11 ng/dL*
*50 to 59 years, 6 to 10 ng/dL*
*>60 years, 5 to 9 ng/dL*

Free testosterone levels are the best reflection of physiologically active androgen. Free testosterone levels measure the concentration of testosterone not bound to any plasma protein in the circulation. When compared with young adult men, elderly men experience an almost 20% increase in SHBG-bound testosterone in the circulation. Therefore, elderly men may develop symptoms of hypogonadism despite having serum total testosterone levels near the normal range.

Free testosterone levels are altered by the concentration of SHBG. Thus, free testosterone levels are preferred to assess testosterone adequacy in patients with concurrent illnesses known to alter SHBG, when patients are taking medications that increase or decrease levels of SHBG (Table 25-2), or when a patient has symptoms of hypogonadism but has a serum total testosterone in the equivocal range.[2,7,9] A free testosterone level that is <6.5 ng/dL in the presence of symptoms of hypogonadism strongly suggests that the patient would benefit from testosterone replacement.[19,20]

Free testosterone levels are subject to the same diurnal patterns of total testosterone levels. Therefore, samples should be drawn in the morning.[2,23] The most accurate assay methods for free testosterone are centrifugal ultrafiltration and an

## MINICASE 1

## Erectile Dysfunction and Low Serum Testosterone Levels

John A. is a 60-year-old white man who reports erectile dysfunction and no sexual drive. He feels like he is disappointing his sexual partner because he has no desire for sexual intercourse and cannot seem to perform adequately. He attributes all of this to getting older and wonders if a pill can "make him better."

Cc: John A. has erectile dysfunction and decreased libido.

HPI: John A. reports that the problem has been getting worse over the past 2 years. Initially, he had periodic erectile dysfunction. Now, he has no nocturnal erections and cannot get an erection when he needs it. He still has morning erections.

PMH: Essential hypertension and hypercholesterolemia

Medications: hydrochlorothiazide, valsartan, and atorvastatin

Allergies: None

Physical exam:

ROS: Well-developed, well-nourished man with mild nocturia and some urinary hesitancy, particularly in the morning

Vital signs: blood pressure (BP) 140/87 mg Hg; heart rate (HR) 65 beats/min; respiratory rate (RR) 16 breaths/min; temperature 98.6°F; weight 75 kg; height 5'11"; BMI 23 kg/m²

Genitourinary tract: Normal penis, no curvature; testes, mildly atrophic; anal sphincter tone intact and within normal limits; digital rectal exam reveals mildly enlarged prostate; pedal pulses, PSA 1.2 ng/mL from 1 month ago

Assessment: Suspect late-onset hypogonadism with erectile dysfunction and BPH

QUESTION: A serum total testosterone level is ordered. The result is 200 ng/dL. Is testosterone supplementation indicated?

DISCUSSION: The patient's decreased libido and erectile dysfunction are consistent with late-onset hypogonadism. His serum testosterone is also significantly below the normal range. He is a candidate for testosterone supplementation once the low serum testosterone level is confirmed with a repeat serum testosterone level.

equilibrium dialysis technique. However, such assays are not routinely available, are time-consuming, and are expensive. Thus, many laboratories offer radioimmunoassay for free testosterone levels. Although inexpensive, this method is associated with less accurate results.[24] Also, saliva specimens using a direct luminescence immunoassay can be used to measure free testosterone.[25]

If free testosterone levels cannot be measured using an assay, the level may be estimated (a commonly used calculator is available at http://www.issam.ch/freetesto.htm). By inserting the values for measured serum levels of albumin, SHBG, and total testosterone into the online calculator, the patient's free testosterone level is derived. Estimated values are comparable to measured values by equilibrium dialysis.[26]

### Bioavailable Testosterone

*Normal age-related ranges for adult men as are follows:*
  *20 to 29 years, 83 to 257 ng/dL*
  *30 to 39 years, 72 to 235 ng/dL*
  *40 to 49 years, 61 to 213 ng/dL*
  *50 to 59 years, 50 to 190 ng/dL*
  *60 to 69 years, 40 to 168 ng/dL*
  *>70 years, not established*
It is also expressed as a percentage of total serum testosterone.
  *Normal range, adult men: 12.3% to 63%*
Bioavailable testosterone levels measure the concentration of free testosterone and testosterone loosely bound to albumin, corticosteroid-binding globulin, or orosomucoid in a serum sample.[4,7] Because these plasma proteins have low affinity for and reversibly bind to testosterone, an equilibrium is established

between free testosterone and the fraction that is loosely bound to these plasma proteins. Thus, testosterone loosely bound to these proteins is considered bioavailable and physiologically active.[4,7]

As men age, bioavailable testosterone levels decrease as serum SHBG levels increase. Bioavailable testosterone levels may be preferred when assessing testosterone activity in patients with significant alterations of SHBG or albumin (**Table 25-6**).

**TABLE 25-6.** Comparison of the Percentage of Serum Bioavailable Testosterone in Young Versus Old Men

|  | YOUNG MEN | OLDER MEN |
|---|---|---|
| % of total testosterone, which is free testosterone | 2 | 2 |
| % of total testosterone, which is bound to albumin | 38 | 20 |
| % of total testosterone, which is bound to SHBG | 60 | 78 |
| % of bioavailable testosterone (% free + % albumin-bound) | 40 | 22 |

*Source:* Adapted with permission from Lombardo F, Lupini C, Meola A, et al. Clinical and laboratoristic strategy in late onset hypogonadism. *Acta Biomed.* 2010;81(suppl 1):85–88.

An ammonium sulfate precipitation assay or the concanavalin A method is used to measure bioavailable testosterone.[4] It is expensive and technically challenging to perform. For this reason, this test is not commonly available in clinical laboratories. If bioavailable testosterone levels cannot be measured using an assay, the level may be estimated (a commonly used calculator is available at http://www.issam.ch/freetesto.htm). By inserting the values for measured serum levels of albumin, SHBG, and total testosterone into the online calculator, the patient's bioavailable testosterone level is derived.

# ERECTILE DYSFUNCTION

*Erectile dysfunction* is the consistent inability over a minimum duration of 3 months to achieve a penile erection that is sufficient for satisfactory sexual intercourse and sexual performance and is sexually satisfying.[27,28] The prevalence of erectile dysfunction increases with increasing patient age. According to the Massachusetts Male Aging Study, the prevalence of moderate erectile dysfunction increases in men from the fourth decade of life to the sixth decade of life, from 12% to 46%, respectively.[29] In the health professional follow-up study of men age ≥50 years, the overall prevalence of erectile dysfunction was 33%, with an increased prevalence in patients with risk factors, including cigarette smoking, excessive alcohol intake, sedentary lifestyles, obesity, diabetes mellitus, or cardiovascular disease.[30-32] However, advancing age is not considered an independent risk factor for erectile dysfunction.

The causes of erectile dysfunction are broadly divided into two types: *organic* and *psychogenic*.[27,28] Most patients with erectile dysfunction have the organic type, in which concurrent medical illnesses interfere with one or more physiologic components essential for a penile erection That is, the patient has one or more medical illnesses that impair vascular flow to the corpora cavernosa, impair central or peripheral innervation necessary for a penile erection, or are associated with testosterone insufficiency, in which case the patient develops erectile dysfunction secondary to decreased libido. Other hormonal disorders, including increased estrogen or hyperprolactinemia, may also cause organic erectile dysfunction. **Table 25-7** shows common

**TABLE 25-7.** Common Causes of Organic Erectile Dysfunction

| IMPAIRMENT | HOW IT CAUSES ERECTILE DYSFUNCTION | EXAMPLE DISEASES/CONDITIONS ASSOCIATED WITH THIS TYPE OF IMPAIRMENT |
|---|---|---|
| Vascular | Decreased arterial flow to the corpora cavernosa | Hypertension |
| | | Congestive heart failure |
| | | Coronary artery disease |
| | | Arteriosclerosis |
| | | Smoking |
| | | Obesity |
| | | Peripheral vascular disease |
| | | Chronic, heavy smoking |
| | | Drugs that cause hypotension: antihypertensives, central and peripheral sympatholytic agents |
| Neurologic | Decreased central processing of sexual stimuli or impaired peripheral nerve transmission, which decreases erectogenic reflex responses to tactile stimuli | Stroke |
| | | Diabetes mellitus |
| | | Chronic alcoholism |
| | | Postradical prostatectomy in which pelvic nerve injury has occurred |
| | | Epilepsy |
| | | Multiple sclerosis |
| | | Parkinson disease |
| | | Psychosis |
| | | Major depression |
| | | Pelvic trauma with nerve injury |
| | | Spinal cord injury |
| | | Drugs with anticholinergic effects: antispasmodics, phenothiazines, tricyclic antidepressants, first-generation antihistamines, etc. |

*(continued)*

**TABLE 25-7.** Common Causes of Organic Erectile Dysfunction, cont'd

| IMPAIRMENT | HOW IT CAUSES ERECTILE DYSFUNCTION | EXAMPLE DISEASES/CONDITIONS ASSOCIATED WITH THIS TYPE OF IMPAIRMENT |
|---|---|---|
| Hormonal | Decreased serum testosterone, increased serum estrogen, increased ratio of serum estrogen to serum testosterone, or hyperprolactinemia results in decreased libido; erectile dysfunction is secondary to the decrease in libido | Late-onset hypogonadism<br>Primary or secondary hypogonadism<br>Hypothyroidism/hyperthyroidism<br>Hyperprolactinemia<br>Adrenal gland disorders<br>Drugs with estrogenic effects or that decrease androgen production or action: diethylstilbestrol, LHRH agonists, LHRH antagonists |
| Anatomic | Penile deformity or curvature when erect | Peyronie disease<br>Traumatic injury to the penis |

*Source*: Adapted from references 28,30,32.

**TABLE 25-8.** Comparison of Organic and Psychogenic Erectile Dysfunction

| | ORGANIC | PSYCHOGENIC |
|---|---|---|
| Patient age | Older male | Younger male |
| Onset | Gradual, unless erectile dysfunction is due to traumatic injury | Sudden and complete loss of erectile function |
| Linked to a particular event in the patient's life | No | Yes (eg, divorce, job-related stress, financial stress) |
| Patient has a normal libido | Yes | No |
| Patient has nocturnal erections, which are reflex reactions | No | Yes |
| Patient has erections on awakening | No | Yes |
| Patient has erections with masturbation | No | Yes |
| Patient has erections with foreplay | No | Yes |
| Patient has concurrent medical illnesses that could contribute to erectile dysfunction | Yes | No |
| Patient's partner is perceived to be a problem in the relationship prior to the onset of erectile dysfunction | No | Yes |
| Patient has performance anxiety prior to the onset of erectile dysfunction | No | Yes |

*Source*: Adapted with permission from references 27,30,32.

causes of organic erectile dysfunction.[28,30,32] Psychogenic erectile dysfunction is commonly situational in that the patient is unable to have an erection with a particular person, has performance anxiety, or is recovering from a major life stress (eg, loss of a job, divorce, death in the family).[30] **Table 25-8** contrasts differences in the clinical presentation of organic and psychogenic erectile dysfunction.

Because type 5 phosphodiesterase inhibitors (eg, sildenafil) are effective in up to 70% of patients independent of the etiology of erectile dysfunction, the diagnostic assessment of these patients has been streamlined. These patients are commonly diagnosed in primary care clinics with a comprehensive sexual history to identify the particular type of sexual dysfunction that the patient has (eg, decreased libido, erectile dysfunction, or ejaculation disorder). Details on onset of symptoms are obtained along with a patient's self-assessment of the severity of the problem using a validated, reliable questionnaire (eg, International Index of Erectile Function) and information on expectations for improved sexual function from the patient and from the spouse or significant other.[33,34]

A comprehensive medical history is then performed to identify treatable underlying diseases that may be contributing to erectile dysfunction (Table 25-7).[28,30,32] In addition, because erectile dysfunction may be the first presenting symptom of underlying cardiovascular or metabolic diseases, the clinician will investigate thoroughly for such conditions.[35] For example, blood pressure is measured and, if elevated, is treated. The patient is instructed to discontinue smoking, if applicable. A physical exam is completed to check for signs of hypogonadism. Peripheral pulses are palpated to assess vascular integrity. A thorough urological examination to evaluate the integrity of the lower urinary tract and functional status of the bladder, urethra, and external genitalia is mandatory. A digital rectal exam is conducted on patients who are ≥50 years. This checks for anal sphincter tone, which indicates adequacy of sacral nerve innervation to the corpora cavernosa; prostate enlargement, which could obstruct urinary flow and lead to incontinence (which has been linked to erectile dysfunction); or a nodular or indurated prostate, which is suggestive of prostate cancer. Finally, an examination of the external genitalia identifies the presence of penile deformity or tissue scarring, which may contribute to erectile dysfunction.

For patients age ≥50 years who have a life expectancy of at least 10 years, prostate cancer screening is conducted. If the medical or medication history suggests that the patient has concurrent medical illnesses that may contribute to erectile dysfunction, laboratory tests should be obtained to determine if these medical illnesses require more aggressive treatment. Such laboratory tests include a fasting blood glucose, HbA1c for diabetes mellitus, a lipid profile for hypercholesterolemia, a urinalysis to check for genitourinary tract disorders, serum testosterone levels for hypogonadism, and a serum prolactin level if the patient has erectile dysfunction, decreased libido, and gynecomastia. Specialized clinical testing is reserved for patients who developed erectile dysfunction at a young age, patients with a family history of cardiovascular disease who cannot be treated with first-line oral erectogenic drugs, patients with a history of pelvic trauma with damage to the vascular supply or neurologic innervation to the corpora cavernosa, or patients who are candidates for vascular correction of erectile dysfunction because of lack of response to drug therapy or noninvasive medical devices. **Table 25-9** provides a brief description of some less commonly used tests for erectile dysfunction that require specialists to perform them and interpret results.[28]

## International Index of Erectile Function, Sexual Health Inventory for Men, and Brief Male Sexual Function Inventory

The *International Index of Erectile Function* (IIEF) is a validated self-assessment questionnaire that includes 15 questions. The patient assesses the presence and severity of decreased libido, erectile or ejaculatory dysfunction, diminished orgasm, and overall satisfaction with his sexual performance for the past month.[33] The questionnaire takes approximately 10 to 15 minutes to complete. Total scores for each domain can be calculated, and each of these scores is associated with a severity level. The IIEF is used at baseline to assist the physician in determining

**TABLE 25-9.** Specialized Diagnostic Testing for Erectile Dysfunction

| TEST | DESCRIPTION | PURPOSE OF TEST |
|---|---|---|
| Nocturnal penile tumescence and rigidity testing | Two strain gauges are placed circumferentially on the penile shaft to measure erectile hardness and frequency of erections when the patient is sleeping. | This test is used to distinguish organic from psychogenic erectile dysfunction. If the patient has organic erectile dysfunction, the test should show that the patient gets no erections when sleeping, whereas a patient with psychogenic erectile dysfunction does get erections when sleeping. |
| Intracavernosal injection (ICI) testing | A single dose of alprostadil, papaverine, and phentolamine is administered as an intracavernosal injection. | If a penile erection is induced by ICI, this allows visual assessment of vascular integrity of penile arterial and venous flow |
| Penile duplex ultrasonography | ICI is performed, then ultrasound and Doppler imaging of arterial flow to the corpora cavernosa is performed. | Allows assessment of the flow through the main dorsal artery and the cavernous artery |

*Source*: Adapted with permission from Burnett AL, Nehra A, Breau RH, et al. American Urological Association Erectile dysfunction: AUA Guideline (2018). https://www.auanet.org/gidelines/erectile-dysfunction-(ed)-guideline#x8057.

the severity of erectile dysfunction. Once treatment is initiated, the patient is asked to complete the IIEF questionnaire again so that the physician can assess the level of improvement in erectile function. The IIEF is summarized in **Table 25-10**.[28]

A shorter self-assessment questionnaire is an abridged IIEF, which includes five of the 15 questions from the original survey that focus on erectile dysfunction; the last question concerns the patient's overall satisfaction with his sexual performance. This is known as the Sexual Heath Inventory for Men.[36] Some clinicians consider this shorter questionnaire to be more practical than the original IIEF. Other commonly used tools are the Brief Male Sexual Function Inventory[37] or the Erection Hardness Scale.[38] **Table 25-11** summarizes the differences among these three self-assessment questionnaires.

## Prolactin

*Normal range, adult men: 0 to 15 ng/mL or 0 to 15 mcg/L*
*(0 to 652 pmol/L)*

The precise role of prolactin in men is unclear; however, it has been hypothesized that high circulating prolactin levels suppress LH and FSH, thereby decreasing testosterone production, decreasing semen volume and spermatogenesis.[39] It also is known that hyperprolactinemia decreases libido, which may lead to erectile dysfunction.

Prolactin is secreted by the lactotroph cells of the anterior pituitary gland in multiple pulses during the day. The normal daily production rate is 200 to 536 mcg/m² total body surface

**TABLE 25-10.** Domains and Maximum Score for Each Domain of the IIEF

| | NUMBER OF QUESTIONS RELATED TO THE DOMAIN | RANGE OF SCORES FOR QUESTION | MAXIMUM TOTAL SCORE FOR THE DOMAIN |
|---|---|---|---|
| Erectile function[a] | 6 | 0–5 | 30 |
| Orgasmic function | 2 | 0–5 | 10 |
| Sexual desire | 2 | 0–5 | 10 |
| Intercourse satisfaction | 3 | 0–5 | 15 |
| Overall satisfaction | 2 | 0–5 | 10 |

[a]This focus area allows for quantitation of ED severity. Score range for erectile function ranges from 0 to 30. A score <10 implies severe dysfunction; 11 to 17 implies moderate dysfunction; 18 to 25 implies mild dysfunction; 26 to 30 implies no dysfunction.
*Source*: Adapted with permission from Rosen RC, Riley A, Wagner G, et al. The international index of erectile function (IIEF): a multidimensional scale for assessment of erectile dysfunction. *Urology*. 1997;49(6):822–830.

**TABLE 25-11.** Summary of Self-Assessment Tools for Patients with Erectile Dysfunction

| | SEXUAL HEALTH INVENTORY FOR MEN (SHIM)[36] | BRIEF MALE SEXUAL FUNCTION INVENTORY[37] | ERECTION HARDNESS SCALE[38] |
|---|---|---|---|
| Number of questions in the tool | 5 | 11 | 1 |
| Focus of questions | Erectile dysfunction | Sexual drive, erection, ejaculation, perception of problems with sexual function, overall satisfaction | Erection hardness |
| Assessment scale | Each item is rated on a 5-point scale; the score for each item ranges from 1–5; total score for the survey characterizes the severity of erectile dysfunction, such that 5–7 equals severe dysfunction; 8–11 equals moderate dysfunction; 12–16 equals mild-to-moderate dysfunction; 17–21 equals mild dysfunction; 22–25 equals no dysfunction | Each item is rated on a 5-point scale; the point scale; the score for each item ranges from 0–4 and each score has an individualized anchor descriptor; total score for the survey ranges from 0–44 and correlates with the patient's overall perception of sexual function and sexual satisfaction. A total score of 0 implies that sexual dysfunction is a big problem, a total score of 22 implies that sexual dysfunction is somewhat of a problem, and a total score of 44 implies that sexual dysfunction is no problem | Scale ranges from 0–4. 0 = penis does not enlarge; 1 = penis enlarges when patient is aroused but is not hard; 2 = penis is enlarged and hard but not hard enough for vaginal penetration; 3 = penis is hard enough for penetration but not completely hard; 4 = penis hard and fully rigid |

area. Although some prolactin circulates in inactive dimeric form (also known as *big prolactin*) or in a less active form complexed to IgG immunoglobulin (also known as *big, big prolactin* or *macroprolactin*), 85% to 95% exists as monomeric prolactin, which is physiologically active hormone.[40] Its pulsatile secretion is predominately controlled by prolactin inhibitory factor, which is thought to be a dopamine$_2$-like substance secreted by the hypothalamus in response to high levels of prolactin in the systemic or hypophyseal portal circulation. A prolactin stimulatory factor also may regulate prolactin secretion; however, its chemical structure still needs to be identified. It may be similar to vasoactive intestinal polypeptide or thyrotropin-releasing hormone, which both simulate prolactin secretion.[40] Prolactin follows a diurnal pattern of secretion, with highest serum levels occurring when the patient sleeps at night. Nadir levels occur between 10:00 a.m. and 12:00 p.m. Prolactin is excreted renally.

True hyperprolactinemia occurs in 1% to 2% of men who present with decreased libido, erectile dysfunction, and gynecomastia and is characterized by the presence of high levels of monomeric prolactin. Medical conditions and medications that can produce hyperprolactinemia are included in **Table 25-12**. They can be broadly classified as disorders of the hypothalamus or pituitary gland, neoplastic conditions, metabolic disorders, or medication-related causes. Whereas hypothalamic (eg, craniopharyngioma), pituitary (eg, large prolactinoma), and paraneoplastic syndromes can cause significant increases in serum prolactin levels exceeding 250 ng/mL,[42] systemic diseases, medications, sleep, pain, or meals cause smaller increases in serum prolactin level that rarely exceed 200 ng/mL.[42-44]

Hypoprolactinemia in a man is a rare condition. The clinical significance of this finding is unknown as it is not associated with symptoms or disease.

Indications for assessing serum prolactin levels include (1) a patient who is <50 years and reports decreased libido, erectile dysfunction, infertility, and gynecomastia or has low serum testosterone levels; (2) a patient who is >50 years and reports gynecomastia; (3) a patient with late-onset hypogonadism and erectile dysfunction whose symptoms are not corrected with a testosterone replacement regimen; and (4) a patient with symptoms consistent with prolactinoma (ie, persistent headache, cranial nerve palsies, and visual field defects). Of note, prolactin levels should not be routinely obtained in patients who present with erectile dysfunction.

It is recommended that blood specimens be collected 3 or 4 hours after the patient has awakened and fasted overnight. Prior to the blood draw, it is recommended that the patient rest for at least 20 to 30 minutes.[40] A diagnosis of hyperprolactinemia generally requires documentation of two elevated prolactin levels.[39]

Assay techniques for prolactin measurement include immunoassays using chemiluminescent, fluorescent, or radioactive labels. To minimize interference of prolactin assays by meals and stress, both of which can increase prolactin levels, and to distinguish macroprolactin from prolactin, polyethylene glycol extraction and centrifugal ultrafiltration assay methods can be used.[41,42] Although simple to perform, the assay methods are sensitive but not specific.

**TABLE 25-12.** Medical Conditions and Medications Associated with Increased or Decreased Prolactin Levels

| INCREASED PROLACTIN LEVELS | DECREASED PROLACTIN LEVELS |
| --- | --- |
| Pituitary adenoma (nonprolactinoma) | Panhypopituitarism |
| Pituitary prolactinoma | Pituitary infarction |
| Acromegaly | Extended critical illness |
| Severe head trauma | Medications: carbamazepine, phenytoin, valproic acid, bromocriptine, clonidine, ergot alkaloids, levodopa, pergolide, nifedipine, rifampin, tamoxifen |
| Craniopharyngioma | |
| Paraneoplastic syndrome with ectopic production of prolactin | |
| Primary hypothyroidism | |
| Renal failure, chronic | |
| Liver cirrhosis | |
| Addison disease | |
| Idiopathic pituitary hyperprolactinemia | |
| Stress provoked by surgery, hypoglycemia, myocardial infarction | |
| Sarcoidosis | |
| Chest wall trauma | |
| Seizures | |
| Epilepsy | |
| Anorexia nervosa | |
| Sexual intercourse | |
| Medications: phenothiazines, butyrophenones, thioxanthenes, buspirone, olanzapine, risperidone, haloperidol, loxapine, pimozide, tricyclic antidepressants, selective serotonin reuptake inhibitors, molindone, quetiapine, monoamine oxidase inhibitors, oral contraceptives, estrogens, megestrol, opiates, methadone, cocaine, tetrahydrocannabinol, antihistamines, ranitidine, cimetidine, metoclopramide, pimozide, reserpine, methyldopa, verapamil, labetalol, phenytoin | |

*Source:* Adapted from references 41–46.

Big prolactin and big, big prolactin (macroprolactin), which are the less active or inactive forms of prolactin, cross-react with prolactin in immunoassays.[45] Macroprolactinemia is diagnosed when the majority of the circulating prolactin is of the macroprolactin form. Separating patients with macroprolactinemia from those with true hyperprolactinemia is important to avoid expensive diagnostic testing and unnecessary or invasive treatment of the former, which is a benign disease. Gel filtration chromatography is considered the gold standard assay.[41,45]

Extremely high serum levels of prolactin may saturate the ability of immunoassays to measure correct levels. This is known as the *hook effect*. Because larger size prolactinomas are associated with higher amounts of prolactin secretion, it may be necessary to dilute the blood specimens of these patients to 1:100 before assaying for prolactin.[41,42,46]

# BENIGN PROSTATIC HYPERPLASIA

*Benign prostatic hyperplasia* (BPH) is an enlargement of the prostate gland that occurs in all men as they age. The histologic disease prevalence is 80% in men 70 to 79 years.[47] Furthermore, 50% of men with a histologic diagnosis of BPH develop clinical symptoms of at least moderate severity.[48] Beginning at approximately age 40 years in men, the prostate gland undergoes a second growth spurt, which is stimulated by DHT, and the prostate grows from a normal adult size of 15 to 20 g to a much larger size that can exceed 100 g. The local complications of BPH include obstructive and irritative voiding symptoms. Collectively, these symptoms are often referred to as *lower urinary tract symptoms* (LUTS); however, they are not specific for BPH and may be due to other genitourinary tract disorders (eg, neurogenic bladder, prostate cancer, urethral stricture, prostatitis, and urinary tract infection).[49] Obstructive symptoms include a slow urinary stream, difficulty emptying urine out of the bladder, hesitancy, dribbling, a sensation of incomplete bladder emptying, and straining to void. Such symptoms can be due to the enlarged prostate, which produces an anatomic block of the bladder neck. In time, this causes hypertrophy of the bladder muscle and increased intravesical pressure, which translates to urgency, frequency, nocturia, and urge incontinence. These symptoms are referred to as irritative voiding symptoms. If untreated, progressive increased resistance at the bladder outlet will result in decompensation and residual urine, and then total urinary retention and overflow incontinence. Other complications of untreated, severe BPH include recurrent urinary tract infection, urosepsis, recurrent or intermittent gross hematuria, urolithiasis (primarily bladder stones), and chronic renal failure.

The symptoms of BPH are most often the driver that brings the patient to medical attention. Nocturia, which interferes with sleeping, and urgency-associated incontinence, which curbs social activity, can significantly reduce quality of life. Thus symptom assessment is crucial in evaluating the disorder. Symptom assessment is typically completed by having the patient use a validated questionnaire such as the American Urological Association Symptom Index (AUA-SI) score or the International Prostate Symptom Score (IPSS).[48,49]

Signs of disease are evaluated by the physician using clinical procedures that can be performed easily in an outpatient setting. A careful medical history is taken to identify any concurrent medical illnesses or medications (eg, α-adrenergic agonists, anticholinergic agents, or androgens, etc., that may cause or worsen LUTS). A physical examination should be performed to check for bladder distention and neurologic innervation of the lower urinary tract. A digital rectal exam is performed to assess prostate gland size, shape, and consistency as well as anal sphincter tone. In addition, to rule out other common causes of urinary frequency and urgency, physicians should obtain a urinalysis. Microscopic examination of the spun sediment for white blood cells (WBCs) and bacteria and a dipstick check for leukocyte esterase and nitrite help identify urinary tract infection as a cause for the patient's symptoms. If gross or microscopic hematuria is present and the patient has a past or current history of smoking, urine is sent for cytologic assessment. Bladder neoplasms typically shed cancer cells into the urine. For patients in whom the urinalysis is suspicious for renal impairment (eg, protein or casts are detected) or cancer or in whom surgical treatment of BPH is being considered, specialized testing is performed. Serum creatinine level may be assessed to check for evidence of chronic renal disease. If present, such patients have a higher risk of postoperative complications than patients with normal renal function, 25% versus 17%, respectively, and of worsening renal function due to radiographic contrast media if used during imaging to assess renal function and anatomy.[48] In such high-risk patients, a renal ultrasound would be a better test for evaluation of renal anatomy.

Routine objective testing includes uroflowmetry and post-void residual urine volume; both are discussed later. In addition, cystoscopy may be performed. Cystoscopy requires that an endoscope be passed transurethrally so that the urologist can visualize the urethra, bladder neck, and bladder. In patients with BPH, the classic findings are muscular changes in the bladder wall (specifically, smooth muscle hypertrophy) secondary to prolonged bladder neck obstruction. BPH gives the appearance that the three sidewalls of the prostatic urethra bulge out and appear to "kiss" each other.

## American Urological Association Symptom Index, International Prostate Symptom Score, and Benign Prostatic Hyperplasia Impact Index

The AUA-SI is a validated survey instrument administered to the patient. It includes seven questions about the severity of obstructive and irritative voiding symptoms.[48-50] For each question, the patient rates symptom severity on a scale of 1 to 5, where 0 is not at all bothersome and 5 is almost always bothersome. Thus, the lowest total score is 0 and the maximum total score is 35. Scores are interpreted according to the following ranges:

- No or mild symptoms, score of 0 to 7
- Moderate symptoms, score of 8 to 19
- Severe symptoms, score of 20 to 35

The AUA-SI is administered to establish a baseline and then is repeated at regular intervals for patients with mild symptoms to determine if symptoms are worsening over time and deserve medical or surgical treatment.[48] Similarly, once specific treatment for moderate or severe symptoms of bladder outlet obstruction is initiated, the AUA-SI is repeated several weeks after treatment is started to determine if the treatment is effective in relieving symptoms. An effective treatment should reduce the AUA-SI score by 30% to 50% or decrease the score by at least three points[51] (**Minicase 2**).

The IPSS is a survey tool that includes all seven questions in the AUA-SI plus one additional question about the impact of the patient's voiding symptoms on overall quality of life. The last question is not included in the total score. Therefore, the total score ranges from 0 to 35, with 0 indicating that the patient has no symptoms and 35 indicating that the patient has severe symptoms.

Both the AUA-SI score and the IPSS may not correlate with the actual severity of the patient's obstruction. This is partly because some patients deny the presence of LUTS and attribute their symptoms to getting older. Furthermore, the AUA-SI score and the IPSS do not always correlate with prostate gland size, urinary flow rate, or postvoid residual urine volume. However, patients with a high AUA-SI score and a high IPSS generally show significant improvement with surgical treatment for BPH.[49]

The BPH Impact Index is a four-question tool. For the first three questions, the patient rates voiding symptoms on a scale of 0 (not bothersome) to 3 (causes a lot of bother). The fourth question focuses on the impact of the patient's voiding symptoms on daily activities, which is rated on a scale of 0 (no impact) to 4 (impacts my activities all of the time). The BPH Impact Index may be used in conjunction with the AUA-SI to correlate symptoms with quality of life.[52]

## MINICASE 2

### Lower Urinary Tract Symptoms and an Enlarged Prostate

Sam B. is a 70-year-old white man who reports poor-quality sleep. He feels tired all the time when he is awake. He falls asleep when he is driving. He says that he "can't live like this."

Cc: Sam B. has to urinate three times a night, sometimes four, and he cannot get a good night's sleep. His nocturia began about 4 months ago. He has reduced caffeine intake and stopped drinking fluids in the evening to control his symptoms, but he has noticed minimal improvement.

HPI: Sam B. reports that over the last 4 years, his symptoms gradually worsened. He used to get up only once a night to urinate, but over time, the number of nighttime voidings has increased. Now he hardly falls asleep before he has the urge to urinate. He reports no urinary incontinence or blood in his urine. He also states that he has not been treated for urinary tract infections. The last visit to his urologist was 1 year ago, and he was told to reduce caffeine intake and withhold fluids 3 hours before bedtime. No medications were prescribed. At that time, the urologist told him that his problem was a natural part of getting old, that his prostate was big, and that he should not worry.

Sam B. remembers that the urologist ran some tests, but he does not remember the results.

PMH: Diabetes mellitus, type II

Medications: metformin

Allergies: ampicillin (skin rash, all over his trunk)

Physical exam:

ROS: Well-developed, well-nourished male with nocturia × 3

Vital signs: BP 138/85 mm Hg; HR 70 beats/min; RR 15 breaths/min; temperature 98.6°F; weight 80 kg; height 5'10"

Genitourinary tract: Normal penis, no curvature; testes, mildly atrophic; anal sphincter tone intact

and within normal limits; digital rectal exam reveals enlarged, symmetric, soft prostate, approximately 40 g, no nodules or induration; pedal pulses +3, bilaterally

Laboratory results: SMA-6 all results are within normal limits; HbA1c 5.5%; PSA (from 2 weeks ago) 2.5 ng/mL

Urinalysis: No bacteria, WBCs, RBCs, or crystals on microscopic examination

Assessment: Nocturia and urinary urgency most likely due to an enlarged prostate; patient is not taking any medications that would exacerbate LUTS; diabetes mellitus is well controlled and is probably not contributing to LUTS

Plan: Conduct assessments to determine the severity of the patient's lower urinary tract symptoms.

QUESTION: From the test results below, how would you assess the severity of this patient's disease?

AUA-SI score: 30

Peak urinary flow rate: 7 mL/sec

Postvoid residual urine volume: 300 mL

DISCUSSION: The AUA-SI score indicates that the patient perceives his voiding symptoms as severe. The peak urinary flow rate is below the normal range, which indicates that he has significant obstruction to urinary outflow from the bladder. He retains a significant amount of urine in his bladder after voiding, as the postvoid residual urine volume is high. This is consistent with bladder outlet obstruction. The patient also reports that he has not been treated for urinary tract infections. In addition, the digital rectal exam reveals a large prostate with no signs consistent with prostate cancer. His PSA is below the age-related normal range, which is consistent with the digital rectal exam findings of an enlarged but noncancerous prostate gland. Thus, this patient has severe lower urinary tract symptoms, most likely due to benign prostatic hypertrophy. He requires symptomatic treatment.

## Digital Rectal Exam of the Prostate

*Normal size in adult men, 15 to 20 g or 15 to 20 cm³*

Because of its location below the urinary bladder, the prostate is difficult to examine directly. Instead, it must be examined indirectly by having a physician insert a gloved index finger into the anus and then digitally palpating the prostate through the rectal wall. This is a simple physical examination procedure that can be performed without any local anesthetic or bowel preparation. The prostate is assessed for its size, shape, consistency, and mobility. A normal prostate is 15 to 20 g in size, is heart-shaped and symmetric, has a soft consistency similar to the thenar eminence of the hand with no areas of nodularity or induration, and should be moveable when pushed with the finger. Patients with BPH have an enlarged, symmetric, rubbery, mobile gland with a smooth surface. In contrast, a patient with prostate cancer could have a variable size (normal-sized or enlarged), asymmetric gland with a nodular or indurated surface on palpation. If the cancer has locally extended to surrounding periprostatic tissue, the prostate becomes fixed in place and is no longer mobile.

The physician can estimate the size of the gland based on the degree to which the examiner's finger can reach up to the base and over the border of the prostate gland. The accuracy of the prostate size assessment by digital rectal exam is dependent on the expertise of the clinician who is conducting the exam. Because of skill variability among clinicians for this physical assessment technique, a transrectal ultrasound (TRUS) is often performed to better assess the volume of an enlarged gland and to check for nodules or induration. TRUS may reveal hyperechoic, hypoechoic, or isoechoic areas of the prostate. By so doing, targets for needle biopsy can be better identified.[48,53]

An accurate prostate size assessment is useful for identifying patients at high risk for developing complications of BPH who would most benefit from treatment with 5α-reductase inhibitors. These agents are most effective in patients with prostates that are least 40 g in size. Treatment can reduce the risk for acute urinary retention, slow BPH progression, and delay the need for surgery.[54,55] In addition, the size of the prostate helps determine the best surgical approach (ie, transurethral versus open) for large prostate glands.

Estimated prostate size does not correlate with the severity of voiding symptoms or degree of bladder neck obstruction.[49] This can be explained by the existence of at least two mechanisms for obstructive voiding symptoms in patients with BPH. In some patients, the obstructive voiding symptoms are caused by the anatomic blockade of the urethra caused by the enlarged prostate gland. In other patients, obstructive voiding symptoms may be due to excessive α-adrenergic stimulation of receptors in the smooth muscle fibers of the prostate and bladder neck, which decreases the caliber of the urethral lumen. Despite the absence of a significantly enlarged prostate gland, the patient may develop significant symptoms.

Alternatively, some patients with BPH have enlargement of the median lobe of the prostate, which grows inside the bladder and produces a ball-valve obstruction of the bladder neck. In this case, the enlarged gland is not palpable on digital rectal exam but must be identified by TRUS.

Finally, during a digital rectal exam, anal sphincter tone is also assessed. The anus is innervated by branches of the pudendal nerve, which emanates from the sacral plexus at S2-S4 and is responsible for bladder contraction and emptying.

## Peak Urinary Flow Rate

*Peak urinary flow rate, normal range: ≥25 mL/sec in young men; ≥10 to 15 mL/sec, minimum, in older men*

The *peak urinary flow rate* refers to the speed with which urine is emptied out of a full bladder. It is assessed as a simple outpatient procedure. The patient is instructed to drink water until his bladder is full and is then instructed to urinate into the uroflowmetry measuring device until he feels empty. The peak urinary flow rate is the maximum flow rate using the time period limited to the interval when the bladder volume was at least 150 mL.[48] The average urinary flow rate is calculated from the total volume (milliliters) of urine collected divided by the total time (seconds) that it took to empty his bladder.

Although there is no absolute cutoff for urinary flow rate that identifies a patient with clinically significant urinary obstruction, a low peak urinary flow rate is suggestive of bladder outlet obstruction, particularly when the peak urinary flow rate is <10 to 12 mL/sec.[48] In addition, a patient with a peak urinary flow rate of <10 mL/sec is more likely to benefit from surgical correction of BPH than a patient with a higher flow rate.[48] However, there is no direct correlation between voiding symptom severity and urinary flow rate, which is likely due to a patient's attribution of voiding difficulty to advancing age (and not due to a prostate disorder) or denial of the presence of symptoms.[48]

In patients with BPH, the urinary flow rate is typically used along with the AUA-SI score and the absence or presence of complications secondary to bladder neck obstruction to assess the severity of the patient's disease.[48] The choice of therapy is influenced by patient perception of symptom severity in addition to objective measures of disease.

A limitation of uroflowmetry testing is intrapatient variability of results from test to test. That is, even if repeated on the same day, the urinary flow rate may not be the same in the same patient.[48] Also, a low flow rate is not specific for BPH. Low flow rates may be due to urethral stricture, meatal stenosis, or neurogenic bladder secondary to detrusor muscle hypotonicity.[48] The latter occurs in patients with diabetes mellitus, peripheral neuropathy, or spinal cord injury.[48]

## Postvoid Residual Urine Volume

*Normal range: <50 mL*

*Postvoid residual urine volume* refers to the amount of urine left in the bladder after a patient empties his bladder and voids a minimum volume of 120 to 150 mL. In a normal person, the postvoid residual urine volume should be 0, usual range 0.09 to 2.24 mL, but may be as high as 12 mL.[56] In patients with BPH, the enlarged prostate at the bladder neck causes an obstruction that makes it difficult to empty urine completely from the bladder. Chronic retention of large volumes of urine increases the risk of urinary tract infections in men with BPH and can lead to decompensation of the detrusor muscle fibers of the urinary bladder, which can result in urinary frequency, overflow incontinence, or urinary retention.

A noninvasive determination of the postvoid residual urine volume with abdominal ultrasonography is inexpensive, readily available, and commonly used.[48] Less frequently, postvoid residual urine volume is measured manually. That is, the patient is asked to empty his urinary bladder. Then a small-bore urethral catheter is inserted up the urethra and into the urinary bladder to drain any residual urine. The urine is collected and the volume is measured. This method is invasive and associated with some risk of urethral injury and pain secondary to catheter insertion.

A specific postvoid residual urine volume has not been identified as a critical value that necessitates treatment, although in clinical practice, a persistent postvoid residual urine volume of ≥50 mL is cause for concern.[48] Although a high postvoid residual urine volume correlates with decreased peak urinary flow rate, the former may not correlate with the patient's reported symptom severity.[48] However, effective drug or surgical treatment that improves symptoms of BPH generally reduces a high postvoid residual urine volume. As a result, clinicians generally evaluate elevated postvoid residual urine volumes in the context of the patient's medical history of recurrent urinary tract infections.

A high postvoid residual urine volume is not specific for BPH or bladder outlet obstruction.[48,57] It is also found in patients with peripheral neuropathies secondary to severe diabetes mellitus, spinal cord injury, or chronic alcoholism.

## PROSTATE CANCER

*Prostate cancer* is the most common cancer of American men and the second leading cause of cancer-related death among American men.[58] The prevalence is highest in men ≥50 years, and the median age at diagnosis is 66 years.[58] The clinical presentation of prostate cancer is variable. In some patients, prostate cancer is slow growing and may or may not be associated with localized symptoms, such as voiding difficulty. Such patients are more likely to die of other concurrent medical illnesses and not prostate cancer. In other patients, prostate cancer spreads quickly, follows a progressive course, and produces many systemic symptoms. Such patients are more likely to die of complications of prostate cancer and its treatment. Today, because of increased screening for prostate cancer, most patients with this disease are diagnosed when their cancer is localized and at an early stage, and the 5-year survival is 100% with surgery or radiation therapy.[59]

The symptoms of prostate cancer are associated with cancer invasion of the prostate gland or tumor spread to metastatic sites. Tumor in the prostate gland generally causes glandular enlargement, which can lead to obstructive voiding symptoms (eg, decreased force of urinary stream, inability to completely empty the bladder, and overflow urinary incontinence, similar to BPH). Tumor spread to bone can cause bone pain and anemia; spread to the vertebral bodies can lead to spinal cord compression resulting in peripheral neuropathies, urinary or fecal incontinence, or difficulty walking; spread to the lymph nodes can cause lymphadenopathy, lower extremity peripheral edema, or ureteral obstruction; and spread to the rectum can cause rectal bleeding.[60]

When a patient has an elevated PSA and a suspicious finding on a digital rectal exam, an ultrasound-guided (or an ultrasound-guided biopsy combined with magnetic resonance imaging) prostate needle biopsy is performed. A tissue diagnosis of prostate cancer confirms the presence of the tumor. Based on the Gleason score of the tumor specimen, PSA, digital rectal exam, transrectal ultrasound of the prostate, and a variety of other tests to check for extraprostatic spread (**Table 25-13**), the clinical stage of disease can be determined and a risk assessment for tumor recurrence can be performed. If a patient has low volume disease on biopsy confined to the prostate, a PSA <10 ng/mL, and a Gleason score ≤6, he is considered to be at

**TABLE 25-13.** Clinical Tests Used to Stage Prostate Cancer

| AREA TO CHECK FOR METASTASES | INITIAL CLINICAL TEST | ADDITIONAL CLINICAL TESTS IF INITIAL CLINICAL TEST IS POSITIVE |
|---|---|---|
| Bone | Bone scan | Bone survey (radiograph of entire bony skeleton) MRI of bone |
| Lung | Chest radiograph | CT of the chest |
| Liver | Liver function tests | CT of the abdomen |
| Lymph nodes | PSA >20 ng/mL or Gleason score of 8–10; or peripheral edema on physical exam; or high-volume disease on prostate needle biopsy | CT of the pelvis MRI of the pelvis Lymph node biopsy |
| Periprostatic tissue (eg, seminal vesicles, fat tissue) | Digital rectal exam of the prostate, TRUS of the prostate, or MRI with ultrasound fusion biopsy | |

CT = computed tomography; MRI = magnetic resonance imaging; TRUS = transrectal ultrasound.

low risk of tumor recurrence and is a candidate for active surveillance, which includes PSA testing every 6 months, a digital rectal exam annually, and a prostate needle biopsy every 1 to 3 years.[60] On the other hand, if the patient has localized disease but is at high risk for tumor recurrence, aggressive treatment that includes surgery and/or radiation therapy with androgen deprivation therapy is indicated for clinically significant disease.

Screening for prostate cancer is recommended for men with at least a 10-year life expectancy. In the past, such screening was performed annually, but it resulted in overdiagnosis of prostate cancer such that patients were subjected to unnecessary and repeated prostate needle biopsies and overaggressive surgical or radiation treatment of a slow-growing, noninvasive, or indolent tumor. Not only are these measures associated with adverse effects but they are also costly to the healthcare system.[61] Finally, screening is associated with improved life expectancy in only about 20% to 32% of patients.[61]

As a result, many professional organizations took a conservative position on who should be screened, when screening should begin, and how often screening procedures should be repeated. Despite differing recommendations for prostate cancer screening among various professional organizations (a sampling of which is shown in **Table 25-14**), the following statements are commonly held:

- Although PSA has been used alone as a prostate cancer screening tool, its specificity is improved when it is combined with a digital rectal examination, performed by an experienced examiner.[70]

- Lengthening the interval between repeat PSA tests from 1 to 2 or more years increases the specificity of PSA when used for prostate cancer screening and reduces the potential harms of screening. This is particularly applicable to patients with very low PSA levels (<1 ng/mL).

- PSA screening should be offered only to men with a life expectancy of at least 10 to 15 years.

- The decision to start prostate cancer screening should be a joint decision of the patient and his physician.[64,67]

- Patients at high risk of prostate cancer include black or African American men and those with a first-degree relative (father or brother) with prostate cancer. These patients should be screened starting at age 40 to 45 years, depending on the national guideline.

- Patients with low-stage, low-grade prostate cancer do not require immediate treatment for prostate cancer. However, they should be managed by active surveillance with repeat PSA testing, digital rectal exams, and prostate biopsies at regular intervals to check for upstaging or upgrading of the disease.[60,62,64,67]

- Patients vary in terms of the value they place on diagnosing and treating prostate cancer early, which should impact joint decision-making by the patient and physician as to the timing and frequency of prostate cancer screening for an individual patient.[60,62]

Currently, there is a focus on the development of new laboratory tests to identify additional tools that can distinguish patients with clinically significant prostate cancer who are at high risk for tumor invasiveness and deserve early aggressive treatment from patients who do not need additional prostate biopsies, frequent PSA testing, or treatment. **Table 25-15** includes some biomarker tests using tissue or urine specimen.[71-74] Some of these tests have not been validated in large-scale clinical trials with long-term follow up of patients, are much more expensive than PSA, may not be covered by insurance plans, and may not be available from all clinical laboratories.[73]

Clinical tests to stage prostate cancer (Table 25-13) fail to identify approximately one-third of patients with low-volume prostate cancer that has spread outside of the prostate gland. Thus, the search continues for improved diagnostic tools. For example, ProstaScint is a type of scan that uses [111]In capromab pendetide, a monoclonal antibody against prostate specific membrane antigen, to detect prostate cancer cells that may have spread to soft tissue outside of the prostate gland.[75] Initial evaluation shows that ProstaScint may be useful for detecting tumor recurrence or identifying patients with disease that has spread locally outside the prostate.

## Prostate-Specific Antigen

*Non–age-related normal range: <4 ng/mL or <4 mcg/L*
*Age-related normal ranges:*
  *40 to 49 years, 0 to 2.5 ng/mL (0 to 2.5 mcg/L)*
  *50 to 59 years, 0 to 3.5 ng/mL (0 to 3.5 mcg/L)*
  *60 to 69 years, 0 to 4.5 ng/mL (0 to 4.5 mcg/L)*
  *≥70 years, 0 to 6.5 ng/mL (0 to 6.5 mcg/L)*

*Prostate-specific antigen* (PSA) is a glycoprotein produced by the androgen-dependent glandular epithelial cells that line the acini and ducts in the transition zone of the prostate gland.[76] PSA is produced by both normal cells and prostate cancer cells. Small amounts also are produced by breast tissue, parotid glands, and periurethral glands. In normal, healthy men, 20 to 45 years of age, mean plasma PSA levels are undetectable or at the low end of the normal range, usually <1.14 ng/mL in white men and <1.37 ng/mL in African American men. PSA is undetectable in younger men because it is carried out of the prostate through ducts to the urethra, where it is passed out of the body in the ejaculate during coitus. PSA liquefies semen after ejaculation. However, once the prostate gland becomes cancerous, the duct system in neoplastic tissue is disrupted. As the gland grows, PSA production increases and it leaks into the circulation, which results in elevated plasma PSA levels.

In the bloodstream, PSA exists in two forms: free PSA (fPSA) and complexed PSA (cPSA). Of the total PSA level measured in plasma, 30% is fPSA, and 70% is complexed to α1-antichymotrypsin (ACT) and α2-macroglobulin (A2M).[76] Free PSA is renally excreted, while cPSA is hepatically catabolized. The plasma half-life of PSA is 2 to 3 days.

In the bloodstream, fPSA exists in several forms. ProPSA is the inactive precursor of PSA and is associated with prostate cancer.[77] It may be modified or clipped to produce two different inactive forms; however, most of it is converted to active (also known as intact) PSA. Active PSA can be converted to inactive PSA or benign PSA (BPSA), which is produced by BPH tissue, as opposed to normal prostate tissue.[76] High levels of BPSA are associated with high-volume BPH and obstructive voiding

**TABLE 25-14.** Comparison of Prostate Cancer Screening Recommendations by Selected Professional Organizations

| ORGANIZATION | AGE (YEAR) AT WHICH SCREENING SHOULD START FOR HIGH-RISK PATIENTS | AGE (YEAR) AT WHICH SCREENING SHOULD START FOR AVERAGE RISK PATIENTS | AGE (YEAR) AT WHICH SCREENING IS NO LONGER RECOMMENDED | RECOMMENDED FREQUENCY OF PSA SCREENING |
|---|---|---|---|---|
| National Comprehensive Cancer Network[60] | 40, if African American or with BRCA-1 or BRCA-2 mutations | 45 | If life expectancy is <10 yr | If PSA >1 ng/mL, repeat every 1–2 yr  If PSA <1 ng/mL, repeat every 2–4 yr |
| American Cancer Society[64] | 40, if male with one first-degree relative with prostate cancer at an early age  45, if black or African American male with first-degree relative diagnosed with prostate cancer at age <65 yr | 50 | If life expectancy is <10 yr | If PSA is 2.5 ng/mL or higher, repeat annually  If PSA is <2.5 ng/mL, repeat every 2 yr |
| U.S. Preventive Services Task Force[65] | The U.S. Preventive Services Task Force recommends discussing with men age 55–69 yr the potential benefits and harms of PSA-based screening for prostate cancer. Screening offers a small potential benefit of reducing the chance of dying of prostate cancer. However, many men experience potential harms: false-positive results that require additional testing and possible prostate biopsy, overdiagnosis, and overtreatment and treatment complications such as incontinence and impotence. Individualized decision-making about screening is recommended.  Patients who are unwilling to be screened or are older than 70 years of age should not be screened. | 55 | 70 | No specific recommendation, periodic screening per patient preference |
| National Cancer Institute[66] | Insufficient evidence to recommend PSA or digital rectal exam | No specific recommendation, periodic screening per patient preference | No specific recommendation, periodic screening per patient preference | No specific recommendation, periodic screening per patient preference |
| American Urological Association[67] | 40, if African American male with family history of metastatic or lethal adenocarcinomas affecting multiple generations and multiple first-degree relatives developed cancers at a younger age | 55; shared decision-making recommended | 70 or if life expectancy is <10–15 yr | Every 2 yr for average-risk patients |
| American College of Physicians[68] | American College of Physicians: 40–45, if African American race and a first degree relative with prostate cancer, or a man with multiple first-degree family members with prostate cancer before age 65 years | 50; shared decision-making recommended | 70 or if life is <10–15 yr | If PSA is ≥ 2.5 ng/dL, repeat annually |
| Canadian Urological Association[69] | Canadian Urological Association: 45–49, with a family history of prostate cancer in a first or second-degree relative. | 50 | If age 60 and PSA is <1 ng/mL, or if age 70 and life expectancy is <10 yr | If PSA is 1–3 ng/mL, repeat every 2 yr  If PSA is >3 ng/mL, repeat more frequently |

BRCA-1 or BRCA-2 = two different mutations of the breast cancer gene.

**TABLE 25-15.** Prostate Tissue and Urine-Based Laboratory Tests for Prostate Cancer Management

| | PROSTATE TISSUE TESTS | | |
|---|---|---|---|
| BRAND NAME OF TEST | HOW TEST IS ASSESSED | IS TEST COMBINED WITH OTHER PARAMETERS? | PURPOSE OF TEST |
| Prolaris® | 46 different genes | Yes. Combined with PSA and Gleason score to produce Prolaris score. | This test helps to predict disease progression in patients with localized disease, which can be used to help decide on the most appropriate treatment or active surveillance. Prolaris score ranges from 0–10. The higher the score, the more aggressive the tumor, and the patient is at high risk of metastases and cancer-specific mortality. |
| ProstaVysion™ | ERG gene fusion (found in aggressive prostate tumors) and PTEN suppressor gene (found in 60% of prostate cancer metastases) | No | If test is positive, it is associated with an aggressive tumor and an unfavorable prognosis. |
| Oncotype DX® | 17 genes necessary for growth and survival of prostate tumor | Yes. Genomic prostate score (GPS) is based on results of this assay, PSA, Gleason score, and NCCN clinical stage of prostate cancer. | If positive, it predicts a patient's risk of cancer-related death and metastases within 10 yr. |
| Decipher® | 22 selected messenger RNA markers | No | Test results are converted to genomic classifier (GC) scores, which predict the rate of metastases within 5 yr. A GC score <0.4 is associated with a 2.4% probability of metastases in 5 yr; whereas a GC score of 0.6 has a 22.5% probability of metastases in 5 yr. This can be used to help with treatment decisions for a patient. |
| ProMark® | 8 protein biomarkers | No | Test generates a personalized score that relates to the aggressiveness of the tumor. Score ranges from 1–100 with higher scores associated with more aggressive tumors. This can be used to help with treatment decisions for a patient. |
| ConfirmMDx® | 3 genes for DNA methylation | No | Used to predict future biopsy results after an initial negative biopsy. If positive, it indicates that the prostate tumor is aggressive. If the patient has an elevated PSA, but has a negative prostate biopsy, this test can detect occult cancer. |
| Mitomic Prostate Core Test™ (MPCT) | Mitochondrial DNA deletion | Yes. Combined with PSA >4 ng/mL, PSADT <3 mo, life expectancy >10 yr, family history, and black race | Used for men with at least one negative biopsy. Results classify patients into two groups. If MPCT negative, patient is at low risk of undiagnosed prostate cancer. If MPCT positive, patient is at high risk of undiagnosed prostate cancer. |

**TABLE 25-15.** Prostate Tissue and Urine-Based Laboratory Tests for Prostate Cancer Management, cont'd

| PROSTATE TISSUE TESTS | | | |
|---|---|---|---|
| **BRAND NAME OF TEST** | **HOW TEST IS ASSESSED** | **IS TEST COMBINED WITH OTHER PARAMETERS?** | **PURPOSE OF TEST** |
| **Urine Tests** | | | |
| SelectMDx® | 2 genes: DLX1 (associated with tumor progression) and HOXC6 (associated with cell proliferation) | Yes. Combined with patient age, PSA, prostate volume, and digital rectal exam | Used in patients prior to first biopsy or after a negative biopsy. Test results stratify patients into two groups: those at increased risk of a Gleason score 7 (aggressive tumor) or higher prostate tumor and those at low risk for an aggressive tumor. |
| ExoDx™ Prostate Test (EPI) | Exosomes and RNA from tumor cells that are shed in urine | No | Used for patient with a negative biopsy. Measurement results in EPI score, range 0–100. Cut off score is 15.6. If score is >15.6, the patient is at higher risk for having a clinically significant prostate tumor. If the score is <15.6, the patient is at low risk of having a clinically significant tumor and this reduces unnecessary additional biopsies. |

EPI = ExoDx Prostate Test; ERG gene = erythroblast transformation specific-related gene; PTEN gene = phosphatase and tensin gene; MPCT = Mitomic Prostate Core Test; NCCN = National Comprehensive Cancer Network.
*Source*: Adapted with permission from references 71–74.

**TABLE 25-16.** Age-Specific Median and Normal Value Ranges for PSA in Adult Men of Various Races

| PATIENT AGE (yr) | OVERALL MEDIAN (ng/mL) | WHITE (ng/mL) | ASIAN (ng/mL) | AFRICAN AMERICAN (ng/mL) |
|---|---|---|---|---|
| 40–49 | 0.7 | 0–2.5 | 0–2.0 | 0–2.0 |
| 50–59 | 0.9 | 0–3.5 | 0–3.0 | 0–4.0 |
| 60–69 | 1.3 | 0–4.5 | 0–4.0 | 0–4.5 |
| >70 | 1.7 | 0–6.5 | 0–5.0 | 0–5.5 |

*Source*: Adapted with permission from references 76,79.

symptoms.[77] Preliminary studies are being conducted to evaluate the diagnostic usefulness of measuring ProPSA, clipped forms of ProPSA, and BPSA. Currently, these forms of fPSA are largely used as research tools.

For the current cutoff value of 4 ng/mL, the specificity of PSA decreases as men age[8] because PSA normally increases as men age and develop BPH. Thus, to minimize the risk of interpreting an increased PSA as due only to prostate cancer, age-related normal value ranges (which have been further delineated for Asian and African American men), as shown in **Table 25-16**, are often provided by clinical laboratories.[76,79] An advantage of age-related normal value ranges is that they increase the likelihood of prostate cancer detection in young men. However, a disadvantage is that they delay biopsies in older men, which can delay the diagnosis of prostate cancer.[76,79]

In some published literature, the normal value of total PSA is considered to be <2.5 ng/dL, particularly in men <60 years.

Thus, patients with a total PSA of ≥2.5 ng/dL would undergo a prostate needle biopsy. This should avoid missing that subgroup of patients with organ-confined prostate cancer who have PSA values in the range of 2.5 to 4 ng/dL.[80] However, lowering the normal value of PSA also is likely to increase the number of biopsies that are negative.

False-negative PSA test results can lead to misdiagnosis and undertreatment. The Prostate Cancer Prevention Trial showed no threshold PSA below which the absence of prostate cancer is guaranteed. Men with PSAs ≤0.5 ng/mL, 0.6 to 1 ng/mL, 1.1 to 2 ng/mL, 2.1 to 3 ng/mL, and 3.1 to 4 ng/mL had a 6.6%, 10%, 17%, 23.9%, and 26.9% prevalence of histologically confirmed prostate cancer, respectively. Of these cases, 10% to 25% had high-grade tumors, which generally carried a worse prognosis than low-grade tumors.[73,76,81]

A 20% biological variation in measured PSA levels has been documented when the PSA ranges from 0.1 to 20 ng/mL.

For this reason, it is common practice to repeat a single elevated PSA and not take action based on a single elevated value.[76,82]

A radioimmunoassay is commonly used to measure total and fPSA levels. Assays are quick to perform and commonly available. Newer commercially available assay kits allow for measurement of PSA concentrations that are <0.1 ng/mL. Several different immunoassays are available, and results are not interchangeable among them. Therefore, it is recommended that the same assay methodology be used when interpreting serial PSA results in an individual patient.[83]

### Four Uses of PSA

As a tumor marker, PSA has several uses: (1) as a diagnostic screening test for prostate cancer, (2) in combination with other clinical tests to determine the clinical stage of disease, (3) to assess a patient's prognosis or likelihood of disease recurrence, and (4) to assess a patient's response to treatment.

As a diagnostic screening test, PSA has high sensitivity (70% to 80%) but low specificity (50%) for prostate cancer when used alone. The positive predictive value of PSA to diagnose prostate cancer is directly related to the PSA value such that the higher the PSA value, the higher the positive predictive value. In the range of 2.5 to 4 ng/mL, PSA has a positive predictive value of 18%. In the range of 4 to 10 ng/mL, PSA has a positive predictive value of 20% to 25%. Above 10 ng/mL, PSA has a positive predictive value of 42% to 64%.[84] PSA is commonly used in combination with a digital rectal examination of the prostate for prostate cancer screening because the combination has better sensitivity and specificity than either test alone. When used in combination with a digital rectal exam, the sensitivity of PSA increases to 85% to 90% and the positive predictive value for a PSA cutoff of 4 ng/mL increases from 32% to 49%.[85]

Although the PSA level increases with the size of the tumor, there is a poor correlation between the PSA level and the actual size of the prostate tumor. However, a semiquantitative relationship exists between the PSA level and the degree of prostate cancer spread such that a PSA level <10 ng/mL suggests that the tumor is confined to the prostate, a PSA level of >20 ng/mL suggests extracapsular spread, and a PSA level of ≥ 80 ng/mL suggests advanced disease[86] (**Minicase 3**).

Pretreatment PSA is used along with the Gleason score of prostate tissue and the clinical stage of disease to predict the patient's posttreatment risk of disease recurrence.[87-89] This information is then used to guide treatment selection for individual patients. Although multiple risk-stratification schemes have been devised,[87,88] the National Comprehensive Cancer Network stratification guideline is commonly used (**Table 25-17**).[60]

When used to assess a patient's response to treatment for prostate cancer, an elevated PSA prior to treatment should be reduced to the normal range or at least exhibit a 2-fold reduction in PSA level, with effective treatment. For patients with localized prostate cancer, the PSA should be undetectable after a successful radical prostatectomy.

**TABLE 25-17.** Example of National Comprehensive Cancer Center Stratification of Risk for Disease Progression Based on Disease Stage, PSA, and Gleason Score

| RISK CATEGORY FOR DISEASE PROGRESSION | STAGE OF PROSTATE CANCER[a] | PSA (ng/mL) | GLEASON SCORE | TREATMENT OPTIONS |
|---|---|---|---|---|
| Very Low | T1C | <10 | ≤6 | Active surveillance if life expectancy <10 yr; surgery or radiation therapy if life expectancy ≥10 yr |
| Low | T1 to T2A | <10 | ≤6 | Active surveillance if life expectancy <10 yr; surgery or radiation therapy if life expectancy ≥10 yr |
| Intermediate, favorable | T2B to T2C | 10–20 | 7 | Active surveillance if life expectancy <10 yr; radiation therapy with or without androgen deprivation therapy, or surgery with or without androgen deprivation therapy if life expectancy ≥10 yr. |
| High | T3A | >20 | 8–10 | Radiation therapy with or without androgen deprivation therapy, or surgery with or without androgen deprivation therapy if life expectancy ≥10 yr. |

[a]Stages T1 and T2 refer to localized to the prostate. Stage T3 refers to cancer that has directly extended to periprostatic tissue or seminal vesicles. Stage T4 is metastatic to lymph nodes, bone, or soft tissues distant from the prostate. The alphabetic letter refers to the volume of the prostate cancer tissue. A = one focus; B = two foci; and C = multiple foci of tumor.

*Source:* Adapted with permission from National Comprehensive Cancer Network (NCCN) guideline version 2. Prostate cancer early detection; 2019. www2.tri-kobe.org/nccn/guideline/urological/English/prostate_detection.pdf.

## MINICASE 3

## Interpreting Prostate-Specific Antigen in a Patient with Prostate Cancer

Robert R. is a 70-year-old black man with cancer of the prostate diagnosed 2 years ago. At that time, his disease was localized to the prostate, and he was offered active surveillance with PSA testing every 6 months and an annual digital rectal exam. However, his most recent three PSAs show an upward trend.

HPI: On a routine annual physical exam, Robert R. has an abnormal digital rectal exam. The prostate is enlarged and asymmetric. A 1-cm indurated area is palpated and subsequently biopsied; it shows adenocarcinoma, Gleason grade 8 in 60% of the biopsy specimens. Three PSA tests, conducted 1 month apart prior to the prostate needle biopsy, showed the following results:

January: 10 ng/mL

February: 20 ng/mL

March: 25 ng/mL

The patient's liver function tests, blood urea nitrogen, and serum creatinine are all normal.

PMH: Hypertension; leg cramps occasionally at night

Medications: lisinopril 20 mg orally once a day; aspirin 325 mg orally once a day

Allergies: None

Vital signs: BP 135/80 mg Hg; HR 80 beats/min; RR 15 breaths/min; weight 190 lb

QUESTION: What does the patient's PSA suggest about his disease? What additional tests should be performed to confirm the stage of prostate cancer?

DISCUSSION: This patient's PSADT is less than 3 months and is associated with prostate cancer recurrence. This is not unexpected based on his most recent prostate biopsy result, which showed Gleason grade 8 prostate cancer in most of the specimen. That finding suggests that the patient is at high risk of tumor metastasis. To determine if tumor has spread outside the prostate, additional testing should include liver enzymes, bone scan, magnetic resonance imaging of the prostate, computed tomography of the pelvis, and chest radiograph.

### Factors That Alter Prostate-Specific Antigen Levels

Prostate-specific antigen serum levels are affected by several patient factors (**Table 25-18**).[90,91] Decreased PSA levels are associated with obesity. It has been postulated that obese patients have larger circulating plasma volumes, which dilute PSA concentrations in the bloodstream.[94] Decreased PSA also is seen in hypogonadism, which results in shrinkage of the prostate gland—the major site of PSA production. Increased PSA levels are observed in some elderly patients because BPH occurs with a high prevalence, and the increased prostate volume results in an increased volume of glandular epithelial tissue. Also, increased PSA normal range levels are reported in African American men <60 years.[95] The reason for this is unknown. Inflammatory disorders of the prostate, including prostatitis, or manipulation of the prostate during a digital rectal exam or massage may increase PSA.

### Medications That May Alter Prostate-Specific Antigen Levels

Of importance, the 5α-reductase inhibitors (eg, finasteride [Proscar] and dutasteride [Avodart]), generally produce an average 50% reduction in PSA after 6 months of continuous treatment. This has been reported with usual daily doses of both finasteride and dutasteride daily for treatment of BPH and also with the lower daily dose of finasteride used for androgenetic alopecia.[96-98] To preserve the usefulness of PSA as a tumor marker in patients who are taking 5α-reductase inhibitors, it is essential to obtain a pretreatment PSA as a baseline. When PSA levels are repeated after at least 6 months of treatment, it is recommended to double the measured PSA level before

interpreting it. If a patient has a PSA level that is significantly higher than baseline after 6 months of treatment, it is recommended that the patient be evaluated for causes of the abnormal PSA level, including prostate cancer. If the patient has not experienced a 50% decrease in measured PSA level after 6 months of treatment, it is recommended that the patient be questioned as to his adherence with the prescribed regimen.

Another interesting aspect of the effect of finasteride on PSA levels is that when finasteride was used to prevent prostate cancer, it appeared to increase the sensitivity of PSA as a screening test for prostate cancer and to improve the ability of the prostate needle biopsy to detect prostate cancer.[97] It is likely that because finasteride shrinks the prostate, it is easier to locate a suspicious nodule or area of induration when performing a digital rectal exam or prostate biopsy.

An increase in PSA can occur for up to 14 weeks after docetaxel treatment of castration-resistant prostate cancer or 17 to 18 months after radiation therapy for prostate cancer.[99,100] This phenomenon is known as *PSA bounce* or *PSA flare*. Such increases in PSA should not be interpreted as biochemical evidence of disease relapse or should not be used to decide additional treatment for the patient. Instead, in the face of metastatic prostate cancer, other objective signs of disease progression should be used to make treatment-related decisions.

To minimize the impact of noncancerous conditions on PSA, it is recommended to allow an adequate interval after the condition has resolved before measuring PSA. Consideration of PSA's plasma half-life of 2 to 3 days along with the time it takes the condition to resolve affects the time interval. For example, following transurethral prostatectomy, it is recommended to wait

**TABLE 25-18.** Diseases, Procedures, and Medications That Increase or Decrease (Total) PSA

| INCREASE PSA | DECREASE PSA |
|---|---|
| BPH | Obesity |
| Prostatitis, infectious or inflammatory | Hypogonadism |
| Prostate trauma (eg, massage, biopsy, digital rectal exam) | Medications: 5α-inhibitors (eg, finasteride, dutasteride), HMG-CoA reductase inhibitors (eg, statins), aspirin, thiazide diuretics |
| | Herbals: saw palmetto |
| Prostate surgery or procedures[a] | |
| Urethral catheterization | |
| Acute urinary retention | |
| Urinary tract infection | |
| Ejaculation | |
| Exercising on a bicycle for 30 min | |
| Medications: parenteral testosterone supplements | |
| PSA bounce after radiation treatment for prostate cancer | |

HMG-CoA = 3-hydroxy-3-methylglutaryl-coenzyme A.
[a]Procedures that have minimal effect on (total) PSA: digital rectal exam, transrectal ultrasound of the prostate, cystoscopy, and urethral catheterization.
*Source*: Adapted with permission from references 76,92,93.

6 weeks before obtaining a PSA, whereas following ejaculation, it is recommended to wait only 2 days. Prostatitis produces sustained elevations in PSA until the infection or inflammation is resolved; therefore, it is recommended that PSA testing be held for up to 8 weeks after symptom resolution. Also, in a patient with PSA levels in the gray zone of 4 to 10 ng/mL who has a normal digital rectal exam and no evidence of infection on urinalysis, a short 3-week treatment course of antibiotics (to treat a presumptive prostate infection) has been used before repeating the PSA. In some cases, the PSA returns to the normal range. This strategy has been used to avoid unnecessary biopsies; however, it is considered a controversial measure at this time.[101]

### PSA Gray Zone

The total PSA range of 4 to 10 ng/mL is a gray-zone range because the increase in PSA in many cases is due to BPH and not prostate cancer. Thus, to improve the usefulness of total PSA as a screening test when the digital rectal exam is normal, to

reduce the number of unnecessary prostate biopsies, or to better assess prognosis of patients, the following strategies have been recommended by some investigators[72,102]:

- PSA density (PSAD). The PSAD is increased in patients with prostate cancer as compared with patients with BPH. The PSAD is calculated by dividing the total PSA by the prostate volume as determined by TRUS. A normal PSAD is <0.15 ng/mL/cm³. If the PSAD is ≥0.15 ng/mL/cm³, it suggests that the patient's increased PSA is due to prostate cancer, and this patient should undergo additional diagnostic testing. However, this cutoff value has only 50% sensitivity, and it misses many patients with prostate cancer.[103] In addition, to derive PSAD, a TRUS must be performed. This adds an extra cost and is usually uncomfortable for the patient. Finally, a TRUS measurement of prostate volume is difficult to reproduce in the same patient.[76]

- PSA velocity. The PSA velocity refers to the rate of increase in PSA values over time and is based on the concept that a faster rate of rise is suggestive of the presence of prostate cancer. To determine PSA velocity, the patient must have at least three PSA tests performed, one at least 3 to 6 months apart; alternatively, the patient must have three PSA tests performed over a 1.5-year period.[72,103,104] A PSA velocity of >0.75 ng/mL/yr suggests that the patient has prostate cancer and should undergo additional diagnostic testing. A PSA velocity that is >0.75 ng/mL/yr has a sensitivity of 90% to 100% and a specificity of 95% as a screening test for prostate cancer. In men <60 years whose lifespans are potentially more severely impacted by aggressive prostate cancer, it is suggested that a PSA velocity >0.4 ng/mL/yr be used as a threshold value.[104] PSA velocity is affected by the intrapatient variation of PSA values. That is, a PSA value may fluctuate 10% to 25% from day to day in the same patient. For this reason, it may be difficult to derive a consistent PSA velocity value for a patient. Thus, some recommend that the trend of an increase in PSA values over a 1.5-year period be considered as suggestive of prostate cancer in place of the 0.75-ng/mL/yr cutoff.[76] However, the long period of time needed to collect enough PSA measurements to determine PSA velocity is a significant disadvantage of using this strategy. It also should be noted that a recent analysis of more than 5,500 men in the Prostate Cancer Prevention Trial showed no advantage of PSA velocity over PSA in clinical practice.[105,106]

- PSA doubling time (PSADT). The PSADT is the length of time it takes for the PSA level to double. The preoperative PSADT has been used to indicate the presence of a more aggressive tumor and predict cancer recurrence after radical prostatectomy. A preliminary study suggests that a PSADT of <3 months indicates that the patient probably has tumor recurrence, has metastatic disease, and is at high risk of prostate cancer–related death; a PSADT <12 months suggests that the patient is at risk for tumor recurrence.[72,107] In the past, a disadvantage to using PSADT was the absence of a standardized number and timing of specimen collections for PSA. However, more recently, the Prostate Specific Antigen Working Group has standardized the determination of PSADT by establishing the following criteria: (1) PSA levels should be at least 0.2 ng/L (0.2 mcg/L); (2) PSA levels should be obtained every 4 weeks for 3 consecutive months; (3) the same clinical laboratory should run all the PSA assays using the same method; and (4) the serum testosterone level should be stable during the PSA measurement period.[107]

- Percentage of fPSA (%fPSA). Prostate cancer is associated with a decreased %fPSA and an increased %cPSA because cPSA produced by prostate cancer cells resists normal intracellular proteolytic processing.[72,74]

  If the %fPSA is <25%, the patient has up to a 56% probability of having prostate cancer (**Table 25-19**).[108,109] One study showed that in the PSA range of 2.5 to 10 ng/mL, the %fPSA cutoff of 25% had more than a 90% sensitivity for screening for organ-confined prostate cancer and reduced unnecessary biopsies by 20%.[109] These findings have been confirmed by other clinical studies.[110,111] Thus, prostate needle biopsy is performed on patients with a %fPSA of <10%; patients with a fPSA of 10% to 25% would be advised to have a prostate needle biopsy. %fPSA levels also identify patients with aggressive prostate cancer. In one study, men 50 to 58 years old had a 2.4-fold increased risk of aggressive prostate cancer when the %fPSA was <20% when compared with men in the same age group with %fPSA percentages >20%.[112]

  Free PSA is renally excreted; therefore, in patients with renal failure, the fPSA level increases.[113] Free PSA increases after digital rectal exam of the prostate, prostate needle biopsy, and ejaculation. 5α-reductase inhibitors decrease fPSA and cPSA but do not affect the ratio of the two; therefore, fPSA percentages are not affected by these medications. Free PSA blood specimens are subject to degradation if stored for long periods of time at ambient temperature. It is recommended that specimens for fPSA be stored at –70°C or assayed within 3 hours of specimen collection.

- cPSA. As previously mentioned, prostate cancer is associated with an increased fraction of cPSA. With this assay, the concentration of PSA complexed to ACT and A2M is measured. Using the PSA normal value of 4 ng/mL, the cPSA normal value is 3.1 ng/mL. Although cPSA assays appear to be comparable in sensitivity to but have higher specificity than total PSA assays, cPSA assays have not replaced PSA assays.[114]

- Prostate Health Index (PHI). The PHI is mathematically calculated from three laboratory test values for total PSA, fPSA, and proPSA. The PHI is used to distinguish patients with prostate cancer from those with benign prostate disorders, identify patients who likely have clinically significant high-grade prostate cancer and should undergo prostate biopsy, and identify patients who were undergoing active surveillance but should be offered treatment.[73,74,115,116] A PHI of ≥30 to 35 is associated with a clinically significant prostate tumor as defined by a Gleason score of ≥7. A meta-analysis of eight studies showed that PHI has a sensitivity for detecting prostate cancer of 90% and a specificity of 31.6%.[117] When the PHI is <25.0 to 28.6, it implies that the increased PSA is probably not due to prostate cancer; therefore, prostate biopsy is not necessary. Using this PHI cut off score reduces 40% of unnecessary prostate biopsies but misses a prostate cancer diagnosis in approximately 5% to 10% of patients.[73,75,117-120]

- 4K Score. The *4K score* is based on measurement of four blood tests: total PSA, fPSA, intact PSA, and hK2, an enzyme known as human kallikrein that is thought to promote cancer growth. These lab values are combined with patient age, digital rectal exam findings, and previous prostate biopsy findings to produce a 4K score that estimates a patient's risk of having high grade prostate cancer (ie, with a Gleason score of ≥7) and the need for aggressive treatment.[119,121] A score of ≥7.5% is associated with a sensitivity of 94% in identifying patients at high risk of a clinically significant tumor and high risk of prostate cancer-related death. A score <7.5% is associated with a low likelihood of prostate cancer metastases and low risk of prostate cancer–related death.[72,74,121,122]

## Gleason Scoring of a Prostate Biopsy Specimen

A needle biopsy of the prostate is used to establish a tissue diagnosis of prostate cancer. It may be performed transrectally in one of three ways: digitally guided, guided by TRUS, or guided by real-time ultrasound fused to magnetic resonance imaging.[123,124]

The false-negative rate is 20% to 25% when four to six biopsy specimens are obtained from the base lateral midportion and apex of the prostate gland.[125] To reduce the false-negative rate, the number of random biopsy specimens is increased from six to 8 to 20.[126,127] With the increase in tissue sampling, the false-negative rate is only 4%.[128] **Table 25-20** shows the probability of

**TABLE 25-19. Estimated Probability of Prostate Cancer Depending on the Percentage of Free PSA**

| FREE PSA RANGE (%) | PROBABILITY OF PROSTATE CANCER (%) |
|---|---|
| 0–10 | 56 |
| 10–15 | 28 |
| 15–20 | 20 |
| 20–25 | 16 |
| >25 | 8 |

*Source*: Adapted with permission from references 108,109.

**TABLE 25-20. Common Interpretation of Increased PSA Laboratory Values as They Relate to Prostate Needle Biopsy for Prostate Cancer**

| | |
|---|---|
| 0–3.9 ng/mL | Normal range |
| 4–9 ng/mL | Biopsy is recommended (the probability of detecting prostate cancer is 25% to 30%) |
| ≥10 ng/mL | Biopsy is recommended (the probability of prostate cancer is at least 50%) |

detecting prostate cancer from a prostate needle biopsy based on the patient's prebiopsy PSA.

All biopsy specimens are sent to the pathologist for examination. If prostate cancer is detected microscopically, the sample is graded histologically. The *Gleason scoring* system is used to grade the pattern of glandular differentiation of the prostate tumor. Two grades are assigned: one for the dominant pattern of glandular differentiation and one for the less prevalent pattern. Uniform, round, well-formed cells would be graded as 1 or 2, whereas solid sheets of tumor cells without gland formation would receive a grade of 5. Transition between these two extremes would be graded as 3 or 4. Two grades are assigned if two patterns of infiltration are identified. If only one pattern of infiltration is evident, the same number is assigned twice. The two numbers are then added to give the Gleason score, which can range from 6 to 10. The Gleason score correlates with progression of the tumor and the patient's prognosis; the higher the score, the worse the prognosis. A single tissue specimen score of 4 or more or a total score of ≥7 suggests that the patient is at intermediate or high risk of developing metastatic disease (Table 25-17).

Prostate needle biopsy is an invasive procedure. It can be painful and result in minor bleeding and infection. Severe adverse effects requiring hospitalization can occur in 1% of patients.

## PCA3 Score (Progensa)

Unlike PSA, which is secreted by both normal prostate and prostate cancer cells, *PCA3* (also known as *DD3 prostate-specific gene* or *differential display code 3*) is a long noncoding RNA marker that is expressed 10- to 100-fold higher in prostate cancer cells when compared with noncancerous prostate tissues.[73] PCA3 regulates the survival of prostate cancer cells by directing protein transcription and chromosomal remodeling.[73] PCA3 is measured from prostate cancer cells shed in a 20- to 30-mL sample of urine collected approximately 1 hour after a prostate massage, in which each lobe of the prostate is stroked three times.[74] PCA3 does not increase with patient age or prostate volume.[129]

A PCA3 score is mathematically calculated from the ratio of PCA3 RNA copies to PSA RNA copies. A PCA3 score is used in a patient >50 years with one or more negative prostate biopsies for prostate cancer and a PSA of 2.5 to 4 ng/mL. The score is used to guide decision-making regarding the need for a repeat prostate biopsy (because it would likely be negative) in a patient. The cutoff PCA3 score is 25. If the PCA3 score is <25, it is considered a negative test, which is interpreted that it is unlikely for the patient to have a positive biopsy if a biopsy were to be repeated. If the PCA3 score is ≥25, it is considered a positive test, which is interpreted that it is likely that the patient will have a positive biopsy if a biopsy is performed. Using this cutoff score in patient sample, the PCA3 score exhibits a sensitivity of 77.5% and specificity of 57.1%.[74,129]

The PCA3 assay should not be used in patients when the most recent prostate biopsy shows atypical small acinar proliferation or when a patient's current biopsy is <3 months old or >7 years after the last biopsy or to interpret the first prostate needle biopsy of a patient.[130] PCA3 assay results may be altered by radiation therapy to the prostate, prostatectomy, or 5α-reductase inhibitor use.

The PCA3 assay appears to be comparable to PHI but better than PSA or %fPSA as a tool to assist the physician in reducing the number of repeat biopsies that would most likely show low-grade prostate cancer.[72,118] However, collecting the urine specimen after prostate massage for PCA3 is more time-consuming and inconvenient than the blood testing needed for PHI. Additional studies to enhance the sensitivity and specificity of PCA3 scores to detect high grade prostate cancer by combining PCA3 score with a patient's age, race, and PSA, and digital rectal exam findings appear promising.[129,130]

## PROSTATITIS

*Prostatitis* is the most common genitourinary tract disorder among men <50 years. The lifetime prevalence is 15% to 16%.[131-133] Prostatitis is an inflammatory condition of the prostate gland due to an infection or a noninfectious cause. Risk factors for prostatitis include BPH, lower urinary tract infection, sexually transmitted diseases, and stress.[132] The National Institutes of Health (NIH) has stratified patients with prostatitis into four unique categories (**Table 25-21**).[134] Of these, only the first two categories—acute and chronic prostatitis—have infection as the etiology and are generally responsive to antibiotic treatment. For the other two categories—chronic pelvic pain syndrome and asymptomatic inflammatory prostatitis—the etiology is unclear, which accounts for the low response rates to existing treatments. Chronic pelvic pain syndrome can be inflammatory or noninflammatory (ie, inflammation is evidenced by the presence of WBCs in the expressed prostate secretion [EPS], semen, or tissue removed from the prostate during prostatectomy or biopsy).[133]

Differentiation among the types of prostatitis is largely determined by clinical presentation of the patient, digital rectal exam of the prostate, and the laboratory analysis of EPS (Table 23-22). Digital exam of the inflamed prostate is described as boggy or having a softer consistency than usual. Because of the concern that prostate massage could expel bacteria from the prostate into the bloodstream, prostate massage is not performed in patients with suspected acute prostatitis. Instead, symptoms and blood and urine cultures are used to diagnose the disease. EPS is key for diagnosing chronic bacterial prostatitis, chronic pelvic pain syndrome, and asymptomatic inflammatory prostatitis. It is collected after a prostate massage in which the prostate is stroked from side to side and then from top to bottom during a digital rectal exam for 2 to 3 minutes (the resulting fluid is collected as it drips out of the urethral meatus).[134]

To assess symptoms and their severity, the NIH has devised a Chronic Prostatitis Symptom Index, which is a self-assessment tool comprised of 13 questions: eight questions focus on the quality and intensity of the patient's pain, two questions focus on urinary voiding symptoms, and three questions focus on the impact of the symptoms on the patient's quality of life. The total score ranges from 0 to 43; the higher the score, the worse the symptoms.

**TABLE 25-21.** National Institutes of Health Categories of Types of Prostatitis

| CATEGORY | SYMPTOMS/SIGNS | PROSTATITIS CASES (%) | INFECTIOUS ETIOLOGY | RESULTS OF FOUR-GLASS SPECIMEN COLLECTION METHOD |
|---|---|---|---|---|
| Acute bacterial prostatitis | Acute onset of urinary frequency, urgency, dysuria; perineal or suprapubic pain; and urinary retention; may be associated with fever, chills, rigors nausea, vomiting, malaise, myalgia, lower abdominal or suprapubic discomfort perineal or rectal pain; swollen, warm, tense, boggy, tender prostate on palpation; urinalysis shows significant WBCs and bacteria; blood cultures are often positive, urine culture is positive | 2–5 | Yes | VB1 and VB2 are positive for infection |
| Chronic bacterial prostatitis | History of recurrent urinary tract infection; episodes of perineal, penile, suprapubic pain; frequency, urgency, and dysuria, which are separated by asymptomatic periods; symptoms are present for a minimum of 3 mo duration; prostate may be normal on digital rectal exam, may be mildly tender and boggy, or focally indurated with crepitation; urinalysis shows significant WBCs; prostatic fluid is purulent | 2–5, up to 15% in some studies | Yes | EPS and VB3 are positive for infection<br><br>There is a 10-fold or more increase in bacteria in VB3 when compared with VB1 or VB2<br><br>WBCs are present in EPS and VB3 |
| Chronic pelvic pain syndrome that can be classified as inflammatory or noninflammatory | Waxing and waning dull aching perineal, suprapubic, scrotal or penile pain; pain on ejaculation, may be associated with frequency, urgency, and dysuria; minimum of 3 mo duration; digital rectal exam is unremarkable; this is stratified into inflammatory and noninflammatory disease | 90–95 | No | All specimens are negative for infection; patients with inflammatory disease have WBCs in EPS, VB3, and semen; patients with noninflammatory disease have no WBCs or bacteria in EPS, VB3, or semen |
| Asymptomatic inflammatory prostatitis | No symptoms; this is incidentally diagnosed on histologic review of a prostate tissue biopsy specimen; digital rectal exam is unremarkable | Unknown | No | WBCs in EPS, VB3, or semen |

VB1 = first 10 mL of urine voided; VB2 = midstream urine collection; VB3 = first 5–10 mL of urine after prostate massage.
*Source*: Adapted with permission from Nickel JC. Classification and diagnosis of prostatitis: a gold standard? *Andrologia*. 2003;35(3):160–167.

A subscore for pain and urinary symptoms also can be calculated. The subscore range is 0 to 31, with 0 to 9 indicating mild symptoms, 10 to 18 indicating moderate symptoms, and 19 to 31 indicating severe symptoms. This tool is used for a baseline assessment and then repeated at regular intervals during the course of the patient's care. This symptom survey is considered a reliable and valid instrument and is commonly used in practice to assess a patient's response to treatment or disease progression.[133,135]

Chronic pelvic pain syndrome is associated with a plethora of symptoms, and treatment is directed at specific symptoms.[136] As a tool for selecting specific treatments for symptomatic relief, UPOINT is a clinical classification system for a patient's symptoms. Six symptom domains are used: urinary, psychosocial, organ specific, infection, neurologic/systemic, and tenderness. Based on the symptom classification of a particular patient, specific treatments are indicated.[137,138]

## Four-Glass Versus Two-Glass Method of Specimen Collection

The gold standard classic method for collecting a specimen to diagnose chronic prostatitis is the four-glass specimen collection method.[131,132]

- Glass 1 or voided bladder (VB1) specimen (first 10 mL of urine): This represents the urethral specimen.
- Glass 2 or VB2 specimen (a midstream urine collection): This represents the bladder specimen.
- Glass 3 or EPS: After 1 to 3 minutes of prostate massage, EPS drips out of the urethra over the next few minutes. This represents the prostate specimen.
- Glass 4 or VB3 (first 5 to 10 mL of urine after the prostate massage): This sample includes any residual EPS in the urethra. This represents the prostate specimen as well.

Although the four-glass specimen collection method has been considered the standard for diagnosis, it should be noted that the method has not been validated for accuracy.[139] The diagnosis of chronic bacterial prostatitis is made when the bacterial culture in EPS or urine specimen after the prostate massage (VB3) has a 10-fold greater bacterial count as compared with the urethral (VB1) and bladder specimens (VB2).

In addition to sending all specimens for bacterial culture, EPS and VB3 are checked for the presence of WBCs. A drop of EPS is applied to a glass side, a cover slip is placed on top, and the specimen is examined under high power on the microscope. VB3 specimens are typically centrifuged for 5 minutes first, and the sediment is examined in a similar fashion. The presence of >5 to 10 WBCs per high power field is considered significant for inflammation. Twenty or more WBCs per high power field or a VB3 with a WBC count of ≥1,000/µL or more is diagnostic of chronic bacterial prostatitis.[135,140] Finally, it should be noted that when chronic prostatitis is strongly suspected but EPS cultures are negative, semen specimens have been used as a substitute for EPS. However, semen cultures are only positive in approximately 50% of men with chronic bacterial prostatitis.[141,142]

Because of the complexity and time-consuming nature of the four-glass specimen collection method, many clinicians use only a two-glass method (which also is known as the *Nickel premassage and postmassage test*), collecting a VB2 and VB3 specimen premassage and postmassage, respectively. The two-glass method produces results that are comparable to the four-glass method and has a sensitivity and specificity of at least 90% and is 96% to 98% as accurate as the four-glass method.[140] A positive test result is indicated by a 10-fold greater bacterial count in the VB3 specimen compared with the VB2 specimen.

## SUMMARY

This chapter reviews common clinical tests and laboratory tests used for diagnosing and monitoring treatment for common urologic disorders in elderly men, including late-onset hypogonadism, erectile dysfunction, BPH, prostate cancer, and prostatitis. Many of these disorders are managed with tests other than laboratory tests.

## LEARNING POINTS

1. *How does a clinician differentiate between serum total testosterone levels and free testosterone levels?*

   ANSWER: Testosterone circulates in the bloodstream in several forms: free testosterone and testosterone bound to proteins. Most protein-bound testosterone is tightly bound to SHBG and only a small portion is loosely and reversibly bound to albumin, corticosteroid-binding globulin, and orosomucoid. The free testosterone fraction is physiologically active. When a clinician orders a testosterone serum level, the level reflects the total testosterone concentration in the bloodstream, which includes free and protein-bound testosterone. A free testosterone serum level reflects only the unbound portion of testosterone in the bloodstream. A free testosterone level may be measured or calculated. Free testosterone serum levels are indicated in patients in whom the concentration of SHBG is decreased or increased. In such patients, a free testosterone serum level is a better indicator of the concentration of physiologically active testosterone. Increased SHBG is associated with cirrhosis, hyperthyroidism, old age, and drug treatment with estrogens or anticonvulsants. Decreased SHBG is associated with hypothyroidism, obesity, or drug treatment with excessive doses of testosterone supplements.

2. *A 60-year-old man reports urinary frequency and nocturia. He wakes up four times every night to urinate. The patient has a slow urinary stream and incomplete bladder emptying. A transrectal ultrasound of the prostate reveals a 30-g prostate with no nodules or induration. The patient's AUA symptom score is 18. His peak urinary flow rate is 9 mL/sec. How would you assess the severity of this patient's BPH?*

   ANSWER: Based on the patient's AUA symptom score, his voiding symptoms are moderately severe. This is consistent with his reports of urinary frequency and nocturia, slow urinary stream, feeling of incomplete bladder emptying, and urinary flow rate <10 mL/sec.

3. *A patient has symptomatic metastatic prostate cancer and is started on androgen-deprivation therapy with leuprolide and bicalutamide. One month after the start of treatment, the patient reports feeling so much better. His bone pain, tiredness, appetite, and urinary difficulty have all improved. He says that he has gained 5 lb since starting treatment. Before the start of treatment, the patient's PSA was 50 ng/mL. What change in PSA is expected 1 month after the start of treatment?*

   ANSWER: Effective treatment should result in a return to the normal range (ie, PSA <4 ng/mL) or at least a 2-fold reduction in PSA level (ie, PSA 12.5 ng/mL).

4. *A patient with a history of chronic prostatitis and dull rectal pain presents with new-onset dysuria. He has completed a 6-month course of daily therapeutic dosing regimen of trimethoprim-sulfamethoxazole. The results*

*of a four-glass method of specimen collection are as follows:*

- VB1: mixed flora
- VB2: *Streptococcus faecalis* 10⁵ colony forming units/mL
- VB3: no growth
- VB4: no growth

5. *When interpreting the results of the four-glass method of specimen collection, does this patient have recurrence of chronic prostatitis?*

**ANSWER:** The VB2 is a midstream urine collection and shows significant bacterial growth, which suggests that the patient has cystitis. Because the VB3 and VB4, which represent EPS, are negative, chronic prostatitis is ruled out. The VB1 shows mixed flora or contamination of the specimen. No conclusion can be drawn as to whether the patient has urethritis.

## REFERENCES

1. Harman SM, Metter EJ, Tobin JD, et al. Longitudinal effects of aging on serum total and free testosterone levels in healthy men. *J Clin Endocrinol Metab*. 2001;86(2):724-731.PubMed

2. Kanakis GA, Tsametis CP, Goulis DG. Measuring testosterone in women and men. *Maturitas*. 2019;125:41-44.PubMed

3. Conners WP 3rd, Morgentaler A. The evaluation and management of testosterone deficiency: the new frontier in urology and men's health. *Curr Urol Rep*. 2013;14(6):557-564.PubMed

4. Goldman AL, Bhasin S, Wu FCW, et al. A reappraisal of testosterone's binding in circulation: physiological and clinical implications. *Endocr Rev*. 2017;38(4):302-324.PubMed

5. Sandher RK, Aning J. Diagnosing and managing androgen deficiency in men. *Practitioner*. 2017;261(1803):19-22.

6. Hsieh A, DiGiorgio L, Fakunle M, Sadeghi-Nejad H, et al. Management strategies in opioid abuse and sexual dysfunction: a review of opioid-induced androgen deficiency. *Sex Med Rev*. 2018;6(4):618-623.PubMed

7. Lombardo F, Lupini C, Meola A, et al. Clinical and laboratoristic strategy in late onset hypogonadism. *Acta Biomed*. 2010;81(suppl 1):85-88.PubMed

8. Yeap BB, Wu FCW. Clinical practice update on testosterone therapy for male hypogonadism: contrasting perspectives to optimize care. *Clin Endocrinol (Oxf)*. 2019;90(1):56-65.PubMed

9. Rastrelli G, Maggi M, Corona G. Pharmacological management of late-onset hypogonadism. *Expert Rev Clin Pharmacol*. 2018;11(4):439-458.PubMed

10. Bremner WJ, Vitiello MV, Prinz PN. Loss of circadian rhythmicity in blood testosterone levels with aging in normal men. *J Clin Endocrinol Metab*. 1983;56(6):1278-1281.PubMed

11. Morley JE, Perry HM 3rd, Kevorkian RT, et al. Comparison of screening questionnaires for the diagnosis of hypogonadism. *Maturitas*. 2006;53(4):424-429.PubMed

12. Blümel JE, Chedraui P, Gili SA, et al. Is the Androgen Deficiency of Aging Men (ADAM) questionnaire useful for the screening of partial androgenic deficiency of aging men? *Maturitas*. 2009;63(4):365-368.PubMed

13. Moore C, Huebler D, Zimmermann T, et al. The Aging Males' Symptoms scale (AMS) as outcome measure for treatment of androgen deficiency. *Eur Urol*. 2004;46(1):80-87.PubMed

14. Salonia A, Rastrelli G, Hackett G, et al. Paediatric and adult-onset male hypogonadism. *Nat Rev Dis Primers*. 2019;5(1):38 10.1038/s41572-019-0087-y.PubMed

15. Sigalos JT, Pastuszak AW, Khera M. Hypogonadism-therapeutic risks, benefits, and outcomes. *Med Clin North Am*. 2018;102(2):361-372. PubMed

16. Qaseem A, Horwitch CA, Vijan S, et al. Testosterone treatment in adult men with age-related low testosterone: a clinical guideline from the American College of Physicians. *Ann Intern Med*. 2020;172(2):126-133. PubMed

17. Ramasamy R, Wilken N, Scovell JM, et al. Hypogonadal symptoms are associated with different serum testosterone thresholds in middle-aged and elderly men. *Urology*. 2014;84(6):1378-1382.PubMed

18. Wang C, Nieschlag E, Swerdloff R, et al. Investigation, treatment, and monitoring of late-onset hypogonadism in males: ISA, ISSAM, EAU, EAA, and ASA recommendations. *J Androl*. 2009;30(1):1-9.PubMed

19. Dean JD, McMahon CG, Guay AT, et al. The International Society for Sexual Medicine's process of care for the assessment and management of testosterone deficiency in adult men. *J Sex Med*. 2015;12(8):1660-1686.PubMed

20. Lunenfeld B, Mskhalaya G, Kalinchenko S, et al. Recommendations on the diagnosis, treatment and monitoring of late-onset hypogonadism in men: a suggested update. *Aging Male*. 2013;16(4):143-150.PubMed

21. Rosner W, Auchus RJ, Azziz R, et al. Position statement: Utility, limitations, and pitfalls in measuring testosterone: an Endocrine Society position statement. *J Clin Endocrinol Metab*. 2007;92(2):405-413.PubMed

22. Field HP. Tandem mass spectrometry in hormone measurement. *Methods Mol Biol*. 2013;1065:45-74.PubMed

23. Antonio L, Wu FCW, O'Neill TW, et al. Low free testosterone is associated with hypogonadal signs and symptoms in men with normal total testosterone. *J Clin Endocrinol Metab*. 2016;101(7):2647-2657.PubMed

24. Van Uytfanghe K, Stöckl D, Kaufman JM, et al. Validation of 5 routine assays for serum free testosterone with a candidate reference measurement procedure based on ultrafiltration and isotope dilution-gas chromatography-mass spectrometry. *Clin Biochem*. 2005;38(3):253-261.PubMed

25. Goncharov N, Katsya G, Dobracheva A, et al. Diagnostic significance of free salivary testosterone measurement using a direct luminescence immunoassay in healthy men and in patients with disorders of androgenic status. *Aging Male*. 2006;9(2):111-122.PubMed

26. Morales A, Collier CP, Clark AF. A critical appraisal of accuracy and cost of laboratory methodologies for the diagnosis of hypogonadism: the role of free testosterone assays. *Can J Urol*. 2012;19(3):6314-6318.PubMed

27. McMahon CG. Current diagnosis and management of erectile dysfunction. *Med J Aust*. 2019;210(10):469-476.PubMed

28. Burnett AL, Nehra A, Breau RH, et al. American Urological Association Erectile dysfunction: AUA Guideline (2018). https://www.auanet.org/gidelines/erectile-dysfunction-(ed)-guideline#x8057. Accessed September 22, 2020.

29. Feldman HA, Goldstein I, Hatzichristou DG, et al. Impotence and its medical and psychosocial correlates: results of the Massachusetts Male Aging Study. *J Urol*. 1994;151(1):54-61.PubMed

30. Mobley DF, Khera M, Baum N. Recent advances in the treatment of erectile dysfunction. *Postgrad Med J*. 2017;93(1105):679-685.PubMed

31. Bacon CG, Mittleman MA, Kawachi I, et al. Sexual function in men older than 50 years of age: results from the health professionals follow-up study. *Ann Intern Med*. 2003;139(3):161-168.PubMed

32. Bacon CG, Mittleman MA, Kawachi I, et al. A prospective study of risk factors for erectile dysfunction. *J Urol*. 2006;176(1):217-221.PubMed

33. Rosen RC, Riley A, Wagner G, et al. The international index of erectile function (IIEF): a multidimensional scale for assessment of erectile dysfunction. *Urology*. 1997;49(6):822-830.PubMed

34. Rosen RC, Cappelleri JC, Smith MD, et al. Development and evaluation of an abridged, 5-item version of the International Index of Erectile Function (IIEF-5) as a diagnostic tool for erectile dysfunction. *Int J Impot Res*. 1999;11(6):319-326.PubMed

35. Inman BA, Sauver JL, Jacobson DJ, et al. A population-based, longitudinal study of erectile dysfunction and future coronary artery disease. *Mayo Clin Proc*. 2009;84(2):108-113.PubMed

36. Cappelleri JC, Rosen RC. The Sexual Health Inventory for Men (SHIM): a 5-year review of research and clinical experience. *Int J Impot Res*. 2005;17(4):307-319.PubMed

37. Mykletun A, Dahl AA, O'Leary MP, et al. Assessment of male sexual function by the Brief Sexual Function Inventory. *BJU Int.* 2006;97(2):316-323.PubMed

38. Mulhall JP, Levine LA, Junemann KP. Erection hardness: a unifying factor for defining response in the treatment of erectile dysfunction. *Urology* 2006 Sept;68(3A suppl):17-25.

39. Lotti F, Corona G, Maseroli E, et al. Clinical implications of measuring prolactin levels in males of infertile couples. *Andrology.* 2013;1(5):764-771.PubMed

40. Huang W, Molitch ME. Evaluation and management of galactorrhea. *Am Fam Physician.* 2012;85(11):1073-1080.PubMed

41. Suliman AM, Smith TP, Gibney J, et al. Frequent misdiagnosis and mismanagement of hyperprolactinemic patients before the introduction of macroprolactin screening: application of a new strict laboratory definition of macroprolactinemia. *Clin Chem.* 2003;49(9):1504-1509.PubMed

42. Chanson P, Maiter D. The epidemiology, diagnosis and treatment of prolactinomas: the old and the new. *Best Pract Res Clin Endocrinol Metab.* 2019;33(2):101290.

43. Ajmal A, Joffe H, Nachtigall LB. Psychotropic-induced hyperprolactinemia: a clinical review. *Psychosomatics.* 2014;55(1):29-36.PubMed

44. Kim S, Park YM. Serum prolactin and macroprolactin levels among outpatients with major depressive disorder following the administration of selective serotonin-reuptake inhibitors: a cross-sectional pilot study. *PLoS One.* 2013;8(12):e82749.

45. Kasum M, Oreskovic S, Zec I, et al. Macroprolactinemia: new insights in hyperprolactinemia. *Biochem Med (Zagreb).* 2012;22(2):171-179.PubMed

46. Melmed S. Pituitary-tumor endocrinopathies. *N Engl J Med.* 2020;382(10):937-950.PubMed

47. Glynn RJ, Campion EW, Bouchard GR, et al. The development of benign prostatic hyperplasia among volunteers in the Normative Aging Study. *Am J Epidemiol.* 1985;121(1):78-90.PubMed

48. McVary KT, Roehrborn CG, Avins AL, et al. American Urological Association guideline: management of benign prostatic hyperplasia (BPH); 2010. https://www.auanet.org/guidelines/benign-prostatic-hyperplasia-(bph)-guideline/benign-prostatic-hyerplasia-(2010-reviewed-and-validity-confirmed-2014. Accessed June 25, 2020.

49. Bosch JL, Hop WC, Kirkels WJ, et al. The International Prostate Symptom Score in a community-based sample of men between 55 and 74 years of age: prevalence and correlation of symptoms with age, prostate volume, flow rate and residual urine volume. *Br J Urol.* 1995;75(5):622-630. PubMed

50. Blankstein U, Van Asseldonk B, Elterman DS. BPH update: medical versus interventional management. *Can J Urol.* 2016;23(suppl 1):10-15.PubMed

51. Barry MJ, Williford WO, Chang Y, et al. Benign prostatic hyperplasia specific health status measures in clinical research: how much change in the American Urological Association symptom index and the benign prostatic hyperplasia impact index is perceptible to patients? *J Urol.* 1995;154(5):1770-1774.PubMed

52. Kingery L, Martin ML, Naegeli AN, et al. Content validity of the Benign Prostatic Hyperplasia Impact Index (BII); a measure of how urinary trouble and problems associated with BPH may impact the patient. *Int J Clin Pract.* 2012;66(9):883-890.PubMed

53. Roehrborn CG, Girman CJ, Rhodes T, et al. Correlation between prostate size estimated by digital rectal examination and measured by transrectal ultrasound. *Urology.* 1997;49(4):548-557.PubMed

54. McConnell JD, Roehrborn CG, Bautista OM, et al. The long-term effect of doxazosin, finasteride, and combination therapy on the clinical progression of benign prostatic hyperplasia. *N Engl J Med.* 2003;349(25):2387-2398.PubMed

55. Roehrborn CG, Barkin J, Siami P, et al. Clinical outcomes after combined therapy with dutasteride plus tamsulosin or either monotherapy in men with benign prostatic hyperplasia (BPH) by baseline characteristics: 4-year results from the randomized, double-blind Combination of Avodart and Tamsulosin (CombAT) trial. *BJU Int.* 2011;107(6):946-954.PubMed

56. Kolman C, Girman CJ, Jacobsen SJ, et al. Distribution of post-void residual urine volume in randomly selected men. *J Urol.* 1999;161(1):122-127.PubMed

57. Mochtar CA, Kiemeney LA, van Riemsdijk MM, et al. Post-void residual urine volume is not a good predictor of the need for invasive therapy among patients with benign prostatic hyperplasia. *J Urol.* 2006;175(1):213-216.PubMed

58. American Cancer Society. Key statistics for prostate cancer. Atlanta, GA: American Cancer Society. www.cancer.org/cancer/prostate-cancer/about/key-statistics.html. Accessed June 25, 2020.

59. American Cancer Society. Survival rates for prostate cancer. Atlanta, GA: American Cancer Society. https://www.cancer.org/cancer/prostate-cancer/detection-diagnosis-staging/survival-rates.html?_ga=2.56837485.676794644.1593436497-1131046557.1593436497. Accessed June 25, 2020.

60. National Comprehensive Cancer Network (NCCN) guideline version 2. Prostate cancer early detection; 2019. www2.tri-kobe.org/nccn/guideline/urological/English/prostate_detection.pdf. Accessed June 24, 2020.

61. Smith RA, Manassaram-Baptiste D, Brooks D, et al. Cancer screening in the United States, 2015: a review of current American Cancer Society guidelines and current issues in cancer screening. *CA Cancer J Clin.* 2015;65(1):30-54.PubMed

62. Kim EH, Andriole GL. Prostate-specific antigen-based screening: controversy and guidelines. *BMC Med.* 2015;13:6.PubMed

63. Holt JD, Gerayli F. Prostate cancer screening. *Prim Care.* 2019;46(2):257-263.PubMed

64. American Cancer Society. Recommendations for prostate cancer early detection. https://www.cancer.org/cancer/prostate-cancer/detection-diagnosis-staging/acs-recommendations.html Accessed June 23, 2020.

65. Grossman DC, Curry SJ, Owens DK, et al. Screening for prostate cancer: US Preventive Services Task Force recommendation statement. *JAMA.* 2018;319(18):1901-1913.PubMed

66. National Cancer Institute. Prostate cancer screening (PDQ)-health professional version. https://www.cancer.gov/types/prostate/hp/prostate-screening-pdq. Accessed June 23, 2020.

67. Carter HB, Albertsen PC, Barry MJ, et al. American Urological Association early detection of prostate cancer; 2018. https://www.auanet.org/guidelines/prostate-cancer-early-detection-guideline. Accessed June 23, 2020.

68. Qaseem A, Barry MJ, Denberg TD, et al. Screening for prostate cancer: a guidance statement from the Clinical Guidelines Committee of the American College of Physicians. *Ann Intern Med.* 2013;158(10):761-769. PubMed

69. Rendon RA, Mason RJ, Marzouk K, et al. Canadian Urological Association recommendations on prostate cancer screening and early diagnosis. *Can Urol Assoc J.* 2017;11(100):298-309.PubMed

70. Catalona WJ, Richie JP, Ahmann FR, et al. Comparison of digital rectal examination and serum prostate specific antigen in the early detection of prostate cancer: results of a multicenter clinical trial of 6,630 men. *J Urol.* 1994;151(5):1283-1290.PubMed

71. Olleik G, Kassouf W, Aprikian A, et al. Evaluation of new tests and interventions for prostate cancer management: a systematic review. *J Natl Compr Canc Netw.* 2018;16(11):1340-1351.PubMed

72. Duffy MJ. Biomarkers for prostate cancer: prostate-specific antigen and beyond. *Clin Chem Lab Med.* 2020;58(3):326-339.PubMed

73. Liu J, Li Y, Yang D, et al. Current state of biomarkers for the diagnosis and assessment of treatment efficacy of prostate cancer. *Discov Med.* 2019;27(150):235-243.PubMed

74. Carneiro A, Priante Kayano P, Gomes Barbosa ÁR, et al. Are localized prostate cancer biomarkers useful in the clinical practice? *Tumour Biol.* 2018;40(9):1010428318799255.PubMed

75. Rieter WJ, Keane TE, Ahlman MA, et al. Diagnostic performance of In-111 capromab pendetide SPECT/CT in localized and metastatic prostate cancer. *Clin Nucl Med.* 2011;36(10):872-878.PubMed

76. Gjertson CK, Albertsen PC. Use and assessment of PSA in prostate cancer. *Med Clin North Am.* 2011;95(1):191-200.PubMed

77. Shariat SF, Semjonow A, Lilja H, et al. Tumor markers in prostate cancer I: blood-based markers. *Acta Oncol.* 2011;50(suppl 1):61-75.PubMed

78. Loeb S, Roehl KA, Antenor JA, et al. Baseline prostate-specific antigen compared with median prostate-specific antigen for age group as predictor of prostate cancer risk in men younger than 60 years old. *Urology.* 2006;67(2):316-320.PubMed

79. Catalona WJ, Southwick PC, Slawin KM, et al. Comparison of percent free PSA, PSA density, and age-specific PSA cutoffs for prostate cancer detection and staging. *Urology.* 2000;56(2):255-260.PubMed

80. Catalona WJ, Smith DS, Ornstein DK. Prostate cancer detection in men with serum PSA concentrations of 2.6-4.0 ng/mL and benign prostate examination: enhancement of specificity with free PSA measurements. *JAMA.* 1997;277(18):1452-1455.PubMed

81. Thompson IM, Pauler DK, Goodman PJ, et al. Prevalence of prostate cancer among men with a prostate-specific antigen level ≤4.0 ng per milliliter. *N Engl J Med.* 2004;350(22):2239-2246.PubMed

82. Soletormos G, Semjenow A, Sibley PE, et al. Biological variation of total prostate specific antigen: a survey of published estimates and consequences for clinical practice. *Clin Chem.* 2005;51(8):1342-1351.

83. Stephan C, Klaas M, Müller C, et al. Interchangeability of measurements of total and free prostate-specific antigen in serum with 5 frequently used assay combinations: an update. *Clin Chem.* 2006;52(1):59-64. PubMed

84. American College of Physicians. Screening for prostate cancer. *Ann Intern Med.* 1997;126(6):480-484.PubMed

85. Bell N, Connor Gorber S, Shane A, et al. Recommendations on screening for prostate cancer with the prostate-specific antigen test. *CMAJ.* 2014; 186(16):1225-1234.PubMed

86. Montironi R, Egevad L, Bjartell A, et al. Role of histopathology and molecular markers in the active surveillance of prostate cancer. *Acta Oncol.* 2011;50(suppl 1):56-60.PubMed

87. Humphrey PA. Gleason grading and prognostic factors in carcinoma of the prostate. *Mod Pathol.* 2004;17(3):292-306.PubMed

88. Sanda MG, Cadeddu JA, Kirkby E, et al. Clinically localized prostate cancer: AUA/ASTRO/SUO Guideline. Part I: risk stratification, shared decision making, and care options. *J Urol.* 2018;199(3):683-690. PubMed

89. D'Amico AV, Renshaw AA, Sussman B, et al. Pretreatment PSA velocity and risk of death from prostate cancer following external beam radiation therapy. *JAMA.* 2005;294(4):440-447.PubMed

90. Oesterling JE, Jacobsen SJ, Chute CG, et al. Serum prostate-specific antigen in a community-based population of healthy men: establishment of age-specific reference ranges. *JAMA.* 1993;270(7):860-864.PubMed

91. Gelmann EP, Chia D, Pinsky PF, et al. Relationship of demographic and clinical factors to free and total prostate-specific antigen. *Urology.* 2001;58(4):561-566.PubMed

92. Tchetgen MB, Song JT, Strawderman M, et al. Ejaculation increases the serum prostate-specific antigen concentration. *Urology.* 1996;47(4): 511-516.PubMed

93. Shi Y, Fung KZ, Freedland SJ, et al. Statin medications are associated with a lower probability of having an abnormal screening prostate-specific antigen result. *Urology.* 2014;84(5):1058-1065.PubMed

94. Bañez LL, Hamilton RJ, Partin AW, et al. Obesity-related plasma hemodilution and PSA concentration among men with prostate cancer. *JAMA.* 2007;298(19):2275-2280.PubMed

95. Fowler JE Jr, Bigler SA, Kilambi NK, et al. Relationships between prostate-specific antigen and prostate volume in black and white men with benign prostate biopsies. *Urology.* 1999;53(6):1175-1178.PubMed

96. Andriole GL, Marberger M, Roehrborn CG. Clinical usefulness of serum prostate specific antigen for the detection of prostate cancer is preserved in men receiving the dual 5alpha-reductase inhibitor dutasteride. *J Urol.* 2006;175(5):1657-1662.PubMed

97. Thompson IM, Chi C, Ankerst DP, et al. Effect of finasteride on the sensitivity of PSA for detecting prostate cancer. *J Natl Cancer Inst.* 2006;98(16):1128-1133.PubMed

98. D'Amico AV, Roehrborn CG. Effect of 1 mg/day finasteride on concentrations of serum prostate-specific antigen in men with androgenic alopecia: a randomised controlled trial. *Lancet Oncol.* 2007;8(1):21-25.PubMed

99. Karzai FH, Madan RA, Figg WD. Beyond PSA: managing modern therapeutic options in metastatic castration-resistant prostate cancer. *South Med J.* 2015;108(4):224-228.PubMed

100. Naghavi AO, Strom TJ, Nethers K, et al. Clinical implications of a prostate-specific antigen bounce after radiation therapy for prostate cancer. *Int J Clin Oncol.* 2015;20(3):598-604.PubMed

101. Kaygisiz O, Uğurlu O, Koşan M, et al. Effects of antibacterial therapy on PSA change in the presence and absence of prostatic inflammation in patients with PSA levels between 4 and 10 ng/ml. *Prostate Cancer Prostatic Dis.* 2006;9(3):235-238.PubMed

102. Moradi A, Srinivasan S, Clements J, et al. Beyond the biomarker role: prostate-specific antigen (PSA) in the prostate cancer microenvironment. *Cancer Metastasis Rev.* 2019;38(3):333-346.PubMed

103. Routh JC, Leibovich BC. Adenocarcinoma of the prostate: epidemiological trends, screening, diagnosis, and surgical management of localized disease. *Mayo Clin Proc.* 2005;80(7):899-907.PubMed

104. Loeb S, Roehl KA, Catalona WJ, et al. Prostate specific antigen velocity threshold for predicting prostate cancer in young men. *J Urol.* 2007;177(3):899-902.PubMed

105. Vickers AJ, Till C, Tangen CM, et al. An empirical evaluation of guidelines on prostate-specific antigen velocity in prostate cancer detection. *J Natl Cancer Inst.* 2011;103(6):462-469.PubMed

106. Vickers AJ, Savage C, O'Brien MF, et al. Systematic review of pretreatment prostate-specific antigen velocity and doubling time as predictors for prostate cancer. *J Clin Oncol.* 2009;27(3):398-403.PubMed

107. Arlen PM, Bianco F, Dahut WL, et al. Prostate Specific Antigen Working Group guidelines on prostate specific antigen doubling time. *J Urol.* 2008;179(6):2181-2185, discussion 2185-2186.PubMed

108. Catalona WJ, Smith DS, Wolfert RL, et al. Evaluation of percentage of free serum prostate-specific antigen to improve specificity of prostate cancer screening. *JAMA.* 1995;274(15):1214-1220.PubMed

109. Catalona WJ, Partin AW, Slawin KM, et al. Use of the percentage of free prostate-specific antigen to enhance differentiation of prostate cancer from benign prostatic disease: a prospective multicenter clinical trial. *JAMA.* 1998;279(19):1542-1547.PubMed

110. Roddam AW, Duffy MJ, Hamdy FC, et al. Use of prostate-specific antigen (PSA) isoforms for the detection of prostate cancer in men with a PSA level of 2-10 ng/ml: systematic review and meta-analysis. *Eur Urol.* 2005;48(3):386-399, discussion 398-399.PubMed

111. Huang Y, Li ZZ, Huang YL, et al. Value of free/total prostate-specific antigen (f/t PSA) ratios for prostate cancer detection in patients with total serum prostate-specific antigen between 4 and 10ng/mL: A meta-analysis. *Medicine (Baltimore).* 2018;97(13):e0249.PubMed

112. Vickers AJ, Ulmert D, Sjoberg DD, et al. Strategy for detection of prostate cancer based on relation between prostate specific antigen at age 40-55 and long term risk of metastasis: case-control study. *BMJ.* 2013;346:f2023 10.1136.bmj.f2023.PubMed

113. Pruthi RS. The dynamics of prostate-specific antigen in benign and malignant diseases of the prostate. *BJU Int.* 2000;86(6):652-658.PubMed

114. Stenman UH, Leinonen J, Alfthan H, et al. A complex between prostate-specific antigen and alpha 1-antichymotrypsin is the major form of prostate-specific antigen in serum of patients with prostatic cancer: assay of the complex improves clinical sensitivity for cancer. *Cancer Res.* 1991;51(1):222-226.PubMed

115. Lepor A, Catalona WJ, Loeb S. The Prostate Health Index: its utility in prostate cancer detection. *Urol Clin North Am.* 2016;43(1):1-6.PubMed

116. Filella X, Foj L. Novel biomarkers for prostate cancer detection and prognosis. *Adv Exp Med Biol.* 2018;1095:15-39.PubMed

117. Filella X, Giménez N. Evaluation of [-2] proPSA and Prostate Health Index (phi) for the detection of prostate cancer: a systematic review and meta-analysis. *Clin Chem Lab Med.* 2013;51(4):729-739.PubMed

118. Osses DF, Roobol MJ, Schoots IG. Prediction medicine: biomarkers, risk calculators and magnetic resonance imaging as risk stratification tools in prostate cancer diagnosis. *Int J Mol Sci*. 2019;20(7):1637.PubMed

119. Zhuang L, Johnson MT. How precisely can prostate cancer be managed. *Int Neurourol J*. 2016;20(suppl 2):S120-S130.PubMed

120. Loeb S, Sanda MG, Broyles DL, et al. The prostate health index selectively identifies clinically significant prostate cancer. *J Urol*. 2015;193(4):1163-1169.PubMed

121. Szeliski K, Adamowicz J, Gastecka A, et al. Modern urology perspectives on prostate cancer biomarkers. *Cent European J Urol*. 2018;71(4):420-426.PubMed

122. Parekh DJ, Punnen S, Sjoberg DD, et al. A multi-institutional prospective trial in the USA confirms that the 4Kscore accurately identifies men with high-grade prostate cancer. *Eur Urol*. 2015;68(3):464-470.PubMed

123. Srigley JR, Delahunt B, Samaratunga H, et al. Controversial issues in Gleason and International Society of Urological *Pathology* (ISUP) prostate cancer grading: proposed recommendations for international implementation. *Pathology*. 2019;51(5):463-473.PubMed

124. Siddiqui MM, Rais-Bahrami S, Turkbey B, et al. Comparison of MR/ultrasound fusion-guided biopsy with ultrasound-guided biopsy for the diagnosis of prostate cancer. *JAMA*. 2015;313(4):390-397.PubMed

125. Stroumbakis N, Cookson MS, Reuter VE, et al. Clinical significance of repeat sextant biopsies in prostate cancer patients. *Urology*. 1997;49(3A suppl):113-118.

126. Presti JC Jr, Chang JJ, Bhargava V, et al. The optimal systematic prostate biopsy scheme should include 8 rather than 6 biopsies: results of a prospective clinical trial. *J Urol*. 2000;163(1):163-167.PubMed

127. Yamamoto S, Ito T, Aizawa T, et al. Does transrectal ultrasound guided eight-core prostate biopsy improve cancer detection rates in patients with prostate-specific antigen levels of 4.1-10 ng/mL? *Int J Urol*. 2004;11(6):386-391.PubMed

128. Descazeaud A, Rubin M, Chemama S, et al. Saturation biopsy protocol enhances prediction of pT3 and surgical margin status on prostatectomy specimen. *World J Urol*. 2006;24(6):676-680.PubMed

129. Wei JT, Feng Z, Partin AW, et al. Can urinary PCA3 supplement PSA in the early detection of prostate cancer? *J Clin Oncol*. 2014;32(36):4066-4072.PubMed

130. Tan GH, Nason G, Ajib K, et al. Smarter screening for prostate cancer. *World J Urol*. 2019;37(6):991-999.PubMed

131. Zaidi N, Thomas D, Chughtai B. Management of chronic prostatitis. *Curr Urol Rep*. 2018;19(11):88.PubMed

132. Khan FU, Ihsan AU, Khan HU, et al. Comprehensive overview of prostatitis. *Biomed Pharmacother*. 2017;94:1064-1076.PubMed

133. Doiron RC, Shoskes DA, Nickel JC. Male CP/CPPS: where do we stand? *World J Urol*. 2019;37(6):1015-1022.PubMed

134. Nickel JC. Classification and diagnosis of prostatitis: a gold standard? *Andrologia*. 2003;35(3):160-167.PubMed

135. Litwin MS, McNaughton-Collins M, Fowler FJ Jr, et al. The National Institutes of Health chronic prostatitis symptom index: development and validation of a new outcome measure. *J Urol*. 1999;162(2):369-375.PubMed

136. DeWitt-Foy ME, Nickel JC, Shoskes DA. Management of chronic prostatitis/chronic pelvic pain syndrome. *Eur Urol Focus*. 2019;5(1):2-4.

137. Shoskes DA, Nickel JC, Dolinga R, et al. Clinical phenotyping of patients with chronic prostatitis/chronic pelvic pain syndrome and correlation with symptom severity. *Urology*. 2009;73(3):538-543.PubMed

138. Tran CN, Li J, Shoskes DA. An online UPOINT tool for phenotyping patients with chronic prostatitis. *Can J Urol*. 2014;21(2):7195-7200.PubMed

139. Meares EM Jr, Stamey TA. Bacteriologic localization patterns in bacterial prostatitis and urethritis. *Invest Urol*. 1968;5(5):492-518.PubMed

140. Nickel JC, Shoskes DA, Wang Y, et al. How does the pre-massage and post-massage 2-glass test compare with pain syndrome? *J Urol*. 2006;176(1):119-124.PubMed

141. Wagenlehner FME, Pilatz A, Bschleipfer T, et al. Bacterial prostatitis. *World J Urol*. 2013;31(4):711-716.PubMed

142. Ramakrishnan K, Salinas RC. Prostatitis: acute and chronic. *Prim Care*. 2010;37(3):547-563, viii-ix.PubMed

## QUICKVIEW | Testosterone

| PARAMETER | DESCRIPTION | COMMENTS |
|---|---|---|
| **Reference range** | | |
| Adult, men | 280–1,100 ng/dL (9.7–38.17 nmol/L) | Normal range exhibits variability among laboratories |
| | | Largely due to the immunoassay method, which is commonly used |
| | | It is recommended that each laboratory establish its own normal range |
| **Critical values** | <200–230 ng/dL (<6.94–7.98 nmol/L) is generally associated with symptomatic hypogonadism | Extremely high or low values should be reported quickly |
| | ≤50 ng/dL (≤1.74 nmol/L) is associated with surgical or medical castration for prostate cancer | |
| | Residual serum testosterone levels reflect continuing adrenal androgen production | |
| **Inherent action?** | Yes | Exerts different physiologic effects at different stages of life in men (Table 25-1) |
| **Location** | | |
| Production | Testosterone is produced in the testes | The testes produce 95% of circulating androgen; the rest is produced by the adrenal glands |
| Storage | It is not stored | |
| Secretion/excretion | Testosterone is activated to DHT intracellularly in some target tissues by 5α-reductase; in adipose tissue, excess testosterone is converted to estrogen | In some target tissues (eg, brain) testosterone is active; in other target tissues (eg, prostate and scalp) testosterone must be activated to DHT to exert an effect; peripheral conversion of testosterone to estrogen results in gynecomastia |
| **Causes of abnormal values** | | |
| High | Hyperthyroidism, adrenal tumors, adrenal hyperplasia, testicular tumors, precocious puberty, anabolic steroids, excessive testosterone supplementation | |
| Low | Primary or secondary hypogonadism, late-onset hypogonadism, primary or secondary hypopituitarism, Klinefelter syndrome, orchiectomy, traumatic injury to testicles, mumps, maldescent of testicles, hepatic cirrhosis, prolactinoma, high-dose corticosteroids, LHRH antagonists, LHRH agonists, estrogens, cytotoxins, high dose ketoconazole | |

*Continued*

## QUICKVIEW | Testosterone (cont'd)

| PARAMETER | DESCRIPTION | COMMENTS |
|---|---|---|
| **Signs and symptoms** | | |
| High level | Increased libido, mood swings | |
| Low level | Absent or depressed libido, lack of energy, decreased sense of well-being, erectile dysfunction, gynecomastia, small testicles, decreased body hair, decreased muscle strength, visceral obesity, hot flashes | |
| **After event, time to...** | | |
| Initial evaluation | After orchiectomy, serum testosterone levels decrease to ≤50 ng/dL (≤.74 nmol/L) in several hours | Orchiectomy is indicated for symptomatic management of metastatic prostate cancer |
| Peak values | After depot LHRH agonist injection, serum testosterone levels decrease to ≤50 ng/dL (≤1.74 nmol/L) in 2–3 wk | LHRH agonists are alternatives to orchiectomy for symptomatic management of metastatic prostate cancer |
| Normalization | With testosterone supplementation for late-onset hypogonadism, an adequate clinical trial is 3 mo in length | Depending on the dosage formulation of testosterone supplement, supraphysiologic serum testosterone concentrations may be produced after administration |
| | After supplementation is started, serum testosterone should be repeated every 3–4 mo during the first year | This occurs with intramuscular depot injections |
| | A low baseline serum testosterone level should return to the normal range with adequate supplementation | In contrast, with other dosage formulations (eg, testosterone transdermal patches or buccal patch systems), only physiologic serum testosterone concentrations are produced after drug administration |
| | | The clinical significance of this difference is not known |
| **Causes of spurious results** | Excessive testosterone supplementation | |
| **Additional information** | Testosterone bound to SHBG is inactive; therefore, conditions which significantly alter the concentration of SHBG can increase or decrease the concentration of free testosterone, which is physiologically active (refer to Table 25-2 for a listing of such conditions) | In such patients, a calculated or measured free or bioavailable testosterone level would be preferred over a total serum testosterone level |

## QUICKVIEW | Prostate-Specific Antigen[a]

| PARAMETER | DESCRIPTION | COMMENTS |
| --- | --- | --- |
| **Reference range** | | |
| Adult men | <4 ng/mL (<4 mcg/L) | This cutoff value misses 27% of patients with organ-confined prostate cancer; as a result, some experts recommend using age-related normal ranges (Table 25-16), %fPSA, PSA velocity, or PSA doubling time, instead |
| **Critical values** | ≥10 ng/mL is highly suggestive of prostate cancer | Extremely high values should be reported to the physician quickly |
| **Inherent action?** | Yes | Responsible for liquefying semen after ejaculation |
| **Location** | | |
| Production | PSA is produced by the prostate | Blood levels of PSA are usually very low; however, in patients with prostate cancer or other diseases of the prostate, the normal prostatic architecture of ducts is not intact |
| Storage | It is not stored | |
| Secretion/ excretion | PSA normally passes out of the body in the ejaculate; it liquefies semen | Instead of passing out of the body, PSA enters the bloodstream, which results in elevated blood levels |
| **Causes of abnormal values** | | |
| High | Prostate cancer | Noncancerous causes of high results include BPH, prostatitis, prostate trauma, prostate surgery, acute urinary retention, ejaculation, exercise bicycling, exogenous testosterone supplements |
| Low | Low laboratory results are normal | |
| **Signs and symptoms** | | |
| High level | This disease is commonly asymptomatic until the prostate cancer is large enough to cause voiding symptoms, or until the tumor has metastasized; in the latter case, the patient may complain of bone pain, shortness of breath, or leg weakness due to bone, lung, or spinal cord metastases, respectively | |
| Low level | Not applicable | |
| **After insult, time to...** | | |
| Initial evaluation | After prostate manipulation, the PSA levels increase within hours and remain elevated for the duration of the prostatic inflammation; for example, after prostate massage, PSA may return to the normal range within days, whereas after transurethral prostatectomy, it may take weeks | |
| Peak values | No maximum value | |

*Continued*

## QUICKVIEW | Prostate-Specific Antigen[a] (cont'd)

| PARAMETER | DESCRIPTION | COMMENTS |
|---|---|---|
| **Causes of spurious results** | | |
| | As patients age, PSA normally increases BPH and organ-confined prostate cancer show overlap in PSA levels | |
| | Refer to Table 25-18 for other conditions that increase or decrease PSA | |

[a]Percentage of fPSA, PSA velocity, PSA density, and PSA doubling time are additional types of PSA tests used to improve the usefulness of PSA as a tumor marker for prostate cancer screening and monitor treatment response.

**APPENDIX A.** Therapeutic Ranges of Drugs in Traditional and SI Units[a]

| DRUG | THERAPEUTIC RANGE, TRADITIONAL UNITS | CONVERSION FACTOR[b] | THERAPEUTIC RANGE, SI UNITS |
|---|---|---|---|
| Acetaminophen | 4–18 mg/dL<br>>140 mg/dL at 4 hours<br>Post ingestion - toxic | 66.16 | 264–1191 µmol/L<br>9,262 µmol/L at 4 hours<br>Post ingestion - toxic |
| N-acetylprocainamide | 5–30 mg/L | 3.606 | 18–108 µmol/L |
| Amikacin | Trough 5–10 mcg/mL<br>Peak 20–30 mcg/mL<br>*range applies to traditional dosing (every 8–12 hrs) | 1.708 | 8.5–17 µmol/L<br>34–51 µmol/L |
| Amiodarone | 0.5–2.5 mcg/mL | 1.55 | 0.8–3.9 µmol/L |
| Amitriptyline | 120–250 ng/mL | 3.605 | 433–901 nmol/L |
| Carbamazepine | 4–12 mg/L | 4.23 | 17–51 µmol/L |
| Desipramine | 115–350 ng/mL | 3.754 | 431–1314 nmol/L |
| Digoxin | 0.5–2.2 ng/mL | 1.281 | 0.64–2.8 nmol/L |
| Ethosuximide | 40–100 mg/L | 7.084 | 280–710 µmol/L |
| Flucytosine | 20–100 mg/L | 7.745 | 155–775 µmol/L |
| Gentamicin | Trough: <1 mcg/mL<br>Peak: 6–10 mcg/mL<br>*range applies to traditional dosing (every 8–12 hrs) | 2.09 | <2.09 µmol/L<br>12.5–21 µmol/L |
| Imipramine | 180–350 ng/mL | 3.566 | 642–1248 nmol/L |
| Isoniazid | >3 mg/L toxic | 7.291 | >22 µmol/L toxic |
| Itraconazole | 0.5–1 mg/L | 1.417 | 0.71–1.42 µmol/L |
| Lidocaine | 1.5–5 mg/L | 4.267 | 6.4–21.3 µmol/L |
| Lithium | 0.5–1.5 mEq/L | 1 | 0.5–1.5 mmol/L |
| Nortriptyline | 50–150 ng/mL | 3.797 | 190–570 nmol/L |
| Pentobarbital | 1–5 mcg/mL | 4.439 | 4–22 µmol/L |
| Phenobarbital | 10–40 mg/L | 4.306 | 43–172 µmol/L |
| Phenytoin | 10–20 mg/L | 3.964 | 40–80 µmol/L |
| Posaconazole | 0.7–1.8 mg/L | 1.427 | 1–2.6 µmol/L |
| Primidone | 5–12 mg/L | 4.582 | 23–55 µmol/L |

*(continued)*

DOI 10.37573/9781585286423.APP

## APPENDIX A. Therapeutic Ranges of Drugs in Traditional and SI Units[a], cont'd

| DRUG | THERAPEUTIC RANGE, TRADITIONAL UNITS | CONVERSION FACTOR[b] | THERAPEUTIC RANGE, SI UNITS |
|---|---|---|---|
| Procainamide | 4–8 mg/L *up to 12 mg/L may be appropriate in some scenarios | 4.249 | 17–34 µmol/L *up to 51 µmol/L may be appropriate in some scenarios |
| Salicylate | 150–300 mcg/mL | 7.24 | 1086–2172 µmol/L |
| Tacrolimus | 5–20 mcg/mL | 1.217 | 6.1–24.3 µmol/L |
| Theophylline | 5–15 mg/L | 5.55 | 28–83 µmol/L |
| Tobramycin | Trough <2 mcg/mL Peak 5–10 mcg/mL *range applies to traditional dosing (every 8–12 hrs) | 2.139 | <4.3 µmol/L 10.7–21 µmol/L |
| Valproic acid | 50–125 mg/L | 6.934 | 347–867 µmol/L |
| Vancomycin | Trough: 10–20 mcg/mL *range for traditional trough-based monitoring | 0.69 | 6.9–13.8 µmol/L |
| Voriconazole | 1–6 mg/L | 2.863 | 2.9–17.2 |

[a]Also see Table 5-3 in Chapter 5.
[b]Traditional units are multiplied by conversion factor to get SI units.
These traditional and SI units are examples and do not necessarily represent current best practice monitoring techniques.
See the chapters discussing the specific medications for more detailed information.

## APPENDIX B. Nondrug Reference Ranges for Common Laboratory Tests in Traditional and SI Units[a,b]

| LABORATORY TEST | REFERENCE RANGE TRADITIONAL UNITS | CONVERSION FACTOR | REFERENCE RANGE SI UNITS | COMMENT |
|---|---|---|---|---|
| Alanine aminotransferase (ALT) | 7–41 IU/L | 0.01667 | 0.12–0.68 µkat/L | SGPT |
| Albumin | 3.5–5 g/dL | 10 | 35–50 g/L | |
| Alkaline phosphatase | 33–96 units/L | 0.0167 | 0.55–1.6 µkat/L | |
| Ammonia (as nitrogen) | 19–60 mcg/dL | 0.714 | 13.6–43 µmol/L | |
| Aspartate aminotransferase (AST) | 12–38 IU/L | 0.01667 | 0.2–0.63 µkat/L | SGOT |
| Bilirubin (direct) | 0.1–0.4 mg/dL | 17.1 | 1.7–6.8 µmol/L | |
| Bilirubin (total) | 0.3–1.3 mg/dL | 17.1 | 5–22 µmol/L | |
| Calcium (total) | 9.2–11 mg/dL | 0.25 | 2.3–2.8 mmol/L | |
| Carbon dioxide ($CO_2$) total content | 22–30 mEq/L | 1 | 22–30 mmol/L | Serum bicarbonate |
| Chloride | 95–106 mEq/L | 1 | 95–106 mmol/L | |
| Cholesterol (HDL) | >40 mg/dL | 0.026 | >1.05 mmol/L | Desirable |
| Cholesterol (LDL) | <130 mg/dL | 0.026 | <3.36 mmol/L | Desirable |

**APPENDIX B.** Nondrug Reference Ranges for Common Laboratory Tests in Traditional and SI Units[a,b]

| LABORATORY TEST | REFERENCE RANGE TRADITIONAL UNITS | CONVERSION FACTOR | REFERENCE RANGE SI UNITS | COMMENT |
|---|---|---|---|---|
| Creatine kinase (CK) | 55–170 IU/L | 0.01667 | 0.92–2.84 µkat/L | Males |
| | 30–135 IU/L | | 0.5–2.25 µkat/L | Females |
| Creatinine, serum (SCr) | 0.6–1.2 mg/dL | 88.4 | 53–106 µmol/L | Adults |
| Creatinine clearance (CrCl) | 90–140 mL/min/1.73 m$^2$ | 0.017 | 1.53–2.38 mL/sec/1.73 m$^2$ | |
| Folic acid | 5–25 ng/mL | 2.266 | 11.33–56.65 nmol/L | |
| γ-glutamyl transpeptidase | 9–58 units/L (but varies) | 0.01667 | 0.15–0.97 µkat/L (but varies) | GGT/GGTP |
| Glucose (fasting) | 70–110 mg/dL | 0.056 | 3.9–6.1 mmol/L | |
| Hemoglobin (Hgb) | 14–18 g/dL | 0.621 | 8.7–11.2 mmol/L | Males |
| | 12–16 g/dL | 0.621 | 7.4–9.9 mmol/L | Females |
| | | 10 | 140–180 g/L | Males |
| | | 10 | 120–160 g/L | Females |
| Iron | 50–150 mcg/dL | 0.179 | 9–26.9 µmol/L | |
| Lactate (arterial), serum | 0.5–2 mEq/L | 1 | 0.5–2 mmol/L | Lactic acid |
| Lactate (venous), serum | 0.5–1.5 mEq/L | 1 | 0.5–1.5 mmol/L | Lactic acid |
| Lactate dehydrogenase (LDH) | 115–221 IU/L | 0.01667 | 1.92–3.68 µkat/L | |
| Magnesium | 1.3–2.1 mEq/L | 0.5 | 0.65–1.05 mmol/L | |
| 5' nucleotidase | 0–11 units/L (but varies) | 0.01667 | 0–0.18 µkat/L (but varies) | |
| Phosphate | 2.3–4.7 mg/dL | 0.3229 | 0.7–1.52 mmol/L | |
| Potassium | 3.5–5 mEq/L | 1 | 3.5–5 mmol/L | |
| Sodium | 136–145 mEq/L | 1 | 136–145 mmol/L | |
| Thyroxine (T$_4$), total serum | 5–12 mcg/dL | 12.87 | 64–154 nmol/L | Total T$_4$ |
| Total iron-binding capacity (TIBC) | 250–410 mcg/dL | 0.179 | 45–73 µmol/L | |
| Triglycerides | <150 mg/dL | 0.0113 | <1.69 mmol/L | Adults >20 yr |
| Triiodothyronine (T$_3$), total serum | 80–200 ng/dL | 0.0154 | 1.2–3 nmol/L | Total T$_3$ |
| Urea nitrogen, blood (BUN) | 8–23 mg/dL | 0.357 | 2.9–8.2 mmol/L | BUN |
| Uric acid (serum) | 2.7–8.5 mg/dL | 59.48 | 161–506 µmol/L | |

SGOT = serum glutamic oxaloacetic transaminase; SGPT = serum glutamic pyruvic transaminase.
The values listed in this table may vary depending by testing site, so always refer to site-specific ranges.
[a]Some laboratories are maintaining traditional units for enzyme tests.
[b]For more extensive listing, refer to www.amamanualofstyle.com/page/si-conversion-calculator (accessed 2021 Dec 9).

*Note*: Page numbers followed by *f* refer to figures; those followed by *t* refer to tables; those followed by *b* refer to boxes.

DOI 10.37573/9781585286423.IDX